PLURAL+PLUS

COMPANION WEBSITE

Purchase of *Preclinical Speech Science: Anatomy, Physiology, Acoustics, and Perception, Third Edition* comes with access to supplementary student and instructor materials on a PluralPlus companion website.

The companion website is located at:
http://www.pluralpublishing.com/publication/pss3e

STUDENTS:

To access the **student** materials, you must register on the companion website and log in using the access code below.*

Access Code: **PSS3E-AYKFL67**

INSTRUCTORS:

To access the **instructor** materials, you must contact Plural Publishing, Inc. to be verified as an instructor and receive your access code.

Email: information@pluralpublishing.com
Tel: 866-758-7251 (toll free) or 858-492-1555

Note for students: If you have purchased this textbook used or have rented it, your access code will not work if it was already redeemed by the original buyer of the book. Plural Publishing does not offer replacement access codes for used or rented textbooks.

PRECLINICAL SPEECH SCIENCE

PRECLINICAL SPEECH SCIENCE

Anatomy, Physiology, Acoustics, and Perception

THIRD EDITION

Thomas J. Hixon
Gary Weismer
Jeannette D. Hoit

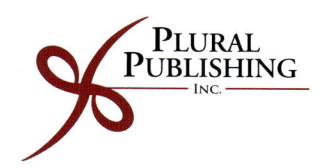

PLURAL PUBLISHING INC.

PLURAL PUBLISHING
INC.

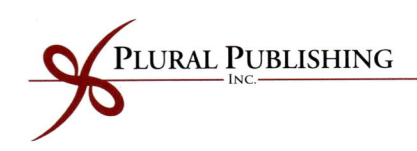

5521 Ruffin Road
San Diego, CA 92123

e-mail: info@pluralpublishing.com
website: http://www.pluralpublishing.com

Copyright © 2020 by Plural Publishing, Inc.

Typeset in 10/12 Palatino by Flanagan's Publishing Services, Inc.
Printed in South Korea through Four Colour Print Group

All rights, including that of translation, reserved. No part of this publication may be reproduced, stored in a retrieval system, or transmitted in any form or by any means, electronic, mechanical, recording, or otherwise, including photocopying, recording, taping, Web distribution, or information storage and retrieval systems without the prior written consent of the publisher.

For permission to use material from this text, contact us by
Telephone: (866) 758-7251
Fax: (888) 758-7255
e-mail: permissions@pluralpublishing.com

Every attempt has been made to contact the copyright holders for material originally printed in another source. If any have been inadvertently overlooked, the publishers will gladly make the necessary arrangements at the first opportunity.

Library of Congress Cataloging-in-Publication Data

Names: Hixon, Thomas J., 1940-2009, author. | Weismer, Gary, author. | Hoit,
　Jeannette D. (Jeannette Dee), 1954- author.
Title: Preclinical speech science : anatomy, physiology, acoustics, and
　perception / Thomas J. Hixon, Gary Weismer, Jeannette D. Hoit.
Description: Third edition. | San Diego, CA : Plural Publishing, [2020] |
　Includes bibliographical references and index.
Identifiers: LCCN 2018018596 | ISBN 9781635500615 (alk. paper) | ISBN
　1635500613 (alk. paper)
Subjects: | MESH: Speech--physiology | Speech Perception | Speech Disorders |
　Respiratory System--anatomy & histology
Classification: LCC QP306 | NLM WV 501 | DDC 612.7/8--dc23
LC record available at https://lccn.loc.gov/2018018596

Contents

PREFACE	xix
ACKNOWLEDGMENTS	xxi
REVIEWERS	xxiii

1 INTRODUCTION — 1
Focus of the Book — 1
Domain of Preclinical Speech Science — 1
  Levels of Observation — 1
  Subsystems of Speech Production and Swallowing — 3
  Applications of Data — 4
Domain of Preclinical Hearing Science — 4
  Levels of Observation — 4
  Subsystems of the Auditory System — 5
  Applications of Data — 6
Review — 7

2 BREATHING AND SPEECH PRODUCTION — 9
Introduction — 9
Anatomy of the Breathing Apparatus — 9
  Skeletal Framework — 9
  Breathing Apparatus and Its Subdivisions — 10
    Pulmonary Apparatus — 10
    Chest Wall — 12
    Pulmonary Apparatus–Chest Wall Unit — 12
Forces of Breathing — 13
  Passive Force — 13
  Active Force — 14
    Muscles of the Rib Cage Wall — 14
    Muscle of the Diaphragm — 17
    Muscles of the Abdominal Wall — 17
  Summary of Passive and Active Forces — 20
  Realization of Passive and Active Forces — 22
Movements of Breathing — 22
  Movements of the Rib Cage Wall — 22
  Movements of the Diaphragm — 23
  Movements of the Abdominal Wall — 25
  Relative Movements of the Rib Cage Wall and Diaphragm–Abdominal Wall — 25
  Forces Underlying Movements — 25
Control Variables of Breathing — 27
  Lung Volume — 27
  Alveolar Pressure — 28

Chest Wall Shape	31
Neural Control of Breathing	34
Control of Tidal Breathing	34
Control of Special Acts of Breathing	36
Peripheral Nerves of Breathing	37
Ventilation and Gas Exchange During Tidal Breathing	38
Breathing and Speech Production	40
Extended Steady Utterances	40
Running Speech Activities	44
Variables That Influence Speech Breathing	49
Body Position	49
Extended Steady Utterances in the Supine Body Position	50
Running Speech Activities in the Supine Body Position	52
Speech Breathing in Other Body Positions	54
Body Type	55
Age	55
Sex	57
Ventilation and Drive to Breathe	57
Cognitive-Linguistic and Social Variables	58
Review	59
References	60

3 LARYNGEAL FUNCTION AND SPEECH PRODUCTION   63

Introduction	63
Anatomy of the Laryngeal Apparatus	63
Skeletal Framework	63
Thyroid Cartilage	63
Cricoid Cartilage	64
Arytenoid Cartilages	65
Epiglottis	66
Hyoid Bone	66
Laryngeal Joints	66
Cricothyroid Joints	68
Cricoarytenoid Joints	69
Internal Topography	72
Laryngeal Cavity	72
Vocal Folds	72
Ventricular Folds	75
Laryngeal Ventricles	75
Ligaments and Membranes	75
Forces of the Laryngeal Apparatus	77
Intrinsic Laryngeal Muscles	78
Extrinsic Laryngeal Muscles	82
Supplementary Laryngeal Muscles	83
Infrahyoid Muscles	83
Suprahyoid Muscles	85
Summary of the Laryngeal Muscles	85
Movements of the Laryngeal Apparatus	86
Movements of the Vocal Folds	86
Vocal Fold Abduction	86

Vocal Fold Adduction	87
Vocal Fold Length Change	89
Movements of the Ventricular Folds	89
Movements of the Epiglottis	91
Movements of the Laryngeal Housing	91
Control Variables of Laryngeal Function	91
Laryngeal Opposing Pressure	92
Laryngeal Airway Resistance	92
Glottal Size and Configuration	93
Stiffness of the Vocal Folds	94
Effective Mass of the Vocal Folds	95
Neural Substrates of Laryngeal Control	95
Laryngeal Functions	97
Degree of Coupling Between the Trachea and Pharynx	97
Protection of the Pulmonary Airways	98
Containment of the Pulmonary Air Supply	98
Sound Generation	98
Laryngeal Function in Speech Production	98
Transient Noise Production	99
Sustained Turbulence Noise Production	99
Sustained Voice Production	100
Vocal Fold Vibration	101
Fundamental Frequency	104
Sound Pressure Level	106
Fundamental Frequency–Sound Pressure Level Profiles	107
Spectrum	107
Voice Registers	108
Running Speech Activities	111
Fundamental Frequency	111
Sound Pressure Level	112
Spectrum	113
Articulation	113
Variables that Influence Laryngeal Function During Speech Production	113
Age	113
Sex	116
Review	118
References	119

4 VELOPHARYNGEAL-NASAL FUNCTION AND SPEECH PRODUCTION — 127

Introduction	127
Anatomy of the Velopharyngeal-Nasal Apparatus	127
Skeletal Framework	127
Pharynx	130
Velum	132
Nasal Cavities	133
Outer Nose	134
Forces of the Velopharyngeal-Nasal Apparatus	135
Muscles of the Pharynx	135
Muscles of the Velum	139
Muscles of the Outer Nose	142

Movements of the Velopharyngeal-Nasal Apparatus	143
Movements of the Pharynx	143
Movements of the Velum	144
Movements of the Outer Nose	145
Control Variables of Velopharyngeal-Nasal Function	145
Velopharyngeal-Nasal Airway Resistance	145
Velopharyngeal Sphincter Compression	146
Velopharyngeal-Nasal Acoustic Impedance	147
Neural Substrates of Velopharyngeal-Nasal Control	148
Velopharyngeal-Nasal Functions	149
Coupling Between the Oral and Nasal Cavities	149
Coupling Between the Nasal Cavities and Atmosphere	150
Ventilation and Velopharyngeal-Nasal Function	151
Nasal Valve Modulation	151
Nasal Cycling (Side-to-Side)	152
Nasal-Oral Switching	152
Velopharyngeal-Nasal Function and Speech Production	152
Sustained Utterances	152
Running Speech Activities	154
Variables that Influence Velopharyngeal-Nasal Function	156
Body Position	156
Age	157
Sex	159
Review	160
References	161

5 PHARYNGEAL-ORAL FUNCTION AND SPEECH PRODUCTION   165

Introduction	165
Anatomy of the Pharyngeal-Oral Apparatus	165
Skeletal Framework	165
Maxilla	165
Mandible	166
Temporomandibular Joints	167
Internal Topography	170
Pharyngeal Cavity	170
Oral Cavity	170
Buccal Cavity	172
Mucous Lining	172
Forces of the Pharyngeal-Oral Apparatus	172
Muscles of the Pharynx	172
Muscles of the Mandible	173
Muscles of the Tongue	175
Muscles of the Lips	178
Movements of the Pharyngeal-Oral Apparatus	182
Movements of the Pharynx	183
Movements of the Mandible	183
Movements of the Tongue	184
Movements of the Lips	184
Control Variables of Pharyngeal-Oral Function	186
Pharyngeal-Oral Lumen Size and Configuration	186

Pharyngeal-Oral Structural Contact Pressure	188
Pharyngeal-Oral Airway Resistance	188
Pharyngeal-Oral Acoustic Impedance	189
Neural Substrates of Pharyngeal-Oral Control	190
Pharyngeal-Oral Functions	191
Degree of Coupling Between the Oral Cavity and Atmosphere	191
Chewing and Swallowing	191
Sound Generation and Filtering	191
Speech Production: Articulatory Descriptions	192
Vowels	192
Place of Major Constriction	192
Degree of Major Constriction	194
Lip Rounding	194
Diphthongs	194
Consonants	194
Manner of Production	195
Place of Production	195
Voicing	195
Speech Production Stream: Articulatory Processes	195
Coarticulation	196
Traditional Theory of Coarticulation (Feature Spreading)	196
Problems with the Traditional Theory of Coarticulation	200
Articulatory Phonology or Gesture Theory	200
Variables That Influence Pharyngeal-Oral Function	202
Age	202
Sex	206
Review	207
References	208

6 SPEECH PHYSIOLOGY MEASUREMENT AND ANALYSIS — 213

Introduction	213
Measurement and Analysis of Breathing	213
Spirometry	213
Chest Wall Surface Tracking	215
Manometry	218
Measurement and Analysis of Laryngeal Function	219
Endoscopy	219
Electroglottography	222
Aeromechanical Observations	224
Measurement and Analysis of Velopharyngeal-Nasal Function	227
Nasendoscopy	227
Aeromechanical Observations	227
Measurement and Analysis of Pharyngeal-Oral Function	230
Structural and Functional Imaging	230
X-Ray Imaging	230
Magnetic Resonance Imaging	231
Ultrasonic Imaging	232
Articulatory Tracking	232
X-Ray Microbeam Imaging	232
Electromagnetic Sensing (Articulography)	234

Optoelectronic Tracking	234
Electropalatographic Monitoring	235
Aeromechanical Observations	235
Health Care Professionals and Clinical Measurements	237
Review	240
References	241

7 ACOUSTICS — 247

Introduction	247
Pressure Waves	247
The Motions of Vibrating Air Molecules Are Governed by Simple Forces	247
The Motions of Vibrating Air Molecules Change the Local Densities of Air	250
Pressure Waves, Not Individual Molecules, Propagate Through Space and Vary as a Function of Both Space and Time	250
The Variation of a Pressure Wave in Time and Space Can Be Measured	251
Temporal Measures	251
Spatial Measures	254
Wavelength and Direction of Sound	255
Pressure Waves: A Summary and Introduction to Sinusoids	255
Sinusoidal Motion	256
Sinusoidal Motion (Simple Harmonic Motion) Is Derived from the Linear Projection of Uniform Circular Speed	256
When the Linear Projection of Uniform Circular Speed Is Stretched Out in Time, the Result Is a Sine Wave	257
Sinusoidal Motion Can Be Described by a Simple Formula and Has Three Important Characteristics: Frequency, Amplitude, and Phase	258
Sinusoidal Motion: A Summary	259
Complex Acoustic Events	259
Complex Periodic Events Have Waveforms That Repeat Their Patterns Over Time and Are Composed of Harmonically Related Frequency Components	259
A Complex Periodic Waveform Can Be Considered as the Sum of the Individual Sinusoids at the Harmonic Frequencies	261
Complex Aperiodic Events Have Waveforms in Which No Repetitive Pattern Can Be Discerned, and Frequency Components That Are Not Harmonically Related	264
Complex Acoustic Events: A Summary	264
Resonance	266
Mechanical Resonance	267
A Spring-Mass Model of Resonance	267
The Relative Values of Mass (M) and Elasticity (K) Determine the Frequency of Vibration of the Spring-Mass Model	268
The Effects of Mass and Stiffness (Elasticity) on a Resonant System: A Summary	270
Acoustic Resonance: Helmholtz Resonators	270
The Neck of the Helmholtz Resonator Contains a Column, or Plug of Air, That Behaves Like a Mass When a Force Is Applied to It	270
The Bowl of a Resonator Contains a Volume of Air That Behaves Like a Spring When a Force Is Applied to It	271
Acoustic Resonance: Tube Resonators	273
Resonance in Tubes: A Summary	276
Resonance Curves, Damping, and Bandwidth	277
Energy Loss (Damping) in Vibratory Systems Can Be Attributed to Four Factors	277

  Time- and Frequency-Domain Representations of Damping in Acoustic Vibratory Systems   278
  An Extension of the Resonance Curve Concept: The Shaping of a Source by the Acoustic   280
   Characteristics of a Resonator
 Resonance, Damping, Bandwidth, Filters: A Summary   282
Review   282
References   283
Appendix 7–A: The Decibel Scale   284

8   ACOUSTIC THEORY OF VOWEL PRODUCTION   289

Introduction   289
What Is the Precise Nature of the Input Signal Generated by the Vibrating Vocal Folds?   290
 The Time Domain   290
 The Frequency Domain   293
  The Periodic Nature of the Waveform   294
  The Shape of the Waveform   295
  The Ratio of Open Time to Closed Time   297
 Nature of the Input Signal: A Summary   297
Why Should the Vocal Tract Be Conceptualized as a Tube Closed at One End?   297
 The Response of the Vocal Tract to Excitation   298
 How Are the Acoustic Properties of the Vocal Tract Determined?   299
 Area Function of the Vocal Tract   301
How Does the Vocal Tract Shape the Input Signal? (How Is the Source Spectrum   303
 Combined with the Theoretical Vocal Tract Spectrum to Produce a Vocal
 Tract Output?)
 Formant Bandwidths   307
 Acoustic Theory of Vowel Production: A Summary   308
What Happens to the Resonant Frequencies of the Vocal Tract When the Tube Is   309
 Constricted at a Given Location?
 The Three-Parameter Model of Stevens and House   314
  Tongue Height   316
  Tongue Advancement   316
  Configuration of the Lips   318
 Importance of the Stevens and House Rules: A Summary   319
  The Connection Between the Stevens and House Rules and Perturbation Theory   320
  Why Are the Stevens and House Rules Important?   322
  Another Take on the Relationship Between Vocal Tract Configuration and Vocal Tract Resonances   323
Confirmation of the Acoustic Theory of Vowel Production   324
 Analog Experiments   325
 Human Experiments   325
Review   326
References   326

9   THEORY OF CONSONANT ACOUSTICS   329

Introduction   329
Why Is the Acoustic Theory of Speech Production Most Accurate and Straightforward   329
 for Vowels?
The Acoustics of Coupled (Shunt) Resonators and Their Application to Consonant Acoustics   330
 Nasal Murmurs   330
  Energy Loss in the Nasal Cavities, Antiresonances, and the Relative Amplitude of   334
   Nasal Murmurs

Nasal Murmurs: A Summary	335
Nasalization	335
Nasalization: A Summary	338
The Importance of Understanding Nasalization	338
Coupled (Shunt) Resonators in the Production of Lateral Sounds	339
Coupled (Shunt) Resonators in the Production of Obstruent Sounds	339
What Is the Theory of Fricative Acoustics?	341
Fluid Flow in Pipes and Source Types	341
Aeromechanic/Acoustic Effects in Fricatives: A Summary	344
A Typical Fricative Waveform and Its Aeromechanical Correlates	345
Mixed Sources in Fricative Production	346
Shaping of Fricative Sources by Vocal Tract Resonators	346
Measurement of Fricative Acoustics	349
Spectral Measurements	349
Temporal Measurements	350
The Acoustic Theory of Fricatives: A Summary	351
What Is the Theory of Stop Acoustics?	351
Intervals of Stop Consonant Articulation: Aeromechanics and Acoustics	353
Closure (Silent) Interval	353
Release (Burst) Interval	354
Frication and Aspiration Intervals	355
Voice-Onset Time	356
Shaping of Stop Sources by Vocal Tract Resonators	356
The Nature of Stop Sources	357
The Shaping of Stop Sources	357
Measurement of Stop Acoustics	358
Spectral Measurements	359
Temporal Measurements	359
Stop Consonants: A Summary	359
What Is the Theory of Affricate Acoustics?	360
Acoustic Contrasts Associated with the Voicing Distinction in Obstruents	360
Review	361
References	361

10 SPEECH ACOUSTIC MEASUREMENT AND ANALYSIS — 363

Introduction	363
A Historical Prelude	363
The Sound Spectrograph: History and Technique	369
The Original Sound Spectrograph: Summary	372
Interpretation of Spectrograms: Specific Features	373
Axes	373
Glottal Pulses	375
Formant Frequencies	375
Silent Intervals and Stop Bursts	376
Aperiodic Intervals	378
Segmentation of Spectrograms	379
Speech Acoustics Is Not All About Segments: Suprasegmentals	382
Digital Techniques for Speech Analysis	384
Speech Analysis by Computer: From Recording to Analysis to Output	384
Sampling Rate	385

Filters	385
Bits	385
Analysis and Display	386
Review	388
References	388

11 ACOUSTIC PHONETICS DATA — 391

Introduction	391
Vowels	391
Vowel Acoustics: Dialect and Cross-Language Phonetics	398
Within-Speaker Variability in Formant Frequencies	401
Summary of Vowel Formant Frequencies	403
A Note on Vowel Formant Frequencies Versus Formant Trajectories	404
Vowel Durations	406
Intrinsic Vowel Durations	406
Extrinsic Factors Affecting Vowel Durations	407
Diphthongs	409
Diphthongs: Two Connected Vowels or a Unique Phoneme?	410
Diphthong Duration	412
Nasals	412
Nasal Murmurs	412
Nasal Place of Articulation	415
Nasalization	418
Semivowels	421
Constriction Interval	421
Formant Transitions	422
Semivowel Acoustics and Speech Development	423
Semivowel Durations	424
Fricatives	425
Sibilants Versus Nonsibilants: Spectral Characteristics	425
Quantification of Fricative Spectra	426
Formant Transitions and Fricative Distinctions	431
Fricative Duration	432
Laryngeal Devoicing Gesture and Fricative Duration	435
/h/ Acoustics	436
Stops	438
Closure Interval and Burst	439
Closure Interval Duration	439
Flap Closures	440
Closure Duration and Place of Articulation	441
Stop Voicing: Some Further Considerations	441
Laryngeal Devoicing Gesture, Stop Closures, and Voice Onset Time	441
Bursts	445
Acoustic Invariance for Stop Place of Articulation	446
Acoustic Invariance and Theories of Speech Perception	449
Locus Equations	450
Acoustic Invariance at the Interface of Speech Production and Perception	452
Affricates	453
Acoustic Characteristics of Prosody	454
Phrase-Level F0 Contours	454

Phrase-Level Intensity Contours	456
Stress	457
Rhythm	458
Review	459
References	460

12 SPEECH PERCEPTION — 467

Introduction	467
Early Speech Perception Research and Categorical Perception	467
The /ba/-/da/-/ga/ Experiment	468
Categorical Perception: General Considerations	471
Labeling Versus Discrimination	472
Categorical Perception: So What?	472
Speech Perception Is Species Specific	474
The Motor Theory of Speech Perception: Proofs and Falsifications	474
Categorical Perception of Stop Place of Articulation Shows the "Match" to Speech Production	474
Duplex Perception	475
Acoustic Invariance	479
The Competition: General Auditory Explanations of Speech Perception	482
Sufficient Acoustic Invariance	482
Replication of Speech Perception Effects Using Nonspeech Signals	483
Animal and Infant Perception of Speech Signals	485
The Competition: Direct Realism	486
Vowel Perception	488
Motor Theory (Original and Revised)	488
Auditory Theories	488
Normalization	489
Direct Realism	490
A Summary of Speech Perception Theories	490
Speech Perception and Word Recognition	491
Speech Intelligibility	493
"Explanatory" Speech Intelligibility Tests	495
Scaled Speech Intelligibility	496
Phonetic Transcription	498
Why Should Speech-Language Pathologists and Audiologists Care About Speech Perception?	499
Review	501
References	501

13 ANATOMY AND PHYSIOLOGY OF THE AUDITORY SYSTEM — 505

Introduction	505
Temporal Bone	505
Peripheral Anatomy of the Auditory System	507
Outer Ear (Conductive Mechanism)	508
Pinna (Auricle)	508
External Auditory Meatus (External Auditory Canal)	509
Tympanic Membrane (Eardrum)	511
Middle Ear (Conductive Mechanism)	512
Chambers of the Middle Ear	512
Ossicles and Associated Structures	513

Ligaments of the Middle Ear	515
Muscles of the Middle Ear	516
Auditory (Eustachian) Tube	517
Medial and Lateral Wall Views of the Middle Ear: A Summary	518
Transmission of Sound Energy by the Conductive Mechanism	519
Inner Ear (Sensorineural Mechanism)	521
Vestibular System	522
Semicircular Canals	523
Vestibule: Saccule and Utricle	524
Summary: Vestibular Structures and Mechanisms	524
Cochlea	525
Fluid Motion within the Scalae: A Broad View	527
Hair Cells and Associated Structures	527
Traveling Waves	530
The Traveling Wave Is Transformed to Action Potentials	533
Auditory Nerve and Auditory Pathways (Neural Mechanism)	533
Auditory Nerve and Associated Structures	534
Efferent Auditory System	534
"Tuning" of the Peripheral Frequency Response	535
Ascending Auditory Pathways	536
Acoustic Reflex	538
Review	540
References	541

14 AUDITORY PSYCHOPHYSICS   543

Auditory Psychophysics	543
Psychophysics of Loudness	543
Auditory Thresholds	543
Equal Loudness Contours for Sinusoids	546
The Psychophysical Function Relating SPL to Scaled Loudness of Sinusoids	546
Phons	547
Sones	547
Loudness of Complex Sounds	550
The Peripheral Auditory System Is a Series of Bandpass Filters	550
The Critical Band Concept and the Loudness of Complex Sounds	556
Sensitivity of the Auditory System to Loudness Change	556
Psychophysics of Pitch	558
Pitch of Sinusoids	559
Sensitivity of the Auditory System to Pitch Change	561
Pitch of Complex Acoustic Events	563
Pitch of Complex Periodic Events	564
Pitch of Complex Aperiodic Events	565
Psychophysics of Timbre	566
Psychophysics of Time	566
Psychophysics of Sound Localization	568
Interaural Cues to Sound Location	570
Auditory Objects and Auditory Scene Analysis	572
Review	575
References	577

15 NEURAL STRUCTURES AND MECHANISMS FOR SPEECH, LANGUAGE, AND HEARING — 579

Introduction	579
The Nervous System: An Overview and Concepts	579
Central Versus Peripheral Nervous System	579
Autonomic Nervous System	580
Anatomical Planes and Directions	581
White and Gray Matter, Tracts and Nuclei, Nerves and Ganglia	584
Gray Matter and Nuclei	584
White Matter and Fiber Tracts	585
Ganglia	585
Efferent and Afferent	585
Neurons and Synapses	586
Lateralization and Specialization of Function	586
Cerebral Hemispheres and White Matter	589
Cerebral Hemispheres	589
Frontal Lobe	590
Parietal Lobe	593
Temporal Lobe	594
Occipital Lobe	596
Insula	596
Limbic System (Limbic Lobe)	597
Cerebral White Matter	597
Association Tracts	598
Striatal Tracts	601
Commissural Tracts	601
Descending Projection Tracts	602
Ascending Projection Tracts	606
Subcortical Nuclei and Cerebellum	607
Basal Ganglia	607
Cortico-Striatal-Cortical Loop	610
Role of Basal Ganglia	611
Thalamus	612
Cerebellum	612
Cortico-Cerebellar-Cortical Loop	613
Role of Cerebellum	613
Cerebellum and Basal Ganglia: New Concepts	614
Brainstem and Cranial Nerves	615
Surface Features of the Brainstem: Ventral View	615
Ventral Surface of Midbrain	616
Ventral Surface of Pons	617
Ventral Surface of Medulla	617
Surface Features of the Brainstem: Dorsal View	617
Dorsal Surface of Midbrain	617
Dorsal Surface of Pons	619
Dorsal Surface of Medulla	619
Cranial Nerves and Associated Brainstem Nuclei	619
Cranial Nerve I (Olfactory)	622
Cranial Nerve II (Optic)	622

Cranial Nerve III (Oculomotor)	622
Cranial Nerve IV (Trochlear)	622
Cranial Nerve V (Trigeminal)	623
Cranial Nerve VI (Abducens)	624
Cranial Nerve VII (Facial)	625
Cranial Nerve VIII (Auditory-Vestibular Nerve)	626
Cranial Nerve IX (Glossopharyngeal)	627
Cranial Nerve X (Vagus)	628
Cranial Nerve XI (Spinal Accessory Nerve)	629
Cranial Nerve XII (Hypoglossal)	629
Cortical Innervation Patterns	630
Why Innervation Patterns Matter	631
The Cranial Nerve Exam and Speech Production	633
Spinal Cord and Spinal Nerves	633
Spinal Cord	633
Spinal Nerves	635
Nervous System Cells	636
Glial Cells	636
Neurons	636
Cell Body (Soma)	637
Axon and Terminal Button	639
Synapses	639
Resting Potential, Action Potential, and Neurotransmitters	640
Resting Potential	640
Action Potential	642
Synaptic Transmission and Neurotransmitters	644
Neuromuscular Junction	645
Meninges, Ventricles, Blood Supply	647
Meninges	647
Dura Mater	648
Arachnoid Mater	649
Pia Mater	649
Meninges and Clinically Relevant Spaces	650
Ventricles	650
Lateral Ventricles	651
Third Ventricle	651
Cerebral Aqueduct, Fourth Ventricle, and Other Passageways for CSF	652
Production, Composition, and Circulation of CSF	652
Blood Supply of Brain	652
Anterior Circulation	652
Posterior Circulation	654
Circle of Willis	654
MCA and Blood Supply to the Dominant Hemisphere	655
Blood–Brain Barrier	658
Speech and Language Functions of the Brain: Possible Sites and Mechanisms	659
Network View of Brain Function	659
DIVA	659
DIVA: Speech Sound Map (lvPMC)	661
DIVA: Articulatory Velocity/Position Maps (PMC)	662

DIVA: Auditory and Somatosensory Processing: Parietal Cortex and Frontal-Parietal 663
   Association Tracts
DIVA: Where Is Aphasia, Where Are Dysarthria Types? 664
Review 665
References 666

16 SWALLOWING 669

Introduction 669
Anatomy 670
   Breathing, Laryngeal, Velopharyngeal-Nasal, and Pharyngeal-Oral Structures 670
   Esophagus 671
   Stomach 671
Forces and Movements of Swallowing 673
   Oral Preparatory Phase 674
   Oral Transport Phase 676
   Pharyngeal Phase 676
   Esophageal Phase 677
   Overlap of Phases 678
Breathing and Swallowing 678
Neural Control of Swallowing 681
   Role of the Peripheral Nervous System 681
   Role of the Central Nervous System 682
Variables That Influence Swallowing 683
   Bolus Characteristics 683
      Consistency and Texture 683
      Volume 683
      Taste 684
   Swallowing Mode 684
      Single Versus Sequential Swallows 684
      Cued Versus Uncued Swallows 685
   Body Position 686
   Development 686
   Aging 687
   Sex 688
Measurement and Analysis of Swallowing 688
   Videofluoroscopy 688
   Endoscopy 689
   Manometry 690
   Surface Electromyography 692
   Ultrasonography 692
   Aeromechanical Observations 692
   Client Self-Report 694
Health Care Professionals 694
Review 695
References 697

NAME INDEX 703
SUBJECT INDEX 715

Preface

The third edition of *Preclinical Speech Science* is a carefully revised and expanded version of the second edition of the textbook. The revised parts include line-by-line edits of all chapters from the second edition for greater clarity, removal of certain sections (several of which are available as supplementary materials on the textbook companion website, including the scenarios of the previous edition), and addition of new material to chapters from the second edition, including text, figures, and recent references from the research literature.

This new edition also contains three new chapters, including Chapter 6 ("Speech Physiology Measurement and Analysis"), Chapter 13 ("Auditory Anatomy and Physiology"), and Chapter 14 ("Auditory Psychophysics"). Chapter 6 was added to complement Chapter 10 ("Speech Acoustic Measurement and Analysis") and Chapters 13 and 14 were added in response to suggestions made by colleagues and students, that this textbook would benefit from chapter-length material on Hearing Science. With the inclusion of these two chapters on hearing science, perhaps a more accurate title for the textbook would be *Preclinical Speech and Hearing Science*. Because this is the third edition of the text, we have chosen to retain the original title to be consistent with the previous editions.

The Workbook accompanying the third edition of this textbook has also been updated with complete sets of problems and exercises for the three new chapters, and revised exercises for all other chapters. The Workbook is a self-study resource, complete with answers to the problems and exercises.

A PluralPlus companion website also accompanies this new edition of *Preclinical Speech Science*. The website has supplementary text and figures, sound files, study guides, and instructor lecture slides.

Acknowledgments

The formulation, writing, and production of this textbook has benefited from the talents, advice, and generosity of many people. First and foremost, we acknowledge and thank Maury Aaseng, the talented, kind, and wise creator of the beautiful images that are such an integral part of the text. Maury is our friend and colleague of these past dozen years, and hopefully of many years to come.

We acknowledge the following people, for reading and commenting on parts of the text, for discussions concerning presentation of material in the text and pointing us to relevant papers in the literature, for generosity in allowing us to use their outstanding figures in this book, and for funding significant time devoted to the preparation of the text. Thank you: Kate Bunton, Michelle Ciucci, Jim Hillenbrand, Corinne Jones, Joel Kahane, David Kuehn, Rosemary Lester-Smith, Bob Lutfi, Tim McCulloch, The Oros family, Robin Samlan, and Brad Story.

Finally, we thank the staff of Plural Publishing, especially Valerie Johns, Kalie Koscielak, and Linda Shapiro, for their invaluable assistance and, most of all, their patience.

GW & JH

Reviewers

Plural Publishing, Inc. and the authors would like to thank the following reviewers for taking the time to provide their valuable feedback during the development process:

Andrew Stuart, PhD, CCC-A, Aud(C)
Professor
Department of Communication Sciences and Disorders
East Carolina University
Greenville, North Carolina

Rosalie M. Uchanski, PhD
Assistant Professor
Program in Audiology and Communication Sciences
Washington University in St. Louis
St. Louis, Missouri

Deborah R. Welling, AuD, CCC/A, FAAA
Associate Professor
Department of Speech-Language Pathology
Seton Hall University
South Orange, New Jersey

For Nevi, Solly, and Isla:
Love thinking, reading, and knowing
You'll learn just what you don't know.
Know this way you are growing
By knowing what you don't know.

And for Tom, Pauline and Sadanand.
You know why.

Introduction

Welcome to *Preclinical Speech Science: Anatomy, Physiology, Acoustics, and Perception, Third Edition*. Two preliminaries are offered here. One is a discussion of the focus of the book, the other a discussion of the domains of preclinical speech science and preclinical hearing science.

FOCUS OF THE BOOK

Preclinical Speech Science: Anatomy, Physiology, Acoustics, and Perception is designed as an introduction to the fundamentals of speech and hearing science that are important to aspiring and practicing clinicians. The text is suitable for courses that cover the anatomy and physiology of speech production and swallowing, the anatomy and physiology of the hearing mechanism and auditory psychophysics, the acoustics and perception of speech, and general neuroanatomy and neurophysiology and its relevance for speech and hearing. It also includes sidetracks of clinical and historical interest, considerations of the scientific bases of clinical protocols and methodologies, and discussions of clinical personnel involved in the evaluation and management of disorders of speaking, hearing, and swallowing. This book provides up-to-date coverage of the science of speech and hearing, is user friendly to beginning students, yet integrative and translational for graduate students and practicing speech-language pathologists and audiologists. It is an outgrowth of the three authors' many years of teaching experience with several thousand undergraduate and graduate students.

The illustrations, done by the extremely talented artist Maury Aaseng, are a key feature of this book. These original illustrations, largely in full color, are supplemented by a small number of illustrations from other sources. The original illustrations were carefully chosen and drafted to convey only salient features, an approach in line with the written text.

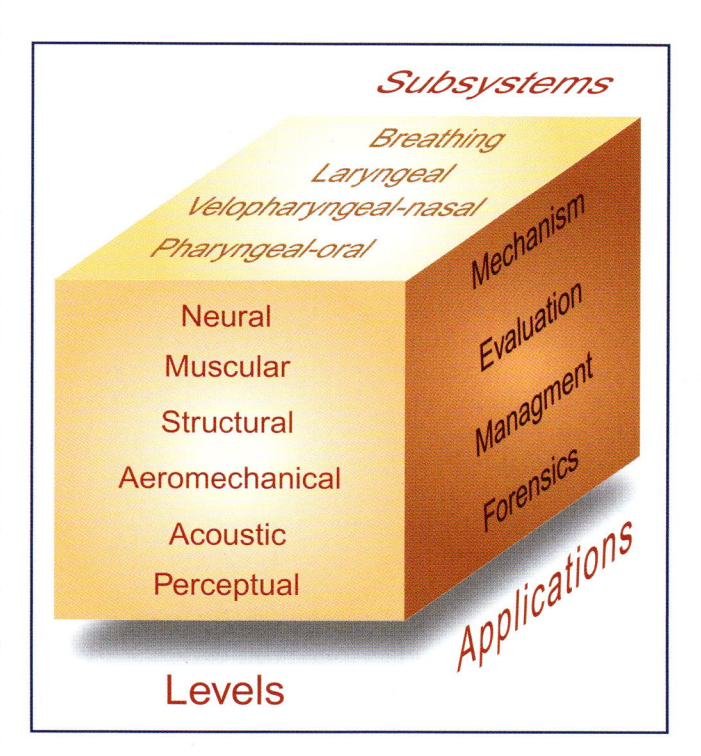

DOMAIN OF PRECLINICAL SPEECH SCIENCE

The domain of preclinical speech science is portrayed in Figure 1–1. This domain encompasses speech production, speech acoustics, speech perception, and swallowing. Within this domain, consideration is given to levels of observation, subsystems of speech production and swallowing, and applications of data.

Levels of Observation

Speech production and swallowing are processes. They result in acoustic products (more so for speech

Figure 1-1. Domain of preclinical speech science.

than swallowing) and perceptual experiences. These processes, products, and experiences involve different levels of observation. Six such levels are represented in Figure 1–1: (a) neural, (b) muscular, (c) structural, (d) aeromechanical, (e) acoustic, and (f) perceptual. These levels of observation are not completely separate entities but have important interactions. These interactions are not shown in the figure but are discussed in subsequent chapters.

The neural level of observation encompasses nervous system events during speech production and swallowing. These include all events that qualify as motor planning and execution and all forms of afferent and sensory information that influence the ongoing control of speech production and swallowing. The neural level of observation pertains to the parts of the brain, spinal cord, and cranial and spinal nerves important to speech production and swallowing and to all underlying neural mechanisms, some voluntary and some automatic, some that involve awareness, and some that do not. Neural data are often derived from physical or metabolic imaging methods that reflect patterns of activation of different regions of the brain. Activation at the neural level can also be inferred from events associated with other (downstream) levels of observation.

The muscular level of observation is concerned with the influence of muscle forces on speech production and swallowing. Muscle forces are responsible for powering these two processes. Muscles are effectors that respond to control signals from the nervous system. The muscular events of speech production and swallowing are manifested in mechanical pulls and are often indexed at the periphery through the electrical activities associated with muscle contractions. Inferences about muscle activities are also made from measurements of the forces or movements generated by different parts of the speech production apparatus and swallowing apparatus. Nevertheless, there are ambiguities introduced when attempting to infer individual muscle activities from forces or movements because forces and movements are usually accomplished by groups of muscles working together. Such inferences, if they can be made at all, require a detailed knowledge of anatomy and physiology.

The structural level of observation deals with anatomical structures and movements of the speech production apparatus and swallowing apparatus. This level of observation is concerned not only with the many muscular and non-muscular structures that make up the speech apparatus, including bone, muscle, ligaments, and membranes, but also with the displacements, velocities, and accelerations/decelerations of structures and how they are timed in relation to the movements of other structures. Certain structural observations can be made with the naked eye, whereas others are hidden from view or are too rapid to be followed with the naked eye and require the use of instrumental monitoring. To the person on the street, the structural level of observation is public evidence of speech production and swallowing. Speech reading (lip reading) has its roots at this level of observation.

The structural movements of speech production and swallowing give rise to an aeromechanical level of observation. It is at this level that air comes into play. Movements of structures impart energy to the air by compressing and decompressing it and causing it to flow from one region to another. The raw airstream generated in association with the aeromechanical level is modified by structures of the speech production apparatus and swallowing apparatus that lie along various passageways. The products of the aeromechanical level are complex, rapid, and nearly continuous changes in air pressures, airflows, and air volumes. These products are usually "invisible," especially for swallowing. However, those who speak and smoke at the same time or who speak in subfreezing temperatures often provide the observer with the opportunity to visualize certain aeromechanical events.

The acoustic level of observation is fully within the public domain. Although certain aspects of swallowing may be accompanied by sounds, primacy at this level pertains to the generation of speech sounds. The raw material of the acoustic level is the sonorous, buzzlike, hisslike, and poplike sounds that result from the speaker's valving of the airstream in different ways and at different locations within the speech production apparatus. This raw material is filtered and conditioned by its passage through the apparatus and radiates from the mouth or nose, or both, in the form of very fast and nearly continuous air pressure changes experienced as sound waves. These sound waves propagate from the speaker's mouth and can be coded in terms of frequency, sound pressure level, and time and are what constitute speech, the acoustic representation of spoken language. The acoustic level is important in face-to-face communication and in the use of telephones, radios, televisions, hearing aids and cochlear implants, and various forms of recording. It is this level that makes it possible to communicate effectively around corners, through obstacles, in the dark, and over long distances.

The perceptual level of observation has somewhat different manifestations for speech and swallowing. For speech, auditory analysis of the speech (acoustic) signal allows the listener to recognize phonetic cues that are consistent with the listener's knowledge of the sound system of a language. The speaker is also a perceiver of her own speech acoustic signal, using it to check that the signal she intended is the one she produced. Visual information is another source of information for the perception of speech. Listeners, even those with normal hearing, are known to combine acoustic and visual information for the most effective perception of speech. In contrast, swallowing relies less on auditory and visual information, but is highly dependent on the more subconscious experiences of kinesthesia and proprioception (awareness of position and movement characteristics of body structures, such as the tongue and jaw). Swallowing is also guided by touch and pressure sensations (as in awareness of contact of the tongue with the hard palate), which originate in sensory receptors embedded in the skin and muscles. Taste, which is detected by specialized taste receptors on the tongue and other oral structures, and consistency of food, which is detected by tactile receptors in the pharyngeal-oral component of the speech apparatus, can also serve as perceptual information for swallowing. Of course, cognitive processes contribute to the perceptual level of observation for both speech and swallowing. Cognitive processes in speaking, swallowing and hearing are not treated in detail in this text.

Subsystems of Speech Production and Swallowing

The activities of speech production and swallowing share many of the same structural and functional components. These components can be divided, somewhat arbitrarily, into subsystems. Speech production subsystems may differ when chosen by a linguist versus a speech scientist versus a speech-language pathologist; and swallowing subsystems may differ when chosen by a swallowing scientist versus a gastroenterologist versus a speech-language pathologist. For the purposes of this book, four subsystems are used for speech production and swallowing. As illustrated in Figure 1–1, these include the (a) breathing apparatus, (b) laryngeal apparatus, (c) velopharyngeal-nasal apparatus, and (d) pharyngeal-oral apparatus. The functional significance of each of the four subsystems differs between speech production and swallowing, but each subsystem is critically important to its respective behaviors and each manifests clinical signs that can reveal abnormality.

The breathing apparatus is defined in the present context to include structures below the larynx within the neck and torso. These are, most importantly, the pulmonary apparatus (pulmonary airways and lungs) and chest wall apparatus (rib cage wall, diaphragm, abdominal wall, and abdominal content). During speech production, the breathing apparatus provides the necessary driving forces while simultaneously serving the functions of ventilation and gas exchange. During swallowing, the breathing apparatus engages in a period of apnea (breath holding) to protect the pulmonary airways and lungs from the intrusion of unwanted substances (food and liquid). The breathing apparatus is the largest of the subsystems and its role in speech production and swallowing is fundamentally important.

The laryngeal apparatus lies between the trachea (windpipe) and the pharynx (throat) and adjusts the coupling between the two. At times, the laryngeal airway is open to allow air to move in and out of the breathing apparatus, whereas at times it is adjusted to obstruct or constrict the airway. Very rapid to and fro movements of the vocal folds within the larynx create voiced sounds and give the laryngeal apparatus its colloquial label "voice box." The larynx can also produce noisy sounds, like whisper. During swallowing, the laryngeal apparatus is active in closing the laryngeal airway to protect the pulmonary airways. Food and liquid are then able to pass over and around the larynx and into the esophagus on their way to the stomach.

The velopharyngeal-nasal apparatus consists of the upper pharynx, velum, nasal cavities, and outer nose. It is important to include the nasal portion of this subsystem because it can have a significant influence on the aeromechanical and acoustic levels of the speech production process. When breathing through the nose, the velopharyngeal-nasal airway is open. When speaking, the size of the velopharyngeal port varies, depending on the nature of the speech produced. For example, consonant sounds that require high oral air pressure are typically associated with airtight closure of the velopharyngeal port, whereas nasal consonants are produced with an open velopharyngeal port. Function of the velopharyngeal-nasal apparatus during swallowing is concerned mainly with keeping the velopharynx sealed airtight. This prevents the passage of food and liquid into the nasal cavities while substances are moved backward and downward through the oropharynx.

The pharyngeal-oral apparatus comprises the middle and lower pharynx, oral cavity, and oral vestibule. During running speech production, the apparatus is typically open during inspiration and makes different adjustments for consonant and vowel productions during expiration, including the generation of transient, voiceless, and voiced sounds and the filtering of those sounds. During swallowing, the pharyngeal-oral apparatus prepares food and liquid and propels it to the esophagus.

Applications of Data

There are many applications of data obtained about speech production and swallowing. These applications depend on who selects and defines the data and what the goals are for collecting and analyzing them. Figure 1–1 shows four important applications of data: (a) understanding mechanism, (b) evaluation, (c) management, and (d) forensics.

One application of data is the understanding of mechanism. This use provides the foundational bases for knowing how speech is produced and how swallowing is performed. Such foundational bases are important for their heuristic value in elucidating fundamental processes and principles and for differentiating normal from abnormal.

Another application of data is their use in evaluation. This use is usually practical in nature and involves quantitative determinations of the status and functional capabilities of an individual's speech production, speech, and swallowing. Evaluation first enables a determination as to whether or not abnormality exists. If abnormality does exist, then appropriate evaluation may contribute to: (a) making a diagnosis, (b) developing a rational, effective, and efficient management plan, (c) monitoring progress during the course of management, and (d) providing a reasonable prognosis as to the extent and speed of improvement to be expected. For example, a specific use of subsystems analysis in the evaluation of speech production is the determination of how individual subsystems contribute to deficits in speech intelligibility. Two individuals may have equivalent intelligibility problems as determined by formal tests but have different subsystems "explanations" for their deficits. The careful evaluation of subsystems performance can point to which parts of the speech production apparatus may be most responsible for speech intelligibility deficits and how those parts should be addressed in management. The subsystems approach to evaluation cannot be applied effectively without solid knowledge of normal structures and functions, as described in this text.

A third application of data is management. Different management strategies may be based on any of the six levels of observation and include any of the four subsystems of speech production and swallowing. Strategies may include adjusting individual variables or combinations of variables, staging the order of different interventions, and providing feedback about speech production and swallowing processes, products, and experiences. Management data provide information about outcomes and whether or not interventions are effective, efficient, and long lasting. Management data can also be used to compare and contrast different interventions to arrive at optimal choices.

The remaining application of data is their use in forensics. This application is concerned with scientific facts and expert opinion as they relate to legal issues. The speech scientist and speech-language pathologist are sometimes called on to give legal depositions or to testify in courts of law in a variety of forensic contexts. Forensic uses of data may include issues pertaining to speaker identification, speaker status under the influence of drugs or alcohol, and speaker intent at deceit, among others. Forensic uses of data may also relate to personal injury claims or malpractice claims. These may involve speech production, speech, or swallowing alone, or in different combinations, and may include adversarial depositions and testimonies of other experts. Under such circumstances, the status and capabilities of the individuals claiming personal injury or malpractice may be considered from the perspective of underlying mechanism, evaluation, and management.

DOMAIN OF PRECLINICAL HEARING SCIENCE

The domain of preclinical hearing science is portrayed in Figure 1–2. This domain encompasses audition, which serves the purpose of hearing and recognizing environmental sounds, music, speech acoustic signals, and electronically transmitted signals (as in the case of hearing aids and cochlear implants). Like the domain of preclinical speech science, consideration is given to levels of observation, subsystems, and applications of data.

Levels of Observation

Figure 1–2 shows levels of observation for audition. They include: (a) acoustic (pressure waves), (b) aeromechanical, (c) structural, (d) muscular, (e) mechanosensory, and (f) neural. This is consistent with the idea of speech production as the output and audition as the input of the speech communication process.[1]

---

[1] It is recognized that other forms of communication can be conceptualized in terms of output-input levels and processes. This includes sign language (gesture as output, vision as input), communication devices (e.g., language boards as output, vision as input), and speech synthesizers (synthesized speech as output, audition as input). Other examples can be imagined. This textbook does not cover these forms of communication in detail.

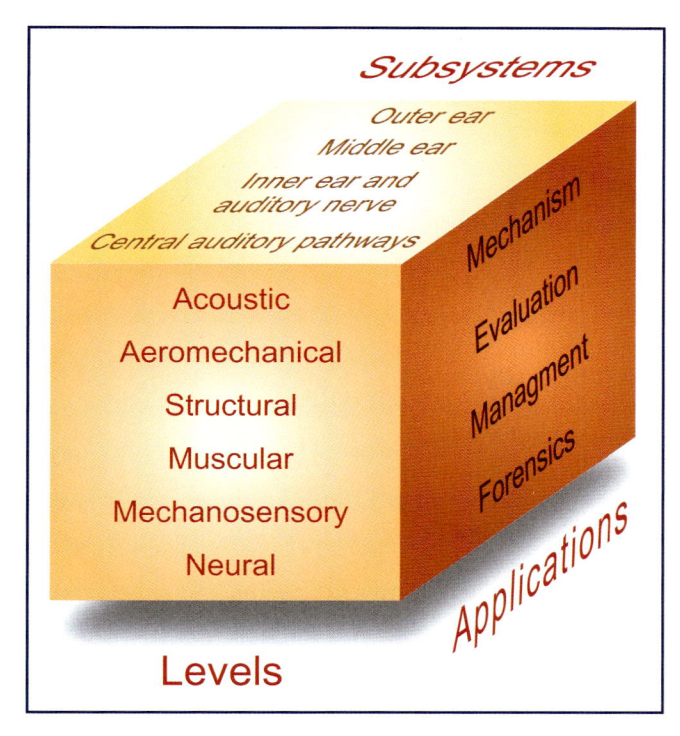

Figure 1-2. Domain of preclinical hearing science.

The acoustic level refers to the frequencies, amplitudes, and temporal characteristics of pressure waves that enter the ear at its opening to the atmosphere. As in the case of the acoustic level of speech production, the acoustic level is public. The signal can be analyzed by sophisticated instruments to extract and modify the spectral content and the way in which it varies over time. This level of observation is relevant to establishing the analysis capabilities of the human auditory system, both normal and disordered.

The aeromechanical level is important because the auditory system responds to the acoustic pressure wave (the "aero" part of the term) with mechanical vibrations of auditory structures. These structures include the tympanic membrane (the eardrum) and the ossicles, which are three tiny bones within the middle ear cavity. These mechanical vibrations replicate the vibrations in air that create pressure waves, but only to a point. The differences between auditory analysis of frequency, amplitude, and temporal characteristics and these characteristics in pressure waves reveal the analysis capabilities of the human ear.

The structural level includes the anatomy of the auditory system as well as the physiology of hearing. As in the case of the structural level of speech science, the anatomy of the auditory system is complex and interesting, and well suited to transmitting vibratory energy from the outer ear to the inner ear. Many of these structures are moving components, such as the tympanic membrane, the ossicles, the fluid within the cochlea (inner ear), and within the fluid a special membrane on which the auditory sense organs are located. A peripheral nerve is dedicated to transmission of auditory information from the cochlea to the central nervous system, and within the central nervous system complex pathways carry auditory information from the brainstem to the cortex.

The muscular level of the auditory system is simple compared with the speech production system, but still critical to hearing processes. A few muscles may cause subtle movements of the pinna (the structure attached to the head and most visible as an auditory structure), but in humans this ability has mostly disappeared. Contraction of two muscles in the middle ear, an air-filled cavity behind the tympanic membrane, stiffens the ossicles and tympanic membrane, and in doing so reduces the transmission of sound energy from the air to the cochlea. One of the muscles plays a primary role in a reflex that minimizes the possibility of damage to the cochlea when the auditory system is exposed to extremely intense sounds.

The mechanosensory level refers to the transduction of mechanical energy to neurochemical energy that is observed when fluid displacements within the cochlea (the mechanical part of the level) are transformed into neurochemical energy (the sensory part). This transformation takes place at the hair cells within the cochlea: fluid movements bend the hair cells, which cause the electrical potential of hair cells to change, which in turn releases a neurotransmitter that initiates firing of nerve fibers in the auditory nerve. The hair cells are the sensory receptors of audition, much like rods and cones within the retina are the sensory receptors for vision.

The neural level of audition includes the auditory nerve, a peripheral nerve that emerges from the cochlea and inserts into the brainstem. Inside the brainstem the fibers travel to brainstem nuclei (clusters of neuronal cell bodies), which send fibers to increasingly higher levels of the central nervous system until they reach cell bodies in the cortex. These fibers, called tracts, constitute the central auditory pathways. Fibers within the auditory nerve and nuclei and tracts that compose the auditory pathways have a tonotopic arrangement, meaning specific fibers and cells respond selectively depending on the frequencies of the incoming acoustic stimulus.

Subsystems of the Auditory System

The idea of subsystems is not frequently used to describe audition, but the concept can be easily adapted for a parallel to the speech production system. As shown in Figure 1–2, the auditory subsystems include: (a) the outer ear, (b) the middle ear, (c) the inner ear and auditory nerve, and (d) the central auditory pathways.

The outer ear includes the pinna (also called the auricle) and the external auditory meatus (the external ear canal). The structures that make up the pinna are variable across humans, and when exposed to sound pressure waves emphasize energy at certain frequencies and de-emphasize energy at other frequencies. The pinna may play a role in the localization of sound sources.

The middle ear is an air-filled cavity. It includes: (a) one surface of the three-layer tympanic membrane (eardrum), the entire membrane vibrating in response to sound energy conducted down the external ear canal, (b) the three connected ossicles (bones) that transmit vibrations of the tympanic membrane to the cochlea (an inner ear structure), (c) the opening of the auditory tube that leads to a closed tube (opened intermittently) in the pharynx, (d) two muscles that contract to stiffen the ossicles and in doing so make the transmission of sound energy from the tympanic membrane to the cochlea less efficient, and (e) segments of several nerves and blood vessels.

The inner ear contains the bony, fluid-filled cochlea, the ganglia, and cranial nerve VIII, which is composed of the auditory and vestibular nerves. Inside the snail-shaped cochlea is a membrane containing the sensory organs of hearing. This membrane and its complex structures are displaced by movement of the fluid caused by vibration of the ossicles. The inner ear also contains the vestibule where the sensory apparatus for balance is located. Vestibular structures are similar but not identical to those of the cochlea.

The central auditory pathways include a series of nuclei (the cell bodies of neurons) and fiber tracts that connect these nuclei to other parts of the brain. The pathways are dedicated to the transmission of auditory information from the brainstem to the auditory cortex. Within the cortex, several regions of cells perform increasingly complex analysis of auditory information, including the analysis resulting in the perception of speech.

Like the subsystems of speech production, the auditory subsystems are not independent and can be organized in different ways. For example, a commonly used organization includes three auditory subsystems: (a) the conductive component, (b) the sensorineural component, and (c) the central auditory pathways. The conductive component includes the outer and middle ears, the sensorineural component the cochlea and auditory nerve, and the central component the auditory pathways described above.

Applications of Data

Like speech production, the applications of data on audition serve many purposes. These purposes include: (a) understanding mechanism, (b) evaluation, and (c) management. A forensic application of audition can also be proposed, although it is clearly part of evaluation.

As stated above for speech production, knowledge of the structure and function of the auditory system is required to distinguish normal from abnormal. In addition, the knowledge is basic to the everyday professional life of speech-language pathologists and audiologists. Professionals who evaluate, diagnose, and manage communication disorders must be able to communicate with allied professionals who are not well versed in the structure and function of the auditory system and need coherent explanations of the basis of a hearing deficit. Similarly, clients and their family members are often interested in knowing the underlying science of a hearing disorder. The speech-language pathologist and audiologist who have mastered auditory structure and function can provide this information in a clear and simplified way.

The second application of data about audition is the evaluation of hearing disorders. Often the first phase of evaluation is performed by audiologists who use a variety of tests to determine the magnitude of hearing loss and the probable structure(s) responsible for the loss. Hearing disorders take many forms, which are often correlated with specific auditory subsystems. For example, an audiologist uses a range of pure tones (single-frequency acoustic events) to document the magnitude of hearing loss as a function of frequency. Depending on the pattern of hearing loss across frequencies, follow-up tests are performed to determine if the loss is in the conductive part of the mechanism, the sensorineural part, or a combination of the two. Sometimes a client shows very little hearing loss by these tests but has difficulty understanding speech. This often suggests a problem in the auditory nerve and/or central auditory pathways, and there are special tests to evaluate this possibility. These tests, and their results, cannot be understood in the absence of detailed knowledge of auditory structure and function.

The third application is management. Management of hearing problems includes the restoration, to the degree possible, of hearing function for those who have suffered hearing loss as children or adults; it also includes the provision of auditory stimulation to those born deaf or deafened by disease or accident. Hearing aids and cochlear implants are the two most common devices used in managing acquired hearing loss in children and adults (or in children who are born with hearing loss but are not deaf), and providing auditory stimulation in children born deaf or older individuals who have lost all hearing. These devices must be programmed with settings that depend on the structure and function of the diseased auditory system. The most effective programming emerges from expert knowledge of how damage to different auditory structures results in different magnitudes and patterns of hearing loss. In addition, the programming must take account of the acoustic properties of speech and how they relate to the ability to understand speech. This is because the primary purpose of any hearing device is to facilitate the understanding of speech.

Finally, an application of forensics in audition is the use of clinical tests that can detect functional hearing skills in persons who claim extensive or complete hearing loss due to accidents, disease, or other factors. This is part of the evaluation component of audition, but the potential legal implications (insurance fraud or compensation from an employer) justifies the use of the "forensic" label for this aspect of auditory evaluation.

REVIEW

Preclinical Speech Science: Anatomy, Physiology, Acoustics, and Perception is intended as an introduction to speech science and hearing science, both of fundamental importance to aspiring clinicians and practicing clinicians.

The text is suitable for different courses that cover anatomy and physiology of speech production and swallowing, hearing science, and the acoustics and perception of speech.

The material in the text is integrative and translational, applicable to both undergraduate and graduate students, and a source of continuing education and reference for practicing speech-language pathologists and audiologists.

The domain of preclinical speech and hearing science encompasses different levels of observation, different subsystems, and different applications of data.

Levels of observation in speech science include the neural, muscular, structural, aeromechanical, acoustic, and perceptual levels.

For hearing science, the levels of observation include the acoustic, structural, aeromechanical, muscular, mechanosensory, and neural.

Subsystems of speech production and swallowing include the breathing apparatus, laryngeal apparatus, velopharyngeal-nasal apparatus, and pharyngeal-oral apparatus.

Subsystems of hearing science include the outer ear, middle ear, inner ear and auditory nerve, and central auditory pathways, although an alternative and clinical set of subsystems includes the conductive, sensorineural, and auditory pathways components of the hearing mechanisms.

Applications of data include the understanding of mechanism, evaluation, management, and forensics.

Sidetracks

Throughout the book you'll find a series of sidetracks. These are short asides that relate to topics being discussed in the main text. Many of the sidetracks in the book are a bit less formal and a bit more lighthearted than the main text they complement. This is intended to enhance your reading enjoyment and to put some fun in your study of the material. We hope you enjoy reading these sidetracks as much as we enjoyed writing them.

2

Breathing and Speech Production

INTRODUCTION

The breathing apparatus moves air into and out of the body for the purpose of sustaining life as well as for performing other important functions such as speaking. It includes an energy source and passive components that couple this source to the air it moves.

This chapter begins with detailed consideration of the anatomical bases of breathing, forces and movements of breathing, control variables of breathing, neural control of breathing, and ventilation and gas exchange during tidal breathing. The latter part of the chapter is dedicated to speech breathing and selected variables that influence it.

ANATOMY OF THE BREATHING APPARATUS

The breathing apparatus is located within the torso (body trunk). A skeleton of bone and cartilage forms the framework for the breathing apparatus. This skeletal framework and the subdivisions of the breathing apparatus are considered here. The muscles of the breathing apparatus are covered under Forces of the Breathing Apparatus.

Skeletal Framework

The skeletal framework of the breathing apparatus is depicted in Figure 2–1. At the back of the torso, 34 irregularly shaped vertebrae (bones) form the vertebral column or backbone. The uppermost 7 of these vertebrae are termed cervical (neck), the next lower 12 are called thoracic (chest), and the next three lower groups of 5 each are referred to as lumbar, sacral, and coccygeal (collectively, abdominal). The vertebral column constitutes a back centerpost for the torso.

The ribs make up most of the upper skeletal framework. They are 12 flat, arch-shaped bones on each side of the body. The ribs slope downward from back to front along the sides of the torso, forming the rib cage and giving roundness to the framework. At the front, most of the ribs attach to bars of costal (rib) cartilage, which, in turn, attach to the sternum or breastbone. The sternum serves as a front centerpost for the rib cage. The typical rib cage includes upper pairs of ribs attached to the sternum by their own costal cartilages, lower pairs that share cartilages, and the lowest two pairs that float without front attachments.

The remainder of the upper skeletal framework is formed by the pectoral girdle (shoulder girdle). This structure is near the top of the rib cage. The front of the pectoral girdle is formed by the two clavicles (collar bones), each of which is a strut extending from the sternum over the first rib toward the side and back of the rib cage. At the back, the clavicles attach to two triangularly shaped plates, the scapulae (shoulder blades). The scapulae cover most of the upper back portion of the rib cage.

Two large, irregularly shaped coxal (hip) bones are located in the lower skeletal framework. These two bones, together with the sacral and coccygeal vertebrae, form the pelvic girdle (bony pelvis). The pelvic

---

Coming to Terms

Terms can either enlighten you or get you into verbal quagmires. Respiratory physiologists have gone out of their way to be precise in their use of terms. They've even held conventions to iron out their differences in language. It's a good idea to take a little extra time and care when reading the early sections of this chapter. Let the lexicon of the respiratory physiologist take firm root. Don't be tempted to skip over parts just because the words in the headings look familiar to you. You may be surprised to find that a term you thought you understood actually has an entirely different meaning to a respiratory physiologist.

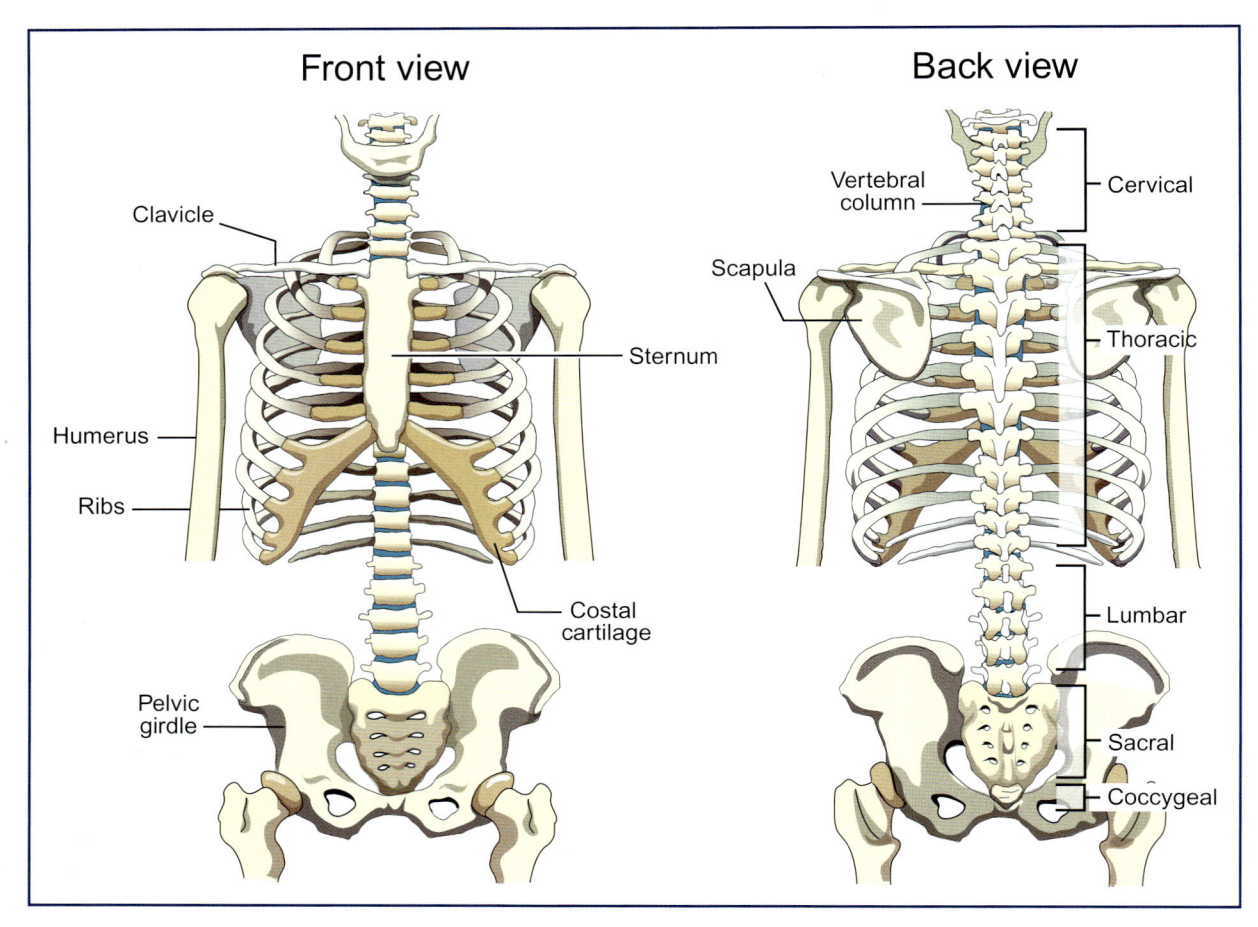

Figure 2–1. Skeletal framework of the breathing apparatus consisting of the clavicles, ribs, sternum, pelvic girdle, scapulae, and vertebral column.

girdle comprises the base, lower back, and sides of the lower skeletal framework.

Breathing Apparatus and Its Subdivisions

The breathing apparatus (breathing pump) and its subdivisions are depicted in Figure 2–2. The torso, which houses the apparatus, consists of upper and lower cavities that are partitioned by the diaphragm. The upper cavity is called the thorax (or colloquially the chest) and is almost totally filled with the heart and lungs; the lower cavity, called the abdomen (or colloquially the belly), contains much of the digestive system and other organs and glands. The structures of the breathing apparatus form two major subdivisions: the pulmonary apparatus and chest wall. These subdivisions are concentrically arranged, with the chest wall surrounding the pulmonary apparatus.

Pulmonary Apparatus

The pulmonary apparatus, portrayed in Figure 2–3, is the air-containing, air-conducting, and gas-exchanging part of the breathing apparatus. It provides oxygen to the cells of the body and removes carbon dioxide from them. The pulmonary apparatus can be subdivided into two components: the pulmonary airways and lungs.

Pulmonary Airways. The pulmonary airways constitute a complex network of flexible tubes through which air can be moved to and from the lungs and between different parts of the lungs. These tubes are arranged like the branches of an inverted deciduous tree. The network, in fact, is commonly referred to as the pulmonary tree.

The trunk of the pulmonary tree (the top part) is the trachea (windpipe). The trachea is a tube attached to the bottom of the larynx (voice box). It runs down through the neck into the torso. The trachea is com-

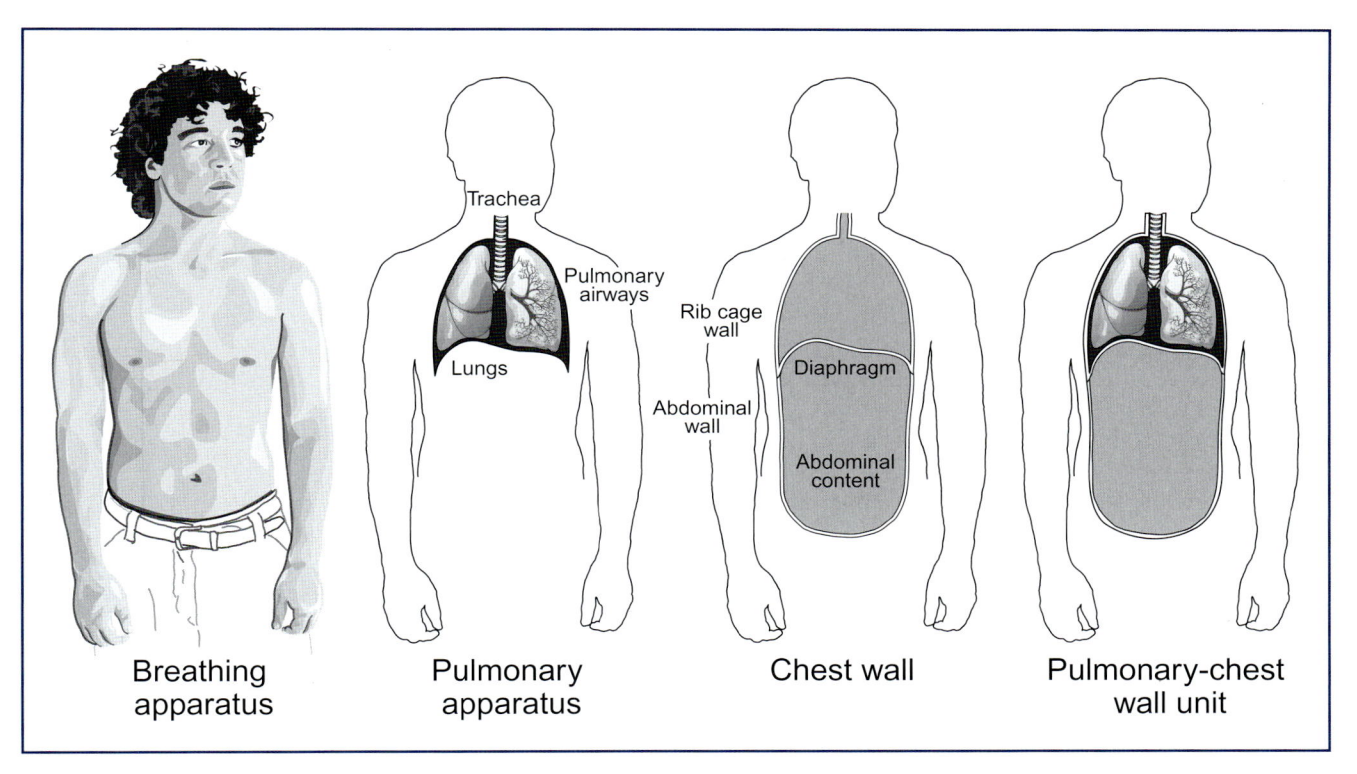

Figure 2–2. Breathing apparatus and its subdivisions: the pulmonary apparatus (lungs and airways) and the chest wall (rib cage wall, diaphragm, abdominal wall, and abdominal content). From *Evaluation and management of speech breathing disorders: Principles and methods* (p. 13), by T. Hixon and J. Hoit, 2005, Tucson, AZ: Redington Brown. Copyright 2005 by Thomas J. Hixon and Jeannette D. Hoit. Modified and reproduced with permission.

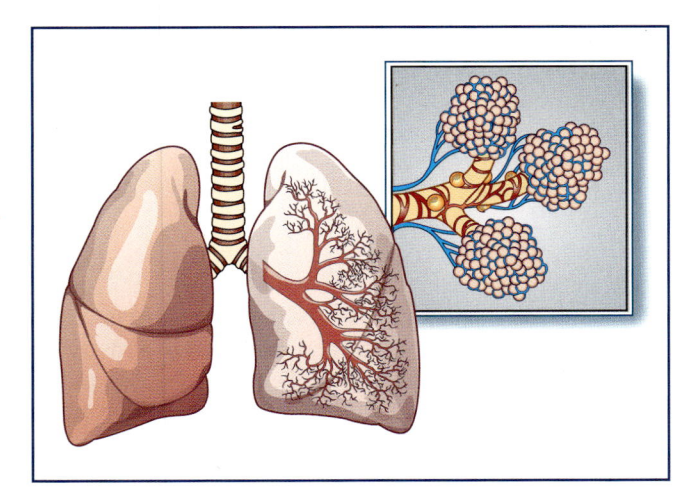

Figure 2–3. The pulmonary apparatus consisting of the airways (trachea, main-stem bronchi, lobar bronchi, segmental bronchi, subsegmental bronchi, small bronchi, terminal bronchi, bronchioles, terminal bronchioles, respiratory bronchioles, alveolar ducts, alveolar sacs, and alveoli) and lungs (spongy structures that surround the pulmonary airways).

posed of a series of C-shaped cartilages whose open ends face toward the back where the structure is completed by a flexible wall shared with the esophagus (the muscular tube leading to the stomach). At its lower end, the trachea divides into two smaller tubes, one running to the left lung and one running to the right lung. These two tubes, called the main-stem bronchi, branch into what are called lobar bronchi, tubes that run to the five lobes of the lungs (two lobes on the left and three on the right). The five lobar bronchi branch and their offspring also branch, and so on, through more than 20 generations. Each successive branching leads to smaller and less rigid structures. These include, in succession, segmental bronchi, subsegmental bronchi, small bronchi, terminal bronchi, bronchioles, terminal bronchioles, respiratory bronchioles, alveolar ducts, alveolar sacs, and alveoli. The last of these, the alveoli, are extremely small cul de sacs filled with air. They number more than 300 million and are the sites where oxygen and carbon dioxide are exchanged. The total surface area of the alveoli, if laid out flat, is said to approximate the size of a tennis court.

Lungs. The lungs are the organs of breathing. They are a pair of cone-shaped structures that are porous and spongy. Each lung contains an abundance of resilient elastic fibers and behaves like a stretchable bag. The outer surfaces of the lungs are covered with a thin airtight membrane, called the visceral pleura. A similar membrane, the parietal pleura, covers the inner surface of the chest wall where it contacts the lungs. Together these two membranes form a double-walled sac that encases the lungs. Both walls of this sac are covered with a thin layer of liquid that lubricates them and enables them to move easily upon one another. The same layer of liquid links the visceral and parietal membranes together, in the way a film of water holds two glass plates together. This is called *pleural linkage*. Thus, the lungs and chest wall tend to move as a unit—where one goes, the other follows.

Chest Wall

The chest wall encases the pulmonary apparatus. There are four parts to the chest wall: the rib cage wall, diaphragm, abdominal wall, and abdominal content.

Rib Cage Wall. The rib cage wall surrounds the lungs and is shaped like a barrel. The rib cage framework includes the thoracic segments of the vertebral column, the ribs, the costal cartilages, the sternum, and the pectoral girdle. The remainder of the rib cage wall is formed by muscular and nonmuscular tissues that fill the spaces between the ribs and cover their inner and outer surfaces.

Diaphragm. The diaphragm forms the convex floor of the thorax and the concave roof of the abdomen. The diaphragm separates the thorax and abdomen, and thus, gets its name—diaphragm meaning *the fence between*. The diaphragm is dome-shaped, like an inverted bowl. The left side of the diaphragm is positioned slightly lower than the right (to accommodate the heart above and the liver below). At its center, the diaphragm consists of a tough sheet of inelastic tissue, called the central tendon. The remainder of the structure is formed by a sheet of muscle that rises as a broad rim from all around the lower portion of the inside of the rib cage and extends upward to the edges of the central tendon.

Abdominal Wall. The abdominal wall provides a casing for the lower half of the torso. This casing is shaped like an oblong tube and runs all the way around the torso. The lower portion of the skeletal framework of the torso forms the structure around which the abdominal wall is built. This includes a back centerpost of 15 vertebrae (lumbar, sacral, and coccygeal) that extends from near the bottom of the rib cage to the tailbone and pelvic girdle. Much of the abdominal wall consists of two broad sheets of connective tissue and several large muscles. The two sheets of connective tissue cover the front and back of the abdominal wall and are called the abdominal aponeurosis and lumbodorsal fascia, respectively. Muscles are located all around the abdominal wall—front, back, and flanks (sides)—and combine with the abdominal aponeurosis, lumbodorsal fascia, vertebral column, and pelvic girdle to form its encircling casing.

Abdominal Content. The abdominal content is everything in the abdominal cavity. This includes the stomach, intestines, and various other internal structures. This content is close to unit density (the density of water) and constitutes a relatively homogeneous mass. This mass is suspended from above by a suction force at the undersurface of the diaphragm and is held in place circumferentially and at its base by the casing of the abdominal wall. Together, the abdominal cavity and the abdominal content are the mechanical equivalent of an elastic bag filled with water.

Pulmonary Apparatus–Chest Wall Unit

The pulmonary apparatus and chest wall are linked by pleural membranes (pleural linkage) to form a single

---

Ribbit, Ribbit

Ever watch a frog breathe? Did you notice how its cheeks moved? Frogs don't have a diaphragm to pull air into their lungs. They push the air in using their mouths like pistons. Frogs are positive pressure breathers. People are negative pressure breathers. A frog doesn't have the ability to emulate us (except, perhaps, Kermit) if its positive pressure pump fails. But we have the ability to emulate the frog if our negative pressure pump fails by doing what is called glossopharyngeal breathing. And what would you suppose is the common name for such breathing? Well, it's "frog breathing." In frog breathing, the tongue and throat are used to pump air into the lungs. Air is gulped in small portions (mouthfuls), each held in place by closing the larynx as a one-way valve. Frog breathing isn't difficult to learn and once mastered can be used to fill the lungs in a stepwise fashion all the way to the top.

functional unit. As illustrated in Figure 2–4, the resting positions of the pulmonary apparatus and chest wall when linked as a unit are different from their individual resting positions. When the pulmonary apparatus is removed from the chest wall, its resting position is a collapsed state in which it contains very little air. This is represented as a collapsed spring in the figure (lower left). In contrast, the resting position of the chest wall, with the pulmonary apparatus removed, is a more expanded state, represented as a stretched spring in the figure (lower middle). With the pulmonary apparatus and chest wall held together by pleural linkage, the breathing apparatus assumes

Laundry Starch

The stiffness of the breathing apparatus changes across life. The term that pertains to this is *compliance* and it refers to the tendency to yield to an applied force. In the lexicon of the respiratory physiologist, compliance is quantified in terms of how much volume is displaced for the pressure applied. We are reminded of laundry starch when we think of this concept. You get a little more starch in the "fabric" of your breathing apparatus as time goes by. The compliance of the breathing apparatus of a newborn is relatively high and somewhat like that of a dishrag. In contrast, the compliance of the breathing apparatus of a senescent adult is relatively low and somewhat like that of a plastic garbage can lid. Thus, we start out life being relatively floppy and end up life being relatively stiff (no pun intended on the stiff part, honestly).

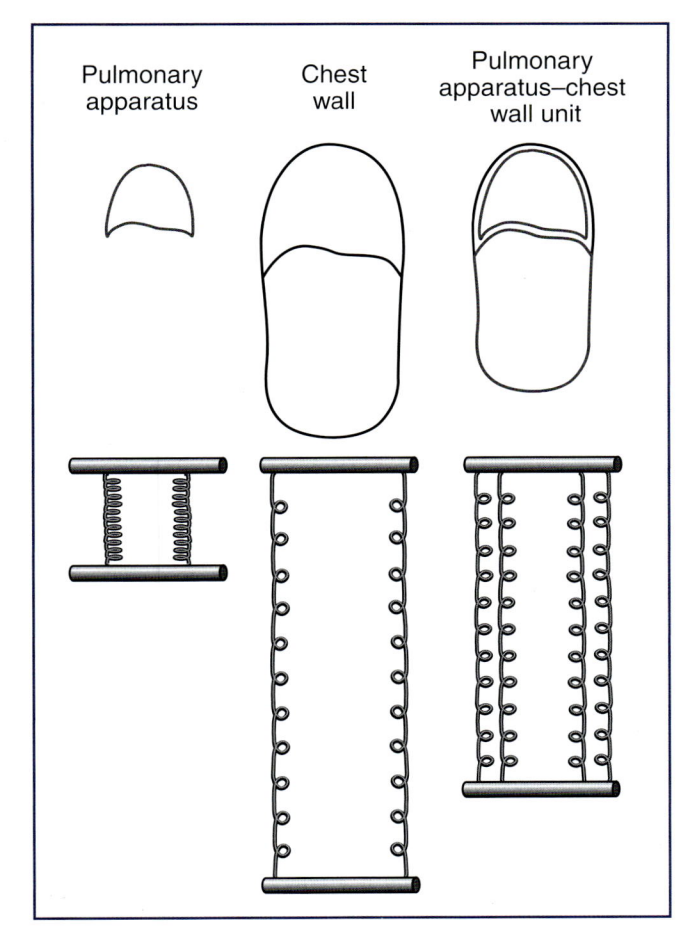

Figure 2–4. Resting positions of the pulmonary apparatus, chest wall, and pulmonary apparatus–chest wall unit (breathing apparatus). Note that when the pulmonary apparatus and chest wall are linked (*right side of figure*), the resting size of the pulmonary apparatus is larger and the resting size of the chest wall is smaller than when they are separated. When linked, the forces of the pulmonary apparatus and chest wall are equal and opposite and the pulmonary–chest wall unit assumes a mechanically neutral (balanced) state.

a resting position between these two positions such that the pulmonary apparatus is somewhat expanded and the chest wall is somewhat compressed. This resting position of the linked pulmonary apparatus–chest wall unit is a mechanically neutral or balanced state in which the force of the pulmonary apparatus to collapse is opposed by an equal and opposite force of the chest wall to expand. The linked pulmonary apparatus–chest wall unit (breathing apparatus) is represented as a combined spring in Figure 2–4 (lower right).

FORCES OF BREATHING

Both passive and active forces operate on the breathing apparatus. Passive force is inherent and always present. Active force, in contrast, is applied willfully by skeletal (voluntary) muscles.

Passive Force

The passive force of breathing can be substantial. It comes from: (a) the natural recoil of muscles, cartilages, ligaments, and lung tissue, (b) the surface tension of alveoli, and (c) the pull of gravity. Passive force causes the breathing apparatus to behave like a coil spring (like that illustrated in the lower right of Figure 2–4), which, when stretched or compressed, tends to recoil toward its resting length.

The sign (inspiratory or expiratory) and magnitude of passive force depends on the amount of air in the breathing apparatus. When the apparatus contains more air than it does at rest, it recoils toward a smaller size (expires), like the release of a stretched spring. The more air contained in the breathing apparatus, the greater the recoil force to expire. In contrast, when the apparatus contains less air than it does at rest, it recoils toward a larger size (inspires), like the release of a compressed spring. The less air in the apparatus, the greater the recoil force to inspire. Thus, like a coil spring, the more the breathing apparatus is deformed from its resting size, whether in the inspiratory (stretched) or expiratory (compressed) direction, the greater the passive recoil force it generates.

Active Force

The active force of breathing comes from the actions of muscles of the chest wall. The sign (inspiratory or expiratory) and magnitude of this force depend on which muscles are active and in what combinations. Active force also depends on the amount of air in the breathing apparatus. The more air in the apparatus, the greater the active force that can be generated to expire; and the less air in the apparatus, the greater the active force that can be generated to inspire.

The roles of individual muscles in generating active force are described below for the rib cage wall, diaphragm, and abdominal wall. These descriptions assume that only the muscle under consideration is active and that it is shortening during contraction. It should be noted, however, that several factors might influence the contribution of an individual muscle, including the actions of other muscles, the mechanical status of different parts of the chest wall, and the breathing activity being performed.

Muscles of the Rib Cage Wall

The muscles of the rib cage wall are defined to include muscles of the neck and rib cage. These muscles are depicted in different views in Figure 2–5.

The *sternocleidomastoid* muscle is a broad, thick structure positioned on the front and side of the neck. It originates in two subdivisions, one at the top and front of the sternum and the other at the top of the sternal end of the clavicle. Fibers from these subdivisions pass upward and backward and insert into the bony skull behind the ear. When the head is fixed in position, contraction of the *sternocleidomastoid* muscle results in elevation of the sternum and clavicle. The force generated is transmitted to the ribs through their connections to the sternum and clavicle. Consequently, the ribs are also elevated.

The *scalenus anterior*, *scalenus medius*, and *scalenus posterior* muscles are three separate muscles that form a functional group. These are positioned on the side of the neck. The *scalenus anterior* muscle originates from the third through sixth cervical vertebrae and runs downward and toward the side to insert along the inner border of the top of the first rib. The *scalenus medius* muscle arises from the lower six cervical vertebrae and descends along the side of the vertebral column to insert into the first rib behind the point of insertion of the *scalenus anterior* muscle. And the *scalenus posterior* muscle originates from the lower two or three cervical vertebrae and passes downward and toward the side to attach to the outer surface of the second rib. When the head is fixed in position, contraction of the *scalenus anterior* and/or *scalenus medius* muscles results in elevation of the first rib, whereas contraction of the *scalenus posterior* muscle results in elevation of the second rib.

The *pectoralis major* muscle is a broad, fan-shaped muscle positioned on the upper front wall of the rib cage. This muscle has a complex origin that includes the front surface of the upper costal cartilages, sternum, and inner half of the clavicle. Fibers run across the front of the rib cage wall and converge to insert into the humerus (the major bone of the upper arm).

Rib Torque

Sounds like leftovers. Actually, it refers to rotational stress produced when one end of a rib is twisted out of line with the other. Some have suggested that when the ribs are elevated during resting tidal inspiration, they're twisted outward (placed under positive torque) and store energy, which is then supposedly released during expiration. Not so. The ribs are actually twisted inward (and are under negative torque) at the resting tidal end–expiratory level because the lungs are pulling inward on the rib cage wall at that level. The ribs untwist during resting tidal inspiration, but do not reach neutral (zero torque) until the 60 %VC (percent vital capacity) level is attained (when in an upright body position). Because resting tidal inspiration involves only about a 10% increase in vital capacity, rib torque actually opposes resting tidal expiration rather than assists it. The only thing leftover about rib torque in this context is the folklore.

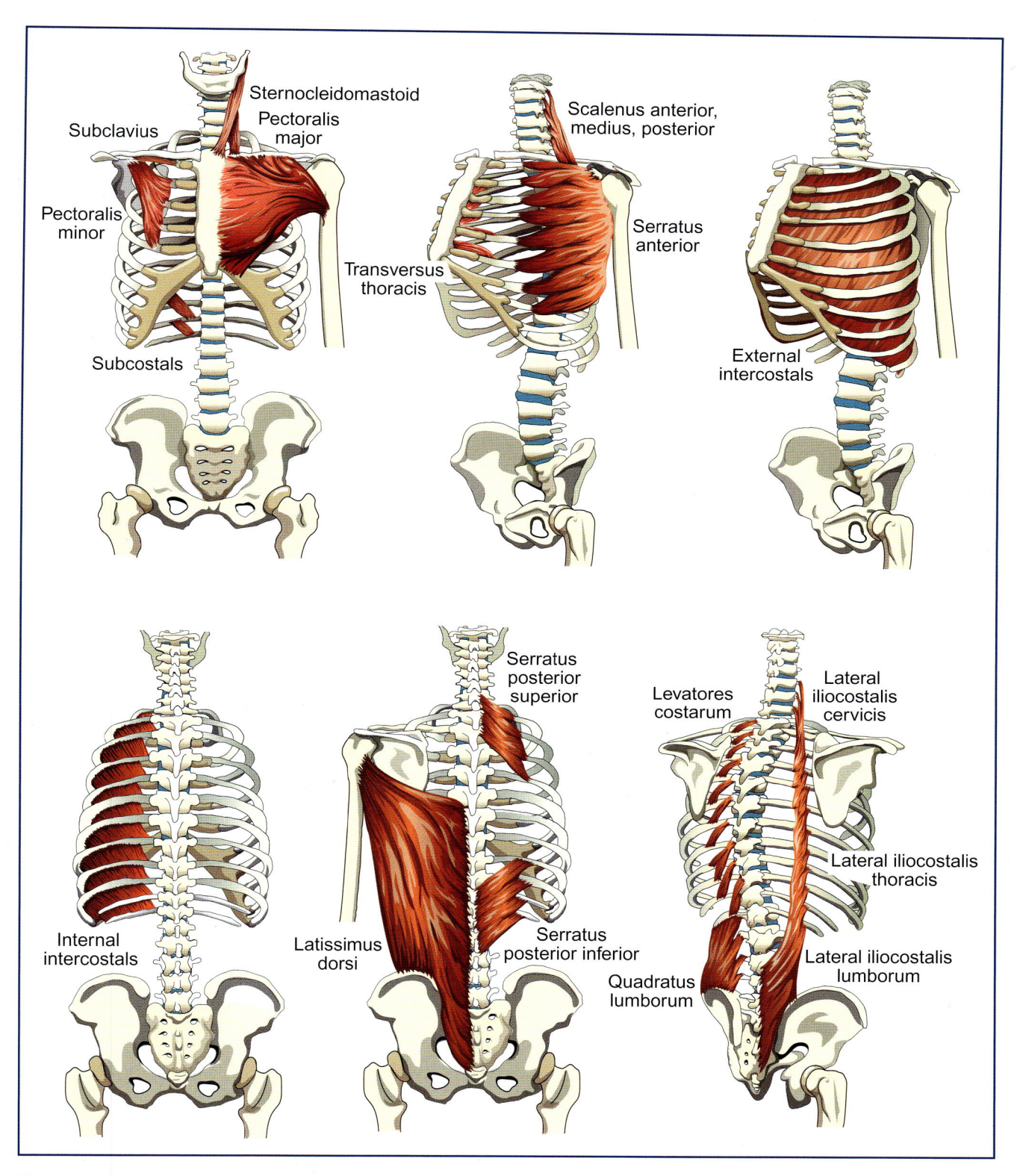

Figure 2-5. Muscles of the rib cage wall. From *Evaluation and management of speech breathing disorders: Principles and methods* (pp. 19–20), by T. Hixon and J. Hoit, 2005, Tucson, AZ: Redington Brown. Copyright 2005 by Thomas J. Hixon and Jeannette D. Hoit. Modified and reproduced with permission.

When the humerus is held in position, contraction of the *pectoralis major* muscle pulls the sternum and ribs upward.

The *pectoralis minor* muscle is a relatively large, thin muscle that lies underneath the *pectoralis major* muscle. Its fibers originate from the second through fifth ribs near their cartilages. From there, they extend upward and toward the side, where they insert into the front surface of the scapula. When the scapula is fixed in position, contraction of the *pectoralis minor* muscle elevates the second through fifth ribs.

The *subclavius* muscle is a small muscle that originates from the undersurface of the clavicle. It runs slightly downward and toward the midline, where it attaches at the junction of the first rib and its cartilage. When the clavicle is braced, contraction of the *subclavius* muscle elevates the first rib.

The *serratus anterior* muscle is a large muscle positioned on the side of the rib cage wall. It originates from the outer surfaces of the upper eight or nine ribs. Fibers pass backward around the side of the rib cage, where they converge and insert into the front of the scapula. When the scapula is fixed in position, contraction of the *serratus anterior* muscle results in elevation of the upper ribs.

The *external intercostal* muscles are 11 muscles that fill the outer portions of the rib interspaces. Each is a thin layer of muscle that runs between adjacent ribs. The fibers of the muscles are oriented forward and downward. Together, the 11 muscles form a large sheet of muscle that links the ribs to one another. This sheet of muscle is anchored from above to the first rib, the cervical vertebrae, and the base of the skull. When the muscle in any rib interspace contracts, it elevates the rib immediately below and, perhaps, other ribs below through their linkage to the sheet of muscle. The *external intercostal* muscles may activate individually in different rib interspaces or they may activate collectively. En masse activation causes the ribs to move upward as a unit. Muscle activation also stiffens the tissue-filled rib interspaces. This prevents them from being sucked inward and pushed outward as internal pressure is lowered and raised, respectively.

The *internal intercostal* muscles are 11 muscles that lie in the inner portions of the rib interspaces. They are located underneath the *external intercostal* muscles and extend from around the sides of the rib cage to the sternum. The *internal intercostal* muscles do not fill the rib interspaces at the back of the rib cage. Fibers of the *internal intercostal* muscles run downward and backward and at a right angle to those of the *external intercostal* muscles. The *internal intercostal* muscles form a large sheet of muscle that links the ribs to one another and to the pelvic girdle through other muscles, especially those of the abdominal wall. When muscle in a rib interspace contracts, it pulls downward on the rib immediately above and, perhaps, on other ribs above through the linkage created by the muscle sheet. The *internal intercostal* muscles may activate individually in any rib interspace or they may activate collectively. When they activate collectively, the ribs tend to move downward as a unit. Muscle contraction stiffens the tissue-filled rib interspaces and prevents them from being sucked inward and bulged outward with changes in internal pressure.

The portion of the *internal intercostal* muscles that lies between the costal cartilages (the *intercartilaginous internal intercostal* muscles) is arranged such that the muscle tissue exerts an upward pull on the rib cage wall rather than the downward pull exerted by the portion of the muscle that lies between the bony ribs (the *interosseous internal intercostal* muscles). Thus, the *internal intercostal* muscles play a functional role in the intercartilaginous region that is similar to that played by their companion *external intercostal* muscles throughout the rib cage wall. Stated otherwise, the two layers of *intercostal* muscles (external and internal) function similarly toward the front of the rib cage, but dissimilarly at other locations.

The *transversus thoracis* muscle is a fan-shaped structure located on the inside, front wall of the rib cage. It originates at the midline on the inner surface of the lower sternum and fourth or fifth through seventh costal cartilages. From there, it fans out across the rib cage and inserts into the inner surface of the costal cartilages and bony ends of the second through sixth ribs. The upper fibers of the muscle run nearly vertically, whereas the intermediate and lower fibers course at other angles. When the *transversus thoracis* muscle contracts, it exerts a downward pull on the second through sixth ribs.

The *latissimus dorsi* muscle is a large muscle positioned on the back of the body. It has a complex origin from the lower six thoracic, lumbar, and sacral vertebrae, along with the back surfaces of the lower three or four ribs. Fibers run upward across the back of the lower torso at different angles to insert into the humerus. When the humerus is fixed in position, contraction of the fibers of the *latissimus dorsi* muscle that insert into the lower ribs will elevate them. Contraction of the muscle as a whole, in contrast, compresses the lower portion of the rib cage wall. Thus, the *latissimus dorsi* muscle is capable of generating active force of different signs (inspiratory and expiratory).

The *serratus posterior superior* muscle is located on the upper back portion of the rib cage wall. It is a thin muscle that originates from the back of the vertebral column. Points of origin include the seventh cervical and first three or four thoracic vertebrae. Fibers course downward across the back of the rib cage and insert into the second through fifth ribs. When the ***serratus posterior superior*** muscle contracts, it pulls upward on the second through fifth ribs.

The ***serratus posterior inferior*** muscle is a thin muscle positioned on the lower back portion of the rib cage wall. It arises from the lower two thoracic and upper two or three lumbar vertebrae and slants upward across the back of the rib cage where it inserts into the lower borders of the lower four ribs. Contraction of the ***serratus posterior inferior*** muscle results in a downward pull on the lower four ribs.

The ***lateral iliocostalis*** muscle group includes three muscles located on the back of the torso. These are positioned to the side of the vertebral column and extend between the cervical and lumbar regions. The ***lateral iliocostalis cervicis*** muscle originates from the outer surfaces of the third through sixth ribs and courses upward and toward the midline to insert into the fourth through sixth cervical vertebrae. The ***lateral iliocostalis thoracis*** muscle arises from the upper edges of the lower six ribs and courses upward to insert into the lower edges of the upper six ribs. And the ***lateral iliocostalis lumborum*** muscle originates from the lumbodorsal fascia, lumbar vertebrae, and back surface of the coxal bone. It courses upward and toward the side to insert into the lower edges of the lower six ribs. Contraction of the ***lateral iliocostalis cervicis*** muscle causes elevation of the third through sixth ribs, whereas contraction of the ***lateral iliocostalis lumborum*** muscle results in depression of the lower six ribs. Contraction of the ***lateral iliocostalis thoracis*** muscle stabilizes large segments of the back of the rib cage wall and makes them move in concert with either the rib elevation or depression caused by the cervical and lumbar elements of the muscle group, respectively.

The ***levatores costarum*** muscles are 12 small muscles positioned on the back of the rib cage wall. Their origin is from the seventh cervical and upper eleven thoracic vertebrae and they extend downward and slightly outward to insert into the back surface of the rib immediately below the vertebra of origin. When an individual muscle of the ***levatores costarum*** muscle group contracts, it elevates the ribs into which it inserts. When the muscle group contracts collectively, its action is similar to that effected by collective contraction of the ***external intercostal*** muscles (the ribs elevate as a unit).

The ***quadratus lumborum*** muscle is a flat, quadrilateral sheet of muscle located on the back of the torso. It arises from the top of the coxal bone and runs upward and toward the midline where it inserts into the first four lumbar vertebrae and lower border of the inner half of the lowest rib. When the ***quadratus lumborum*** muscle contracts, it pulls downward on the lowest rib.

The ***subcostal*** muscles comprise a group of thin muscles located on the inside back wall of the rib cage. They differ in number from person to person and are most often located and best developed in the lower portion of the rib cage wall. The ***subcostal*** muscles originate near the vertebral column on the inner surfaces of ribs and course upward and toward the side where they insert into the inner surfaces of ribs immediately above, or skip a rib or two and insert into higher ribs. When the ***subcostal*** muscles contract, they pull downward on the ribs into which they are inserted.

Muscle of the Diaphragm

The muscular features of the diaphragm are portrayed in Figure 2–6. The ***diaphragm*** muscle is a large, complex muscle that subdivides the torso into two compartments: the thorax (upper cavity) and abdomen. It originates around the internal circumference of the lower rib cage, including the bottom of the sternum, the lower six ribs and their cartilages, and the first three or four lumbar vertebrae. From this internal rim, muscle fibers radiate upward to insert into the circumference of the central tendon, a broad sheet of inelastic tissue that forms the centermost portion of the diaphragm.

When the ***diaphragm*** muscle contracts, it can effect two actions. One of these is to pull the central tendon downward and forward, thus enlarging the thorax vertically; the other is to enlarge the thorax circumferentially through elevation of the lower six ribs. The actions of lowering the base of the thorax and expanding its circumference occur in patterns that depend on the relative stiffness (compliance) of the rib cage wall and abdominal wall.

Muscles of the Abdominal Wall

The muscles of the abdominal wall are depicted in Figure 2–7. They are located on the front and sides of the abdominal wall.

The ***rectus abdominis*** muscle is a ribbon-like structure located on the front of the lower rib cage wall and abdominal wall just off the midline. It arises from the upper, front edge of the coxal bone and runs upward vertically to insert into the outer surfaces of the fifth, sixth, and seventh costal cartilages and lower sternum. The ***rectus abdominis*** muscle is compartmentalized into four or five short segments by tendinous breaks. The entire muscle is encased in a fibrous sheath formed by the abdominal aponeurosis. The muscle and sheath form a centerpost along the front of the abdominal wall that is a continuation of the front centerpost formed by the sternum on the rib cage wall. When the ***rectus abdominis*** muscle contracts, it pulls the lower ribs and sternum downward and forces the front of the abdominal wall inward. The compartmentalized segments of the muscle are also capable of independent contraction.

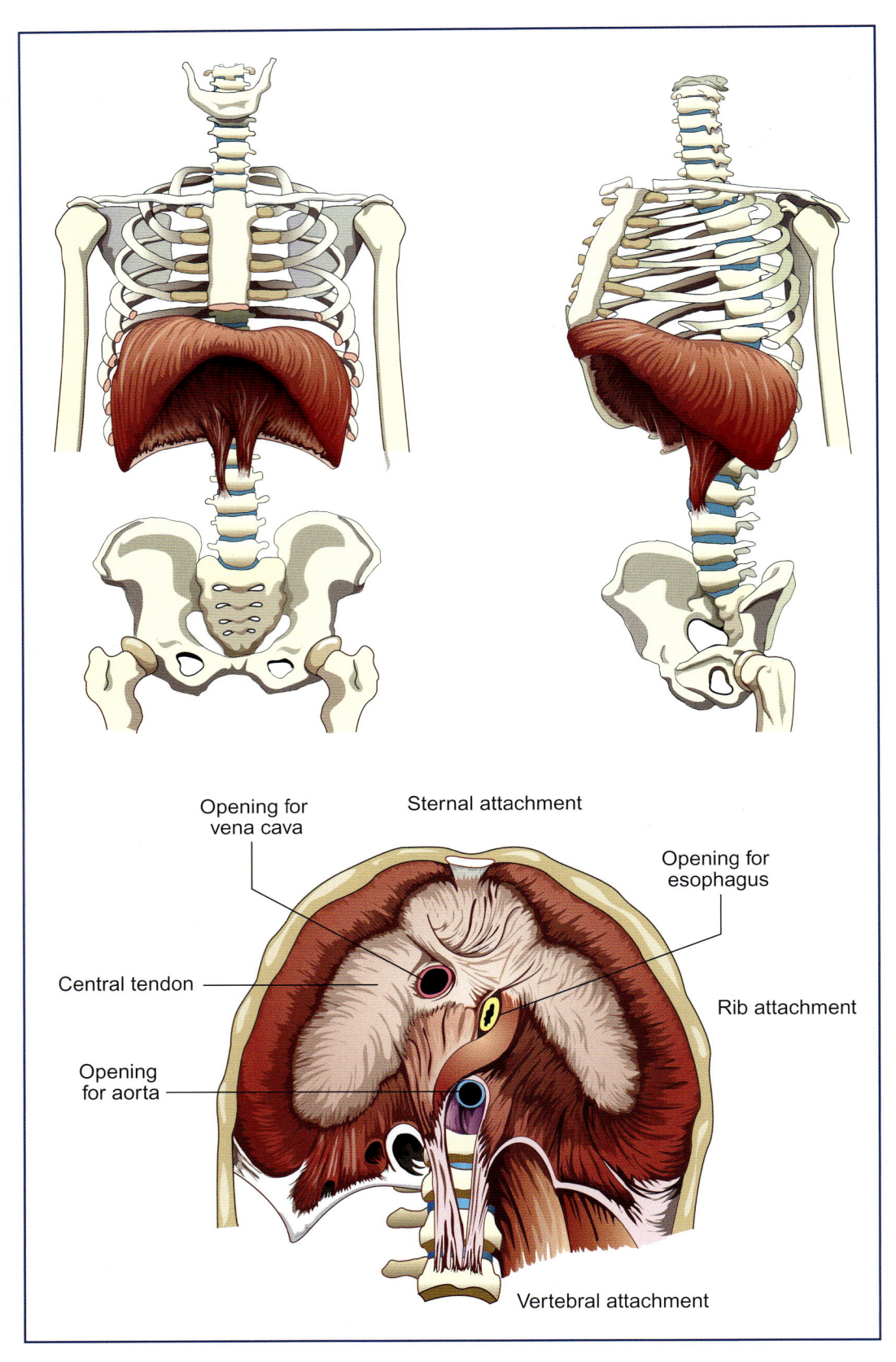

Figure 2–6. Muscle of the diaphragm shown from different views. Upper panels from *Evaluation and management of speech breathing disorders: Principles and methods* (p. 25), by T. Hixon and J. Hoit, 2005, Tucson, AZ: Redington Brown. Copyright 2005 by Thomas J. Hixon and Jeannette D. Hoit. Modified and reproduced with permission.

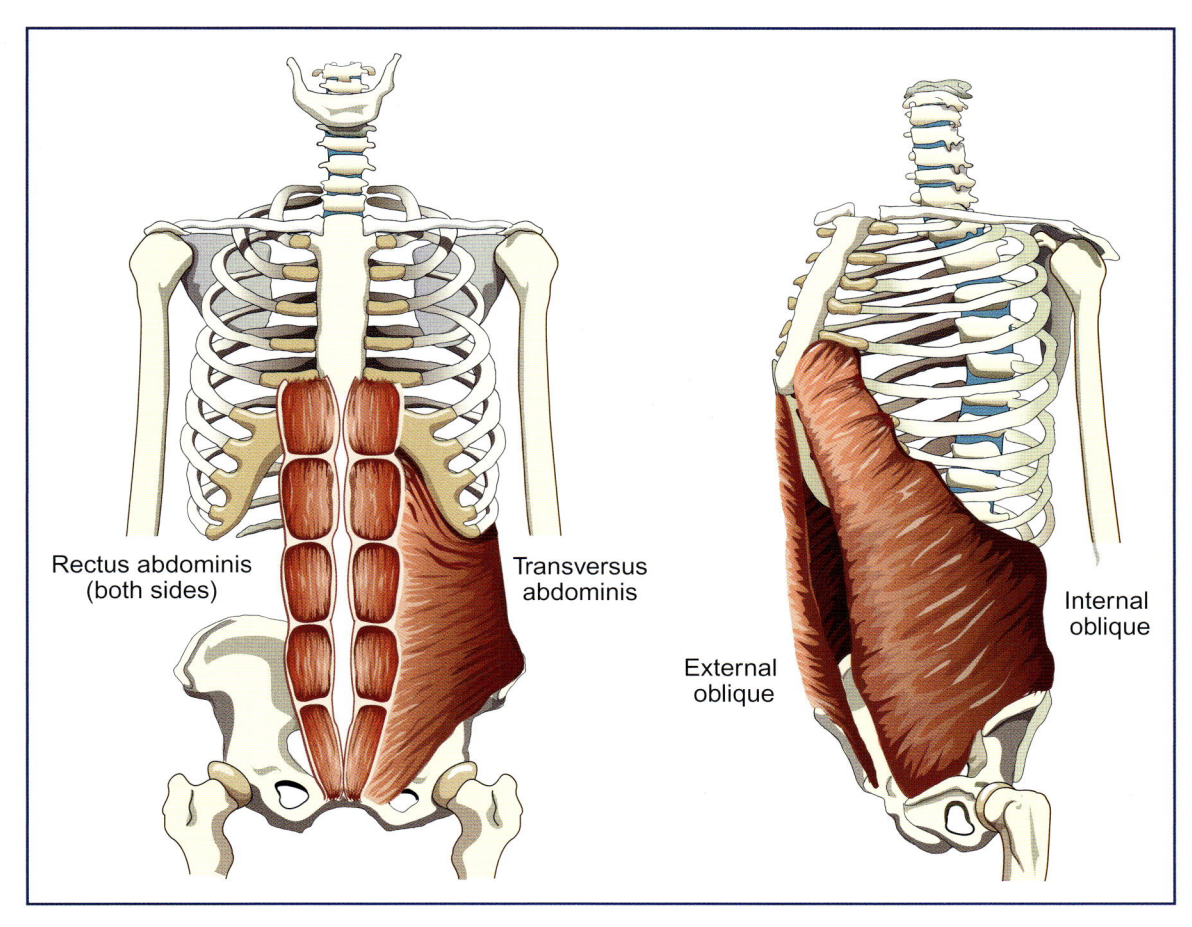

Figure 2–7. Muscles of the abdominal wall. From *Evaluation and management of speech breathing disorders: Principles and methods* (p. 26), by T. Hixon and J. Hoit, 2005, Tucson, AZ: Redington Brown. Copyright 2005 by Thomas J. Hixon and Jeannette D. Hoit. Modified and reproduced with permission.

The *external oblique* muscle is a broad structure located on the side and front of the lower rib cage wall and abdominal wall. It originates from the upper surface of the coxal bone and abdominal aponeurosis near the midline. Fibers course upward across the abdominal wall at various angles. The most prominent course is upward and toward the side, with insertions being on the outer surfaces and lower borders of the lower eight ribs. When the *external oblique* muscle contracts, it pulls the lower ribs downward and forces the front and side of the abdominal wall inward.

The *internal oblique* muscle is a large muscle positioned on the side and front of the lower rib cage wall and abdominal wall. It lies underneath the *external oblique* muscle. The *internal oblique* muscle originates from the upper surface of the coxal bone and lumbodorsal fascia. Its fibers fan out across the abdominal wall to insert into the abdominal aponeurosis and the lower borders of the costal cartilages of the lower three or four ribs. The fibers of the *internal oblique* muscle run at a right angle to those of the *external oblique* muscle. When the *internal oblique* muscle contracts, it pulls the lower ribs downward and forces the front and side of the abdominal wall inward. Thus, its functional potential is similar to that of the *external oblique* muscle.

The *transversus abdominis* muscle is a broad structure located on the front and side of the abdominal wall. It lies underneath the *internal oblique* muscle. The *transversus abdominis* muscle has a complex origin that includes the upper surface of the coxal bone, lumbodorsal fascia, and inner surfaces of the costal cartilages of ribs seven through twelve. Fibers of the muscle run horizontally around the abdominal wall and insert at the front into the abdominal aponeurosis. The paired left and right *transversus abdominis* muscles encircle the abdominal wall. When the *transversus abdominis* muscle contracts, it forces the front and side of the abdominal wall inward.

The four muscles just described are routinely referred to as "the abdominal muscles." However, the abdominal wall runs all the way around the torso and includes more than just its front and sides. Three other muscles traverse the abdominal wall at the back and are as much a part of the abdominal wall as the muscles just discussed. These are the *latissimus dorsi*, *lateral iliocostalis lumborum*, and *quadratus lumborum* muscles, described above in the context of the rib cage wall muscles. These muscles do not effect major displacements of the abdominal wall; rather, they brace the abdominal wall at the back and alter its stiffness.

Summary of Passive and Active Forces

The breathing apparatus can exert passive and active forces that are both inspiratory and expiratory. Figure 2–8 summarizes the passive and active forces for the different parts of the breathing apparatus—the pulmonary apparatus, chest wall, and the individual components of the chest wall that contain muscles (rib cage wall, diaphragm, and abdominal wall). Negative and positive signs in the figure represent forces that tend to inspire (−) and expire (+) the breathing apparatus.

The pulmonary apparatus exerts only passive force. Specifically, it recoils toward a smaller size, like a stretched coil spring. Thus, it operates in the expiratory direction only.

The chest wall can exert both passive and active force. At large chest wall sizes, it recoils inward (expiratory) and at small sizes it recoils outward (inspiratory). Muscles of the chest wall can generate active force to either inspire or expire the breathing apparatus at any chest wall size. Muscles that inspire the apparatus are located in the rib cage wall and diaphragm, and

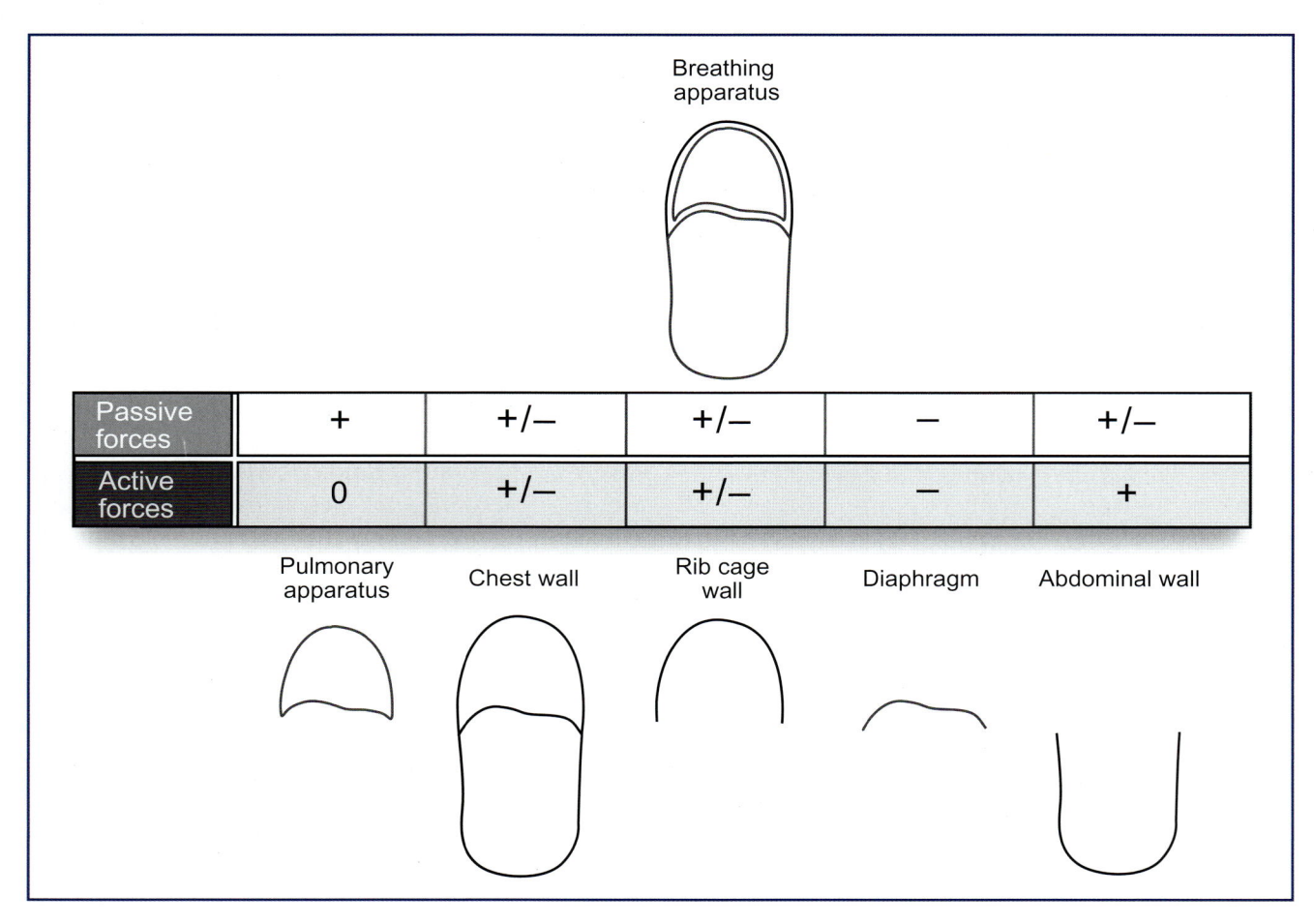

Figure 2–8. Passive and active forces of breathing. The pulmonary apparatus has only passive expiratory (+) force, whereas the chest wall (composed of the rib cage wall, diaphragm, and abdominal wall) has both passive and active forces that produce both inspiratory (−) and expiratory (+) force. From *Evaluation and management of speech breathing disorders: Principles and methods* (p. 31), by T. Hixon and J. Hoit, 2005, Tucson, AZ: Redington Brown. Copyright 2005 by Thomas J. Hixon and Jeannette D. Hoit. Modified and reproduced with permission.

muscles that expire the apparatus are located in the rib cage wall and abdominal wall. Active force available to inspire the breathing apparatus is greater at small chest wall sizes, and active force available to expire the apparatus is greater at large chest wall sizes. This is because the inspiratory and expiratory muscles of the chest wall are on more favorable portions of their length-force characteristics at small and large chest wall sizes, respectively.

The rib cage wall can contribute both passively and actively to adjustments of the breathing apparatus. It recoils inward at large sizes and outward at small sizes in most body positions. Muscles of the rib cage wall can generate active inspiratory and expiratory force. Those muscles responsible for inspiratory force are generally located in superficial layers of the rib cage wall and those responsible for expiratory force are generally located in deep layers of the wall. Active inspiratory force is greater at small rib cage wall sizes and active expiratory force is greater at large rib cage wall sizes, due to more favorable length–force characteristics for the inspiratory and expiratory muscles at small and large rib cage wall sizes, respectively. The smallest muscles of the breathing apparatus are located in the rib cage wall and provide it with the capability for fast and precise action.

The diaphragm has both passive and active force capabilities. When displaced footward, as it is at large lung volumes, it develops no recoil. In contrast, when displaced headward, as it is at small lung volumes, it recoils in the inspiratory direction. The diaphragm can generate active force in the inspiratory direction only.

The abdominal wall can produce both passive and active force. It recoils in the expiratory direction at large abdominal wall volumes and in the inspiratory direction at small abdominal wall volumes in most body positions. The abdominal wall can generate active force in only the expiratory direction, with greater expiratory force being generated at large abdominal wall volumes because its muscles are on more favorable portions of their length-force characteristics.

The chest wall muscles that exert active force on the breathing apparatus are summarized in Table 2–1. Activation of these muscles can change the volume of

Table 2-1. Muscles of the Chest Wall and Their Potential Actions on the Thorax

CIRCUMFERENCE INCREASERS	CIRCUMFERENCE DECREASERS
Sternocleidomastoid	Internal intercostal (interosseus)
Scalenes (anterior, medius, posterior)	Transverse thoracis
Pectoralis major	Latissimus dorsi
Pectoralis minor	Serratus posterior inferior
Subclavius	Lateral iliocostalis lumborum
Serratus anterior	Lateral iliocostalis thoracis
External intercostal	Quadratus lumborum
Internal intercostal (intercartilaginous)	Subcostal
Latissimus dorsi	Rectus abdominis
Serratus posterior superior	External oblique abdominis
Lateral iliocostalis cervicis	Internal oblique abdominis
Lateral iliocostalis thoracis	
Levatores costarum	
Diaphragm	
VERTICAL LENGTH INCREASER	**VERTICAL LENGTH DECREASERS**
Diaphragm	Rectus abdominis
	External oblique abdominis
	Internal oblique abdominis
	Transverse abdominis

Note. Those muscles that increase the circumference or increase the vertical length of the thorax are considered *inspiratory* muscles and those that decrease the circumference or decrease the vertical length of the thorax are considered *expiratory* muscles.

the pulmonary apparatus (pulmonary airways and lungs) by increasing or decreasing the circumference of the thorax, increasing or decreasing the vertical length of the thorax (by lowering or raising its floor), or both. Increasing thoracic size (and, thus, increasing the volume of the pulmonary apparatus) is an inspiratory action, and decreasing thoracic size is an expiratory action.

Realization of Passive and Active Forces

Forces of breathing are realized in two ways. One way is through pulls on structures and the other way is through pressures developed at various locations. Pulling forces are distributed in a complex fashion. Fortunately, they are uniformly distributed at certain points where they manifest as pressures. The locations of the most important of these pressures are shown in Figure 2–9.

Included among these pressures are alveolar pressure, pleural pressure, abdominal pressure, and transdiaphragmatic pressure. Alveolar pressure is the pressure inside the lungs; pleural pressure is the pressure inside the thorax but outside the lungs (between the pleural membranes); abdominal pressure is the pressure inside the abdominal cavity; and transdiaphragmatic pressure is the difference in pressure across the diaphragm (the difference between pleural pressure and abdominal pressure). Although all of these pressures are critical to the function of the breathing apparatus, the pressure of greatest primacy to the understanding of speech production is alveolar pressure.

MOVEMENTS OF BREATHING

Breathing is accomplished through movements of the individual parts of the chest wall—rib cage wall, diaphragm, and abdominal wall. These movements can be described for each part individually, as they are below. Nevertheless, the forces that underlie these movements are not necessarily easy to determine. This is because the interactions among the different parts of the chest wall are quite complex.

Movements of the Rib Cage Wall

The rib cage wall is able to move because of two sets of joints, those between the ribs and sternum (costosternal joints) and those between the ribs and the vertebral column (costovertebral joints). Actual movement differs somewhat from rib to rib, owing to differences in the lengths and shapes of individual ribs. Nevertheless, two types of rib movements are typical and are illustrated in Figure 2–10. One type of rib movement is a vertical excursion of its front (sternal) end and is either upward and forward or downward and backward, resulting in an increase or decrease, respectively, in the front-to-back diameter of the rib cage. Each rib rotates through the axis of its neck (at the back near the vertebral column) in a movement pattern that resembles the raising and lowering of the handle on a water pump.

The other type of rib movement is vertical excursion along the side of the rib cage that involves a rotation of the rib around an axis extending between its two ends. The rotation is either upward and outward or downward and inward, the result being an increase or decrease, respectively, in the side-to-side (transverse) diameter of the rib cage. Such movement is similar to the raising and lowering of the handle on a water bucket.

These two types of rib movement occur together and in phase. Thus, the circumference of the rib cage wall increases and decreases along with increases and decreases in its two diameters (front-to-back and side-to-side).

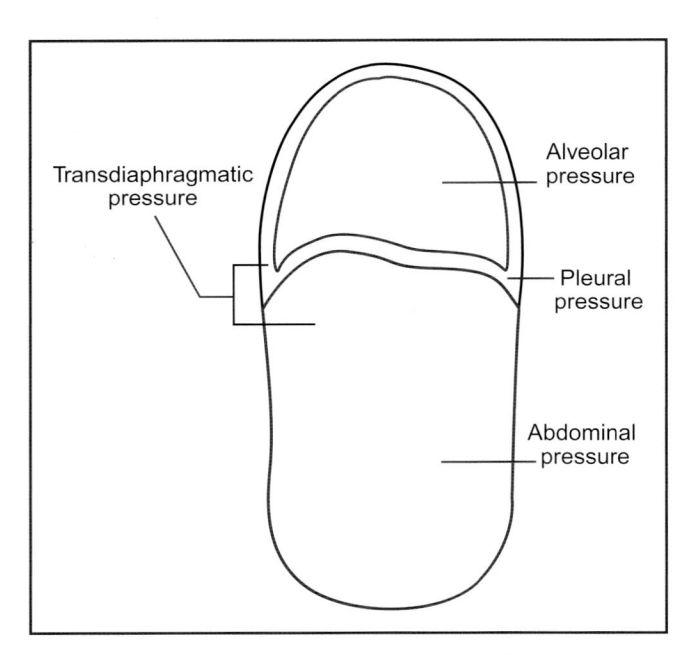

Figure 2–9. Pressures of the breathing apparatus. Alveolar pressure is the pressure inside the lungs. Pleural pressure is the pressure between the pleural (visceral and parietal) membranes. Abdominal pressure is the pressure inside the abdomen. Transdiaphragmatic pressure is the difference between the pleural and abdominal pressures.

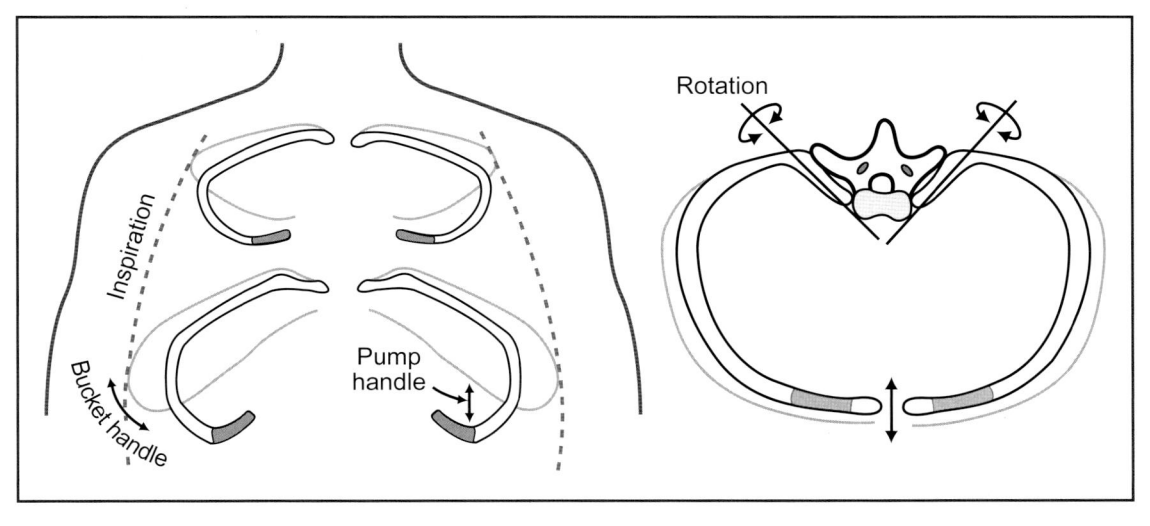

Figure 2–10. Two types of rib movements. They are (1) upward and forward/downward and backward (like the handle on a water pump) and (2) upward and outward/downward and inward (like a bucket handle).

Not Doing What Comes Naturally

The initiation and execution of voluntary breathing movements come naturally for most of us. But, for some individuals with maldeveloped or damaged brains, these may not be easy, or even possible, to do. Their problem is praxis or action. They have dyspraxia when they have difficulty with action, and apraxia when they are unable to carry out action at all. One of the most perplexing clients we ever encountered was a young man who showed difficulties with breathing actions following a traumatic brain injury. When he attempted to initiate voluntary inspirations or expirations on command, he often became frozen in position. Occasionally, his attempt resulted in movement in the opposite direction (he breathed in when trying to breathe out). He knew exactly what he wanted to do, but just couldn't do it. Imagine the depth of his frustration.

Movements of the Diaphragm

The diaphragm can enlarge the thorax vertically by pulling down on the central tendon or it can enlarge the thorax circumferentially by elevating the lower ribs. It can also do both simultaneously, as depicted in Figure 2–11.

The actions of the diaphragm (Figure 2–11), as well as the actions of the rib cage wall and abdominal wall, can change the configuration of the diaphragm such that it can flatten or become more highly domed, as illustrated in Figure 2–12. Flattening is accompanied by descent of the central tendon and/or elevation of the lower ribs; doming of the diaphragm is accompanied by elevation of the central tendon and/or descent of the lower ribs. In general, the more highly domed the diaphragm, the more active (inspiratory) force it is able to exert. This is because its muscle fibers are stretched and are on more favorable portions of their length–force characteristics.

Movements of the diaphragm are hidden from view and must be inferred from movements of more superficial structures of the chest wall. Diaphragm movements are manifested in changes in the radius of its curvature and depend on the relative fixation of the lower ribs and central tendon. When the rib cage is fixed in position, the movement of the diaphragm is reflected superficially in movement of the abdominal

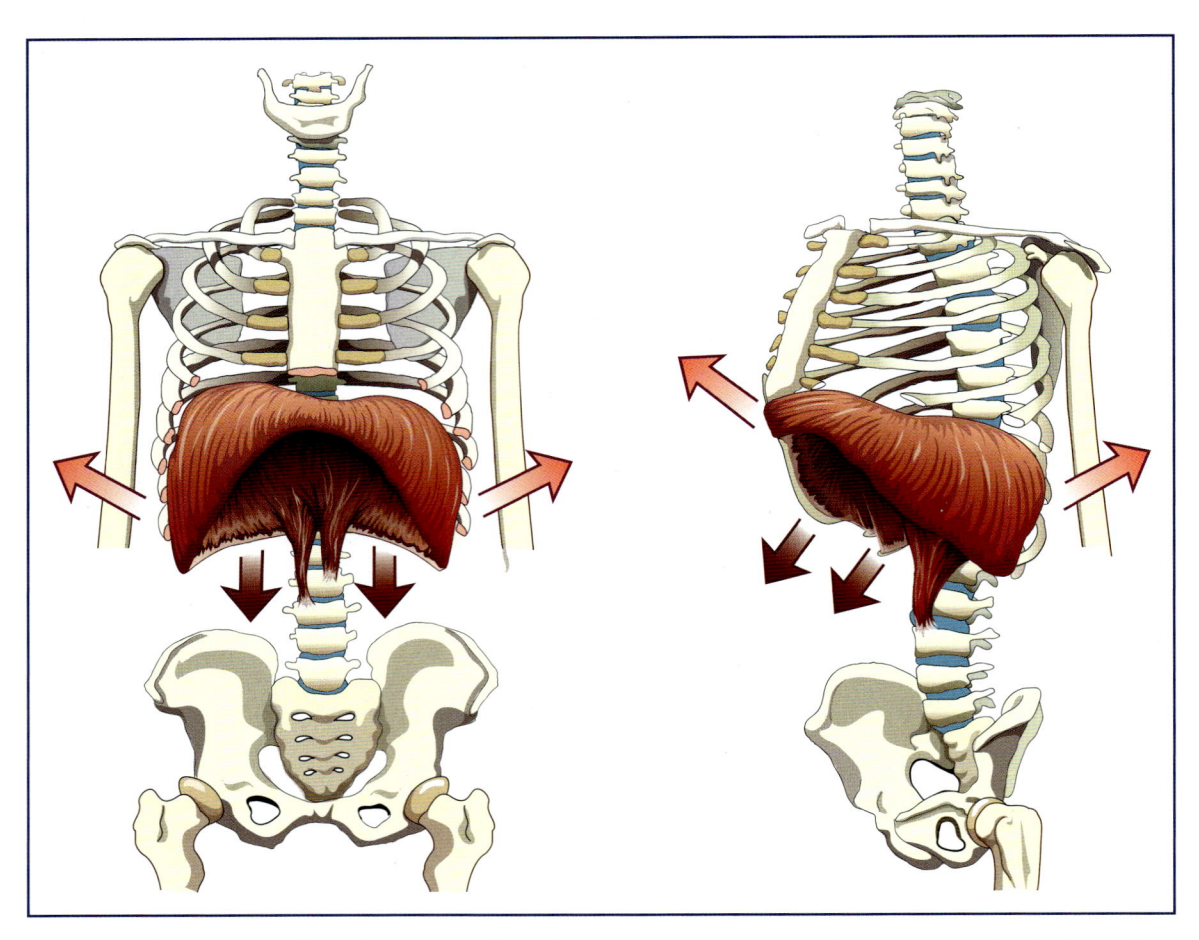

Figure 2-11. Actions of the diaphragm. The diaphragm can enlarge the thorax vertically by pulling the central tendon downward and forward (*downward pointing arrows*) and it can expand the thorax circumferentially by lifting the lower ribs (*upward pointing arrows*). Structural features from *Evaluation and management of speech breathing disorders: Principles and methods* (p. 25), by T. Hixon and J. Hoit, 2005, Tucson, AZ: Redington Brown. Copyright 2005 by Thomas J. Hixon and Jeannette D. Hoit. Modified and reproduced with permission.

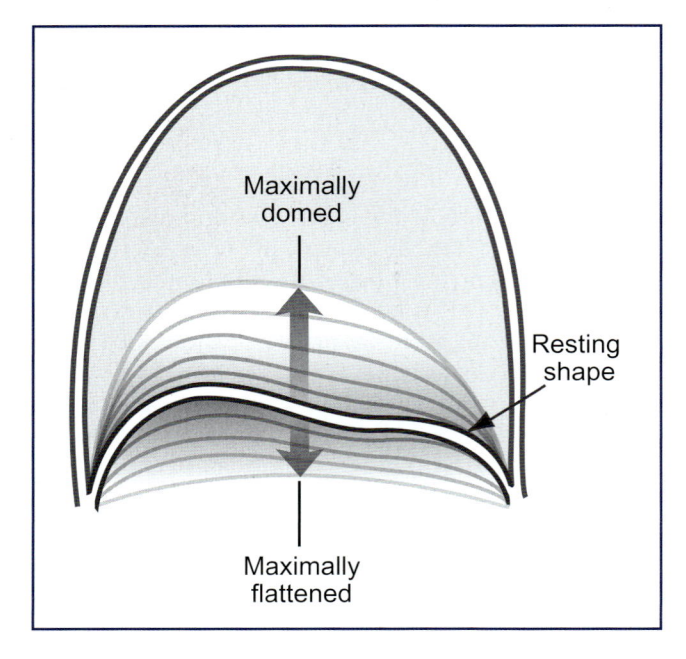

Figure 2-12. Configurations of the diaphragm. The diaphragm can assume a flattened configuration by descent of the central tendon and/or lifting of the lower ribs, and a domed configuration by elevation of the central tendon and/or descent of the lower ribs.

wall; when the central tendon is fixed in position, the movement of the diaphragm is reflected in movement of the rib cage wall.

Movements of the Abdominal Wall

When at rest in an upright position, the lower abdominal wall is distended somewhat because the pressure inside the abdomen is greater near the bottom than near the undersurface of the diaphragm. This pressure pushes the lower abdominal wall outward. Inward movement flattens the abdominal wall and outward movement increases the degree to which the abdominal wall is protruded. Most movement occurs in the anteroposterior dimension, as depicted in Figure 2–13.

Relative Movements of the Rib Cage Wall and Diaphragm–Abdominal Wall

The rib cage wall contacts about three-fourths of the surface of the pulmonary apparatus, whereas the diaphragm–abdominal wall unit contacts only about one-fourth of the surface area. This means that a small movement of the rib cage wall can move a substantial amount of air into or out of the pulmonary apparatus or cause a major pressure change within the pulmonary apparatus. In contrast, the diaphragm–abdominal wall unit must move a much greater distance to displace the same amount of air or create the same pressure change. The relative consequences of rib cage wall movement versus diaphragm–abdominal wall movement on pulmonary volume and pressure are illustrated in Figure 2–14.

Forces Underlying Movements

The breathing apparatus can exert forces that may cause movements, pressure changes, or both. Some of these are confined to the parts of the chest wall in which they

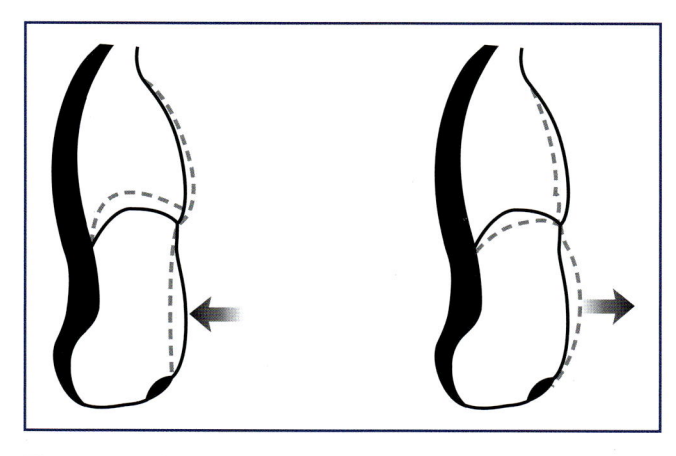

Figure 2-13. Inward and outward movement of the abdominal wall.

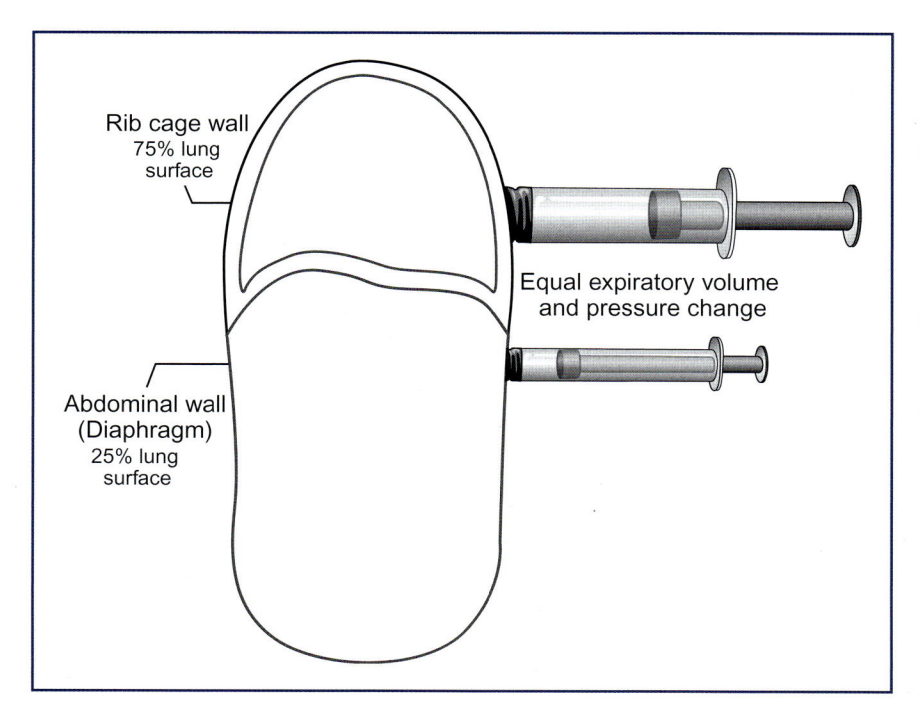

Figure 2-14. Relative movements of the rib cage wall and diaphragm–abdominal wall. The different-sized plungers represent the fact that a small movement of the rib cage wall can cause a large volume and pressure change within the pulmonary apparatus when compared with the same movement of the diaphragm–abdominal wall. This is because the rib cage wall covers approximately three times as much surface area of the pulmonary apparatus compared with the diaphragm–abdominal wall.

occur. Others are the result of actions between different parts of the chest wall. Thus, it is possible for one part of the breathing apparatus to cause movements and/or pressure changes in other parts of the apparatus, as illustrated in Figure 2–15 and discussed in the following examples.

Figure 2–15A represents active expansion of the rib cage wall (using inspiratory rib cage wall muscles) and quiescent diaphragm and abdominal wall muscles. In this situation, rib cage wall expansion lowers pleural pressure and pulls the diaphragm headward and the abdominal wall inward. This action is like pulling liquid up a drinking straw (hence the phrase "sucking it in" when referring to the resulting inward movement of the abdominal wall). The opposite situation is shown in Figure 2–15B, where actively compressing the rib cage wall (using expiratory rib cage wall muscles) causes pleural pressure to rise and pushes the diaphragm footward and the abdominal wall outward.

Actions of the diaphragm can move the rib cage wall, abdominal wall, or both, depending on the mechanical status of these two chest wall parts. When the rib cage wall is fixed in position, as depicted in Figure 2–14C, contraction of the diaphragm causes it to move footward and pushes the abdominal wall outward. In contrast, when the abdominal wall is fixed in position, as in Figure 2–14D, diaphragm contraction is resolved into headward displacement (expansion) of

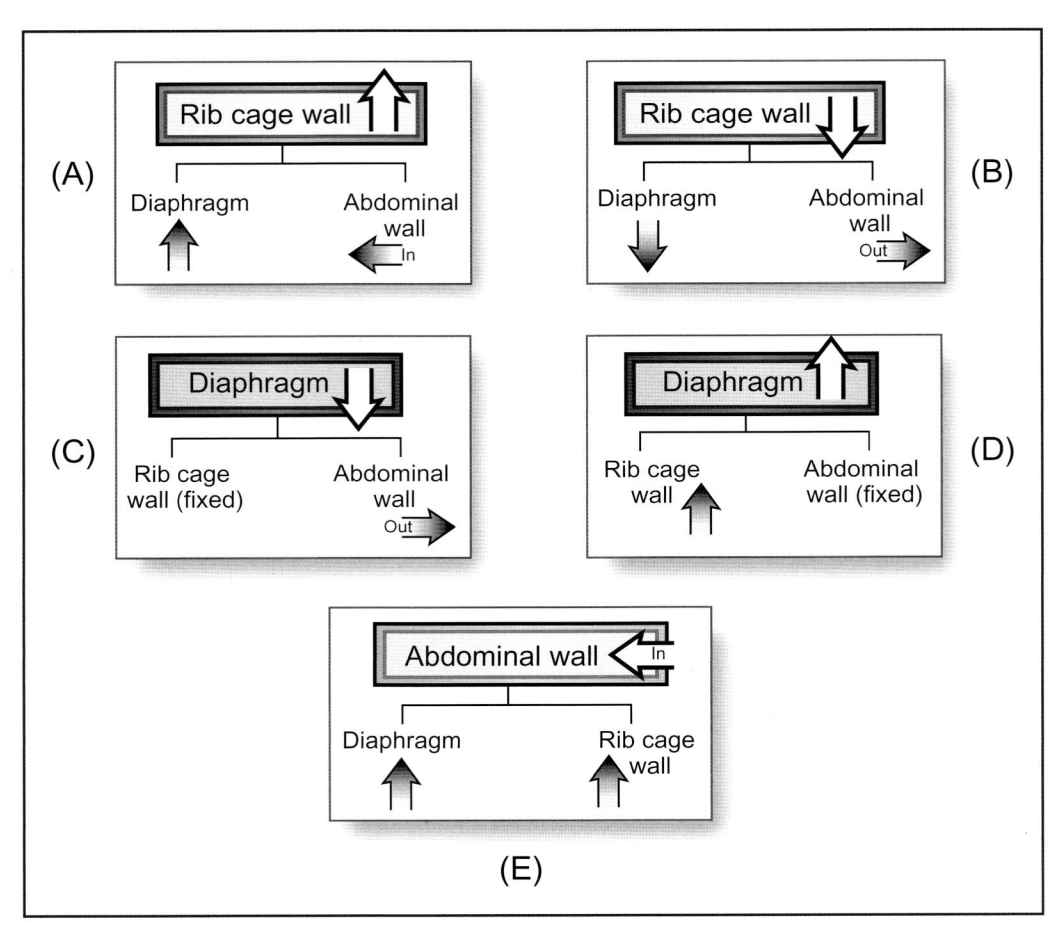

Figure 2–15. Examples of how the rib cage wall, diaphragm, and abdominal wall can affect one another. The white arrow in each example indicates which chest wall component is active; the filled arrows represent the effects on the other chest wall components. **A.** Expansion of the rib cage wall can pull the diaphragm headward and the abdominal wall inward through the lowering of pleural pressure. **B.** Compression of the rib cage wall can push the diaphragm footward and the abdominal wall outward through the raising of pleural pressure. **C.** Contraction of the diaphragm can push the abdominal wall outward, if the rib cage wall is fixed. **D.** Contraction of the diaphragm can lift the rib cage wall upward and outward, if the abdominal wall is fixed. **E.** Inward displacement of the abdominal wall can push the diaphragm headward and lift and expand the rib cage wall.

the rib cage wall. Usually, neither the rib cage wall nor abdominal wall is rigidly positioned, so that both move in accordance with their relative compliance (stiffness).

Actions of the abdominal wall can cause adjustments in both the rib cage wall and diaphragm. When the muscles of the abdominal wall contract, they force the abdominal wall inward and raise abdominal pressure. As depicted in Figure 2–14E, this action forces the lower rib cage wall outward and the diaphragm headward. The combination of these two effects causes a passive lifting of the rib cage wall.

Actions of the breathing apparatus often seem deceptively simple and can be erroneously ascribed as being caused only by the parts of the apparatus in which the movement is observed. Thus, when observing movements of the rib cage wall, it should not be assumed that the rib cage wall necessarily moved itself. Similarly, movement of the abdominal wall may or may not be ascribed to activation of abdominal wall muscles.

CONTROL VARIABLES OF BREATHING

The breathing apparatus controls a number of variables, some of which are particularly important to speech production. These variables are lung volume, alveolar pressure, and chest wall shape.

Lung Volume

Volume is defined as the size of a three-dimensional object or space. The volume of interest here is the volume of air inside the pulmonary apparatus. This volume is termed the lung volume and it reflects the size of the breathing apparatus. Movements of the breathing apparatus can change lung volume by moving air into or out of the pulmonary apparatus. Such movement, sometimes called volume displacement, can occur only if the larynx and upper airway are open.

The volume variable can be partitioned into what are called lung volumes and lung capacities. As shown in Figure 2–16, volume can be displayed in a spirogram, a record of lung volume change over time obtained from a spirometer (a device that records volume displacement; see Chapter 6).

There are four lung volumes. Each covers a portion of the lung volume range that is mutually exclusive of the others.

The *tidal volume* (TV) is the volume of air inspired or expired during the breathing cycle. When recorded in the resting individual, this volume is termed the resting tidal volume.

The *inspiratory reserve volume* (IRV) is the maximum volume of air that can be inspired from the tidal end–inspiratory level (the peak of the tidal volume cycle).

The *expiratory reserve volume* (ERV) is the maximum volume of air that can be expired from the tidal end–expiratory level (the trough of the tidal volume cycle).

The *residual volume* (RV) is the volume of air remaining in the pulmonary apparatus at the end of a maximum expiration. This volume cannot be measured directly.

There are four lung capacities. Each capacity includes two or more of the lung volumes defined above.

The *inspiratory capacity* (IC) is the maximum volume of air that can be inspired from the resting tidal end–expiratory level. It is the sum of the tidal volume and the inspiratory reserve volume.

The *vital capacity* (VC) is the maximum volume of air that can be expired following a maximum inspiration (or inspired following a maximum expiration). It includes the inspiratory reserve volume, the tidal volume, and the expiratory reserve volume.

The *functional residual capacity* (FRC) is the volume of air in the pulmonary apparatus at the resting tidal end–expiratory level. This capacity includes the expiratory reserve volume and the residual volume.

Where Did That Come From?

We have seen many young children with cerebral palsy and breathing disorders. Many of these children, especially those who are quadriplegic and show major signs of spasticity, seem to have a governor on them. That is, they behave like there's a device that is limiting the degree to which they can willfully adjust the breathing apparatus. When asked to perform an inspiratory capacity maneuver ("Take in all the air you can"), they may only be able to inspire to their resting tidal end–inspiratory level. Try it over and over again and the same thing happens. Then, out of the blue, the child shows you a gaping yawn of boredom and takes in an enormous breath. The breath may actually be several times the size the child could generate during voluntary inspiration. Now, you're faced with a dilemma. What do you record as the child's inspiratory capacity? Think about it, carefully.

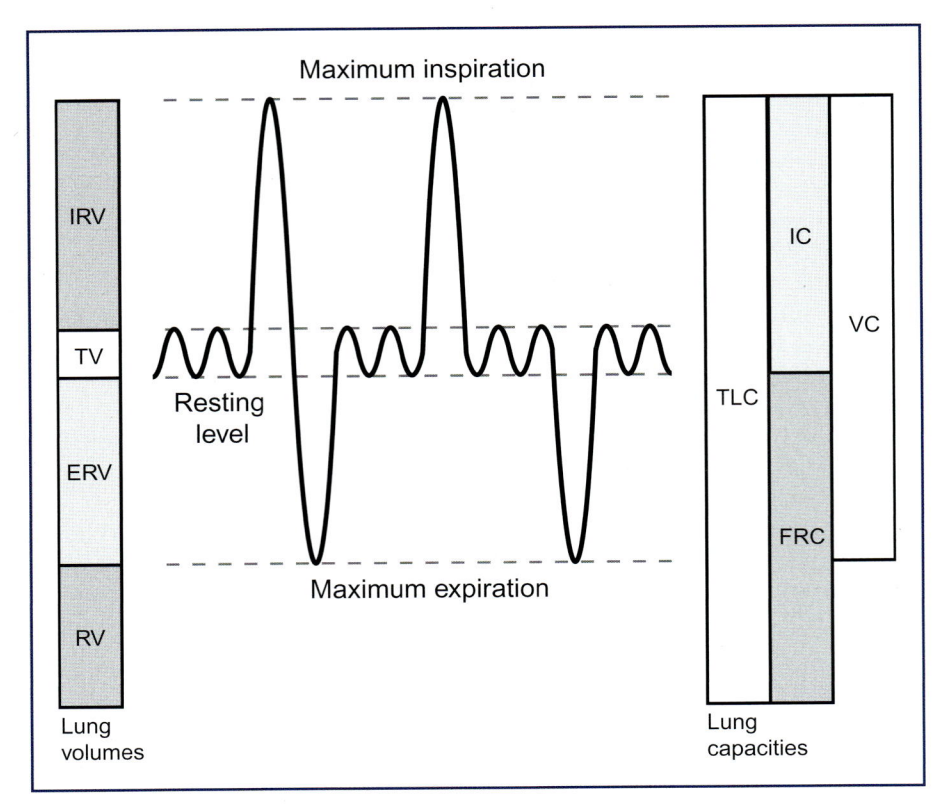

Figure 2–16. A spirogram showing lung volumes and lung capacities. The lung volumes are tidal volume (TV), inspiratory reserve volume (IRV), expiratory reserve volume (ERV), and residual volume (RV). The lung capacities are inspiratory capacity (IC), vital capacity (VC), functional residual capacity (FRC), and total lung capacity (TLC). From *Evaluation and management of speech breathing disorders: Principles and methods* (p. 36), by T. Hixon and J. Hoit, 2005, Tucson, AZ: Redington Brown. Copyright 2005 by Thomas J. Hixon and Jeannette D. Hoit. Modified and reproduced with permission.

Because this includes the residual volume, it cannot be measured directly.

The *total lung capacity* (TLC) is the volume of air in the pulmonary apparatus at the end of a maximum inspiration. It includes the inspiratory reserve volume, the tidal volume, the expiratory reserve volume, and the residual volume. This lung capacity cannot be measured directly because it includes the residual volume.

The lung volumes used in a number of everyday breathing activities are shown in Figure 2–17. Here, lung volume is expressed in percent vital capacity (%VC), a common way of expressing breathing events because it allows for comparisons across people of different sizes. Note that in this figure the volume of the breathing apparatus at the end of a resting tidal expiration is shown as 40 %VC. This is a typical resting level for someone in an upright (sitting or standing) body position.

Alveolar Pressure

Pressure is defined as a force distributed over a surface (pressure = force/area). The most important pressure for present purposes is the pressure inside the lungs, the alveolar pressure. Alveolar pressure represents the sum of all the passive and active forces operating on the breathing apparatus.

Alveolar pressure is generated by the collision of air molecules within the pulmonary apparatus. When air molecules are more crowded, more collisions occur and pressure is higher. In contrast, when air molecules are less crowded, fewer collisions occur and alveolar pressure is lower. When the larynx and/or upper air-

[Figure 2-17 diagram showing lung volume change (%VC) with labels:]
- 100 — Maximum inspiration
- 95 — Inspiration during vigorous yawning
- 90 — Inspiration during classical singing
- 85
- 80 — Inspiration during loud reading
- 75
- 70
- 65
- 60 — Inspiration during conversational speaking
- 55
- 50 — Resting tidal inspiration
- 45
- 40 — Resting tidal expiration
- 35
- 30
- 25
- 20
- 15 — Expiration during vigorous laughing
- 10
- 5
- 0 — Maximum expiration

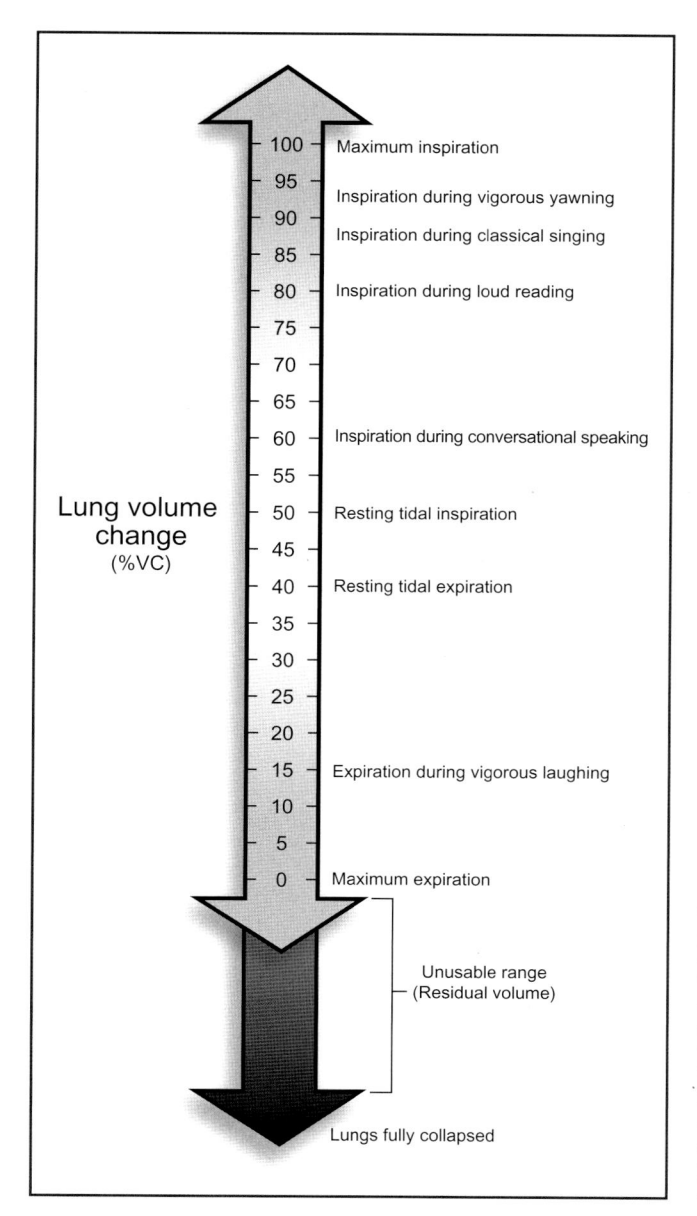

Unusable range (Residual volume)
Lungs fully collapsed

Figure 2–17. Lung volumes used in some everyday activities expressed in percent vital capacity (%VC) and performed in an upright body position. Some of these volumes shift when performed in other body positions.

Always Under Pressure

The zero pressure seen on breathing diagrams really doesn't mean zero. It actually represents atmospheric pressure, the pressure we are under all the time. Far from zero, atmospheric pressure has a magnitude of 1.01325×10^5 newtons per square meter (N/m²). That's roughly 1000 cmH$_2$O, a unit of pressure measurement often used by respiratory physiologists. When we blow our hardest, we might (on a good day) develop 225 cmH$_2$O of alveolar pressure. That's interesting. We blow as hard as we possibly can and we can only increase our alveolar pressure to about one-fourth the magnitude of the pressure that is operating on us as we just sit there. Most of us probably aren't even aware that we have 1000 cmH$_2$O of pressure continuously trying to squash us. But, in fact, we're always under pressure.

way are closed, lung volume and alveolar pressure are inversely related. That is, in a closed system, a halving of volume causes a doubling of pressure, and a doubling of volume causes a halving of pressure (provided temperature remains constant). This is called Boyle's law. Boyle's law does not apply when the larynx and upper airway are open.

One way to display alveolar pressure is in a pressure-volume diagram, such as that shown in Figure 2–18. The vertical axis of the diagram represents lung volume (in %VC) and the horizontal axis represents alveolar pressure (in centimeters of water, cmH$_2$O). The light horizontal line represents the resting level of the breathing apparatus (resting tidal end-expiration), shown to be 40 %VC in this diagram. The light vertical line represents atmospheric pressure (zero, by convention). Points to the left of this line represent pressures that are below atmospheric (negative, by convention), and points to the right of this line represent pressures that are above atmospheric (positive, by convention). The middle, curved line labeled "Relaxation" represents the volume-pressure relation when the muscles of the breathing apparatus are completely quiescent and the larynx or upper airway is closed.

The relaxation pressure is the pressure produced entirely by the passive force of the breathing apparatus. As shown in Figure 2–18, the relaxation pressure varies with lung volume. Relaxation pressure is positive at lung volumes larger than the resting level of the breathing apparatus (40 %VC in the figure), and negative at lung volumes smaller than the resting level. The greatest positive relaxation pressure is generated at the largest lung volume, and the greatest negative relaxation pressure is generated at the smallest lung volume. In the midrange of the vital capacity, the relaxation pressure changes nearly in direct proportion to lung volume change, whereas at the extremes of the vital capacity, pressure changes more abruptly with volume change. This is because the breathing apparatus is stiffer at very large and very small lung volumes.

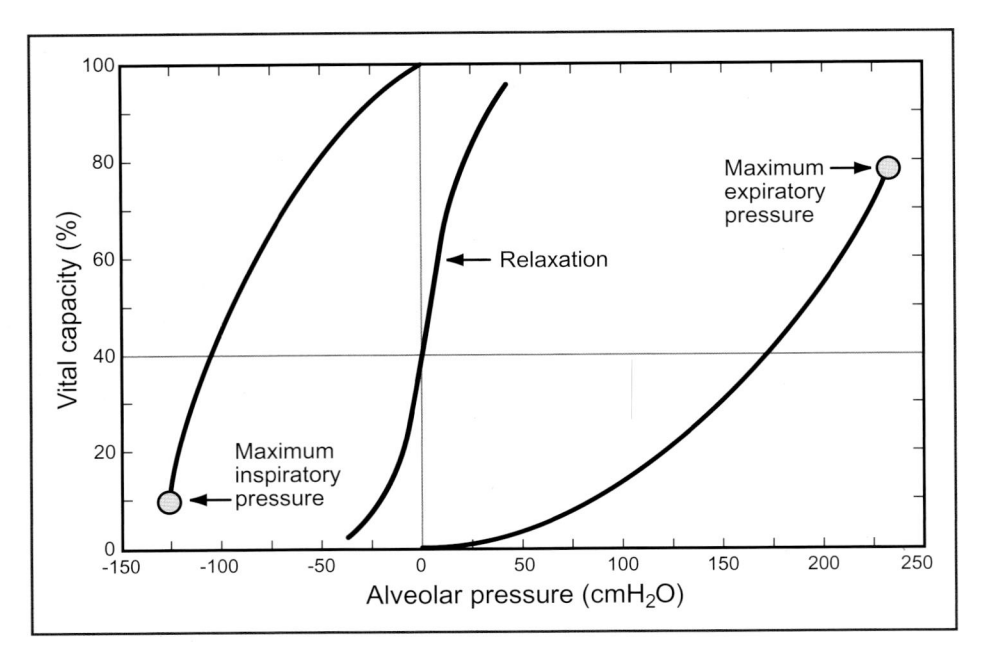

Figure 2-18. Pressure-volume diagram (for an upright body position). Volume is shown on the vertical axis (in percent vital capacity, % VC) ranging from 0 to 100%. Alveolar pressure is on the horizontal axis (in centimeters of water, cmH$_2$O) ranging from negative to positive pressures. Alveolar pressure is 0 (atmospheric) at 40% VC in this diagram. Relaxation pressure (*curved line in the middle of diagram*) is the passive pressure generated in the absence of active muscular pressure and is negative (inspiratory) at small lung volumes (smaller than 40% VC in this diagram) and positive (expiratory) at large lung volumes (larger than 40% VC in this diagram). Maximum inspiratory pressure is generated with passive plus maximum active inspiratory muscular pressure at the prevailing lung volume and is represented by the curved line to the left of the Relaxation line. The lower left circle represents the greatest negative (inspiratory) pressure achievable. Maximum expiratory pressure is generated with passive plus maximum active expiratory muscular pressure at the prevailing lung volume and is represented by the curved line to the right of the relaxation line. The upper right circle represents the greatest positive (expiratory) pressure achievable. Modified from *Evaluation and management of speech breathing disorders: Principles and methods* (p. 38), by T. Hixon and J. Hoit, 2005, Tucson, AZ: Redington Brown. Copyright 2005 by Thomas J. Hixon and Jeannette D. Hoit. Modified and reproduced with permission.

Departures from the relaxation pressure require active muscular pressure. A net inspiratory muscular pressure is needed to generate pressure that is lower than the relaxation pressure (to the left of the volume-pressure relaxation curve) at the prevailing lung volume. In contrast, a net expiratory muscular pressure is needed to generate pressure that is higher than the relaxation pressure (to the right of the relaxation curve) at the prevailing lung volume. When net is specified, as it is here, it means that both inspiratory and expiratory muscular pressures may be operating simultaneously, but one or the other is predominating. When pressure is equal to the relaxation pressure, this may mean that all the muscles of the breathing apparatus are relaxed, or it may mean that equal inspiratory and expiratory muscular pressures are being exerted so that they cancel one another.

Maximum inspiratory and expiratory pressure characteristics are also depicted in Figure 2-18. The maximum inspiratory pressure that can be generated by the breathing apparatus (with the larynx or upper airway closed) is represented by the leftmost curve in the figure. Note that the maximum inspiratory pressure is greater (more negative) at smaller lung volumes than larger lung volumes and that the greatest inspiratory pressure is generated near the bottom of the vital capacity (see the circle labeled "Maximum inspiratory pressure"). This is because negative relaxation pressure is more forceful at smaller lung volumes, and because the inspiratory muscles are operating under more favorable length-force conditions at smaller lung volumes.

The maximum expiratory pressure that can be generated by the breathing apparatus (with the larynx or upper airway closed) is represented by the rightmost curve in Figure 2–18. The maximum expiratory pressure is greater (more positive) at larger lung volumes than smaller lung volumes and the greatest expiratory pressure is generated near the top of the vital capacity (see the circle labeled "Maximum expiratory pressure"). This is because positive relaxation pressure is more forceful at larger lung volumes and because the expiratory muscles are operating under more favorable length-force conditions at larger lung volumes.

Figure 2–19 shows the range of achievable alveolar pressures (in cmH$_2$O) that might be generated by a young healthy man. Shown along the pressure scale is a list of activities and typical alveolar pressures associated with those activities.

Chest Wall Shape

Shape is the configuration of an object, independent of its volume (size). The shape of interest in the present context is the shape of the chest wall. Chest wall shape refers to the surface configuration of the rib cage wall and abdominal wall, the two parts of the chest wall that can be observed externally. Shape is important because it provides information about the prevailing mechanical advantages of different parts of the chest wall and clues about what muscle groups might be activated.

One convention for illustrating shape is to display the relative sizes of the rib cage wall and abdominal wall against one another, as portrayed in Figure 2–20. In this figure, the size of the rib cage wall is on the vertical axis, increasing upward, and the size of the abdominal wall is on the horizontal axis, increasing rightward. The actual size measurement may be a circumference or anteroposterior diameter, depending on the type of instrumentation used.

The dashed line in Figure 2–20 represents the relaxation characteristic of the chest wall. This is the shape assumed by the chest wall at different lung volumes when the breathing muscles are completely relaxed. The open circle at the top of the relaxation characteristic represents the total lung capacity, and the open circle at the bottom of the characteristic represents the residual volume. The filled circle represents the resting level of the breathing apparatus (recall the resting spring analogy represented in Figure 2–4, bottom right). The circumscribed area in the diagram depicts the full range of shapes that the chest wall can assume. Each point

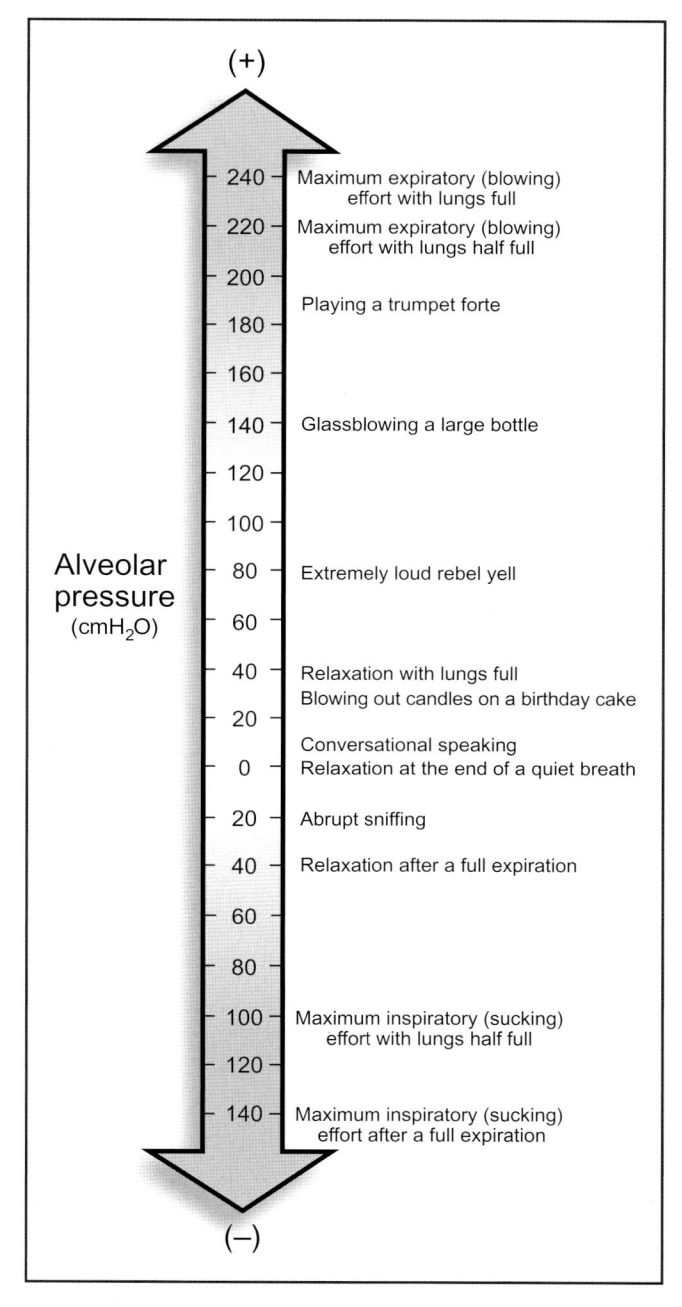

Figure 2-19. Alveolar pressures (in cmH$_2$O) used for different activities. The range of values shown here approximate those of a young healthy man.

within the circumscribed area represents a unique combination of chest wall shape and lung volume.

Figure 2–21 shows the range of achievable chest wall shapes (in relative terms) and activities associated with those shapes. A chest wall shape near the bottom of the arrow is characterized by a larger than relaxed abdominal wall and a smaller than relaxed rib cage

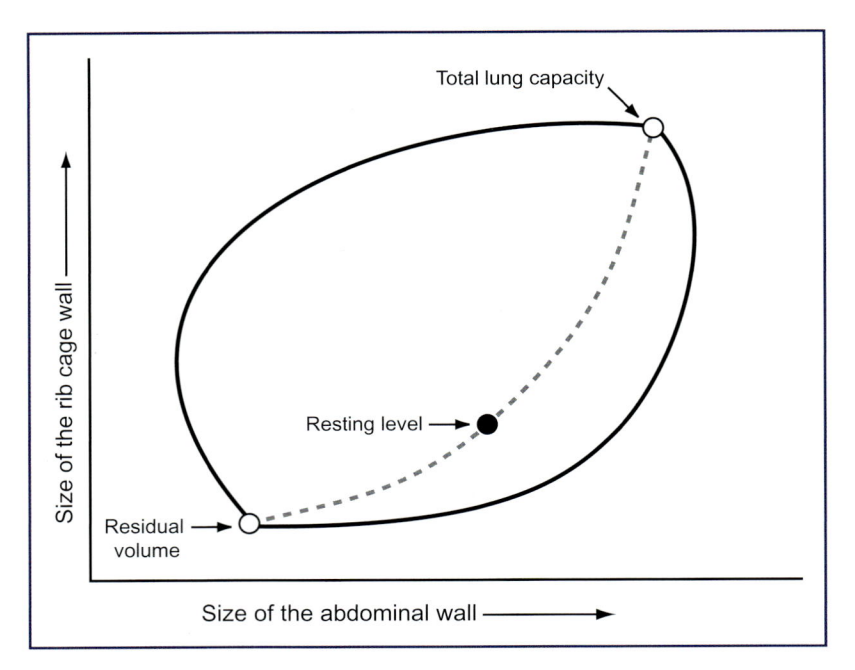

Figure 2–20. Relative size diagram of the rib cage wall and abdominal wall to represent chest wall shape. Rib cage wall size is shown as increasing upward on the vertical axis and abdominal wall size is shown as increasing rightward on the horizontal axis. The dashed line represents the continuum of chest wall shapes assumed during relaxation (no muscle activity) throughout the vital capacity. The solid lines represent the most extreme chest wall shapes that can be assumed (using muscle activity) at different lung volumes throughout the vital capacity (from residual volume to total lung capacity). The resting level of the lung volume (resting end expiration) is shown as a filled circle at approximately 40 %VC in this figure (as is typical in upright body positions). Modified from *Evaluation and management of speech breathing disorders: Principles and methods* (p. 41), by T. Hixon and J. Hoit, 2005, Tucson, AZ: Redington Brown. Copyright 2005 by Thomas J. Hixon and Jeannette D. Hoit. Modified and reproduced with permission.

wall; this shape would be represented to the right of the relaxation characteristic in Figure 2–20. Conversely, a chest wall shape characterized by a smaller than relaxed abdominal wall and a larger than relaxed rib cage wall (top part of arrow in Figure 2–21) would be represented to the left of the relaxation characteristic in Figure 2–20.

Figure 2–22 illustrates how chest wall shape can be used to make inferences about what muscle groups might be active. Points along the relaxation characteristic in Figure 2–22 represent either complete relaxation of the muscles of the chest wall or equal expiratory muscular pressures of the rib cage wall and abdominal wall that cancel one another (+RC = +AB). Points that are not on the relaxation characteristic can only be achieved using active muscular pressure. Points to the left of the relaxation characteristic (dark gray area) can be achieved using: (a) a net inspiratory rib cage wall pressure (–RC), (b) an expiratory abdominal wall pressure (+AB), (c) a net inspiratory rib cage wall pressure and an expiratory abdominal wall pressure (–RC, +AB), or (d) a net expiratory rib cage wall pressure and a greater expiratory abdominal wall pressure (+RC < +AB). Points to the right of the relaxation characteristic (light gray area) can be achieved using: (a) a net expiratory rib cage wall pressure (+RC) or (b) a net expiratory rib cage wall pressure and a lesser expiratory abdominal wall pressure (+RC > +AB). Thus, chest wall shape measurements can be used to infer possible muscular mechanisms by comparing the chest wall shape during an activity (such as speaking) with the chest wall shape during relaxation at the same lung volume.

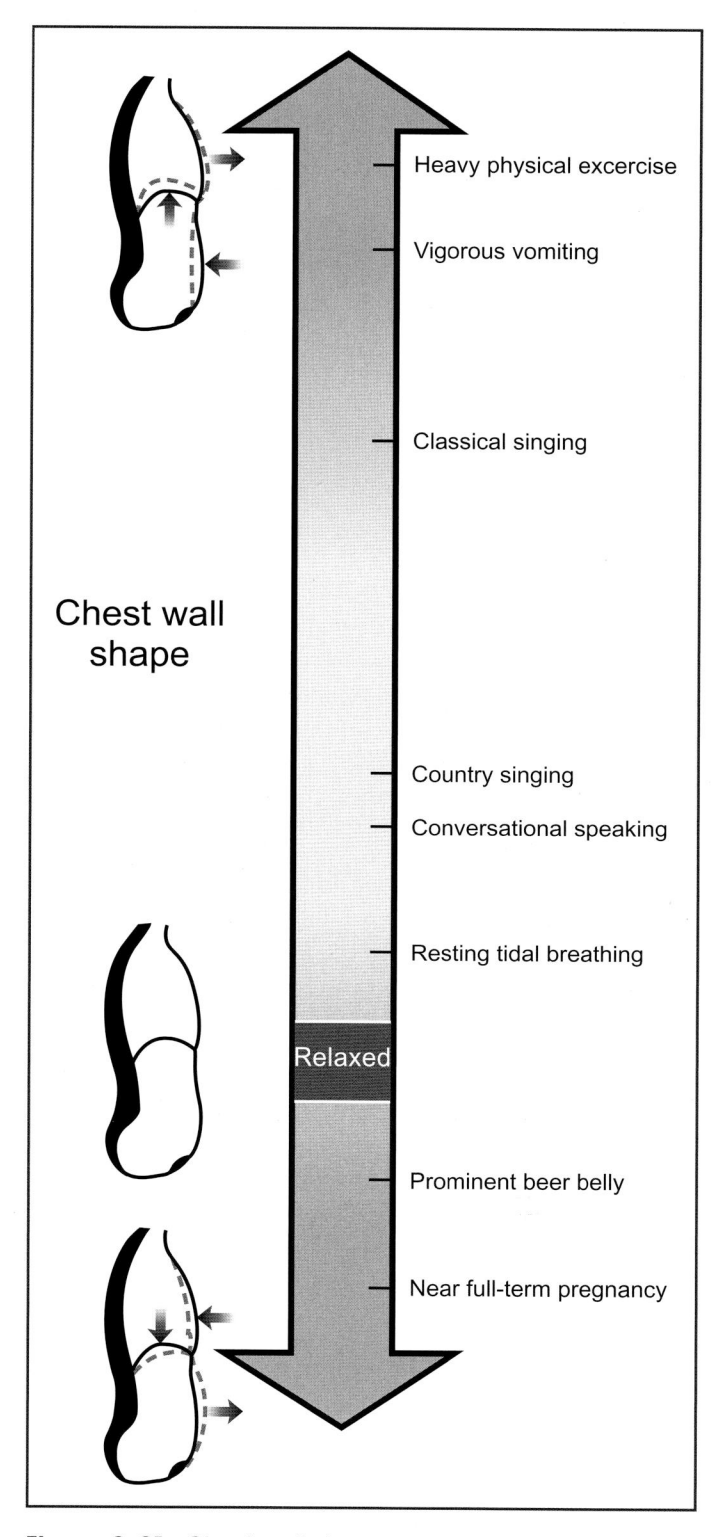

Figure 2-21. Chest wall shapes characteristic of different events and conditions. Shapes range from a larger-than-relaxed abdominal wall and a smaller-than-relaxed rib cage wall (*bottom part of arrow*) to a smaller-than-relaxed abdominal wall and a larger-than-relaxed rib cage wall (*top part of arrow*).

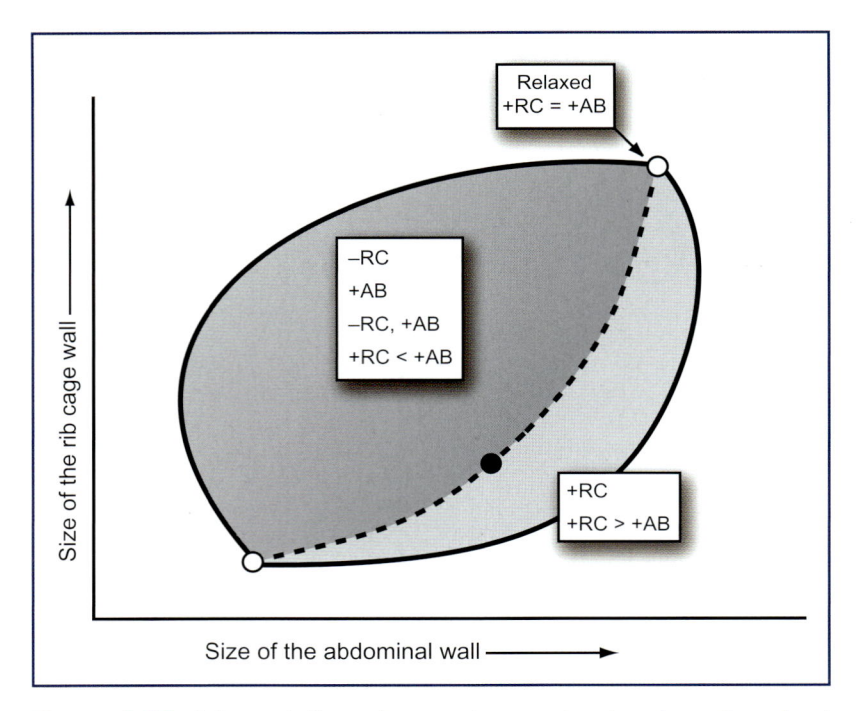

Figure 2–22. Interpretation of muscular mechanism from the chest wall shape diagram. Points along the dotted line are achieved by total relaxation or equal expiratory muscular pressures of the rib cage wall and abdominal wall. Points to the left of the dotted line can be achieved with inspiratory rib cage wall pressure (–RC); abdominal wall pressure (+AB); combined inspiratory rib cage wall pressure and abdominal wall pressure (–RC, +AB); or expiratory rib cage wall and abdominal wall muscular pressure, with the latter predominating (+RC < +AB). Points to the right of the dotted line can be achieved with expiratory rib cage wall pressure (+RC) or expiratory rib cage wall and abdominal wall muscular pressure, with the former predominating (+RC > +AB).

NEURAL CONTROL OF BREATHING

Breathing is controlled by the nervous system. The parts of the nervous system that participate in the control of breathing are located within the central nervous system (brain and spinal cord) and selected nerves within the peripheral nervous system (cranial and spinal nerves), as illustrated in Figure 2–23. The brainstem (lower part of the brain) is responsible for the control of tidal breathing, and higher brain centers are responsible for controlling special acts of breathing. Control of all breathing-related activities is played out through peripheral nerves.

Provided here is foundational information about the control of tidal breathing and special acts of breathing and the peripheral nerves that send control commands to muscles. Detailed coverage of the nervous system is provided in Chapter 15.

Control of Tidal Breathing

Tidal breathing, the most common form of breathing, is sometimes called automatic breathing, metabolic breathing, or involuntary breathing. The control of tidal breathing is vested in the brainstem, primarily in structures located in the medulla, the lowest region of the brainstem that is contiguous with the spinal cord. These structures contain a network of neurons that generate a rhythmic pattern of breathing and regulate gas levels (oxygen and carbon dioxide) in arterial blood by adjusting ventilation. This network is often called the central pattern generator for breathing. It can run breathing on its own automatically without input from higher brain centers.

Signals from the brainstem travel via peripheral nerves to reach the muscles of the chest wall. For example, signals from the brainstem reach the *diaphragm* muscle via the phrenic nerve and cause its fibers to

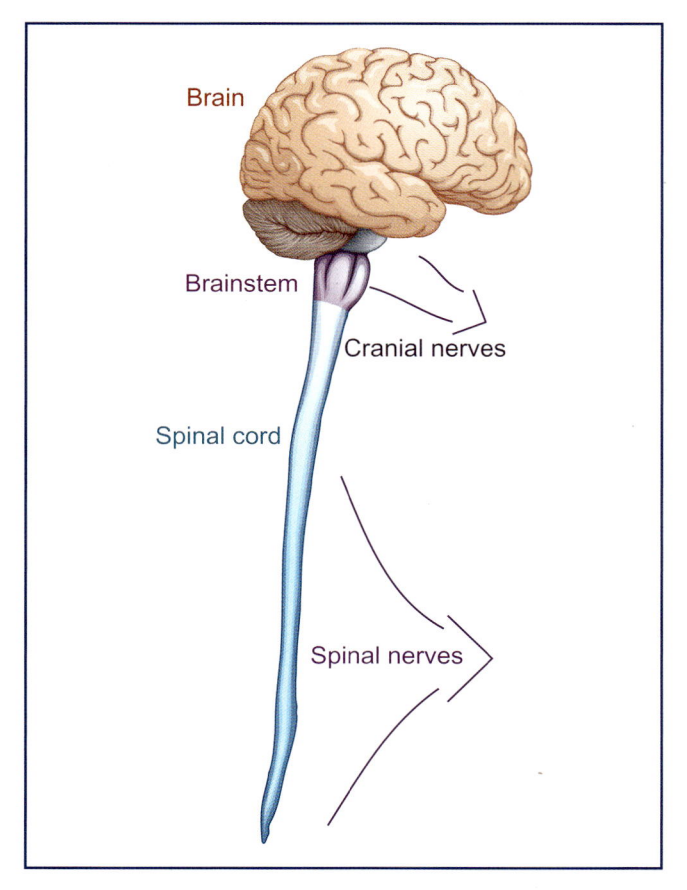

Figure 2–23. The central nervous system (brain and spinal cord) and peripheral nervous system (cranial and spinal nerves). Control of tidal breathing is vested in the brainstem and control of special acts of breathing is vested in higher brain centers. Control commands are sent to muscles through peripheral nerves. From *Evaluation and management of speech breathing disorders: Principles and methods* (p. 43), by T. Hixon and J. Hoit, 2005, Tucson, AZ: Redington Brown. Copyright 2005 by Thomas J. Hixon and Jeannette D. Hoit. Modified and reproduced with permission.

contract for inspiration. Signals may also travel to the *external intercostal* muscles, causing them either to stiffen the rib cage wall (during resting tidal inspiration) or to assist the diaphragm as a supplemental prime mover (during more forceful tidal inspiration). Signals are sent simultaneously through cranial nerves to enlarge the laryngeal airway and stiffen the tissues of the upper airway to make it less likely that the airways will be sucked inward, thereby minimizing resistance to inspiratory airflow.

The breathing pattern generated by the brainstem is strongly conditioned by afferent (incoming) information from a variety of sources. Most of the time, this afferent information is received and processed unconsciously. Sometimes, however, afferent information is processed to a level of awareness (sensation) or to a level of meaning and association (perception). At such times, individuals may begin to consciously attend to their breathing and to develop breathing-related perceptions having to do with forces, movements, and feelings of breathing comfort or discomfort.

The most important afferent information comes from chemoreceptors and mechanoreceptors. Chemoreceptors are sensitive to chemical status and those most relevant to breathing are called central and peripheral chemoreceptors. As illustrated in Figure 2–24, central chemoreceptors are located on the front and side surfaces of the medulla, and peripheral chemoreceptors are located in the carotid bodies at the bifurcation of the common carotid arteries, near the major blood supply to the brain. Central chemoreceptors respond primarily to changes in the amount of carbon dioxide in cerebral spinal fluid, and peripheral chemoreceptors are the primary oxygen receptors for the body, although they also respond to changes in the level of carbon dioxide and balance of acidity-alkalinity (pH, or potential of hydrogen) in arterial blood. Central and peripheral chemoreceptors generally act synergistically to stimulate adjustments in breathing by providing moment-to-moment updates on the concentration of gas in the blood. For example, an increase in carbon dioxide or a decrease in oxygen stimulates the brainstem to send signals through the peripheral nerves to the chest wall muscles to increase breathing.

Mechanoreceptors are sensitive to mechanical changes and those of special importance to the control of tidal breathing are located in the pulmonary apparatus and chest wall. Those in the pulmonary apparatus respond to stimuli that include the stretching of smooth muscles (such as occurs with an increase in lung volume), airway irritants (such as smoke, dust, chemicals, cold air), and distortions of the alveolar wall (such as might occur when excess fluid surrounds the alveoli). Signals from these pulmonary mechanoreceptors reach the central nervous system by way of cranial nerve X (vagus). Mechanoreceptors in the chest wall respond to changes in muscle length (such as occur with changes in rib cage wall or abdominal wall volume) or changes in force (such as occur with changes in inspiratory or expiratory muscular efforts). Their afferent signals reach the central nervous system via spinal nerves.

Other afferent input can also influence tidal breathing. For example, afferent signals from mechanoreceptors located in the larynx and upper airway and signals from cranial nerves that transmit visual and auditory information (cranial nerves II and VIII, respectively) can affect breathing. Thus, tidal breathing can be

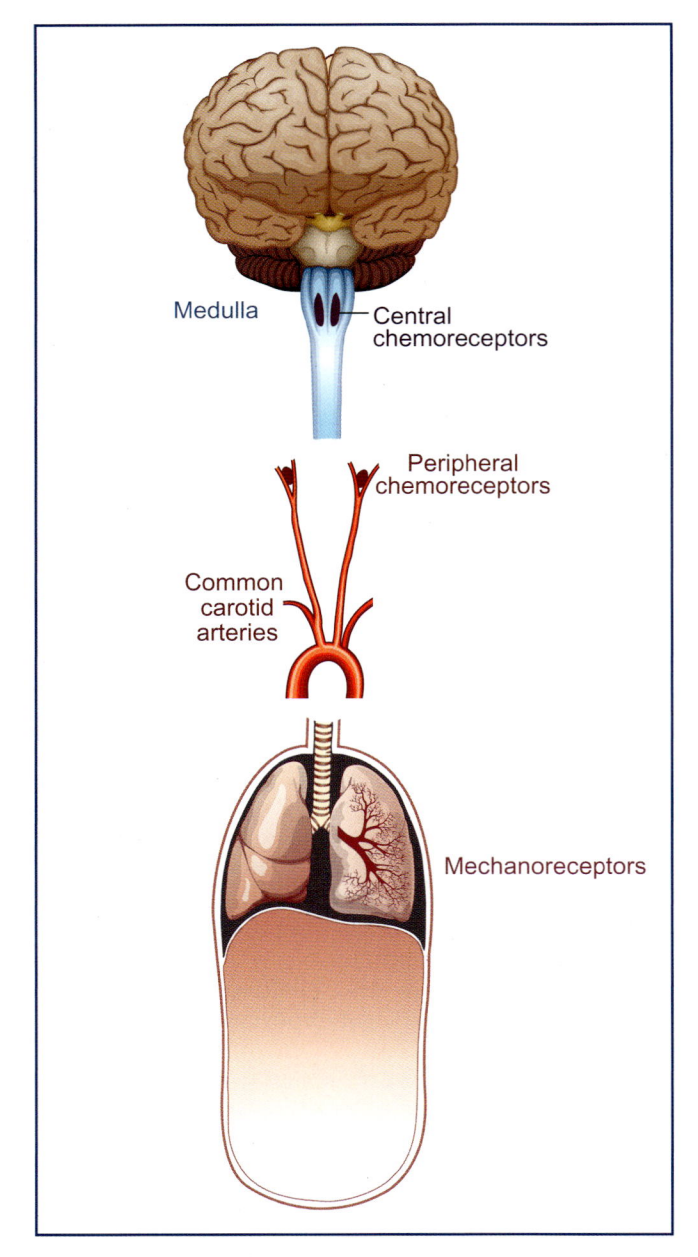

Figure 2-24. Central and peripheral chemoreceptors and mechanoreceptors. The central chemoreceptors are located in the medulla of the brainstem and the peripheral chemoreceptors are located in the carotid bodies at the bifurcation of the common carotid arteries. They are sensitive to changes in gas composition in the blood and cerebral spinal fluid. Mechanoreceptors are found in the pulmonary apparatus; these are sensitive to stretch, irritants, and alveolar distortion. Mechanoreceptors are also found in the chest wall; these are sensitive to muscle length and force changes. From *Evaluation and management of speech breathing disorders: Principles and methods* (p. 43), by T. Hixon and J. Hoit, 2005, Tucson, AZ: Redington Brown. Copyright 2005 by Thomas J. Hixon and Jeannette D. Hoit. Modified and reproduced with permission.

altered by the presence of an irritant in the larynx or upper airway, by images in an action-packed movie, or by musical rhythms (Shea, Walter, Pelley, Murphy, & Guz, 1987; Wyke, 1974).

Tidal breathing can also be influenced by internally generated activity from brain areas outside the brainstem (Mador & Tobin, 1991; Shea, 1996; Shea, Murphy, Hamilton, Benchetrit, & Guz, 1988; Western & Patrick, 1988). For example, cognitive activity (originating from cortical areas), such as that associated with the performance of mental arithmetic, can change tidal breathing. In fact, merely being consciously aware of breathing can change its pattern. Emotional influences (originating from limbic areas) can also have a profound influence on tidal breathing. Feelings of excitement, anger, or fear, for example, can be associated with hyperventilation, breath holding, or erratic breathing. Changes in tidal breathing can even be a primary sign (and feelings of breathlessness a primary symptom) of certain psychogenic disorders, such as anxiety disorder or panic disorder. These types of disorders have been so strongly linked to breathing that they are sometimes classified as hyperventilation disorders (Gardner, 1996).

Control of Special Acts of Breathing

Special acts of breathing can be defined as acts of breathing that are not effected for the primary purpose of maintaining homeostasis of arterial blood gases (Shea, 1996). They are controlled by higher brain centers that either override or bypass activity of the lower (brainstem) center for breathing. Special acts of breathing can be voluntary (highly conscious), such as breath holding or performing a guided breathing exercise. Or they can be learned and well-practiced and require little conscious control—for example, breathing associated with glass blowing, wind-instrument playing, singing, or speaking. Neural commands from higher brain centers can be integrated at the brainstem level such that they override the central pattern generator for breathing, or they can be routed directly from the cortex to spinal nerves, bypassing the brainstem altogether (Corfield, Murphy, & Guz, 1998). Other special acts of breathing, such as laughing or crying, are driven primarily by emotions and by the limbic system, a phylogenetically old part of the brain.

It is common for the nervous system to manage multiple breathing-related drives simultaneously, and often these drives compete with one another. Voluntary breath holding is one example. Breath holding is controlled by the cerebral cortex and is a clear demonstration of the ability of the cortex to override the brainstem's control of breathing. Nevertheless, cortical

Breathing as a Laughing Matter

Breathing plays a huge role in laughter. Much of laughter, especially the hearty type, goes on within the expiratory reserve volume. Laughter also often involves large movements of the abdominal wall. This is probably the reason our folk language is riddled with statements like, "I busted a gut laughing," "We laughed 'til our sides hurt," and "What a hearty belly laugh he has!" The neural mechanisms that underlie laughter are different from those that underlie speech breathing. This is illustrated dramatically in persons who can't move the abdominal wall on command or use it for speech production, but show vigorous movement of the wall during involuntary laughter. Thus, even if someone appears to be paralyzed, it's always wise to ask the question, "Paralyzed for what activity?"

Table 2–2. Summary of the Segmental Origins of the Motor Nerve Supply to the Muscles of the Chest Wall

MUSCLE	SPINAL NERVE
RIB CAGE WALL	
Sternocleidomastoid*	C1–C5
Scalenus group	C2–C8
Pectoralis major	C5–C8
Pectoralis minor	C5–C8
Subclavius	C5–C6
Serratus anterior	C5–C7, T2–T3
External intercostals	T1–T11
Internal intercostals	T1–T11
Transversus thoracis	T2–T6
Latissimus dorsi	C6–C8
Serratus posterior superior	T2–T3
Serratus posterior inferior	T9–T12
Lateral iliocostals group	C4–L2
Levatores costarum	C8–T11
Quadratus lumborum	T12–L2
Subcostals	T1–T11
DIAPHRAGM	
Diaphragm	C3–C5
ABDOMINAL WALL	
Rectus abdominis	T7–T12
External oblique	T8–L1
Internal oblique	T8–L1
Transversus abdominis	T7–T12
Latissimus dorsi	C6–C8
Lateral iliocostal lumborum	T7–L2
Quadratus lumborum	T12–L2

*Innervation of the **sternocleidomastoid** muscle comes from the spinal portion of the spinal accessory nerve, which is considered to be a cranial nerve (cranial nerve XI, see Chapter 15). The spinal accessory nerve also innervates the **trapezius** muscle; however, this muscle is not included in this chapter because it does not have a breathing function.

C = cervical, T = thoracic, L = lumbar.

Source: Based on Dickson and Maue-Dickson (1982).

control must eventually give way to brainstem control as danger signals from chemoreceptors make it impossible to continue to inhibit inspiration. Less dramatic examples of competing drives occur frequently and include situations such as attempting to speak while exercising, or playing a wind instrument while experiencing stage fright.

Peripheral Nerves of Breathing

The peripheral nervous system connects the central nervous system with different parts of the breathing apparatus via cranial and spinal nerves. Four cranial nerves participate in the control of breathing: cranial nerves IX (glossopharyngeal), X (vagus), and XII (hypoglossal) innervate muscles that dilate the larynx and stiffen the upper airway during inspiration, and cranial nerve IX (accessory) innervates the *sternocleidomastoid* muscle that elevates the sternum, clavicle, and rib cage.

Twenty-two spinal nerves contribute to the control of breathing. These are listed in Table 2–2 along with the muscles they innervate. As shown there, the spinal nerves relevant to breathing include the 8 cervical (C) nerves, the 12 thoracic (T) nerves, and the first 2 lumbar (L) nerves. Successively lower spinal nerves generally provide motor nerve supply to successively lower regions of the breathing apparatus. An exception is the diaphragm, which derives its motor nerve supply from C3 to C5, a collection of motor nerves designated as the phrenic nerve. Table 2–2 lists only the motor nerve supply to the muscles of the chest wall. The sensory nerve supply to the chest wall is generally similar in pattern to its motor nerve supply, a notable exception being the sensory supply of the diaphragm, which is vested in the phrenic nerve and lower thoracic nerves.

The Young(er) and the Reckless

Young men contribute mightily to the statistics on spinal cord injury. They tend to engage in activities that involve fast movement and in which collision may occur. And they are often less concerned about taking risks than are their opposite sex counterparts or their elders. No wonder insurance companies charge them higher premiums. There are over 300,000 people in the United States with spinal cord injury (a number equal to the population of St. Louis, Missouri). Each year about 17,000 new cases are added to the roll. More than 80% of people with spinal cord injury are men. Automobile crashes lead the way as the cause, followed by falls, violent acts (such as gunshot wounds), and sports injuries. Although several decades ago the average age was 29 years, the average has now risen to over 40. It looks like the approach of middle age is no longer quelling the desire to engage in the risk-taking behaviors or that people are living longer after their spinal cord injury.

Pink Puffers and Blue Bloaters

No, we're not talking about exotic tropical fish. Pink puffers and blue bloaters are terms that refer to people with chronic obstructive pulmonary disease. Pink puffers suffer mainly from emphysema. Their blood is relatively well saturated with oxygen, making their complexion pink. The puffer part comes from their compensatory expiration through pursed lips. They have decreased lung recoil, decreased vital capacity, increased residual volume, and increased total lung capacity. Blue bloaters suffer mainly from chronic bronchitis. They have associated heart problems with cyanosis and edema. Thus, their bodies turn blue and become bloated. They show decreased vital capacity and increased residual volume. Chronic obstructive pulmonary disease can be nasty and debilitating. Bronchitis may be reversible. Emphysema usually is not.

VENTILATION AND GAS EXCHANGE DURING TIDAL BREATHING

Tidal breathing is the most common type of breathing. Its name comes from the ebb and flow of air that resembles the ebb and flow of an ocean tide. Tidal breathing is driven by the need to ventilate (to move air in and out of the pulmonary apparatus) for the purpose of gas exchange (to deliver oxygen, O_2, to the body and remove carbon dioxide, CO_2, from it).

Figure 2–25 depicts the process of gas exchange during tidal breathing. Air, which consists of approximately 21% oxygen, enters the alveoli during tidal breathing. Oxygen then leaves the alveoli and enters the bloodstream to travel to tissues throughout the body. Tissues absorb oxygen from the blood and

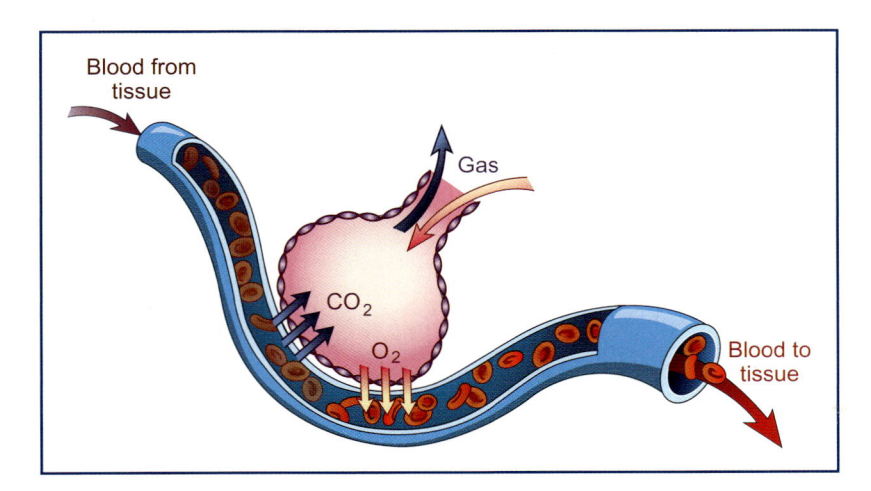

Figure 2–25. Process of gas exchange during tidal breathing. Oxygen is delivered to the blood and carbon dioxide is removed from the blood via the alveoli.

return carbon dioxide (a byproduct of metabolism) to the blood. The carbon dioxide then travels through the bloodstream and eventually reaches the alveoli, where it is released. When metabolic demand increases, as with increased physical or mental activity, more oxygen is consumed and more carbon dioxide is produced.

Tidal breathing at rest is associated with a relatively regular inspiration-expiration pattern, as shown in the top panel of Figure 2–26. A tidal breath begins and ends at the resting size of the breathing apparatus (shown as "0" lung volume in the figure). During inspiration, the chest wall expands, causing the lungs to expand and alveolar pressure to fall. This creates a pressure gradient, with the pressure inside the pulmonary apparatus being lower than that outside the apparatus (see bottom panel of Figure 2–26). As a result, air flows into the pulmonary apparatus and lung volume increases. When equilibration is reached (the pressures outside and inside the pulmonary apparatus are equal), inspiratory airflow ceases (where the dashed line intersects both the upper and lower panels of Figure 2–26).

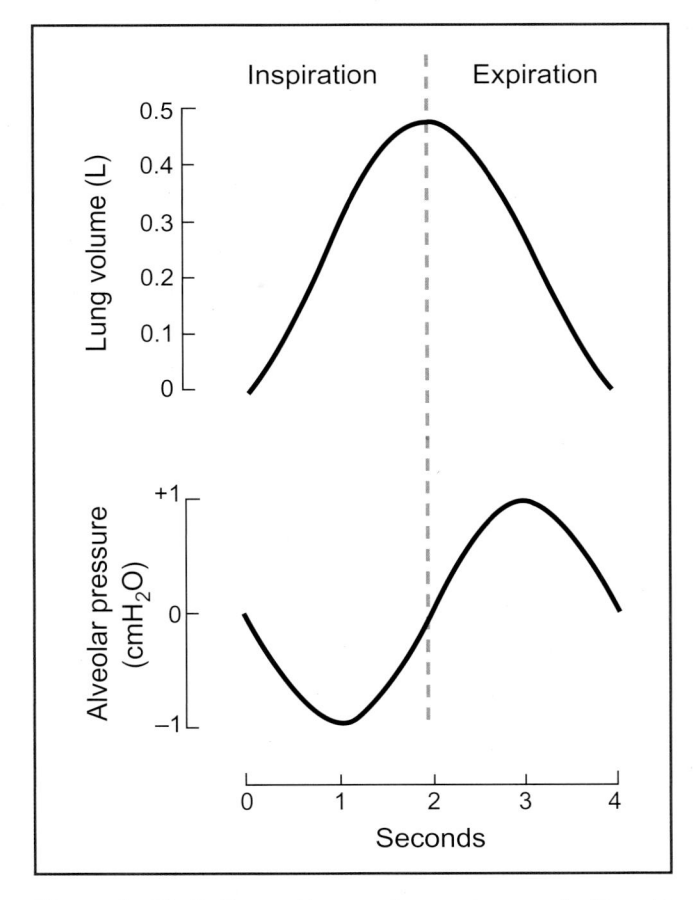

Figure 2–26. Pattern of lung volume change (in liters, L) and alveolar pressure change (in cmH$_2$O) during resting tidal breathing.

Expiration begins as the lungs compress and alveolar pressure becomes slightly positive (relative to atmosphere). Expiration continues until the resting level of the breathing apparatus is reached and alveolar pressure returns to 0 cmH$_2$O (atmospheric). These patterns of lung volume and alveolar pressure change are generally the same across body positions, except that the absolute lung volume range differs with body position. For example, resting tidal breathing ranges from about 40 to 50 %VC in upright body positions and from about 20 to 30 %VC in the supine (lying on one's back, facing upward) body position.

Resting tidal breathing is driven by a combination of passive and active forces that are somewhat dependent on body position. These forces are summarized graphically in Figure 2–27 for two body positions: upright and supine. During inspiration, essentially all of the active force comes from the diaphragm. This is true for all body positions. In the upright body position, some rib cage wall muscles and abdominal wall muscles are also active during inspiration (Hixon, Goldman, & Mead, 1973; Loring & Mead, 1982). Rib cage wall muscle activity stiffens the rib cage wall to prevent it from being sucked inward when the diaphragm contracts. Abdominal wall muscle activity usually causes the abdominal wall to move inward slightly. When the abdominal wall moves inward, the rib cage wall is lifted and the diaphragm is pushed slightly headward. This stretches the fibers of the diaphragm so that they are placed on more favorable portions of their length-force characteristics for contraction. In the supine body position, as in the upright body position, the rib cage wall muscles are slightly active to stiffen the rib cage wall. However, in contrast to upright body positions, the abdominal wall muscles are relaxed. This is because the abdominal wall is already pulled inward and the diaphragm is already pushed headward by the force of gravity.

During resting tidal expiration, the passive (recoil) pressure of the breathing apparatus moves the rib cage wall and abdominal wall inward. Thus, resting tidal expiration is primarily a passive event. Nevertheless, in the upright body position, the abdominal wall muscles remain active throughout the resting tidal breathing cycle.

Although resting tidal breathing shares general features across individuals, its specific details differ from person to person. In fact, each person has what might be thought of as a signature resting tidal breathing pattern that remains relatively unchanged over the years (Benchetrit, Shea, Pham Dinh, Bodocco, Baconnier, & Guz, 1989; Dejours, 1996; Shea & Guz, 1992; Shea, Horner, Benchetrit, & Guz, 1990; Shea, Walter, Murphy, & Guz, 1987).

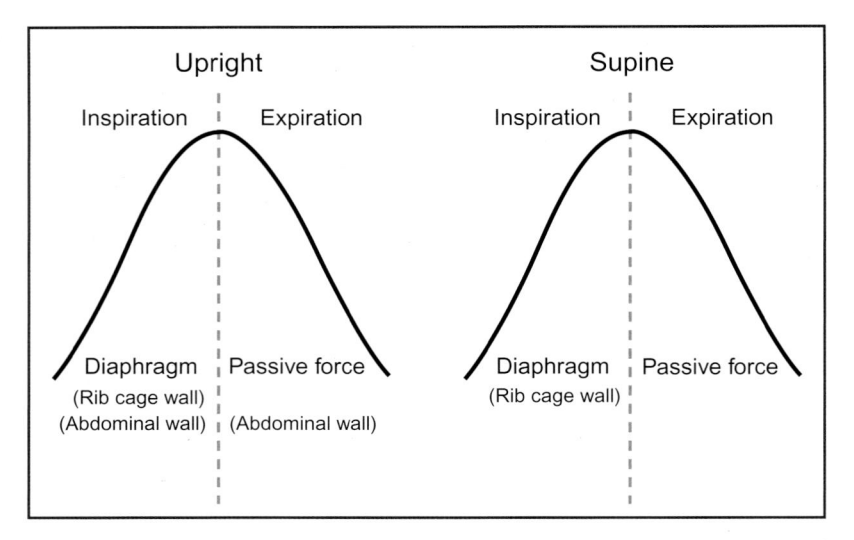

Figure 2-27. Passive and active forces of resting tidal breathing in upright and supine body positions. In both body positions, the diaphragm is the primary muscle of inspiration. In upright, the rib cage wall and abdominal wall muscles are also tonically (continuously) active, but only to enhance the mechanical conditions for diaphragm contraction. In supine, the force of gravity supplants the need for the abdominal wall muscles to activate. Expiration is driven by passive force (recoil of the breathing apparatus) in both body positions, though the abdominal muscles usually remain active in upright.

BREATHING AND SPEECH PRODUCTION

The breathing apparatus provides the driving forces that generate speech. Actions of the breathing apparatus contribute to the control of speech intensity (loudness), voice frequency (pitch), linguistic stress (emphasis), and the segmentation (division) of speech into units (syllables, words, phrases). At the same time it performs these speech-related functions, the breathing apparatus continues to serve its primary functions of ventilation and gas exchange.

This section describes two forms of speech breathing—extended steady utterances and running speech activities—as performed in the upright body position (standing or seated erect). These are based on the conceptualizations and elaborations of Hixon (1973), Hixon et al. (1973), Hixon, Mead, and Goldman (1976), Weismer (1985), and Hixon and Hoit (2005).

Extended Steady Utterances

An extended steady utterance is an utterance that is produced throughout most of the vital capacity. It begins after taking the deepest inspiration possible and continues until the air supply is depleted. Such

---

Thomas J. Hixon (1940–2009)

What is this? An author writing a sidetrack about himself? No, it's the other two authors writing about Tom Hixon, who left us too early to help with the second and third editions of this book, because we want you to know something about him. At age 25, Tom burst onto the scene, having already completed his master's degree (in one year) and his PhD (in two years!) from the University of Iowa. His intense fascination of speech breathing led him to Harvard, where, under the tutelage of Jere Mead, Tom learned about respiratory mechanics. He spent hours each day in Countway Library poring over articles on respiratory physiology and then more hours poring over data in the laboratory. He immersed himself for years, doing the experiment again and again, until he understood beyond doubt exactly how the respiratory system works for speech production. He completely revolutionized our understanding of this complicated system, and then presented it with elegant simplicity in this text. You can thank Tom for everything you know about speech breathing.

an utterance might be a sustained vowel, a series of repeated syllables of equal stress, or a sung note.

Figure 2–28 shows the lung volume and alveolar pressure events associated with a sustained vowel produced at a usual and steady loudness, pitch, and voice quality. As can be seen in the figure, lung volume decreases at a constant rate throughout the vital capacity as the utterance progresses. In contrast, alveolar pressure rises abruptly, remains steady throughout the utterance, and falls abruptly as the utterance ends.

Both relaxation pressure and active muscular pressure contribute to extended steady utterance production. This is illustrated in Figure 2–29 for the same sustained vowel as that depicted in Figure 2–28. In the top panel of Figure 2–29, alveolar pressure (in cmH$_2$O) is plotted on the horizontal axis, ranging from negative (inspiratory) to positive (expiratory). Lung volume (in %VC) is plotted on the vertical axis, with 40 %VC representing the resting level of the breathing apparatus. Recall that the resting level is the level (or size) at which the breathing apparatus is in a mechanically neutral position and alveolar pressure is the same as atmospheric pressure (zero). Note that the relaxation pressure is positive at lung volumes larger than the resting level and negative at lung volumes smaller than the resting level. This is because at large lung volumes the breathing apparatus is expanded from its resting size and wants to collapse inward to its resting level; in contrast, at small lung volumes it is compressed from its resting size and wants to expand outward to its resting level. The target alveolar pressure for producing the vowel is shown to be constant throughout the lung volume (this is analogous to the pressure tracing from Figure 2–28, oriented vertically instead of horizontally).

The middle panel of Figure 2–29 shows the active muscular pressure required to achieve the target alveolar pressure. At large lung volumes (near the beginning of the utterance), a negative (inspiratory) muscular pressure is required to counteract the high positive (expiratory) relaxation pressure. In the mid-lung-volume range, a slight positive muscular pressure is required to achieve the target alveolar pressure. And, at small lung volumes (near the end of the utterance), increasingly greater positive muscular pressure is required. By studying the top two panels of Figure 2–29, it should

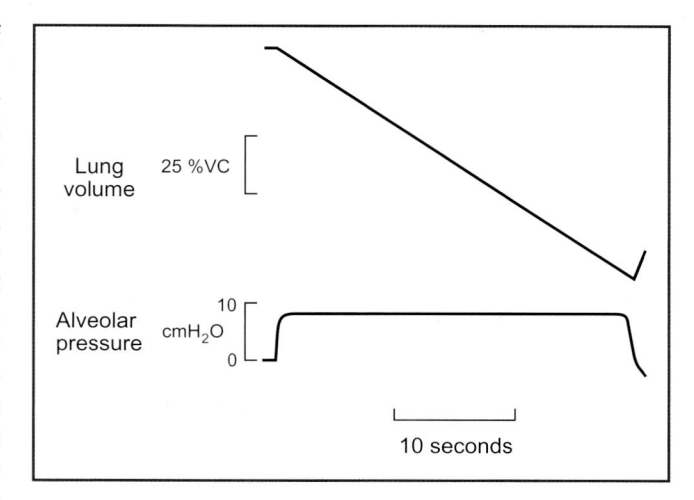

Figure 2–28. Lung volume (in %VC) and alveolar pressure (in cmH$_2$O) events for an extended steady utterance (sustained vowel) produced in the upright body position. Only expiration (vowel production) is represented. From *Evaluation and management of speech breathing disorders: Principles and methods* (p. 57), by T. Hixon and J. Hoit, 2005, Tucson, AZ: Redington Brown. Copyright 2005 by Thomas J. Hixon and Jeannette D. Hoit. Modified and reproduced with permission.

be clear that it is possible to specify the required muscular pressure by knowing the target alveolar pressure and the relaxation pressure at the prevailing lung volume. In this example, the target alveolar pressure for an extended steady utterance of normal loudness is 8 cmH$_2$O. The target alveolar pressure would be higher for louder utterances and lower for softer utterances. For a higher target alveolar pressure (louder speech), less negative muscular pressure is required at large lung volumes and more positive muscular pressure is required at small lung volumes. In contrast, for lower target alveolar pressures (softer speech), more negative muscular pressure is required at large lung volumes and less positive muscular pressure is required at small lung volumes.

The bottom panel of Figure 2–29 illustrates the activities of the different components of the breathing apparatus in the generation of muscular pressure.[1] The solid horizontal bars indicate when the different

---

[1]This panel is based on the work of Hixon, Mead, and Goldman (1976) and was distilled by Hixon and Hoit (2005) into the simple graphic display shown. The actions of the rib cage wall, diaphragm, and abdominal wall portrayed in the panel are based on strain-stress (volume-pressure) analyses, which enabled the determination of the individual muscular pressure contributions of different components of the chest wall. The data required for these analyses included rib cage wall volume, abdominal wall volume, and lung volume (estimated via respiratory magnetometers—devices described in Chapter 6), as well as pleural pressure, abdominal pressure, and transdiaphragmatic pressure (estimated from catheter-balloon devices swallowed into the esophagus and stomach and connected to pressure transducers). The data of Hixon et al. do not specify how individual muscles contribute to the muscular pressure generated by each chest wall part (except for the diaphragm, where there is only a single muscle in the part). Such data as are available on how individual muscles function have come from the use of electromyography, a method that senses the electrical activity of muscles through the use of metal electrodes placed over

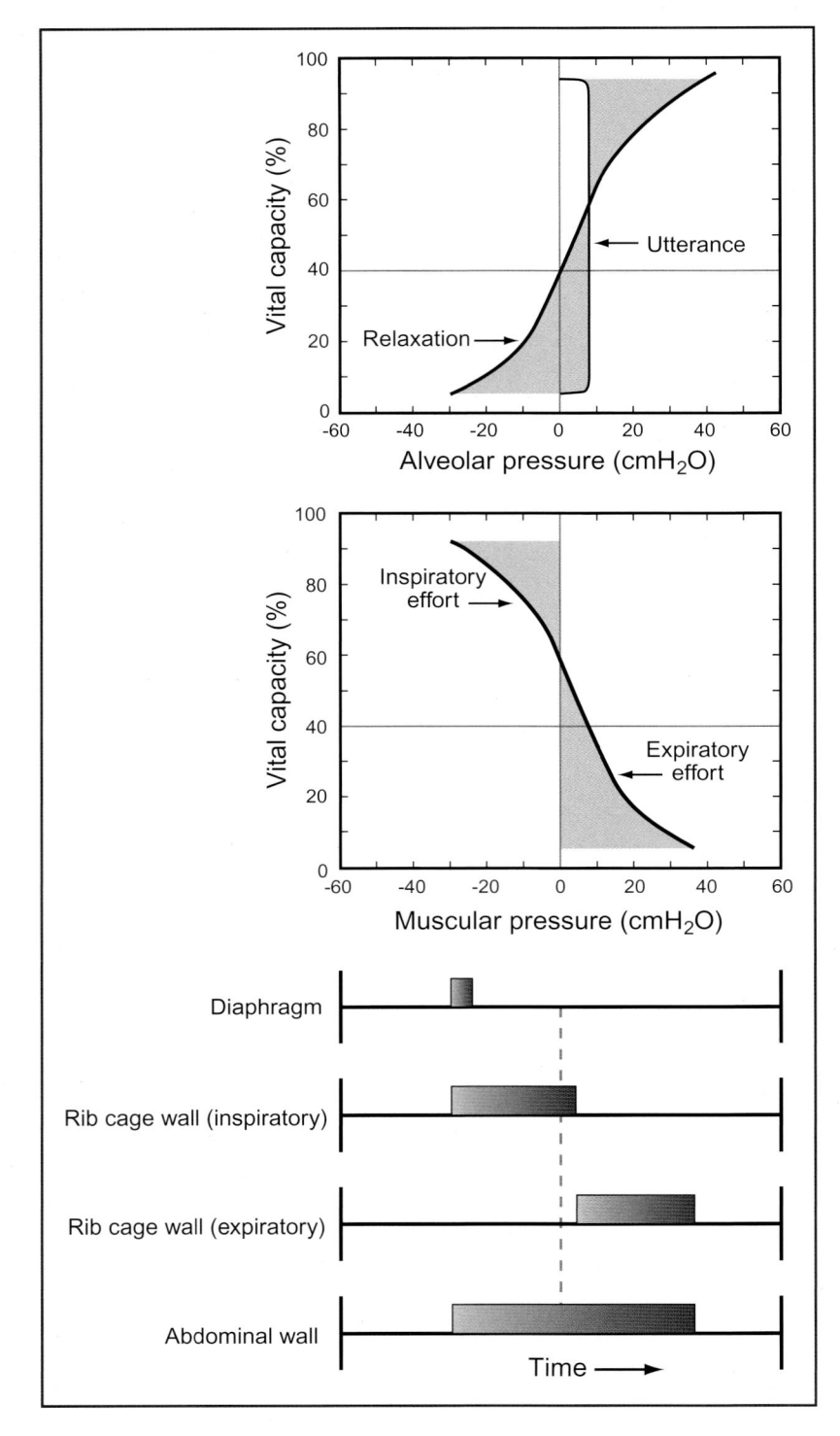

Figure 2–29. Relaxation pressure, target alveolar pressure, muscular pressure, and temporal activity of chest wall components for a sustained vowel produced in the upright body position. Only expiration (vowel production) is represented. The top panel depicts the relaxation pressure and the target alveolar pressure (8 cmH$_2$O) for the vowel. The horizontal line at 40 %VC represents the resting level of the breathing apparatus. As depicted in the middle panel, inspiratory braking is required at the beginning to produce the target pressure, but as the vowel proceeds, the need for inspiratory braking ceases and expiratory muscular effort is required and continues to increase in magnitude through the expiratory reserve volume. The bottom panel depicts the activation of muscle groups, with the inspiratory rib cage wall muscles doing most of the inspiratory braking (with some initial contribution from the diaphragm) and the expiratory rib cage wall and abdominal muscles providing the expiratory muscular pressures. From *Evaluation and management of speech breathing disorders: Principles and methods* (p. 59), by T. Hixon and J. Hoit, 2005, Tucson, AZ: Redington Brown. Copyright 2005 by Thomas J. Hixon and Jeannette D. Hoit. Modified and reproduced with permission.

components of the chest wall are active. The darker the shading within the bars, the greater the muscular pressure being generated. Reading from left to right, the panel shows that the diaphragm (inspiratory), the inspiratory rib cage wall component, and the abdominal wall (expiratory) component are active

---

them or inserted directly into them. Available data of this type are piecemeal, incomplete, and, in some cases, known to be invalid (Hixon & Weismer, 1995).

at the beginning of the utterance. The diaphragm and the inspiratory rib cage wall component generate the negative pressure required to counteract the positive relaxation pressure in this large lung volume range. However, the diaphragm shuts off very quickly and the inspiratory rib cage wall component alone assumes the role of inspiratory braking (sometimes called inspiratory checking) against the high expiratory relaxation pressure. At the instant the inspiratory rib cage wall component shuts off, the expiratory rib cage wall component becomes active and remains active until the end of the utterance. Note that the abdominal wall is active throughout the utterance.

Thus, extended steady utterance is produced using a continuously changing combination of relaxation pressure and muscular pressure, and a continuously changing activation of different chest wall components. Relaxation pressure goes from substantially positive to substantially negative, whereas muscular pressure follows an opposite pattern, going from substantially negative to substantially positive. The inspiratory muscles of the rib cage wall do nearly all of the inspiratory work (braking) at large lung volumes and the expiratory muscles of the rib cage wall and abdominal wall muscles do all of the expiratory work. Interestingly, the abdominal wall muscles are active throughout the utterance, even at times when a net negative pressure is required.

The reason that the inspiratory muscles of the rib cage wall do most of the inspiratory braking in upright is because it is a mechanically efficient strategy. As illustrated in Figure 2–30, when the inspiratory muscles of the rib cage wall contract (and the diaphragm is inactive), the rib cage wall expands and pleural and abdominal pressures decrease. The decrease in abdominal pressure causes the liquid-filled abdominal content to place a downward hydraulic pull on the undersurface of the diaphragm. This hydraulic pull creates a stable base against which the inspiratory muscles of the rib cage wall can contract. In effect, the hydraulic pull of the abdominal content enables the inspiratory muscles of the rib cage wall to simultaneously elevate the rib cage wall and pull downward on the diaphragm, without the diaphragm having to contract to stay in position. This mechanism works in the upright body position, but not in the supine body position, as discussed below.

Another interesting observation is that the abdominal wall muscles remain active throughout extended steady utterance, even when a net inspiratory muscular pressure is required (at large lung volumes near the beginning of the utterance). This appears to be a strategy for enhancing the precision and control of speech breathing. When the diaphragm is inactive (as it is throughout almost all of an extended steady utterance production), any pressure change is manifested identically across both the rib cage wall and abdominal wall (the breathing apparatus becomes a single compartment functionally). Whether such pressure resolves into movement of the rib cage wall, abdominal wall,

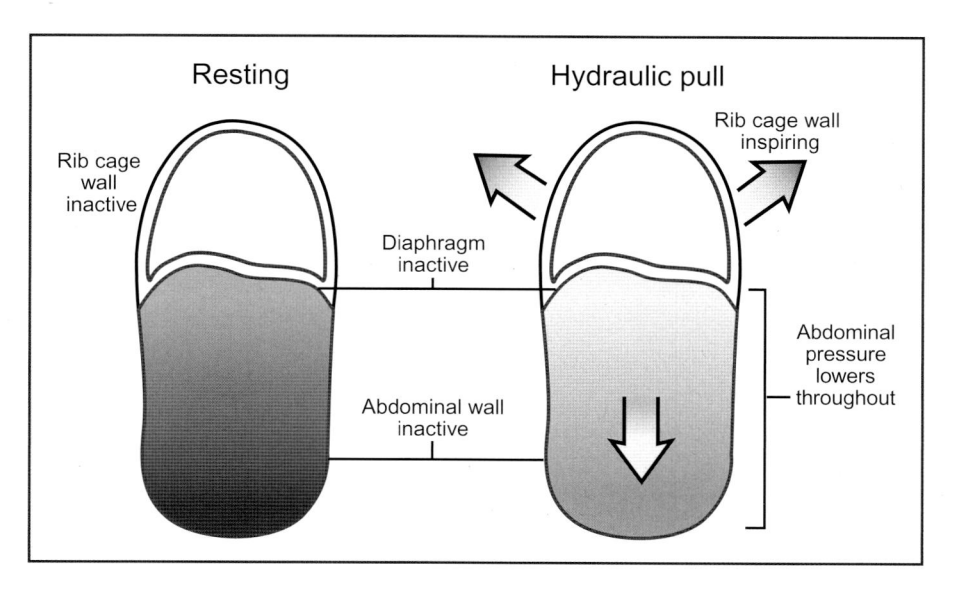

Figure 2–30. Mechanism of hydraulic pull of the abdominal content on the diaphragm. This mechanism explains why, in upright positions, the inspiratory rib cage wall muscles do almost all the inspiratory braking to counteract the large positive relaxation pressures that prevail at large lung volumes.

or both depends on the relative impedance of the two structures. If one part has relatively high impedance (due to muscle activation) and the other has relatively low impedance (due to absence of muscle activation), then alveolar pressure change will initially result in movement of the low impedance part.

A simple analogy, depicted in Figure 2–31, can help illustrate the concept just discussed (Hixon & Hoit, 2005). The figure on the left shows a balloon being held by two hands. The balloon represents the air-containing pulmonary apparatus, the lower hand represents the abdominal wall muscles, the upper hand represents the expiratory rib cage wall muscles, and the squeaker in the neck of the balloon represents the larynx. The figure in the middle depicts the upper hand (expiratory rib cage muscles) squeezing without the help of the lower hand. This causes the lower half of the balloon (the abdomen) to be pushed outward. Thus, the efforts of the rib cage wall expiratory muscles are first resolved into outward (paradoxical) abdominal wall movement before effecting the desired increase in balloon (alveolar) pressure to drive the squeaker (vocal folds within the larynx). Paradoxical in this context means that the abdomen is moving in the opposite direction to the flow of air; that is, the abdominal wall is moving in the inspiratory direction as the air is flowing in the expiratory direction. The figure on the right shows both hands (rib cage wall and abdominal wall) squeezing simultaneously and most closely resembles the way that extended steady utterances are produced. The squeezing of the lower hand (abdominal wall muscles) prohibits the unproductive outward movement of the lower half of the balloon (abdominal wall) and allows all squeezing (expiratory) efforts to be resolved into pressure change. In this way, control over the pressure within the balloon (or within the pulmonary apparatus) can be more precisely controlled.

Running Speech Activities

Running speech activities—such as reading aloud, extemporaneous speaking, and conversational speaking—present different demands and require a different

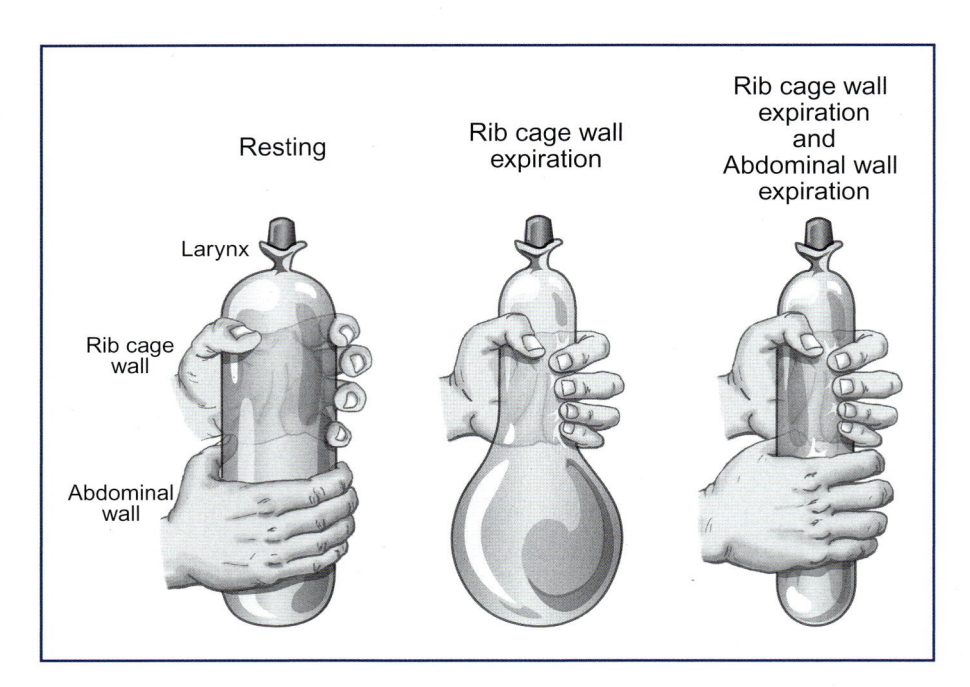

Figure 2–31. Balloon analogy of breathing apparatus control. The balloon represents the pulmonary apparatus, the hands represent the rib cage wall expiratory muscles (*upper hand*) and abdominal wall muscles (*lower hand*), and the squeaker in the neck of the balloon represents the larynx containing the vocal folds. When only the upper hand (rib cage wall) squeezes, depicted in the middle figure, the lower part of the balloon is pushed outward before the pressure within the balloon can rise to drive the squeaker. When both hands are squeezing (rib cage wall and abdominal wall), as shown in the right figure, pressure can rise immediately and any unproductive outward (paradoxical) movement of the abdominal wall is prevented.

set of muscular strategies than those used for extended steady utterances. Volume and pressure events are much more varied than those associated with extended steady utterances. This is because running speech is characterized by variations in phonetic content (sounds that differ in voicing and manner of production), prosody (utterances that differ in rate, intonation, loudness variation, and linguistic stress), and voice quality (utterances that differ in relative breathiness).

Volume events during running speech activities usually occur in the midrange of the vital capacity. As illustrated in the top panel of Figure 2–32, breath groups (expiratory phases of speech breathing cycles) during running speech production generally start at twice resting tidal breathing depth (or less) and continue to near the resting level of the breathing apparatus, although at times they may encroach upon the expiratory reserve volume. There are mechanical advantages to speaking in this lung volume range. To begin, the breathing apparatus is not as stiff and the relaxation pressure is not as extreme as at very large and very small lung volumes. Furthermore, the relaxation pressure is positive for most running speech production (because relaxation pressure is positive at lung volumes larger than the resting level of the breathing apparatus) and this positive pressure is used to supplement the positive muscular pressure required. When speech production encroaches upon the expiratory reserve volume, muscular pressure must be exerted against a negative relaxation pressure.

Volume change during inspiration is much quicker (that is, airflow is much faster) during running speech breathing than during resting tidal breathing. This is represented in Figure 2–32 (top panel) as a steeper inspiratory (upward) volume slope. In contrast, volume change during expiration is slower than during resting tidal breathing, as indicated by a shallower downward slope. The slower average expiratory airflow can be explained by the valving of the airstream

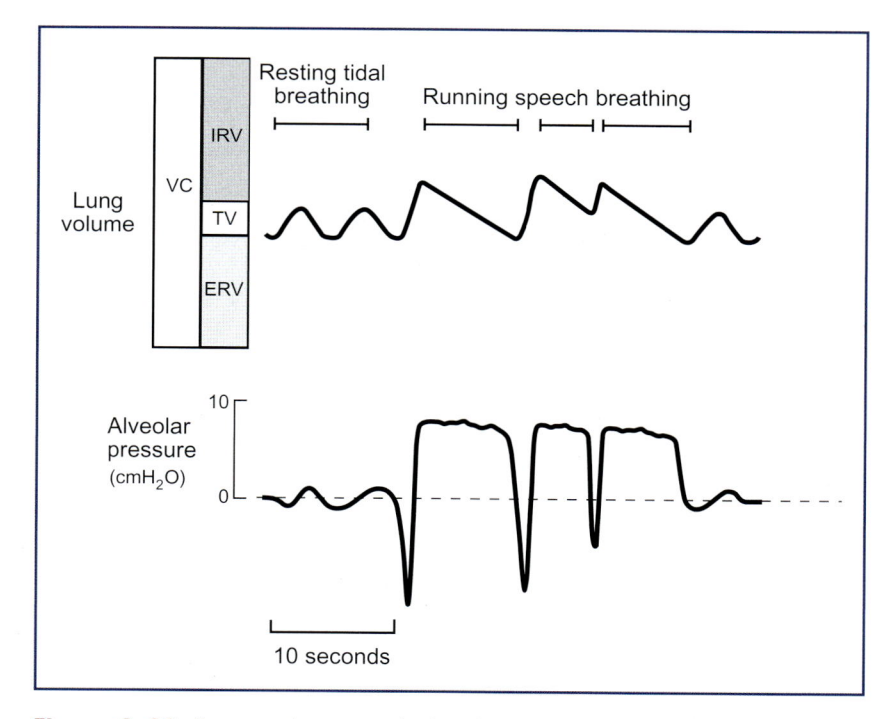

Figure 2–32. Lung volume and alveolar pressure events during resting tidal breathing and running speech breathing (such as reading aloud). Running speech breathing occurs within the midrange of the vital capacity, ranging from about twice tidal depth to near the resting expiratory level. Inspirations are faster (*steeper volume slope*), requiring a negative alveolar pressure, and expirations are slower (*shallower volume slope*), requiring a positive alveolar pressure, during running speech breathing compared with resting tidal breathing. Expiration volume and duration varies from breath to breath, depending on the length of the phrase, and alveolar pressure during speaking varies somewhat, depending on variations in linguistic stress and loudness.

by the larynx and the upper airway articulators that create the sounds of speech.

Alveolar pressure during running speech breathing, depicted in the lower panel of Figure 2–32, is negative during inspiration and positive during expiration. During speaking (expiration) alveolar pressure varies somewhat (in contrast to extended steady utterance production during which loudness is meant to remain constant). Specifically, alveolar pressure often declines near the end of breath groups (thus loudness declines) and it often increases momentarily to produce stressed (relatively more prominent) syllables.

Chest wall shape events during running speech production are depicted in Figure 2–33 (note that only expiration is shown in this figure). This is a relative volume (size) graph with rib cage volume on the vertical axis and abdominal volume on the horizontal axis, and the addition of a third axis depicting lung volume (details about how to calibrate for lung volume and the theory underlying these measurements are beyond the scope of this book). The relaxation characteristic (dashed line) and the resting lung volume level (filled circle and the line extending from it) are also shown (as in Figure 2–20). The lines marked "speech" indicate the continuum of shapes produced for three individual breath groups.

As can be seen by examining the speech lines in Figure 2–33, rib cage wall and abdominal wall volumes decrease (that is, they move downward and leftward on the graph) throughout the breath group. In most people, rib cage wall volume decreases more and at a much faster rate than abdominal wall volume; this can be seen in the slope of the speech lines (nearly vertical). Recall that the rib cage wall covers a much larger surface of the lungs than does the abdominal wall (indirectly, through the diaphragm). Thus, the rib cage wall is well suited for effecting lung volume change during running speech production.

Figure 2–33 also shows that running speech production begins at lung volumes that are larger than the resting level and ends at lung volumes near the resting level. This typical lung volume range is also illustrated in other graphic forms in this chapter (see Figures 2–17 and 2–32).

The speech lines in Figure 2–33 are to the left of the relaxation characteristic (dashed line). This placement on the graph provides clues as to potential muscular mechanisms that could have produced these lines (see Figure 2–22). Empirical evidence has shown that the muscular mechanism that is actually used for speaking is a combination of expiratory rib cage wall and abdominal wall muscular pressures,

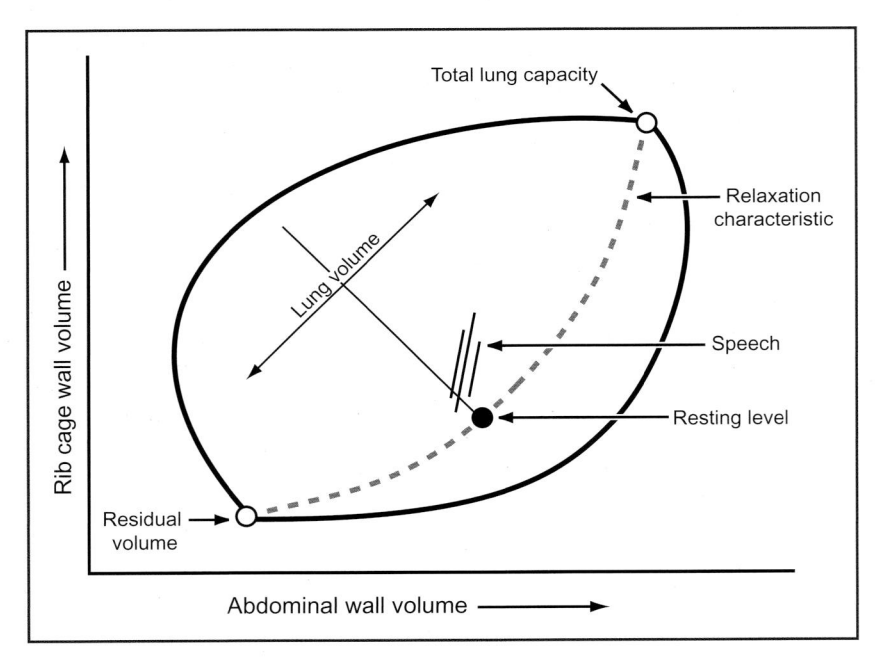

Figure 2-33. Relative volume graph showing chest wall shape lines for three individual breath groups. Note that these breath groups (speech lines) are: (a) nearly vertical, indicating much greater rib cage wall movement than abdominal wall movement, (b) almost entirely above the resting level (along the diagonal lung volume axis), indicating that speech is produced in the midrange of the vital capacity, and (c) to the left of the relaxation characteristic (dashed line), indicating a limited number of possible muscular strategies (see Figure 2–22).

with the latter predominating (Hixon, Mead, & Goldman, 1976).

Both relaxation pressure and muscular pressure contribute to the production of running speech production, as illustrated in Figure 2–34. As can be seen in the top panel of the figure, the target alveolar pressure (shown to be 8 cmH$_2$O in this case) is usually higher (more positive) than the prevailing relaxation pressure. This means that positive muscular pressure must be added to the relaxation pressure throughout the breath group, as shown in the middle panel of the figure. The magnitude of the positive muscular pressure increases as the breath group proceeds to supplement the progressively decreasing relaxation pressure. There is

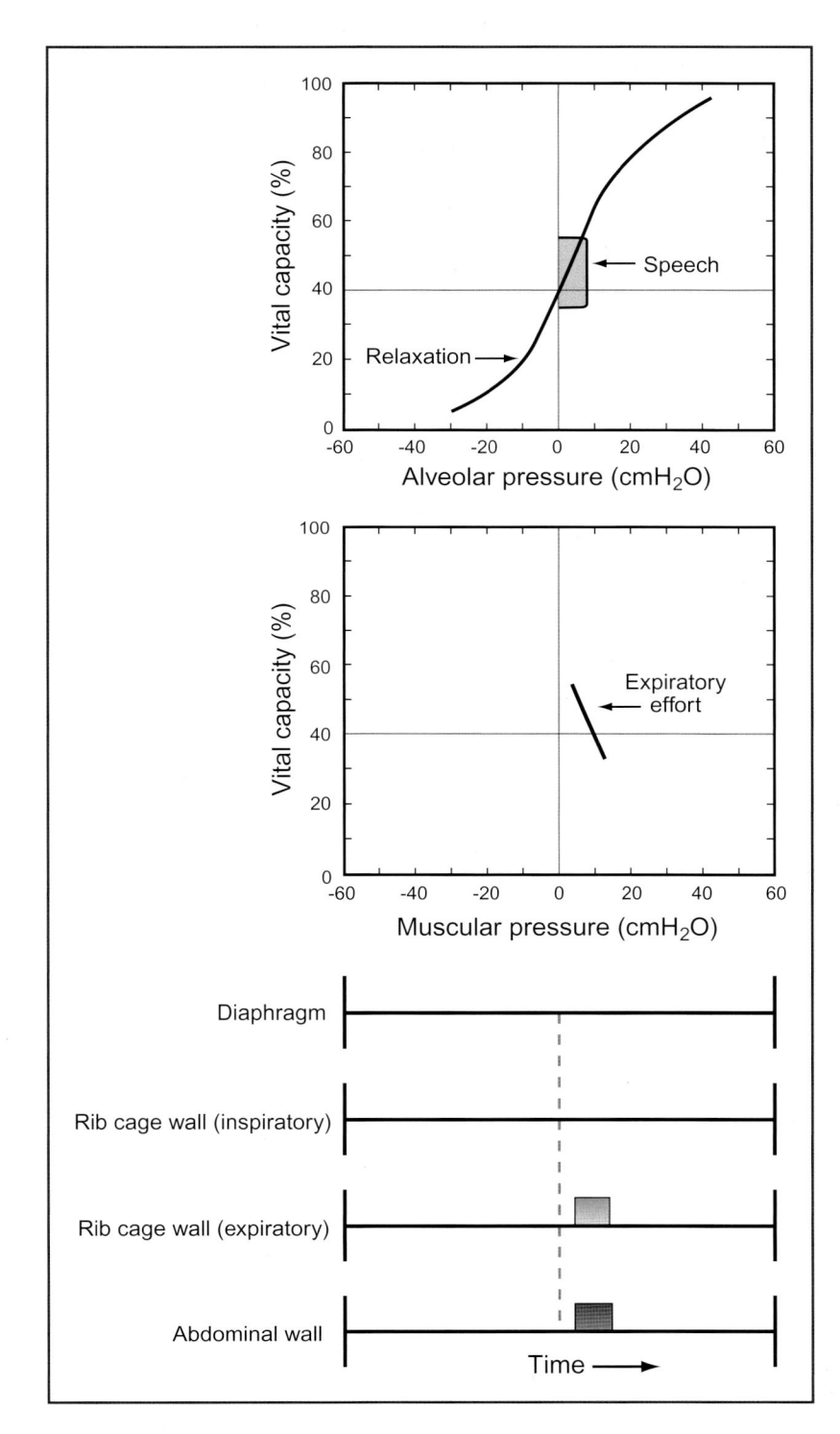

Figure 2–34. Relaxation pressure, target alveolar pressure, muscular pressure, and temporal activity of chest wall components for one breath group of running speech production performed in the upright body position. Only expiration (speaking) is represented. The top panel depicts the relaxation pressure and the target alveolar pressure (8 cmH$_2$O). The horizontal line at 40 %VC represents the resting level of the breathing apparatus. This combination of graphs indicates that running speech is produced near the resting level, that only expiratory muscular pressures are required, that those muscular pressures come from expiratory rib cage wall and abdominal muscles, and that the abdominal muscles contribute more than the expiratory rib cage muscles (represented by the relative darkness of the bars in the lower graph).

almost never a need to use inspiratory muscular pressure during running speech production. Thus, inspiratory braking, such as that required near the beginning of extended steady utterance, is *not* used during running speech production.

The middle panel of Figure 2–34 shows that expiratory muscular pressure is required throughout the breath group and the bottom panel indicates that this expiratory pressure is produced by both the expiratory rib cage wall muscles and abdominal muscles, with the abdominal wall muscles contributing the most (as indicated by the darker bar). These muscular mechanisms are consistent with what is depicted in the shape diagram of Figure 2–33, which shows that running speech is produced to the left of the relaxation characteristic. As discussed above and depicted in Figure 2–22, potential muscular mechanisms for speech produced to the left of the relaxation characteristic include: (a) inspiratory rib cage muscular pressure, (b) (expiratory) abdominal muscular pressure, (c) inspiratory rib cage muscular pressure and (expiratory) abdominal muscular pressure; and (d) expiratory rib cage muscular pressure and abdominal muscular pressure, with the latter predominating. By examining Figure 2–34, it is clear that the muscular mechanism actually used by speakers is the last one: expiratory rib cage wall muscular pressure combined with a greater abdominal wall muscular pressure.

The target alveolar pressure shown in Figure 2–34 (8 cmH$_2$O) is typical for speaking at a conversational loudness level. For running speech activities that are louder than usual, higher alveolar pressures are targeted; for softer than usual speech, lower alveolar pressures are targeted. This means that when speaking within the mid lung volume range, higher than usual muscular pressures are required to produce louder speech and lower than usual muscular pressures are required to produce softer speech. Another way to increase loudness is to speak at larger lung volumes where the prevailing relaxation pressure is greater.

The inspiratory phase of the running speech breathing cycle (not included in Figure 2–34) is driven by the diaphragm. Interestingly, expiratory muscles of the rib cage wall and abdominal wall maintain a low level of activity during inspiration. This enables them to be in a state of readiness to begin driving expiration (speech production) as soon as inspiration has ended.

The abdominal wall plays an extremely important role in running speech breathing produced in an upright body position. As stated above, it generates most of the expiratory muscular pressure during speech production. It is also responsible for imposing the general background configuration assumed by the chest wall throughout the speech breathing cycle (smaller than relaxed abdominal wall and larger than relaxed rib cage wall). As it turns out, there are important advantages to having the abdominal wall play such a prominent role in upright running speech breathing.

Figure 2–35 illustrates these advantages in the context of the shape of the chest wall used for upright running speech activities. Inward displacement of the abdominal wall (by its own muscular action) has important consequences for the diaphragm and rib cage wall. As the abdominal wall moves inward, the diaphragm is pushed headward such that its radius of curvature increases and its principal muscle fibers elongate. This positions the diaphragm so that it can produce the quick and powerful inspirations that are critical for minimizing interruptions during running speech activities. Inward displacement of the abdominal wall also lifts the rib cage wall. This stretches the expiratory muscles of the rib cage wall, thereby increasing their potential for generating the quick expiratory pulses needed to produce linguistic stress and loudness change. Also, with the abdominal wall held firmly inward, expiratory efforts by the rib cage wall can be fully resolved into pressure change. If the abdominal wall were not held firmly in place, expiratory efforts of the

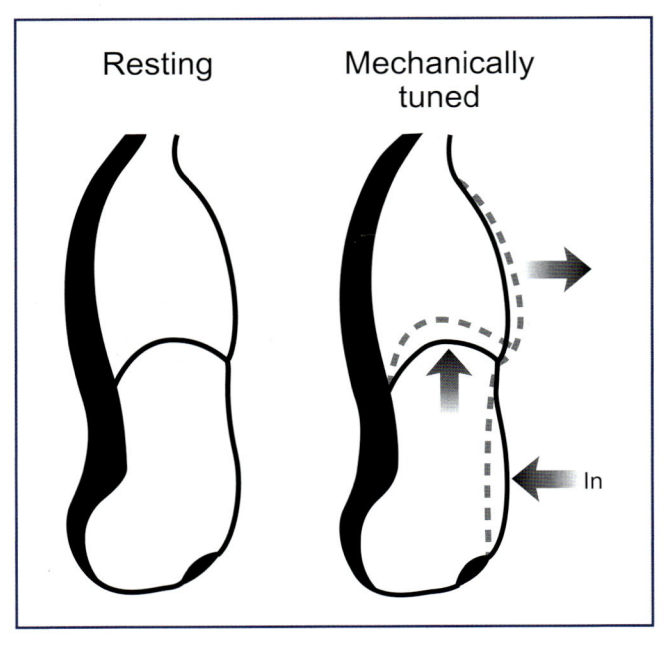

Figure 2–35. Shape of the chest wall for running speech activities in upright body positions. This chest wall shape is characterized by an inwardly displaced abdominal wall that causes the diaphragm to move headward and the rib cage wall to lift. This shape "tunes" the diaphragm to produce quick inspirations and the expiratory rib cage wall muscles to generate quick expiratory pressure changes.

> ### More than One Way to . . .
>
> The text describes how most of us speech breathe most of the time. However, this is not always the way it is—sometimes we have to change our speech breathing to adapt to the circumstances. This is called adaptive control. Adaptive control is not unique to speech breathing, but occurs in essentially all motor control systems. For example, if a violinist breaks a string during a performance, he may decide not to stop, but rather to continue playing by reprogramming his usual fingering (Wolff, 1979). In a skilled violinist, this reprogramming can be done instantly and without much effort. The violinist adapts by allowing the "motor idea" to control the performance. The goal is the important thing, not the way it is attained. In much the same way, our speech breathing can be automatically reprogrammed when we wear a tight-fitting garment that restricts our breathing movements or when we have to speak in an awkward body position. Yup, there is more than one way to . . .

rib cage wall would be resolved into outward movement of the abdominal wall before a pressure change could be effected (recall the balloon analogy provided above). Thus, the activation of abdominal wall muscles and the resultant inward displacement serve to mechanically tune the breathing apparatus for inspiration and expiration during running speech breathing. When the abdominal wall muscles are impaired, speech breathing is impaired.

A good deal of information about volume, pressure, and shape events for running speech activities is carried in the speech (acoustic) signal. Thus, a listener can gather clues about running speech breathing by just listening to a person's speech. To begin, breath group length provides clues about lung volume events. In general, the longer the breath group, the larger the lung volume excursion. Loudness provides clues about alveolar pressure. As a general rule, the louder the speech produced, the higher the alveolar pressure. Finally, inspiratory duration and the rate of loudness change may provide clues about the shape of the chest wall. When the chest wall is configured appropriately for speech production (larger than relaxed rib cage wall and smaller than relaxed abdominal wall), inspirations are short and loudness changes for linguistic stress are quick.

VARIABLES THAT INFLUENCE SPEECH BREATHING

The previous section describes speech breathing produced in an upright body position by a typical young adult and contains the most important foundational concepts for understanding speech breathing. Nevertheless, there are several variables that influence speech breathing that may be relevant to clinical and research applications. These include body position, body type, age, sex, ventilation and drive to breathe, and cognitive-linguistic and social variables.

Body Position

A change in body position alters the mechanical behavior of the breathing apparatus, primarily because gravity has such a strong influence on this massive structure. Thus, with each new body position, a new mechanical solution may need to be found. Most of this section is devoted to discussion of speech breathing in the supine body position (as contrasted to the upright body position discussed above), but other body positions are considered as well.

Figure 2–36 depicts the influence of gravity on different parts of the chest wall in the upright and supine body positions. In the upright body position, gravity acts in the expiratory direction on the rib cage wall, tending to pull it downward and reduce its size, and gravity acts in the inspiratory direction on the abdominal wall, tending to pull it outward and increase its size. In contrast, in the supine body position, gravity acts in the expiratory direction on both the rib cage wall and abdominal wall. This causes the relaxation pressure to be greater at any given lung volume in the supine body position than in the upright body position. In addition, the gravitational force exerted on the abdominal wall pushes the diaphragm headward, causing the resting level of the breathing apparatus to decrease from its upright value (from about 40 %VC in upright to about 20 %VC in supine).

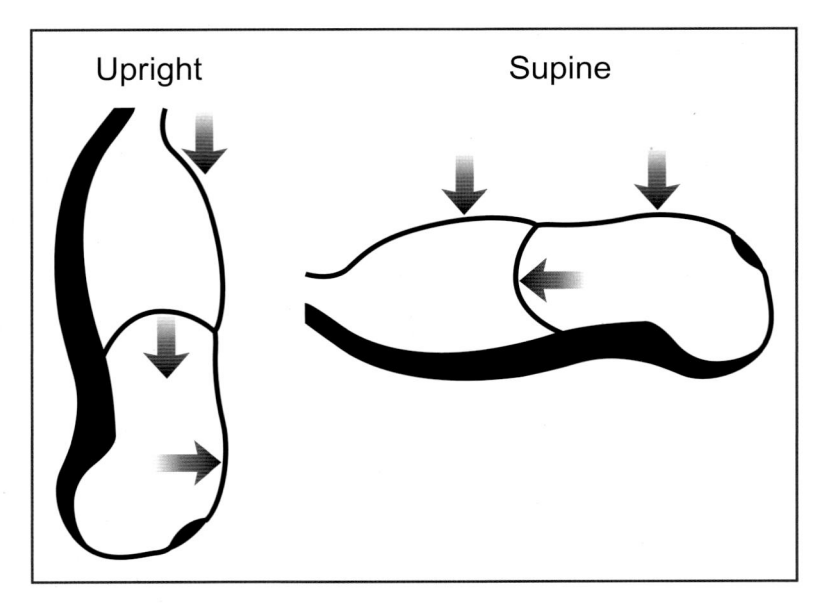

Figure 2–36. Gravitational effects on the breathing apparatus. In upright positions (seated upright or standing), gravity "expires" the rib cage, but "inspires" the abdomen. In supine, gravity expires all parts of the breathing apparatus. This causes the resting lung volume level of the breathing apparatus to be smaller by about 20 %VC in the supine body position compared with upright.

Extended Steady Utterances in the Supine Body Position

Extended steady utterance production in supine requires continuously changing muscle activations to counteract the continuously changing relaxation pressure, just as it does in the upright body position. However, the nature and the time course of those muscle activations are different from those in upright, as depicted in Figure 2–37.

Because gravity has a greater expiratory influence on the breathing apparatus in supine, the relaxation pressure is higher than it is in upright at any given lung volume. This can be visualized by comparing the upright and supine pressure-volume relaxation characteristics (see top panels of Figures 2–29 and 2–37) and noting that the supine characteristic is shifted rightward. This rightward shift of the relaxation characteristic also shifts the point at which the relaxation pressure is zero; that is, it shifts the resting level to a smaller lung volume (to about 20 %VC).

Because the relaxation pressure is shifted rightward (to a greater positive value), to achieve the same target alveolar pressure in the supine body position, a greater inspiratory effort (a greater negative muscular pressure) must be exerted at large lung volumes, and that effort must be continued to a smaller lung volume compared with the upright body position. Stated another way, greater inspiratory braking is required to produce the first part of an extended steady utterance in supine than in upright. Conversely, at small lung volumes (near the end of the extended steady utterance) a less substantial expiratory effort (a lesser positive muscular pressure) is required in supine than in upright. This can be seen in the middle panel of Figure 2–37.

Another way that extended steady utterance production differs in supine and upright is in the muscles used for achieving the target alveolar pressure. Recall that nearly all inspiratory braking in upright is done by the inspiratory rib cage wall muscles. In contrast, as shown in the bottom panel of Figure 2–37, all inspiratory braking in supine is accomplished with diaphragm activation. In fact, the inspiratory rib cage wall muscles are not activated at all during extended steady utterance in supine.

There are mechanical reasons for why the diaphragm performs the inspiratory braking in the supine body position. In supine, there is a substantial influence of gravity on the abdominal wall, causing abdominal pressure to be high; thus, there is no significant hydraulic pull on the undersurface of the diaphragm as there is in the upright body position. Without a significant hydraulic pull, the inspiratory rib cage wall muscles cannot contribute much to the lowering of

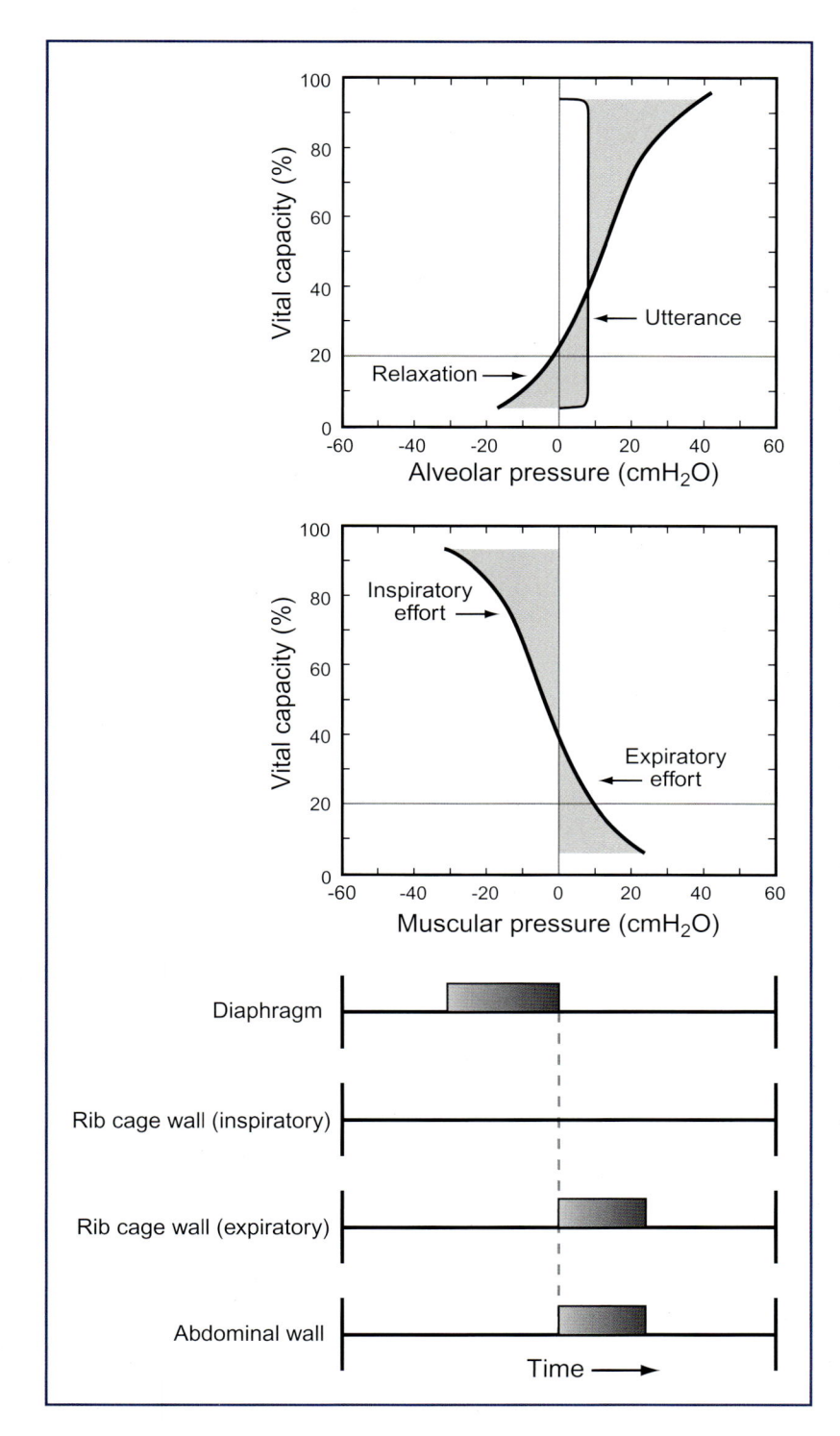

Figure 2-37. Relaxation pressure, target alveolar pressure, muscular pressure, and temporal activity of chest wall components for a sustained vowel produced in the supine body position. Only expiration (vowel production) is represented. The top panel depicts the relaxation pressure and the target alveolar pressure (8 cmH$_2$O) for the vowel. The horizontal line at 20 %VC represents the resting level of the breathing apparatus. As depicted in the middle panel, to produce the target pressure, inspiratory braking is required at the beginning (at large lung volumes), but as the vowel proceeds, the need for inspiratory braking ceases and expiratory muscular effort is required and continues to increase in magnitude through the expiratory reserve volume. The bottom panel depicts the activation of muscle groups, with the diaphragm performing all of the inspiratory braking and the expiratory rib cage wall and abdominal muscles producing the expiratory muscular pressures. From *Evaluation and management of speech breathing disorders: Principles and methods* (p. 59), by T. Hixon and J. Hoit, 2005, Tucson, AZ: Redington Brown. Copyright 2005 by Thomas J. Hixon and Jeannette D. Hoit. Modified and reproduced with permission.

alveolar pressure (because they have nothing to pull against, unless the diaphragm also activates). Thus, contracting the diaphragm is the only efficient way to hold back against the high relaxation pressure at large lung volumes in the supine body position.

Near the end of an extended steady utterance, at lung volumes smaller than the resting level, both expiratory rib cage wall and abdominal wall muscles activate to maintain the target alveolar pressure in the face of the prevailing inspiratory relaxation pressure

> ### Flat Out
>
> Two terms that get more than their fair share of misuse are *supine* and *prone*. Supine means lying on your back (usually face up). The easy way to remember this is to consider the spelling of supine. Take out its second letter and you have *spine*. On your spine is on your back. So-called couch potatoes spend a lot of supine time in front of their television sets. Prone, also called procumbent, means lying on your front (usually face down). Take its first three letters and you have the first three letters of the word *prostrate* (as in face down submission or adoration). Certain yoga poses, such as the sphinx pose, begin by assuming a prone position. The confusion encountered when using the terms supine and prone arises because both involve being flat out. The memory devices suggested here should make it easy to keep the two body positions straight (pun intended).

(bottom panel of Figure 2–37). This is much the same as what occurs in upright body positions.

Running Speech Activities in the Supine Body Position

Breathing during running speech activities also differs in the supine body position compared with the upright body position. These differences can be seen by comparing events associated with supine running speech production, shown in Figure 2–38, with those associated with upright running speech production in Figure 2–34.

As can be seen in the top two panels of Figure 2–38, running speech production starts from about twice resting tidal depth (or less) and continues to near the resting level of the breathing apparatus. This is the same as in the upright body position; however, the actual lung volume range within the vital capacity is different. That is, because the resting level of the breathing apparatus shifts with body position, lung volume events in supine range from about 40 to 20 %VC compared with about 60 to 40 %VC in upright.

As in upright running speech production, both relaxation pressure and muscular pressure contribute to running speech production in the supine body position. Relaxation pressure is slightly positive in the range of lung volumes in which running speech is produced (the 20 %VC above the resting level), but not positive enough to achieve the target alveolar pressure. Therefore, positive muscular pressure is required throughout the breath group, the magnitude of which depends on the desired speech loudness. In supine, expiratory muscular pressure is provided primarily by activation of rib cage wall expiratory muscles, as shown in the bottom panel of Figure 2–38. Only when loud speech is produced or when speech is produced within the expiratory reserve volume do abdominal wall muscles also become active.

Inspiration during running speech production (not shown in Figure 2–38) is driven by the diaphragm, just as it is in the upright body position. The expiratory muscles of the rib cage wall remain active during inspiration, as they do for running speech activities in the upright body position, so that no time is lost in reactivating them for expiration (speaking).

The muscular strategy for the abdominal wall is quite different for supine compared with upright running speech activities. Recall that in upright, abdominal wall muscle activation plays a critical role during speech production (expiration) as well as during inspiration. In contrast, it plays little or no role for running speech produced in the supine body position. This is because in supine, gravity does what the abdominal wall muscles do in upright; that is, gravity drives the abdominal content and diaphragm headward, stretching the muscle fibers of the diaphragm and positioning them to be able to generate forceful and rapid inspirations. Gravity also forces the rib cage wall somewhat headward and positions its expiratory muscles for quicker actions. Because the breathing apparatus is mechanically tuned by gravity in supine, the expiratory rib cage wall muscles are generally sufficient to produce the required muscular pressures for speaking.

Chest wall shape during supine running speech production is unlike that assumed in upright running speech production. Whereas speech in the upright body position is produced with the abdominal wall displaced inward and the rib cage wall elevated, the opposite chest wall shape is used in the supine body position. That is, the abdominal wall is pushed outward and the rib cage wall is smaller relative to their relaxed positions at the prevailing lung volume during speaking.

Table 2–3 summarizes the major differences between upright and supine running speech breathing. They are as follows:

a. Although the size of breath groups is the same in the two body positions (about 20 %VC on average), lung volume events occur at smaller lung volumes in supine (40 to 20 %VC) than in upright (60 to 40 %VC). This is because the resting level is smaller

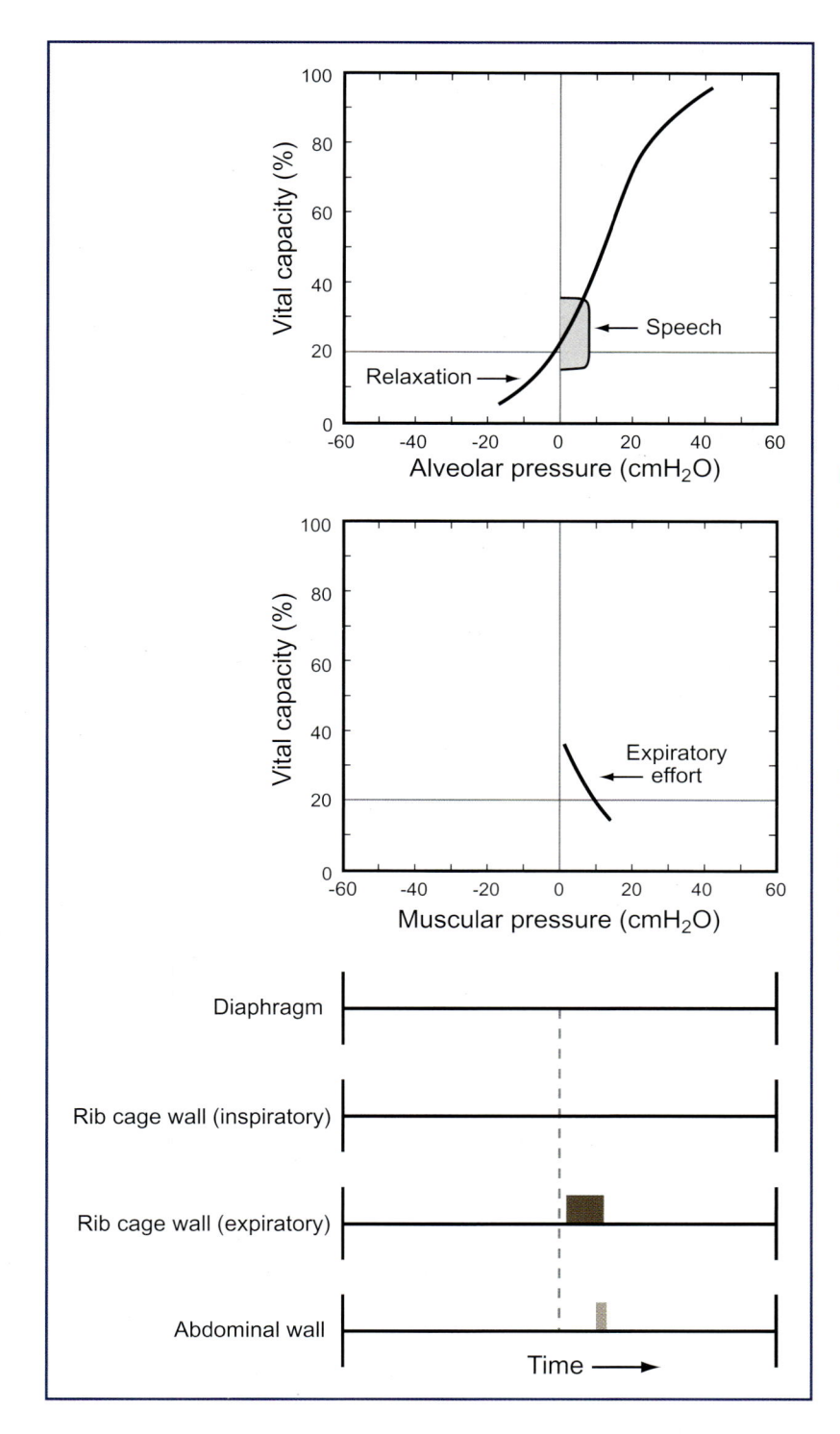

Figure 2-38. Relaxation pressure, target alveolar pressure, muscular pressure, and temporal activity of chest wall components for one breath group of running speech production performed in the supine body position. Only expiration (speaking) is represented. The top panel depicts the relaxation pressure and the target alveolar pressure (8 cmH2O). The horizontal line at 20 %VC represents the resting level of the breathing apparatus. This combination of graphs indicates that running speech is produced near the resting level, that only expiratory muscular pressures are required, and that those muscular pressures come primarily from expiratory rib cage wall muscles (as indicated by the relative darkness and the length of the bars in the lower graph).

in supine and speech breathing tends to follow the resting level.

b. Alveolar pressure is the same in the two body positions for speech of normal loudness and is generally in the range of 5 to 10 cmH$_2$O.

c. In upright body positions, the shape of the chest wall is characterized by an abdominal wall that is displaced inward and a rib cage wall that is elevated. In contrast, chest wall shape is just the opposite in supine running speech production: the rib cage wall is displaced inward and the abdominal wall is displaced outward.

Table 2–3. Differences Between Running Speech Breathing of Normal Loudness Produced in Upright Versus Supine Body Position

BREATHING VARIABLE	UPRIGHT	SUPINE
Lung volume range	Begins near 60 %VC and ends near 40 %VC	Begins near 40 %VC and ends near 20 %VC
Alveolar pressure	5 to 10 cmH$_2$O	5 to 10 cmH$_2$O
Chest wall shape	Smaller than relaxed AB Larger than relaxed RC	Larger than relaxed AB Smaller than relaxed RC
Muscular mechanisms: expiration	+RC < +AB	+RC
Muscular mechanisms: inspiration	–DI, +AB	–DI

Note. VC = vital capacity; AB = abdominal wall; RC = rib cage wall; DI = diaphragm; + = expiratory muscle activity; – = inspiratory muscle activity.

d. Upright running speech is produced with a combination of expiratory rib cage wall and abdominal wall muscular pressure, with the latter predominating. In contrast, supine running speech is usually produced with only expiratory rib cage wall muscular pressure. There are times when abdominal muscular pressure may also contribute to the generation of alveolar pressure, such as during loud speaking or speaking at small lung volumes.

e. Inspiration is driven by the diaphragm in both upright and supine body positions. The primary difference is that the abdominal (expiratory) muscles remain active for upright inspirations to help the diaphragm maintain a mechanical advantage by stretching its fibers and providing a more solid base against which it can contract.

Speech Breathing in Other Body Positions

The number of body positions is limitless and the mechanical solution to each is different. Nevertheless, there are some overarching principles that apply across body positions.

One principle is that the resting level of the breathing apparatus changes as body position changes. This is illustrated in Figure 2–39 for several different body positions. Much of the change in resting level can be attributed to the influence of gravity on the abdominal content and the resultant axial displacement of the diaphragm. As the diaphragm is pushed headward, air moves out of the pulmonary apparatus and shifts the resting level to a smaller lung volume. Conversely, as the diaphragm is pulled footward, air moves into the pulmonary apparatus and shifts the resting level to a larger lung volume. Of particular importance in the present context is that lung volume events for running speech production are determined primarily by the resting level of the breathing apparatus (as shown by the several sets of vertical lines in Figure 2–39, each line representing a single breath group).

A second principle is that the relaxation pressure for any given lung volume increases as the body is tilted from upright toward supine. This means that a different muscular pressure is required to achieve a given alveolar pressure target at a specified lung volume.

A third principle is that different chest wall components assume different roles in generating muscular pressure as body position changes. In particular, the abdominal wall muscles are highly active during speaking in more upright body positions, whereas they are increasingly less active as the body is tilted toward supine. Also, in those rare cases in which running speech is produced at very large lung volumes (but something that commonly occurs during extended steady utterance), the inspiratory muscles of the rib cage wall do most of the inspiratory braking in upright, whereas the diaphragm takes over this role as the body is tilted toward supine.

The fourth principle is that the expiratory rib cage muscles almost always participate in running speech production, regardless of body position. The rib cage wall has the mechanical advantage of covering a much larger area of the lungs than does the diaphragm–abdominal wall (recall Figure 2–14) and of containing small and fast-acting muscles. These features make the rib cage wall well suited for moving lung volume and generating muscular pressure change for speech production in all body positions.

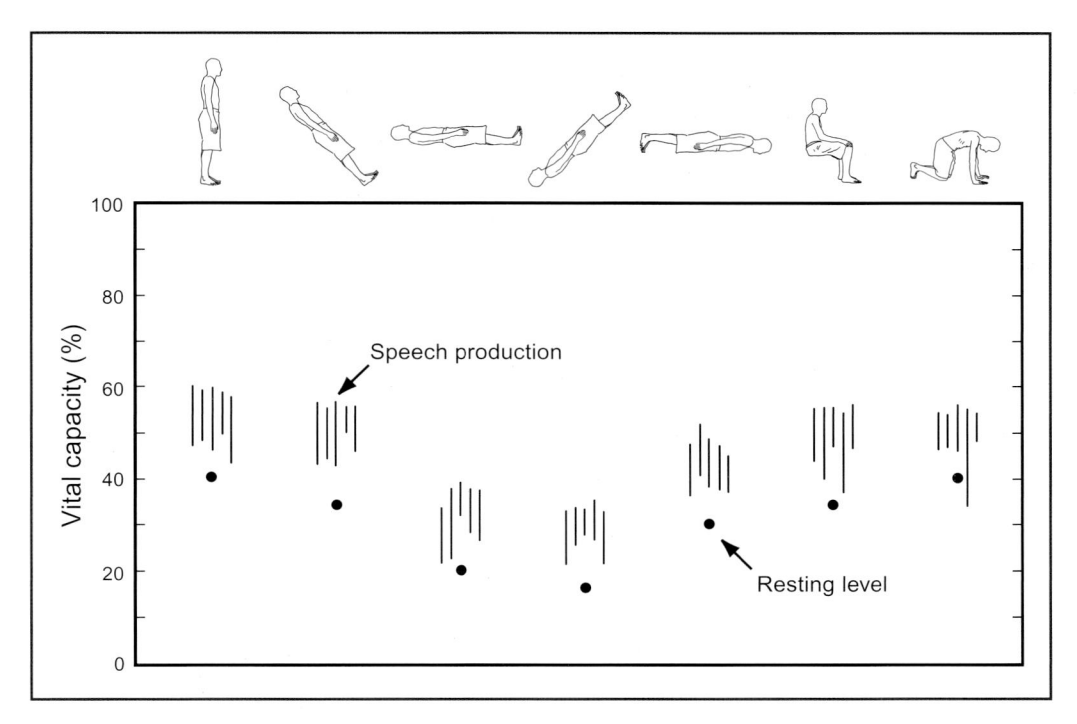

Figure 2–39. Breath groups during running speech production in different body positions. Each vertical line represents a single breath group (expiration containing speech). Note that breath groups are produced just above the resting level of the breathing apparatus (*represented by filled dots*) in all body positions. From *Evaluation and management of speech breathing disorders: Principles and methods* (p. 77), by T. Hixon and J. Hoit, 2005, Tucson, AZ: Redington Brown. Copyright 2005 by Thomas J. Hixon and Jeannette D. Hoit. Modified and reproduced with permission.

Body Type

People come in many different sizes, shapes, and compositions, or so-called body types. Because the breathing apparatus makes up a large portion of the body, it is not surprising that those differences influence the way the breathing apparatus functions for speech breathing.

Figure 2–40 illustrates men with three very different body types (from left to right): highly endomorphic (high in relative fatness), highly mesomorphic (high in musculoskeletal development), and highly ectomorphic (high in relative linearity). The most striking difference in speech breathing among young men with these body types is that endomorphic men tend to pull the abdominal wall inward farther and move it a greater distance during speaking than ectomorphic men (Hoit & Hixon, 1986). This is probably because the diaphragm is flattened by the downward pull of the large abdominal mass in an endomorphic person (when in an upright body position). By actively moving the abdominal wall inward, the diaphragm can assume a more domed configuration and produce more forceful inspirations, such as those required during speech breathing. The ectomorphic person, with his flat abdominal wall, already has a well-positioned diaphragm and has no need to move the abdominal wall during speech breathing.

Age

Thus far, this chapter has discussed speech breathing from the perspective of a young adult (fully mature) system. However, speech breathing develops over time, as do all other motor (movement) behaviors. Developmental changes during infancy, childhood, and adolescence can be linked to changes in the size of the breathing apparatus, musculoskeletal geometry, chest wall compliance, pressure generation capability, neural control, linguistic sophistication, and many other factors.

Developmental trends in speech breathing have been identified for early infancy through the mid-teenage years (Boliek, Hixon, Watson, & Jones, 2009; Boliek, Hixon, Watson, & Morgan, 1996, 1997; Connaghan, Moore, & Higashakawa, 2004; Hoit, Hixon,

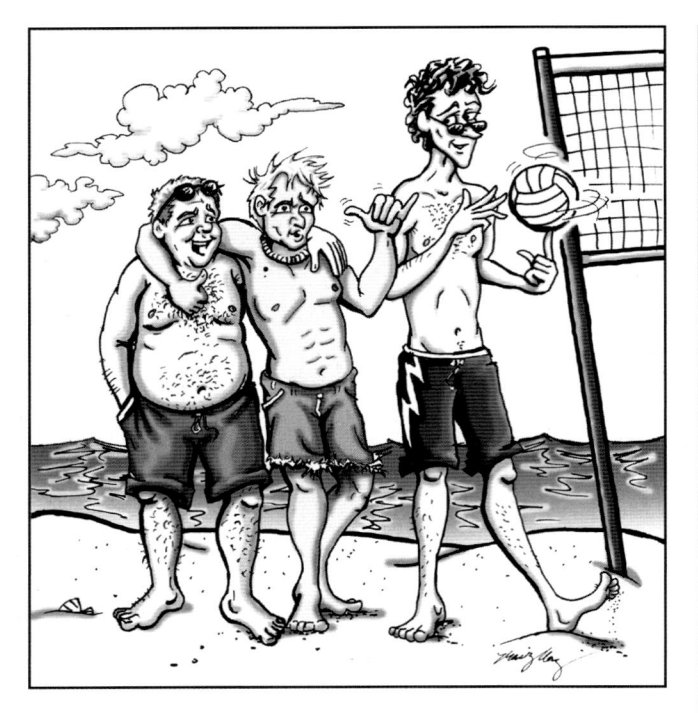

Figure 2–40. Cartoon of three teammates of different body types. The endomorph (*left*) is high in relative fatness; the mesomorph (*middle*) is particularly muscular; and the ectomorph (*right*) is lean and linear with little fat and muscle.

Rock-a-Bye Baby

Lullabies tend to put infants to sleep and change their breathing patterns. A supine infant who is awake breathes with in-phase movements of the rib cage wall and abdominal wall. The two structures rise and fall together in a gentle rhythm. But if the same infant falls asleep, there may be an abrupt change in breathing pattern. During rapid eye movement sleep the pattern may change to out-of-phase movements of the rib cage wall and abdominal wall. One structure rises while the other falls. The reason is that, during sleep, structures in the pharyngeal-oral airway relax and the tongue falls toward the back of the infant's throat. This increases the airway resistance through which the breathing apparatus must work. One consequence is that pleural pressure must be lowered more during each inspiration, causing the floppy rib cage wall to be sucked inward. So, it's rock-a-bye baby, but bye-bye in-phase movements.

Watson, & Morgan, 1990; Moore, Caulfield, & Green, 2001; Parham, Buder, Oller, & Boliek, 2011) and include the following: (a) in general, the amount of air expired per breath becomes increasingly larger as the size of the child increases and (b) speech breathing becomes less variable as children grow older. Unlike adults, who tend to be rather consistent in their speech breathing across time, infants and toddlers seem to use a different strategy for each vocalization (different lung volumes, different chest wall shapes, and different relative volume contributions of the rib cage wall and abdominal wall to lung volume change), as though they are experimenting with the breathing apparatus to see what works best. Other speech breathing features seem to be nearly adult like from the beginning. For example, infants and toddlers, whether 5 weeks or 3 years of age, usually initiate breath groups within the midrange of the vital capacity, in the same way adults do. Also, as early as 18 months of age, inspirations preceding vocalization are quicker than inspirations associated with tidal breathing.

When volume measures are normalized to take into account age-related size differences, speech breathing is essentially adult like in most features by 10 years of age (before puberty). The only major difference seen beyond age 10 years is an increase in the amount of speech per breath group, reflecting changes in linguistic skill and sophistication. It is also notable that young children use relatively high alveolar pressures when speaking (Bernthal & Beukelman, 1979; Netsell, Lotz, Peters, & Schulte, 1994; Stathopoulos & Sapienza, 1993, 1997; Stathopoulos & Weismer, 1985); these pressures eventually decrease to adult-like values.

Speech breathing remains relatively stable throughout adulthood until the seventh or eighth decade of life when it begins to change (Hoit & Hixon, 1987; Hoit, Hixon, Altman, & Morgan, 1989; Huber, 2008; Huber, Darling, Francis, & Zhang, 2012; Huber & Darling-White, 2017; Sperry & Klich, 1992). In a senescent person, breath groups start from larger lung volumes, encompass more of the vital capacity, and contain less speech when compared with breath groups of a younger adult. This means that senescent speakers tend to expend more air per syllable and take deeper breaths before speaking, probably in anticipation of the increased air loss. This air loss appears to be due to uneconomical valving by downstream structures. Subsequent research pointed to the larynx as the valve most responsible for the air wastage exhibited by senescent speakers, although the mechanism of wastage appears to differ for men and women. In men, air wastage has been attributed to an age-related decrease in laryngeal airway resistance during phonation (Melcon, Hoit,

& Hixon, 1989), whereas in women the air wastage appears to be related to nonspeech expirations before or after spoken utterances (Hoit & Hixon, 1992; Sperry & Klich, 1992). Of course, it is possible that age-related changes in speech breathing and laryngeal function are more tightly linked to biological age (health status and physical fitness) than to chronological age.

Sex

There is a pervasive myth that males and females breathe differently. This myth might also be applied to speech breathing, except that there is substantial evidence that contradicts it (Boliek et al., 1996, 1997, 2009; Hodge & Rochet, 1989; Hoit et al., 1989, 1990). From infancy through senescence, speech breathing is generally the same in the two sexes. The one exception is that after puberty, the absolute lung volumes associated with speech breathing are generally larger in boys than girls (and men than women) because boys are generally taller and, therefore, have larger airways. Nevertheless, when volume measures are normalized to take into account differences in size, there are no sex-related differences in speech breathing to be found.

Ventilation and Drive to Breathe

Most of the time, ventilation (the rate at which air moves in and out of the breathing apparatus) matches the gas exchange (metabolic) needs of the body. For example, ventilation is lower when sleeping (low metabolic need) than when exercising (high metabolic need). Sometimes, however, ventilation is higher or lower than the metabolic need, resulting in hyperventilation or hypoventilation, respectively.

Under normal circumstances, speech breathing is associated with hyperventilation (Abel, Mottau, Klubendorf, & Koepchen, 1987; Bunn & Mead, 1971; Hoit & Lohmeier, 2000; Meanock & Nicholls, 1982; Warner, Waggener, & Kronauer, 1983). That is, ventilation is greater and carbon dioxide levels are lower when we speak than when we sit quietly. The degree of hyperventilation is dictated, in part, by the nature of the speaking activity. Ventilation is greater during continuous speaking (such as lecturing) than during intermittent speaking (such as conversing, wherein both speaking and listening occur). In addition, ventilation is greater when the speech is heavily loaded with high-flow sounds (such as voiceless consonants) than if it contains all-voiced sounds.

When the drive to breathe is strong, such as at a high elevation or during vigorous exercise, speaking can become a struggle (Figure 2–41). In such situations, there arises an awareness of having to balance the need to breathe with the desire to speak.

Speech breathing under conditions of high drive differs substantially from speech breathing under usual (resting) conditions. Speech breathing in high drive has been studied using two general approaches: one is to have people speak while exercising (walking on a

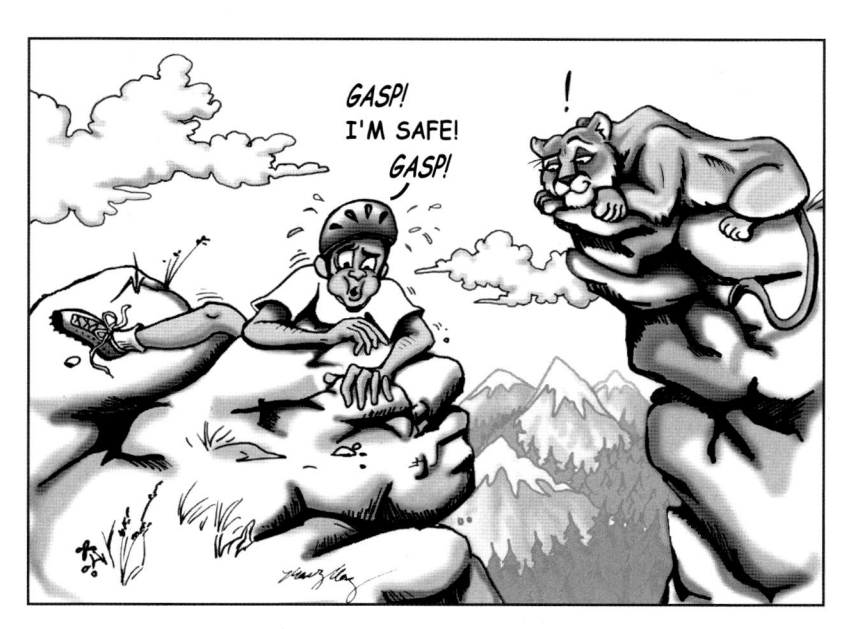

Figure 2–41. Cartoon depicting elevation, exercise, and speaking as a triple challenge to ventilation.

treadmill or riding a stationary bicycle) and the other is to alter the gas composition of the blood, usually by having people breathe air containing high concentrations of carbon dioxide (Bailey & Hoit, 2002; Baker, Hipp, & Alessio, 2008; Bunn & Mead, 1971; Doust & Patrick, 1981; Hale & Patrick, 1987; Hoit, Lansing, & Perona, 2007; Meanock & Nicholls, 1982; Otis & Clark, 1968; Phillipson, McClean, Sullivan, & Zamel, 1978).

The most robust characteristic of speech breathing in high drive is perhaps the least surprising: ventilation increases with the magnitude of the stimulus (exercise or carbon dioxide levels). Increases in ventilation are accomplished by larger tidal volumes, faster breathing frequencies, or both. It is interesting to note, however, that although ventilation increases when a person is speaking under high drive, it does not increase as much as it does if the person is not speaking. This suggests that the act of speaking tends to suppress (or override) the full response to a high-drive stimulus.

Less speech is produced per breath group when speaking under high drive, apparently to help maximize ventilation. This is done using two commonly adopted strategies. The first is to blow off air. When people use this strategy, they may produce a few syllables and then expire the remainder of the breath without speaking or they may expire at the beginning of the breath group and then speak. The second strategy for increasing ventilation is to produce breathy speech. When people use this strategy, they use high airflow while speaking so that air is expired more quickly. This usually means that the airflow through the larynx is higher during productions of voiced-speech segments and that airflow associated with voiceless consonant productions is also higher. Often, people use a combination of these two strategies.

When speaking under high drive, people tend to adjust the size and shape of the breathing apparatus. Specifically, they tend to begin and end breath groups at larger-than-usual lung volumes, so that the breathing apparatus is larger overall than it is when they are speaking under usual conditions. They also make large and fast chest wall shape changes when speaking in high drive. These adjustments in size and shape may reflect physiological strategies to help relieve the discomfort (dyspnea) that accompanies a high drive to breathe.

Finally, there seems to be one speech breathing behavior that is relatively resistant to change under high drive conditions. This is the coordination of inspirations with the linguistic content of speech. Even when people attempt to speak while "gasping for air," they tend to pause (to blow off air, inspire, or both) at linguistically appropriate junctures, such as sentence, clause, or phrase boundaries, at least when reading aloud. This illustrates the strong influence of linguistic factors on speech breathing, even when the drive to breathe is very strong.

Cognitive-Linguistic and Social Variables

Cognitive-linguistic demands differ widely, depending on whether one recites a well-memorized poem, reads aloud a simple paragraph, converses with a friend, or delivers an extemporaneous speech on a complex topic. Of these four speaking activities, speaking extemporaneously on a complex topic generally carries the highest cognitive-linguistic load.

Cognitive-linguistic factors affect certain details of the inspiratory and expiratory limbs of the speech breathing cycle. Inspirations are most likely to occur at linguistic structural boundaries (sentence, clause, and phrase boundaries), especially during reading aloud and, to a lesser degree, when speaking extemporaneously (Bailey & Hoit, 2002; Conrad, Thalacker, & Schönle, 1983; Grosjean & Collins, 1979; Henderson, Goldman-Eisler, & Skarbek, 1965; Hixon et al., 1973; Sugito, Ohyama, & Hirose, 1990; Wang, Green, Nip, Kent, & Kent, 2010; Winkworth, Davis, Adams, & Ellis, 1995; Winkworth, Davis, Ellis, & Adams, 1994). Also, inspirations tend to be larger (deeper) when followed by longer breath groups and smaller (shallower) when followed by shorter breath groups (Denny, 2000; Horii & Cooke, 1978; Huber & Darling, 2011; McFarland & Smith, 1992; Sperry & Klich, 1992; Whalen & Kinsella-Shaw, 1997; Winkworth et al., 1994, 1995).

Expirations, too, are influenced by cognitive-linguistic factors. The number of speech units (syllables) produced during expiration generally dictates where within the vital capacity the breath group stops. Expirations containing more speech units tend to end at smaller lung volumes than those containing fewer speech units (Hodge & Rochet, 1989; Wilder, 1983; Winkworth et al., 1994, 1995). However, the most powerful cognitive-linguistic influence on expirations relates to silent pausing. Silent pauses (moments of silence that last at least 200 to 250 milliseconds) are believed to reflect the time needed to formulate the upcoming spoken message (Goldman-Eisler, 1956; Greene, 1984; Greene & Cappella, 1986; Henderson et al., 1965; Lay & Paivio, 1969; Reynolds & Paivio, 1968; Rochester, 1973; Taylor, 1969). Silent pauses that are accompanied by breath holding seem to be associated with particularly high cognitive-linguistic demands, but those that are accompanied by nonspeech expirations are more common (Mitchell, Hoit, & Watson, 1996; Webb, Williams, & Minifie, 1967). Because nonspeech expirations "waste air," there tends to be less speech produced per breath when cognitive-linguistic demands are high than when they are low.

Although several features of the inspiratory and expiratory phases of speech breathing are influenced by cognitive-linguistic factors, the general mechanical behavior of the breathing apparatus does not appear to be affected. Whether reading aloud or speaking extemporaneously, speech breathing tends to be produced within the midrange of the vital capacity, at lung volumes larger than the resting level, using a larger-than-relaxed rib cage wall and smaller-than-relaxed abdominal wall, and engaging predictable muscular strategies (Hixon et al., 1973, 1976; Hodge & Rochet, 1989; Hoit & Hixon, 1986, 1987; Hoit et al., 1989, 1990; Mitchell et al., 1996).

Social variables may also come into play, especially during conversational interchange wherein the speech breathing patterns, or rhythms, of one conversational partner may influence the behavior of the other conversational partner. There is substantial evidence that people tend to entrain their intrinsic biological and behavioral rhythms with people with whom they are interacting and that the most enjoyable interactions are those in which individual rhythms entrain easily to one another (Chapple, 1970).

Different types of rhythms have been identified in conversational speech breathing (McFarland, 2001; Warner et al., 1983). Long-term rhythms (oscillations), ranging from as short as a minute to as long as several minutes, have been identified in which ventilation and speaking activity wax and wane relatively cyclically during conversation (Warner et al., 1983). Short-term rhythms are characterized by synchrony between the breathing movements of conversational partners in which the breathing movements during listening resemble the speech breathing movements of the conversational partner. For example, when listening to the speech of a conversation partner, inspiratory movements are quicker and expiratory movements are slower (more like speech breathing) than when not listening to someone speak (McFarland, 2001; Rochet-Capellan & Fuchs, 2014).

Turn-taking during conversation seems to be strongly linked to breathing. The most successful turn-taking attempts appear to occur immediately following an inspiration, and unsuccessful attempts are more likely to occur during late expiration (Rochet-Capellan & Fuchs, 2014). This suggests that breathing is an active component of turn-taking during conversational interchange.

Thus, speech breathing produced in the context of conversational interchange appears to have emergent properties. Its nature is complex and is determined by the speaker, the conversational partner(s), and interactions between the speaker and conversational partner(s).

REVIEW

The breathing apparatus is a mechanical pump that includes an energy source and passive components that couple this source to the air it moves.

The breathing apparatus is formed around a skeletal framework and consists of the pulmonary apparatus and chest wall (linked together as a unit), the former including the pulmonary airways and lungs and the latter including the rib cage wall, diaphragm, abdominal wall, and abdominal content.

The forces of breathing are passive and active, the former arising from the natural recoil of tissues, surface tension within alveoli, and gravity, and the latter being vested in more than 20 muscles of the chest wall.

Muscles of the rib cage wall include the *sternocleidomastoid, scalenus anterior, scalenus medius, scalenus posterior, pectoralis major, pectoralis minor, subclavius, serratus anterior, external intercostal, internal intercostal, transversus thoracis, latissimus dorsi, serratus posterior superior, serratus posterior inferior, lateral iliocostalis cervicis, lateral iliocostalis thoracis, lateral iliocostalis lumborum, levatores costarum, quadratus lumborum,* and *subcostal*.

The *diaphragm* muscle divides the torso into two compartments: the thorax (upper cavity) and abdomen.

Muscles of the abdominal wall include the *rectus abdominis, external oblique, internal oblique,* and *transversus abdominis* at the front and the *latissimus dorsi, lateral iliocostalis lumborum,* and *quadratus lumborum* at the back.

The forces of the breathing apparatus are realized as pulls on structures and pressures developed at various locations, with the most important pressure for speech production being alveolar pressure.

The movements of breathing occur within the rib cage wall, diaphragm, and abdominal wall, with each component part having its own movement capabilities.

Movement of the rib cage wall has the potential to create greater volume and pressure change than movement of the abdominal wall because it covers a greater surface area of the pulmonary apparatus.

Movements of the breathing apparatus are effected by passive and active forces that come from different parts of the apparatus, making it difficult to specify what forces are responsible for any given movement.

The control variables of breathing include lung volume, alveolar pressure, and chest wall shape.

The nervous system controls different acts of breathing through a group of lower and higher brain centers that mediate breathing movements and related perceptions during tidal breathing and special acts of breathing.

Ventilation (the movement of air into and out of the pulmonary apparatus) supports the life-sustaining process of oxygen and carbon dioxide exchange and is characterized by patterns that are relatively individualized across people.

Speech breathing is the process by which driving forces are supplied to generate the sounds of speech, while simultaneously serving the functions of ventilation and gas exchange.

Speech breathing, whether it be during extended steady utterance or during running speech activities, is achieved through the combining of relaxation pressure and muscular pressure, the muscular pressure required at any moment depending on the relaxation pressure available at the prevailing lung volume and the target alveolar pressure of the utterance.

The activity of individual parts of the chest wall (rib cage wall, diaphragm, and abdominal wall) may differ for the generation of utterances involving different alveolar pressures at different lung volumes.

The control strategy for running speech activities is distinct from that for other forms of breathing and serves to enhance function during both the inspiratory and expiratory phases of the speech breathing cycle.

Speech breathing is influenced by body position, mainly because gravity affects relaxation pressure, the resting level of the breathing apparatus, and the mechanical advantages of different parts of the chest wall.

Body type affects speech breathing, with the most dramatic contrasts existing between people who are endomorphic and ectomorphic, the former showing a much higher degree of abdominal wall participation.

Speech breathing develops during childhood, becoming adult like in many ways by 10 years of age, and then changes again around the seventh or eighth decade of life, due, at least in part, to factors believed to be related to laryngeal valving economy and air wastage.

Despite the pervasive myth that the two sexes breathe differently, there is no evidence to support this notion, and, in the case of speech breathing, substantial evidence to contradict it.

People naturally hyperventilate when speaking and reorganize their speech breathing behaviors under conditions of high drive so as to relieve breathing discomfort.

Cognitive-linguistic factors influence both the inspiratory and expiratory phases of speech breathing, as do social interactions between conversational partners.

REFERENCES

Abel, H., Mottau, B., Klubendorf, D., & Koepchen, H. (1987). Pattern of different components of the respiratory cycle and autonomic parameters during speech. In G. Sieck, S. Gandevia, & W. Cameron (Eds.), *Respiratory muscles and their neuromotor control* (pp. 109–113). New York, NY: Alan R. Liss.

Bailey, E., & Hoit, J. (2002). Speaking and breathing in high respiratory drive. *Journal of Speech, Language, and Hearing Research, 45*, 89–99.

Baker, S., Hipp, J., & Alessio, H. (2008). Ventilation and speech characteristics during submaximal aerobic exercise. *Journal of Speech, Language, and Hearing Research, 51*, 1203-1214.

Benchetrit, G., Shea, S., Pham Dinh, T., Bodocco, S., Baconnier, P., & Guz, A. (1989). Individuality of breathing patterns in adults assessed over time. *Respiration Physiology, 75*, 199–210.

Bernthal, J., & Beukelman, D. (1978). Intraoral air pressure during the production of /p/ and /b/ by children, youths, and adults. *Journal of Speech and Hearing Research, 21*, 361–371.

Boliek, C., Hixon, T., Watson, P., & Jones, P. (2009). Refinement of speech breathing in healthy 4- to 6-year-old children. *Journal of Speech, Language, and Hearing Research, 52*, 990–1007.

Boliek, C., Hixon, T., Watson, P., & Morgan, W. (1996). Vocalization and breathing during the first year of life. *Journal of Voice, 10*, 1–22.

Boliek, C., Hixon, T., Watson, P., & Morgan, W. (1997). Vocalization and breathing during the second and third years of life. *Journal of Voice, 11*, 373–390.

Bunn, J., & Mead, J. (1971). Control of ventilation during speech. *Journal of Applied Physiology, 31*, 870–872.

Chapple, E. (1970). *Culture and biological man.* New York, NY: Holt, Rinehart, and Winston.

Connaghan, K., Moore, C., & Higashakawa, M. (2004). Respiratory kinematics during vocalization and nonspeech respiration in children from 9 to 48 months. *Journal of Speech, Language, and Hearing Research, 47*, 70–84.

Conrad, B., Thalacker, S., & Schönle, P. (1983). Speech respiration as an indicator of integrative contextual processing. *Folia Phoniatrica, 35*, 220–225.

Corfield, D., Murphy, K., & Guz, A. (1998). Does the motor cortical control of the diaphragm "bypass" the brain stem respiratory centres in man? *Respiratory Physiology, 114*, 109–117.

Dejours, P. (1996). *Respiration.* New York, NY: Oxford University Press.

Denny, M. (2000). Periodic variation in inspiratory volume characterizes speech as well as inspiration. *Journal of Voice, 10,* 23–38.

Dickson, D., & Maue-Dickson, W. (1982). *Anatomical and physiological bases of speech.* Boston, MA: Little, Brown and Company.

Doust, J., & Patrick, J. (1981). The limitation of exercise ventilation during speech. *Respiration Physiology, 46,* 137–147.

Feldman, J., & McCrimmon, D. (1999). Neural control of breathing. In M. Zigmond, F. Bloom, S. Landis, J. Roberts, & L. Squire (Eds.), *Fundamental neuroscience* (pp. 1063–1090). New York, NY: Academic Press.

Gardner, W. (1996). The pathophysiology of hyperventilation disorders. *Chest, 109,* 516–534.

Goldman-Eisler, F. (1956). The determinants of the rate of speech output and their mutual relations. *Journal of Psychosomatic Research, 1,* 137–143.

Greene, J. (1984). Speech preparation processes and verbal fluency. *Human Communication Research, 11,* 61–84.

Greene, J., & Capella, J. (1986). Cognition and talk: The relationship of semantic units to temporal patterns of fluency in spontaneous speech. *Language and Speech, 29,* 141–157.

Grosjean, F., & Collins, M. (1979). Breathing, pausing, and reading. *Phonetica, 36,* 98–114.

Hale, M., & Patrick, J. (1987). Ventilatory patterns during human speech in progressive hypercapnia. *Journal of Physiology, 394,* 60P.

Henderson, A., Goldman-Eisler, F., & Skarbek, A. (1965). Temporal patterns of cognitive activity and breath control in speech. *Language and Speech, 8,* 236–242.

Hertegård, S., Gauffin, J., & Lindestad, P-Å. (1995). A comparison of subglottal and intraoral pressure measurements during phonation. *Journal of Voice, 9,* 149–155.

Hixon, T. (1973). Respiratory function in speech. In F. Minifie, T. Hixon, & F. Williams (Eds.), *Normal aspects of speech, hearing, and language* (pp. 75–125). Englewood Cliffs, NJ: Prentice-Hall.

Hixon, T., Goldman, M., & Mead, J. (1973). Kinematics of the chest wall during speech production: Volume displacements of the rib cage, abdomen, and lung. *Journal of Speech and Hearing Research, 16,* 78–115.

Hixon, T., & Hoit, J. (2005). *Evaluation and management of speech breathing disorders: Principles and methods.* Tucson, AZ: Redington Brown.

Hixon, T., Mead, J., & Goldman, M. (1976). Dynamics of the chest wall during speech production: Function of the thorax, rib cage, diaphragm, and abdomen. *Journal of Speech and Hearing Research, 19,* 297–356.

Hixon, T., & Weismer, G. (1995). Perspectives on the Edinburgh study of speech breathing. *Journal of Speech and Hearing Research, 38,* 42–60.

Hodge, M., & Rochet, A. (1989). Characteristics of speech breathing in young women. *Journal of Speech and Hearing Research, 32,* 466–480.

Hoit, J., & Hixon, T. (1986). Body type and speech breathing. *Journal of Speech and Hearing Research, 29,* 313–324.

Hoit, J., & Hixon, T. (1987). Age and speech breathing. *Journal of Speech and Hearing Research, 30,* 351–366.

Hoit, J., & Hixon, T. (1992). Age and laryngeal airway resistance during vowel production in women. *Journal of Speech and Hearing Research, 35,* 309–313.

Hoit, J., Hixon, T., Altman, M., & Morgan, W. (1989). Speech breathing in women. *Journal of Speech and Hearing Research, 32,* 353–365.

Hoit, J., Hixon, T., Watson, P., & Morgan, W. (1990). Speech breathing in children and adolescents. *Journal of Speech and Hearing Research, 33,* 51–69.

Hoit, J., Lansing, R., & Perona, G. (2007). Speaking-related dyspnea in healthy adults. *Journal of Speech, Language, and Hearing Research, 50,* 361–374.

Hoit, J., & Lohmeier, H. (2000). Influence of continuous speaking on ventilation. *Journal of Speech, Language, and Hearing Research, 43,* 1240–1251.

Horii, Y., & Cooke, P. (1978). Some airflow, volume, and duration characteristics of oral reading. *Journal of Speech and Hearing Research, 21,* 470–481.

Huber, J. (2008). Effects of utterance length and vocal loudness on speech breathing in older adults. *Respiratory Physiology and Neurobiology, 164,* 323–330.

Huber, J., & Darling, M. (2011). Effect of Parkinson's disease on the production of structured and unstructured speaking tasks: Respiratory physiologic and linguistic considerations. *Journal of Speech, Language, and Hearing Research, 54,* 33–46.

Huber, J., Darling, M., Francis, E., & Zhang, D. (2012). Impact of typical aging and Parkinson's disease on the relationship among breath pausing, syntax, and punctuation. *American Journal of Speech-Language Pathology, 21,* 368–379.

Huber, J., & Darling-White, M. (2017). Longitudinal changes in speech breathing in older adults with and without Parkinson's disease. *Seminars in Speech and Language, 38,* 200–209.

Lay, C., & Paivio, A. (1969). The effects of task difficulty and anxiety on hesitations in speech. *Canadian Journal of Behavioral Sciences, 1,* 25–37.

Loring, S., & Mead, J. (1982). Abdominal muscle use during quiet breathing and hyperpnea in uninformed subjects. *Journal of Applied Physiology, 52,* 700–704.

Mador, J., & Tobin, M. (1991). Effect of alterations in mental activity on the breathing pattern in healthy subjects. *American Review of Respiratory Disease, 144,* 481–487.

McFarland, D. (2001). Respiratory markers of conversational interaction. *Journal of Speech, Language, and Hearing Research, 44,* 128–143.

McFarland, D., & Smith, A. (1992). Effect of vocal task and respiratory phase on prephonatory chest wall movements. *Journal of Speech and Hearing Research, 35,* 971–982.

Meanock, C., & Nichols, A. (1982). The effect of speech on the ventilatory response to carbon dioxide or to exercise. *Journal of Physiology, 325,* 16P–17P.

Melcon, M., Hoit, J., & Hixon, T. (1989). Age and laryngeal airway resistance during vowel production. *Journal of Speech and Hearing Disorders, 54,* 282–286.

Mitchell, H., Hoit, J., & Watson, P. (1996). Cognitive-linguistic demands and speech breathing. *Journal of Speech and Hearing Research, 39,* 93–104.

Moore, C., Caulfield, T., & Green, J. (2001). Relative kinematics of the rib cage and abdomen during speech and nonspeech behaviors of 15-month-old children. *Journal of Speech, Language, and Hearing Research, 44,* 80–94.

Netsell, R., Lotz, W., Peters, J., & Schulte, L. (1994). Developmental patterns of laryngeal and respiratory function for speech production. *Journal of Voice, 8,* 123–131.

Otis, A., & Clark, R. (1968). Ventilatory implications of phonation and phonatory implications of ventilation. In A. Bouhuys (Ed.), *Sound production in man* (pp. 122–128). New York, NY: Annals of the New York Academy of Sciences.

Parham, D., Buder, E., Oller, D. K., & Boliek, C. (2011). Syllable-related breathing in infants in the second year of life. *Journal of Speech, Language, and Hearing Research, 54,* 1039–1050.

Phillipson, E., McClean, P., Sullivan, C., & Zamel, N. (1978). Interaction of metabolic and behavioral respiratory control during hypercapnia and speech. *American Review of Respiratory Disease, 117,* 903–909.

Reynolds, A., & Paivio, A. (1968). Cognitive and emotional determinants of speech. *Canadian Journal of Psychology, 22,* 164–175.

Rochester, S. (1973). The significance of pauses in spontaneous speech. *Journal of Psycholinguistic Research, 2,* 51–81.

Rochet-Capellan, A., & Fuchs, S. (2014). Take a breath and take the turn: How breathing meets turns in spontaneous dialogue. *Philosophical Transactions of the Royal Society B, 369.* http://dx.doi.org/10.1098/rstb.2013.0399.

Shea, S. (1996). Behavioural and arousal-related influences on breathing in humans. *Experimental Physiology, 81,* 1–26.

Shea, S., & Guz, A. (1992). Personnalite ventilatoire: An overview. *Respiration Physiology, 52,* 275–291.

Shea, S., Horner, R., Benchetrit, G., & Guz, A. (1990). The persistence of a respiratory "personality" into stage IV sleep in man. *Respiration Physiology, 80,* 33–44.

Shea, S., Murphy, K., Hamilton, R., Benchetrit, G., & Guz, A. (1988). Do the changes in respiratory pattern and ventilation seen with different behavioural situations reflect metabolic demands? In C. von Euler & M. Katz-Salamon (Eds.), *Respiratory psychophysiology* (pp. 21–28). Basingstoke, UK: Macmillan Press.

Shea, S., Walter, J., Murphy, K., & Guz, A. (1987). Evidence for individuality of breathing patterns in resting healthy men. *Respiration Physiology, 68,* 331–344.

Shea, S., Walter, J., Pelley, C., Murphy, K., & Guz, A. (1987). The effect of visual and auditory stimuli upon resting ventilation in man. *Respiration Physiology, 68,* 345–357.

Sperry, E., & Klich, R. (1992). Speech breathing in senescent and younger women during oral reading. *Journal of Speech and Hearing Research, 35,* 1246–1255.

Stathopoulos, E., & Sapienza, C. (1993). Respiratory and laryngeal measures of children during vocal intensity variation. *Journal of the Acoustical Society of America, 94,* 2531–2543.

Stathopoulos, E., & Sapienza, C. (1997). Developmental changes in laryngeal and respiratory function with variations in sound pressure level. *Journal of Speech, Language, and Hearing Research, 40,* 595–614.

Stathopoulos, E., & Weismer, G. (1985). Oral airflow and air pressure during speech production: A comparative study of children, youths, and adults. *Folia Phoniatrica, 37,* 152–159.

Sugito, M., Ohyama, G., & Hirose, H. (1990). A preliminary study on pauses and breaths in reading speech materials. *Annual Bulletin of the Research Institute of Logopedics and Phoniatrics, 24,* 121–130.

Taylor, I. (1969). Content and structure in sentence production. *Journal of Verbal Learning and Verbal Behavior, 8,* 170–175.

Wang, Y-T., Green, J., Nip, I., Kent, R., & Kent, J. (2010). Breath group analysis for reading and spontaneous speech in healthy adults. *Folia Phoniatrica et Logopaedica, 62,* 297–302.

Warner, R., Waggener, T., & Kronauer, R. (1983). Synchronized cycles in ventilation and vocal activity during spontaneous conversational speech. *Journal of Applied Physiology, 54,* 309–317.

Webb, R., Williams, F., & Minifie, F. (1967). Effects of verbal decision behavior upon respiration during speech production. *Journal of Speech and Hearing Research, 10,* 49–56.

Weismer, G. (1985). Speech breathing: Contemporary views and findings. In R. Daniloff (Ed.), *Speech science* (pp. 47–72). San Diego, CA: College-Hill Press.

Western, P., & Patrick, J. (1988). Effects of focusing attention on breathing with and without apparatus on the face. *Respiration Physiology, 72,* 123–130.

Whalen, D., & Kinsella-Shaw, J. (1997). Exploring the relationship of inspiration duration to utterance duration. *Phonetica, 54,* 138–152.

Wilder, C. (1983). Chest wall preparation for phonation in female speakers. In D. Bless & J. Abbs (Eds.), *Vocal fold physiology: Contemporary research and clinical issues* (pp. 109–123). San Diego, CA: College-Hill Press.

Winkworth, A., Davis, P., Adams, R., & Ellis, E. (1995). Breathing patterns during spontaneous speech. *Journal of Speech and Hearing Research, 38,* 124–144.

Winkworth, A., Davis, P., Ellis, E., & Adams, R. (1994). Variability and consistency in speech breathing during reading: Lung volumes, speech intensity, and linguistic factors. *Journal of Speech and Hearing Research, 37,* 535–556.

Wolff, P. (1979). Theoretical issues in the development of motor skills. *Symposium on developmental disabilities in the pre-school child.* Chicago, IL: Johnson and Johnson Baby Products.

Wyke, B. (1974). Respiratory activity of intrinsic laryngeal muscles: An experimental study. In B. Wyke (Ed.), *Ventilatory and phonatory control systems* (pp. 408–429). New York, NY: Oxford University Press.

3

Laryngeal Function and Speech Production

INTRODUCTION

The larynx is an air valve located within the front of the neck. This valve is positioned vertically between the trachea (windpipe) and pharynx (throat) and can be adjusted to vary the amount of coupling between the two. The larynx serves a variety of functions, including speech production (inclusive of voice production).

This chapter begins with description of the anatomy of the laryngeal apparatus followed by discussion of its forces and movements, control variables, neural control, and general functions. Focus then turns to laryngeal function during speech production and variables that influence that function.

ANATOMY OF THE LARYNGEAL APPARATUS

The skeleton of the larynx, its joints, and its internal topography are considered in this section. The muscles of the larynx are discussed in the next section, Forces of the Laryngeal Apparatus.

Skeletal Framework

Figure 3–1 depicts the skeletal framework of the laryngeal apparatus. This framework consists of cartilage, bone, ligament, and tendon. The flexibility of this framework changes with age, being soft and pliable in childhood and hard and more rigid in adulthood.

Thyroid Cartilage

The thyroid cartilage is the largest of the laryngeal cartilages and forms most of the front and sides of the laryngeal skeleton. This cartilage provides a shield-like housing for the larynx and offers protection for many of its structures.

Figure 3–2 shows the thyroid cartilage from four different views. Two quadrilateral plates, called the thyroid laminae, are fused together at the front of

---

Sizing Things Up

There's a tendency when viewing anatomical drawings, photographs, and video images of structures of the larynx to overestimate their size. The trachea looks long and large in cross-section. The glottis seems to be a big hole. The vocal folds appear to be massive lips. The vocal ligaments look like pencils. And the vibratory movements of the vocal folds (when slowed down) give the impression of a flag blowing in a stiff wind. Some calibration may be helpful. Your trachea is about as long and big around as your middle finger. Your wide-open glottis is about the size of a dime. Your approximated vocal folds have a surface area about the size of your thumbnail (well trimmed). The vocal ligaments are about as thick as wooden matchsticks. And your vocal folds only move about the length of the cuticle on your thumbnail. If you're like us, you'll find this to be surprisingly small. Yes?

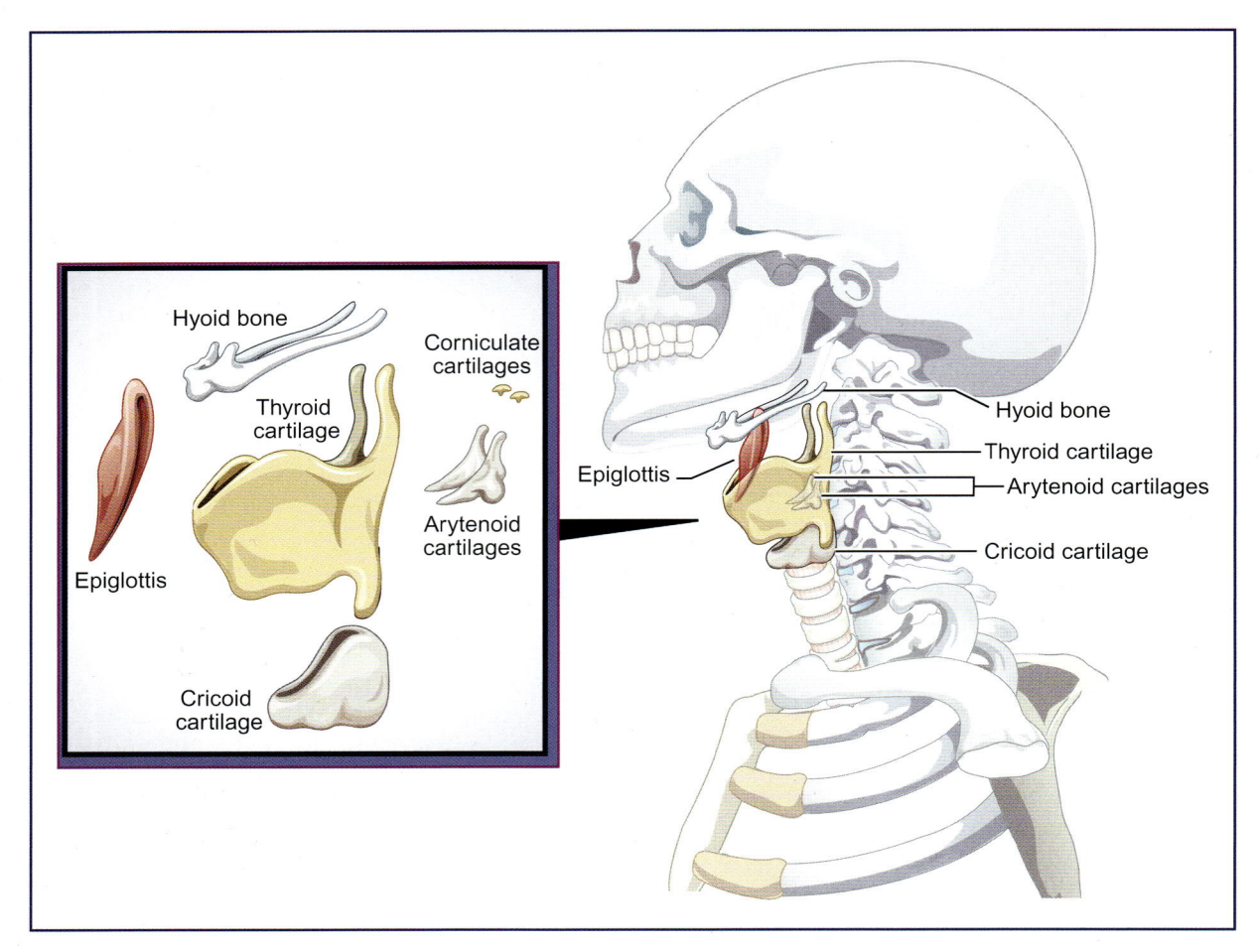

Figure 3-1. Skeletal framework of the laryngeal apparatus. This framework is composed of two paired cartilages (arytenoid cartilages and corniculate cartilages), three unpaired cartilages (thyroid cartilage, cricoid cartilage, and epiglottis), and one bone (hyoid bone).

the thyroid cartilage and diverge widely (more so in women than in men) toward the back. The configuration of the two thyroid laminae resembles the bow of a ship. The line of fusion between the two plates is called the angle of the thyroid. The upper part of the structure contains a prominent V-shaped depression termed the thyroid notch that can be palpated at the front of the neck. This notch is located just above the most forward projection of the cartilage, an outward jutting called the thyroid prominence or Adam's apple.

The back edges of the thyroid laminae extend upward into two long horns, called the superior cornua, and downward into two short horns, called the inferior cornua. The superior cornua are coupled to the hyoid bone. The inferior cornua have facets (areas where other structures join) on their lower inside surfaces that form joints with the cricoid cartilage. The inferior cornua straddle the cricoid cartilage like a pair of legs (see Figure 3-1).

Cricoid Cartilage

The cricoid cartilage forms the lower part of the laryngeal skeleton. It is a ring-shaped structure located above the trachea. As shown in Figure 3-3, the cricoid cartilage has a thick plate at the back, the posterior quadrate lamina, which resembles a signet on a finger ring. A semicircular structure, called the anterior arch, forms the front of the cricoid cartilage and is akin to a band on a finger ring.

Four facets are located on the cricoid cartilage. The lower two facets, one on each side at the same level, are positioned near the junction of the posterior quadrate lamina and anterior arch. Each of these facets articulates with a facet on one of the inferior cornua

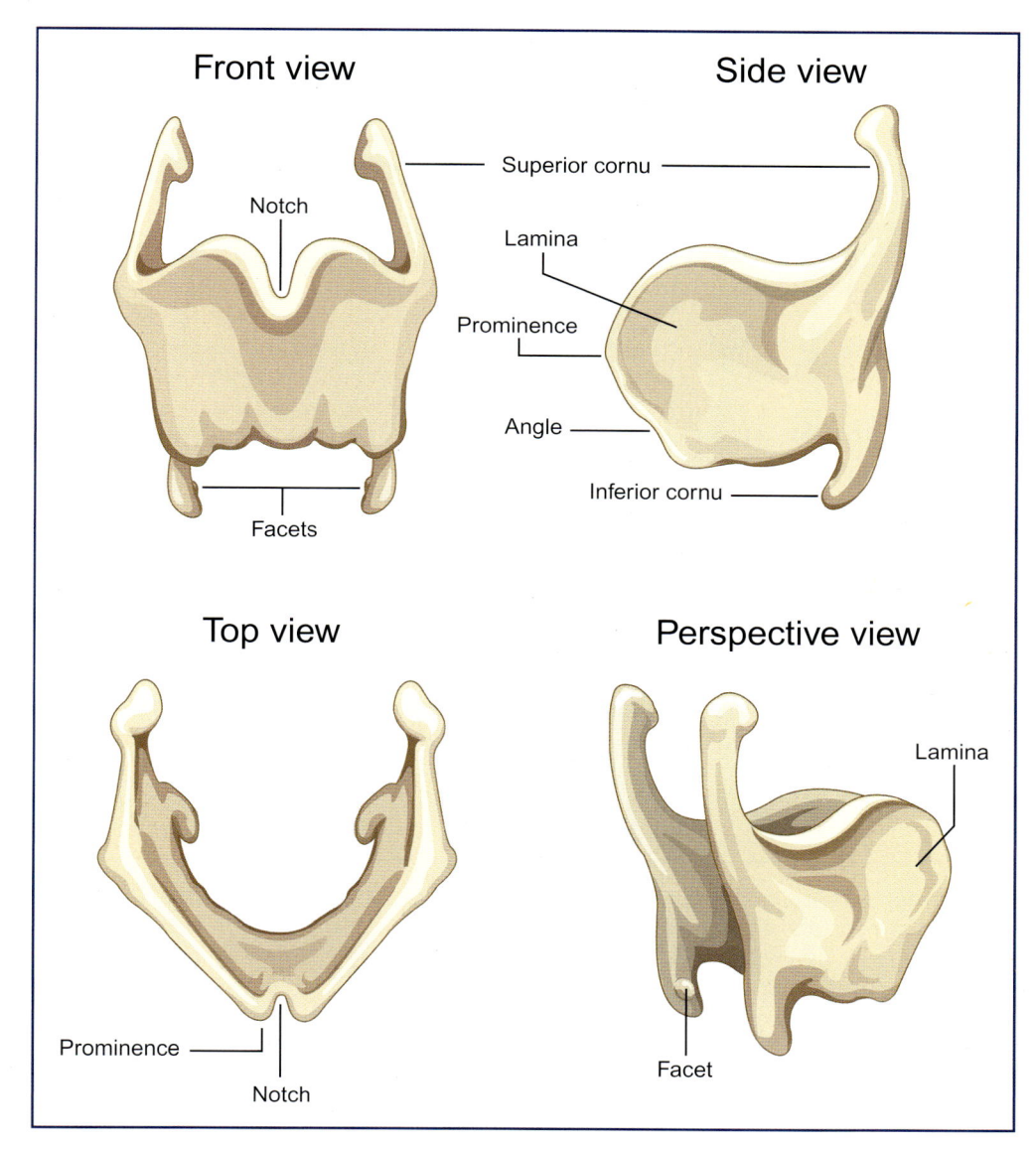

Figure 3–2. Thyroid cartilage from four different views. The thyroid prominence is also called the Adam's apple.

of the thyroid cartilage. The upper two facets of the cricoid cartilage, one on each side at the same level, are located on the sloping rim of the posterior quadrate lamina. Each of these facets articulates with a facet on the undersurface of one of the arytenoid cartilages.

Arytenoid Cartilages

There are two arytenoid cartilages. Each is located atop one side of the sloping rim of the posterior quadrate lamina of the cricoid cartilage. As shown in Figure 3–4, each arytenoid cartilage has a complex shape that includes an apex, base, and three sides. The apex of each cartilage is capped with another small cone-shaped cartilage called a corniculate cartilage that is often fused to the arytenoid cartilage. The base of each arytenoid cartilage has a flexible pointed projection that extends toward the front and is designated the vocal process. The base also includes a rounded stubby projection that extends toward the back and side and is referred to as the muscular process. The undersurface of each muscular process has a facet that articulates with one of the upper facets of the cricoid cartilage.

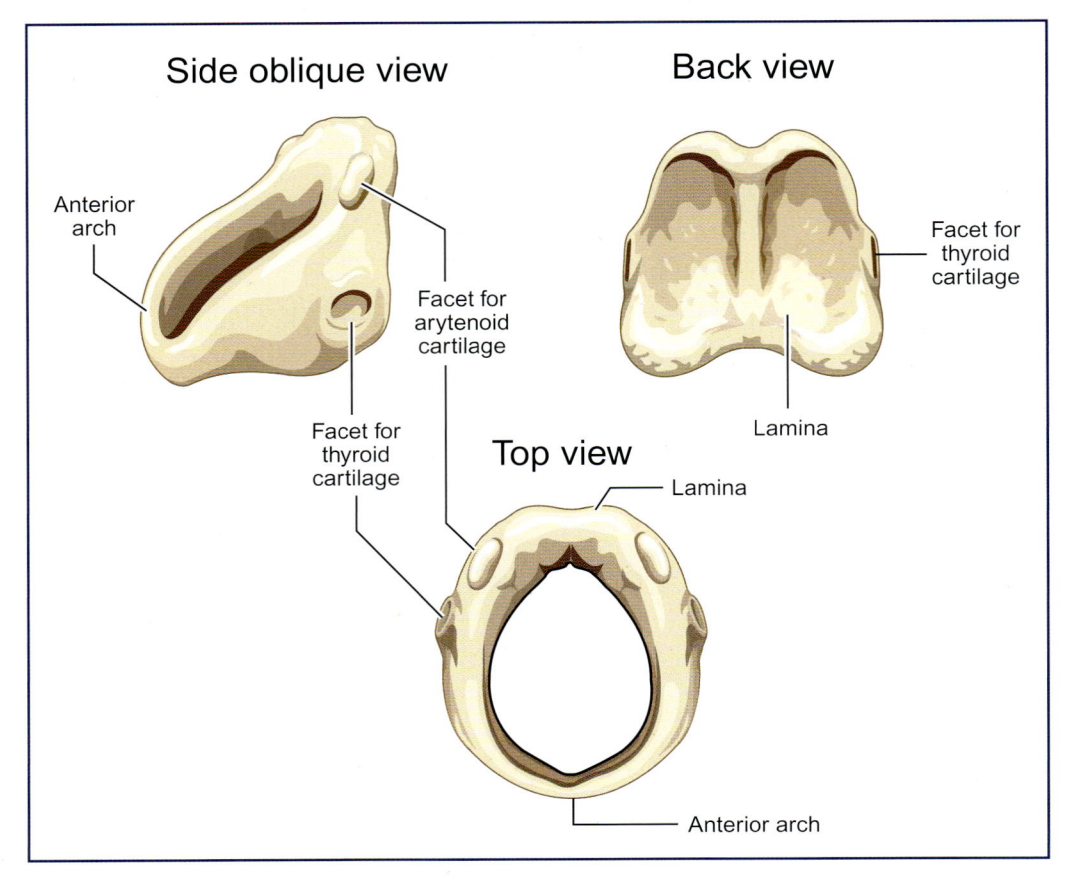

Figure 3–3. Cricoid cartilage from three different views. This cartilage is often described as having the shape of a signet ring.

Epiglottis

Figure 3–5 depicts the epiglottis. The epiglottis is a single cartilage that is positioned behind the hyoid bone and root of the tongue. The upper part of the epiglottis, its body, is broad and resembles the distal end of a forward-curving shoehorn. The front and back surfaces of this part of the structure are referred to as its lingual (tongue) and laryngeal (larynx) surfaces, respectively. The lingual surface attaches to the hyoid bone. The lower part of the cartilage tapers downward into a stalk called the petiolus (little leg) and attaches to the inside of the thyroid cartilage just below the thyroid notch.

Hyoid Bone

Figure 3–6 depicts the hyoid bone (tongue bone). Technically, the hyoid bone is not a part of the larynx. Nevertheless, it serves as an integral component in many laryngeal functions. Thus, it is commonly afforded a prominent place in discussion of the laryngeal skeleton. The hyoid bone is described as free-floating in the sense that it is not attached to any other bone. It is a U-shaped structure that is positioned horizontally within the neck, its open end facing toward the back. The hyoid bone consists of a body and two pairs of greater and lesser horns (cornua) that project upward. The greater cornua are located toward the back of the structure and join with the superior cornua of the thyroid cartilage. The lesser cornua extend from the body of the structure and may be capped by tiny cone-shaped cartilages. The hyoid bone is positioned at the top of the larynx and suspends it from above through various connections.

Laryngeal Joints

There are two pairs of joints in the larynx. One pair is between the cricoid and thyroid cartilages on each side. The other pair is between the cricoid and arytenoid cartilages on each side. Movements at these joints are

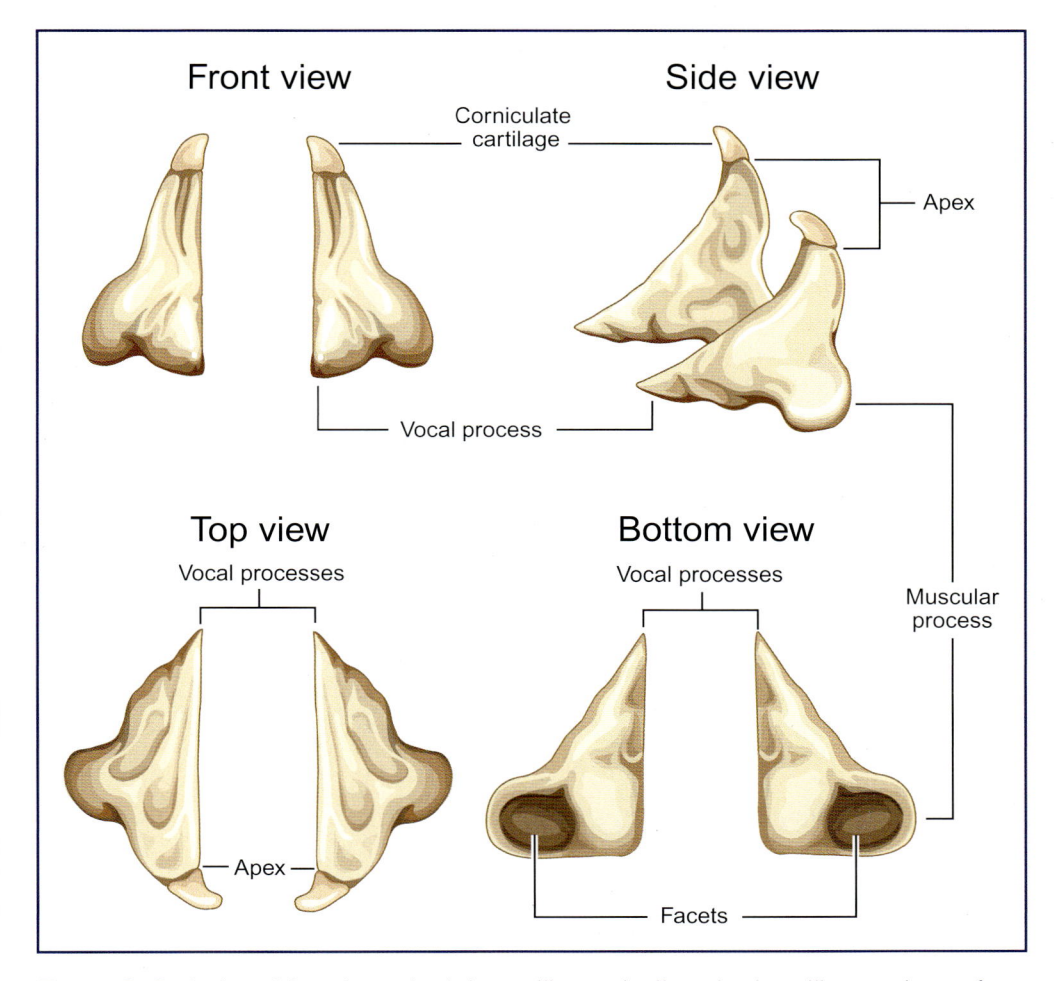

Figure 3-4. Arytenoid and corniculate cartilages, both paired cartilages, shown from four different views.

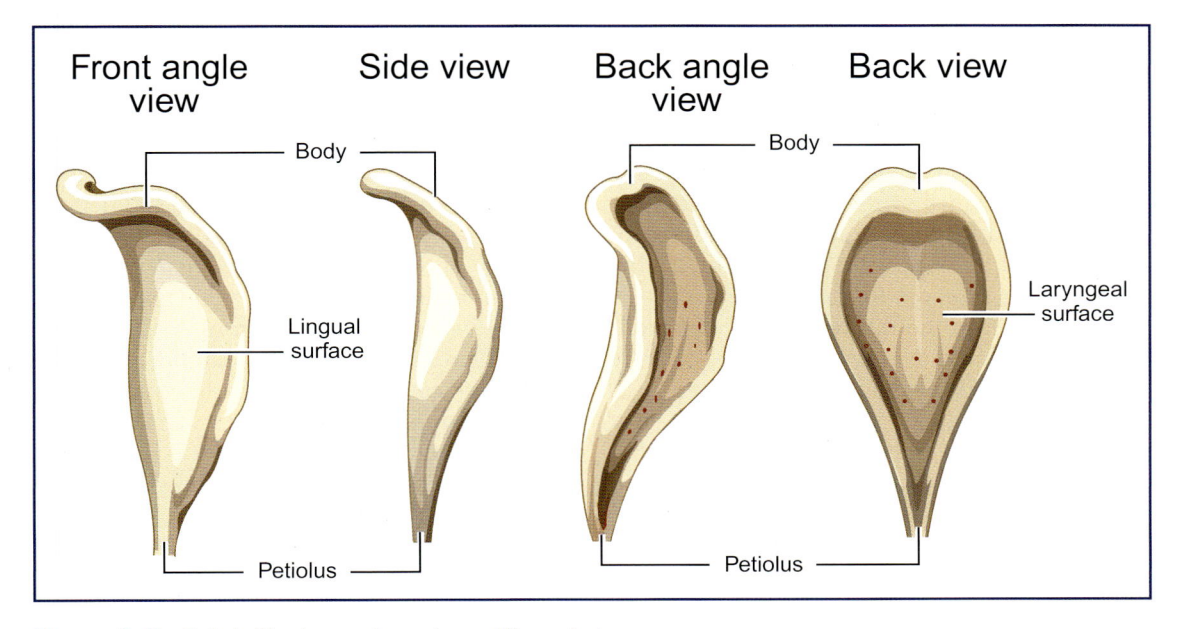

Figure 3-5. Epiglottis shown from four different views.

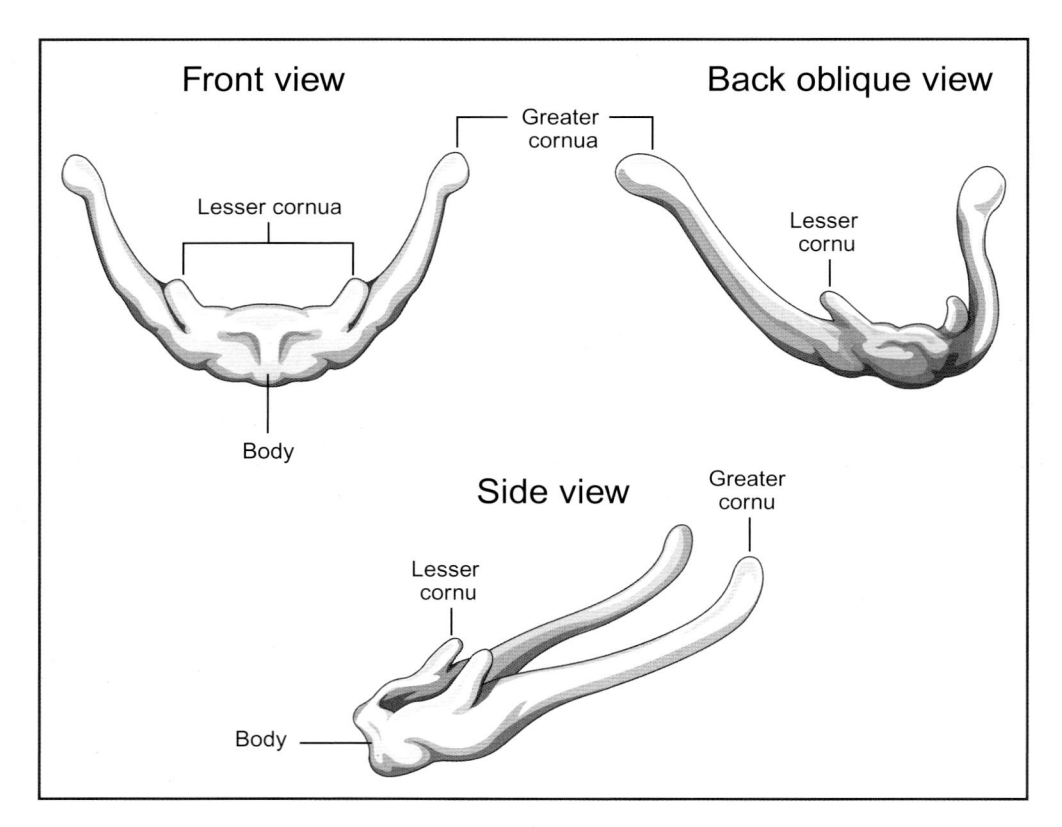

Figure 3–6. Hyoid bone from three different views. The hyoid bone, often described as horseshoe-shaped, has the special status of being the only free-floating bone in the body, meaning that it does not directly articulate with any other bones. The hyoid bone is not technically part of the larynx.

conditioned by the nature of the facets on their articulating cartilages and the arrangement of surrounding ligaments.

Cricothyroid Joints

Figure 3–7 depicts the cricothyroid joints. These joints are positioned on the sides of the larynx and involve articulations between facets on the inner surfaces of the inferior cornua of the thyroid cartilage (see A in the figure) and the outer surfaces of the lower part of the cricoid cartilage (see B in the figure). The cricothyroid joints are encapsulated by membranes that secrete synovial fluid. This fluid serves as a lubricant.

Facets on the cricoid and thyroid cartilages vary from larynx to larynx and from side to side within the same larynx (Dickson & Maue-Dickson, 1982). Those on the cricoid cartilage generally face upward, toward the side, and backward. They are usually round or oval in shape and are concave. Facets on the thyroid cartilage typically face downward, toward the midline, and forward. They are usually round in shape and are convex. Occasionally a larynx will have cricothyroid joint facets that are rudimentary. Then the articulation between the cricoid and thyroid surfaces is formed by fibrous connective tissue (Zemlin, 1998).

Three ligaments extend between the side and back surfaces of the cricoid cartilage and the lower outside surfaces of the inferior cornu of the thyroid cartilage on each side. These three ligaments encircle most of the corresponding cricothyroid joint and are referred to as the anterior, lateral, and posterior ceratocricoid (*cerato* meaning horn) ligaments. The anterior ligament extends backward into the front surface of the inferior cornu. The lateral ligament extends upward into the lower surface of the cornu. And the posterior ligament extends forward into the back surface of the cornu. Together the three ligaments bind the corresponding cricothyroid joint and place restrictions on the movements of the cricoid and thyroid cartilages.

The movements at the cricothyroid joints are of two types—rotating and sliding—as portrayed in Figure 3–8. The most significant movements are rotational and occur about a lateral axis extending through the

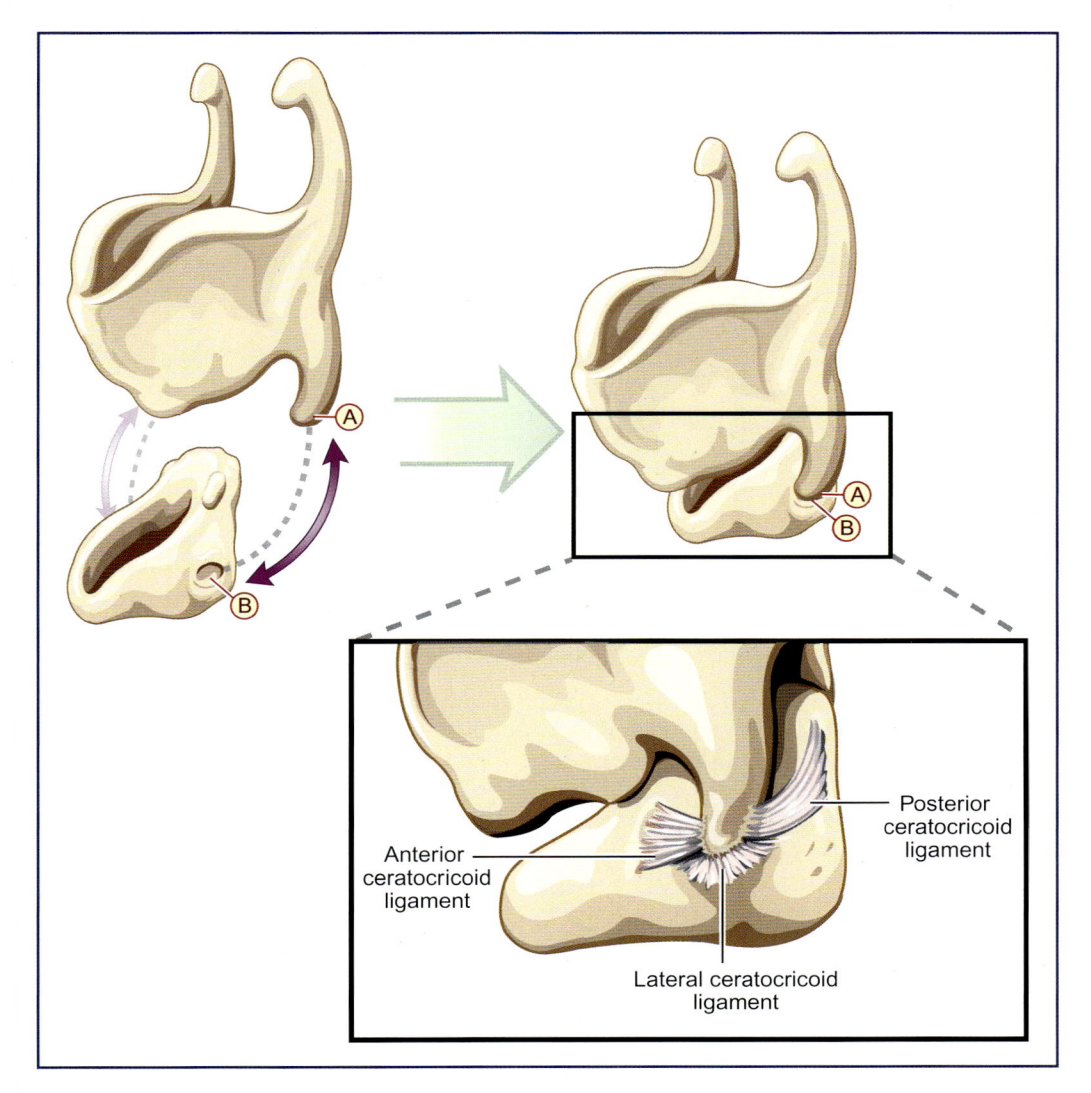

Figure 3–7. Cricothyroid joints. These two joints, one on each side, are created by articulations between convex facets on the inner surface of the inferior cornu of the thyroid cartilage (A) and concave facets on the outer surface of the cricoid cartilage (B). The anterior, lateral, and posterior ceratocricoid ligaments secure the joints and restrict their movements.

two joints. Either or both the cricoid and thyroid cartilages can rotate about this axis (Mayet & Muendnich, 1958; Takano & Honda, 2005; Vennard, 1967; Zemlin, 1998). One consequence of rotation is a change in the distance between the top of the anterior arch of the cricoid cartilage and the bottom of the laminae of the thyroid cartilage at the front. This is analogous to rotating the chin guard (representing the anterior arch of the cricoid cartilage) and the visor (representing the laminae of the thyroid cartilage) on a motorcycle helmet.

Secondary movements at the cricothyroid joints are of a sliding nature and can occur in those larynges that have oval-shaped cricoid facets. These movements are small and occur along the long axes of the cricoid facets (Takano & Honda, 2005; Titze, 1994; van den Berg, Vennard, Berger, & Shervanian, 1960).

Cricoarytenoid Joints

The cricoarytenoid joints are illustrated in Figure 3–9. These joints are positioned near the top of the larynx and involve articulations between the facets on the undersurfaces of the arytenoid cartilages (A in the figure) and sloping rims of the cricoid cartilage (B in the

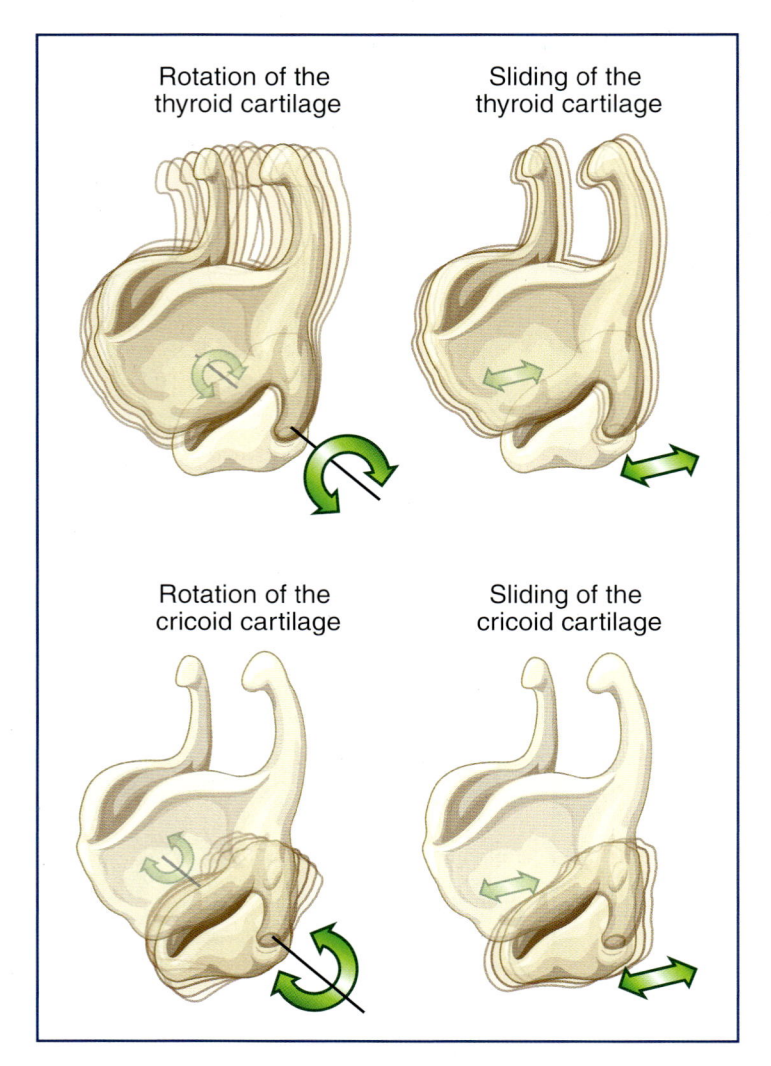

Figure 3-8. Cricothyroid joint movements. These movements are primarily rotational. They can also be of a sliding nature.

figure). Synovial membranes encapsulate these joints and lubricate them.

Facets on the cricoid and arytenoid cartilages are relatively uniform in characteristics from larynx to larynx and from side to side within a larynx (Dickson & Maue-Dickson, 1982). Facets on the cricoid cartilage face upward, toward the side, and forward. These facets are usually oval in shape and are convex. Facets on the arytenoid cartilages face downward, toward the midline, and backward. They are usually round in shape and are concave (Frable, 1961; Zemlin, 1998).

Two ligaments, the anterior and posterior cricoarytenoid ligaments, influence the function of each cricoarytenoid joint by binding it and restricting its movements. The anterior cricoarytenoid ligament extends from the side of the cricoid cartilage to the front and side of the arytenoid cartilage. The ligament runs upward and backward and limits the degree to which the arytenoid cartilage can be moved backward. The posterior cricoarytenoid ligament extends upward and toward the side from the back of the cricoid cartilage to the back of the arytenoid cartilage. This ligament limits the degree to which the arytenoid cartilage can be moved forward.

Figure 3–10 depicts the movements at the cricoarytenoid joints. These can be of two types, rocking and sliding, the most significant of which is rocking. Rocking movements involve the arytenoid cartilages moving at right angles to the long axes of their articulating cricoid facets (Ardran & Kemp, 1966; Selbie, Zhang, Levine, & Ludlow, 1998; Sellars & Keen, 1978; Sonesson, 1959; von Leden & Moore, 1961). This means that

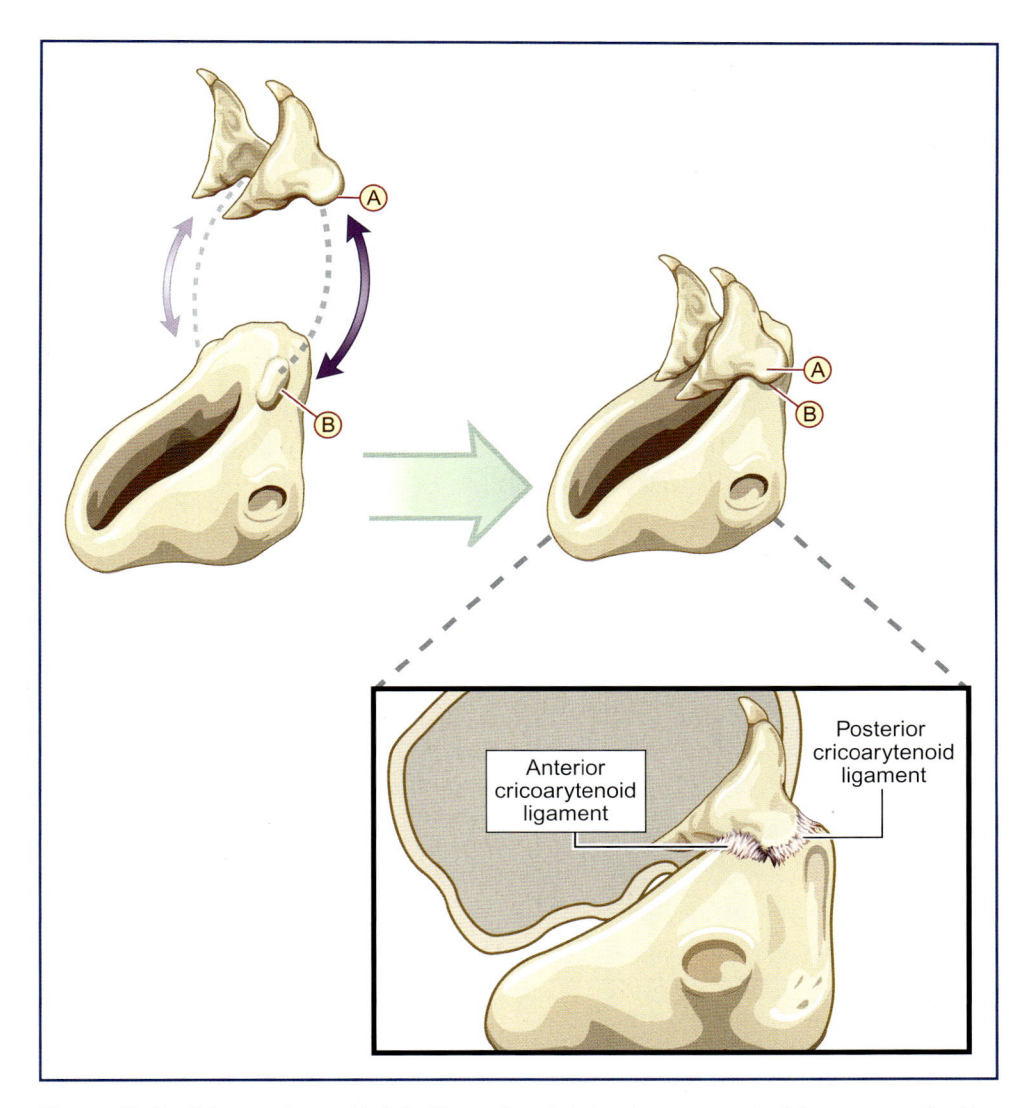

Figure 3-9. Cricoarytenoid joints. These two joints, one on each side, are created by articulations between concave facets on the arytenoid cartilages (A) and convex facets on the cricoid cartilage (B). The anterior and posterior cricoarytenoid ligaments secure the joints and restrict their movements.

Being One with Your Larynx

Many aspects of laryngeal measurement show an uncanny "oneness" with the metric system. Titze (1994) suggested that this realization is helpful in making calculations off the top of your head when you don't have references at hand. A partial listing of items that he recommends be committed to memory are that (a) the mass of a vocal fold is about 1 g, (b) the length of a vibrating vocal fold is about 1 cm, (c) the excursion of a vibrating vocal fold is about 1 mm, (d) the shortest period of vocal fold vibration is about 1 ms, (e) the surface wave velocity on a vibrating vocal fold is about 1 m/s, (f) the maximum peak-to-peak airflow through a vibrating larynx is about 1 L/s, (g) the maximum acceleration of airflow through a vibrating larynx is about 1 m^3/s^2, and (h) the maximum aerodynamic power generated by a vibrating larynx is about 1 J/s. We suggest you make it a goal to memorize these before you go to sleep tonight.

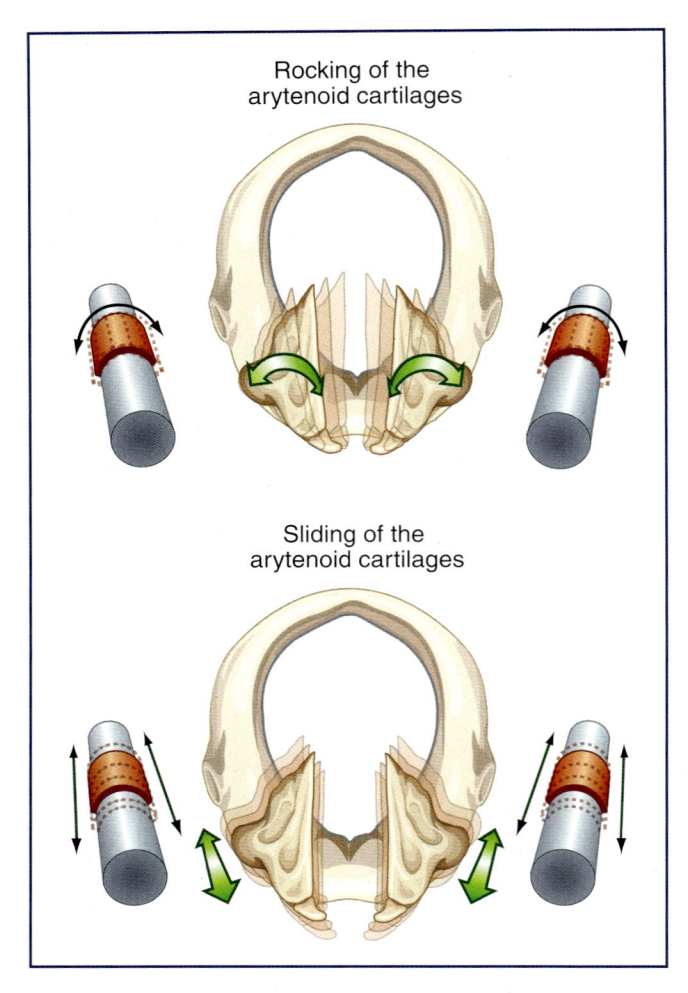

Figure 3–10. Cricoarytenoid joint movements. These are primarily rocking movements, although they can also be of a sliding nature.

as the arytenoid cartilages rock on the cricoid cartilage their vocal processes move either upward and outward or downward and inward.

Limited sliding movements can also occur along the cricoid facets. These movements involve small upward and inward or downward and outward adjustments of the arytenoid cartilages that follow the courses of the long axes of the cricoid facets (Fink, Basek, & Epanchin, 1956; Pressman, 1942; von Leden & Moore, 1961; Wang, 1998).

Internal Topography

The interior of the larynx defines the boundaries of the laryngeal airway. Figure 3–11 depicts the structures that form these boundaries and lie immediately deep to them.

Laryngeal Cavity

The laryngeal cavity extends from a lower opening formed by the base of the cricoid cartilage to an upper opening designated as the laryngeal aditus. The laryngeal aditus forms a collar at the top of the larynx. The rim of this collar comprises the tops of the arytenoid cartilages (and corniculate cartilages), sides of the epiglottis, and the aryepiglottic folds. The aryepiglottic folds run between the arytenoid cartilages and the epiglottis and envelop the *aryepiglottic* muscles (discussed below) and a pair of small cuneiform (wedge-shaped) cartilages. The cuneiform cartilages stiffen the aryepiglottic folds and help to maintain the upper opening (collar entrance) into the larynx.

The upper region of the laryngeal cavity (sometimes called the supraglottal region) is bounded below by the ventricular folds and above by the laryngeal aditus (upper opening into the larynx). This region is also called the laryngeal vestibule (cavity approaching a cavity). The configuration of the vestibule is roughly that of a funnel, the lumen of which increases in size toward its upper end. The lower region of the laryngeal cavity (sometimes called the subglottal region) is bounded below by the lower margin of the cricoid cartilage and above by the vocal folds. This region is cone-shaped and converges toward the undersurface of the vocal folds.

Vocal Folds

The vocal folds are two prominent shelf-like structures that extend from the sidewalls of the laryngeal cavity into the laryngeal airway. Each vocal fold has a front attachment near the midline of the thyroid cartilage and a rear attachment to the vocal process of the arytenoid cartilage on the same side.

The vocal folds are not structurally homogeneous, but are made up of muscle covered by several layers of tissue. Figure 3–12 shows a frontal section through the midlength of an adult vocal fold that exemplifies this characteristic layering. Up to five layers are recognized (Hirano, 1974; Hirano & Sato, 1993) and include: (a) a thin stiff capsule of squamous epithelium that determines the outer shape of the vocal fold, (b) a superficial layer of lamina propria (subflooring) that consists of loose fibrous matrix that resembles soft gelatin and is anchored to the epithelium through a region called the basement membrane zone, (c) an intermediate layer of lamina propria that contains elastic fibers and is likened to a bundle of soft rubber bands, (d) a deep layer of lamina propria that contains collagen fibers and bears analogy to a bundle of cotton thread, and (e) muscle fibers that form the inner vocal fold and are

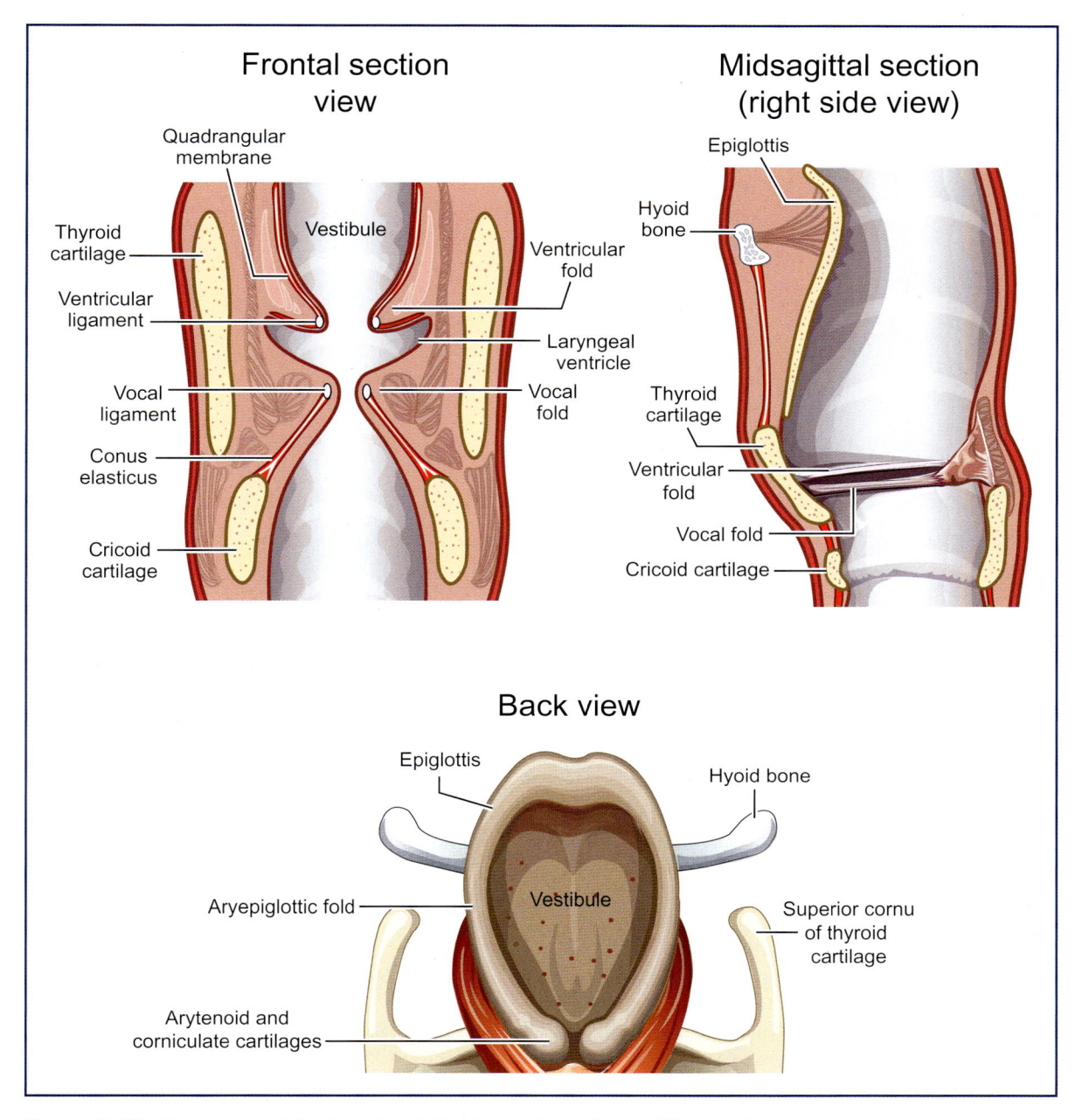

Figure 3–11. Structures of the interior of the larynx from three different views.

the equivalent of a bundle of stiff rubber bands. The combined epithelium and superficial layer of the lamina propria make up what is called the mucosa. The combined intermediate and deep layers of the lamina propria make up what is called the vocal ligament, a ligament that runs along the inner edge of the vocal folds from front to back.

Although the layering shown in Figure 3–12 is typical at the midlength of the vocal folds, it may be quite different at other locations because the layers of the lamina propria change in their relative proportions along the length of the vocal fold. For example, toward the ends of each vocal fold, elastic fibers and then collagenous fibers predominate. These masses of elastic and collagenous fibers act to cushion and protect those areas of the vocal folds from stresses. There are also differences in the cellular structure and concentration of other constituents at other locations within the lamina propria (Catten, Gray, Hammond, Zhou, & Hammond, 1998; de Melo et al., 2003; Ishii, Zhai, Akita, & Hirose,

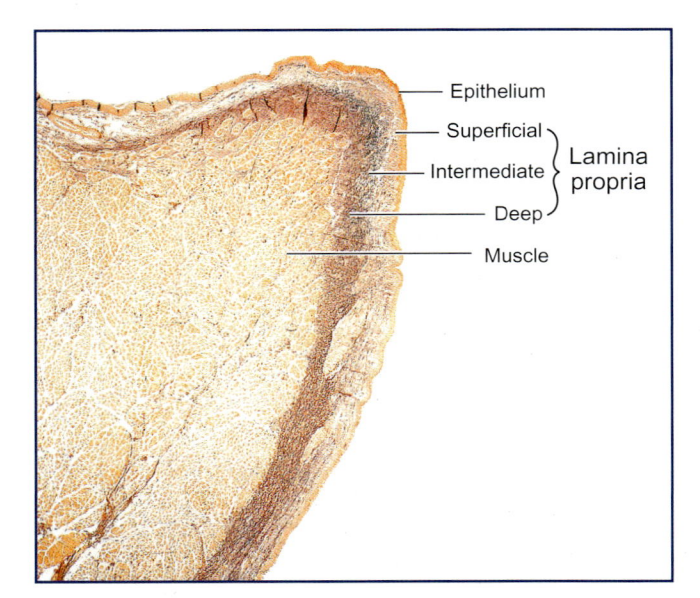

Figure 3–12. Frontal section through the mid-length of the membranous adult vocal fold. This section shows the five layers of the vocal folds. The epithelium and superficial layer of the lamina propria make up the mucosa and the intermediate and deep layers of the lamina propria make up the vocal ligament. From *Histological Color Atlas of the Human Larynx,* (1st ed., p. 45), by M. Hirano and K. Sato, 1993, Belmont, CA: Delmar Learning. Copyright 1993 by Delmar Learning, a division of Thomson Learning: http://www.thomsonrights.com. Fax: 800-730-2215. Modified and reproduced with permission.

Figure 3–13. Subgroupings of the five layers of the vocal folds into the body and the cover. The body of the vocal folds consists of the muscle and deep layer of the lamina propria (L. P.) and the cover consists of the intermediate and superficial layers of the lamina propria and the epithelium. This subgrouping is helpful to understanding the mechanical behavior of the vocal folds during phonation.

1996; Obrebowski, Wojnowski, & Obrebowski-Karsznia, 2006; Strocchi et al., 1992).

It is common practice to subgroup the five layers of the vocal folds into a so-called *body* and *cover*. The vocal fold body comprises muscle fibers and the deep layer of the lamina propria; the vocal fold cover comprises the intermediate and superficial layers of the lamina propria and the epithelium. This two-layered scheme, depicted in Figure 3–13, is significant because it helps to explain certain aspects of the mechanical behavior of the vocal folds during phonation.

When viewed from above, the medial borders of the vocal folds diverge from front to back when at rest, as illustrated in Figure 3–14. Between the vocal folds is a triangularly shaped opening called the glottis. The front part of the glottis is termed the membranous glottis and occupies about 60% of the length of the vocal folds. It lies between the thyroid cartilage and the tips of the vocal processes of the arytenoid cartilages and courses along the vocal ligaments. The back part of the glottis is called the cartilaginous glottis. It occupies about 40% of the length of the vocal folds and lies between the tips of the vocal processes of the ary-

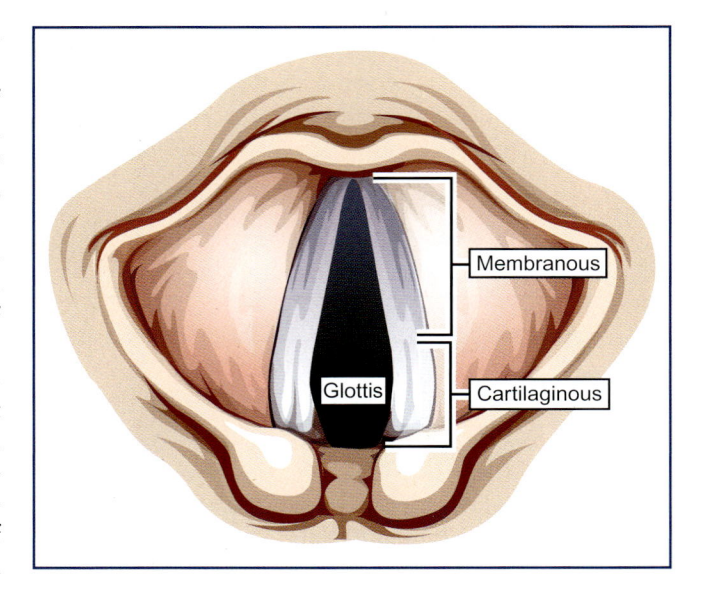

Figure 3–14. The vocal folds as viewed from above (with the front of the larynx at the top). The glottis (opening between the vocal folds) is bounded in the front by the membranous vocal folds and in the back by the vocal processes of the arytenoid cartilages.

tenoid cartilages and the most rearward points on their medial surfaces.

Ventricular Folds

As shown in Figure 3–11 (upper images), another set of shelf-like structures extends from the sidewalls of the laryngeal cavity into the laryngeal airway. These structures lie above the vocal folds (but are less prominent) and are referred to as the ventricular folds or false vocal folds. These folds attach to the thyroid cartilage at the front and to the fronts and sides of the arytenoid cartilages at the back. Each fold contains a ventricular ligament that runs from front to back near its medial edge. Muscular tissue is sparse within the ventricular folds. The opening between the ventricular folds is referred to as the false glottis and is nearly always wider than the glottis between the vocal folds.

Laryngeal Ventricles

The vocal folds and ventricular folds have a sinus (depression) between them (see Figure 3–11, upper left image). This sinus is called the laryngeal ventricle and constitutes a horizontal pouch in each sidewall of the laryngeal tube. The laryngeal ventricles extend most of the length of the vocal folds. Toward the front of the larynx they course upward into saccules that are richly endowed with mucous glands. These glands contain mucus that lubricates the vocal folds.

Ligaments and Membranes

Laryngeal ligaments and membranes help to bind the laryngeal structures to one another as well as to structures outside the larynx. The ligaments that bind the joints of the larynx are discussed above and depicted in Figures 3–7 and 3–9. These are the anterior, lateral, and posterior ceratocricoid ligaments, for the cricothyroid joints, and the anterior and posterior cricoarytenoid ligaments, for the cricoarytenoid joints. Most of the other intrinsic and extrinsic ligaments and membranes are depicted in Figure 3–15 and discussed below.

Intrinsic Ligaments and Membranes. The intrinsic ligaments and membranes of the larynx are those that connect laryngeal cartilages to one another. These ligaments and membranes are important in regulating the extent and direction of movement of the laryngeal cartilages in relation to one another. Most of the intrinsic ligaments and membranes of the larynx arise from a common sheet of connective tissue called the elastic membrane. This sheet lines the entire laryngeal airway, except for the part that lies between the vocal and ventricular ligaments on each side. This discontinuity enables the mucous glands in the laryngeal saccules to be expressed into the laryngeal cavity as lubricant.

The part of the elastic membrane that lines the region between the lower margin of the cricoid cartilage and the vocal folds connects the cricoid, arytenoid, and thyroid cartilages to one another and is designated as the conus elasticus. This membrane gives rise to a middle cricothyroid ligament, two lateral cricothyroid membranes, and two vocal ligaments. The middle cricothyroid ligament extends between the top of the anterior arch of the cricoid cartilage and the bottom of the thyroid cartilage in the region of the angle of the thyroid cartilage. This ligament limits the degree to which the cricoid cartilage and thyroid cartilage can be separated vertically at the front. The two lateral cricothyroid membranes are thinner than the middle cricothyroid ligament and extend upward from the upper border of the anterior arch of the cricoid cartilage at the sides. They, like the middle cricothyroid ligament, restrict the separation of the cricoid and thyroid cartilages toward the front. The lateral cricothyroid membranes thicken significantly toward the top of the conus elasticus and are continuous with the paired vocal ligaments. The vocal ligaments extend between the angle of the thyroid cartilage and the vocal processes of the arytenoid cartilages and lie near the free margins of the vocal folds. These ligaments restrict the degree to which the thyroid and arytenoid cartilages can be separated from front to back.

The part of the elastic membrane that lines the region from the ventricular folds to the laryngeal aditus connects the epiglottis, thyroid cartilage, arytenoid cartilages, and corniculate cartilages to one another and is referred to as the quadrangular membrane. This membrane is paired left and right and thickens significantly toward the bottoms of the pair to form the ventricular (false vocal fold) ligaments. These ligaments extend the length of the ventricular folds near their free margins and attach to the thyroid and arytenoid cartilages. The ventricular ligaments place limits on the degree to which the thyroid and arytenoid cartilages can be separated from front to back. The remaining intrinsic ligament of the larynx is the thyroepiglottic ligament. This ligament extends between the bottom of the epiglottis and the inside of the angle of the thyroid cartilage, just beneath the thyroid notch, and functions as a fastener.

Extrinsic Ligaments and Membranes. Extrinsic ligaments and membranes of the larynx connect laryngeal cartilages to structures outside the larynx and provide support and stability for the laryngeal housing. The cricotracheal membrane (sometimes called the cricotracheal ligament) comprises the lowermost extrinsic

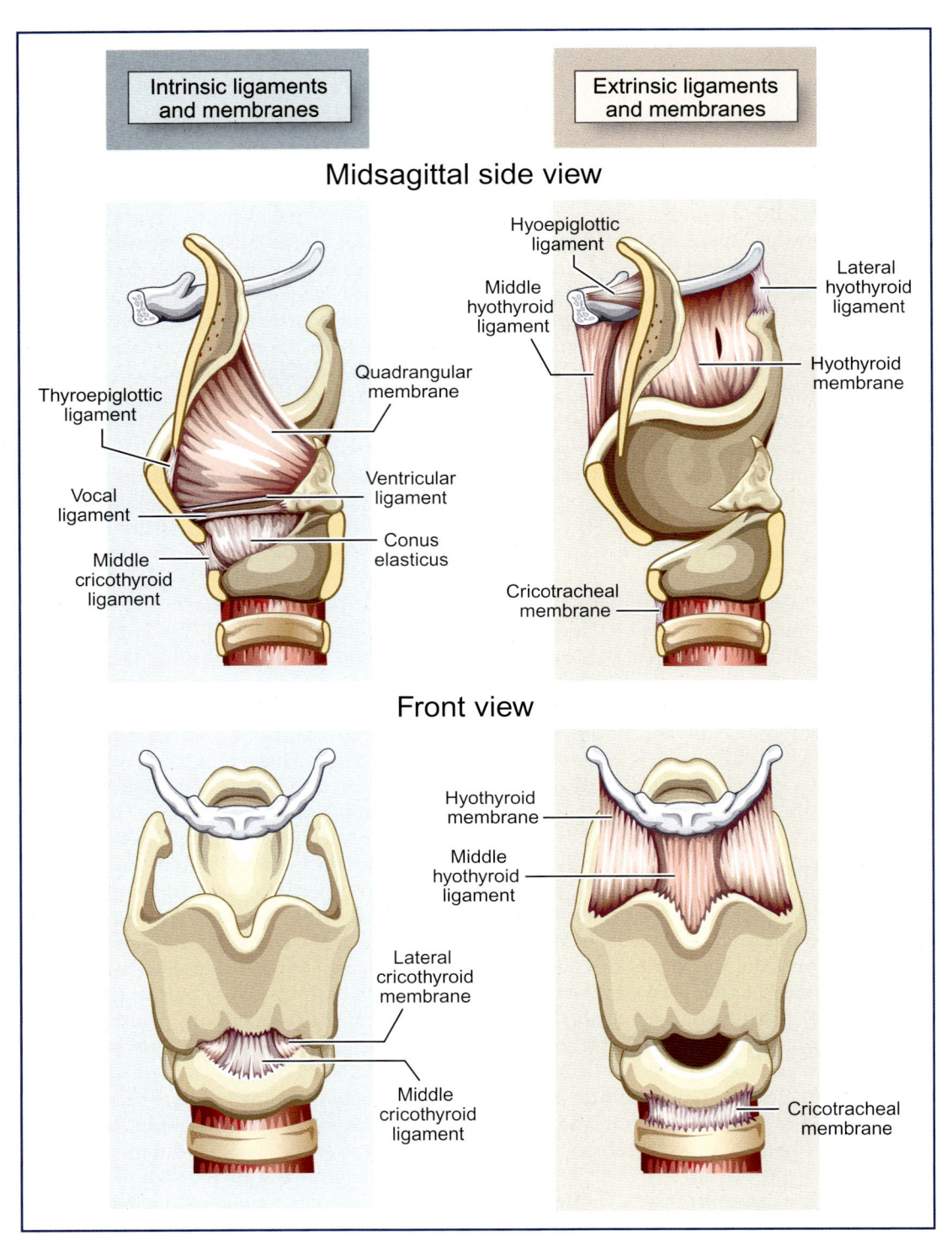

Figure 3-15. Intrinsic and extrinsic laryngeal ligaments and membranes. The intrinsic ligaments (middle cricothyroid, vocal, ventricular, and thyroepiglottic ligaments) and membranes (conus elasticus, lateral cricothyroid, and quadrangular membranes) connect laryngeal cartilages to one another. Extrinsic ligaments (hyoepiglottic and middle and lateral hyothyroid ligaments) and membranes (cricotracheal and hyothyroid membranes) connect laryngeal cartilages to structures outside the larynx. Mucous membrane (not shown) lines the entire laryngeal cavity.

connection to the larynx. This membrane extends around the bottom of the larynx between the first tracheal ring and the lower margin of the cricoid cartilage. The cricotracheal membrane is somewhat more extensive than the connective tissue between successive tracheal rings, the first tracheal ring being somewhat larger than the rest. The hyoepiglottic ligament extends between the upper back surface of the body of the hyoid bone and the lingual surface of the epiglottis. This ligament limits the degree to which these two structures can be separated from front to back. The hyothyroid (also called the thyrohyoid) ligaments and membrane form a large interconnection between the hyoid bone and the upper margin of the thyroid cartilage of the larynx. This interconnection gives the appearance that the laryngeal housing proper is suspended from the hyoid bone. The hyothyroid membrane thickens toward the midline of the larynx at the front and is designated in that location as the middle hyothyroid ligament. The same membrane also thickens toward the back in the space between the greater cornua of the hyoid bone and the superior cornua of the thyroid cartilage. These thickenings are referred to as the lateral hyothyroid ligaments. Often embedded within each of these lateral ligaments is a small triticeal (grain of wheat) cartilage.

Mucous Membrane. The entire internal laryngeal cavity is lined by a mucous membrane, like the trachea below it and the pharynx above it. This lining is covered by columnar epithelium, except for the inner edges of the vocal folds and ventricular folds and the upper half of the epiglottis, which are covered with squamous epithelium.

FORCES OF THE LARYNGEAL APPARATUS

Two types of force, passive and active, operate on the larynx. Passive force is inherent within the apparatus. Active force is applied in accordance with the will and ability of the individual.

The passive force of the larynx comes from several sources. These include the natural recoil of muscles, cartilages, and connective tissues (ligaments and membranes), the surface tension between structures in apposition (vocal folds, ventricular folds, epiglottis and aryepiglottic folds, and/or tongue), and the pull of gravity. The distribution, sign, and magnitude of passive force depend on the mechanical milieu, including the positions, deformations, and levels of muscle activity (if applicable) of different parts of the laryngeal apparatus.

The active force of the laryngeal apparatus results from activation of laryngeal muscles. Laryngeal muscles can be categorized as intrinsic, extrinsic, or supplementary. Muscles categorized as intrinsic have both ends attached within the larynx, whereas muscles categorized as extrinsic have one end attached within the larynx and one end attached outside the larynx. Muscles categorized as supplementary do not attach to the larynx directly but influence it by way of attachments to the neighboring hyoid bone.

The function described below for individual muscles assumes that the muscles of interest are engaged in shortening (concentric) contractions, unless otherwise specified as being engaged in lengthening (eccentric) contractions or fixed-length (isometric) contractions. The influence of individual muscle actions may also be conditioned by whether or not other muscles are active.

Two Worlds

Technical and colloquial definitions of terms can sometimes be quite different. Take, for example, the term "elastic." In a physical sense, something that's elastic returns to its original shape following deformation. Throw a golf club on the floor and it will deform and then return to its original shape. And you can predict what that shape will be. But consider the waistband of your underwear. Throw your underwear on the floor and its waistband will not assume a shape you can predict. That's because, in a physical sense, it's inelastic—it doesn't return to its original shape following deformation. So, although you might think of the waistband of your underwear as being elastic, a physicist would think just the opposite. Both of you are right in your uses of the term "elastic," but you need to know which world you're talking in (colloquial or technical) before you consider something to be "elastic" or not.

> **Motorboat**
>
> Probably as a child you played "motorboat" with friends by rapidly pounding your fists on their chests or backs while they sustained "ah." The variation in loudness that sounded to you like an idling motorboat was caused by rapid changes in alveolar pressure. Pound on someone's chest or back and with each blow their lungs compress a small amount and the air pressure inside them goes up momentarily. Pound at different rates and you change the perceived speed of your imaginary motor noise. The basis of all this fun is that the laryngeal apparatus and the voice are sensitive to adjustments in the breathing apparatus. You don't necessarily need to have a friend pounding on you to appreciate this sensitivity. Try to talk while driving a car down a cross-rutted dirt road or while sitting atop a trotting horse. The road and the horse will effectively do the pounding for you by bouncing your gut up and down and changing your alveolar pressure.

Intrinsic Laryngeal Muscles

Figure 3–16 depicts the intrinsic muscles of the larynx. These muscles are responsible for changing the position and mechanical status of structures that form the walls of the laryngeal cavity. They are the *thyroarytenoid*, *posterior cricoarytenoid*, *lateral cricoarytenoid*, *arytenoid*, and *cricothyroid* muscles.

The *thyroarytenoid* muscle forms most of each vocal fold. This muscle extends between the inside surface of the thyroid cartilage (near the angle) and the arytenoid cartilage on the corresponding side. The front attachment of the muscle lies to the side of the front attachment of the corresponding vocal ligament. Fibers run generally parallel to the vocal ligament to insert on the front and outer sides of the arytenoid cartilage. Upper fibers run a straight course from front to back, whereas lower fibers twist in their course and swing off in an outward, backward, and upward direction (Broad, 1973; Zemlin, 1998). A small number of

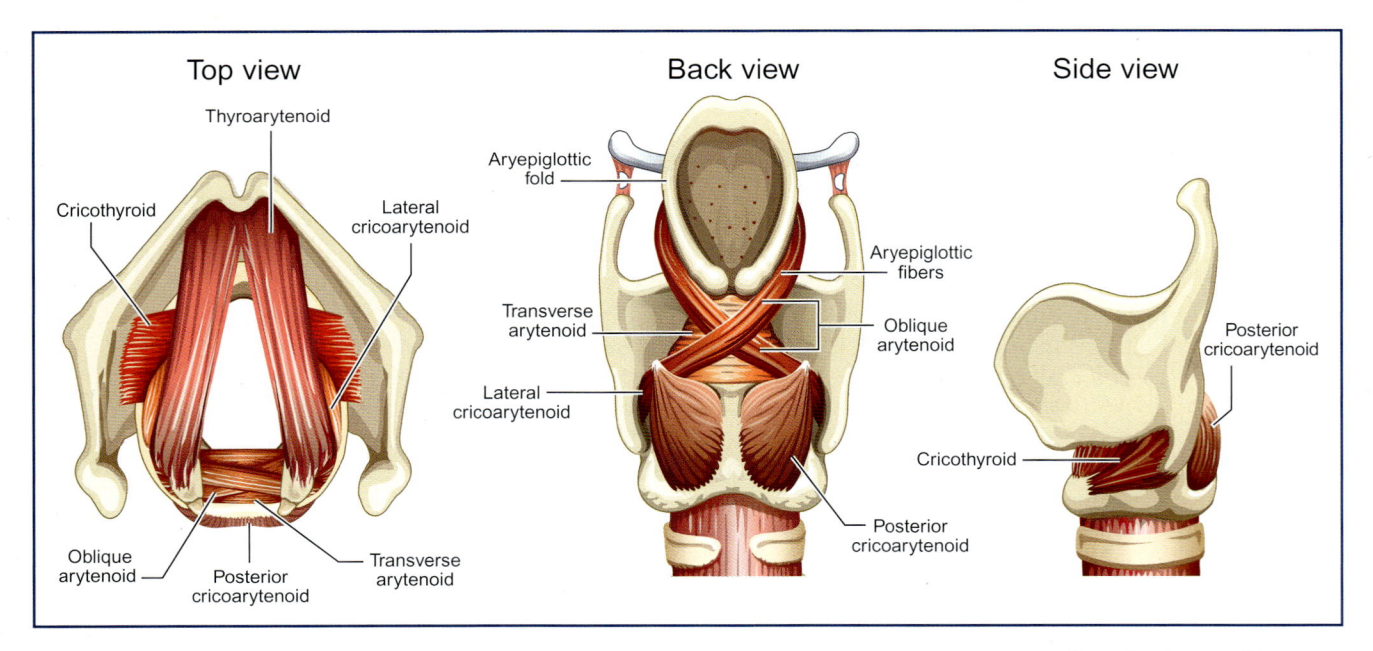

Figure 3–16. Intrinsic muscles of the larynx. Intrinsic muscles have both ends attached within the larynx. They are the **thyroarytenoid**, **posterior cricoarytenoid**, **lateral cricoarytenoid**, **arytenoid** (**transverse** and **oblique**), and **cricothyroid** muscles.

fibers toward the side of the muscle depart from the predominant front-to-back orientation of the others and course upward to the aryepiglottic fold, the side of the epiglottis, and into the region of the ventricular fold on the same side (Zemlin, 1998). The effects of contraction of the *thyroarytenoid* muscle are portrayed in Figure 3–17. Contraction of its longitudinal fibers shortens it and reduces the distance between the thyroid and arytenoid cartilages. The reduction in distance between the two cartilages is typically effected as a forward pull on the arytenoid cartilage that rocks it toward the midline. Fixed-length (isometric) or lengthening (eccentric) contractions of the *thyroarytenoid* muscle (with other intrinsic muscles opposing) increase its internal tension (force per unit length). Contraction of vertical fibers of the *thyroarytenoid* muscle near the sidewall of the larynx may have an influence on the position and configuration of the corresponding ventricular fold (Reidenbach, 1998; not illustrated in Figure 3–17).

The *thyroarytenoid* muscle is sometimes described as having two distinct parts (Dickson & Maue-Dickson, 1982; van den Berg & Moll, 1955; Wustrow, 1953): the *thyromuscularis* muscle (sometimes called the *external thyroarytenoid*) and the *thyrovocalis* or *vocalis* muscle (sometimes called the *internal thyroarytenoid*). As depicted schematically in Figure 3–18, the *thyromuscularis* muscle lies nearest the laryngeal wall and to the side of the *thyrovocalis* muscle. The *thyrovocalis* muscle and the vocal ligament are sometimes referred to as the vocal cord, as distinguished from the vocal fold (which also includes the *thyromuscularis* muscle); however, the terms "vocal cord" and "vocal fold" are also used interchangeably. The term "vocal fold" is more descriptive of the entire shelf-like structure and is generally preferred (Hall, Cobb, Kapoor, Kuchai, & Sandhu, 2017).

The notion of a two-part *thyroarytenoid* muscle, although embraced by many, is not accepted universally. Some argue that dissections have failed to reveal a separating fascial sheath within the *thyroarytenoid* muscle that would support the notion of two distinct anatomical parts (Mayet, 1955; Zemlin, 1998). Others argue that, with or without such a separating fascial sheath, the *thyroarytenoid* muscle is capable of differential actions in what are conceptualized to be its *thyromuscularis* and *thyrovocalis* subdivisions (Broad, 1973; Sonesson, 1960). These presumed differential actions (discussed below in another section) are believed by some to have salience in the control of voice production (Kahane, 2007; Orlikoff & Kahane, 1996; Sanders, Rai, Han, & Biller, 1998; Titze, 2006a).

The *posterior cricoarytenoid* muscle is fan-shaped and located on the back surface of the cricoid cartilage. The muscle originates on the cricoid lamina and courses upward and toward the side in a converging

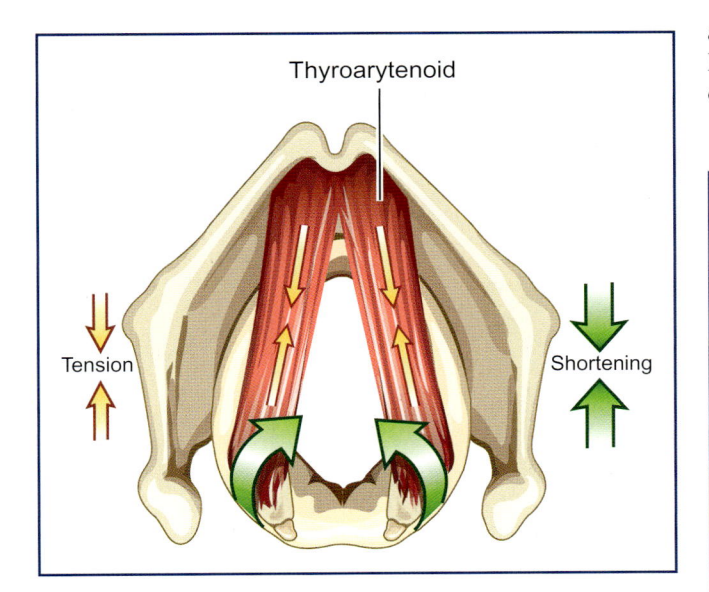

Figure 3-17. Effects of contraction of the **thyroarytenoid** muscles. Contraction of the longitudinal fibers shortens the muscle (*straight green arrows*) and reduces the distance between the thyroid and arytenoid cartilages. This contraction also rocks the arytenoid cartilages toward the midline (*curved green arrows*). If the contraction is isometric (*fixed length*) and is opposed by other muscle forces, the internal tension of the muscle is increased (*yellow arrows*).

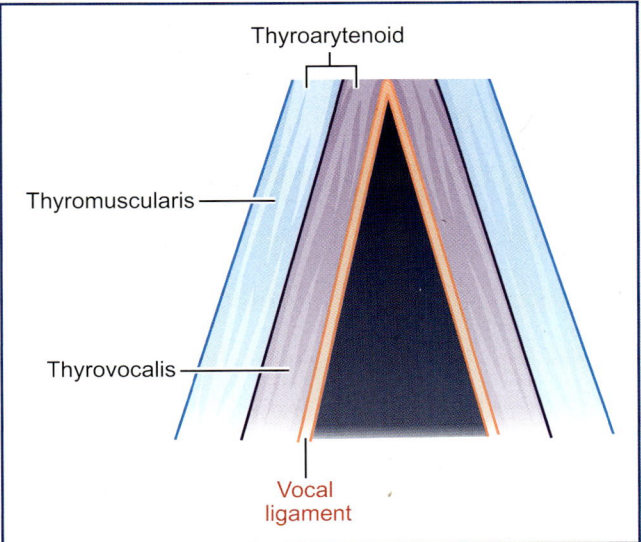

Figure 3-18. **Thyromuscularis** and **thyrovocalis** (or **vocalis**) subdivisions of the **thyroarytenoid** muscle. The vocal ligament runs along the internal edge of the **thyrovocalis** muscle.

pattern to insert on the upper and back surfaces of the muscular process of the arytenoid cartilage. As illustrated in Figure 3–19, contraction of the *posterior cricoarytenoid* muscle rocks the arytenoid cartilage away from the midline. This rocking is effected mainly by fibers located laterally within the muscle and that insert on the upper surface of the muscular process. Forceful contraction of these fibers may also slide the arytenoid cartilage upward and backward along the sloping rim of the cricoid cartilage. Fibers in the medial part of the *posterior cricoarytenoid* muscle insert on the back surface of the muscular process and contract to stabilize the arytenoid cartilage against other forces that are directed forward (Zemlin, Davis, & Gaza, 1984).

The *lateral cricoarytenoid* is a small fan-shaped muscle that originates from the upper rim of the cricoid cartilage. Fibers of this muscle extend upward and backward to insert on the muscular process and front surface of the arytenoid cartilage. As depicted in Figure 3–20, contraction of the *lateral cricoarytenoid* muscle rocks the arytenoid cartilage toward the midline. Activation of the *lateral cricoarytenoid* muscle may also slide the arytenoid cartilage forward and toward the side along the downward sloping path of the long axis of the cricoid facet of the cricoarytenoid joint.

The *arytenoid* (also called the *interarytenoid*) muscle extends from the back surface of one arytenoid cartilage to the back surface of the other arytenoid cartilage. The *arytenoid* muscle has two distinct and separate subdivisions: the *transverse arytenoid* muscle and the *oblique arytenoid* muscle. The *transverse arytenoid* muscle arises from the back surface and side of one arytenoid cartilage and courses horizontally to insert on the back surface and side of the other arytenoid cartilage. Those muscle fibers that insert on the sides of the arytenoid cartilages interdigitate with fibers of the *thyroarytenoid* muscles. The *oblique arytenoid* muscle overlies the transverse component of the muscle and diagonally crosses the back surface of the two arytenoid cartilages. The muscle originates from the back and side surface and muscular process of one arytenoid cartilage and courses upward to insert near the apex of the other arytenoid cartilage. Some muscle fibers of the *oblique arytenoid* muscle extend around the side of the apex of the arytenoid cartilage and course upward and forward to insert into the side of the epiglottis. This

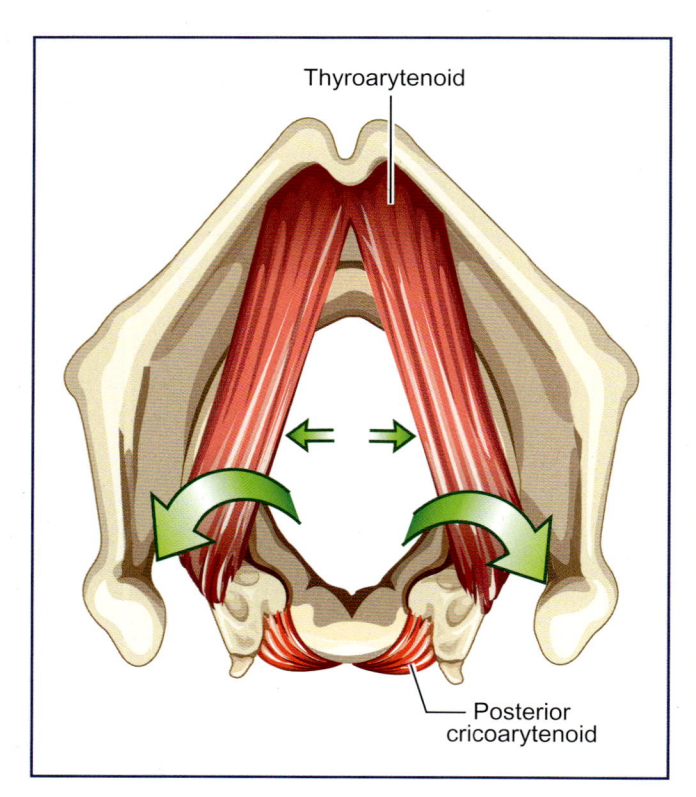

Figure 3–19. Effects of contraction of the *posterior cricoarytenoid* muscles. Their contraction rocks the arytenoid cartilages rock away from the midline and also moves the vocal folds (which contain the *thyroarytenoid* muscles) away from the midline.

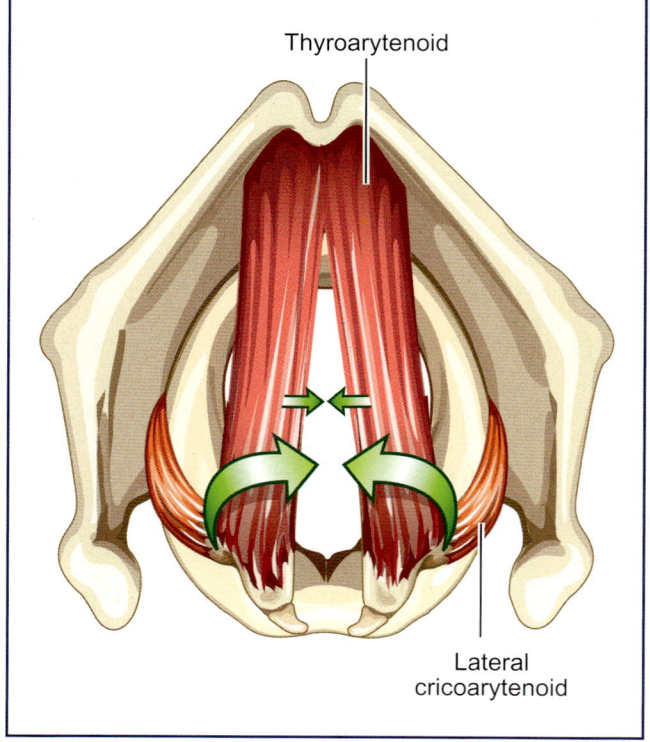

Figure 3–20. Effects of contraction of the *lateral cricoarytenoid* muscles. Their contraction rocks the arytenoid cartilages toward the midline and moves the vocal folds (which contain the *thyroarytenoid* muscles) toward the midline.

part of the muscle is given its own name, the *aryepiglottic* muscle. As illustrated in Figure 3–21, contraction of different components of the *arytenoid* muscle has different effects. Contraction of the *transverse arytenoid* muscle pulls the arytenoid cartilages toward one another. This is manifested through an upward, inward, and backward sliding movement along the long axis of each cricoarytenoid joint. Contraction of

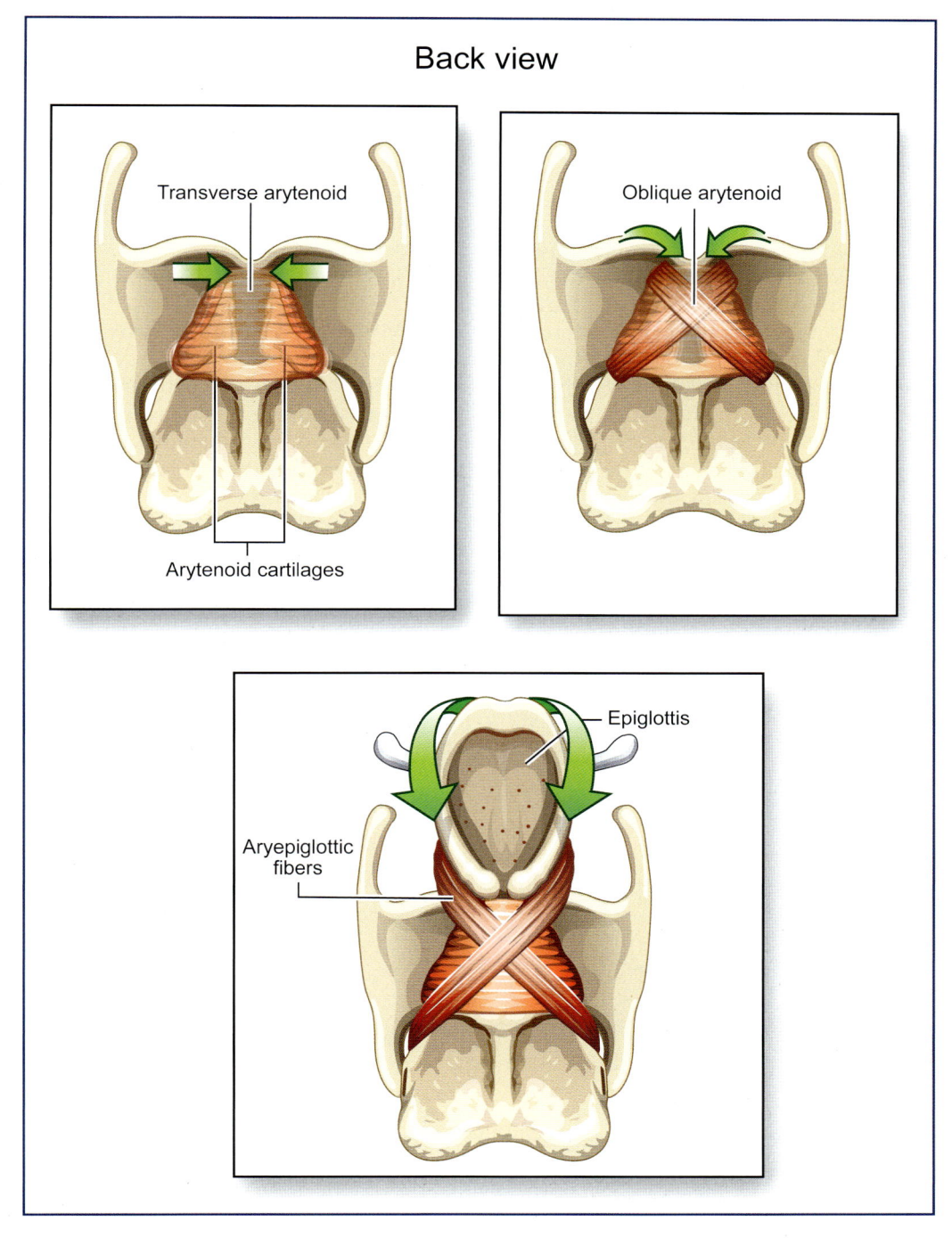

Figure 3–21. Effects of contractions of different parts of the *arytenoid* muscles. Contraction of the *transverse arytenoid* muscle pulls the arytenoid cartilages toward one another. Contraction of the *oblique arytenoid* muscle tips the arytenoid cartilages toward one another. Contraction of the *aryepiglottic* muscle (an extension of the *oblique arytenoid* muscle) pulls the epiglottis backward and downward.

the *oblique arytenoid* muscle pulls one arytenoid cartilage toward the other in a tipping action that occurs in accordance with the movement permitted at the cricoarytenoid joint. And contraction of the *aryepiglottic* muscle pulls the epiglottis backward and downward to cover the upper opening into the larynx.

The *cricothyroid* muscle extends between the outer front and side of the anterior arch of the cricoid cartilage and the outer front and side of the lower border of the lamina and inferior cornu of the thyroid cartilage. The muscle is fan-shaped with its fibers diverging as they course from the cricoid cartilage to the thyroid cartilage. Two subdivisions of the muscle are most often recognized, a vertical component toward the front called the *par rectus*, and an upward sloping component toward the back called the *pars oblique* (Zemlin, 1998). A third subdivision, the *pars media*, is occasionally noted. Its fibers lie underneath and closer to the midline than the fibers of the *pars rectus* (Charpied & Shapshay, 2004), although some consider the *pars media* to be an anatomical variation of the *cricothyroid* muscle proper (Kucinski, Okrazewska, & Piszcz, 1979). As illustrated in Figure 3–22, contraction of the *cricothyroid* muscle increases the distance between the thyroid and arytenoid cartilages and decreases the distance between the upper border of the cricoid cartilage and the lower border of the thyroid cartilage at the front of the larynx (decreases the angle formed between the two cartilages). These distance changes result from a rotation of the thyroid cartilage on the cricoid cartilage and/or a rotation of the cricoid cartilage on the thyroid cartilage. Rotation is effected through activation of both the **pars rectus** and **pars oblique** components of the *cricothyroid* muscle. Activation of the **pars oblique** component also results in a secondary movement that increases the distance between the thyroid and arytenoid cartilages. This movement causes a limited forward sliding of the thyroid cartilage, backward sliding of the cricoid cartilage, or both (Arnold, 1961; Takano & Honda, 2005; van den Berg et al., 1960).

Extrinsic Laryngeal Muscles

Figure 3–23 depicts the extrinsic laryngeal muscles. These muscles have a role in supporting and stabilizing the larynx and in changing its position within the neck. They include the *sternothyroid*, *thyrohyoid*, and *inferior constrictor* muscles.

The *sternothyroid* is a long muscle located toward the front and side of the larynx. It originates from the

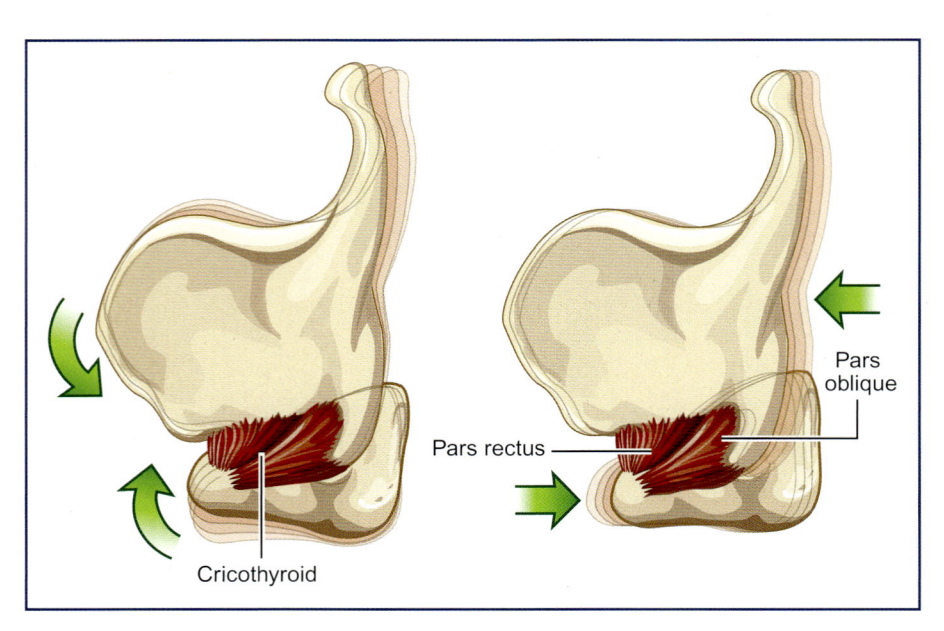

Figure 3–22. Effects of contractions of the *cricothyroid* muscles. Contraction of the *cricothyroid* muscles (*pars rectus* and *pars oblique*) rotates the thyroid cartilage on the cricoid cartilage (or vice versa). This rotation increases the distance between the thyroid and arytenoid cartilages at the back and decreases the distance between the thyroid and cricoid cartilages at the front. The *pars oblique* component can also cause the thyroid cartilage to slide forward and/or the cricoid cartilage to slide backward.

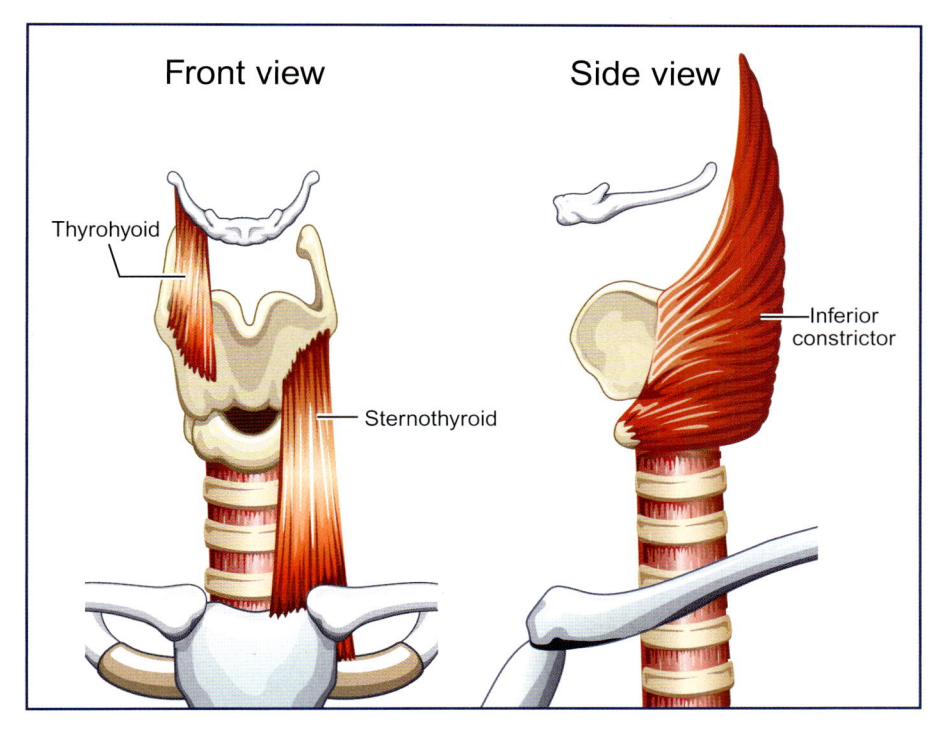

Figure 3–23. Extrinsic muscles of the larynx. Extrinsic muscles have one attachment inside the larynx and one attachment outside the larynx. The extrinsic laryngeal muscles are the **sternothyroid**, **thyrohyoid**, and **inferior constrictor** muscles.

back surface of the top of the sternum (breastbone) and the first costal (rib) cartilage. Fibers of the muscle course upward and slightly toward the side to insert on the outer surface of the thyroid cartilage. Contraction of the *sternothyroid* muscle pulls the thyroid cartilage downward. This action may also enlarge the pharynx by drawing the larynx forward and downward (Zemlin, 1998).

The *thyrohyoid* muscle is located on the front and side of the larynx. It extends between the outer surface of the thyroid cartilage and the lower edge of the greater cornu of the hyoid bone. The course of its fibers is essentially vertical. Contraction of the *thyrohyoid* muscle decreases the distance between the thyroid cartilage and the hyoid bone. Relative fixation of the thyroid cartilage and hyoid bone determines the extent to which the structures may move toward one another.

The *inferior constrictor* muscle (discussed in more detail in Chapter 4) is the lowest of the group of three muscles that forms the back and sidewalls of the pharynx. Fibers of the *inferior constrictor* muscle extend forward from the median raphe (seam) at the back of the pharynx to insert on the sides of the cricoid and thyroid cartilages. Contraction of the *inferior constrictor* muscle moves the sidewall of the lower pharynx inward and decreases the size of the pharyngeal lumen (tubular cavity). Its activation also serves to stabilize the position of the laryngeal housing.

Supplementary Laryngeal Muscles

Some muscles do not attach on the larynx, but are nonetheless important in influencing its position and stability. These muscles, depicted in Figure 3–24, are referred to as supplementary muscles of the larynx. Most of them attach to the hyoid bone and are subdivided into those that originate below the hyoid bone, the so-called infrahyoid muscles, and those that originate above the hyoid bone, the so-called suprahyoid muscles.

Infrahyoid Muscles

The infrahyoid muscles include the *sternohyoid* and *omohyoid* muscles. These two muscles apply forces that can influence the positioning of the hyoid bone from below.

The *sternohyoid* muscle is a flat structure that courses vertically along the front surface of the neck and overlies the *sternothyroid* muscle (an extrinsic laryngeal muscle). The *sternohyoid* muscle originates from the back surface of the top of the sternum and

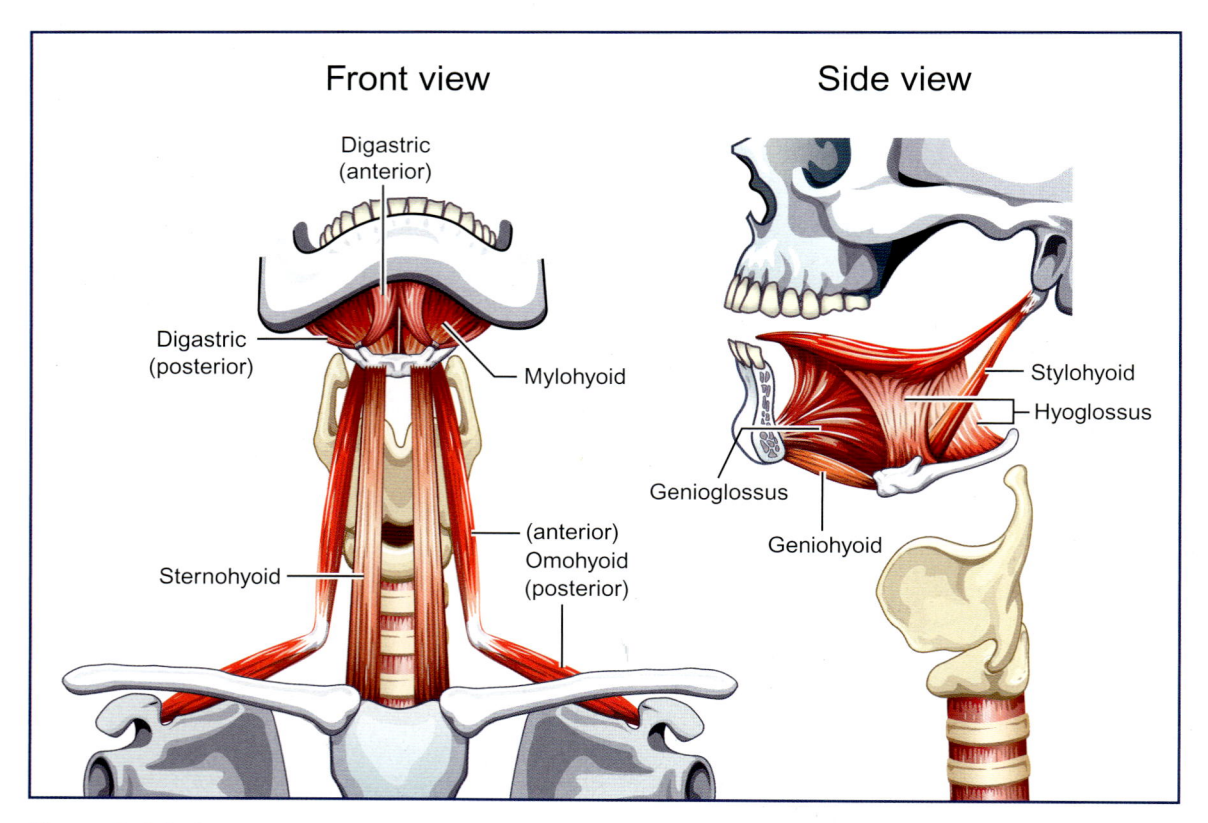

Figure 3–24. Supplementary muscles of the larynx. Supplementary muscles do not attach directly to the larynx, but exert indirect influences through attachments to the hyoid bone. Infrahyoid muscles (**sternohyoid** and **omohyoid** muscles) originate below the hyoid bone, and suprahyoid muscles (**digastric**, **stylohyoid**, **mylohyoid**, **geniohyoid**, **hyoglossus**, and **genioglossus** muscles) originate above the hyoid bone.

They Didn't Quite Get It

She had a beautiful coloratura soprano voice and after years of formal training was just about to begin an operatic career. It ended abruptly on a ski slope when a careless youngster crashed into her and slammed her headfirst into a tree. She suffered facial lacerations, blunt trauma to the larynx, and temporomandibular joint damage. She never again had full singing ability. Jaw movement was difficult and very painful. She could no longer meet the demands of operatic roles. Forensic testimony concluded that she was 100% impaired because she could not perform a full operatic role. The career for which she had prepared was lost. The jury decided otherwise and awarded her little more than her medical expenses. The twisted logic was revealed in an interview with the foreman of the jury following the trial. "We didn't see why she couldn't just sing country songs instead. They're short and not as demanding." They didn't quite get it.

---

the inner end of the clavicle (collar bone). Fibers course upward and insert on the lower edge of the body of the hyoid bone. Contraction of the *sternohyoid* muscle places a downward pull on the hyoid bone. This downward pull lowers the hyoid bone, or it can anchor the hyoid bone in position if the downward pull is counterbalanced by other forces.

The *omohyoid* (shoulder-to-hyoid bone) muscle is located on the front and side of the neck. It is a narrow muscle that has two long bellies. The *posterior* (lower) belly arises from the upper edge of the scapula (shoulder blade) and courses horizontally inward and forward to attach to an intermediate tendon positioned near the sternum. The *anterior* (upper) belly arises from the opposite end of the same intermediate tendon and runs vertically and toward the midline to attach to the lower edge of the greater cornu of the hyoid bone. Contraction of the *omohyoid* muscle places a downward and backward pull on the hyoid bone. Contraction also tenses the supporting fascia in the region and prevents the neck from being sucked inward during forceful inspiration.

Suprahyoid Muscles

The suprahyoid muscles apply forces that can influence the positioning of the hyoid bone from above. They are the *digastric, stylohyoid, mylohyoid, geniohyoid, hyoglossus*, and *genioglossus* muscles.

The *digastric* is a two-bellied sling of muscle in which the two bellies are joined end-to-end by an intermediate tendon that attaches to the top of the hyoid bone. The *anterior* belly originates inside the lower border of the mandible (jaw) and courses downward and backward to the intermediate tendon. The *posterior* belly originates from the mastoid process of the temporal bone of the skull and courses downward and forward to the intermediate tendon. Contraction of the *digastric* muscle pulls upward on the hyoid bone and/or downward on the mandible. The relative movement of the hyoid bone and mandible is dependent on the degree to which the two structures are fixed in position by other muscles. Of interest here are influences on the hyoid bone. Contraction of the *anterior* belly of the muscle moves the hyoid bone upward and forward, whereas contraction of the *posterior* belly of the muscle moves the hyoid bone upward and backward. Contraction of the two bellies of the *digastric* muscle at the same time pulls the hyoid bone upward and forward or upward and backward at any angle, depending on the forces generated by the two bellies.

The *stylohyoid* muscle runs a course somewhat parallel to the *posterior* belly of the *digastric* muscle. The *stylohyoid* muscle originates from the back and side surfaces of the styloid process of the temporal bone of the skull and courses downward and forward to the hyoid bone. The muscle divides into two bundles that pass on either side of the intermediate tendon of the *digastric* muscle before inserting at the junction of the body and greater cornu of the hyoid bone. Contraction of the *stylohyoid* muscle places an upward and backward pull on the hyoid bone. The action is similar to that which results from contraction of the *posterior* belly of the *digastric* muscle.

The *mylohyoid* muscle contributes to the formation of the floor of the oral cavity. Fibers of this muscle originate along much of the inner surface of the body of the mandible and course inward, backward, and downward. They join with fibers of their paired mate of the opposite side at a tendinous midline raphe (a seam running down the center of the floor of the oral cavity). Fibers toward the rear of the oral cavity attach directly into the front surface of the body of the hyoid bone. Contraction of the *mylohyoid* muscle results in an upward and forward pull on the hyoid bone. Contraction can also result in elevation of the floor of the oral cavity and tongue. With the hyoid bone fixed in position, contraction of the *mylohyoid* muscle may lower the mandible.

The *geniohyoid* is a cylindrical muscle that lies above the *mylohyoid* muscle. This muscle extends from the inner surface of the front of the mandible to the front surface of the body of the hyoid bone. Its fibers extend backward and downward in a diverging pattern. The muscle bundle runs above and nearly parallel to the fiber course of the *anterior* belly of the *digastric* muscle. Contraction of the *geniohyoid* muscle pulls the hyoid bone upward and forward. Its functional potential is similar to that of the *anterior* belly of the *digastric* muscle.

The *hyoglossus* is an extrinsic muscle of the tongue (having attachments within and outside the tongue) that has the potential to exert force on the hyoid bone and move the housing of the larynx. Fibers of this muscle course vertically and extend between the side of the tongue toward the back and the body and greater cornu of the hyoid bone. When the *hyoglossus* muscle contracts, it retracts and depresses the tongue and/or elevates the hyoid bone. If the tongue is relatively more fixed than the hyoid bone, the hyoid bone will rise within the neck.

The *genioglossus* is also an extrinsic muscle of the tongue and is the largest and strongest of such extrinsic muscles. This muscle has the potential to exert force on both the tongue and the hyoid bone. Fibers of the *genioglossus* muscle extend from the inner surface of the mandible and course complexly to insert into the entire undersurface of the tongue and body of the hyoid bone. Contraction of the *genioglossus* muscle can have a variety of influences on the positioning of the tongue and/or hyoid bone. Its major influence on the hyoid bone is to draw it upward and forward.

Summary of the Laryngeal Muscles

The laryngeal muscles are categorized as intrinsic, extrinsic, and supplemental, depending on the locations of their attachments (inside or outside the larynx).

> **Donation and a Growing Cause**
>
> Two interesting developments hold promise for those with severe laryngeal injury or disease. One is laryngeal transplantation, in which a donor larynx from another individual is transferred to an individual whose larynx is no longer viable. The results of initial efforts in transplantation are somewhat encouraging, although only two laryngeal transplants have been reported in the medical literature to date. More promising is the regeneration and reconstruction of new laryngeal tissue through the use of tissue engineering. Tissue engineering has advanced to the stage where successful growth of new laryngeal tissue has been accomplished in humans. New cell therapies combined with new techniques for scaffold construction, such as 3D printing, hold great promise for those with damaged or diseased larynges (Hertegård, 2016). Imagine, one day we may be able to grow an entirely new larynx!

Actions of the intrinsic laryngeal muscles (those with both attachments inside the larynx) have a direct and profound influence on the vocal folds. Specifically, they can abduct (move apart), adduct (move together), shorten, lengthen, and tense the vocal folds. Actions of the extrinsic and supplemental laryngeal muscles (those with at least one attachment outside the larynx) serve to stabilize the larynx and can change its position within the neck. In general, contractions of muscles with attachments below the larynx can lower the larynx, and contractions of those with attachments above the larynx can raise the larynx. These laryngeal movements and their associated forces are detailed in the next two sections.

MOVEMENTS OF THE LARYNGEAL APPARATUS

Movements of the laryngeal apparatus allow it to function as a valve. These movements include those of the vocal folds, ventricular folds, epiglottis, and laryngeal housing.

Movements of the Vocal Folds

The vocal folds are movable and flexible. Changes can be effected in their vertical and side-to-side positioning and in their shape and length.

Each vocal fold can go through vertical and side-to-side position changes as its corresponding arytenoid cartilage rocks at a right angle to the long axis of its associated cricoid facet. When the rocking movement is downward and inward, the back end of the vocal fold moves downward and toward the midline. When rocking movement is upward and outward, the back end of the vocal fold moves upward and toward the side. Under normal circumstances, the two arytenoid cartilages move simultaneously and similarly so that the two vocal folds move in similar trajectories.

The cross-sectional shape of each vocal fold can change. Changes in shape mainly constitute a thinning or thickening of the vocal fold toward its free margin such that the free margin may be relatively sharp or blunt in cross section toward the airway. The vocal fold may also appear to be somewhat tilted in its configuration.

The vocal folds can be lengthened or shortened considerably. Lengthening is limited by the degree to which the covering tissue of the vocal fold, vocal ligament, and different parts of the *thyroarytenoid* muscle are distensible. Lengthening of the vocal folds is effected when either or both the thyroid and cricoid cartilages are moved away from one another. Shortening of the vocal folds occurs when either or both the thyroid and cricoid cartilages are drawn toward one another.

These movements have functional significance to speech production. Of particular relevance are the movements that effect vocal fold abduction, adduction, and length change.

Vocal Fold Abduction

Vocal fold abduction is the movement of a vocal fold away from the midline (although other meanings are possible; see Figure 3–25 for an example). Abduction is normally simultaneous and symmetric in the two vocal folds. As the vocal folds move toward the side, the glottis (space between them) increases in size. As portrayed in Figure 3–26, full abduction of the vocal folds results in a wide glottis and the condition in which air flows most freely in and out of the pulmonary apparatus. It is the vocal folds that abduct, not the glottis.

Abduction of the vocal folds and concomitant enlargement of the glottis are effected mainly by contractions of the *posterior cricoarytenoid* muscles. These pull on the muscular processes of the arytenoid cartilages to swing the vocal folds upward and outward. Vocal fold abduction can also result from a downward pull on the larynx which places a downward pull on the conus elasticus (lower elastic lining of the larynx). Such a pull tends to tug the free margin of the vocal fold downward and toward the side, thus dilating the laryngeal airway (Zenker, 1964). This can

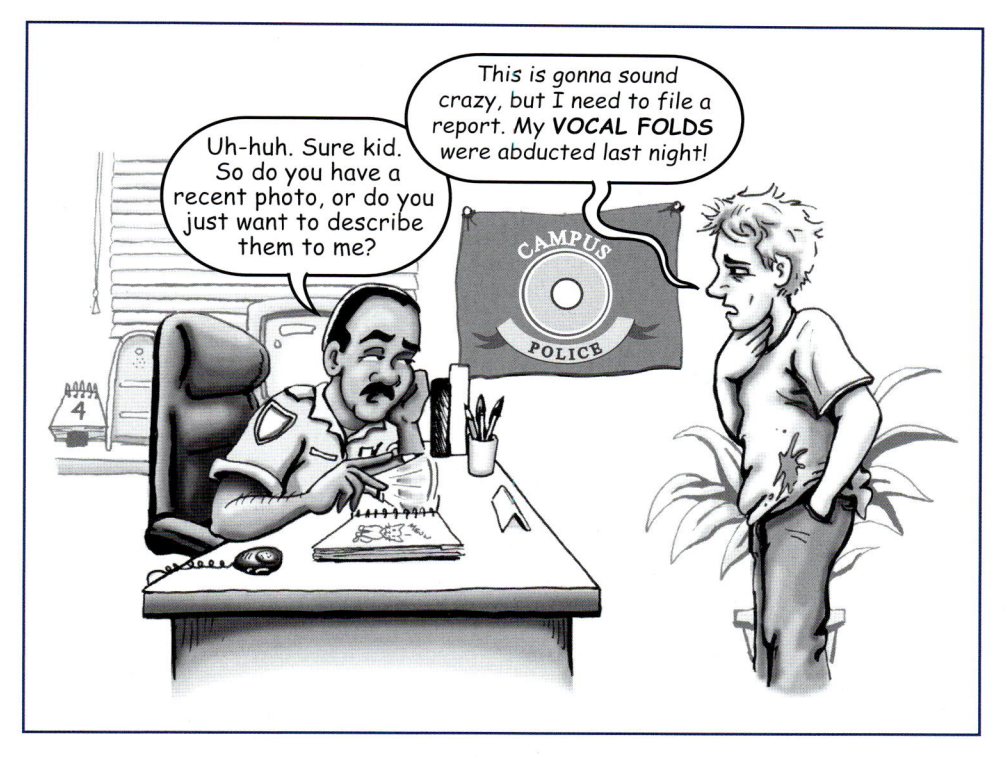

Figure 3-25. Cartoon about vocal fold abduction.

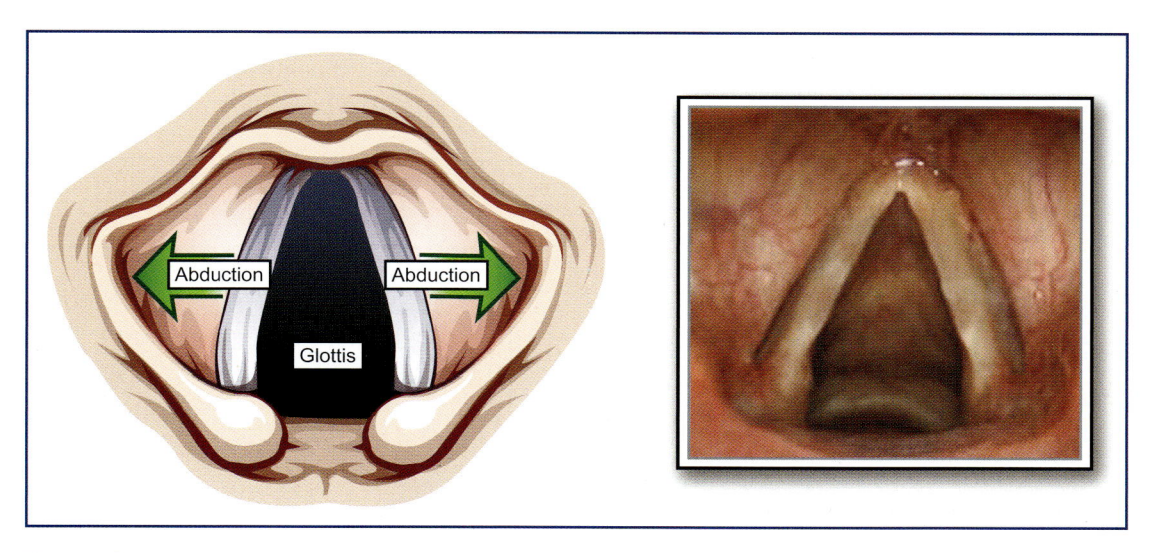

Figure 3-26. Vocal fold abduction and widening of the glottis. Vocal fold abduction is accomplished primarily by contraction of the paired **cricoarytenoid** muscles, though downward force exerted on the larynx can also exert an abductory force on the vocal folds. The image on the right is a photograph of an author's vocal folds (courtesy of Robin Samlan).

happen when the diaphragm contracts footward and pulls downward on the trachea; this is called tracheal tug. The contribution of the *posterior cricoarytenoid* muscles to vocal fold abduction is much greater than that of tracheal tug.

Vocal Fold Adduction

Vocal fold adduction is the movement of a vocal fold toward the midline. During adduction the two vocal folds usually follow similar movement pathways and the glottis decreases in size. As illustrated in Figure 3–27, movement toward the midline may be sufficient to approximate (bring together) the entire free margins of the two vocal folds and close the laryngeal airway. Alternatively, movement toward the midline may be limited to the membranous part of the vocal folds (front 60%), resulting in closure of only that portion of the airway, while leaving the cartilaginous portion (back 40%) of the vocal folds abducted.

Adduction resulting in full approximation of the two vocal folds is caused by the combined contraction of the *lateral cricoarytenoid* muscles and *arytenoid* muscles (*transverse* and *oblique* components), whereas adduction resulting in approximation of only the membranous (front) portions of the vocal folds is caused by contraction of the *lateral cricoarytenoid* muscles alone. Action of the *lateral cricoarytenoid* muscles pulls forward on the muscular processes of the arytenoid cartilages, rocking them over the cricoid cartilage and swinging the vocal folds downward and inward. Action of the *arytenoid* muscles pulls the arytenoid cartilages toward the midline and approximates the cartilaginous (back) portion of the vocal folds.

Once the vocal folds are approximated (fully adducted), the vertical extent of their approximation (amount of contact) and the compressive force (force of contact) can be adjusted. The amount of contact of the cross-sectional thickness through the approximated vocal fold surfaces can be adjusted by contracting the *thyrovocalis* portion of the *thyroarytenoid* muscle. Contraction of the *thyrovocalis* muscle bulges the medial surfaces of the vocal folds toward the midline.

Daniel R. Boone

The Daniel Boone you've heard of may or may not be this one. Both are pioneers. This one wrote a clinical textbook that represented the first comprehensive approach to the topic of voice disorders. In it, he proposed a set of facilitating techniques that were widely adopted by clinicians working with individuals with voice disorders and remain in use today throughout the world—his textbook is in its 9th edition! Boone is a master clinician and an outstanding clinical teacher. He has a knack for cutting to the heart of clinical matters quickly, and few equal him in his compassion for people with serious voice disorders. Boone is a past president of the American Speech-Language-Hearing Association and was instrumental in guiding that association to prominence. He is retired and lives in Tucson, Arizona, but still travels the world lecturing about voice disorders. Boone has a wonderful sense of humor. One of his passions is the card game Hearts.

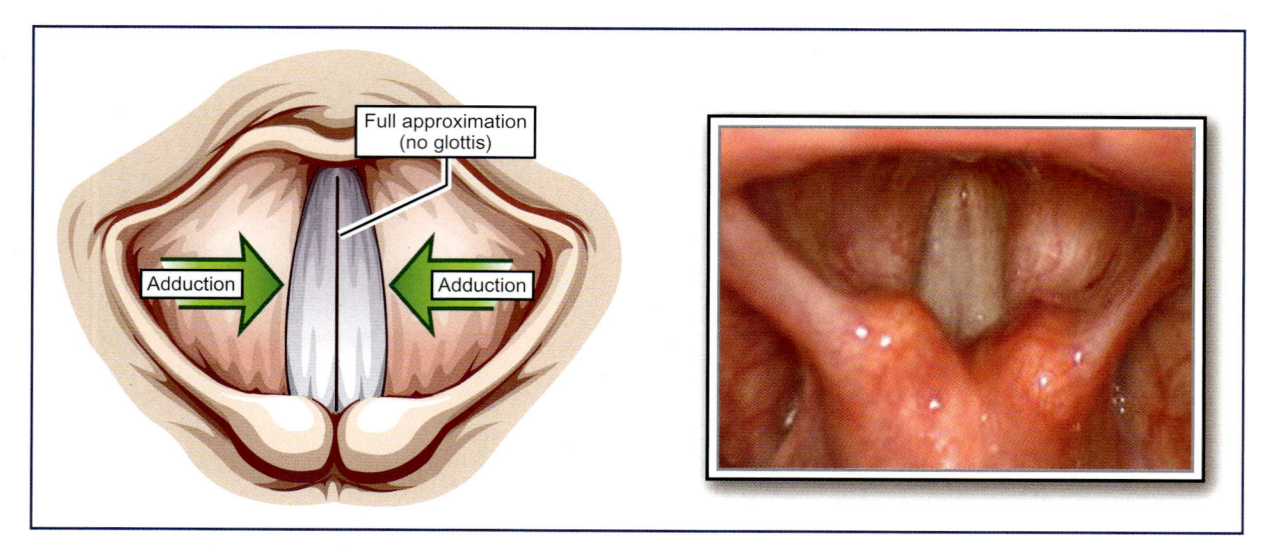

Figure 3–27. Vocal fold adduction. The *lateral cricoarytenoid* muscles adduct the front (membranous) portion of the vocal folds and the *arytenoid* muscles adduct the back (cartilaginous) portion of the vocal folds. The amount of vocal fold contact in the vertical dimension can be adjusted by bulging of the medial surfaces through contraction of the *thyrovocalis* muscles. The image on the right is a photograph of an author's vocal folds (courtesy of Robin Samlan).

The force of contact is adjusted by actions of the *lateral cricoarytenoid* muscles and the *arytenoid* muscles that squeeze the vocal folds together. The squeezing force exerted between the vocal processes of the arytenoid cartilages by the *lateral cricoarytenoid* muscles has been called medial compression (van den Berg et al., 1960). Medial compression can be applied even when the vocal folds are separated along their cartilaginous length.

Vocal Fold Length Change

The length of the vocal folds can be changed through a variety of external and internal adjustments. The length changes that are most important to speech production are mediated through the cricothyroid joints. Length changes can also be mediated through the cricoarytenoid joints.

The vocal fold length changes that are mediated through the cricothyroid joints are best understood in the context of approximated vocal folds, as illustrated in Figure 3–28. Vocal fold lengthening (upper images in Figure 3–28) is achieved by forward directed forces pulling on the front ends of the vocal folds at their points of attachment to the inside of the thyroid cartilage and/or by backward directed forces pulling on the back ends of the vocal folds at their points of attachment to the vocal processes of the arytenoid cartilages. Forward directed forces result from contraction of the *cricothyroid* muscles, which place pulls on the front ends of the thyroid and cricoid cartilages that tend to close the visor angle of the larynx by rocking the thyroid cartilage on the cricoid cartilage and/or rocking the cricoid cartilage on the thyroid cartilage. The consequence of any combination of rocking of the front ends of these two cartilages toward one another is an increase in the distance between the front of the thyroid cartilage and the vocal processes of the arytenoid cartilages and a forward stretching of the vocal folds. Actions of the *cricothyroid* muscles (especially the *pars oblique* portions) can also cause a sliding movement at the cricothyroid joints that increases the distance between the front of the thyroid cartilage and the vocal processes of the arytenoid cartilages and contributes to vocal fold lengthening.

Actions of the *posterior cricoarytenoid* muscles counteract those of the *cricothyroid* muscles and serve to anchor the arytenoid cartilages and their vocal processes from forward tilting and sliding during contractions of the *cricothyroid* muscles. The *posterior cricoarytenoid* muscles may also lengthen the vocal folds somewhat by pulling the arytenoid cartilages backward and upward along the facets on the slope of the cricoid rim. Thus, the *cricothyroid* muscles are responsible for stretching the vocal folds to a greater length in a forward direction, whereas the *posterior cricoarytenoid* muscles are responsible for securing the back ends of the vocal folds or for stretching them to a greater length in a rearward direction.

Shortening of the vocal folds (lower images in Figure 3–28) results from relaxation of the distending muscles just discussed (*cricothyroid* and *posterior cricoarytenoid* muscles) or from concentric contractions of the *thyroarytenoid* muscles. Because the *thyroarytenoid* muscles constitute the main mass of the vocal folds, their contraction shortens the vocal folds and their internal fibers. If unopposed by actions of other muscles of the larynx, *thyroarytenoid* muscle contractions serve to draw the thyroid and arytenoid cartilages toward one another (pull the two ends of the vocal folds toward their respective centers lengthwise).

Vocal fold length changes also occur during abduction and adduction (see Figures 3–26 and 3–27) and are mediated through the cricoarytenoid joints. These length changes are the result of rocking and sliding of the arytenoid cartilages on the cricoid cartilage, which carries the tips of the vocal processes of the arytenoid cartilages upward, backward, and outward or downward, forward, and inward. Upward, backward, and outward movement of the vocal processes, as mediated through activation of the *posterior cricoarytenoid* muscles, abducts the vocal folds and lengthens them; downward, forward, and inward movement of the processes, as mediated through activation of the *lateral cricoarytenoid* muscles, adducts the vocal folds and shortens them.

Movements of the Ventricular Folds

The ventricular folds can move and change shape. Although the ventricular folds are usually widely separated and rounded toward the airway, under certain circumstances they may extend well into the airway to form a roof over the vocal folds. The ventricular folds may also tilt downward toward the vocal folds and even come in contact with them.

The muscular mechanisms underlying ventricular fold movements are not well understood. One suggestion is that the actions of other muscles in the vicinity of the ventricular folds combine to effect sphincter-like folding and unfolding of the interior of the larynx that moves and shapes the passive ventricular folds (Fink, 1975; Zemlin, 1998). Fibers of the *thyromuscularis* portions of *thyroarytenoid* muscles that course upward along the sidewalls of the larynx above the vocal folds may serve a special role in the enfolding influence on the ventricular folds (Reidenbach, 1998).

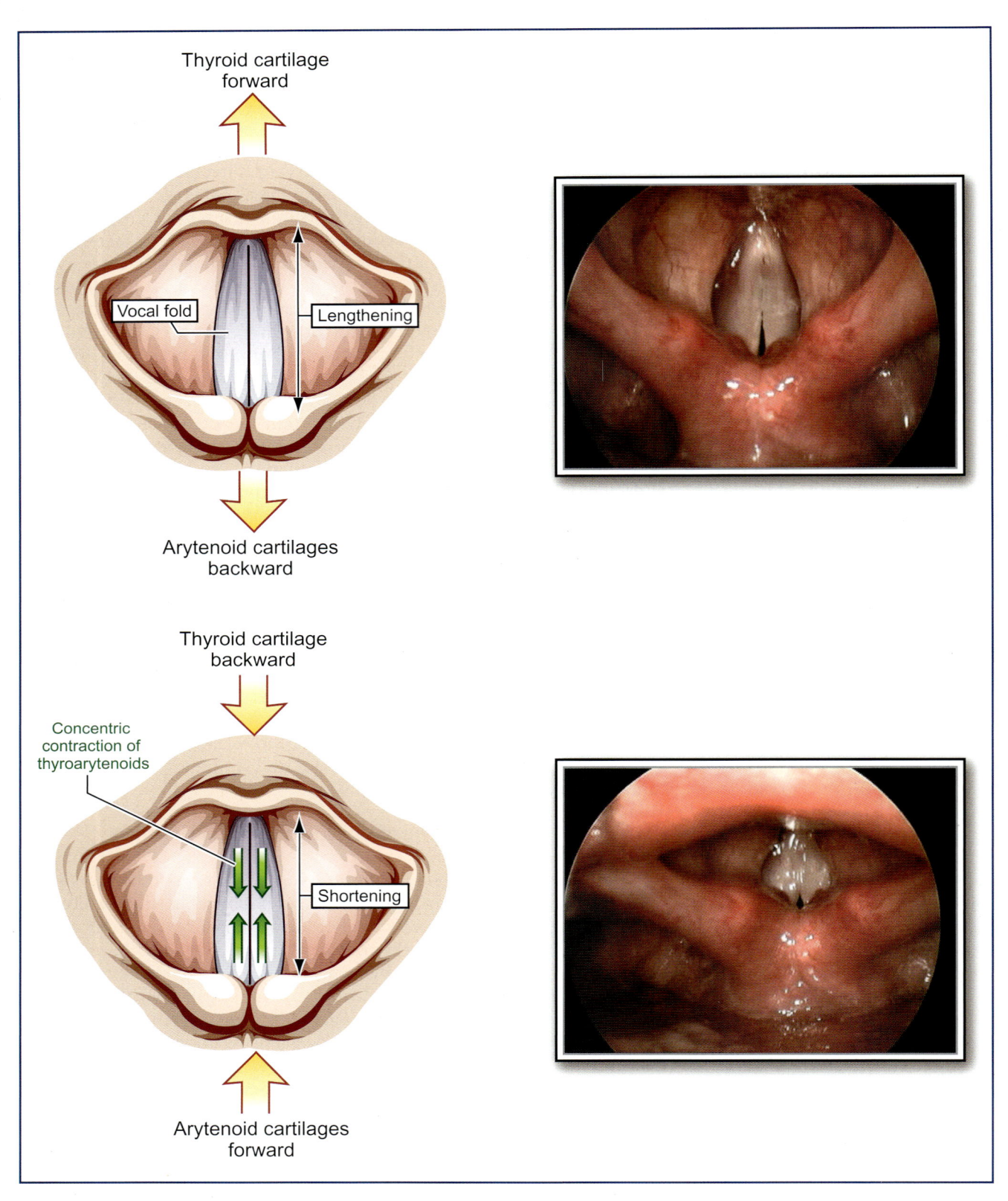

Figure 3-28. Vocal fold length changes mediated through the cricothyroid joints. Active vocal fold lengthening (*upper images*) is accomplished primarily by forward directed forces through contraction of the **cricothyroid** muscles (with possibly backward-directed forces exerted by the **posterior cricoarytenoid** muscles). Active vocal fold shortening (*lower images*) is accomplished primarily by contraction of the **thyroarytenoid** muscles. The images on the right are photographs of actual vocal folds (courtesy of Robin Samlan).

Movements of the Epiglottis

The epiglottis is usually oriented upright. From this position, it can be moved backward and downward to horizontal or beyond and thereby cover the laryngeal aditus. Downward movement of the epiglottis can also be segmental, such that just the upper third can be folded backward over the laryngeal aditus.

The epiglottis is cartilage only and has no motive force other than its own recoil properties and gravity and therefore its movements and shape changes are effected by external mechanisms. One mechanism is contraction of the *aryepiglottic* muscles, which can lower the epiglottis and/or alter its configuration by folding it inward upon itself from top-to-bottom and/or across. The other mechanism is elevation of the laryngeal housing, which forces the front of the epiglottis against the base of the tongue, compressing it backward and downward over the upper opening to the larynx. This action helps to protect the laryngeal airway and prevent the aspiration of food or liquid into the pulmonary apparatus during swallowing.

Movements of the Laryngeal Housing

The housing of the larynx can move within the neck. Although it can move in nearly all directions, the most important movement is vertical. The laryngeal housing can also be shifted forward or backward within the neck, having a potential for greater forward than backward movement from its resting position.

Extrinsic and supplementary laryngeal muscles are responsible for moving and stabilizing the laryngeal housing. These muscles act by direct pulls on the larynx as well as indirect pulls through insertions on the hyoid bone, as illustrated in Figure 3–29.

Upward movements of the laryngeal housing can be brought about by activation of one or a combination of muscles that includes the *thyrohyoid, digastric (anterior* and *posterior* bellies), *stylohyoid, mylohyoid, geniohyoid, hyoglossus,* and *genioglossus* muscles, and downward movements can result from activation of one or a combination of muscles that includes the *sternothyroid, sternohyoid,* and *omohyoid (anterior* and *posterior* bellies) muscles. Forward movements of the laryngeal housing can result from activation of one or a combination of muscles that includes the *sternothyroid, digastric (anterior* belly), *mylohyoid, geniohyoid,* and *genioglossus* muscles, and backward movements of the housing can be brought about through activation of one or a combination of muscles that includes the *omohyoid (anterior* and *posterior* bellies), *digastric (posterior* belly), and *stylohyoid* muscles.

Harry Hollien

Hollien has been a champion of the study of laryngeal function in the context of experimental phonetics for more than half a century. He pioneered the quantification of vocal fold correlates of voice fundamental frequency change, one of his most clever endeavors being his work on stroboscopic laminagraphy (phase-advanced frontal x-rays). He also contributed significantly to our understanding of factors influencing speech intelligibility in deep-water divers. Well known for his forensic studies on speaker identification, Hollien is widely considered the most celebrated expert witness in the world in matters involving the use of voice in the commission of crime. Hollien founded the American Association of Phonetic Sciences and has fostered the careers of many outstanding speech and voice scientists. A colorful and outspoken advocate for his professional passions, Hollien is one of the key figures in the history of experimental phonetics.

The larynx can also be fixed in position through different combinations of counteractive forces exerted by the muscles listed above. Fixation may include activation of the *inferior constrictor* muscle of the pharynx, which can stabilize the larynx against forward directed forces.

CONTROL VARIABLES OF LARYNGEAL FUNCTION

Several control variables are important in laryngeal function. Their relative significance depends on the particular activity being performed, whether it is breathing, speaking, singing, laughing, whistling, swallowing, coughing, panting, bearing down, weight-lifting, or wind instrument playing. For example, singing requires certain fine adjustments based on acoustic goals, whereas swallowing does not; stiffness of the vocal folds may be important for adjusting fundamental frequency (pitch) of the voice, but inconsequential for whistling.

Discussion is devoted to five control variables that influence laryngeal function. These are: (a) laryngeal opposing pressure, (b) laryngeal airway resistance, (c) glottal size and configuration, (d) stiffness of the vocal folds, and (e) effective mass of the vocal folds.

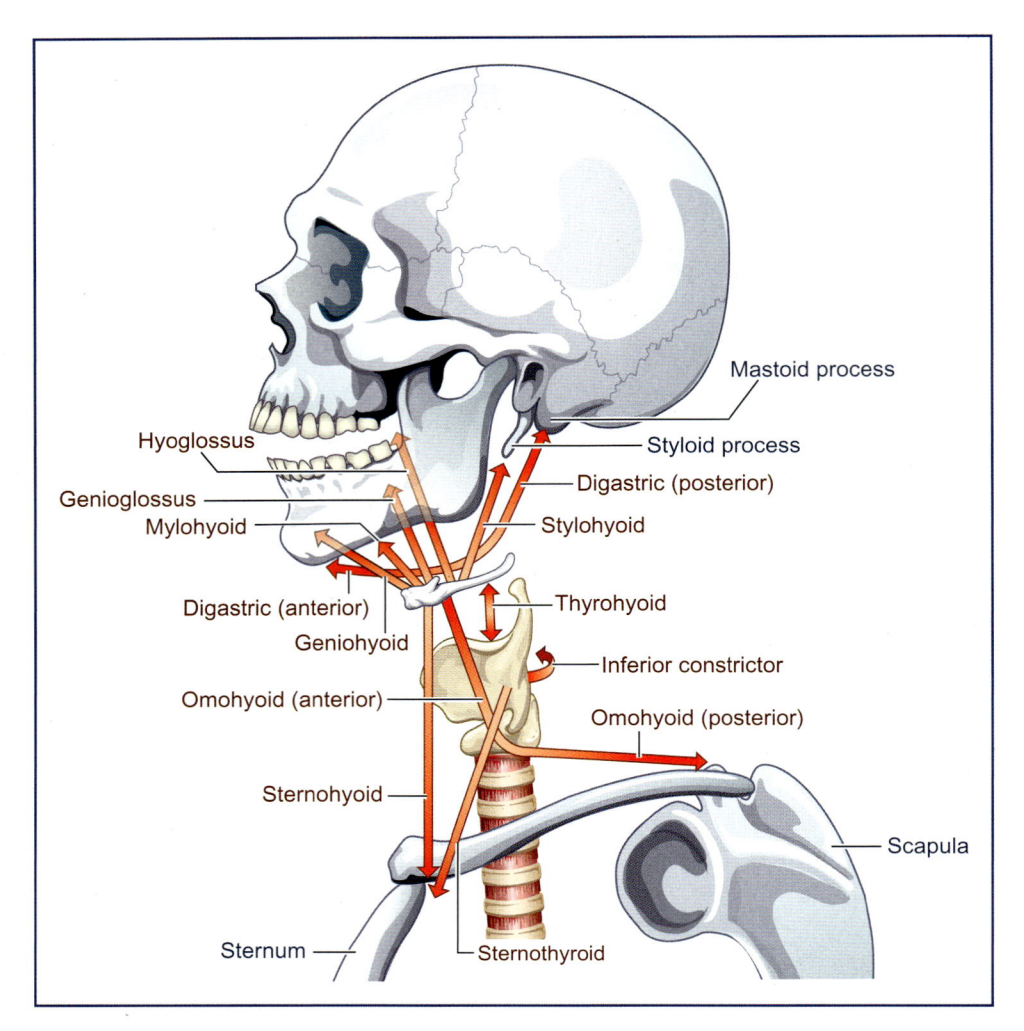

Figure 3–29. Actions of extrinsic and supplementary laryngeal muscles on the laryngeal housing. These actions, alone or in combination, can move the larynx upward, downward, forward, and/or backward. They can also fix the larynx in position through counteractive forces.

Laryngeal Opposing Pressure

Laryngeal opposing pressure is a measure of the opposition provided by the larynx to translaryngeal air pressure (the air pressure difference between the trachea and pharynx) when the larynx is closed airtight (Hixon & Minifie, 1972). This opposition is represented by the force provided at the level of the larynx to maintain it in a closed configuration despite positive or negative aeromechanical forces that tend to either blow or suck it open. As illustrated in Figure 3–30, laryngeal opposing pressure is the net opposing pressure and has three components: (a) compressive muscular pressure that "squeezes" the closed larynx and holds the vocal folds together, (b) surface tension between the apposed surfaces of the moist vocal folds that holds them together, and (c) gravity that weighs down the vocal folds and influences them differently in different body positions (or different gravity fields). Of these three, compressive muscular pressure by far is the greatest contributor to laryngeal opposing pressure. The laryngeal opposing pressure required to effect airtight closure of the larynx can range from low to high, depending on the nature of the activity.

Laryngeal Airway Resistance

Laryngeal airway resistance is a measure of the opposition provided by the larynx to airflow through it. Such

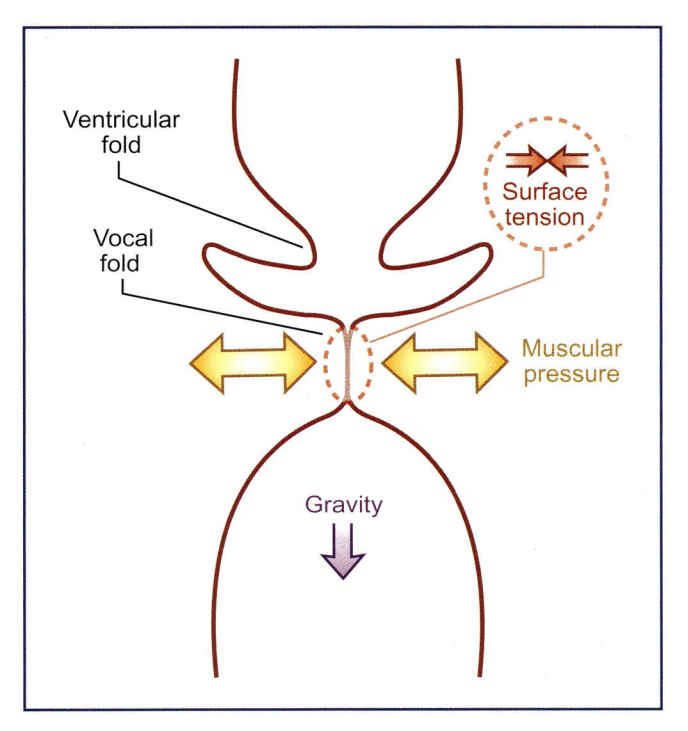

Figure 3–30. Laryngeal opposing pressure has three components. These are muscular pressure (by far the greatest contributor to laryngeal opposing pressure), surface tension between the surfaces of the moist vocal folds, and gravity.

resistance is a property of the airway itself. Because the main constriction within the larynx is at the level of the vocal folds, this region of the larynx is the foremost contributor to laryngeal airway resistance. The ventricular folds are a secondary contributor. Thus, by adjusting the cross-sectional area and/or length of the internal larynx in the region of the vocal folds and ventricular folds, the laryngeal airway resistance will likely change. Resistance increases with increasing constriction and length of constriction. It also is important to note that laryngeal airway resistance is airflow dependent. This means that even at a fixed cross-sectional area and/or length of the laryngeal airway, resistance is influenced by how fast air is moving (van den Berg, Zantema, & Doornenbal, 1957). Laryngeal airway resistance is not measurable, but is calculated from the quotient of translaryngeal air pressure to translaryngeal airflow (see Chapter 6 for description of calculation). Laryngeal airway resistance can range from a very low resistance (wide open airway) to infinity (airtight closure of the airway) as illustrated in Figure 3–31.

Glottal Size and Configuration

The glottis can be adjusted to change length, diameter, area, and shape as shown in Figure 3–32. Maximum

Needling the Teacher

One way to tap tracheal pressure is to puncture the trachea with a hypodermic needle. We know someone whose tracheal pressure was studied this way. The physician inserted the needle (attached to a syringe), but had difficulty on the first attempt. He withdrew the needle and made a successful second insertion. After the study, the person went off to teach. Shortly into the lecture, a pea-size bump rose on his neck. As the lecture continued, the bump enlarged to walnut size. Seeing it continue to grow, a student told the teacher what was happening. In the emergency room, it was discovered that the teacher had emphysema (air inflation) within the interstices (spaces) inside his neck. Some air had apparently been pumped into the interstices during attempts at needle insertion. When the teacher raised internal pressures to speak, this air was forced to the surface and made his neck balloon. Never again did he allow himself to be needled.

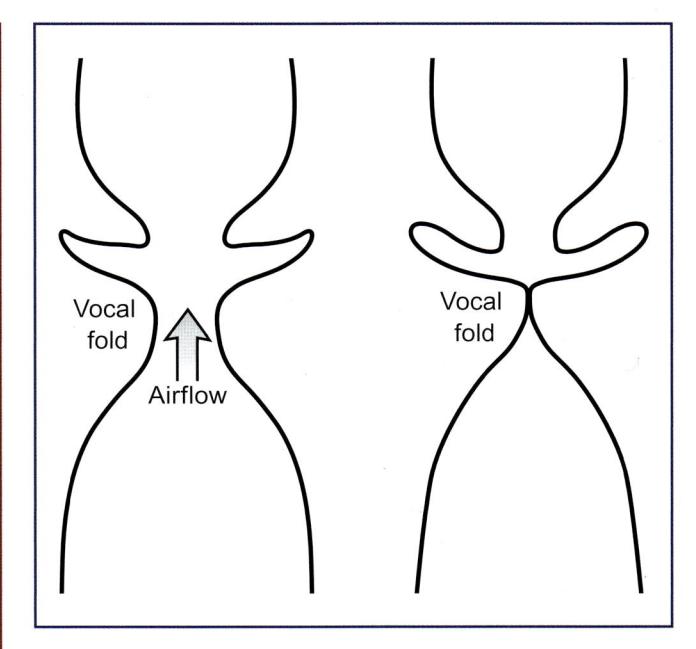

Figure 3–31. Laryngeal airway resistance, a calculated quantity that reflects the opposition provided by the larynx to airflow through it. It can range from very low (*left figure*) to infinite (*right figure*).

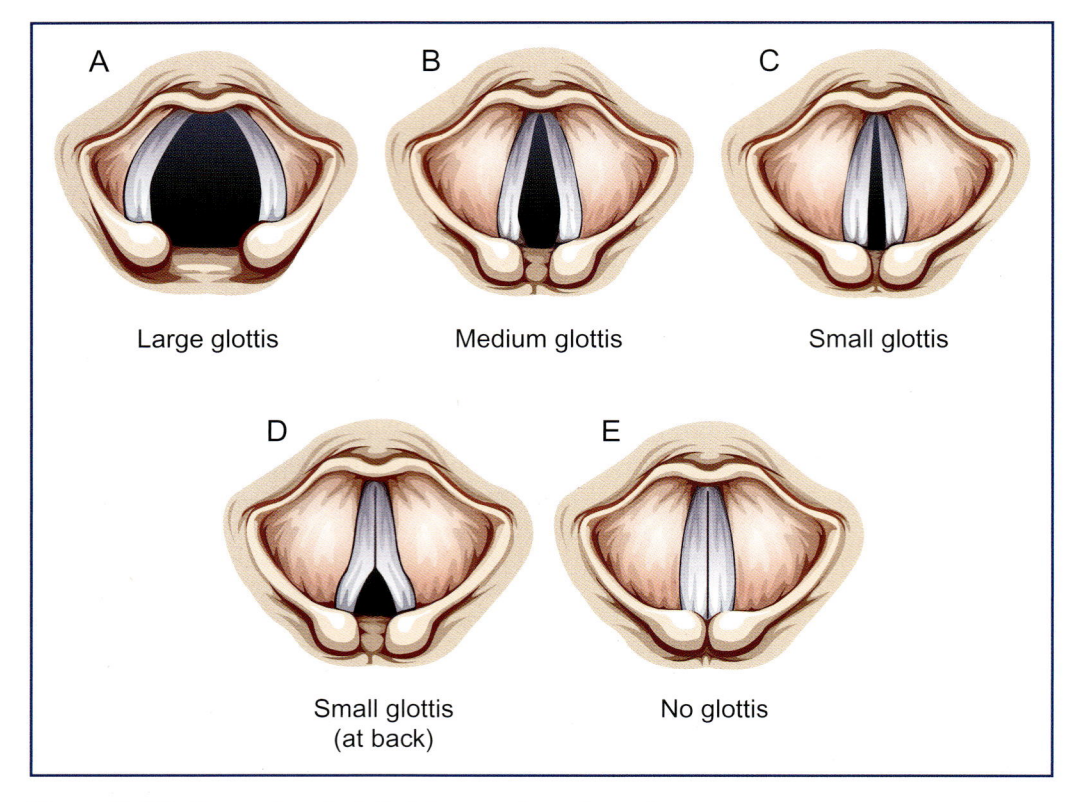

Figure 3–32. Examples of glottal sizes and configurations.

glottal size (A in the figure) can be achieved during a very deep inspiration following panting (Sekizawa, Sasaki, & Takishima, 1985). This is achieved mainly from contraction of the *posterior cricoarytenoid* muscles. A glottis of medium size (B in the figure) might be associated with resting tidal breathing. A small glottis may be achieved by simultaneous contraction of the *lateral cricoarytenoid* muscles and the *arytenoid* muscles (*transverse* and *oblique* subdivisions) to form a narrow glottis along the length of the vocal folds (C in the figure) or a small gap at the posterior part of the larynx (D in the figure) if just the *lateral cricoarytenoid* muscles are activated. Stronger activation of the *lateral cricoarytenoid* and *arytenoid* muscles can bring the vocal folds in full contact with one another so that the airway is closed airtight and there is no glottis (E in the figure).

Stiffness of the Vocal Folds

Stiffness of the vocal folds is an indication of their rigidity or tautness. Stiffness is the reciprocal of compliance and in physical terms conveys how much the vocal folds move for a given force applied to them. The stiffness of the vocal folds may differ somewhat from one location to another within the vocal folds. For example, the folds may be stiffer nearer their points of attachment to the thyroid and arytenoid cartilages than at their midpoints.

Vocal fold stiffness is adjusted primarily by lengthening the vocal folds (Titze, 1994). Vocal fold lengthening is accomplished primarily by contracting the *cricothyroid* muscles to increase their longitudinal tension, as illustrated on the left side of Figure 3–33. This is similar to the stretching of a guitar string by the turning of its tuning peg to tighten and tense the string. The tensile strength of the vocal ligaments along the medial edges of the vocal folds is the limiting factor as to how much the vocal folds can be stretched and how much longitudinal tension can be applied.

Vocal fold stiffness can also be changed by contracting muscles within the vocal folds themselves, as illustrated on the right side of Figure 3–33. Contractions of muscle fibers that lie within the lateral portions of the vocal folds (the *thyromuscularis* muscles) mainly stiffen those parts of the vocal folds, and contractions of the muscle fibers that lie within the medial portions of the vocal folds (the *thyrovocalis* muscles) mainly affect those portions. The more forceful the contraction, the greater the stiffness.

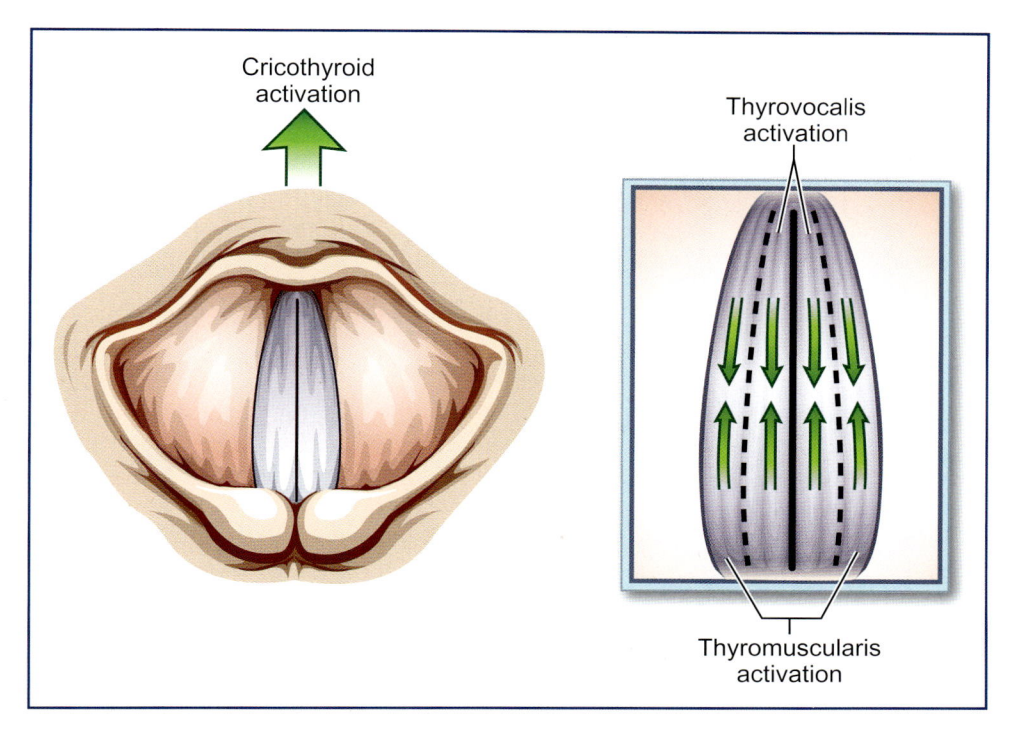

Figure 3–33. Vocal fold stiffness. Stiffness can be increased by contracting the *cricothyroid* muscles (thereby exerting longitudinal tension; *left figure*) and/or by contracting the *thyrovocalis* and *thyromuscularis* muscles (parts of the *thyroarytenoid* muscles) within the vocal folds (*right figure*).

Effective Mass of the Vocal Folds

Although the overall mass of the vocal folds does not change (at least on a moment-to-moment basis), the *effective* mass may change in the sense that only part of the vocal fold mass may participate in a given activity. Full mass and effective mass are the same when the vocal folds are fully abducted and maximally elongated and have unencumbered free margins along their lengths. Full mass and effective mass are different, however, when the vocal folds are partitioned by some action that encumbers them at some intermediate point along their lengths. An example can be seen in Figure 3–34 in the form of adductory adjustments of the vocal folds that are mediated through the cricoarytenoid joints, accomplished by activation of the *lateral cricoarytenoid* muscles, and manifested as medial compression between the tips of the vocal processes of the arytenoid cartilages. When the vocal processes of the arytenoid cartilages are made to toe inward sufficiently, the membranous portions of the vocal folds are approximated and their cartilaginous portions remain separated. Under this circumstance, the vocal folds are partitioned longitudinally into two masses having very different functional potentials. The membranous portion of the configuration impedes the flow of air through the larynx, whereas the cartilaginous portion allows air to pass freely. As medial compression increases (via increased activation of the *lateral cricoarytenoid* muscles), there may be a concomitant decrease in the effective mass of the membranous portions of the vocal folds that are able to vibrate during voice production (see section below on Fundamental Frequency).

NEURAL SUBSTRATES OF LARYNGEAL CONTROL

Laryngeal movement is controlled by the nervous system. The nature of such movement and the nature of its control are different for different activities (for example, coughing, throat clearing, crying, singing, speaking, and swallowing).

All control commands to the laryngeal apparatus are sent through cranial nerves that originate in the brainstem and cervical spinal nerves that originate within the uppermost segments of the spinal cord. These nerves provide motor innervation to the intrinsic, extrinsic, and supplementary muscles of the laryngeal

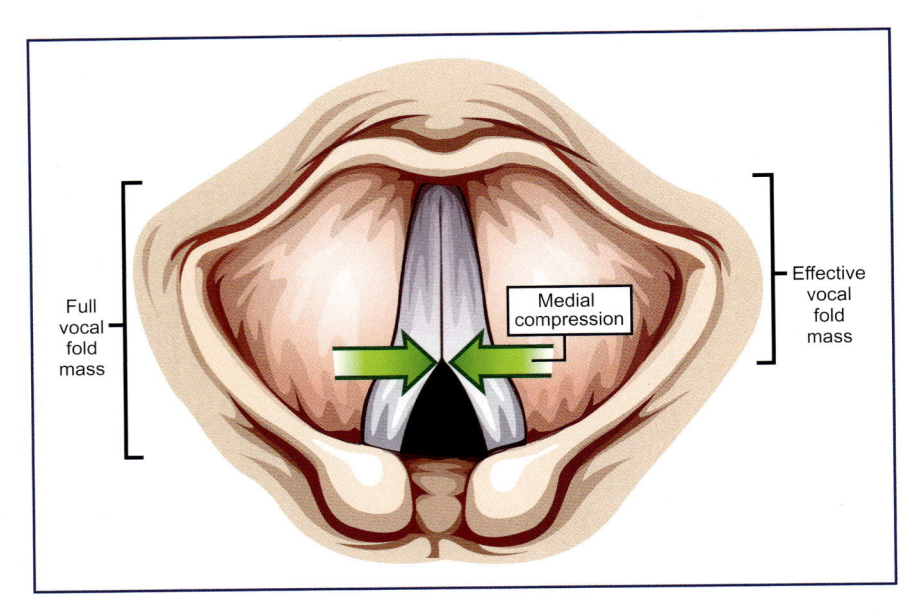

Figure 3–34. Effective vocal fold mass. Forceful medial compression by contraction of the **lateral cricoarytenoid** muscles can reduce the effective mass of the membranous portions of the vocal folds for an activity such as vocal fold vibration.

apparatus. As shown in Table 3–1, motor innervation to the laryngeal apparatus is effected by cranial nerves V (trigeminal), VII (facial), X (vagus), and XII (hypoglossal) and cervical spinal nerves C1, C2, and C3.

Innervation to the five intrinsic muscles of the larynx is through cranial nerve X (vagus). As cranial nerve X leaves the brainstem and descends in the neck it gives off two main branches to innervate intrinsic muscles of the larynx. These are the superior laryngeal nerve and the recurrent laryngeal nerve. The recurrent laryngeal nerve (also called the inferior laryngeal branch) provides motor supply to four intrinsic muscles, the *thyroarytenoid, posterior cricoarytenoid, lateral cricoarytenoid,* and *arytenoid*. The remaining intrinsic muscle of the larynx, the *cricothyroid*, receives its motor supply from the external branch of the superior laryngeal nerve. There is variation among larynges in the way specific nerves branch on their way to the larynx and how they interconnect with other nerves (Sanders, Wu, Mu, & Biller, 1993; Sanudo et al., 1999). For example, the recurrent laryngeal nerve has been shown to bifurcate or trifurcate before entering into the left or right sides of the larynx in more than a third of larynges studied (Beneragama & Serpell, 2006).

Innervation of the three extrinsic muscles of the larynx is provided by cervical spinal nerves for the *sternothyroid* (C1, C2, and C3) and *thyrohyoid* (C1 and C2) muscles, whereas the *inferior constrictor* muscle of the pharynx is supplied by branches of cranial nerve X. The eight supplementary muscles of the laryngeal apparatus receive their motor innervation in various combinations through cranial nerves V, VII, and XII and cervical spinal nerves C1, C2, and C3. The *sternohyoid* and *omohyoid* muscles receive motor supply from C1, C2, and C3; the *geniohyoid* muscle from C1; and the *hyoglossus* and *genioglossus* muscles are supplied by cranial nerve XII. The remaining three supplementary muscles are innervated by cranial nerves V and/or VII. The *digastric* muscle receives motor innervation from both cranial nerves, its *anterior* belly from cranial nerve V and its *posterior* belly from cranial nerve VII (Dickson & Maue-Dickson, 1982). The *stylohyoid* and *mylohyoid* muscles receive motor innervation from cranial nerves VII and V, respectively.

Laryngeal adjustments are not executed without information about their consequences. This is especially true for activities in which rapid and precise movements are at a premium, such as those that are characteristic of vocal fold adjustments. Sensory information is critical to the control of such movements. This information comes from several sources, the relative importance of which depends on the activity being performed. These sources have in common some type of mechanoreceptor that converts a mechanical event into a neural signal that is then transmitted along a sensory nerve to the central nervous system.

Mechanoreceptors are distributed throughout the larynx in its muscles, joints, and mucosal cover-

Table 3–1. Summary of the Cranial and Segmental Origins of the Motor Nerve Supply to the Muscles of the Laryngeal Apparatus

MUSCLE	INNERVATION
INTRINSIC	
Thyroarytenoid	X (recurrent)
Posterior cricoarytenoid	X (recurrent)
Lateral cricoarytenoid	X (recurrent)
Arytenoid	X (recurrent)
Cricothyroid	X (external branch of superior laryngeal nerve)
EXTRINSIC	
Sternothyroid	C1, C2, C3
Thyrohyoid	C1, C2
Inferior constrictor	X
SUPPLEMENTARY	
Sternohyoid	C1, C2, C3
Omohyoid	C1, C2, C3
Digastric	V, VII
Stylohyoid	VII
Mylohyoid	V
Geniohyoid	C1
Hyoglossus	XII
Genioglossus	XII

Note. Cranial nerves include V (trigeminal), VII (facial), X (vagus), and XII (hypoglossal). Spinal nerves include the first three cervical spinal nerves (C1, C2, C3). Cranial nerve X includes a recurrent laryngeal nerve and a superior laryngeal nerve. Muscles are categorized as intrinsic, extrinsic, or supplementary.

ings. Included among these are receptors that provide information about muscle lengths and their rates of length change (Konig & von Leden, 1961b; Okamura & Katto, 1988; Sanders, Han, Wang, & Biller, 1998), joint movements (Jankovskaya, 1959; Kirchner & Wyke, 1965), and mucosal deformations (Kirchner & Suzuki, 1968; Konig & von Leden, 1961a; Sampson & Eyzaguirre, 1964). Such information is used to determine the mechanical status of the larynx and to elicit certain reflexive behaviors. Much remains to be known about the contribution of mechanoreceptors during laryngeal adjustments. Presumably they function as part of an integrated laryngeal feedback system (Orlikoff & Kahane, 1996). For laryngeal adjustments that target sound production, such a system would also have to take into account information provided by another type of mechanoreceptor, hair cells within the cochlea of the auditory system (via cranial nerve VIII).

Less than full agreement exists about which cranial and spinal nerves and branches convey sensory information from different structures of the larynx to the central nervous system (Dickson & Maue-Dickson, 1982). Most agree that the internal branch of the superior laryngeal nerve (part of cranial nerve X) carries sensory information from the mucosa that covers the supraglottal region of the laryngeal cavity, including the base of the tongue, epiglottis, aryepiglottic folds, and backs of the arytenoid cartilages. This nerve is also believed to transmit information from mechanoreceptors in the muscles of the larynx that respond to stretch (Duffy, 2013). There is general agreement that the recurrent laryngeal nerve (part of cranial nerve X) carries sensory information from the mucosa and structures that are located below the vocal folds. Sensory information from the extrinsic and supplementary muscles travels via several different nerves. For example, the *mylohyoid* and *stylohyoid* muscles are served by sensory components of cranial nerves V and VII, respectively, whereas the *digastric* muscle is served by sensory components of both cranial nerves V and VII.

LARYNGEAL FUNCTIONS

The larynx performs a variety of functions. Those considered here relate to the degree of coupling between the trachea and pharynx, protection of the pulmonary airways, containment of the pulmonary air supply, and sound generation.

Degree of Coupling Between the Trachea and Pharynx

Actions of the larynx determine the degree of coupling between the trachea and pharynx. Such coupling is usually adjusted by changing the positions of the vocal folds, though other laryngeal structures may also participate. The trachea and pharynx are fully coupled during tidal breathing when the vocal folds are abducted and the laryngeal airway is open so that air can move easily to and from the pulmonary apparatus. In contrast, they are decoupled during coughing when the laryngeal airway closes momentarily so that tracheal pressure can build before the cough is abruptly released to blow substance away from the trachea and lower airways.

> **Get Thee Out**
>
> Reflexive coughing is our friend. It serves to clear the breathing airway via a powerful and violent explosion or series of such explosions. Your own experience with uncontrollable coughing is evidence of just how dedicated the pulmonary apparatus and laryngeal apparatus are to keeping things out of your lungs. Enormous air pressures and airflows are generated during reflexive coughing that cause violent movements of the vocal folds. Excessive reflexive coughing can be abusive to the larynx, lead to unpleasant symptoms, and result in voice disorders. Less violent coughing done voluntarily and repeatedly over long periods can have similar cumulative effects. Then there is the equally notorious family cousin, the bad habit of continual throat clearing. Less outgoing than its other two relatives (pun intended), frequent throat clearing can be grating on the vocal folds. Abuse not thy larynx.

Protection of the Pulmonary Airways

The pulmonary airways are a major part of the respiratory lifeline and the maintenance of their integrity is critical. The larynx, being positioned at the juncture between the pulmonary airways and the so-called upper airway (pharyngeal cavity, oral cavity, nasal cavities), is strategically located to protect the pulmonary airways from the invasion of foreign matter. Its role is particularly critical during swallowing, given that the main food channel (from the mouth to the esophagus) and the main air channel (from the nose and mouth to the larynx) cross paths just above the larynx. Thus, during swallowing, the laryngeal airway must be closed to prevent food or liquid from entering the trachea. This closure is accomplished by approximation of the vocal folds and other laryngeal structures and includes a brief period of apnea (breath holding).

Containment of the Pulmonary Air Supply

Closure of the laryngeal valve is important to containment of the pulmonary air supply for activities that require the generation of high pressures at different locations within the torso (abdominal, pleural, alveolar, tracheal) and/or the fixation of structures of the torso (rib cage wall, diaphragm, abdominal wall). Closure of the laryngeal valve to raise internal pressure is critical to forceful acts such as defecation, parturition (child birth), and lifting heavy objects.

Sound Generation

Sound generation by the larynx can be of several types, three of which are most relevant to the concerns of this chapter. They are transient (popping) sounds (in which the airstream is momentarily obstructed and then abruptly released), turbulence (hissing) sounds (in which air is forced through a narrowed airway), and quasi-periodic (buzzing) sounds (in which the vocal folds are forced into vibration and move rapidly to and fro to interrupt the airstream repeatedly). The last of these generates voice and is what gives the larynx its popular designation as the "voice box."

LARYNGEAL FUNCTION IN SPEECH PRODUCTION

Laryngeal function in speech production is complex and takes many forms. Four of these forms are discussed here. They are transient noise production, sustained turbulence noise production, sustained voice production, and running speech activities.

> **Tick Tock**
>
> Anyone who has played music to the beat of a metronome knows how maddening it can be. When just learning the music, it's a challenge to keep up. Then, once you have the music mastered, it seems like you have to slow down to be on pace. But something has to set the pace, like a conductor of an orchestra. The larynx usually does this during speech production. It's the metronome of the speech production apparatus. The movements of other speech production structures are constrained by what the larynx does. It does no good to get to a position before the larynx because then you'll just have to wait. And if you arrive at a position later than the time specified by the larynx, you have big problems. It's not quite as simple as we've portrayed, but it's close enough to give you the idea. Maybe you've heard the nursery rhyme "Hickory, dickory, dock, the voice box is the clock." Well, maybe not, because it was just written.

Transient Noise Production

A transient (very brief duration) utterance can be produced at the level of the larynx in the form of a sudden explosive burst. This constitutes a glottal stop-plosive that is analogous to the downstream production of the voiceless stop-plosives consonants /p/, /t/, and /k/. As depicted in Figure 3–35, glottal stop-plosive production involves an initial blockage of the laryngeal airstream by full adduction of the vocal folds. Air pressure then builds up within the tracheal space. This is followed by an abrupt release of the vocal fold adductory force and a simultaneous abrupt release of the pent-up air (Rothenberg, 1968; Stevens, 2000).

The speed with which air flows through the rapidly opening laryngeal airway is very high and gives rise to the generation of a brief burst of noise that excites the pharyngeal-oral airway. The sudden release of pent-up air creates an impulse-like popping sound at the glottis (Broad, 1973) and bears analogy to the discharge of an electrical capacitor through a time-varying resistance (Fant, 1960). The noise excitation during the release causes the pharyngeal-oral airway to vibrate throughout its entire length and to produce a plosive utterance that is distinctly lower in pitch than the pitches associated with other stop-plosives generated by the tongue and lips.

Sustained Turbulence Noise Production

Major constrictions cause air to flow turbulently. This means that air tumbles on itself, forming eddies (back flows), burbles (bubbles), and other irregularities. This agitation of air results in the generation of turbulence (friction) noise that contains a broad range of frequencies. The specific spectrum (frequency and sound pressure level content) of this noise depends on the nature of the interaction between the airstream and the constriction (Fant, 1960; Hixon, 1966; Minifie, 1973; Stevens, 2000).

Sustained noise can be produced by constriction of the laryngeal airway, typically at the level of the vocal folds. A common example is the production of the glottal fricative /h/, as illustrated in Figure 3–36. Glottal fricative production can be achieved by positioning the vocal folds well inward to form a long slit-like constriction.

Another example of sustained noise production is whispering. Whispering can also be accomplished

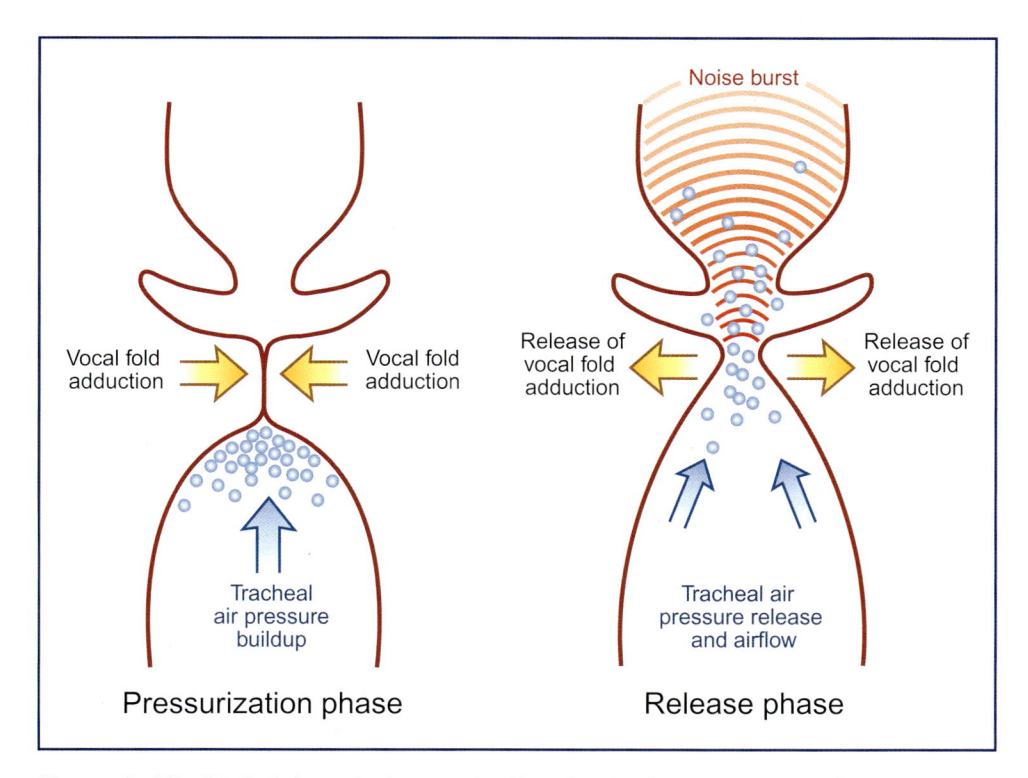

Figure 3–35. Glottal stop-plosive production. Production begins with full adduction of the vocal folds and buildup of tracheal air pressure followed by an abrupt release of the vocal fold adductory force and simultaneous release of tracheal air.

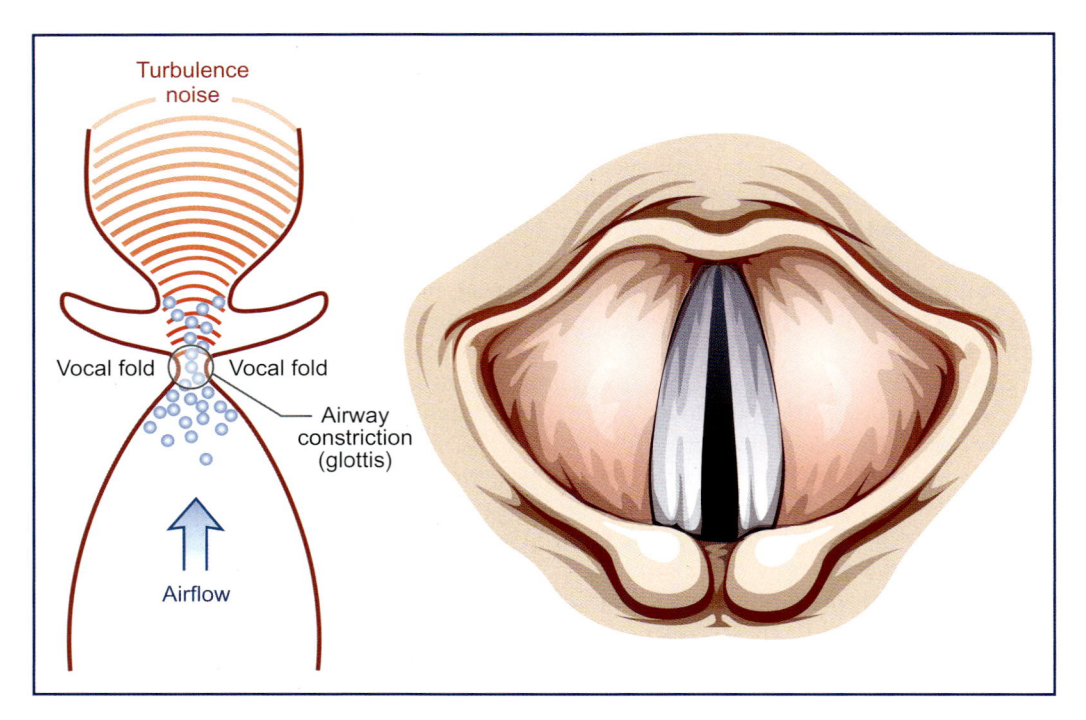

Figure 3–36. Glottal voiceless fricative production. Air is forced through a small laryngeal constriction causing the air molecules to tumble on themselves and create turbulence noise. This form of noise is associated with production of the glottal fricative /h/ and whispering.

with a long slit-like constriction, but is often accompanied by other glottal configurations. One of the most frequent of these is a rearward-facing Y configuration in which the membranous front parts of the vocal folds are firmly approximated (as in Figure 3–32 panel D), loosely approximated, or not approximated at all and the cartilaginous rear parts of the vocal folds are relatively far apart (Monoson & Zemlin, 1984; Rubin, Praneetvataku, Gherson, & Moyer, 2006; Solomon, McCall, Trosset, & Gray, 1989; Zemlin, 1998). This configuration is achieved by contracting the *lateral cricoarytenoid* muscles so that the vocal processes of the arytenoids cartilages toe inward, while leaving the *arytenoid* muscles less active or inactive.

Glottal configuration during whispering does not appear to change with changes in loudness (Solomon et al., 1989). This suggests that it may be the size of the glottis, rather than its specific configuration, that is the more important variable. It also appears that changes in the frequency content and sound pressure level of the whispered noise are most influenced by the magnitude of the tracheal air pressure generated by the breathing apparatus and the resultant flow of air through the larynx (Hixon, Minifie, & Tait, 1967). Quiet whispering, when compared with voicing, has been shown to be produced with relatively low tracheal air pressure, relatively high translaryngeal airflow, and relatively low laryngeal airway resistance (Konnai, Scherer, Peplinski, & Ryan, 2017; Stathopoulos, Hoit, Hixon, Watson, & Solomon, 1991; Sundberg, Scherer, Hess, & Muller, 2010). Loud whispering, compared with quiet whispering, is produced with higher tracheal pressure, higher translaryngeal airflow, and similar laryngeal airway resistance (Konnai et al., 2017).

Sustained Voice Production

Voice (the acoustic product of voice production) results from vibration of the vocal folds. Such vibration modulates (chops up) the airstream. As depicted in Figure 3–37, the repeated, sudden decreases in airflow are what acoustically excite the upper airway (pharyngeal, oral, and nasal cavities) during voice production (Gauffin & Sundberg, 1989; Rothenberg, 1983). This section discusses the nature of vocal fold vibration during sustained voice production and various other aspects of voice, including fundamental frequency, sound pressure level, fundamental frequency-sound pressure level profiles, spectrum, and registers.

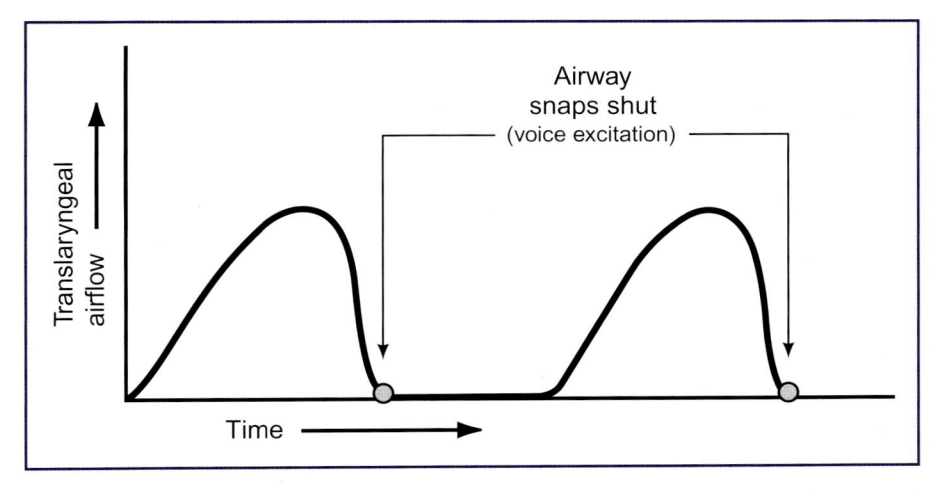

Figure 3–37. Voice source generation. The abrupt closures of the laryngeal airway and sudden airflow declination acoustically excite the upper airway to create voice.

Vocal Fold Vibration

Once vocal fold vibration is established, it proceeds in a relatively steady quasi-periodic fashion. Each vibration consists of lateral and medial excursions of the vocal folds that rapidly and repeatedly valve the expiratory airstream.

Individual vocal fold vibrations are *not* caused by muscular contractions that pull them apart and force them back together again. Rather, movements of the vocal folds are passive and akin to the movements of the lips when air is blown between them. (Try it. Moisten your lips, pucker up slightly, gently blow air through them, and feel them vibrate.) Muscular forces are important, but only in the sense that they set the vocal folds (or lips) in position to be moved passively to and fro by aeromechanical forces. Thus, a key element of the laryngeal adjustment for sustained vocal fold vibration is to position and hold the vocal folds in the airway so that vibration can be established and maintained by air pressures and airflows acting on the vocal folds (van den Berg, 1958). The conditions needed to sustain vocal fold vibration, once established, are a steady source of energy from the breathing apparatus and some form of nonlinear interaction with the structures being vibrated, namely, the vocal folds.

A single cycle of vocal fold vibration is depicted in Figure 3–38. Taking closure of the larynx (full approximation of the edges of the vocal folds) as a starting point, movement begins when the air pressure below

---

To or Fro and To and Fro

Is this title a misprint? No. It's about oscillation and vibration. Many writers use the terms "oscillation" and "vibration" as if they were interchangeable. Some dictionaries do likewise. But, in the strictly correct use of the two terms, they are not synonymous. Your late author, Tom Hixon, was adamant that an oscillation is a movement in one direction (either to or fro), whereas a vibration is a double oscillation in two directions (to and fro). He used as an example the term "oscilloscope," which is a device that can display signal change in one direction (or two, if you like), pointing out that it's not called a vibroscope. He went on to point out that if you read the box that your electrical fan came in, you'll see that it's called a double-oscillation fan (and could just as well be called a single-vibration fan). However, your other two authors are not so convinced. We have found alternative definitions—for example, oscillation is a to and fro movement, whereas vibration is a movement in many directions. Here is another example: oscillation is a repeated variation around a central value, whereas vibration refers specifically to mechanical oscillations. The bottom line is that oscillation and vibration apparently do not mean the same thing. We challenge the reader to figure out what the difference is.

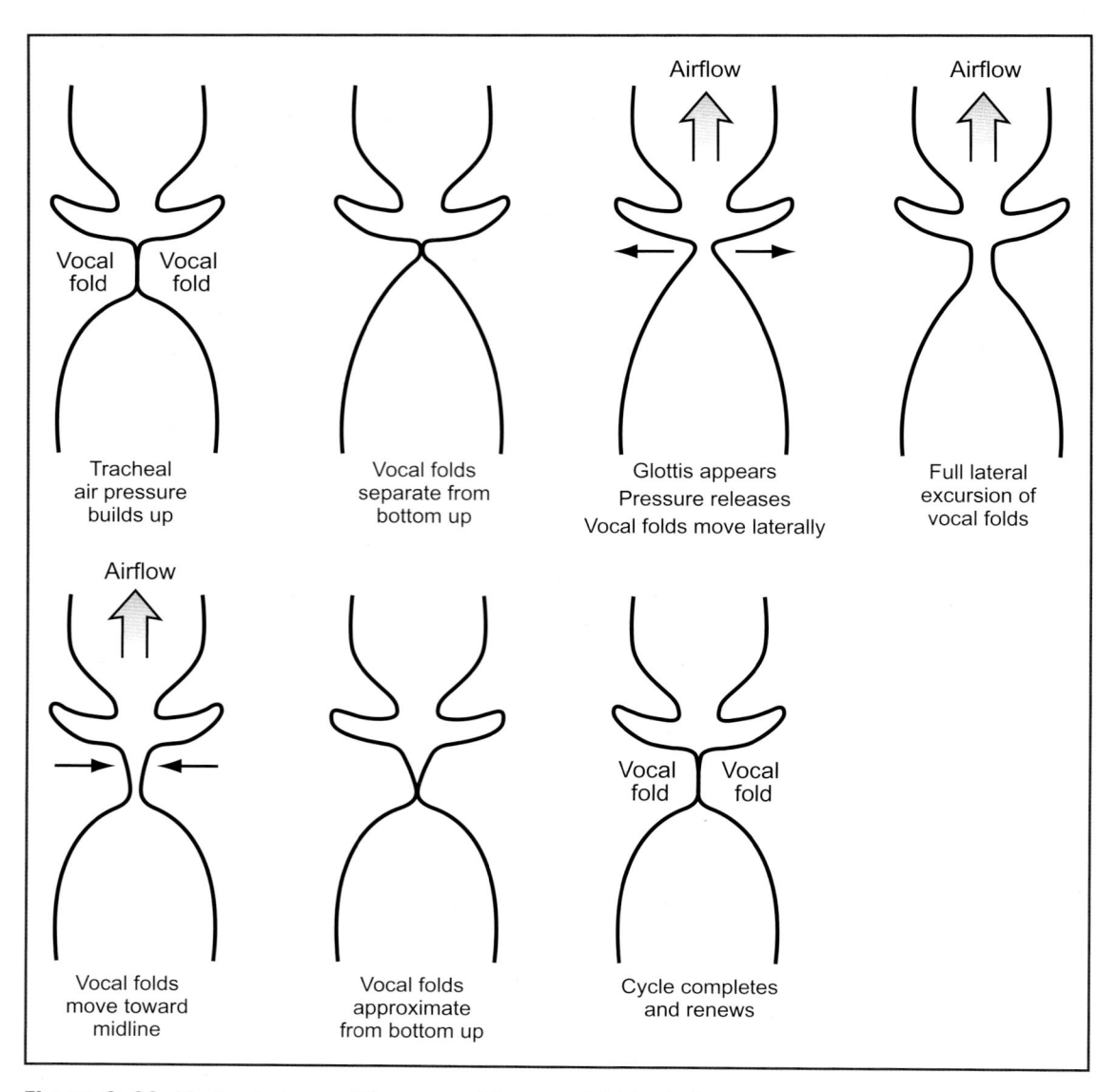

Figure 3-38. Vertical phase difference of the vocal folds during voice production. This figure represents a single vocal fold vibration cycle, beginning with the vocal folds approximated. The vocal folds are separated from bottom to top by air pressure until a glottis appears. Next, the vocal folds move laterally and then medially until they approximate again from bottom to top.

the vocal folds (tracheal air pressure) rises and forces the bottom edges of the two folds apart. This is followed by a forcing apart of the middle and upper parts of the folds. This pattern of lateral excursion of the vocal folds exhibits a so-called *vertical phase difference* in which lower points on the medial surfaces of the vocal folds are displaced earlier than points above them. A vertical phase difference is also manifested as the vocal folds move back together again. That is, lower points on the medial surfaces of the vocal folds move together before points on the upper surfaces move together (Hirano, Yoshida, & Tanaka, 1991; Schonharl, 1960; Timcke, von Leden, & Moore, 1958). These movements of the medial surfaces of the vocal folds occur because the covers of the vocal folds (consisting of the intermediate and superficial layer of the lamina propria and the epithelium; see Figure 3–13) are relatively loosely coupled to their muscular bodies (Story & Titze, 1995). Such movements have been described as vertically propagating mucosal waves (like surface waves on water) that progress within the covers of the vocal folds and whose rippling effects can be seen on the top surfaces of the vocal folds (Berke & Gerratt, 1993; Hirano, Kakita, Kawasaki, Gould, & Lambiase, 1981).

The vertical phase difference of vocal fold vibration has also been conceptualized as two primary modes of movement, one translational and one rotational (Berry & Titze, 1996; Story, 2002). The translational mode is the lateral movement of the vocal folds away from the midline and back again. The rotational mode is the rotation of the vocal fold cover around a pivot point located somewhere between the bottom and top of the medial surface (the location of the pivot point depends on factors such as muscle activation levels and hydration of the tissue). This is illustrated schematically in Figure 3–39.

An even more detailed look at a single cycle of vocal fold vibration is shown in Figure 3–40. When tracheal pressure rises and pushes the lower portion of the vocal folds apart, a convergent-shaped glottis is created (that is, wider at the bottom than the top), as illustrated in (A) in the figure. At this point in the vibratory cycle, the intraglottal air pressure (the pressure within the glottis) is relatively high, higher than the opposing recoil force being exerted by the vocal fold tissues. The intraglottal pressure pushes the vocal folds away from the midline until the restoring force exerted by the vocal folds exceeds the force exerted by the intraglottal pressure. At this point, the vocal folds begin to move inward toward the midline, starting from the bottom and rotating into a divergent-shaped glottis (narrower at the bottom than the top), as shown in (B) of Figure 3–40. As this divergent-shaped glottis is created, intraglottal pressure decreases rapidly because the air column above the vocal folds is continuing to flow toward the airway opening, leaving fewer air molecules within the glottis and just above it. This drop in intraglottal pressure, along with the recoil force of the vocal fold tissue, causes the vocal folds to move medially toward each other relatively rapidly.

Vibration of the vocal folds is self-sustained because the intraglottal pressure is relatively high as the vocal folds are moving outward (away from the midline), and it is relatively low as the vocal folds are moving inward (toward the midline). These conditions are created by two important factors. One factor is the dynamic nature of the glottal geometry, the alternating

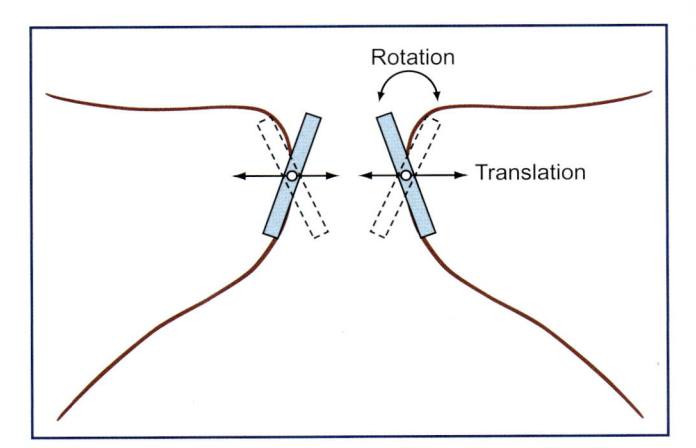

Figure 3-39. Two primary modes of vocal fold vibration. The translational mode constitutes the lateral movement of the vocal folds and the rotational mode is the rotation of the vocal fold cover around a pivot point (*open circle*). Modified after Story (2002).

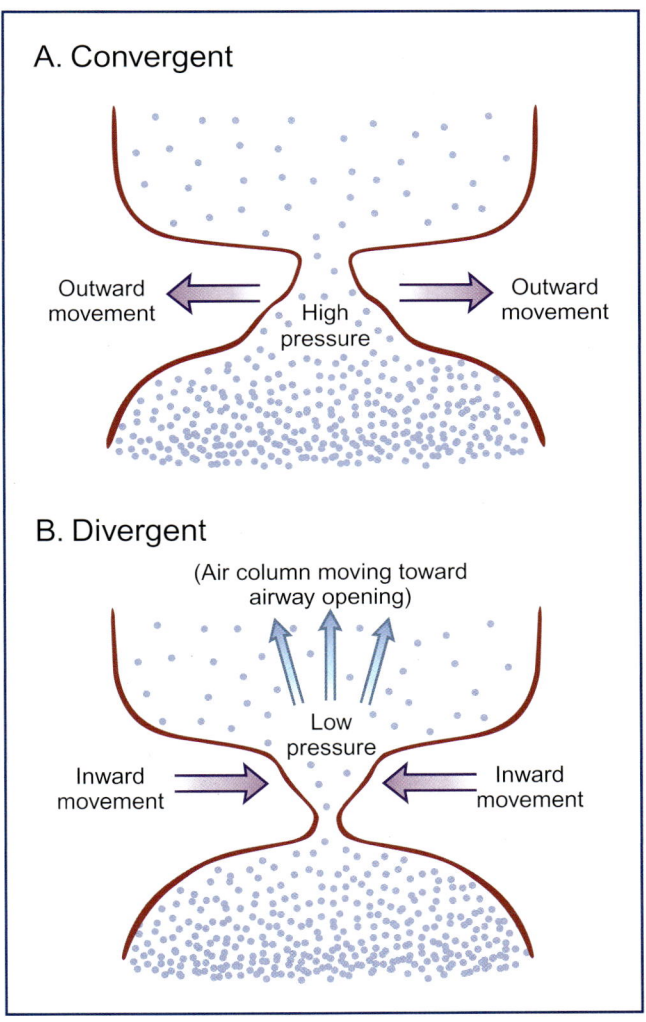

Figure 3-40. Convergent (**A**) and divergent (**B**) glottal shapes and associated intraglottal air pressure (the air pressure within the glottis) and vocal fold movements during a single vibration. When the glottis is in a convergent shape, intraglottal air pressure is high enough to overcome the tissue recoil forces and pushes the vocal folds away from each other. When the glottis is in a divergent shape, intraglottal pressure lowers and tissue recoil pressure moves the vocal folds back together.

> **Every Which Way**
>
> Despite current understanding of how the vocal folds vibrate to produce voice, it was only within the earlier part of the last century that scholars were unenlightened about many aspects of the process. Some scholars argued that voice resulted from up and down movements of the two vocal folds in opposite directions. Others believed that vocal fold movements during voice production were strictly horizontal and akin to stiff shutters that slid together and apart repeatedly. These incorrect guesses about how the vocal folds functioned during voice production were dispelled by data obtained with high-speed motion picture filming of the larynx. This technology enabled the study of the rapid movements of the vocal folds in precise detail. Thus, what earlier in the last century seemed to be "every which way" of vocal fold movement during voice production has settled down to the way they are as described in the adjacent text.

convergent and divergent shaped glottis. The other factor relates to the changes in airflow and air pressure just above the glottis. As the vocal folds move outward away from midline, airflow through the glottis increases and accelerates the column of air above it. This causes the air pressure above the vocal folds to build up and increase the already high intraglottal pressure, thereby driving the vocal folds outward. When the tissue recoil forces reverse the movement of the vocal folds so that they begin to move inward, the airflow through the glottis decreases, but the accelerated air column continues to move upward. This reduces the air pressure just above the vocal folds and helps lower intraglottal air pressure to allow an unimpeded return of the tissue toward midline (see Titze [2006a] for a more detailed explanation).

Fundamental Frequency

The fundamental frequency is the rate at which the vocal folds vibrate. Fundamental frequency can be changed over a very wide range, typically about three octaves (an octave is a doubling or a halving of frequency) for a young adult (Fairbanks, 1960). Fundamental frequency is usually expressed on a continuum in units of cycles per second or hertz (abbreviated Hz). It can also be expressed on a musical scale in semitones (the interval between two adjacent keys on a keyboard instrument) (Baken & Orlikoff, 2000). The average fundamental frequency of the human voice depends in large part on the size of the larynx and the sex of the individual, with men having lower average fundamental frequencies than women, and women having lower average fundamental frequencies than children. Control of change in fundamental frequency is vested primarily in adjustments of the vocal folds. Adjustments of the breathing apparatus have a supporting role in fundamental frequency control.

The strongest auditory-perceptual correlate of fundamental frequency is the pitch of the voice. Pitch is the subjective impression of the relative position of a sound along a musical scale. Sound pressure level and spectral content of the voice also influence the perception of pitch, but to far less important degrees than does the fundamental frequency. Thus, for the most part, a higher fundamental frequency is associated with a higher pitch and a lower fundamental frequency is associated with a lower pitch. In-depth coverage of the psychophysics of pitch perception is found in Chapter 14.

Vocal fold adjustments that influence fundamental frequency (and pitch) are those that determine the stiffness of the vocal folds and their effective vibrating mass, with stiffness generally considered to be the more important of the two factors (Stevens, 2000). The most important mechanisms for increasing vocal fold stiffness operate through external force exerted by the *cricothyroid* muscles and internal force exerted through the *thyroarytenoid* muscles. As discussed above and illustrated in Figure 3–33, contraction of the *cricothyroid* muscles tends to stretch the vocal folds and increase the force per unit length along them, whereas activation of the *thyroarytenoid* muscles (particularly the *thyrovocalis* part) tends to increase the stiffness of the muscular part of the vibrating vocal folds. It is the combined activities of these two pairs of muscles that are primarily responsible for setting the effective stiffness of the vocal folds and for controlling the fundamental frequency (Shipp & McGlone, 1971; Titze, 1994; Titze, Jiang, & Drucker, 1988; Titze, Luschei, & Hirano, 1989).

When moving up the musical scale from lower to higher fundamental frequencies, the relative activations of the *cricothyroid* and *thyroarytenoid* muscles tend to alternate. For example, *cricothyroid* muscle activity may increase the fundamental frequency of the voice by applying an external stretching force to the vocal folds over a limited range of fundamental frequencies and then *thyroarytenoid* muscle activity may further adjust fundamental frequency by exerting an internal force on the vocal folds. Once the upper limit of stiffness is reached, the *cricothyroid* muscle increases its level of activity again to set the next externally generated stiffness range and the *thyroarytenoid* muscle further adjusts internally to meet the stiffness demands of the fundamental frequency target. This alternation of activity is often referred to as a stair-step adjustment of stiffness (Hollien, 1960b).

The relative activations of the *cricothyroid* and *thyroarytenoid* muscles can vary substantially for the production of a given fundamental frequency (Titze & Story, 2002). This is represented in graphic form in Figure 3–41, with the relative activation of the *cricothyroid* muscle increasing upward and the relative activation of the *thyroarytenoid* muscle increasing rightward. This graph illustrates that a given fundamental frequency can be produced by a continuum of different combinations of muscular activities. For example, a fundamental frequency of 120 Hz can be produced by using relatively high activation of the *cricothyroid* muscles combined with relatively low activation of the *thyroarytenoid* muscles; alternatively, the same 120 Hz fundamental frequency can be produced using relatively low activation of the *cricothyroid* muscles and a relatively high activation of the *thyroarytenoid* muscles. Thus, the same fundamental frequency can be produced in many different ways.

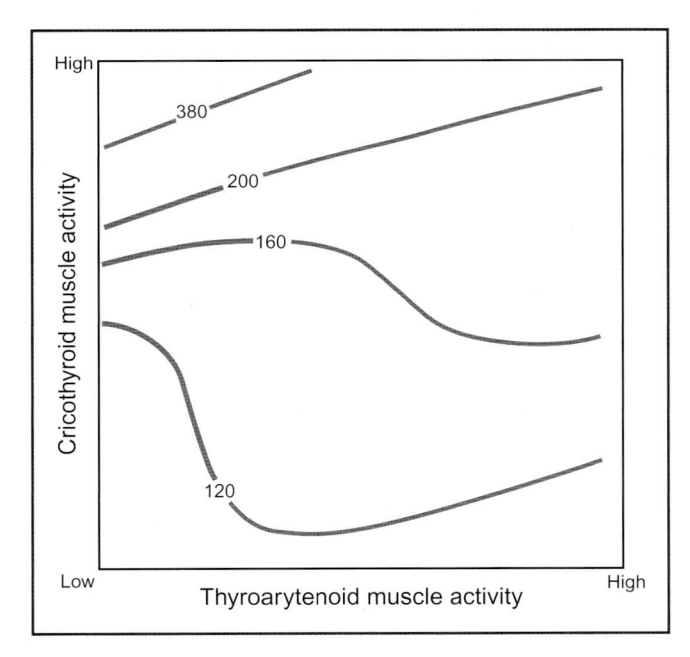

Figure 3–41. Continuum of *cricothyroid* and *thyroarytenoid* muscle activations for the production of selected fundamental frequencies. This graph illustrates that a single fundamental frequency can be produced using a wide range of combinations of relative activations of the *cricothyroid* and *thyroarytenoid* muscles. Based on modeling data from Titze and Story (2002).

Although modification of *cricothyroid* and *thyroarytenoid* muscle activity is the primary mechanism for changing fundamental frequency, it is not the only one. The mechanism of medial compression can also effect changes in the fundamental frequency of the voice. This is done through actions of the *lateral cricoarytenoid* muscles that can adjust the medial compression of the vocal folds in the area of approximation of the tips of the vocal processes (illustrated in Figure 3–34). Studies of air-driven excised larynges, in which medial compression was experimentally manipulated, have shown that increases in medial compression result in increases in fundamental frequency (van den Berg & Tan; 1959; van den Berg et al., 1960). The suspected mechanism is a decrease in the effective vibrating mass of the vocal folds caused by stopping their vibration in the region of the tips of the arytenoid processes (Honda, 1995). This mechanism has been likened to the pressing of a guitar string against a fret so that only the part of the string nearer the sounding box of the guitar is permitted to vibrate (Broad, 1973). Medial compression is considered to be a secondary or ancillary mechanism of fundamental frequency control.

Still another mechanism that influences the fundamental frequency of the voice relates to the elevation of the larynx (sometimes referred to as its vertical height). When high fundamental frequencies are generated, there is a tendency for the larynx to rise in the neck, especially near the upper extreme of the fundamental frequency range. This elevation is probably accomplished by activation of the *thyrohyoid* muscles (Faaborg-Andersen & Sonninen, 1960; Sonninen, 1968). Elevation of the larynx is believed to further increase the stiffness of the vocal folds once major effort has been exerted to increase stiffness through activation of the *thyroarytenoid* and *cricothyroid* muscles. Elevation of the larynx results in a downward pull on the undersurface of the vocal folds mediated through the conus elasticus. This pull stiffens the covers of the vocal folds (especially at the free margins of the vocal folds) by placing a vertical tug on them, and thereby increases the rate at which the vocal folds vibrate (Ohala, 1972). This mechanism is usually the last biomechanical adjustment invoked to reach the highest fundamental frequencies possible. Laryngeal elevation is considered a secondary or ancillary mechanism of fundamental frequency control.

Although nearly all fundamental frequency control is vested in the larynx, the breathing apparatus can adjust tracheal pressure to raise fundamental frequency slightly (Rubin, 1963; van den Berg, 1957); however, typical magnitudes of change are only 2 to 4 Hz in fundamental frequency per cmH$_2$O of air pressure (Hixon, Klatt, & Mead, 1971; Titze, 1989). Changes in tracheal pressure can have a more significant effect on fundamental frequency in the loft register (discussed below).

To lower fundamental frequency from a high value to its usual value, muscle activations may decrease to decrease vocal fold stiffness and/or tracheal air pressure. To lower fundamental frequency below its usual value, other mechanisms may come into play. One mechanism is to reduce vocal fold stiffness by contraction of the *thyromuscularis* (lateral) portions of the *thyroarytenoid* muscles. This contraction shortens the vocal folds and causes a slackening of the vocal ligaments and the *thyrovocalis* (medial) portions of the *thyroarytenoid* muscles (Zemlin, 1998). Another frequency-lowering mechanism entails a lowering of the larynx within the neck, which decreases the stiffness of the vocal folds by removing some of the usual traction placed on their undersurfaces. This is brought about through activation of the *sternothyroid* and *sternohyoid* muscles, which pull downward on the laryngeal housing (Atkinson, 1978; Honda, 1995; Ohala, 1972; Ohala & Hirose, 1970; Zemlin, 1998).

Sound Pressure Level

The sound pressure level (abbreviated as SPL) of speech (the acoustic signal) is a measure of its physical magnitude (Baken & Orlikoff, 2000). This magnitude is related to the amplitude of the sound emanating from the upper airway and is generically referred to as the intensity of the signal (although technically sound pressure level and intensity are different quantities and the latter is more difficult to measure; see Chapter 7 appendix). The sound pressure level of speech is expressed on a continuum in ratio units of decibels (dB) and can be changed over a wide range, typically by about 40 dB for a young adult (Coleman, Mabis, & Hinson, 1977). A vowel produced at a usual loudness level and measured 30 cm from the lips (a standard distance) might be 65 dB, whereas a vowel produced at a shouting level might be in excess of 100 dB. Control of the sound pressure level of speech is vested primarily in adjustments of the breathing apparatus and the laryngeal apparatus, and to a lesser degree the pharyngeal-oral apparatus. These adjustments are usually executed simultaneously across these three subsystems.

The breathing apparatus influences sound pressure level of the voice through changes in tracheal air pressure, which correspond closely to changes in alveolar air pressure. That is, increases and decreases in tracheal air pressure cause increases and decreases in sound pressure level (Cavagna & Margaria, 1965; Hixon & Minifie, 1972; Isshiki, 1964; Ladefoged & McKinney, 1963; Titze, 1994; van den Berg, 1956). A doubling of tracheal air pressure for usual voice production might result in an increase in sound pressure level in the neighborhood of 8 to 12 dB (Broad, 1973; Daniloff, Shuckers, & Feth, 1980; Stevens, 2000). The precise linkage between change in tracheal air pressure and change in sound pressure level depends on the prevailing sound pressure level of the voice. For example, a 1 cmH$_2$O change in tracheal air pressure during the production of a soft voice results in as much as a 3 dB change in sound pressure level, whereas the same change in tracheal air pressure during the production of a loud voice results in only a 0.5 dB change in sound pressure level (Hixon & Minifie, 1972).

Laryngeal adjustments also play a role in changing sound pressure level. Specifically, higher sound pressure levels of the voice are produced with higher laryngeal opposing pressures (Isshiki, 1964; Kunze, 1962), which are effected primarily by increasingly forceful contractions of the *lateral cricoarytenoid* and *arytenoid* muscles. Higher laryngeal opposing pressures are needed to contain the increased tracheal air pressure and prevent it from escaping uselessly (Daniloff et al., 1980).

The combined increase in tracheal pressure and heightened opposition provided by the larynx results in a change in the pattern of vocal fold vibration and excitation of the upper airway. For voice of higher sound pressure level, the vocal folds separate faster, return to the midline faster, and remain in approximation at the midline for a longer period during each cycle of vocal fold vibration (Minifie, 1973).

Rest in Peace

You may wonder why we don't use the term "subglottal pressure" in the text. The reason is that we believe the term has problems. Consider the following. The "sub" part of the term isn't specific to a location. Bronchial and alveolar pressures are also "sub" glottal. The "glottal" part of the term is also troublesome. Glottis means hole. There are times during voice production when the vocal folds are in apposition and the larynx is closed. How during those times can anything be "sub" glottal? You can't be below a hole when there isn't one. Respiratory physiologists use tracheal pressure to refer to the pressure of interest. Tracheal pressure designates the site of the pressure and is accurate regardless of whether the laryngeal airway is open or closed. Using the term "tracheal pressure" also removes ambiguity involved in the use of "sub" as a location. The term "subglottal pressure" should be buried. Rest in peace.

Two underlying features of laryngeal behavior are critically important to how efficiently energy from the breathing apparatus is converted into acoustic energy (Titze, 1988b, 1994, 2006b). One of these is the abruptness with which the vocal folds return to the midline (see Figure 3–37) and airflow declines (referred to as glottal area declination rate and airflow declination rate, respectively). The more abrupt the decline, the greater the acoustic excitation of the upper airway (Dromey, Stathopoulos, & Sapienza, 1992; Holmberg, Hillman, & Perkell, 1988; Titze, 2006b). The other important feature of laryngeal behavior is the size of the glottis. Computer modeling suggests that an average glottal size (versus small or large) is best for generating the optimal acoustic power (Titze, 1994).

Although the breathing apparatus and laryngeal apparatus contribute most to sound pressure level changes, the pharyngeal-oral apparatus also contributes. In general, it tends to blossom open more and more with successive increases in sound pressure level, achieving an effect like a megaphone. The velum (soft palate and uvula) elevates, the mandible lowers, the tongue lowers, and the mouth opening increases (Netsell, 1973; Tucker, 1963), adjustments that lower the radiation impedance of the pharyngeal-oral apparatus so that the sound energy is transmitted more effectively to the atmosphere (Fant, 1960; Flanagan, 1972).

The strongest auditory-perceptual correlate of sound pressure level is loudness. Loudness is the subjective sensation of the relative magnitude of sound that relies mainly on sound pressure level, but is influenced to lesser degrees by the fundamental frequency and spectral content of the sound produced. Generally, the higher the sound pressure level, the greater the magnitude of the perceived loudness (see Chapter 14 for further discussion of the psychophysics of loudness perception).

Fundamental Frequency–Sound Pressure Level Profiles

The term "voice range" is most often used when referring to the lowest and highest values that can be produced in either the fundamental frequency or sound pressure level of the voice. These two variables are not independent of one another in that the fundamental frequency has a different set of lowest and highest values at different sound pressure levels, and the sound pressure level has a different set of lowest and highest values at different fundamental frequencies (Fairbanks, 1960). These relations are illustrated in what are called fundamental frequency–sound pressure level profiles (Coleman et al., 1977; Damste, 1970; Gramming, 1991) or voice range profiles, such as that shown for an adult male in Figure 3–42.

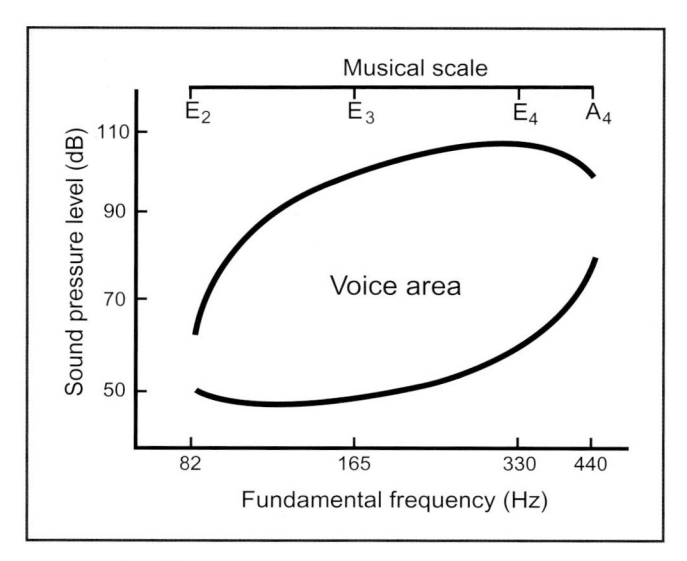

Figure 3-42. Fundamental frequency–sound pressure level profile (also called voice range profile) of an adult male. Note that the largest range of fundamental frequencies can be produced in the midrange of the sound pressure level range and that the largest range of sound pressure levels can be produced in the midrange of the fundamental frequency range.

Figure 3–42 depicts the lowest and highest fundamental frequencies and sound pressure levels attainable (and sustainable for brief durations) across the ranges of fundamental frequency and sound pressure level. This figure illustrates that, in general, lower fundamental frequencies and sound pressure levels can be produced at lower values of the other variable, whereas higher fundamental frequencies and sound pressure levels can be produced at higher values of the other variable. The fundamental frequency range of the voice is greatest in the midrange of sound pressure levels, and the sound pressure level range is greatest in the midrange of fundamental frequencies.

Spectrum

The spectrum of the sound generated by the vibrating larynx is complex and composed of a combination of different frequencies and sound pressure levels (Minifie, 1973; Stevens, 2000). This source signal is discussed in more detail in Chapter 8; however, a brief description is offered here.

The usual laryngeal source spectrum consists of a fundamental frequency and successive odd and even harmonics (whole number multiples of the fundamental frequency) that decrease in sound pressure level with increasing harmonic number at a rate of about 12 dB per octave (each doubling of frequency) above

1000 Hz (Fant, 1960). A wide variety of source spectra can be produced through changes in tracheal air pressure, translaryngeal airflow, and mechanical properties of the vocal folds.

The voice source spectrum changes with fundamental frequency because the spacing of the harmonics depends on the fundamental frequency (as fundamental frequency increases, the spacing between the harmonics increases). The spectrum also changes with sound pressure level (as sound pressure level increases, the energy in the higher frequency region tends to increase). In addition, the spectral content of the voice source is influenced by changes in the vibratory pattern of the vocal folds (Stevens, 2000) and the degree to which the laryngeal airway is constricted. The extremes are embodied in the spectra generated with pressed voice (vocal folds set to be forcefully approximated) and breathy voice (vocal folds set to be easily parted and to allow continuous airflow between them). The breathy voice contains less high frequency energy (that is, the high frequency harmonics are lower in sound pressure level) compared with the pressed voice. In addition, the breathy voice contains more noise (aperiodic sound) than its pressed counterpart.

The voice source generated at the laryngeal level constitutes the raw material of voice production and, when heard in the absence of an upper airway, it sounds like a coarse buzz (see sidetrack called The Cattle Are Lowing). To sound like a human voice, the voice source must be filtered by the air spaces above it (pharyngeal cavity, oral cavity, and in some cases nasal cavity).

Voice Registers

The nature of vocal fold vibration is strongly conditioned by so-called voice registers. Voice registers reflect different modes of vocal fold vibration that result from different mechanical conditions (Titze, 1994) and that give rise to differences in perceived voice quality (Laver, 1991). Accordingly, a voice register can be defined perceptually as a series of consecutive utterances of similar voice quality produced along a pitch scale through application of similar mechanical principles.

The topic of voice registers is controversial, especially in singing pedagogy. The number and nature of voice registers is often argued in the singing literature, as are the mechanisms involved in their generation

---

Listen My Children and You Shall Hear

Some people are loud and then some people are really loud. The conversion of aerodynamic power to acoustic power is better in some than in others and some of the best at it have been listed as celebrities in folk sources. Different hollering, yelling, screaming, shouting, and loud voice champions have been crowned around the world. The *Guinness Book of Records* (Folkard, 2006) lists Jill Drake as the reigning screaming champion at 129 dB and Annalisa Flanagan as the reigning shouting champion at 121.7 dB. Alan Myatt, the town crier of Gloucester, England, once was touted in the *Guinness Book of Records* as having the world's loudest voice, an ear-piercing 112.8 dB. Had Paul Revere been so endowed as a town crier he wouldn't have had to knock on so many doors and he might have been able to awaken all of Lexington, Massachusetts on a single breath. Well, maybe not all, but at least much of the South Side.

The Cattle Are Lowing

An effective method for teaching certain principles of voice production involves the use of an excised cow larynx. The cow larynx is large compared with the human larynx and is different in some respects. The cow larynx does not have false vocal folds, nor is it richly endowed with mucous glands for lubricating the vocal folds. After all, cows don't produce voice for long periods like people do. A cow larynx can be made to vibrate by attaching the blower end of a vacuum cleaner to the tracheal end of the larynx—the vibration sounds like a coarse buzz. If you then manually stretch the vocal folds, change the medial compression, and make other adjustments, you can alter the fundamental frequency, sound pressure level, and source spectrum. If you then place an inverted container (the size of a coffee pot) above the larynx, which roughly simulates the resonance contribution of the missing upper airway, the buzz can be transformed into something that almost sounds like a cow. When all is done right, the experience is both instructive and "moooooving" to students.

(sometimes taken to include both laryngeal and upper airway adjustments). Far less controversy exists about the number and nature of voice registers in the speaking voice, and this section is limited to those.

There are three voice registers in the speaking voice. The general location of these along the fundamental frequency scale is illustrated for men and women in Figure 3–43. They are labeled as the pulse, modal, and loft voice registers and correspond to three different modes of vocal fold vibration encountered in sequence when speaking at an ascending fundamental frequency from the lowest to highest fundamental frequencies within the speaking range (Hollien, 1972, 1974). Each voice register is confined to a restricted range of fundamental frequencies and within each register a particular mode or pattern of vocal fold vibration prevails. The boundary between adjacent registers is determined by raising and lowering the fundamental frequency and noting where an abrupt change in voice quality occurs.

The modal voice register is the middle of the three speaking voice registers and gets its name from the statistical mode, the most often occurring event (in fundamental frequency). The modal register is characteristic of the type of vocal fold vibration described thus far in this chapter and is the voice register typically used during most conversational speech production. Voice production in the modal voice register is characterized by moderate values of vocal fold length, vocal fold thickness, vocal fold stiffness, laryngeal opposing pressure, laryngeal airway resistance, tracheal air pressure, and translaryngeal airflow (Hollien, 1960a, 1960b, 1962; Hollien, Brown, & Hollien, 1971; Hollien & Colton, 1969; Hollien & Curtis, 1960; Hollien & Moore, 1960; Isshiki, 1964; Kunze, 1962; Murry & Brown, 1971b; Shipp & McGlone, 1971; van den Berg, 1956).

The pulse voice register is the lowest of the three speaking voice registers and derives its name from the nature of its pulse-like voice source waveform. The quality of voice produced in this register is sometimes referred to as vocal fry, glottal fry, or creaky voice, and has a certain growl-like quality that some have described as coarse and bubbly (Orlikoff & Kahane, 1996). Voice can be produced continuously in the pulse voice register, although this would be atypical. Pulse register usually manifests intermittently at the ends of breath groups when the voice trails off in sound pressure level and drops in fundamental frequency (comes to a growling halt).

The vibration of the vocal folds in pulse voice register is distinct and is characterized by prolonged approximation of the vocal folds and brief appearances of a small glottis. The pulse produced in association with this short-lived glottis is relatively rich in harmonic structure, but low in sound pressure level. Fundamental frequency and sound pressure level tend to change together in the pulse register and do not have the relative independence found in modal voice register (Murry & Brown, 1971a, 1971b).

Voice production in the pulse voice register is generated with moderate or low values of tracheal air pressure and translaryngeal airflow (Allen & Hollien, 1973; Holmberg, Hillman, & Perkell, 1989; McGlone, 1967; McGlone & Shipp, 1971; Murry, 1971; Murry & Brown, 1971b). The vocal folds are short, thick, slack, and compliant (Allen & Hollien, 1973; Hollien, Damste, & Murry, 1969) and medial compression is moderate (McGlone & Shipp, 1971). Lateral vocal fold movements are moderate and usually not along the entire length of the membranous portion of the vocal folds (Orlikoff & Kahane, 1996) and there is a pronounced vertical phase difference. A prolonged approximation phase of vocal fold vibration results in a near-total damping of upper airway excitation with each pulse of activity (Coleman, 1963; Titze, 1988a; Wendahl, Moore, & Hollien, 1963). The voice source, therefore, is a series of nearly discrete excitations to the upper airway that give the listener the perception that the voice is a string of tiny pops (like those that can be made by applying repeated bursts of pressure behind the lips when they are thickly puckered and gently held together).

The loft voice register, also called the falsetto register, is the highest of the three speaking voice registers and gets its name from its high placement within the fundamental frequency range. The quality of the voice produced in this register is sometimes described as thin, flute-like, and breathy, with acoustic characteristics that resemble a pure tone. In this register excursions of the vocal folds are relatively small, the glottis is narrow, and there is little to no vertical phase difference. Rather, movements are mainly horizontal and confined to the vicinity of the free margins of the vocal folds. Such movements take on the appearance of vibrating strings alternately moving horizontally away from and toward one another. The vocal folds do not have to approximate to produce voice in the loft register, and when they do, contact between them is usually light (low adductory forces). Loft voice contains less high harmonic energy than modal voice (Colton, 1972) and the sound pressure level of the voice is lower in the loft register than in the modal register (Orlikoff & Kahane, 1996).

Voice production in the loft voice register is generated with moderately high tracheal air pressure and translaryngeal airflow (Large, Iwata, & von Leden, 1970; McGlone, 1970; Shipp & McGlone, 1971; Shipp, McGlone, & Morrisey, 1972), elongated and thin vocal folds that are under great longitudinal tension (Hollien

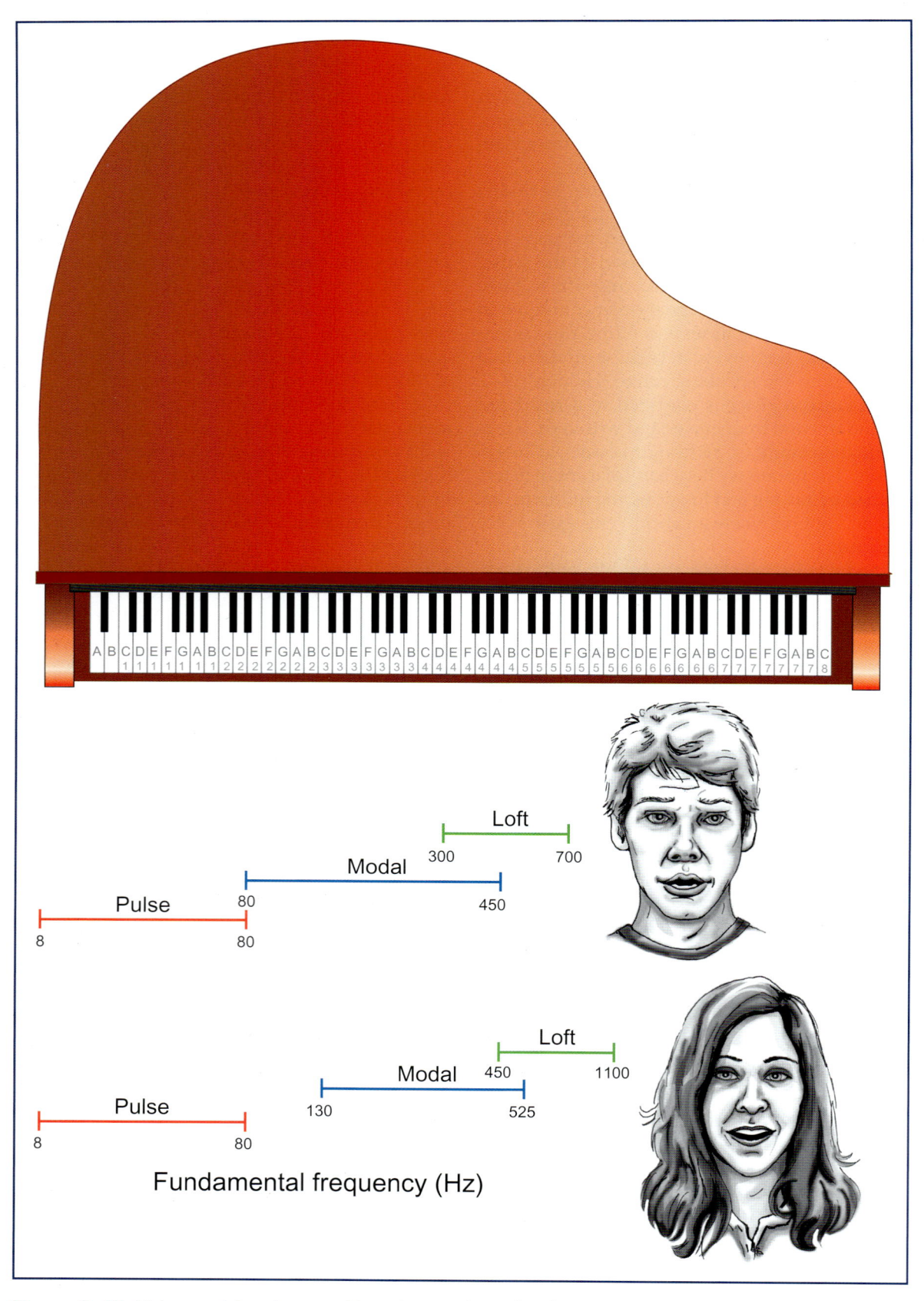

Figure 3–43. Voice registers for speaking shown along the fundamental frequency scale (and corresponding piano scale). The lowest register is pulse, the middle register is modal and is the most often used register, and the highest register is loft.

110

& Moore, 1960), and very high stiffness of the mucosal covers of the vocal folds (Gay, Hirose, Strome, & Sawashima, 1972; Hirano, 1974; Hirano, Vennard, & Ohala, 1970). Changes in fundamental frequency and sound pressure level in the loft register are significantly influenced by changes in tracheal air pressure and airflow through the larynx (Colton, 1973; Isshiki, 1964, 1965; van den Berg et al., 1960; Yanagihara & Koike, 1967), with acoustic variables following directional changes in aeromechanical variables (Hollien, 1972). For example, increases in airflow through the larynx result in increases in both fundamental frequency and sound pressure level of the resulting laryngeal tone (van den Berg et al., 1960).

Running Speech Activities

The larynx is a critical participant in running speech activities. During inspiration, the vocal folds abduct and dilate the laryngeal airway to allow air to flow freely into the pulmonary apparatus. During expiration (speech production), the vocal folds adduct to produce voice and intermittently abduct to allow air pressures and airflows to reach downstream structures for voiceless oral consonant production.

The laryngeal tone is the carrier of speech and has an important influence on speech intelligibility. It also conveys information about the speaker's age, sex, physical stature, health status, emotional status, identity, and other factors. The laryngeal tone can be adjusted in fundamental frequency, sound pressure level, and spectrum to convey meaning, disambiguate certain aspects of the communication, emphasize certain parts of the flow of speech over others, provide information through different voice shadings and nuances, establish certain affects (impressions), and affirm roles in relationships. The larynx also plays an important role in articulation.

Fundamental Frequency

Fundamental frequency change is prominent during running speech activities and can range as much as two octaves (Fairbanks, 1960). Fundamental frequency is often displayed and measured in a tracing called a fundamental frequency contour, which tracks change in fundamental frequency over time. Such a contour is shown in Figure 3–44 for a spoken sentence.

Listening to fundamental frequency change in the voice evokes a perception of time-varying pitch change that is referred to as an intonation contour. Perceptions of intonation contours are influenced by sensitivity to pitch inflections and pitch shifts. Inflections are modu-

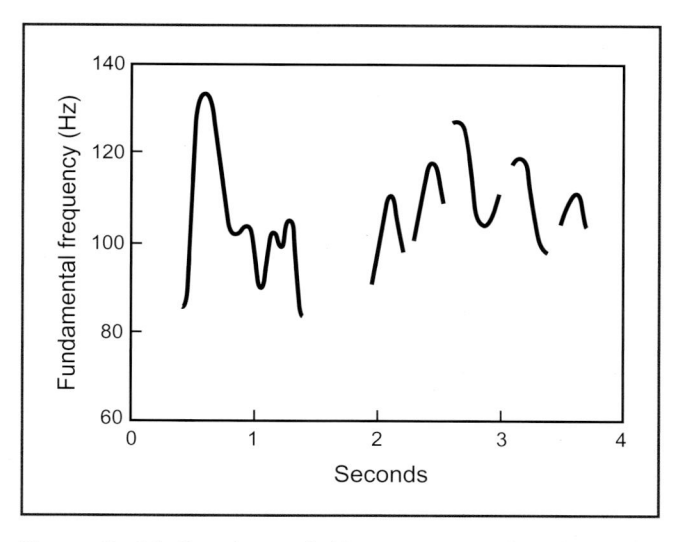

Figure 3-44. Fundamental frequency contour for a sentence spoken by an adult male (courtesy of Brad Story).

lations in pitch during voiced segments, whereas shifts are changes in pitch from the end of one voiced segment to the beginning of the next (Fairbanks, 1960). The intonation contour underlies what the listener comes to consider as the melody or tunefulness of speech. This contour operates around a mode (the most often sensed pitch) that determines what the listener judges to be the characteristic (or habitual) pitch of the voice.

Adjustments in fundamental frequency during running speech activities are vested mainly in laryngeal actions. These laryngeal actions rely, in large part, on interplay between contractions of the *cricothyroid* and *thyroarytenoid* muscles, along with bracing actions of the *posterior cricoarytenoid* muscles, which also adjust the stiffness of the vocal folds (Atkinson, 1978; Gay et al., 1972; Hirano, Ohala, & Vennard, 1969; Netsell, 1969). Actions of the *cricothyroid* muscles are more strongly correlated with the fundamental frequency of the voice than are the actions of other intrinsic muscles of the larynx, as long as the *cricothyroid* muscles are not functioning near their maximum output (Atkinson, 1978; Titze, 1994). Thus, as discussed above for sustained voice production, changes in the longitudinal tension of the vocal folds (via *cricothyroid* muscle activation) and change in internal stiffness of the vocal folds (via *thyroarytenoid* muscle activation) are of prime importance to the control of the fundamental frequency of the voice during running speech events.

Adjustments of the breathing apparatus in the form of changes in pressure and volume can also influence fundamental frequency. Although tracheal pressure remains relatively steady during running speech production, it does fluctuate slightly with linguistic stress. Pulsatile increases in tracheal pressure cause slight increases in the fundamental frequency of the voice (Hixon et al., 1971; Lester & Story, 2013; Titze, 1989), suggesting that pressure fluctuations associated with the production of stressed syllables may contribute to momentary increases in fundamental frequency. Although running speech is generally produced within the midrange of the vital capacity, when it is produced at larger than usual lung volumes, it may be associated with higher than usual fundamental frequencies (Watson, Ciccia, & Weismer, 2003). This may be due to higher tracheal pressure associated with higher expiratory recoil pressures at large lung volumes, or it may be due to a downward pull on the larynx (through its connections to the diaphragm) that could increase vocal fold tension, or both.

Sound Pressure Level

Like fundamental frequency, sound pressure level also changes significantly during running speech activities. This is true of the average sound pressure level associated with different speaking situations (soft, normal, or loud speech) and rapid variations from the average level (such as accompany varying levels of linguistic stress). A routine conversation might find the sound pressure level to swing as much as 25 to 30 dB. The magnitude of sound pressure level and its directional changes can be displayed and measured in a tracing referred to as a sound pressure level contour, one of which is shown for the production of a sentence in Figure 3–45.

Changes in sound pressure level over time give rise to a subjective impression of a loudness contour that embodies percepts of an average loudness and variations about it. Vowels are the main contributors to loudness judgments in running speech activities. Adjustment in vowel and consonant sound pressure levels, while usually moving in the same direction, find vowel sound pressure level to change more than consonant sound pressure level (Hixon, 1966; Stevens, 2000). This is due to a tendency to open up the pharyngeal-oral apparatus to increase sound pressure level for vowels, and a tendency to constrict the apparatus to increase sound pressure level for consonants. These two competing tendencies result in a tradeoff in sound pressure level change, in which the vowel dominates because of its more prominent carrying power (Fairbanks & Miron, 1957).

Perceived loudness contours are strongly related to sound pressure level contours, but do not bear a one-to-one correspondence to them. That is, although certain sounds have intrinsically higher or lower sound pressure levels, they may be perceived as being of equal loudness. For example, when counting from one to ten, the syllables tend to sound equally loud to the listener despite the differences in sound pressure levels across the different vowels in the series.

Control of sound pressure level for running speech activities is conditioned by adjustments of the breathing apparatus, laryngeal apparatus, and pharyngeal-oral apparatus. The most important breathing apparatus adjustment has to do with changing the magnitude of the average tracheal air pressure and with effecting small increases in pressure to emphasize certain speech segments (Netsell, 1969). These background level and pulsatile tracheal air pressure events are the result of muscular pressure adjustments by the chest wall (Hixon, Mead, & Goldman, 1976).

Laryngeal participation in sound pressure level control for running speech activities usually involves heightened vocal fold adductory forces that manifest as increases in the laryngeal opposing pressure. These vocal fold adductory forces enable the buildup of tracheal air pressure and increase as speech becomes progressively louder or contrastive stress levels become greater from one syllable to another (Hirano et al., 1969; Netsell, 1969, 1973). The muscles implicated in heightening vocal fold adductory forces are primarily the *lateral cricoarytenoid* and *arytenoid* muscles, although the *thyroarytenoid* muscles also contribute by bulging the vocal folds toward the midline.

Pharyngeal-oral adjustments that change the acoustic radiation impedance are often associated with changes in the sound pressure level of running speech. That is, the pharyngeal-oral apparatus tends to open more and more with successive increases in the sound pressure level to enhance transmission of acoustic energy generated at the glottis (Daniloff et al., 1980; Netsell, 1973).

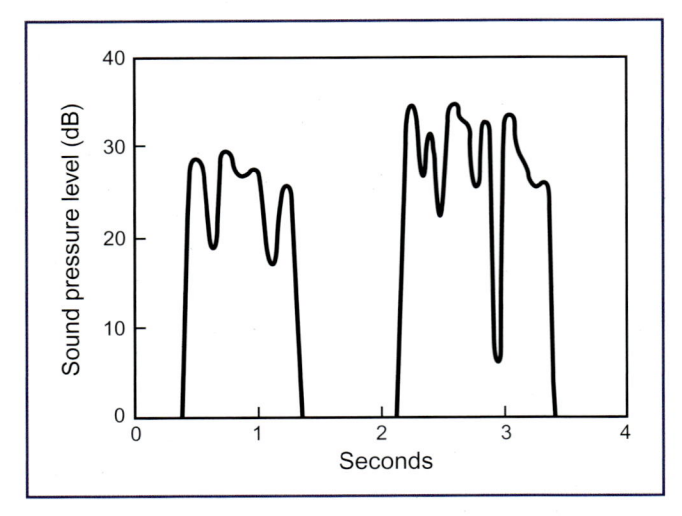

Figure 3–45. Sound pressure level contour for a sentence spoken by an adult male (courtesy of Brad Story).

Spectrum

The spectrum of the laryngeal source changes rapidly and often during running speech activities. Such changes are associated with changes in the fundamental frequency or sound pressure level of the voice and with other changes in the pattern of vocal fold vibration. Slower changes in the spectrum of the laryngeal tone may result from prolonged use of the vocal folds, transient abuse of the vocal folds, illness, aging, or other factors.

Source spectrum changes may give rise to changes in voice quality, a perceptual attribute that pertains to the sound of the voice beyond its pitch and loudness characteristics (Behrman, 2007). Depending on the speaking situation, the spectrum can change in ways that cause the listener to perceive voice qualities that range from breathy to pressed (Minifie, 1973; Stevens, 2000) and include other commonly used descriptors such as roughness and strain (Kempster, Gerratt, Abbott, Barkmeier-Kraemer, & Hillman, 2009).

Articulation

Although the larynx is most strongly associated with generating the voice source, it can also be thought of as an articulator (a movable structure that contributes to the production of speech sounds). The larynx, specifically the vocal folds, are the primary articulators for productions of what are called glottal sounds, which include the glottal stop-plosive consonant and the glottal fricative consonant /h/ (Hirose, 1977; Lofqvist & Yoshioka, 1984; Orlikoff & Kahane, 1996; Sawashima, Abramson, Cooper, & Lisker, 1970; see Figures 3–35 and 3–36). The vocal folds also abduct briefly to produce voiceless consonants such as /p/ or /s/. In the production of the word "pass," for example, the vocal folds abduct briefly during the /p/, adduct for the vowel, and abduct again for the /s/. The movements of the vocal folds toward and away from one another are rapid and precise in their timing, just as rapid and precise as other articulators found in the upper airway (tongue, lips, velum). Further consideration of the larynx as an articulator can be found in Chapter 5.

VARIABLES THAT INFLUENCE LARYNGEAL FUNCTION DURING SPEECH PRODUCTION

To this point in the chapter, discussion has focused on laryngeal structure and function as found in a typical adult. Nevertheless, there are significant changes in the anatomy of the larynx and the nature of voice production that take place during both the developmental period and the aging years. Also, once an individual reaches a certain age, important sex-related differences emerge in laryngeal structure and function. This section provides a brief overview of the influence of age and sex on the larynx.

Age

The larynx changes across a lifespan, most dramatically during the first years of life and more gradually during adulthood. Some of the more important laryngeal changes and the voice alterations that accompany them are considered here.

The larynx of the newborn rides high within the neck with the lower edge of the cricoid cartilage positioned between the third and fourth cervical vertebrae. The epiglottis contacts the velum, a mechanical arrangement that facilitates the nursing needs of the infant while simultaneously ensuring an adequate airway for ventilation (Laitman & Crelin, 1976; Sasaki, Levin, Laitman, & Crelin, 1977). The larynx descends gradually throughout the first two decades of life (Vorperian et al., 2009) until it reaches the region of the seventh cervical vertebra.

The framework of the infant larynx is destined to triple in size during the developmental period (Bosma, 1985), with its growth being more linear in the female than the male and the most rapid changes in the size

---

Donald Duck

Many reading this have breathed in from a helium-filled balloon and then tried to speak. The resulting sound makes people laugh because it reminds them of the voice of the cartoon character Donald Duck. What causes this? Helium is lighter than air, has a different kinematic viscosity, and effectively reduces the acoustic size of the upper airway. This makes the speech production apparatus behave acoustically as if it belonged to a smaller person. Helium results in upper airway resonances that are higher than usual in frequency. It's as if a child's upper airway were being excited by an adult's larynx. As utterance (expiration) proceeds, the inspired helium gives way to a mixture of helium and air and then just air. The sound of the voice gradually returns to normal, all the while simulating the growth of an upper airway that eventually attains its corresponding adult size to go along with its adult-size larynx.

of the male laryngeal framework occurring during the pubertal growth spurt (Dickson & Maue-Dickson, 1982; Kahane, 1978, 1982). At the beginning of life, the laryngeal framework is soft and pliable, becoming firm and less flexible with age (Tucker & Tucker, 1979). Ossification (turning to bone) of the hyoid begins at about 2 years of age, whereas cartilages of the larynx begin to show signs of ossification much later in life (Aronson, 1990). At birth, the thyroid cartilage is contiguous with the hyoid bone and then separates from it vertically. The laminae of the thyroid cartilage are somewhat semicircular in the infant larynx and become more angular in the older child (Kahane, 1975).

The vocal folds double their length during childhood, and puberty adds another growth spurt to the vocal folds, especially in males (Dickson & Maue-Dickson, 1982; Kahane, 1978). This developmental increase in length occurs in both parts of the vocal folds such that the relative lengths of the membranous and cartilaginous portions do not change (Rogers, Setlur, Raol, Maurer, & Hartnick, 2014). Similarly, the weights of the individual intrinsic muscles of the larynx increase with age but remain proportional throughout the developmental period (Kahane & Kahn, 1984).

The composition and resulting mechanical properties of the vocal folds change significantly during development. The larynx of the newborn shows a homogeneous and undifferentiated lamina propria (Hirano & Sato, 1993). This contrasts markedly with the distinctive multilayered structure of the lamina propria of the adult vocal folds (Hirano, 1974, 1981). The vocal ligament does not develop in the child until about 4 years of age (Zemlin, 1998) and the adult-like lamina propria is not apparent until about 16 years of age (Kent, 1997) after the most rapid change in vocal fold length has taken place (Kazarian, Sarkissian, & Isaakian, 1978). The difference in the lamina propria between infancy and adulthood prevents the infant from achieving some of the subtle vocal fold adjustments that are a part of the adult repertoire as well as introduces additional acoustic phenomena, such as increased noise, in the infant voice (Fuamenya, Robb, & Wemke, 2015).

Perhaps the most obvious change in the voice during development is in the fundamental frequency. As portrayed in Figure 3–46, the average fundamental frequency decreases from about 500 Hz (newborns) to about 250 Hz (10 year olds) in both boys and girls, with

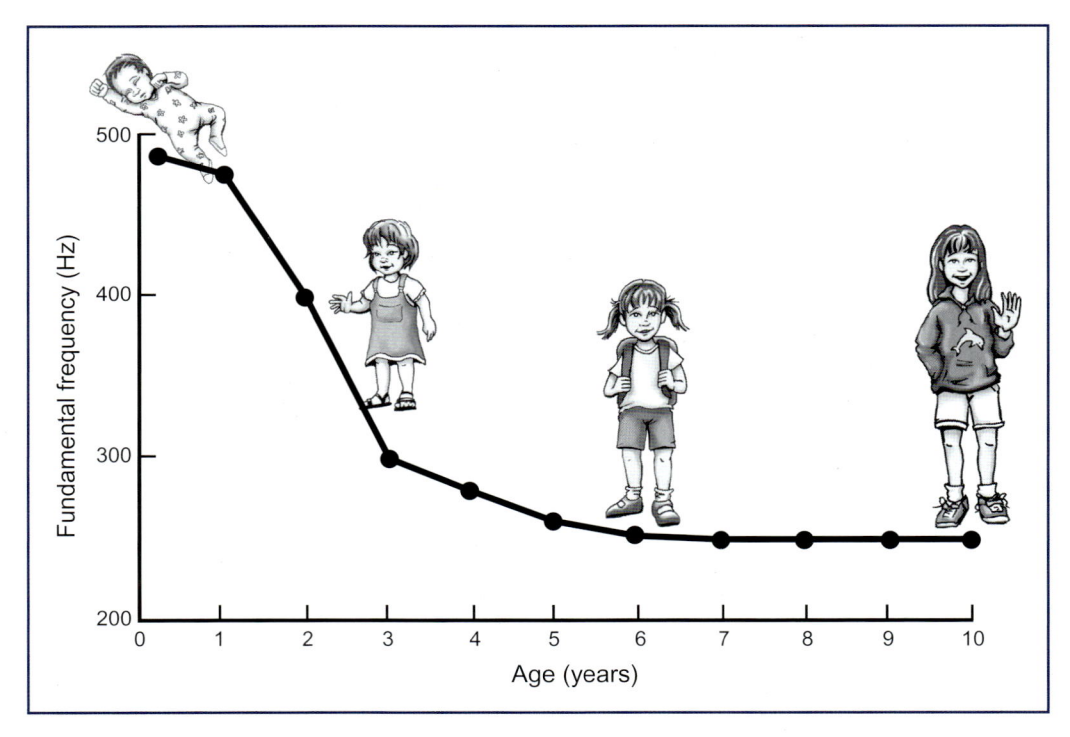

Figure 3-46. Fundamental frequency changes during the first decade of life. Based on data summarized in "Anatomical and neuromuscular maturation of the speech mechanism: Evidence from acoustic studies" (p. 423), by R. Kent, 1976, *Journal of Speech and Hearing Research, 19*, 421–447. Copyright 1976 by the American Speech and Hearing Association. Data summary reproduced with permission.

much of the decrease occurring during the first 3 years (Kent, 1976). Prior to the onset of puberty, males and females have a similar average fundamental frequency and a similar variation in fundamental frequency (Fairbanks, Herbert, & Hammond, 1949; Fairbanks, Wiley, & Lassman, 1949; Wilson, 1979). In cases where differences between boys and girls have been reported, they do not appear to be related to sex, per se, but rather appear to be associated with factors such as height or cultural background (Glaze, Bless, Milenkovic, & Susser, 1988; Hasek, Singh, & Murry, 1980). During and after puberty, fundamental frequency undergoes a large and rapid downward change in males and a much less precipitous downward change in females. The greater downward change in males is a consequence of a greater growth spurt in both the length and thickness of the male vocal folds compared with the female vocal folds. The adolescent voice change that is perceptually prominent in males usually occurs between 12.5 and 14.5 years of age and may be accompanied by pitch breaks and other phenomena that reflect transient instability in the control of the voice (Hollien, Green, & Massey, 1994). The male adolescent voice can also be somewhat breathy, rough, and hoarse (Curry, 1946; Kahane, 1982), probably due to structural changes within the vocal fold covers (Hirano, Kurita, & Nakashima, 1983; Hirano & Sato, 1993).

During the adult years the larynx continues to lower slightly (Wind, 1970). Some of the cartilages of the larynx gradually ossify (turn to bone), whereas others gradually calcify (turn to salt), making the aging adult larynx increasingly stiff and brittle as time goes on (Zemlin, 1998). Ossification is confined to components of the framework that are constituted of a hyaline matrix and manifests sequentially in the thyroid, cricoid, and arytenoid cartilages of the larynx. Ossification begins in these three cartilages during the early decades of adulthood (a little earlier in men than in women) and is relatively complete by the time senescence begins (Hately, Evison, & Samuel, 1965; Zemlin, 1998). Calcification is confined to components of the framework that are formed by an elastic matrix. Such calcification occurs later in senescence (more pronounced in men than in women) and is exhibited in the epiglottis, corniculate cartilages, cuneiform cartilages, and parts of the arytenoid cartilages (Kent & Vorperian, 1995; Malinowski, 1967). The arytenoid cartilages are unique as components of the laryngeal scaffolding because they are made of a hyaline matrix in some parts and an elastic matrix in other parts (Kahane, 1980, 1983; Sato, Kurita, Hirano, & Kiyokawa, 1990). Thus, the arytenoid cartilages are subjected to hardening twice during the aging process, early in adulthood by ossification and late in adulthood by calcification.

The joints of the larynx also change with advancing age in adulthood. The cricoarytenoid joints, for example, undergo modification in both their joint capsules and articular surfaces (Kahane & Hammons, 1987; Kahn & Kahane, 1986; Segre, 1971). Changes at the articular surfaces include abrasion, ossification, erosion, and deformation, all of which influence movements at the joints. Most important is that the movement of the arytenoid cartilages around the cricoarytenoid joints can be reduced in older individuals, which, in turn, can limit the degree to which the vocal folds can be approximated (Kahane, 1988).

The vocal folds undergo modification with advanced age. Such modification includes nerve fiber loss and muscle atrophy that lead to losses in mass and muscle strength (Aronson, 1990; Cooper, 1990; Ferreri, 1959). Other changes include a reduction in tissue elasticity in the vocal folds, dehydration of the laryngeal mucosa, edema, and alteration in the density of different fibers constituting the structural matrices of the vocal folds (Aronson, 1990; Benjamin, 1988; Kahane & Beckford, 1991; Keleman & Pressman, 1955; Kent & Vorperian, 1995; Linville, 1995; Mueller, Sweeney, & Baribeau, 1985). With advanced age, not only is muscle tissue lost within the body of the vocal fold, connective tissue is gained (Kahane, 1983). Simultaneously, the cover of the vocal fold undergoes modification, with different layers of the lamina propria changing in different ways with advancing age (Hirano et al., 1983; Kahane, 1983; Kahane, Stadlin, & Bell, 1979). The superficial layer thickens, becomes swollen with fluid, and declines in fiber density. The intermediate layer thins out as elastic fibers wane in size and number. And the deep layer thickens (especially in males over 50 years of age) as collagenous fibers increase in size and density. These age-related changes in the lamina propria may cause the vocal folds to take on a bowed configuration (Honjo & Isshiki, 1980; Mueller et al., 1985), develop surface irregularities along their free margins (Kahane, 1983), and stiffen (Kent, 1997).

Age-related changes in the structure of the vocal folds may affect the way they function during voice production. In particular, it is common to see a gap between aged vocal folds during phonation (Biever & Bless, 1989; Honjo & Isshiki, 1980; Kahane, 1987; Linville, 1992; Pontes, Yamaski, & Behlau, 2006; Yamauchi et al., 2012) and aperiodicity and asymmetry of vocal fold vibration are also often seen in aged speakers. Around the eighth decade of life, men begin to show a lowering of laryngeal airway resistance during phonation (Holmes, Leeper, & Nicholson, 1994; Melcon, Hoit, & Hixon, 1989), although women do not (Hoit & Hixon, 1992). Whether or not these physiological changes are directly responsible for age-related changes in the sound of the voice is not entirely clear.

Nearly everything known about the influence of aging on laryngeal structure and function is based on the use of chronological age (easy to quantify) as the primary temporal marker (Shipp & Hollien, 1969). However, it may be that physiological age (more difficult to measure) is, in fact, a more relevant temporal marker. It is also important to recognize that health status must be taken into account when attempting to understand voice changes across adulthood (Ramig & Ringel, 1983).

Sex

During infancy and early childhood, the structure and function of the larynx are relatively similar in males and females. Later in childhood, differences between the sexes start to emerge, especially during puberty. The sexual dimorphism of the larynx seen in early adolescence is maintained across the adult life span.

Once fully mature, the most obvious difference between the male and female larynx is its overall size, with the typical male larynx being larger than the typical female larynx (Jotz et al., 2014). There is also a noticeable configuration difference, with the angle formed by the thyroid laminae being narrower in men than women (Glikson, Sagiv, Eyal, Wolf, & Primov-Fever, 2017; Kahane, 1978; Malinowski, 1967). This sharper angle accounts for the fact that men have a larger Adam's apple (thyroid prominence) than women.

Size and configuration differences between the male and female larynx are the primary contributors to sex-related differences in fundamental frequency. Following puberty, males have lower fundamental frequencies than females of similar age, as shown in Figure 3–47. The difference in average fundamental frequency generally increases to about middle age and then decreases in senescence. This is because, as suggested from a collection of cross-sectional studies, older men have somewhat higher fundamental frequencies than younger men (Eichhorn, Kent, Austin, & Vorperian, 2017; Hollien & Shipp, 1972; Honjo & Isshiki, 1980; Mueller et al., 1985; Stathopoulos, Huber,

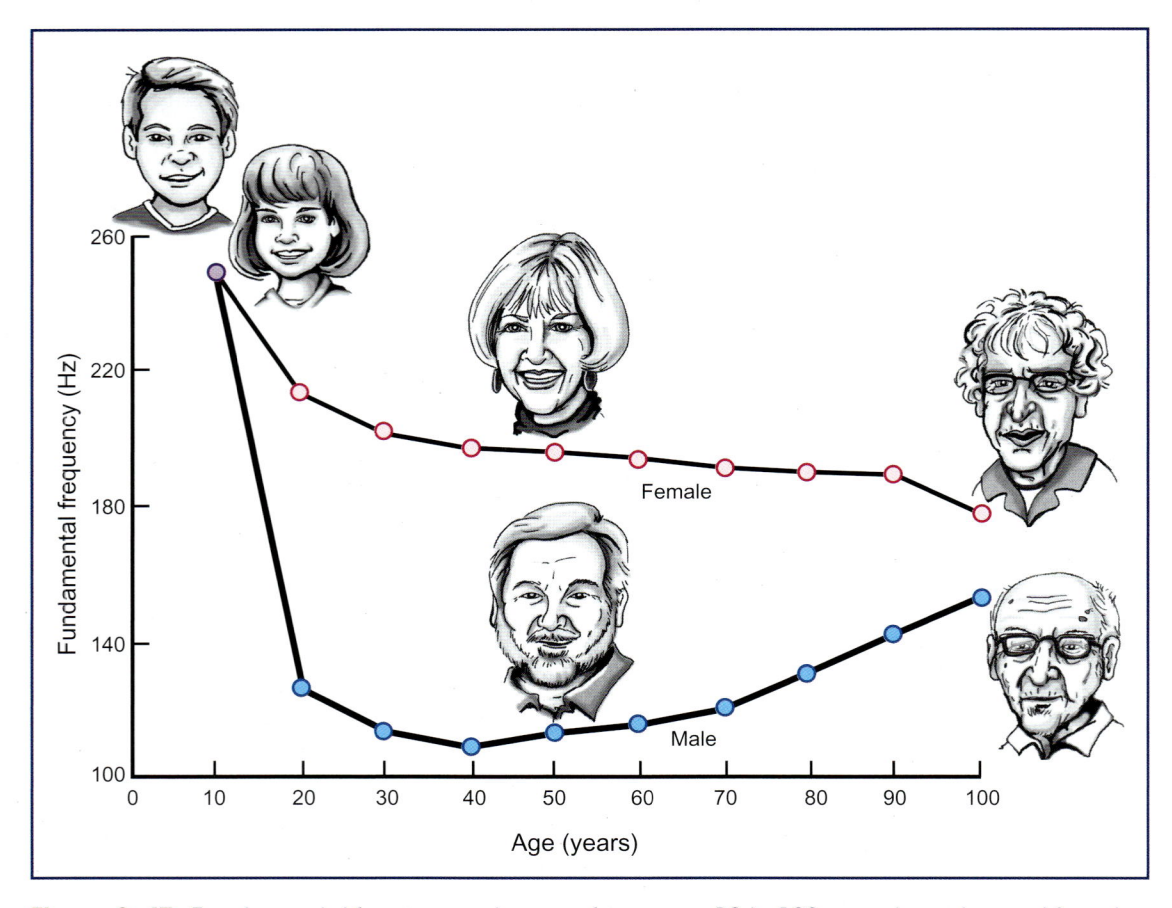

Figure 3–47. Fundamental frequency changes from ages 10 to 100 years in males and females. Data obtained from many published sources (see text) and rounded to the nearest decade for each sex. Note that fundamental frequency tends to decrease with age in females. In contrast, fundamental frequency decreases then increases with age in males.

& Sussman, 2011), whereas older women have lower fundamental frequencies than younger women (Awan & Mueller, 1992; Benjamin, 1981; Eichhorn et al., 2017; Honjo & Isshiki, 1980; Linville, 1987; Linville & Fisher, 1985; Mueller et al., 1985; Russell, Penny, & Pemberton, 1995; Stoicheff, 1981). In men, the increase in fundamental frequency may have roots in muscle atrophy, thinning of the lamina propria, and general loss of mass (Hirano, Kurita, & Sakaguchi, 1989; Kahane, 1987; Segre, 1971), factors that would tend to move the fundamental frequency upward. In women, the decrease in fundamental frequency (very late in life) may have roots in an age-related increase in edema (Ferreri, 1959; Honjo & Isshiki, 1980), a factor that would tend to move the fundamental frequency downward. Fundamental frequency changes with advanced age may help to explain why it is sometimes difficult to tell whether the voice on a telephone is that of a relatively high-pitched elderly man or a relatively low-pitched elderly woman. Life, as conveyed in the voice, would appear to have come full circle to anyone who has struggled to discern whether it is a 6-year-old boy or a 6-year-old girl who just picked up the telephone and said "Hello."

In women, hormonal fluctuations appear to influence fundamental frequency. For example, the menstrual cycle may produce subtle changes in fundamental frequency (and intensity) (Banal, 2017). Menopause may also influence voice, as evidenced by the significantly lower fundamental frequencies found in women who have completed menopause compared with women of the same age who have not completed menopause (Stoicheff, 1981). The effects of menopause on fundamental frequency appear to be offset somewhat by the use of hormone replacement therapy, as postmenopausal women who were using hormone replacement therapy have been found to have higher fundamental frequencies than those who were not (Hamdan et al., 2018).

Sex-related differences may also be seen in the way young adults approximate the vocal folds for voice production. As portrayed in Figure 3–48, many young

He Said—She Said

Male–female differences are inherently interesting. So are male–female differences in voice. Understanding these differences is particularly relevant to speech-language pathologists who work with transgender clients. The number of people who identify as transgender in the United States has substantially increased over the past decade (Flores, Herman, Gates, & Brown, 2016) and with this increase comes more and more people requesting clinical services to help their voices become gender congruent. Voice therapy with transgender clients typically focuses on modification of fundamental frequency and its variation, with trans women striving for a higher-pitched voice and greater pitch variability compared with their previous male voice. Voice quality is also often a target of therapy, usually with a focus on increasing breathiness and changing resonance characteristics as a way to sound more feminine. With the increased demand for speech-language pathology services for transgender clients comes the need for a better understanding of male–female voice differences and stronger evidence upon which to base our clinical services (Oates & Dacakis, 2015).

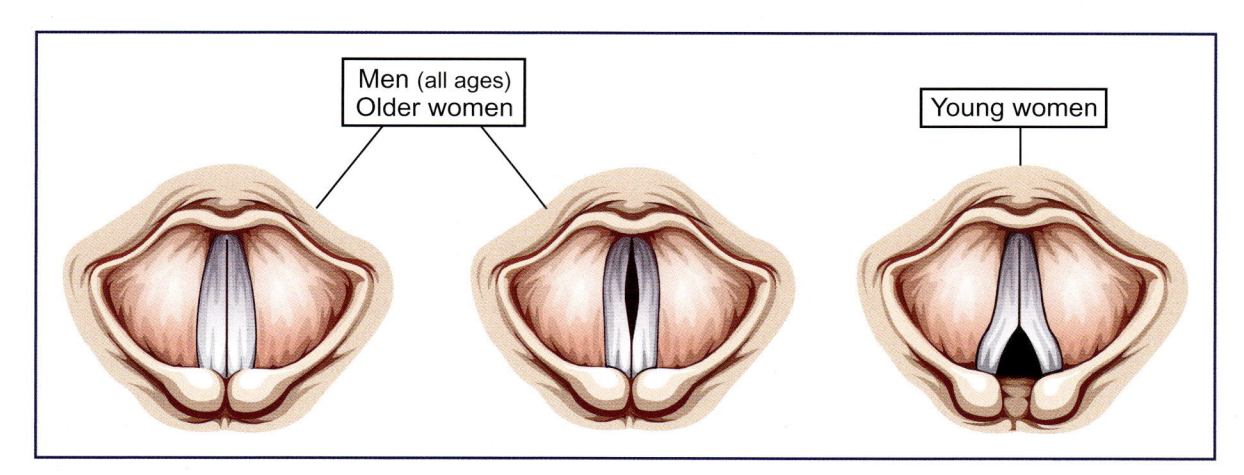

Figure 3–48. Vocal fold approximation during voice production in men and women. Whereas men of all ages and older women tend to either fully approximate the vocal folds or exhibit a spindle-shaped glottis during voice production, young women have a tendency to maintain a posterior glottis.

women show an opening between the vocal folds during voicing, especially in the cartilaginous segment (Behrman, 2007; Biever & Bless, 1989; Sodersten & Lindestad, 1990), whereas men do not. In contrast, men of all ages and older women more often exhibit either full vocal fold approximation or a spindle-shaped opening (Ahmad, Yan, & Bless, 2012; Biever & Bless, 1989; Linville, 1992; Pontes et al., 2006). Reasons for male–female differences in vocal fold approximation are speculative and include sex-related differences in the arrangement of the cricoarytenoid joints, muscle mass of the body of the vocal folds, and covers of the vocal folds (Hirano, Kiyokawa, & Kurita, 1988; Hirano, Kiyokawa, Kurita, & Sato, 1986). Cultural factors may also be at play, with a breathy voice quality being a more desirable characteristic of a female voice than of a male voice (Linville, 1992).

REVIEW

The larynx (voice box) is an air valve positioned between the trachea (windpipe) and the pharynx (throat) that can be adjusted to vary the amount of coupling between the two.

The skeleton of the larynx forms a framework consisting of bone, cartilages, ligaments, and tendons.

Major cartilages of the larynx include the thyroid, cricoid, arytenoids, and epiglottis, which function, along with the hyoid bone, as an integral unit.

Two pairs of joints mediate movements of the interior of the larynx, one between the cricoid and thyroid cartilages on each side, and one between the cricoid and arytenoid cartilages on each side.

Prominent structures within the larynx include the laryngeal cavity, vocal folds, ventricular folds (false vocal folds), laryngeal ventricles, and ligaments and membranes.

The most important laryngeal structures are the vocal folds, which have a muscular body at their core and an intricate outer covering with distinct layers.

Two types of forces operate on the larynx, one passive, which includes the natural recoil of tissues, surface tension between structures in apposition, and the pull of gravity; and one active, which includes intrinsic, extrinsic, and supplementary muscles that are nearly 20 in number and are activated in accordance with will and ability.

Intrinsic muscles of the larynx include the *thyroarytenoid, posterior cricoarytenoid, lateral cricoarytenoid, arytenoid*, and *cricothyroid*.

Extrinsic muscles of the larynx include the *sternothyroid, thyrohyoid*, and *inferior constrictor*.

Supplementary muscles of the larynx are classified as infrahyoid muscles—*sternohyoid* and *omohyoid*—and suprahyoid muscles—*digastric, stylohyoid, mylohyoid, geniohyoid, hyoglossus*, and *genioglossus*.

Movements of the larynx can result in changes in the positioning of the vocal folds (abduction, adduction, and changing length), ventricular folds, epiglottis, and laryngeal housing.

The control variables of laryngeal function include laryngeal opposing pressure, laryngeal airway resistance, glottal size and configuration, stiffness of the vocal folds, and effective mass of the vocal folds.

The neural substrates of laryngeal control are supported by cranial nerves V, VII, X, and XII and cervical spinal nerves C1, C2, and C3, which provide motor supply to the muscles of the larynx and sensory supply that conveys information from mechanoreceptors about muscle lengths, rates of change in muscle length, joint movements, and mucosal deformations.

Laryngeal function is concerned mainly with the degree of coupling between the trachea and pharynx, protection of the pulmonary airways, containment of the pulmonary air supply, and sound generation.

Laryngeal function for speech production includes the generation of transient noise production (glottal stop-plosive), sustained noise production (glottal fricative or whisper), sustained voicing, and running speech activities.

Voice production relies on quasi-periodic vocal fold vibration governed by nonlinear interaction between an energy source (the breathing apparatus) and the structures being vibrated (the vocal folds).

Vocal fold vibration is self-sustaining because certain conditions exist, including alternations in the shape of the glottis (ranging from convergent to divergent), alternations in the intraglottal pressure (ranging from relatively high to relatively low), and the presence of vocal fold tissue recoil force (ranging from lower than intraglottal pressure to higher than intraglottal pressure).

The fundamental frequency of the voice (correlated with the pitch of the voice) is the rate of vocal fold vibration and is controlled primarily by the stiffness of the vocal folds as well as their mass.

Fundamental frequency is manipulated primarily by the *cricothyroid* and *thyroarytenoid* muscles, with additional contributions by other laryngeal muscles.

The sound pressure level of the voice (correlated with the loudness of the voice) is controlled mainly by adjustments of the breathing apparatus (tracheal pressure) and the larynx (primarily laryngeal opposing pressure and laryngeal airflow declination rate) with somewhat less important adjustments of the pharyngeal-oral airway that alter the radiation impedance.

The lowest and highest values that can be produced in fundamental frequency and sound pressure level of the voice are not independent of one another, with the fundamental frequency range being greatest in the midrange of sound pressure levels and the sound pressure level range being greatest in the midrange of fundamental frequencies.

The voice source (tone produced at the larynx) is complex and has a spectrum (combination of frequencies and sound pressure levels) that bears some relation to the quality of the voice.

Pulse, modal, and loft are terms applied to three different voice registers that correspond to three different modes of vocal fold vibration and voice qualities encountered when speaking from the lowest to highest fundamental frequencies within the speaking range.

Laryngeal function during running speech activities is complex in that adjustments are made to control fundamental frequency, sound pressure level, and spectrum of the voice and to control actions of the larynx that constitute articulatory behaviors.

The larynx undergoes relocation and remodeling during a developmental period that extends into adolescence and is characterized by sexual dimorphism and a rapid growth spurt in males that lowers their fundamental frequency significantly in relation to females, whereas the mature larynx undergoes slower modification as a result of aging processes that stiffen it, degrade its joints, decrease its muscle mass, alter its composition, and otherwise make its function somewhat less efficient.

Males and females show laryngeal differences and voice production differences that have roots in structural and hormonal differences, different rates of ossification and calcification of laryngeal cartilages, different patterns of change in the covers of the vocal folds, and different patterns of valving by the vocal folds.

REFERENCES

Ahmad, K., Yan, Y., & Bless, D. (2012). Vocal fold vibratory characteristics of healthy geriatric females—analysis of high-speed digital images. *Journal of Voice, 26,* 751–759.

Allen, E., & Hollien, H. (1973). Vocal fold thickness in pulse (vocal fry) register. *Folia Phoniatrica, 25,* 241–250.

Ardran, G., & Kemp, F. (1966). The mechanism of the larynx, I: The movements of the arytenoid and cricoids cartilages. *British Journal of Radiology, 39,* 641–654.

Arnold, G. (1961). Physiology and pathology of the cricothyroid muscle. *Laryngoscope, 71,* 687–753.

Aronson, A. (1990). *Clinical voice disorders: An interdisciplinary approach* (3rd ed.). New York, NY: Thieme.

Atkinson, J. (1978). Correlation analysis of the physiological factors controlling fundamental voice frequency. *Journal of the Acoustical Society of America, 63,* 211–222.

Awan, S., & Mueller, P. (1992). Speaking fundamental frequency characteristics of centenarian females. *Clinical Linguistics and Phonetics, 6,* 249–254.

Baken, R., & Orlikoff, R. (2000). *Clinical measurement of speech and voice* (2nd ed.). San Diego, CA: Singular.

Banal, I. (2017). Voice in different phases of menstrual cycle among naturally cycling women and users of hormonal contraceptives. *PLoS One, 12.* https://doi.org/10.1371/journal.pone.0183462

Behrman, A. (2007). *Speech and voice science.* San Diego, CA: Plural.

Beneragama, T., & Serpell, J. (2006). Extralaryngeal bifurcation of the recurrent laryngeal nerve: A common variation. *ANZ Journal of Surgery, 76,* 928–931.

Benjamin, B. (1981). Frequency variability in the aged voice. *Journal of Gerontology, 36,* 722–736.

Benjamin, B. (1988). Changes in speech production and linguistic behaviors with aging. In B. Shadden (Ed.), *Communication behavior and aging: A sourcebook for clinicians* (pp. 162–181). Baltimore, MD: Williams & Wilkins.

Berke, G., & Gerratt, B. (1993). Laryngeal biomechanics: An overview of mucosal wave mechanics. *Journal of Voice, 7,* 123–128.

Berry, D., & Titze, I. (1996). Normal modes in a continuum model of vocal fold tissues. *Journal of the Acoustical Society of America, 100,* 3345–3354.

Biever, D., & Bless, D. (1989). Vibratory characteristics of the vocal folds in young adult and geriatric women. *Journal of Voice, 3,* 120–131.

Bosma, J. (1985). Postnatal ontogeny of performance of the pharynx, larynx, and mouth. *American Review of Respiratory Disease, 131,* 10–15.

Broad, D. (1973). Phonation. In F. Minifie, T. Hixon, & F. Williams (Eds.), *Normal aspects of speech, hearing, and language* (pp. 127–167). Englewood Cliffs, NJ: Prentice-Hall.

Catten, M., Gray, S., Hammond, T., Zhou, R., & Hammond, E. (1998). Analysis of cellular location and concentration in vocal fold lamina propria. *Otolaryngology–Head and Neck Surgery, 118,* 663–667.

Cavagna, G., & Margaria, R. (1965). An analysis of the mechanics of phonation. *Journal of Applied Physiology, 20,* 301–307.

Charpied, G., & Shapshay, S. (2004). *Anatomy and histology of the pars media of the cricothyroid muscle: A comparative study.* Paper presented at the International Conference on Voice Physiology and Biomechanics, Marseille, France.

Coleman, R. (1963). Decay characteristics of vocal fry. *Folia Phoniatrica, 15,* 256–263.

Coleman, R., Mabis, J., & Hinson, J. (1977). Fundamental frequency—sound pressure level profiles of adult male and female voices. *Journal of Speech and Hearing Research, 20,* 197–204.

Colton, R. (1972). Spectral characteristics of the modal and falsetto registers. *Folia Phoniatrica, 24,* 337–344.

Colton, R. (1973). Vocal intensity in the modal and falsetto registers. *Folia Phoniatrica, 25,* 62–70.

Cooper, D. (1990). *Maturation, characteristics, and aging of laryngeal muscles.* Paper presented at the Pacific Voice Conference, San Francisco, CA.

Curry, E. (1946). Voice changes in male adolescents. *Laryngoscope, 56,* 795–805.

Damste, H. (1970). The phonetogram. *Practica Oto-RhinoLaryngologica, 32,* 185–187.

Daniloff, R., Shuckers, G., & Feth, L. (1980). *The physiology of speech and hearing.* Englewood Cliffs, NJ: Prentice-Hall.

de Melo, E., Lemas, M., Filho, J., Sennes, L., Saldiva, P., & Tsuji, D. (2003). Distribution of collagen in the lamina propria of the human vocal fold. *Laryngoscope, 113,* 2187–2191.

Dickson, D., & Maue-Dickson, W. (1982). *Anatomical and physiological bases of speech.* Boston, MA: Little, Brown and Company.

Dromey, C., Stathopoulos, E., & Sapienza, C. (1992). Glottal airflow and electroglottographic measures of vocal function at multiple intensities. *Journal of Voice, 6,* 44–54.

Duffy, J. (2013). *Motor speech disorders: Substrates, differential diagnosis, and management* (3rd ed.). New York, NY: Mosby.

Eichhorn, J., Kent, R., Austin, D., & Vorperian, H. (2017). Effects of aging on vocal fundamental frequency and vowel formants in men and women. *Journal of Voice.* Advance online publication. https://doi.org/10.1016/j.jvoice.2017.08.003

Faaborg-Andersen, K., & Sonninen, A. (1960). The function of the extrinsic laryngeal muscles at different pitch: An electromyographic and roentgenologic investigation. *Acta Otolaryngologica, 51,* 89–93.

Fairbanks, G. (1960). *Voice and articulation drillbook.* New York, NY: Harper & Row.

Fairbanks, G., Herbert, E., & Hammond, J. (1949). An acoustical study of vocal pitch in seven- and eight-year-old girls. *Child Development, 20,* 71–78.

Fairbanks, G., & Miron, M. (1957). Effect of vocal effort upon the consonant-vowel ratio within the syllable. *Journal of the Acoustical Society of America, 29,* 621–626.

Fairbanks, G., Wiley, J., & Lassman, F. (1949). An acoustical study of vocal pitch in seven- and eight-year-old boys. *Child Development, 20,* 63–69.

Fant, G. (1960). *Acoustic theory of speech production.* The Hague, Netherlands: Mouton.

Ferreri, G. (1959). Senescence of the larynx. *Italian General Review of Otorhinolaryngology, 1,* 640–709.

Fink, B. (1975). *The human larynx: A functional study.* New York, NY: Raven Press.

Fink, B., Basek, M., & Epanchin, V. (1956). The mechanism of opening of the human larynx. *Laryngoscope, 66,* 410–425.

Flanagan, J. (1972). *Speech analysis, synthesis, and perception.* New York, NY: Springer-Verlag.

Flores, A., Herman, J., Gates, G., & Brown, T. (2016). *How many adults identify as transgender in the United States?* Los Angeles, CA: The Williams Institute

Folkard, C. (2006). *Guinness world records: 2006.* New York, NY: Bantam Books.

Frable, M. (1961). Computation of motion at the cricoarytenoid joint. *Archives of Otolaryngology, 73,* 551–556.

Fuamenya, N., Robb, M., & Wermke, K. (2015). Noisy but effective: Crying across the first 3 months of life. *Journal of Voice, 29,* 281–286.

Gauffin, J., & Sundberg, J. (1989). Spectral correlates of glottal voice source waveform characteristics. *Journal of Speech and Hearing Research, 32,* 556–565.

Gay, T., Hirose, H., Strome, M., & Sawashima, M. (1972). Electromyography of the intrinsic laryngeal muscles during phonation. *Annals of Otology, Rhinology, and Laryngology, 81,* 401–409.

Glaze, L., Bless, D., Milenkovic, P., & Susser, R. (1988). Acoustic characteristics of children's voice. *Journal of Voice, 2,* 312–319.

Glikson, E., Sagiv, D., Eyal, A., Wolf, M., & Primov-Fever, A. (2017). The anatomical evolution of the thyroid cartilage from childhood to adulthood: A computed tomography evaluation. *Laryngoscope, 127,* E354–E358.

Gramming, P. (1991). Vocal loudness and frequency capabilities of the voice. *Journal of Voice, 5,* 144–157.

Hall, A., Cobb, R., Kapoor, K., Kuchai, R., & Sandhu, G. (2017). The instrument of voice: The "true" vocal cord or vocal fold? *Journal of Voice, 31,* 133–134.

Hamdan, A-L., Tabet, G., Fakhri, G., Sarieddine, D., Btaiche, R., & Seoud, M. (2018). Effect of hormonal replacement therapy on voice. *Journal of Voice, 32*(1): 116–121.

Hasek, C., Singh, S., & Murry, T. (1980). Acoustic attributes of children's voices. *Journal of the Acoustical Society of America, 68,* 1252–1265.

Hately, B., Evison, G., & Samuel, E. (1965). The pattern of ossification in the laryngeal cartilages: A radiological study. *British Journal of Radiology, 38,* 585–591.

Hertegård, S. (2016). Tissue engineering in the larynx and airway. *Current Opinion in Otolaryngology Head and Neck Surgery, 24,* 469–476.

Hirano, M. (1974). Morphological structures of the vocal cord as a vibrator and its variations. *Folia Phoniatrica, 26,* 89–94.

Hirano, M. (1981). *Clinical examination of voice.* New York, NY: Springer-Verlag Wien.

Hirano, M., Kakita, Y., Kawasaki, H., Gould, W., & Lambiase, A. (1981). Data from high-speed motion picture studies. In K. Stevens & M. Hirano (Eds.), *Vocal fold physiology* (pp. 85–93). Tokyo, Japan: University of Tokyo Press.

Hirano, M., Kiyokawa, K., & Kurita, S. (1988). Laryngeal muscles and glottal shaping. In O. Fujimura (Ed.), *Vocal physiology: Voice production, mechanisms, and functions* (pp. 49–65). New York: Raven Press.

Hirano, M., Kiyokawa, K., Kurita, S., & Sato, K. (1986). Posterior glottis: Morphological study in excised larynges. *Annals of Otology, Rhinology, and Laryngology, 95,* 576–581.

Hirano, M., Kurita, S., & Nakashima, T. (1983). Growth, development and aging of human vocal folds. In D. Bless & J. Abbs (Eds.), *Vocal fold physiology: Contemporary research and clinical issues* (pp. 22–43). San Diego, CA: College-Hill Press.

Hirano, M., Kurita, S., & Sagaguchi, S. (1989). Aging of the vibratory tissue of the human vocal folds. *Acta Otolaryngologica, 107,* 428–433.

Hirano, M., Ohala, J., & Vennard, W. (1969). The function of the laryngeal muscles in regulating fundamental frequency and intensity of phonation. *Journal of Speech and Hearing Research, 12,* 616–628.

Hirano, M., & Sato, K. (1993). *Histological color atlas of the human larynx.* San Diego, CA: Singular.

Hirano, M., Vennard, W., & Ohala, J. (1970). Regulation of register, pitch and intensity of voice. *Folia Phoniatrica, 22*, 1–20.

Hirano, M., Yoshida, T., & Tanaka, S. (1991). Vibratory behavior of human vocal folds viewed from below. In J. Gauffin & B. Hammarberg (Eds.), *Vocal fold physiology: Acoustic, perceptual, and physiological aspects of voice mechanisms* (pp. 1–6). San Diego, CA: Singular.

Hirose, H. (1977). Laryngeal adjustments in consonant production. *Phonetica, 34*, 289–294.

Hixon, T. (1966). Turbulent noise sources for speech. *Folia Phoniatrica, 18*, 168–182.

Hixon, T., Klatt, D., & Mead, J. (1971). Influence of forced transglottal pressure change on vocal fundamental frequency. *Journal of the Acoustical Society of America, 49*, 105.

Hixon, T., Mead, J., & Goldman, M. (1976). Dynamics of the chest wall during speech production: Function of the thorax, rib cage, diaphragm, and abdomen. *Journal of Speech and Hearing Research, 19*, 297–356.

Hixon, T., & Minifie, F. (1972). *Influence of forced transglottal pressure change on vocal sound pressure level*. Paper presented at the Convention of the American Speech and Hearing Association, San Francisco, CA.

Hixon, T., Minifie, F., & Tait, C. (1967). Correlates of turbulent noise production for speech. *Journal of Speech and Hearing Research, 10*, 133–140.

Hoit, J., & Hixon, T. (1992). Age and laryngeal airway resistance during vowel production in women. *Journal of Speech and Hearing Research, 35*, 309–313.

Hollien, H. (1960a). Some laryngeal correlates of vocal pitch. *Journal of Speech and Hearing Research, 3*, 52–58.

Hollien, H. (1960b). Vocal pitch variations related to changes in vocal fold length. *Journal of Speech and Hearing Research, 3*, 150–156.

Hollien, H. (1962). Vocal fold thickness and fundamental frequency of phonation. *Journal of Speech and Hearing Research, 5*, 237–243.

Hollien, H. (1972). Three major vocal registers: A proposal. In A. Rigault & R. Charbonneau (Eds.), *Proceedings of the Seventh International Congress of Phonetic Sciences* (pp. 320–331). The Hague, Netherlands: Mouton.

Hollien, H. (1974). On vocal registers. *Journal of Phonetics, 2*, 125–143.

Hollien, H., Brown, W., & Hollien, K. (1971). Vocal fold length associated with modal, falsetto and varying vocal intensity phonations. *Folia Phoniatrica, 23*, 66–78.

Hollien, H., & Colton, R. (1969). Four laminagraphic studies of vocal fold thickness. *Folia Phoniatrica, 21*, 179–198.

Hollien, H., & Curtis, J. (1960). A laminagraphic study of vocal pitch. *Journal of Speech and Hearing Research, 3*, 362–371.

Hollien, H., Damste, H., & Murry, T. (1969). Vocal fold length during vocal fry phonation. *Folia Phoniatrica, 21*, 257–265.

Hollien, H., Green, R., & Massey, K. (1994). Longitudinal research on adolescent voice change in males. *Journal of the Acoustical Society of America, 34*, 80–84.

Hollien, H., & Moore, P. (1960). Measurements of the vocal folds during changes in pitch. *Journal of Speech and Hearing Research, 3*, 157–163.

Hollien, H., & Shipp, T. (1972). Speaking fundamental frequency and chronological age in males. *Journal of Speech and Hearing Research, 15*, 155–159.

Holmberg, E., Hillman, R., & Perkell, J. (1988). Glottal airflow and transglottal air pressure measurements for male and female speakers in soft, normal, and loud voice. *Journal of the Acoustical Society of America, 84*, 511–529.

Holmberg, E., Hillman, R., & Perkell, J. (1989). Glottal airflow and transglottal air pressure measurements for male and female speakers in low, normal, and high pitch. *Journal of Voice, 3*, 294–305.

Holmes, L., Leeper, H., & Nicholson, I. (1994). Laryngeal airway resistance of older men and women as a function of vocal sound pressure level. *Journal of Speech and Hearing Research, 37*, 789–799.

Honda, K. (1995). Laryngeal and extra-laryngeal mechanisms of Fo control. In F. Bell-Berti & L. Raphael (Eds.), *Producing speech: Contemporary issues—for Katherine Safford Harris* (pp. 215–245). New York, NY: American Institute of Physics.

Honjo, I., & Isshiki, N. (1980). Laryngoscopic and voice characteristics of aged persons. *Archives of Otolaryngology, 106*, 149–150.

Ishii, K., Zhai, W., Akita, M., & Hirose, H. (1996). Ultra-structure of the lamina propria of the human vocal fold. *Acta Otolaryngologica, 116*, 778–782.

Isshiki, N. (1964). Regulatory mechanism of voice intensity variation. *Journal of Speech and Hearing Research, 7*, 17–29.

Isshiki, N. (1965). Vocal intensity and air flow rate. *Folia Phoniatrica, 17*, 92–104.

Jankovskaya, N. (1959). The receptor innervation of the perichondrium of the laryngeal cartilages. *Arkhiv Anatomii, Gistologii l'Enbriologii, 37*, 70–75.

Jotz, G., Stefani, M., Pereira da Costa Filho, O., Malysz, T., Soster, P., & Leão, H. (2014). A morphometric study of the larynx. *Journal of Voice, 28*, 668–672.

Kahane, J. (1975). *(The developmental anatomy of the human prepubertal and pubertal larynx* (Doctoral dissertation). University of Pittsburgh, Pittsburgh, PA.

Kahane, J. (1978). A morphological study of the human prepubertal and pubertal larynx. *American Journal of Anatomy, 151*, 11–20.

Kahane, J. (1980). Age related histological changes in the human male and female laryngeal cartilages: Biological and functional implications. In V. Lawrence (Ed.), *Transcripts of the Ninth Symposium: Care of the Professional Voice, Part I* (pp. 11–20). New York, NY: The Voice Foundation.

Kahane, J. (1982). Growth of the human prepubertal and pubertal larynx. *Journal of Speech and Hearing Research, 25*, 446–455.

Kahane, J. (1983). A survey of age-related changes in the connective tissue of the human adult larynx. In D. Bless & J. Abbs (Eds.), *Vocal fold physiology: Contemporary research and clinical issues* (pp. 44–49). San Diego, CA: College-Hill Press.

Kahane, J. (1987). Connective tissue changes in the larynx and their effects on voice. *Journal of Voice, 1*, 27–30.

Kahane, J. (1988). Age-related changes in the human cricoarytenoid joint. In O. Fujimura (Ed.), *Vocal physiology: Voice production, mechanisms, and functions* (pp. 145–157). New York, NY: Raven Press.

Kahane, J. (2007). *A description of regional specialization in the human thyroarytenoid muscle.* Paper presented at the 36th Annual Symposium on Care of the Professional Voice, Philadelphia, PA.

Kahane, J., & Beckford, N. (1991). The aging larynx and voice. In D. Ripich (Ed.), *Handbook of geriatric communication disorders* (pp. 165–186). Austin, TX: Pro-Ed.

Kahane, J., & Hammons, J. (1987). Developmental changes in the articular cartilage of the human cricoarytenoid joint. In T. Baer, C. Sasaki, & K. Harris (Eds.), *Laryngeal function in phonation and respiration* (pp. 14–28). San Diego, CA: College-Hill Press.

Kahane, J., & Kahn, A. (1984). Weight measurements of infant and adult intrinsic laryngeal muscles. *Folia Phoniatrica, 36,* 129–133.

Kahane, J., Stadlin, J., & Bell, J. (1979). *A histological study of the aging human larynx.* Scientific exhibit presented at the Convention of the American Speech-Language-Hearing Association, Atlanta, GA.

Kahn, A., & Kahane, J. (1986). India pin prick experiments on surface organization of cricoarytenoid joints (CAJ) articular surfaces. *Journal of Speech and Hearing Research, 29,* 536–543.

Kazarian, A., Sarkissian, L., & Isaakian, D. (1978). Length of the human vocal cords by age. *Zhurnal Eksperimentalnoi I Klinicheskoi Meditsiny, 18,* 105–109.

Keleman, G., & Pressman, J. (1955). Physiology of the larynx. *Physiological Review, 35,* 506–554.

Kempster, G., Gerratt, B., Abbott, K. Barkmeier-Kraemer, J., & Hillman, R. (2009). Consensus auditory-perceptual evaluation of voice: Development of a standardized clinical protocol. *American Journal of Speech-Language Pathology, 18,* 124–132.

Kent, R. (1976). Anatomical and neuromuscular maturation of the speech mechanism: Evidence from acoustic studies. *Journal of Speech and Hearing Research, 19,* 421–447.

Kent, R. (1997). *The speech sciences.* San Diego, CA: Singular.

Kent, R., & Vorperian, H. (1995). Anatomic development of the craniofacial-oral-laryngeal systems: A review. *Journal of Medical Speech-Language Pathology, 3,* 145–190.

Kirchner, J., & Suzuki, M. (1968). Laryngeal reflexes and voice production. *Annals of the New York Academy of Sciences, 155,* 98–109.

Kirchner, J., & Wyke, B. (1965). Articular reflex mechanisms in the larynx. *Annals of Otology, Rhinology, and Laryngology, 74,* 749–768.

Konig, W., & von Leden, H. (1961a). The peripheral nervous system of the human larynx, 1: The mucous membrane. *Archives of Otolaryngology, 73,* 1–14.

Konig, W., & von Leden, H. (1961b). The peripheral nervous system of the human larynx, 2: The thyroarytenoid (vocalis) muscle. *Archives of Otolaryngology, 74,* 153–163.

Konnai, R., Scherer, R., Peplinski, A., & Ryan, K. (2017). Whisper and phonation: Aerodynamic comparisons across adduction and loudness. *Journal of Voice, 31,* 773.e11–773.e20.

Kucinski, P., Okrazewska, E., & Piszcz, W. (1979). Variability of the course of the cricothyroid muscle in humans. *Folia Morphologica, 38,* 391–396.

Kunze, L. (1962). *An investigation of changes in sub-glottal air pressure and rate of air flow accompanying changes in fundamental frequency, intensity, vowels, and voice registers in adult male speakers* (Doctoral dissertation). University of Iowa, Iowa City.

Ladefoged, P., & McKinney, N. (1963). Loudness, sound pressure, and subglottal pressure in speech. *Journal of the Acoustical Society of America, 35,* 454–460.

Laitman, J., & Crelin, E. (1976). Postnatal development of the basiocranium and vocal tract region in man. In J. Bosma (Ed.), *Symposium on development of the basiocranium* (pp. 206–220). Washington, DC: Department of Health, Education, and Welfare.

Large, J., Iwata, S., & von Leden, H. (1970). The primary female register transition in singing: An aerodynamic study. *Folia Phoniatrica, 22,* 385–396.

Laver, J. (1991). The gift of speech. *Papers in the analysis of speech and voice.* Edinburgh, Scotland: Edinburgh University Press.

Lester, R., & Story, B. (2013). Acoustic characteristics of simulated respiratory-induced vocal tremor. *American Journal of Speech-Language Pathology, 22,* 205–211.

Linville, S. (1987). Maximum phonational frequency range capabilities of women's voices with advancing age. *Folia Phoniatrica, 39,* 297–301.

Linville, S. (1992). Glottal gap configurations in two age groups of women. *Journal of Speech and Hearing Research, 35,* 1209–1215.

Linville, S. (1995). Vocal aging. *Current Opinion in Otolaryngology and Head and Neck Surgery, 3,* 183–187.

Linville, S., & Fisher, H. (1985). Acoustic characteristics of perceived versus actual age in controlled phonation by adult females. *Journal of the Acoustical Society of America, 78,* 40–48.

Lofqvist, A., & Yoshioka, H. (1984). Intrasegmental timing: Laryngeal-oral coordination in voiceless consonant production. *Speech Communication, 3,* 279–289.

Malinowski, A. (1967). Shape, dimensions, and process of calcification of the cartilaginous framework of the larynx in relation to age and sex in the Polish population. *Folia Morphologica, 26,* 118–128.

Mayet, A. (1955). Zur functionellen anatomie der menschlichen stimmlippe. *Zeitschrift fur Anatomie und Entwicklungsgeschichte, 119,* 87–111.

Mayet, A., & Muendnich, K. (1958). Beitrag zur anatomie und zur funktion des m. cricothyroideus und der cricothyreiodgelenke. *Acta Anatomica, 33,* 273–288.

McGlone, R. (1967). Air flow during vocal fry. *Journal of Speech and Hearing Research, 10,* 299–304.

McGlone, R. (1970). Air flow in the upper register. *Folia Phoniatrica, 22,* 231–238.

McGlone, R., & Shipp, T. (1971). Some physiologic correlates of vocal fry phonation. *Journal of Speech and Hearing Research, 14,* 769–775.

Melcon, M., Hoit, J., & Hixon, T. (1989). Age and laryngeal airway resistance during vowel production. *Journal of Speech and Hearing Disorders, 54,* 282–286.

Minifie, F. (1973). Speech acoustics. In F. Minifie, T. Hixon, & F. Williams (Eds.), *Normal aspects of speech, hearing, and language* (pp. 236–284). Englewood Cliffs, NJ: Prentice-Hall.

Monoson, P., & Zemlin, W. (1984). Quantitative study of whisper. *Folia Phoniatrica, 36,* 53–65.

Mueller, P., Sweeney, R., & Baribeau, L. (1985). Acoustic and morphologic study of the senescent voice. *Ear, Nose, and Throat Journal, 63,* 71–75.

Murry, T. (1971). Subglottal pressure and airflow measures during vocal fry phonation. *Journal of Speech and Hearing Research, 14,* 544–551.

Murry, T., & Brown, W. (1971a). Regulation of vocal intensity in vocal fry phonation. *Journal of the Acoustical Society of America, 49,* 1905–1907.

Murry, T., & Brown, W. (1971b). Subglottal air pressure during two types of vocal activity: Vocal fry and modal phonation. *Folia Phoniatrica, 23,* 440–449.

Netsell, R. (1969). *A perceptual-acoustic physiological study of syllable stress* (Doctoral dissertation). University of Iowa, Iowa City.

Netsell, R. (1973). Speech physiology. In F. Minifie, T. Hixon, & F. Williams (Eds.), *Normal aspects of speech, hearing, and language* (pp. 211–234). Englewood Cliffs, NJ: Prentice-Hall.

Oates, J., & Dacakis, G. (2015). Transgender voice and communication: Research evidence underpinning voice intervention for male-to-female transsexual women. *Perspectives on Voice and Voice Disorders, 25,* 48–58.

Obrebowski, A., Wojnowski, W., & Obrebowski-Karsznia, Z. (2006). The characteristics of vocal fold molecular structure. *Otolaryngologia Polska, 60,* 9–14.

Ohala, J. (1972). *How is pitch lowered?* Paper presented at the Spring Meeting of the Acoustical Society of America. Buffalo, NY.

Ohala, J., & Hirose, H. (1970). The function of the sternohyoid muscle in speech. *Annual Report of the Institute of Logopedics and Phoniatrics, 4,* 41–44.

Okamura, H., & Katto, Y. (1988). Fine structure of muscle spindle in interarytenoid muscle of the human larynx. In O. Fujimura (Ed.), *Vocal fold physiology: Voice production, mechanisms, and functions* (pp. 135–143). New York, NY: Raven Press.

Orlikoff, R., & Kahane, J. (1996). Structure and function of the larynx. In N. Lass (Ed.), *Principles of experimental phonetics* (pp. 112–181). St. Louis, MO: Mosby.

Pontes, P., Yamasaki, R., & Behlau, M. (2006). Morphological and functional aspects of the senile larynx. *Folia Phoniatrica et Logopaedica, 58,* 151–158.

Pressman, J. (1942). Physiology of the vocal cords in phonation and respiration. *Archives of Otolaryngology, 35,* 355–398.

Ramig, L., & Ringel, R. (1983). Effects of physiological aging on selected acoustic characteristics of voice. *Journal of Speech and Hearing Research, 26,* 22–30.

Reidenbach, M. (1998). The muscular tissue of the vestibular folds of the larynx. *European Archives of Otorhinolaryngology, 255,* 365–367.

Rogers, D., Setlur, J., Raol, N., Maurer, R., & Hartnick, C. (2014). Evaluation of true vocal fold growth as a function of age. *Otolaryngology–Head and Neck Surgery, 151,* 681–686.

Rothenberg, M. (1968). The breath-stream dynamics of simple-released-plosive production. *Bibliotheca Phonetica No. 6.* Basel, Switzerland: S. Karger.

Rothenberg, M. (1983). An interactive model for the voice source. In D. Bless & J. Abbs (Eds.), *Vocal fold physiology: Contemporary research and clinical issues* (pp. 155–165). San Diego, CA: College-Hill Press.

Rubin, A., Praneetvataku, V., Gherson, S., & Moyer, C. (2006). Laryngeal hyperfunction during whispering: Reality or myth? *Journal of Voice, 20,* 121–127.

Rubin, H. (1963). Experimental studies in vocal pitch and intensity in phonation. *Laryngoscope, 72,* 973–1015.

Russell, A., Penny, L., & Pemberton, C. (1995). Speaking fundamental frequency changes over time in women: A longitudinal study. *Journal of Speech and Hearing Research, 38,* 101–109.

Sampson, S., & Eyzaguirre, C. (1964). Some functional characteristics of mechanoreceptors in the larynx of the cat. *Journal of Neurophysiology, 27,* 464–480.

Sanders, I., Han, Y., Wang, J., & Biller, H. (1998). Muscle spindles are concentrated in the superior vocalis subcompartment of the human thyroarytenoid muscle. *Journal of Voice, 12,* 7–16.

Sanders, I., Rai, S., Han, Y., & Biller, H.F. (1998). Human vocalis contains distinct superior and inferior subcompartments: Possible candidates for the two masses of vocal fold vibration. *Annals of Otology, Rhinology & Laryngology, 107,* 826–833.

Sanders, I., Wu, L., Mu, Y., & Biller, H. (1993). Innervation of the human larynx. *Archives of Otolaryngology–Head and Neck Surgery, 119,* 934–939.

Sanudo, J., Maranillo, E., Xavier, L., Mirapeix, R., Orus, C., & Quer, M. (1999). An anatomical study of anastomoses between the laryngeal nerves. *Laryngoscope, 109,* 983–987.

Sasaki, C., Levin, P., Laitman, J., & Crelin, E. (1977). Post-natal descent of the epiglottis in man: A preliminary report. *Archives of Otolaryngology, 103,* 169–171.

Sato, K., Kurita, S., Hirano, M., & Kiyokawa, K. (1990). Distribution of elastic cartilage in the arytenoids and its physiologic significance. *Annals of Otology, Rhinology, and Laryngology, 99,* 363–368.

Sawashima, M., Abramson, A., Cooper, F., & Lisker, L. (1970). Observing laryngeal adjustments during running speech by use of a fiberoptics system. *Phonetica, 22,* 193–201.

Schonharl, E. (1960). *Die stroboskopie in der praktischen laryngologie.* Stuttgart, Germany: Thieme-Verlag.

Segre, R. (1971). Senescence of the voice. *Eye, Ear, Nose, and Throat Monthly, 50,* 223–233.

Sekizawa, K., Sasaki, H., & Takishima, T. (1985). Laryngeal resistance immediately after panting in control and constricted airways. *Journal of Applied Physiology, 58,* 1164–1169.

Selbie, W., Zhang, L., Levine, W., & Ludlow, C. (1998). Using joint geometry to determine the motion of the cricoarytenoid joint. *Journal of the Acoustical Society of America, 103,* 1115–1127.

Sellars, I., & Keen, E. (1978). The anatomy and movements of the cricoarytenoid joint. *Laryngoscope, 88,* 667–674.

Shipp, T., & Hollien, H. (1969). Perception of the aging male voice. *Journal of Speech and Hearing Research, 12,* 704–710.

Shipp, T., & McGlone, R. (1971). Laryngeal dynamics associated with voice frequency change. *Journal of Speech and Hearing Research, 14,* 761–768.

Shipp, T., McGlone, R., & Morrissey, P. (1972). Some physiologic correlates of voice frequency change. In A. Rigault & R. Charbonneau (Eds.), *Proceedings of the 7th International Congress of Phonetic Sciences* (pp. 407–411). The Hague, Netherlands: Mouton.

Sodersten, M., & Lindestad, P. (1990). Glottal closure and perceived breathiness during phonation in normally speaking subjects. *Journal of Speech and Hearing Research, 33,* 601–611.

Solomon, N., McCall, G., Trosset, M., & Gray, W. (1989). Laryngeal configuration and constriction during two types of whispering. *Journal of Speech and Hearing Research, 32,* 161–174.

Sonesson, B. (1959). Die funktionelle anatomie des cricoarytaenoidgelenkes. *Zeitschrift fur Anatomie und Entwicklungsgeschichte, 121,* 292–303.

Sonesson, B. (1960). On the anatomy and vibratory pattern of the human vocal folds. *Acta Otolaryngologica, Supplement 156,* 1–80.

Sonninen, A. (1968). The external frame function in the control of pitch in the human voice. *Annals of the New York Academy of Sciences, 155,* 68–90.

Stathopoulos, E., Hoit, J., Hixon, T., Watson, P., & Solomon, N. (1991). Respiratory and laryngeal function during whisper. *Journal of Speech and Hearing Research, 34,* 761–767.

Stathopoulos, E., Huber, J., & Sussman, J. (2011). Changes in acoustic characteristics of the voice across the life span: Measures from individuals 4–93 years of age. *Journal of Speech, Language, and Hearing Research, 54,* 1011–1021.

Stevens, K. (2000). *Acoustic phonetics.* Cambridge, MA: MIT Press.

Stoicheff, M. (1981). Speaking fundamental frequency characteristics of nonsmoking female adults. *Journal of Speech and Hearing Research, 24,* 437–441.

Story, B., & Titze, I. (1995). Voice simulation with a bodycover model of the vocal folds. *Journal of the Acoustical Society of America, 97,* 1249–1260.

Story, B. (2002). An overview of the physiology, physics and modeling of the sound source for vowels. *Acoustical Science and Technology, 23,* 195–206.

Strocchi, R., De Pasquale, V., Messerotti, G., Raspanti, M., Franchi, M., & Ruggeri, A. (1992). Particular structure of the anterior third of the human true vocal cord. *Acta Anatomica, 145,* 189–194.

Sundberg, J., Scherer, R., Hess, M., & Muller, F. (2010). Whispering—a single-subject study of glottal configuration and aerodynamics. *Journal of Voice, 24,* 574–584.

Takano, S., & Honda, K. (2005). Observation of the cricothyroid joint by high-resolution MRI. *Japanese Journal of Logopedics and Phoniatrics, 46,* 174–178.

Timcke, R., von Leden, H., & Moore, P. (1958). Laryngeal vibrations: Measurements of the glottic wave, I: The normal vibratory cycle. *Archives of Otolaryngology, 68,* 1–19.

Titze, I. (1988a). A framework for the study of vocal registers. *Journal of Voice, 2,* 183–194.

Titze, I. (1988b). Regulation of vocal power and efficiency by subglottal pressure and glottal width. In O. Fujimura (Ed.), *Vocal fold physiology: Voice production, mechanisms, and functions* (pp. 227–238). New York, NY: Raven Press.

Titze, I. (1989). On the relation between subglottal pressure and fundamental frequency in phonation. *Journal of the Acoustical Society of America, 85,* 901–906.

Titze, I. (1994). *Principles of voice production.* Englewood Cliffs, NJ: Prentice-Hall.

Titze, I. (2006a). *The myoelastic aerodynamic theory of phonation.* Iowa City, IA: National Center for Voice and Speech.

Titze, I. (2006b). Theoretical analysis of maximum flow declination rate versus maximum area declination rate in phonation. *Journal of Speech, Language, and Hearing Research, 49,* 439–447.

Titze, I., Jiang, J., & Drucker, D. (1988). Preliminaries to the body-cover theory of pitch control. *Journal of Voice, 1,* 314–319.

Titze, I., Luschei, E., & Hirano, M. (1989). Role of the thyroarytenoid muscle in regulation of fundamental frequency. *Journal of Voice, 3,* 213–224.

Titze, I., & Story, B. (2002). Rules for controlling low dimensional vocal fold models with muscle activation. *Journal of the Acoustical Society of America, 112,* 1064–1076.

Tucker, J., & Tucker, G. (1979). A clinical perspective on the development and anatomical aspects of the infant larynx and trachea. In G. Healy & T. McGill (Eds.), *Laryngotracheal problems in the pediatric patient* (pp. 3–8). Springfield, IL: Charles C. Thomas.

Tucker, L. (1963). *Articulatory variations in normal speakers with changes in vocal pitch and effort* (Master's thesis). University of Iowa, Iowa City.

van den Berg, J. (1956). Direct and indirect determination of the mean subglottic pressure. *Folia Phoniatrica, 8,* 1–24.

van den Berg, J. (1957). Subglottic pressure and vibrations of the vocal folds. *Folia Phoniatrica, 9,* 64–71.

van den Berg, J. (1958). Myoelastic-aerodynamic theory of voice production. *Journal of Speech and Hearing Research, 1,* 227–244.

van den Berg, J., & Moll, J. (1955). Zur anatomie des menschlichen musculus vocalis. *Zeitschrift fur Anatomie und Entwicklungsgeschichte, 118,* 465–470.

van den Berg, J., & Tan, T. (1959). Results of experiments with human larynxes. *Practica Oto-Rhino Laryngologica, 21,* 425–450.

van den Berg, J., Vennard, W., Berger, D., & Shervanian, C. (1960). *Voice production* [black and white 16-mm sound motion picture film]. Utrecht, Netherlands: SFW-UNFI.

van den Berg, J., Zantema, J., & Doornenbal, P. (1957). On the air resistance and the Bernoulli effect of the human larynx. *Journal of the Acoustical Society of America, 29,* 626–631.

Vennard, W. (1967). *Singing: The mechanism and the technic.* New York, NY: Carl Fischer.

von Leden, H., & Moore, P. (1961). The mechanics of the cricoarytenoid joint. *Archives of Otolaryngology, 73,* 541–550.

Vorperian, H., Wang, S., Chung, M.K., Schimek, E.M., Durtschi, R.B., & Kent, R.D. (2009). Anatomic development of the oral and pharyngeal portions of the vocal tract: An imaging study. *Journal of the Acoustical Society of America, 125*, 1666–1678.

Wang, R. (1998). Three-dimensional analysis of cricoarytenoid joint motion. *Laryngoscope, 108*, 1–17.

Watson, P., Ciccia, A., & Weismer, G. (2003). The relation of lung volume initiation to selected acoustic properties of speech. *Journal of the Acoustical Society of America, 113*, 2812–2819.

Wendahl, R., Moore, P., & Hollien, H. (1963). Comments on vocal fry. *Folia Phoniatrica, 15*, 251–255.

Wilson, K. (1979). *Voice disorders in children*. Baltimore, MD: Williams & Wilkins.

Wind, J. (1970). *On the phylogeny and the ontogeny of the human larynx*. Groningen, Netherlands: Wolters-Noordhoff.

Wustrow, F. (1953). Bau und funktion des menshlichne musculus vocalis. *Zeitschrift fur Anatomie und Entwick-lungsgeschichte, 116*, 506–522.

Yamauchi, A., Imagawa, H., Yokonishi, H., Nito, T., Yamasoba, T., Goto, T., . . . Tayama, N. (2012). Evaluation of vocal fold vibration with an assessment form for high-speed digital imaging: Comparative study between healthy young and elderly subjects. *Journal of Voice, 26*, 742–750.

Yanagihara, N., & Koike, Y. (1967). The regulation of sustained phonation. *Folia Phoniatrica, 19*, 1–18.

Zemlin, W. (1998). *Speech and hearing science: Anatomy and physiology*. Boston, MA: Allyn & Bacon.

Zemlin, W., Davis, P., & Gaza, C. (1984). Fine morphology of the posterior cricoarytenoid muscle. *Folia Phoniatrica, 36*, 233–240.

Zenker, W. (1964). Questions regarding the function of external laryngeal muscles. In D. Brewer (Ed.), *Research potentials in voice physiology* (pp. 20–40). Syracuse, NY: State University of New York.

4

Velopharyngeal-Nasal Function and Speech Production

INTRODUCTION

The velopharyngeal-nasal apparatus is located within the head and neck and comprises a system of valves and air passages that interconnects the pharynx (throat) and the atmosphere through the nose. Although most textbooks focus on the velopharyngeal part of this system, this chapter covers the complete velopharyngeal-nasal apparatus as a single functional entity. This is because the nasal part of the apparatus can have a significant influence on speech production, especially when velopharyngeal function is impaired.

This chapter covers the anatomy of the velopharyngeal apparatus, forces and movements of the apparatus, control variables, neural substrates, various functions of the apparatus, especially speech production, and variables that may influence speech production. The chapter concludes with a review.

ANATOMY OF THE VELOPHARYNGEAL-NASAL APPARATUS

The valves and air passages of the velopharyngeal-nasal apparatus are linked together, some arranged in mechanical series (one after another) and some arranged in mechanical parallel (side by side). The superstructure of the velopharyngeal apparatus is the skeletal framework that supports it and this is discussed in the first part in this section. From there, discussion moves to the anatomy of the pharynx, velum, nasal cavities, and outer nose. The muscles of the velopharyngeal-nasal apparatus are covered in the section on forces.

Skeletal Framework

The skeletal framework of the velopharyngeal-nasal apparatus consists of the first six cervical vertebrae and various bones of the skull. The bones of the skull include cranial (braincase) bones and facial (forehead, eyes, nose, mouth, and upper throat) bones. These bones are individually intricate structures that are rigidly joined together and contribute to formation of the walls, floor, and roof of the velopharyngeal-nasal apparatus, as well as provide anchors to which many of the velopharyngeal-nasal muscles attach. The velopharyngeal-nasal apparatus and the pharyngeal-oral apparatus share many bones of the skull. Therefore, the bones discussed in this section pertain to Chapter 5 as well.

Figure 4–1 depicts the cranial bones. Some of these bones are paired and some are not. The eight cranial bones are the temporal (two), parietal (two), occipital (one), frontal (one), sphenoid (one), and ethmoid (one) bones. Each temporal bone includes a narrow prominence called the styloid process to which muscle and ligament attach (other relevant features of the temporal bone are discussed in Chapter 13). The sphenoid bone, a double-winged structure, sits behind the eyes and forms the back wall of the nasal cavities. The ethmoid bone forms the upper sidewalls of the nasal cavities and the upper part of their medial wall.

Figure 4–2 depicts the facial bones, most of which are paired. These 14 bones are the maxillary (two), palatine (two), vomer (one), inferior nasal conchae (two), lacrimal (two), nasal (two), and zygomatic bones (two) and mandible (one). The bones most closely associated with structure of the velopharyngeal-nasal apparatus are the maxillary bones, which form the front of the floor of the nasal cavities; the palatine bones, which form the back of the floor of the nasal cavities; the

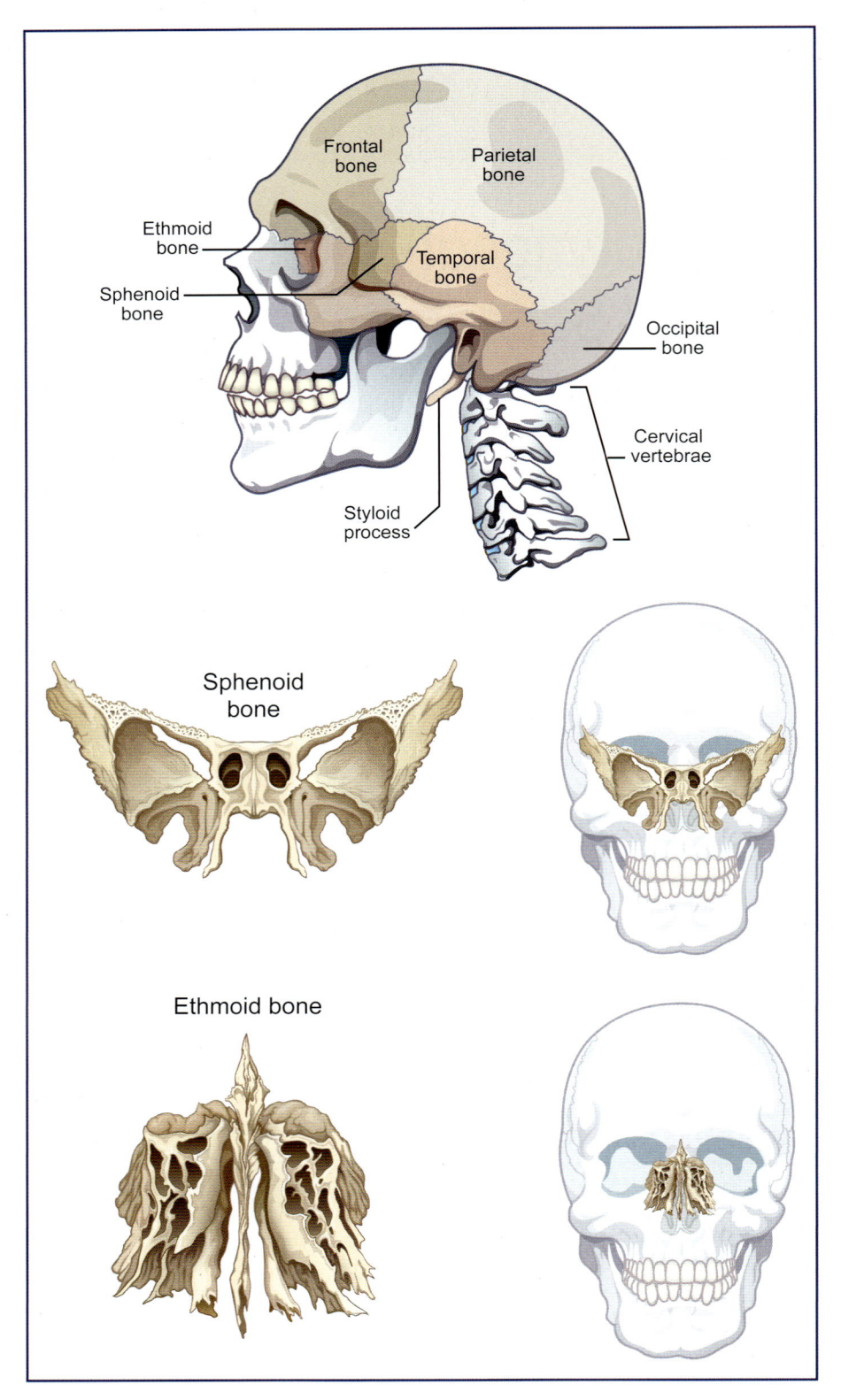

Figure 4-1. The cranial bones of the skull, two of which are paired. They include the temporal (paired), parietal (paired), occipital, frontal, sphenoid, and ethmoid bones.

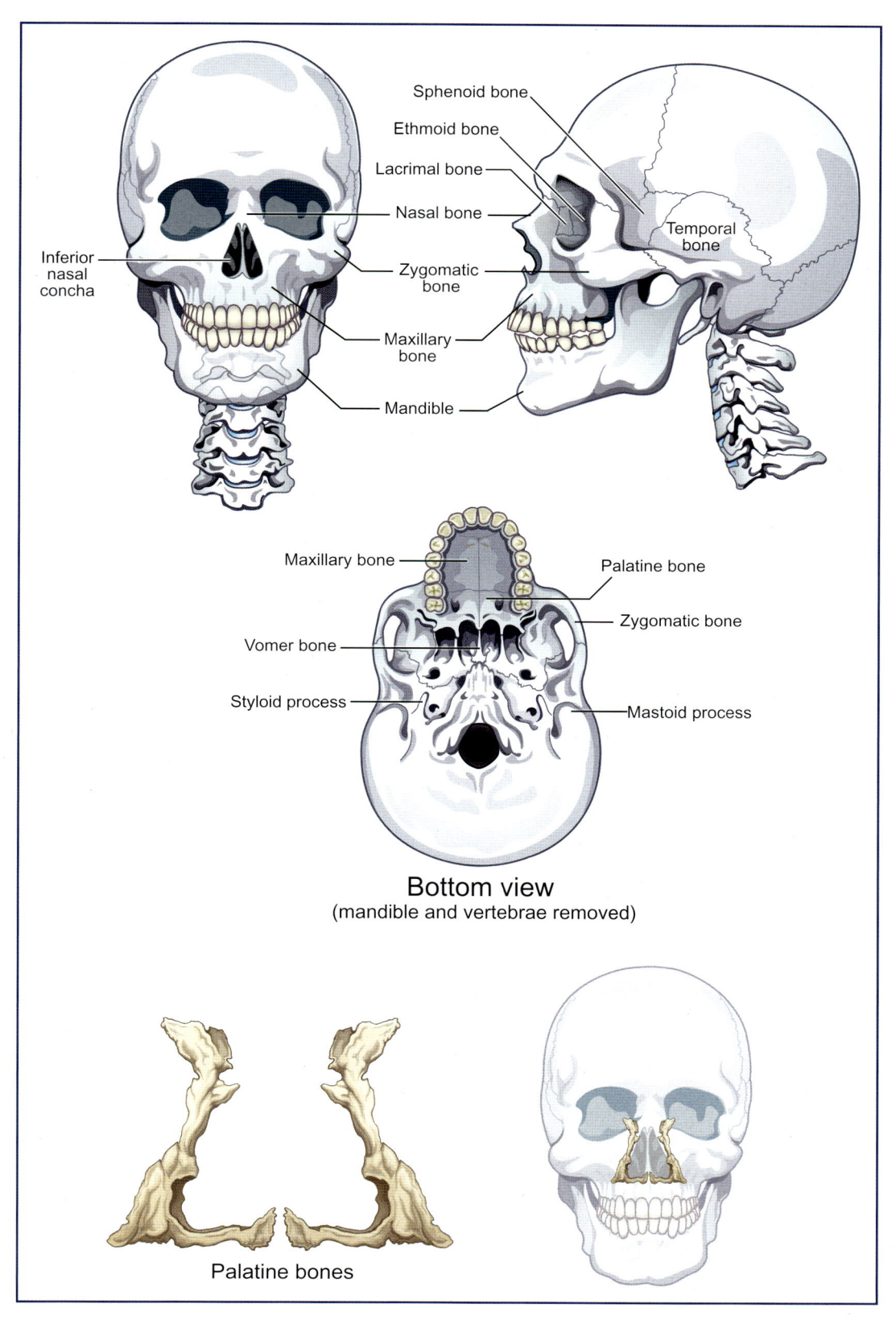

Figure 4-2. The facial bones of the skull, most of which are paired. They are the maxillary (paired), palatine (paired), vomer (single), inferior nasal conchae (paired), lacrimal (paired), nasal (paired), and zygomatic bones (paired) and mandible (single).

> ### Duane C. Spriestersbach (1916–2011)
>
> Spriestersbach had a distinguished career as a clinical investigator of the communication problems of children with cleft palate and craniofacial disorders. "Sprie," as he was affectionately called, served for many years as the program director of a large federally funded research grant on cleft palate at the University of Iowa. His leadership fostered much of the research done over two decades on normal velopharyngeal function for speech production and on the mechanisms involved in control of the velopharyngeal apparatus in individuals with velopharyngeal incompetence. Many of the names in the reference list to this chapter cut their research teeth under his guidance. Spriestersbach was an exceptional thinker. He had an enormous impact on translating the products of research into practical clinical applications for those with speech disorders caused by cleft palate. In his spare time, he took to the stage, where he performed in the Iowa City Community Theatre, and to the card table, where he played a legendary mean hand of poker.

vomer bone, which forms the lower part of the medial wall of the nasal cavities; the inferior nasal conchae (plural for concha), which form the lower sidewalls of the nasal cavities; and the nasal bones, which form the bridge of the outer nose. The zygomatic bones form the prominences of the cheeks and are also called the cheekbones. The small and fragile lacrimal bones form part of the orbit and articulate with the inferior nasal concha, ethmoid, frontal, and maxillary bones. The mandible is a movable facial bone that is discussed in detail in Chapter 5.

Pharynx

The pharynx is a tube of tendon and muscle that extends from the base of the skull to the cricoid cartilage in the front and to the sixth cervical vertebra in the back. The pharyngeal tube is widest at the top and narrows down its length and is oval in cross section, being larger side to side than front to back. As shown in Figure 4–3, the front wall of the pharynx is partially formed by the back surfaces of the velum (defined below), tongue, and epiglottis. Otherwise, the structure

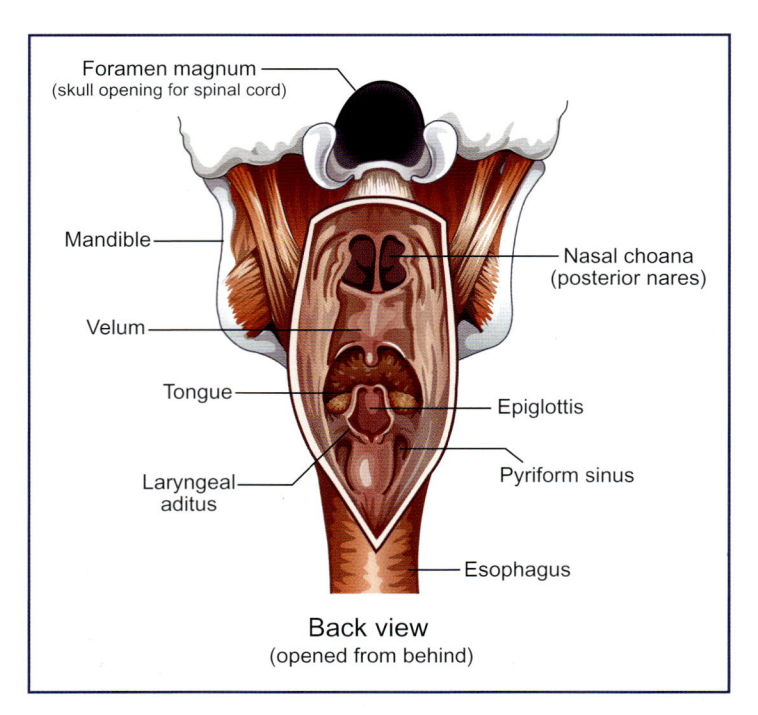

Figure 4-3. Salient features of the pharynx as revealed from a back view in which the posterior pharyngeal wall is opened from behind. The skull and mandible are shown for reference.

is open at the front and connects, from top to bottom, with the nasal cavities, oral cavity, and laryngeal aditus (upper entrance to the larynx).

The mix of tendon and muscle varies along the length of the pharynx. The upper part is made up solely of connective tissue, called the pharyngeal aponeurosis, which effectively suspends the pharyngeal tube from above (the way the rim of a basketball goal suspends the net). Muscular tissue increases in proportion down the length of the pharynx until it predominates. Muscle tissue encircles the pharynx, making its architecture resemble that of a sphincter. In fact, its overall arrangement is similar to that of the gut. This should come as no surprise, given that the pharynx is an active component of the digestive system and its lower part is continuous with the esophagus (gullet), where its front and back walls are in contact. This contact is broken during activities such as swallowing and regurgitation.

The pharynx comprises three cavities that are designated, from top to bottom, as the nasopharynx, oropharynx, and laryngopharynx. The boundaries of these cavities are shown in Figure 4–4. The nasopharynx lies behind the nose and above the velum. Because the velum is mobile, the lower boundary of the nasopharynx is somewhat arbitrary. Thus, a common convention is to specify this boundary by a reference line extending between the upper surface of the hard palate and the most forward point on the uppermost vertebra.

The nasopharynx always remains patent, a feature that distinguishes it from the other subdivisions of the pharynx. The pharyngeal ends of the paired auditory tubes (also called the eustachian tubes) are located on the lateral walls of the nasopharynx. When these tubes open, they allow the pressure to equilibrate between the middle ears and atmosphere. Across the back surface of the nasopharynx, between the pharyngeal orifices of the auditory tubes, lies a large mass of lymphoid tissue called the pharyngeal tonsil. This tissue is also referred to as the nasopharyngeal tonsil and, when abnormally enlarged, is designated as adenoid tissue (or just the adenoids). At the front, the nasopharynx connects to

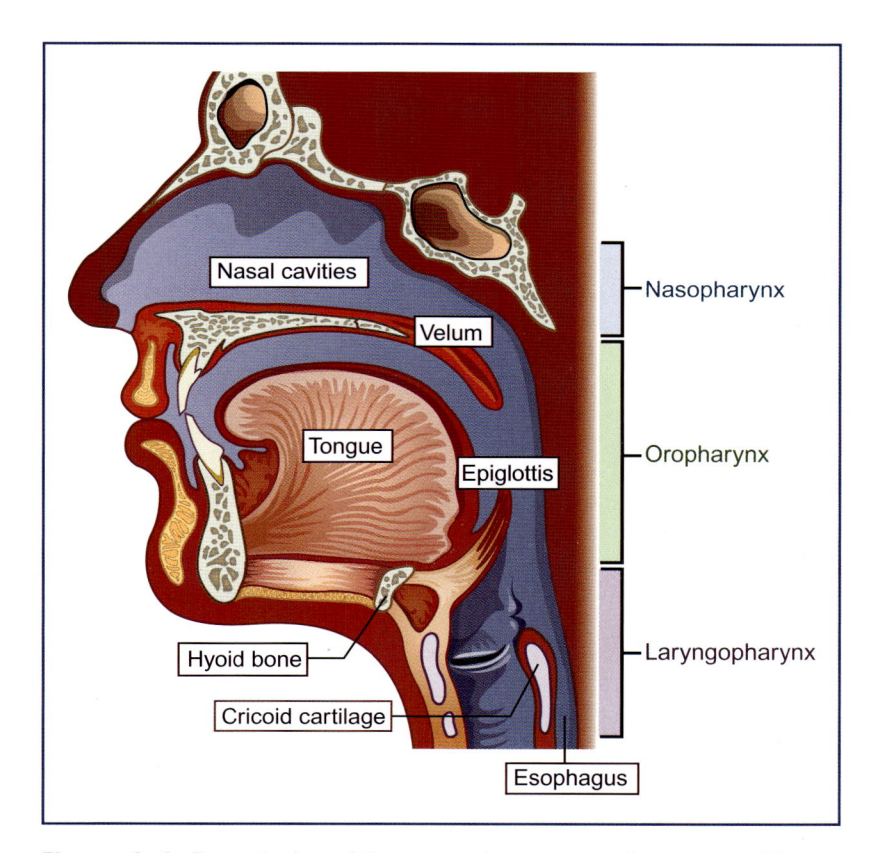

Figure 4–4. Boundaries of the nasopharynx, oropharynx, and laryngopharynx. The boundary between the nasopharynx and oropharynx can be arbitrary; in this figure it is defined by an imaginary line extending backward at the level of the hard palate. The boundary between the oropharynx and laryngopharynx is the hyoid bone, and the lower boundary of the laryngopharynx is the base of the cricoid cartilage.

the nasal cavities through the nasal choanae (funnel-like openings), also called the posterior nares (nostrils) or internal nares. These are two oval-shaped apertures that are about twice as long (top to bottom) as they are wide (side to side) and are oriented in the vertical plane (see Figure 4–3).

The oropharynx forms the middle part of the pharyngeal tube. Its upper boundary is coextensive with the lower boundary of the nasopharynx and its lower boundary is the hyoid bone. As shown in Figure 4–5, the front of the oropharynx opens into the oral cavity through the faucial isthmus (the narrow passage situated between the velum and the base of the tongue). This isthmus is bounded on the left and right sides by the anterior and posterior faucial pillars, pairs of muscular bands that resemble pairs of legs. The palatine tonsils are located between the anterior and posterior faucial pillars on each side of the isthmus. They are also often called the faucial tonsils and are "the" tonsils most often referred to colloquially. The back surface of the tongue is the site of yet another tonsil, the so-called lingual tonsil. This tonsil is a broad aggregate of lymph glands distributed across much of the posterior (root) part of the tongue. The oropharynx is the only subdivision of the pharynx that can be visualized without special equipment. The back wall of the oropharynx is best viewed when the velum is elevated, as in "open your mouth wide and say 'ah.'"

The laryngopharynx constitutes the lowermost part of the pharynx. The upper boundary of the laryngopharynx is the hyoid bone and the lower boundary is the base of the cricoid cartilage, where the pharynx is continuous with the esophagus. At the front, the laryngopharynx is bounded by the back surface of the tongue (and the lingual tonsil), the laryngeal aditus (the opening into the larynx formed by the epiglottis and aryepiglottic folds), and the pyriform sinuses (pear-shaped cavities located lateral to the aryepiglottic folds; see Figure 4–3).

Velum

The velum, which means *curtain*, is a pendulous flap consisting of the soft palate and uvula (meaning *little grape*). In this case, the velum is the curtain that hangs down from the back of the roof of the mouth, as illustrated in Figures 4–4 (side view) and 4–5 (front view). A broad sheet of connective tissue, the palatal aponeurosis, forms a fibrous skeleton for the velum.

Despite a similar surface appearance throughout, the velum is not structurally homogeneous. Four tissue layers have been identified in the velum (Kuehn & Kahane, 1990). These include: (a) a layer toward the under surface (oral surface) that is glandular (secreting) tissue with adipose (fat) tissue at the sides, (b) a

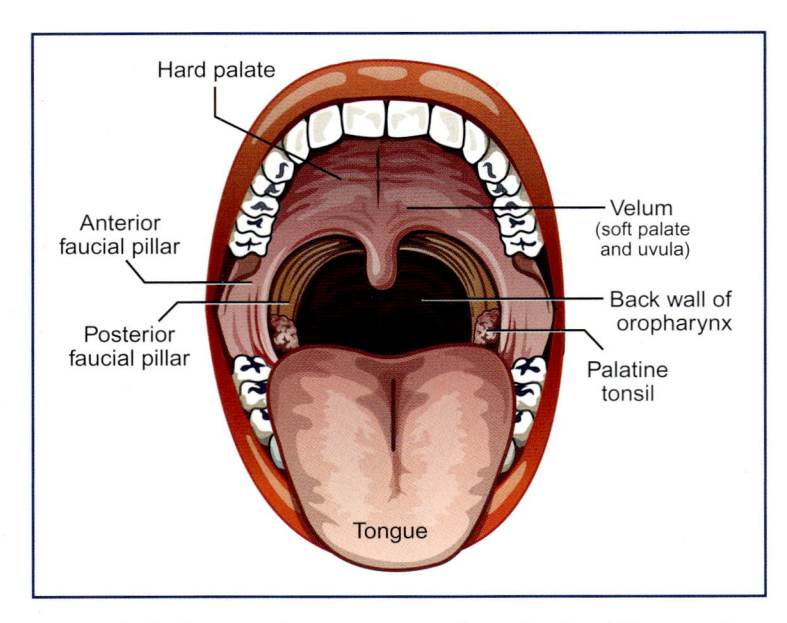

Figure 4–5. The oropharynx as seen from the front. The oropharynx is best viewed when instructed to "open your mouth wide and say 'ah.'" The narrow opening between the velum and the tongue (top to bottom) and between the anterior and posterior faucial pillars (side to side) is called the faucial isthmus.

Show Me Your Hand

They were twin girls. Each had speech that was a dead ringer for the other and was characterized by multiple misarticulations and hypernasality. What was the cause? Had they developed some sort of twin speech? Did one have a problem and the other was imitating it? Oral examinations revealed identical structural anomalies. Each girl had a short velum. Nasoendoscopic examinations further revealed that, for each girl, the velum elevated only occasionally during speech production, but never came close to the posterior pharyngeal wall. The girls' parents were with them and being interviewed by a student clinician and her supervisor. The moment the mother spoke there were suspicions. She had a severe speech disorder characterized by multiple misarticulations and hypernasality, and exhibited pronounced nasal grimacing when speaking. She allowed an oral examination. She had a short velum. It was three of a kind.

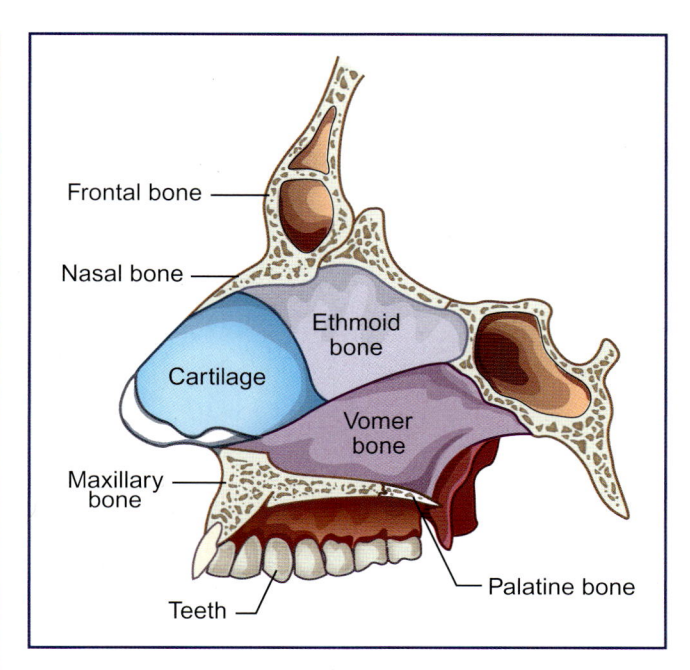

Figure 4-6. Components of the nasal septum (partition between the two nasal cavities). The nasal septum consists of cartilage at the front and bone (ethmoid and vomer) in the back. Selected other bones and teeth are shown for reference.

middle layer of muscle tissue in which fibers run side to side in the central portion of the structure and front to back in its more superficial portion toward the upper surface (nasal surface), (c) an upper front layer consisting of connective tissue (tendon), and (d) a lower back layer consisting largely of glandular tissue.

Patterns of muscle fiber distribution differ along the length of the velum (Kuehn & Moon, 2005). These include: (a) a front portion that is void of muscle fibers, (b) a middle one-third that is rich with muscle fibers that course in various directions (including across the midline) and include insertions into the lateral margins of the structure, (c) a proportioning of muscle fibers that tapers off toward the front and back of the structure, and (d) a uvular (back) portion that is sparsely interspersed with muscle fibers. The uvula also has a richer vascular system than the soft palate, perhaps to prevent excessive cooling of this region (Moon & Kuehn, 2004).

Nasal Cavities

The nasal cavities, also called the nasal fossae (pronounced like posse), lie behind the outer nose. They are two large chambers that run side by side and are separated from each other by the nasal septum (which is often not perfectly vertical). As shown in Figure 4-6, this partition has: (a) a front part composed of cartilage, (b) an upper back part that is the perpendicular plate of the ethmoid bone, and (c) a lower back part that is the vomer bone. The floor of the nasal cavities is broad and slightly concave and is formed by two sets of bones that constitute the hard palate. The palatine processes of the maxillary bones (left and right upper jaws) form the front three-fourths and the horizontal processes of the palatine bones form the back one-fourth of the hard palate (this can be seen in the middle image in Figure 4-2). The roof of the nasal cavities, in contrast to the floor, is quite narrow and formed by part of the ethmoid bone called the cribriform plate. The configuration of the two cavities is similar to the roofline of an A-frame house.

By far the most complex formations within the nasal cavities are located on its lateral walls. These formations are convoluted and labyrinthine and contain many nooks and crannies. Three shell-like structures give rise to this complexity. These structures are portrayed in Figure 4-7 and include the superior, middle, and inferior nasal conchae, also called the nasal turbinates. The nasal conchae extend along the length of the nasal cavities and have corresponding meatuses (passages) named for the conchae with which they are associated. The enfolding structure of the nasal cavities provides a large surface area to the inner nose and has a rich blood supply. Near the front of each nasal cavity is the nasal vestibule, a modest dilation just inside the aperture of the anterior naris.

There are four sinuses (hollows) that surround the nasal cavities. Called the paranasal sinuses, they include the maxillary, frontal, ethmoid, and sphenoid sinuses, each located within the bone of corresponding name. Three of these are shown in Figure 4–8. The sphenoid, not pictured, is located behind and above the superior nasal conchae within the sphenoid bone. They are usually air filled but can become liquid filled when infected. Their relevance to speech is primarily related to their effects on the resonance characteristics of the acoustic signal during nasal sound production (see Chapter 9).

Outer Nose

Unlike the other components of the velopharyngeal-nasal apparatus, the outer nose is familiar to everyone. The outer nose is hard to ignore because it is in the center of the face and projects outward and downward conspicuously. The more prominent surface features of the outer nose include the root, bridge, dorsum, apex,

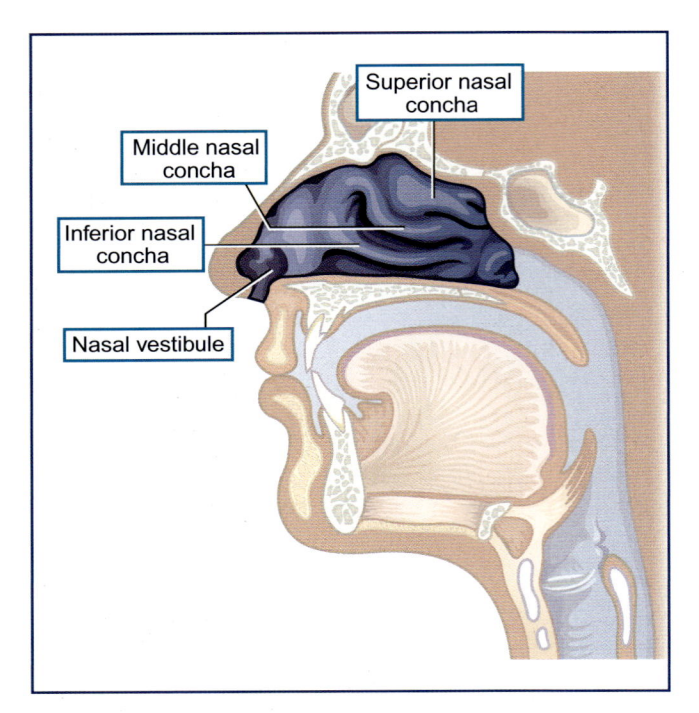

Figure 4–7. Superior, middle, and inferior nasal conchae (also called nasal turbinates). These conchae contain many nooks and crannies and create a large surface area to the inner nose.

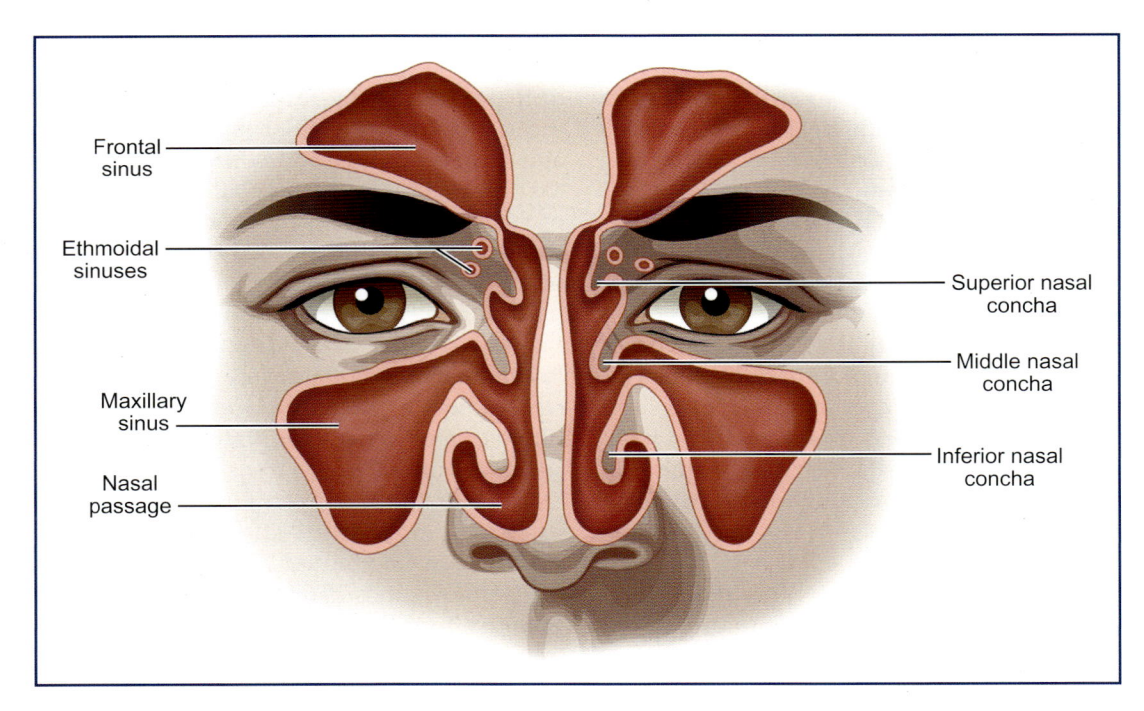

Figure 4–8. The paranasal sinuses. Shown in this figure are the maxillary, frontal, and ethmoid sinuses. Not shown are the paired sphenoid sinuses, which are located behind and above the superior nasal conchae.

> **Disposing of Things**
>
> Mucus (a slimy substance) is formed in the nose to the tune of about half a pint a day (more when you have a cold). Particles filtered by the nose are collected in a blanket of mucus and moved through the nose by the action of cilia (tiny hair cells that collectively form a fringe). Things that get trapped are moved along toward the back of the throat and then swallowed into the stomach. Some material dries before reaching the back of the throat and fractionates into pieces containing filtered particles. This happens at different spots within the nose and in residues of various consistencies. Prim and proper folks refer to these residues as nasal exudates. Most of us refer to them as "boogers." They are best gently blown into a tissue to rid them from the nose, but we all know other manual methods that are commonly practiced.

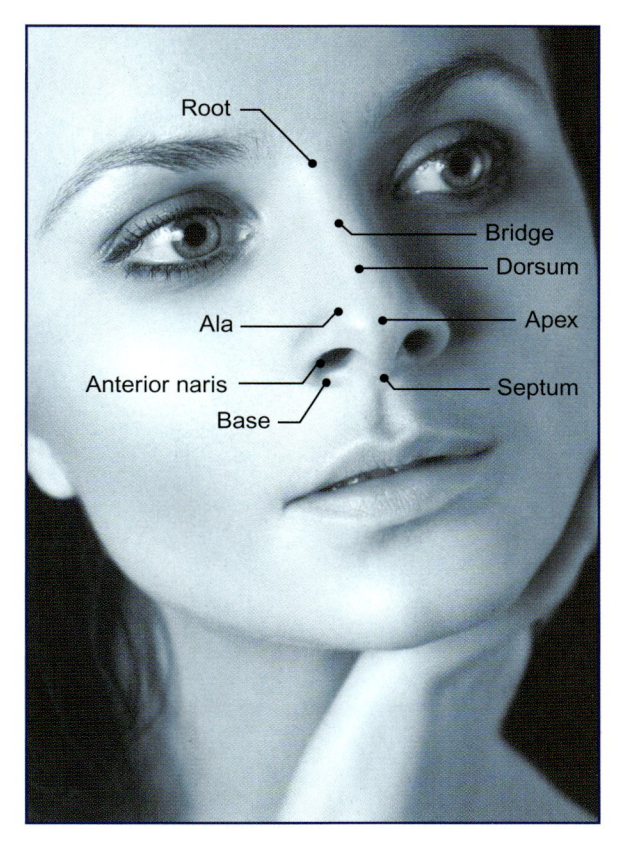

Figure 4–9. Surface features of the outer nose.

alae, base, septum, and anterior nares, as shown in Figure 4–9.

The root (point of attachment) of the outer nose is to the bottom of the forehead. Following downward along the center line are the bridge (upper bony part), dorsum (prominent upper surface), and apex (tip). The alae (wings) form much of the sides of the nose and contribute significantly to its general shape. The base of the nose is partitioned down the middle (more or less) by the lowermost part of the nasal septum and includes the anterior nares (nostrils), also called the external nares. The anterior nares are apertures that are somewhat pear-shaped, typically about twice as long (front to back) as they are wide (side to side). Margins of the anterior nares contain stiff hairs, called vibrissae. These hairs arrest the passage of particles riding on air currents.

FORCES OF THE VELOPHARYNGEAL-NASAL APPARATUS

Both passive and active forces operate on the velopharyngeal-nasal apparatus. Passive force is inherent and always present (although subject to change) and arises from the natural recoil of muscles, cartilages, and connective tissues, the surface tension between structures in apposition, the pull of gravity, and aeromechanical forces. Active force is applied by muscles and depends on the will and ability of the individual. Active force within the velopharyngeal-nasal apparatus comes from muscles of the pharynx, velum, and outer nose.

Muscles of the Pharynx

Figure 4–10 portrays the muscles of the pharynx and Figure 4–11 summarizes their actions. They are the *superior constrictor, middle constrictor, inferior constrictor, salpingopharyngeus, stylopharyngeus,* and *palatopharyngeus* muscles. These muscles influence the size and shape of the lumen (cavity) of the pharyngeal tube. Of course, other structures along the front side of the pharynx can also influence the lumen of the pharynx through their adjustments (velum, tongue, and epiglottis).

The *superior constrictor* muscle is located in the upper part of the pharynx. It is a complex muscle with multiple origins that arise from the front of the pharyngeal tube. Front points of attachment include the medial pterygoid plate of the sphenoid bone, the

Back view | Side view

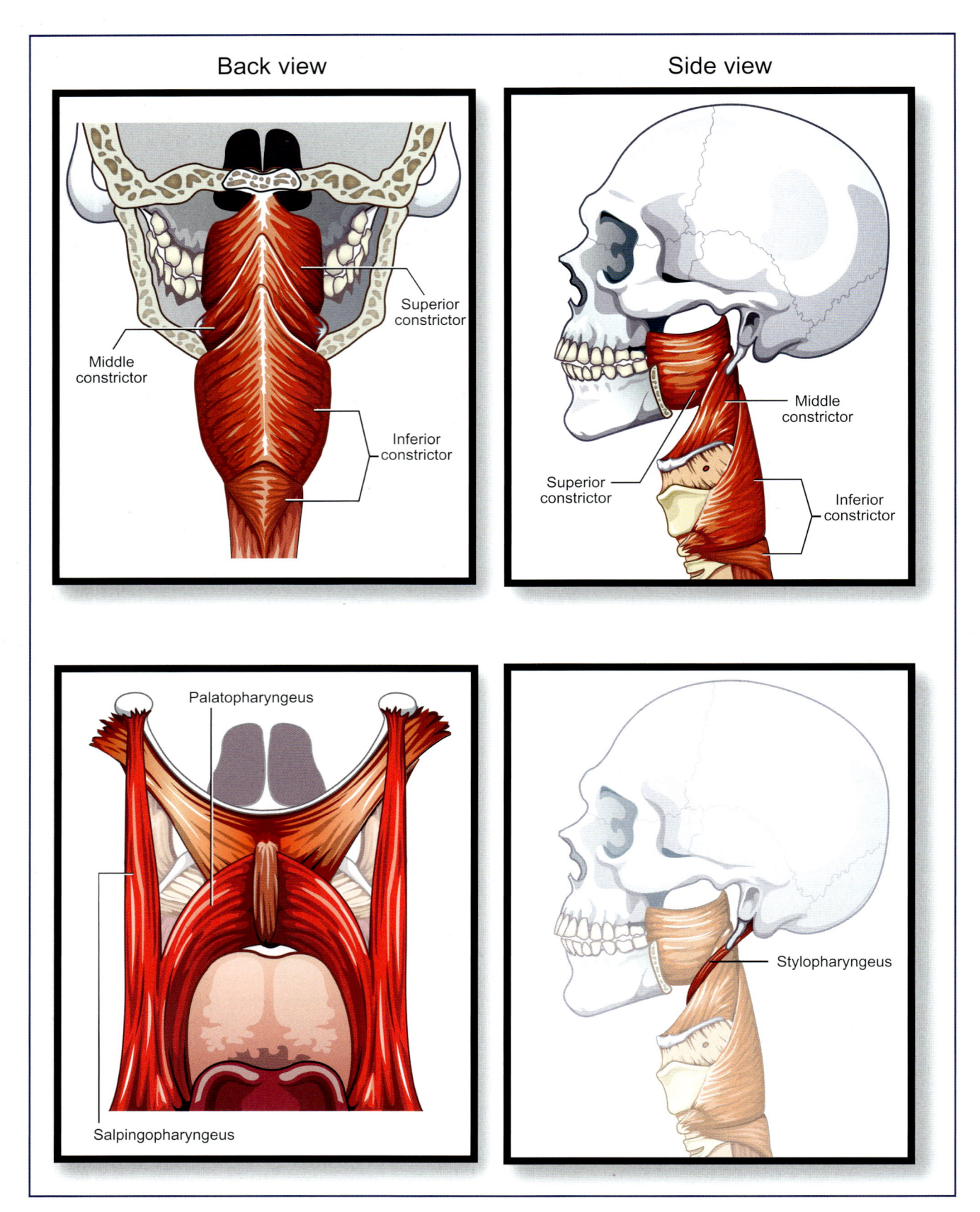

Figure 4-10. Muscles of the pharynx. The *superior constrictor*, *middle constrictor*, *inferior constrictor*, *salpingopharyngeus*, and *palatopharyngeus* muscles constrict the pharynx, whereas the *stylopharyngeus* muscle dilates the pharynx. Some of these muscles can also move the pharynx in other ways (see Figure 4-11).

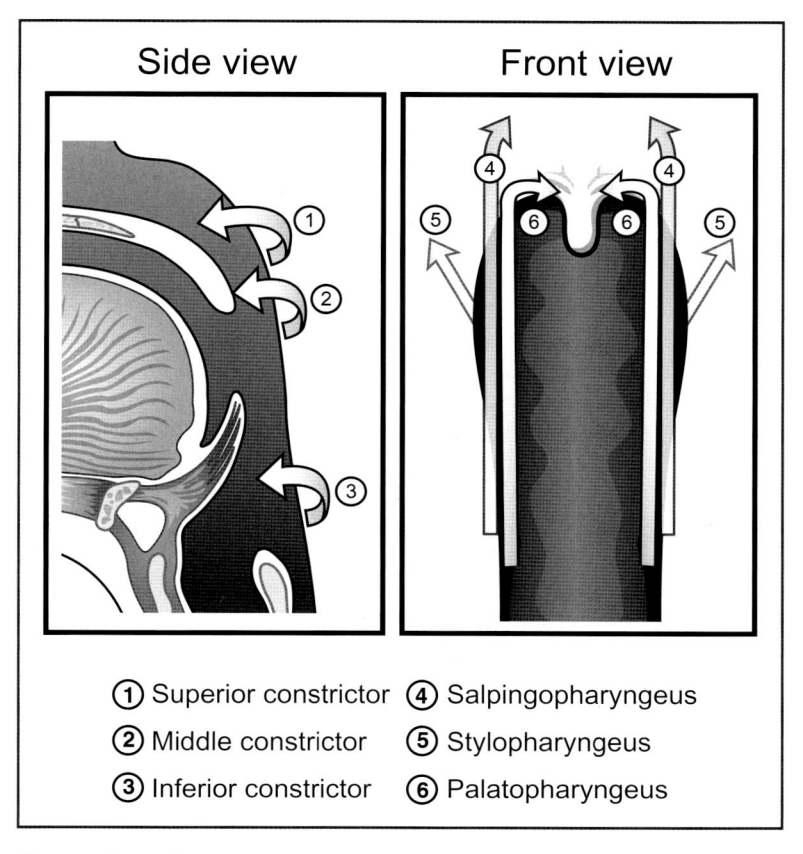

Figure 4–11. Summary of force vectors of the muscles of the pharynx. The muscles that constrict the pharynx are the **superior constrictor** (1), **middle constrictor** (2), and **inferior constrictor** (3) muscles. Muscles that pull both upward and inward on the pharynx are the **salpingopharyngeus** (4) and **palatopharyngeus** (6). The **stylopharyngeus** muscle (5) pulls upward and outward on the pharynx.

pterygomandibular ligament (a tendinous inscription between the *superior constrictor* muscle and the *buccinator* muscle, described in Chapter 5), the mylohyoid line (site of attachment of the *mylohyoid* muscle, described in Chapter 5, on the inner surface of the body of the mandible), and the side of the back part of the tongue. These multiple points of origin are sometimes used as a basis for conceptualizing the *superior constrictor* muscle as a cluster of four individual muscles. From top to bottom, these four are designated as the *pterygopharyngeus*, *buccopharyngeus*, *mylopharyngeus*, and *glossopharyngeus* muscles. Fibers from the multiple origins of the *superior constrictor* muscle course backward, toward the midline, and upward to insert into the fibrous median raphe (seam) of the posterior pharyngeal wall. There, they join with fibers of the paired muscle from the opposite side. The uppermost fibers of the *superior constrictor* muscle are horizontal and located at the level of the velum. When the *superior constrictor* muscle contracts, it reduces the regional cross section of the pharyngeal lumen by forward movement of the posterior pharyngeal wall and forward and inward movement of the lateral pharyngeal wall on the same side. The paired *superior constrictor* muscles encircle the posterior and lateral walls of the upper pharynx so that their simultaneous contraction constricts the lumen of that part of the pharyngeal tube in the manner of a sphincter.

The *middle constrictor* muscle is a fan-shaped structure located midway along the length of the pharyngeal tube. Fibers of the muscle arise from the greater and lesser horns of the hyoid bone and the stylohyoid ligament (which runs between the downward and forward projecting styloid process of the temporal bone and the lesser horn of the hyoid bone) and radiate backward and toward the midline where they insert into the median raphe of the pharynx. The *middle constrictor* muscle is also sometimes conceptualized as comprising two muscles designated as the *chondropharyngeus* and *ceratopharyngeus* muscles. The uppermost fibers of the *middle constrictor* muscle course obliquely upward and overlap the lower fibers of the *superior constrictor* muscle, whereas the lowermost fibers of the muscle run obliquely downward beneath the fibers of the *inferior constrictor* muscle. The middle fibers of the *middle constrictor* muscle run horizontally. The overlapping arrangement of the muscle fibers between the *middle constrictor* and *superior constrictor* muscles and between the *inferior constrictor* and *middle constrictor* muscles is akin to the way in which roof shingles partially overlap. When the *middle constrictor* muscle contracts, it decreases the cross section of the pharynx regionally, by virtue of forward movement of the posterior pharyngeal wall and forward and inward movement of the lateral pharyngeal wall. When the middle *constrictor muscle* acts in conjunction with its paired mate on the opposite side, the pharyngeal lumen is regionally constricted in the manner of a sphincter.

The *inferior constrictor* muscle is the most powerful of the three constrictor muscles of the pharynx. The fibers of this muscle arise from the sides of the thyroid and cricoid cartilages. The *inferior constrictor* muscle is sometimes thought of as consisting of two muscles. These are referred to as the *thyropharyngeus* and *cricopharyngeus* muscles. Fibers of the *inferior constrictor* muscle diverge from their origins in a fanlike configuration and course backward and toward the midline. There, they interdigitate with fibers from the *inferior constrictor* muscle of the opposite side at the median raphe of the pharyngeal tube. The middle and upper fibers of the *inferior constrictor* muscle ascend obliquely, whereas the lowermost fibers run horizontally and downward and are continuous with those of the esophagus. When the *inferior constrictor* muscle contracts, it draws the lower part of the posterior wall of the pharynx forward and pulls the lateral walls of the lower pharynx forward and inward. This action, in conjunction with that of the *inferior constrictor* muscle on the opposite side, constricts the lumen of the lower pharynx.

The *salpingopharyngeus* is a narrow muscle that arises from near the lower border of the pharyngeal orifice of the auditory tube. The fibers of the muscle course downward vertically and insert into the lateral wall of the lower pharynx where they blend with fibers of the *palatopharyngeus* muscle (discussed below). When the *salpingopharyngeus* muscle contracts, it pulls the lateral wall of the pharynx upward and inward. Acting simultaneously with its paired muscle from the opposite side, the effect is to decrease the width of the pharynx.

The *stylopharyngeus* is a slender muscle that runs a relatively long course. It originates from the styloid process of the temporal bone and runs downward, forward, and toward the midline. Most fibers of the muscle insert into the lateral wall of the pharynx at and near the juncture of the *superior constrictor* and *middle constrictor* muscles. Some fibers extend lower in the pharyngeal wall and insert into the thyroid cartilage. When the *stylopharyngeus* muscle contracts, it pulls upward on the pharyngeal tube and draws the lateral wall of the pharynx toward the side. Together with similar action of its paired mate from the opposite side, it widens the lumen of the pharynx in the region where the muscle fibers insert into the lateral walls of the pharynx. There is also an upward pull placed on the pharynx (and larynx) when the *stylopharyngeus* muscles contract.

The *palatopharyngeus* muscle runs the length of the pharynx. It is a pharyngeal muscle as well as a muscle of the soft palate (in that context it is called the *pharyngopalatine* muscle; see sidetrack on this page). The muscle is considered here from the pharyngeal perspective. The *palatopharyngeus* muscle arises mainly from the soft palate. The uppermost fibers are directed horizontally and intermingle with fibers of the *superior constrictor* muscle. A major fiber course is downward and toward the side through the posterior faucial pillar. Below the pillar, the fibers continue into the lower half of the pharynx and spread to the lateral wall of the structure and the thyroid cartilage. Some have suggested that the portion of the muscle

---

Having It Both Ways

A muscle is usually thought of as having an origin and an insertion. The origin is its anchored end and the insertion is its movable end. This is all well and good in textbooks, but in real life things are a bit more complicated. What may be the anchored end of a muscle for one activity may be the movable end of that muscle for another activity. A lot of it has to do with what neighboring muscles are doing. Thus, a muscle's function may change from time to time because various forces cause the mobility of its two ends to change in relation to one another. The convention adopted in this book is to reflect such change by alternately labeling a muscle in accordance with its perceived primary function in a given context. Some purists may not embrace this convention, but it carries instructive power and simply points out that in the busy world of the muscle, turnabout is fair play.

that attaches to the thyroid cartilage be given recognition of its own as the *palatothyroideus* muscle (Cassell & Elkadi, 1995), whereas others disagree (Moon & Kuehn, 2004). When the velum is relatively stable, contraction of the *palatopharyngeus* muscle results in two movements. The uppermost fibers of the muscle draw the lateral pharyngeal wall inward to complement the action of the *superior constrictor* muscle of the pharynx, whereas the lowermost fibers of the muscle pull upward on the lateral pharyngeal wall and elevate the pharynx (attachments to the thyroid cartilage also effect an upward and forward pull on the larynx).

Muscles of the Velum

The muscles of the velum are shown in Figure 4–12. They are the *palatal levator, palatal tensor, uvulus, glossopalatine*, and *pharyngopalatine* muscles. These muscles influence the positioning, configuration, and mechanical status of the velum. Their force vectors are illustrated in Figure 4–13.

The *palatal levator* muscle (also called the *levator veli palatini* muscle) forms much of the bulk of the velum. The *palatal levator* is a flattened cylindrical muscle that arises from the petrous (hard) portion of the temporal bone and from the cartilaginous portion of the auditory tube. From there, it courses downward, forward, and toward the midline, passing on the outside of the posterior naris. Fibers of the *palatal levator* muscle insert into the side of the velum and spread out where they join those of the *palatal levator* muscle from the opposite side. The spread of muscle fibers in each of the *palatal levator* muscles is to the midline and beyond to the other side of the velum (Kuehn & Moon, 2005). Fibers extend from behind the hard palate to the front of the uvula, encompassing approximately the middle 40% of the velum (Boorman & Sommerlad, 1985) or more (Kuehn & Kahane, 1990). The paired *palatal levator* muscles form a muscular sling from their cranial attachments through the velum. Each *palatal levator* muscle inserts into the velum at an angle of about 45°. When the *palatal levator* muscle contracts, it draws the velum upward and backward. Simultaneous

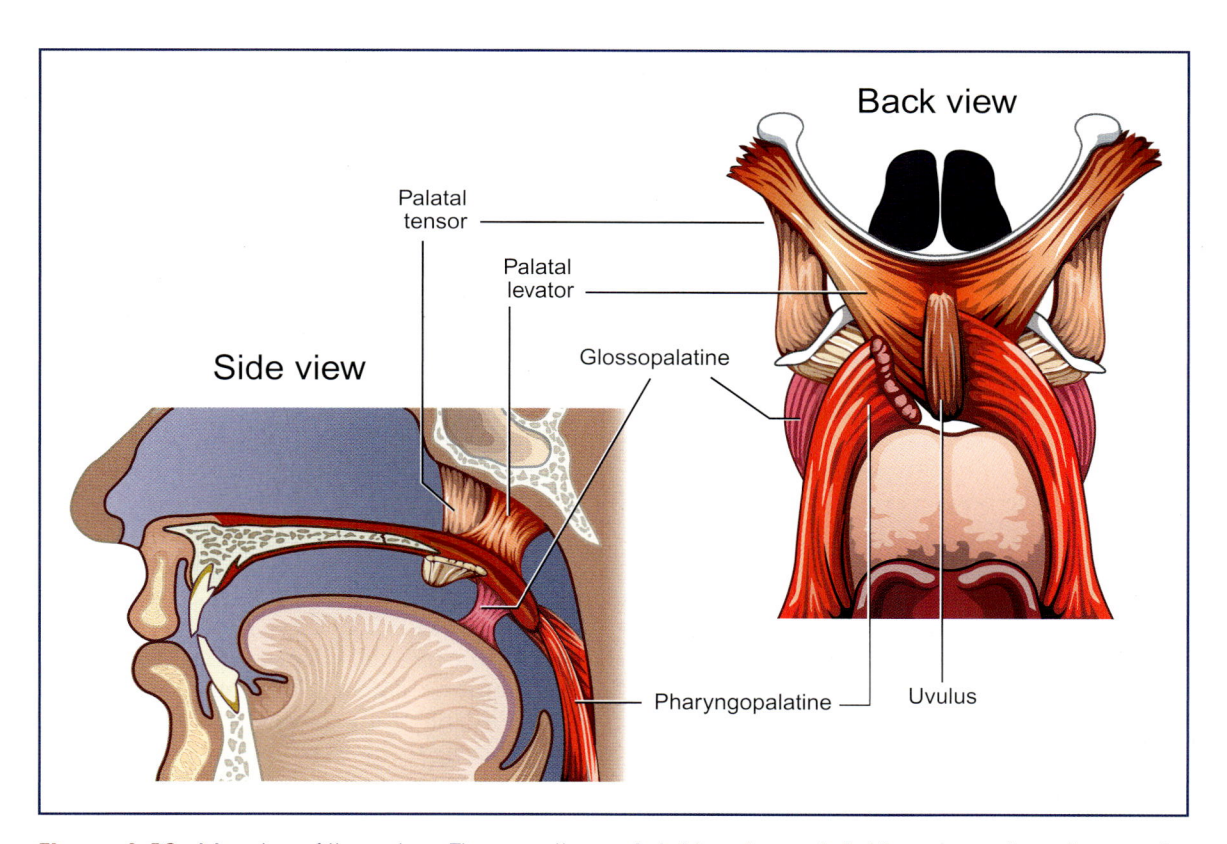

Figure 4–12. Muscles of the velum. They are the ***palatal levator, palatal tensor, uvulus, glossopalatine***, and ***pharyngopalatine*** muscles. Most of these muscles act primarily to move the velum upward and backward and downward and forward. Their individual actions are shown schematically in Figure 4–13.

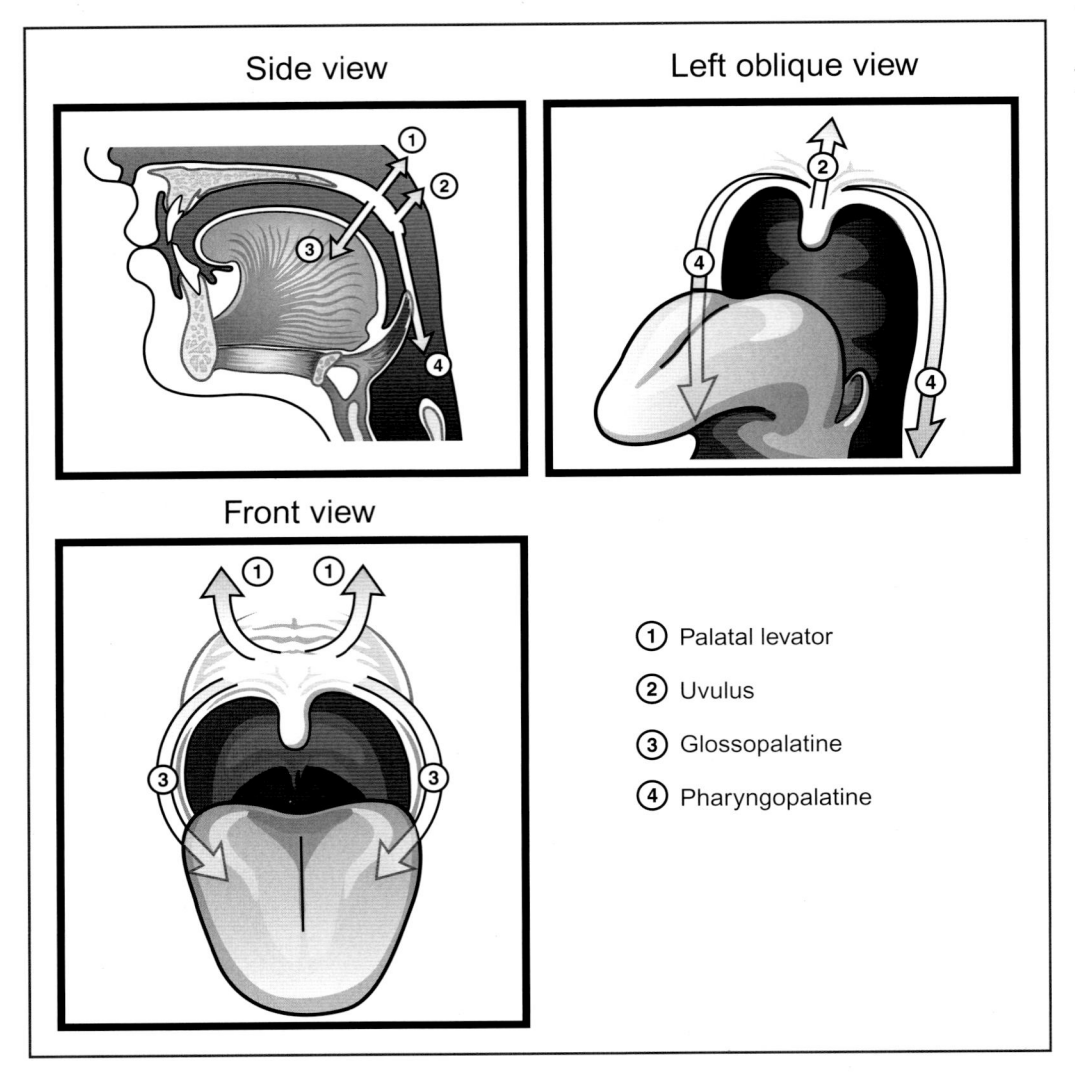

Figure 4-13. Summary of force vectors of the muscles of the velum. The ***palatal levator*** muscle (1) pulls the velum upward and backward. The ***uvulus*** muscle (2) shortens, lifts, and increases the thickness of the velum. The ***glossopalatine*** muscle (3) pulls the velum downward and forward and the ***pharyngopalatine*** muscle (4) pulls the velum downward and backward. The ***palatal tensor*** muscle is not included in this figure because it is not thought to have a significant effect on the velum.

contraction of the paired *palatal levator* muscles lifts the velum toward the posterior pharyngeal wall along an angular trajectory. The velum and the posterior pharyngeal wall come into contact frequently, sometimes with significant contact force. The upper surface of the velum can withstand such forces, in part, because of the stratified squamous epithelium that covers it. Frictional forces can also result from the sliding of the velum up and down the posterior pharyngeal wall. These are mitigated by glandular secretions of the velum which lubricate the contact areas (Kuehn & Moon, 2005).

The *palatal tensor* muscle (also termed the *tensor veli palatini* muscle) lies on the outer side of the *palatal levator* muscle. It arises from the pterygoid and scapular fossae and angular spine of the sphenoid bone as well as the cartilaginous portion of the auditory tube. From there, fibers course vertically downward to terminate in a tendon and insert into the hook-shaped hamulus of the medial pterygoid plate of the sphenoid bone. The tendon of the *palatal tensor* muscle (along with a sparse number of *palatal tensor* muscle fibers) courses inward and inserts into the hard palate and the velum (Barsoumian, Kuehn, Moon, & Canady, 1998).

The *palatal tensor* muscle plays an important role in dilating the auditory (eustachian) tube, possibly in conjunction with other velopharyngeal muscles (Okada et al., 2018). Earlier conceptions of the function of the *palatal tensor* muscle also suggested that its contraction would tense the velum, because it was thought that the muscle itself wrapped around the hamulus to contribute to the horizontal portion of the structure. However, the fact that the *palatal tensor* muscle is now known to insert on the hamulus, with only a few fibers continuing on to insert into the velum, indicates that it does not have the mechanical means to tense the velum to any significant degree. In contrast, the tendon does seem to play an important mechanical role. The prominent size of this tendon suggests that it may relieve stress at the junction between the hard and soft palates, stress induced by frequent up-and-down movements of the velum. The stress-relief function can be thought of as analogous to a reinforced collar at the junction between an electrical plug and the wire extending from it (Kuehn, 1990).

The *uvulus* muscle is the only intrinsic muscle of the velum (both ends of its fibers are within the velum). Fibers of the *uvulus* muscle originate to the side of the posterior nasal spine formed by the palatine bones and behind the hard palate near the sling formed by the *palatal levator* muscles and about a fourth of the way along the length of the soft palate from the front. The muscle courses downward and backward, extending through much of the length of the soft palate. Very few fibers of the *uvulus* muscle actually enter the uvula proper, from which the muscle historically derived its name (Azzam & Kuehn, 1977; Huang, Lee, & Rajendran, 1997). This has prompted some to argue (and seemingly rightfully so) that the designation of this muscle as the *uvulus* muscle is both a misnomer and anatomically misleading (Moon & Kuehn, 2004). The location of the so-called *uvulus* muscle is above the sling formed by the *palatal levator* muscles. Structurally, the paired *uvulus* muscles account for the longitudinal convexity of the upper surface of the velum. This is true even in the region of the uvula, where muscle fibers are sparse, if they exist at all. One reason is that the encapsulating sheath that surrounds each *uvulus* muscle persists into the uvula, providing some cohesiveness between the soft palate and uvula and a girder for the uvula (Kuehn & Moon, 2005). When the *uvulus* muscle contracts, it has several effects that can be realized alone or in combination. These include that it (a) shortens the velum, (b) lifts the velum, and (c) increases the thickness (bulk) of the velum in the third quadrant of its length. Classic thought about the function of the paired *uvulus* muscles focused on the first of these effects, shortening of the velum. More recent conceptualizations, however, have focused on possible effects that involve the control of the stiffness of the upper part of the velum (Kuehn, Folkins, & Linville, 1988). Stiffness effected in the back part of the velum may counteract the deformation imposed on the velum by contraction of the *palatal levator* muscles. This avoids stretching of the top layer of the velum upward rather than moving the overall mass of the structure. It may also be that the *uvulus* muscles act to exert force within the upper part of the velum that causes the curvilinear structure to behave like a flexible beam that rotates the back half of the structure toward the posterior pharyngeal wall (somewhat analogous to extending flexed fingers with the palm of the hand facing downward). In this case, the *uvulus* muscles function as muscles that shorten the distance between the velum and the posterior pharyngeal wall or facilitate contact and/or force of contact between the two.

The *glossopalatine* muscle is both a muscle of the tongue (called the *palatoglossus* muscle in that context) and a muscle of the velum, and is discussed here as a muscle of the velum. Fibers of the *glossopalatine* muscle arise from the side of the tongue where they are closely blended with longitudinal fibers of the dorsum of the tongue. They course upward and inward, forming the substance of the anterior faucial pillar, and insert into the lower surface of the palatal aponeurosis. The location of attachment to the soft palate is reported to vary across individuals, with some having insertions forward near the hard palate and others having insertions rearward near the uvula (Kuehn & Azzam, 1978). When the dorsum of the tongue is relatively fixed, contraction of the *glossopalatine* muscle places a downward and forward pull on the velum. Although the *glossopalatine* muscle has force potential on the velum, that potential is limited in comparison to the force potential of the *pharyngopalatine* muscle (Moon & Kuehn, 2004).

The *pharyngopalatine* muscle (discussed above as the *palatopharyngeus* muscle in the context of the pharynx) is considered here in the context of the velum. Its fibers arise from the lower half of the lateral wall of the pharynx and thyroid cartilage and course upward and toward the midline where they pass through the posterior faucial pillar and insert into the soft palate (also the *superior constrictor* muscle). Its fibers do not approach or cross the midline of the soft palate, but insert more laterally within the structure (Kuehn & Kahane, 1990). One notion of mechanical prominence is that there is a downward directed sling formed by the *pharyngopalatine* muscles that is antagonistic to the upward directed sling provided by the *palatal levator* muscles (Fritzell, 1969; Moon, Smith, Folkins, Lemke, & Gartlin, 1994b). This notion has intuitive appeal but has been questioned on anatomical grounds, given the observation that fibers of the *pharyngopalatine* muscles do not extend to the midline of the velum (Moon & Kuehn, 2004). Dismissal of the notion based on this criticism may be premature, however, because interconnection through other structures of the velum may still effect a functional, if not anatomical, sling that can direct force downward symmetrically as a consequence of action of the paired *pharyngopalatine* muscles. When the pharyngeal attachment of the *pharyngopalatine* muscle is relatively fixed, contraction of its fibers (especially those that are vertically oriented) places a downward and backward pull on the velum. This suggested action is founded on assumed muscle vector pulls inferred from anatomical observations, which may or may not be wholly correct.

Muscles of the Outer Nose

All of the muscles of the outer nose can be used for facial expression to convey meaning. For the purposes of this chapter, however, interest in these muscles is in their potential to influence velopharyngeal-nasal function. Five muscles of the outer nose, shown in Figure 4–14, have this potential.

The *levator labii superioris alaeque nasi* muscle (the muscle with the longest name of any muscle in animals) is a thin structure located at the side of the outer nose between the orbit of the eye and the upper lip. Its origin is from the frontal process and infraorbital margin of the maxilla. From there, the muscle courses downward and toward the side, subdividing into two muscular slips. One slip inserts into the upper lip (blending with the *orbicularis oris* muscle, described in Chapter 5) and the other slip (of more interest here) inserts into the cartilage of the nasal ala (wing at the side of the nose). Contraction of this latter muscular slip draws the ala upward on the same side of the outer nose (like lifting a side flap on a tent) and enlarges the corresponding anterior naris.

The *anterior nasal dilator* muscle is a small muscle positioned on the lower lateral surface of the outer nose. It arises from the lower edge of the lateral nasal cartilage and runs downward and outward. Following a short course, it inserts into the deep surface of the skin near the outer margin of the naris on the same side. Contraction of the *anterior nasal dilator* muscle enlarges the anterior naris on that side of the outer nose.

The *posterior nasal dilator* is a small muscle located on the lower lateral surface of the outer nose. It lies behind the *anterior nasal dilator* muscle. Fibers

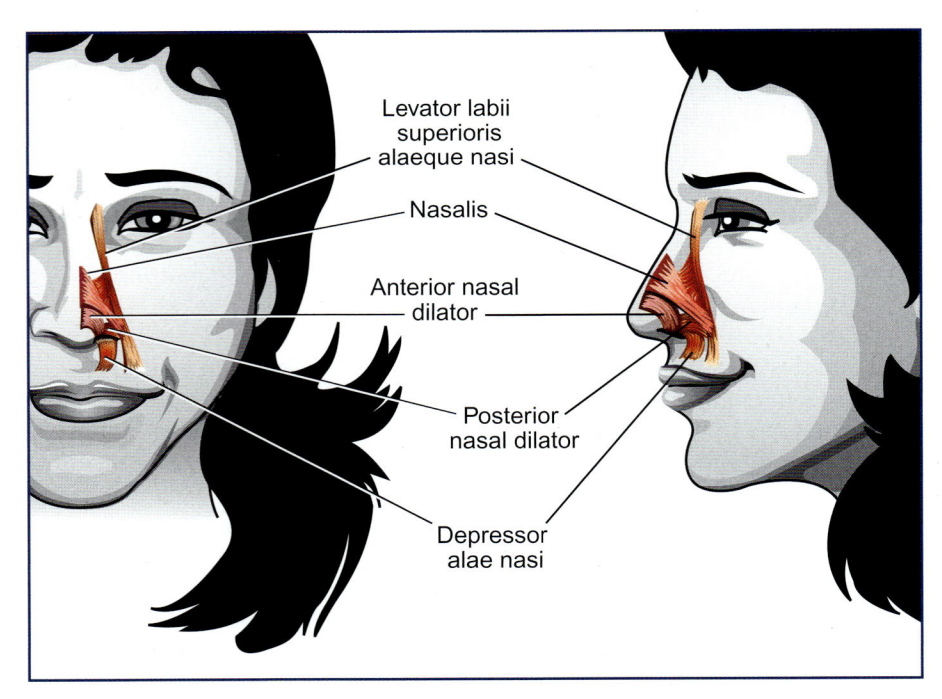

Figure 4–14. Muscles of the outer nose. Three muscles can dilate the nares (*levator labii superioris alaeque nasi*, *anterior nasal dilator*, and *posterior nasal dilator* muscles) and two can constrict the nares (*nasalis* and *depressor alae nasi* muscles) when activated.

of the *posterior nasal dilator* muscle originate from the nasal notch of the maxilla and adjacent cartilages of the outer nose. From this origin, they follow a short course and insert into the skin near the lower part of the alar cartilage along the outer margin of the naris on the same side. Contraction of the *posterior nasal dilator* muscle enlarges the corresponding anterior naris.

The *nasalis* muscle is located on the side of the outer nose. It originates from the maxilla, above and lateral to the incisive fossa (a depression in the maxilla above the incisor teeth). Fibers run upward and toward the midline and insert into an aponeurosis that is continuous with its paired muscle from the opposite side. When the *nasalis* muscle contracts, it draws down the cartilaginous part of the outer nose on the same side (like pulling down a side flap on a tent) and decreases the aperture of the corresponding anterior naris. Strong contraction of this muscle and its counterpart from the opposite side may bring the two alae of the outer nose together or compress them against one another.

The *depressor alae nasi* is a short muscle that originates from the incisive fossa of the maxilla and radiates upward to insert into the back part of the ala and the cartilaginous septum of the outer nose. When the *depressor alae nasi* muscle contracts, it draws the ala of the outer nose downward on the side of action and decreases the aperture of the corresponding naris.

MOVEMENTS OF THE VELOPHARYNGEAL-NASAL APPARATUS

The velopharyngeal-nasal apparatus comprises several movable parts. Movements of the pharynx, velum, and outer nose are considered here.

Movements of the Pharynx

The pharynx is a highly mobile tube. As illustrated in Figure 4–15, this mobility is vested in structures of the pharynx itself and in structures that comprise its lower and front boundaries. These movement capabilities are:

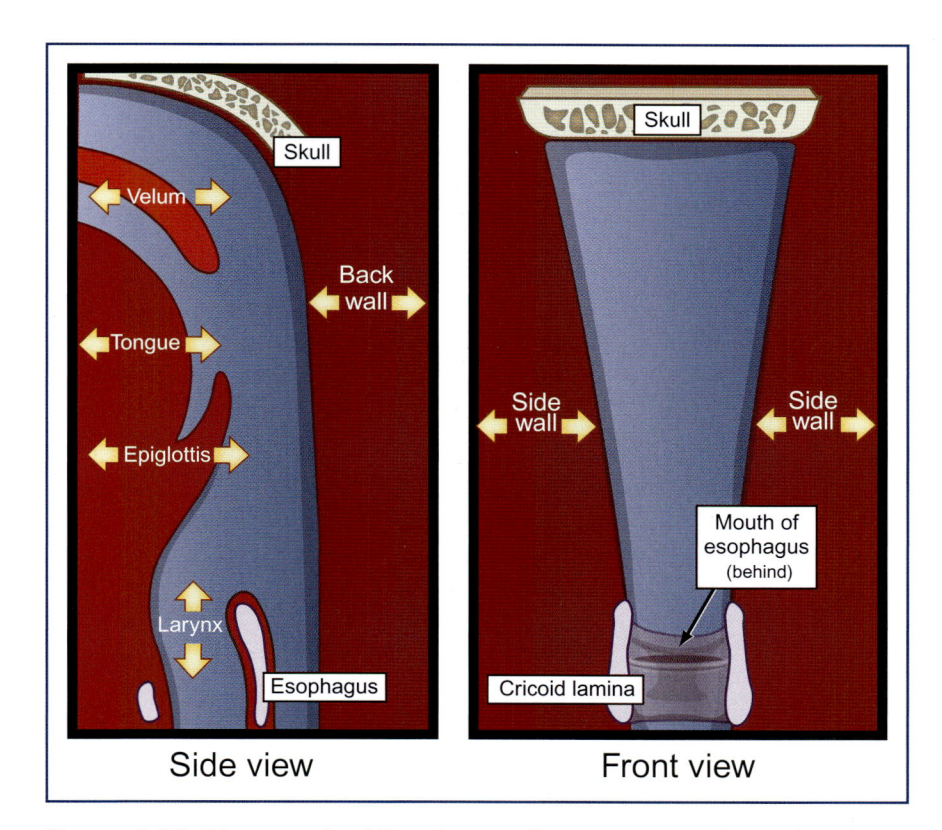

Figure 4–15. Movements of the pharynx. These movements can be downward and upward, inward and outward, and forward and backward and can lengthen, shorten, widen, and constrict the pharyngeal tube. Some of these movements are carried out by parts of the pharynx and others are carried out by nearby structures (velum, tongue, epiglottis, and larynx).

Sonar in a Teacup

Early study of lateral pharyngeal wall movement was problematic because x-ray techniques of the day did not provide good frontal views of the pharynx. Two speech scientists and a medical physicist from the University of Wisconsin provided the first clean data on lateral pharyngeal wall movement through the use of pulsed ultrasound. This technique sounded the depth of a point on the pharyngeal wall (like tracking a submarine). To learn the technique, they attended a short course on obstetrics where the uses of ultrasound were being taught as a pioneering means for scanning the abdomen of pregnant women. The first monitoring of lateral pharyngeal wall movement during speech production was done at that short course on an individual immersed (except for the face) in a water-filled gunner's turret of a bomber (envision an enormous teacup). Gels were just then starting to be used to transmit ultrasound into the body for medical purposes.

ear (Kent, Carney, & Severeid, 1974) or linear (Kuehn, 1976). Maximum upward movement of the velum places the upper surface of the structure within the nasopharynx (above the boundary specified by convention to separate the oropharynx and nasopharynx).

The velum is a flap and in some ways resembles a trapdoor, but it does not move like a trapdoor (as if it were swinging from a hinge). Rather, as depicted in Figure 4–16, the shape of the velum actually changes when it moves. The farther up and back it moves, the more hooked its appearance (as viewed from the side), and the farther down and forward it moves, the more pendulous its appearance (as viewed from the side). This is because the major lifting force that pulls the velum upward (by activation of the *palatal levator* muscles) is applied toward the middle of the velum. The hooked appearance of the velum results in identifiable landmarks during movement. The top of the hook (on the upper surface of the velum) is referred to as the velar eminence (also called the velar knee) and the undersurface of the hook (on the lower surface of the velum) is designated as the dimple of the velum.

(a) lengthening and shortening through downward and upward movements of the larynx, (b) inward and outward movements of the lateral pharyngeal walls, (c) forward and backward movements of the posterior pharyngeal wall, and (d) forward and backward movements of velum, tongue, and epiglottis. These movements, which dilate or constrict the pharynx at multiple sites, can change the size and shape of its internal cavity. In fact, one part of the pharynx may be constricted, another part dilated, and yet another part alternately constricted and dilated during the performance of a given activity. These size and shape changes can have a profound influence on the acoustic signal during speaking. They are also critical to certain phases of the swallowing process.

Movements of the Velum

The velum is a fleshy flap that is largely muscular. Most of the time, it hangs pendulously in the oropharyngeal space, but for many activities it moves substantially. Movements of the velum are mainly along an upward-backward or downward-forward path, in which those in one direction closely trace those in the other. The angular trajectory is reported to be slightly curvilin-

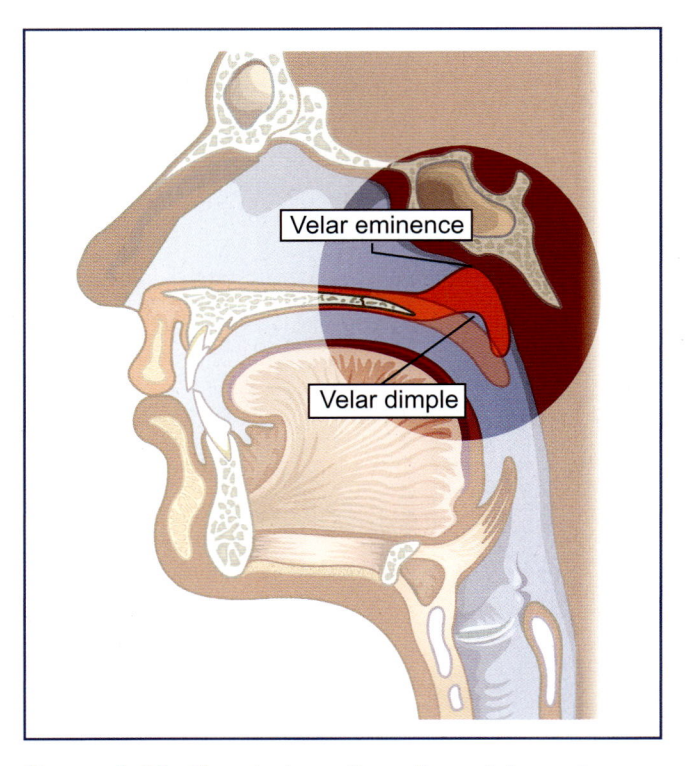

Figure 4-16. Elevated configuration of the velum as viewed from the side. Note its hooked appearance. The upper surface of the hook is called the velar eminence (or velar knee) and the undersurface of the hook is called the velar dimple.

Movements of the Outer Nose

Movements of the outer nose result mainly from outward or inward movements of the nasal alae that may change the cross-sections of the apertures of the anterior nares (nostrils). Under most circumstances, these movements are small. Exceptions occur during certain breathing events, when signaling emotions (disdain, contempt, and anger), and when using the nares to slow the flow of air from the outer nose by increasing resistance at its exit ports.

CONTROL VARIABLES OF VELOPHARYNGEAL-NASAL FUNCTION

Several control variables are important in velopharyngeal-nasal function. Their relative significance depends on the particular activity being performed, whether it is breathing, speaking, singing, blowing, sucking, swallowing, gagging, whistling, wind instrument playing, or glassblowing. For example, control variables for speaking take into account acoustic goals, whereas those for breathing do not. In contrast, both speaking and breathing involve aeromechanical control variables. For persons with a normally functioning velopharyngeal-nasal apparatus, the most significant features of control pertain to the velopharyngeal portion of the apparatus. There are times, however, when control of the outer nose can become important.

Attention is devoted to three control variables that influence aeromechanical and acoustic aspects of velopharyngeal-nasal function. These include: (a) the magnitude of the airway resistance offered by the velopharyngeal-nasal apparatus, (b) the magnitude of the muscular pressure exerted by the velopharyngeal sphincter to accomplish and maintain velopharyngeal closure, and (c) the magnitude of the acoustic impedance offered by the velopharyngeal-nasal apparatus.

Velopharyngeal-Nasal Airway Resistance

Resistance is defined, in a mechanical sense, as opposition to movement and results in a loss of energy through friction (similar to that of direct current in an electrical circuit). Velopharyngeal-nasal airway resistance is the opposition to the mass flow of air (the breath) through structures of the velopharyngeal-nasal airway. This is analogous to the resistance to airflow through the laryngeal apparatus discussed in Chapter 3.

> ### The Flap Flap
>
> Pharyngeal flaps are secondary surgical procedures usually performed on persons with repaired cleft palates who persist with velopharyngeal incompetence or insufficiency following primary surgery. Flaps are constructed using tissue from the posterior pharyngeal wall (peeled away like the skin on a banana) and attaching it to the velum to form a bridge. Flaps have also been used in children with cerebral palsy who have paresis of the velum. They have been found to improve speech in such children, but they also have been found to have a major negative side effect. They may raise the resistance to breathing through the nose and cause some children to switch from nose breathing to mouth breathing. Mouth breathing opens the door (pun intended) to drooling. The negative social consequences of drooling are often judged to outweigh the positive social consequences of improved speech. Thus, flaps have sometimes had to be removed.

Adjustments of the velopharyngeal port, nasal cavities, and/or outer nose can effect a change in airway resistance between the oral cavity and atmosphere through the nasal route, as portrayed in Figure 4–17. Specifically, an increase in velopharyngeal-nasal airway resistance may occur with a decrease in cross-sectional area and/or an increase in length of the velopharyngeal port, engorgement of the nasal cavities, or a decrease in cross-sectional area of the anterior nares. Airflow also alters the resistance because resistance is airflow dependent. That is, resistance increases with increases in airflow, even when the physical dimensions of the velopharyngeal-nasal airway remain unchanged.

Velopharyngeal-nasal airway resistance can range from very low, such as during resting tidal breathing with patent nasal cavities (following administration of a nasal decongestant), to infinite (completely obstructed). Infinite airway resistance is usually effected through airtight closure of the velopharyngeal port. Once airtight velopharyngeal closure is attained, adjustments of the nasal cavities and outer nose have no further influence on the resistance value. Infinite velopharyngeal-nasal airway resistance can also be achieved in the case of an open velopharynx under circumstances where there is complete nasal blockage. This is an example of why it is critical to include the nasal component in this subsystem rather than focus exclusively on the velopharyngeal component.

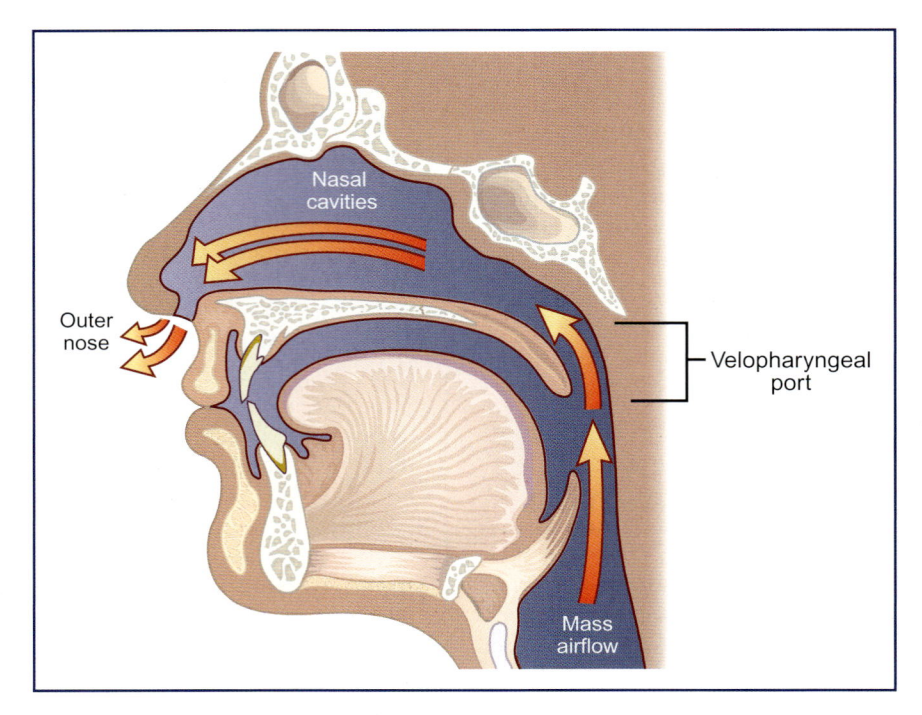

Figure 4–17. Velopharyngeal-nasal airway resistance. The resistance of the velopharyngeal-nasal apparatus to air flowing through it can be altered by adjustments of the velopharyngeal port, the nasal cavities, and the outer nose. Changes in the rate at which air flows through the apparatus can also alter the resistance.

Velopharyngeal Sphincter Compression

Once airtight velopharyngeal closure is attained, the force of that closure can be adjusted to meet the needs of the situation. This force, depicted in Figure 4–18, is represented by the compressive muscular pressure exerted to maintain the velopharyngeal sphincter in a closed configuration. The muscular pressure exerted at any moment must exceed the magnitude of the air pressure difference across the velopharyngeal sphincter (whether it be positive or negative) to prevent the velopharynx from being forced (blown or sucked) open. Thus, only a low compressive force is required to effect airtight velopharyngeal closure for an activity

---

Some Things Are Not Quite What They Seem

There seems to be a relatively large number of musicians who complain of "air leaks out the nose" during wind instrument playing (Malick, Moon, & Canady, 2007; Schwab & Schulze-Florey, 2004). Such complaints are red flags for what might be stress-induced velopharyngeal incompetence, a condition that may require medical intervention such as augmentation of the posterior pharyngeal wall (Koprowski, VanLue, & McCormick, 2018). Sometimes physical measurements confirm that, in fact, the velopharynx is open during sound production. But sometimes physical measurements show that, surprisingly, the velopharynx is closed during sound production, despite what the musician is feeling. Why the mismatch? A study of trombonists may have found the answer. By sensing changes in air pressure at the anterior nares, Bennett and Hoit (2013) discovered that some trombonists open the velopharynx at the beginning of expiration before the sound begins, and then close the velopharynx right as the sound starts. What they felt was correct—the velopharynx was open. But it was not open while they were actually playing. Sometimes the senses play tricks on us.

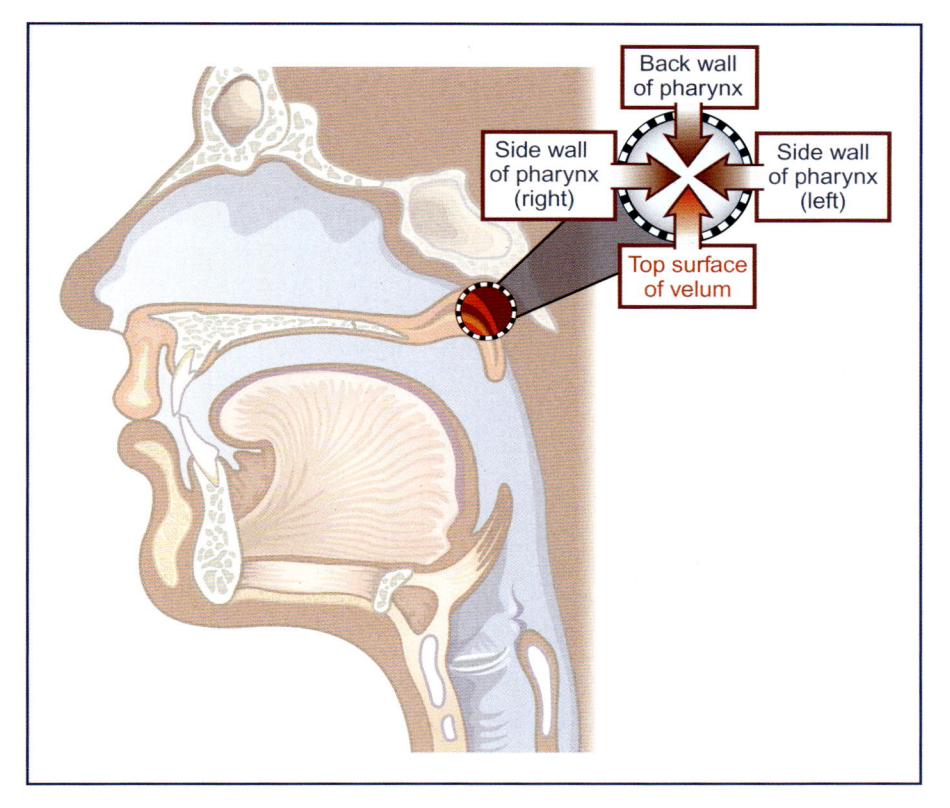

Figure 4–18. Compressive muscular pressure during velopharyngeal closure. The greater the air pressure difference across the velopharynx, the higher the compressive pressure needed to maintain velopharyngeal closure.

involving low oral air pressure, whereas a high compressive force is required for an activity involving high positive oral air pressure.

Velopharyngeal-Nasal Acoustic Impedance

Acoustic (sound) impedance, like airway resistance, is opposition to flow. However, it is opposition to the flow of sound rather than to mass airflow. Thus, the acoustic impedance offered by the velopharyngeal-nasal apparatus pertains to the rapid to-and-fro bumping of air molecules in which each molecule stays in a very restricted region and passes energy on to its neighbors. The opposition to acoustic flow is frequency dependent (similar to that of an alternating current in an electrical circuit). Acoustic impedance influences flow propagation of sound waves (not breath).

As portrayed in Figure 4–19, the velopharyngeal port can be adjusted to influence the degree of coupling between the oral and nasal cavities and thereby change the velopharyngeal-nasal acoustic impedance. The greater proportion of sound energy will be directed through the airway (oral or nasal) having the lower acoustic impedance. When the port is closed (Figure 4–19A), the oral and nasal airways are separated and nearly all of the sound energy passes through the oral airway and mouth. In this case, the acoustic impedance looking into the nasal cavities from their velopharyngeal end is nearly infinite, although a small amount of sound energy may be transmitted through the closed velopharynx via sympathetic vibration, such as when the velum acts like a drumhead. When the velopharyngeal port is open (Figures 4–19B and C), the oral and nasal cavities are free to exchange sound energy and interact with one another acoustically, and sound energy may pass between the outer nose and atmosphere. Changes in the size of the velopharyngeal port are important to determining how sound energy is divided between the oral and nasal cavities. Also important are configurations of the oral and nasal cavities themselves and the extent to which each impedes the flow of sound energy. In the case of the nasal part of the system, degree of engorgement of the nasal cavities and status of the anterior nares are relevant factors.

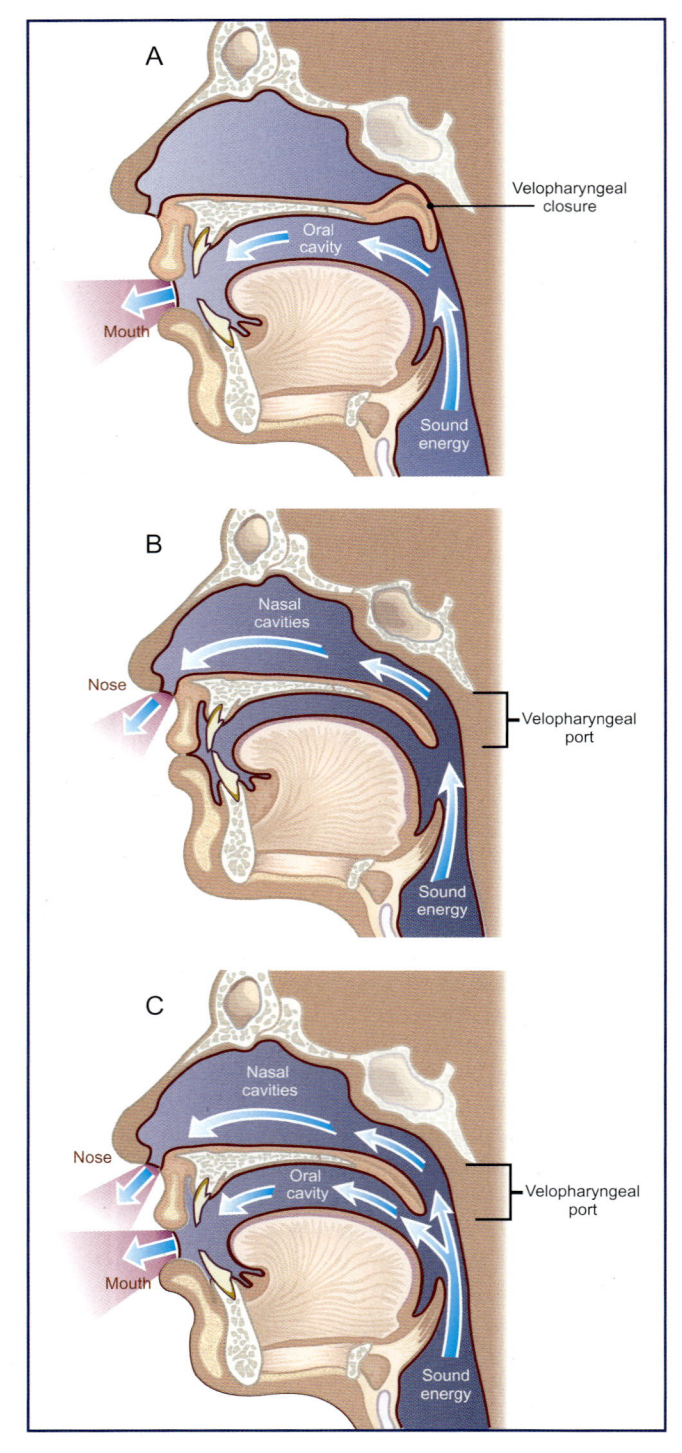

Figure 4–19. Oral-nasal sound wave propagation through the velopharyngeal-nasal pathway (velopharynx, nasal cavities, and outer nose) and oral pathway (oral cavity and mouth). The conditions shown are the velopharynx closed with sound routed through the oral pathway (**A**), the oral pathway closed with sound routed through the velopharyngeal-nasal pathway (**B**), and both pathways open so that sound is routed through both simultaneously (**C**).

Which Hunt

It is often stated that velopharyngeal incompetence or insufficiency allows air to pass into the nasal cavities, thereby causing hypernasality. This is a misconception. Significant quantities of air can pass into the nasal cavities through the velopharynx during utterance production without there being a perception of hypernasality. Also, hypernasality may be heard when no air is passing into the nasal cavities, such as when the tissue covering a submucous cleft palate vibrates and excites the nasal cavities into sympathetic vibration. Flow of air into the nose does not cause hypernasality. In fact, hypernasality may be present when inspiratory speech is produced and airflow is passing through the nasal cavities in the opposite direction from usual. It's instructive to go through written discussions about velopharyngeal dysfunction and see which authors get it right and which authors get it wrong. Think of it as sort of a "which" hunt.

NEURAL SUBSTRATES OF VELOPHARYNGEAL-NASAL CONTROL

Velopharyngeal-nasal movement is controlled by the nervous system, but the nature of that movement and the nature of its control differ with the activity being performed, whether it be sneezing, blowing, swallowing, or speaking. Although different parts of the central nervous system are responsible for the control of different velopharyngeal-nasal activities, control commands are sent through the same set of cranial nerves to muscles. These nerves originate in the brainstem and course outward to provide motor innervation to the pharynx, velum, and outer nose.

As shown in Table 4–1, motor innervation of the pharynx and velum is effected through the pharyngeal plexus, a network that includes fibers from cranial nerves IX (glossopharyngeal), X (vagus), and possibly XI (accessory). An exception is found in the case of the *palatal tensor* muscle, whose motor innervation is provided by cranial nerve V (trigeminal). There may also be additional motor innervation to the pharynx and velum through cranial nerve VII (facial), especially to the *palatal levator* and *uvulus* muscles. Motor innervation to the outer nose is effected by cranial nerve VII.

One might think that information about the motor nerve supply to different parts of the velopharyngeal-nasal apparatus would be straightforward and agreed

Table 4-1. Summary of the Motor and Sensory Nerve Supply to the Pharynx, Velum, and Outer Nose Components of the Velopharyngeal-Nasal Apparatus

	INNERVATION	
COMPONENT	MOTOR	SENSORY
Pharynx[a]	IX, X, (XI)[b]	V, VII, IX, X
Velum[a]	IX, X, (XI) (except **palatal tensor** muscle, which is innervated by V)	V, VII, IX, X
Outer nose	VII	V

Note. Cranial nerves include V (trigeminal), VII (facial), IX (glossopharyngeal), X (vagus), and possibly XI (accessory).

[a]There may be additional motor innervation from cranial nerve VII to certain muscles of the pharynx and velum, especially the **palatal levator** muscle and **uvulus** muscle (Shimokawa, Yi, & Tanaka, 2005).

[b]The branches of cranial nerves IX and X (and possibly XI) that innervate parts of the velopharynx are sometimes called the pharyngeal plexus.

upon. This is, indeed, the case for motor innervation to the outer nose, but not for motor innervation to the pharynx and velum. This is because the linkage between specific cranial nerves and the motor supply to specific muscles is equivocal in some cases (Cassell & Elkadi, 1995; Dickson, 1972; Moon & Kuehn, 2004) and because conducting research on motor nerve function in the velopharyngeal-nasal region of human beings is extremely difficult (Kuehn & Perry, 2008).

Sensory innervation to the pharynx and velum is effected through cranial nerves V, VII, IX, and X, and sensory innervation to the outer nose is effected through cranial nerve V. Neural information traveling along the sensory nerve supply from the pharynx, velum, and outer nose comes from receptors that respond to various types of stimuli, including mechanical stimuli. For example, receptors located in the mucosa of the velum and pharynx respond to light touch and receptors located in and near the velopharyngeal-nasal muscles relay information about muscle length and tension.

Much of the incoming information from the velopharyngeal portion of the velopharyngeal-nasal apparatus is not sensed or perceived. Specifically, the potential for sensing the position of the velum in space (proprioception) and its movement (kinesthesia) is believed to be rudimentary or nonexistent. Empirical evidence for this can be found in studies in which normal speakers have been shown to have difficulty controlling velopharyngeal movements voluntarily (Ruscello, 1982; Shelton, Beaumont, Trier, & Furr, 1978). Thus, it seems likely that control of the velopharyngeal apparatus relies more heavily on other types of infor-

mation, such as that associated with the sensing of air pressure and airflow (Liss, Kuehn, & Hinkle, 1994; Warren, Dalston, & Dalston, 1990) and that associated with the sensing of the acoustic signal (Netsell, 1990) via cranial nerve VIII (auditory-vestibular).

VELOPHARYNGEAL-NASAL FUNCTIONS

The velopharyngeal-nasal apparatus performs many functions, most of which relate to adjusting the degree of coupling between the oral and nasal cavities (through the velopharyngeal port) and between the nasal cavities and atmosphere (through the apertures of the anterior nares). The general nature of these functions is covered here. Oral-nasal coupling as it pertains to speech production is covered in another section of this chapter. Oral-nasal coupling as it pertains to swallowing is covered in Chapter 16.

Coupling Between the Oral and Nasal Cavities

The degree of coupling between the oral and nasal cavities is adjusted by changing the size of the velopharyngeal port (the opening between the oral and nasal cavities). The velopharyngeal port is open most of the time to accommodate nasal breathing. Closure of the port is usually accomplished through action of the velum, often with participation of the pharynx. This closure pattern can be described as a flap-sphincter action, the flap being movement of the velum and the sphincter being movement of the pharynx.

There is no universal pattern for achieving velopharyngeal closure. On the contrary, several movement strategies for achieving closure of the velopharyngeal port have been identified that involve different actions or combinations of actions of the velum, lateral pharyngeal walls, and posterior pharyngeal wall (Croft, Shprintzen, & Rakoff, 1981; Finkelstein et al., 1995; Poppelreuter, Engelke, & Bruns, 2000; Shprintzen, 1992; Skolnik, McCall, & Barnes, 1973). These movement strategies include: (a) elevation of the velum alone, (b) inward movement of the lateral pharyngeal walls with little to no participation of the velum, (c) elevation of the velum combined with inward movement of the lateral pharyngeal walls, and (d) elevation of the velum combined with inward movement of the lateral pharyngeal walls and forward movement of the posterior pharyngeal wall. The prevailing wisdom is that these different movement strategies for achieving velopharyngeal closure are rooted in differences in anatomy (Finkelstein et al., 1995). For example, individuals with smaller front-to-back than side-to-side dimensions of the resting velopharyngeal port may be more likely to use elevation of the velum alone as the strategy for achieving closure. In contrast, those with more equal front-to-back and side-to-side dimensions to the velopharyngeal port may be more likely to incorporate inward movement of the lateral walls of the pharynx in their closure pattern. It should be noted that velopharyngeal closure patterns are not necessarily fixed within an individual, but can change over time, such as during development. Figure 4–20 illustrates a typical pattern of velopharyngeal closure in a normal individual (Croft et al., 1981).

The positioning of the velum for velopharyngeal closure is most often attributed to action of the *palatal levator* muscles (Dickson, 1972). Thought typically has been that lifting of the velum follows from the contractile force provided by the *palatal levator* muscles and accounts for the fact that the midportion of the velum usually attains the highest elevation during closure of the velopharyngeal port (see Figure 4–16) (Bell-Berti, 1976; Fritzell, 1963; Lubker, 1968; Seaver & Kuehn, 1980). Although action of the *palatal levator* muscles seems to be clearly associated with the flap component of the flap-sphincter closure adjustment, correlations between *palatal levator* muscle activity and the elevation of the velum are weaker (albeit positive) than would be expected were the *palatal levator* muscles alone responsible for positioning the velum (Fritzell, 1979; Lubker, 1968). This suggests that other muscles must also be active in positioning the velum. Research, in fact, supports this inference. For example, different combinations of muscle activity among the *palatal levator*, *glossopalatine*, and *pharyngopalatine* muscles have been found to be associated with the same positioning of the velum (Kuehn, Folkins, & Cutting, 1982). This and other evidence (Moon et al., 1994b) suggest that there is a trading relationship among these three muscles that contribute to movements of the velum.

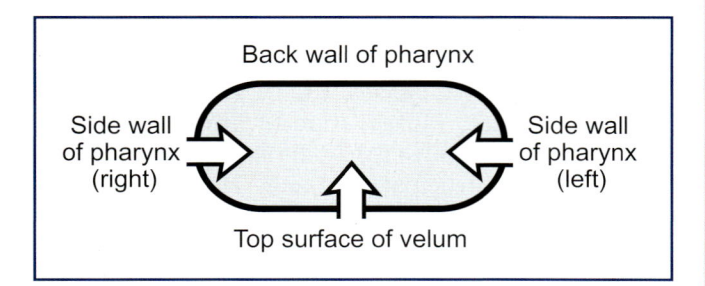

Figure 4–20. A typical pattern of velopharyngeal closure as seen from above. In this pattern, the velum elevates and the lateral pharyngeal walls move inward. Several other closure patterns are possible.

Coupling Between the Nasal Cavities and Atmosphere

The degree of coupling between the nasal cavities and atmosphere can be adjusted by changing the size of the anterior nares. The range of possibilities extends from fully open nares to fully closed nares. It is also possible to have different degrees of coupling for the two nares (one being open more than the other).

The anterior nares, like the velopharynx, are relatively open most of the time to accommodate nasal breathing. The nares can be dilated or constricted through the actions of muscles of the outer nose. Such actions can be either opposed or supplemented by aeromechanical forces associated with breathing. For example, muscles that dilate the anterior nares may activate to resist the tendency of the nares to collapse in response to low air pressures (created by high airflows) in their lumina. The need for such activation can be appreciated by sniffing briskly while watching the outer nose in a mirror: the nares and alae of the outer nose tend to be sucked inward by the lowering of nasal pressures.

Although not a typical pattern, there are times when the anterior nares constrict during expiration as a means of slowing airflow through the nose. An exaggerated version of such constriction is often observed in individuals with velopharyngeal incompetence (those whose velopharynx cannot close) during speech pro-

Where's the Rest?

Many studies have examined the correlation between velopharyngeal incompetence and articulation skill in children with repaired cleft palates. The highest correlation found in these studies is 0.5. Square that number and you find that velopharyngeal incompetence predicts only 25% of the variance in articulation skill. Where's the rest? Some have suggested it's to be found in "learning." We believe 75% is far too much to be attributed to such a notion. Rather, we suspect that the rest is confounded by the fact that the children studied were never categorized with regard to the magnitude of their nasal airway resistance. Not knowing or controlling for this factor would have an important influence on the strength of the correlation obtained between velopharyngeal incompetence and articulation skill. Where's the rest of the variance of interest? We think it's probably in the nose and has been overlooked.

duction. Referred to clinically as "nares constriction," this is often taken as a cardinal sign of velopharyngeal dysfunction and is thought to represent an attempt to valve the airstream to compensate for an inability to valve it at the velopharynx (Warren, Hairfield, & Hinton, 1985).

VENTILATION AND VELOPHARYNGEAL-NASAL FUNCTION

Ventilation (the movement of air in and out of the pulmonary apparatus for the purpose of gas exchange) can be routed through the nose, the mouth, or both. The most common form of ventilation, resting tidal breathing, usually occurs through the nose alone. Three important aspects of ventilation and velopharyngeal-nasal function are discussed here: nasal valve modulation, nasal cycling (side-to-side), and nasal-oral switching.

Nasal Valve Modulation

The nose is a major source of resistance to the flow of air during breathing. This resistance is governed mainly by nasal patency and may be altered by many factors, including infection, trauma, emotion, and air temperature, among others (Bridger, 1970).

In the normal upper airway, the greatest resistance to airflow occurs toward the front ends of the nasal passages in what are called the nasal valves. As portrayed in Figure 4–21, each nasal valve (left and right) comprises two components, an external valve and an internal valve.

The external nasal valve is contained in the vestibule of the nose and constitutes a vault formed by the nasal floor, nasal rim, and nasal septum. The nasal muscles can adjust the external valve in ways that dilate, constrict, and/or change its configuration. Nasal muscles that dilate the anterior nares increase the rigidity of the external valves and make them less likely to collapse when air pressure lowers, such as occurs with high airflows (Bridger, 1970). The external nasal valves dilate during inspiration, an action that parallels active dilation in other parts of the breathing airway, such as the pharynx and larynx (Cole, 1976; Drettner, 1979).

The internal nasal valve is an orifice that forms the transition between the vestibule and the osseous nasal cavity (fossa) on each side just in front of the inferior nasal concha. The cross-sectional area of the internal nasal valve is the smallest found in the nasal airway and accounts for up to two-thirds of the resistance to airflow through the velopharyngeal-nasal apparatus

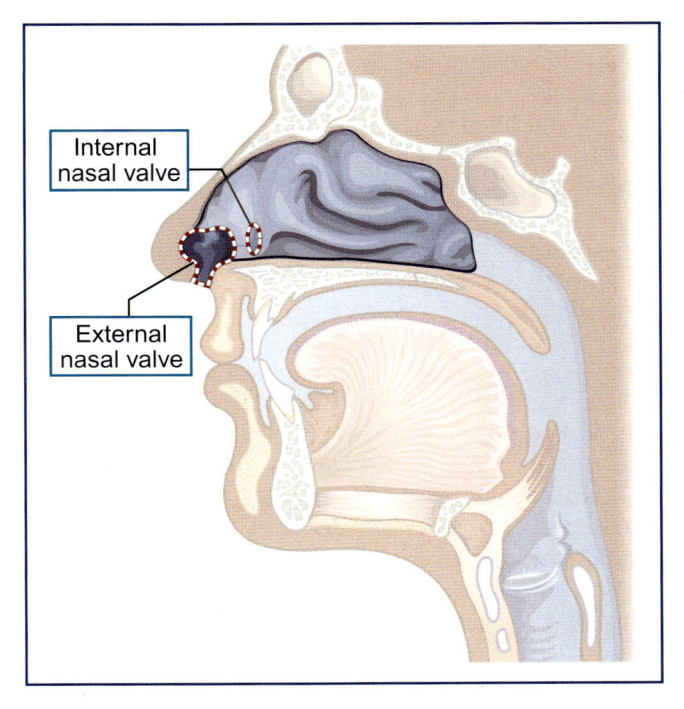

Figure 4–21. Internal and external nasal valves. During nasal breathing, both valves become larger during inspiration and smaller during expiration. The internal nasal valve is the smallest part of the nasal airway and accounts for up to two-thirds of the resistance to airflow during inspiration.

during inspiration (Foster, 1962). Based on its anatomic (Proctor, 1982) and airflow-resistive (Hairfield, Warren, Hinton, & Seaton, 1987) characteristics, this valve is considered to be the main regulator of the nasal airway. The internal nasal valve is an active participant in tidal breathing, becoming larger during inspiration and smaller during expiration (Hairfield et al., 1987). This pattern is maintained even when the external nasal valve is fixed in size, indicating that adjustments of the anterior nares and alae are not responsible for the effect. The precise mechanism of regulation of the internal nasal valve is unknown.

Although the effort it takes to breathe is about three times greater through the nose than through the mouth, the nasal route typically prevails. This is because it provides advantages for both inspiration and expiration. During inspiration, nasal breathing warms, humidifies, and filters the incoming air before it reaches the lungs and lower airways. During expiration, nasal breathing helps ensure adequate alveolar gas exchange (Hairfield et al., 1987). It does so by providing an in-series braking mechanism (Jackson, 1976) to accompany the laryngeal braking mechanism that serves to lengthen expiration and, thereby, enhance alveolar gas exchange (Gautier,

Remmers, & Bartlett, 1973). This may help to explain the paradoxical preference people have for breathing through their nose.

Nasal Cycling (Side-to-Side)

The rhythmic exchange of resting tidal breathing usually goes unnoticed. Also unnoticed, and even unknown, is the fact that the two sides of the nose behave differently during breathing. The fact of the matter is, everybody has two noses.

For most people (estimates range up to 80%) these two noses (one on the left side and one on the right side) go through cycles of concha (turbinate) engorgement and deflation (Principato & Ozenberger, 1970; Stoksted, 1953). These cycles are typically 180° out of phase so that as the left side is congesting (swelling), the right side is decongesting (shrinking), and vice versa. Cycling time varies from person to person and can range from as short as 30 minutes to as long as 5 hours or more. These alternating blockages and returns to patency go on throughout the day and night without awareness on the part of the person breathing (Principato & Ozenberger, 1970), probably because the total resistance to airflow remains relatively constant (Huang et al., 2003).

Nasal-Oral Switching

As mentioned above, most breathing is done through the nose because it: (a) converts the temperature of incoming air to that of the body, (b) adjusts the relative humidity of incoming air to an advantageous 80%, (c) extracts dust, bacteria, and other contaminants from incoming air, and (d) provides airway resistance during expiration that may aid in alveolar gas exchange. Breathing through the mouth at rest is much less common, but it does occur in a small percentage of healthy people (Niinimaa, Cole, & Mintz, 1981; Saibene, Mognoni, & LaFortuna, 1978; Vig & Zajac, 1993; Warren, Drake, & Davis, 1992; Warren, Hairfield, Seaton, & Hinton, 1988).

When ventilation demands exceed those associated with rest, it may become necessary to switch to oral (mouth) breathing or oral combined with nasal breathing. The key factor in such switching appears to be the prevailing nasal resistance. When that resistance exceeds a critical value, the natural tendency is to switch from solely nasal breathing to nasal-oral breathing (Warren, Hairfield, Seaton, Morr, & Smith, 1988). This critical value turns out to be slightly lower than the resistance value that leads to the sensation of breathing discomfort (Warren, Mayo, Zajac, & Rochet, 1996). Thus, the switch from nasal breathing to oral-nasal breathing occurs before awareness of breathing difficulty. This observation is consistent with the established notion that physiological responses to changes in the internal environment generally occur prior to psychophysical recognition of change in all homeostatic systems (Warren, Hairfield, Seaton, & Hinton, 1987).

VELOPHARYNGEAL-NASAL FUNCTION AND SPEECH PRODUCTION

The velopharyngeal-nasal apparatus has two important roles during speech production. One is to manage the airstream to produce certain types of oral consonant sounds (those that require high oral pressure). This requires that the velopharynx be closed, or nearly closed, so that aeromechanical energy be directed through the oral channel. The other role is to manage the flow of acoustic energy into the oral and nasal cavities, which is important for the production of vowels and both oral and nasal consonants. This section considers these roles in the contexts of sustained utterances and running speech activities.

Sustained Utterances

Sustained vowels and consonants are usually produced with relatively stable configurations of the velopharyngeal-nasal apparatus. Slight differences in velopharyngeal function have been observed across different sustained vowels, and obvious differences can be seen in sustained oral consonants when contrasted with sustained nasal consonants.

Observations of the velopharynx (primarily through the use of x-ray and aeromechanical techniques) during sustained vowel production have shown that the velum moves upward and backward toward the posterior pharyngeal wall in anticipation of the upcoming vowel (Bzoch, 1968; Lubker, 1968; Moll, 1962). At the same time, the lateral pharyngeal walls move inward[1]

---

[1]The suggestion has been made (Dickson & Dickson, 1972) that the *palatal levator* muscles are responsible for both elevation of the velum and inward movements of the lateral pharyngeal walls. Those in support of this suggestion contend that inward movements of the lateral pharyngeal walls occur in a region of the pharynx above the fiber course of the *superior constrictor* muscles (Honjo, Harada, & Kumazasa, 1976; Isshiki, Harita, & Kawano, 1985). A contrary viewpoint is that elevation of the velum and inward movements of the lateral pharyngeal

and the posterior pharyngeal wall may move forward slightly (Iglesias, Kuehn, & Morris, 1980). The velum is usually elevated maximally in its midportion during vowel production, and contact with the posterior pharyngeal wall is typically achieved by the third quadrant of the velum (Graber, Bzoch, & Aoba, 1959). There is also a tendency for the velum to be elevated to a higher position when sustained vowels are produced at higher vocal effort levels (Tucker, 1963).

Sustained vowel production may or may not be accompanied by airtight closure of the velopharyngeal port. The probability of airtight closure favors high vowels (such as "ee" in peek) over low vowels (such as "a" in cat) (Moll, 1962). Whether or not airtight velopharyngeal closure is achieved, high vowels and low vowels contrast in still other ways. Compared with low vowel production, high vowel production is associated with: (a) greater velar height, (b) greater extent of velar contact with the posterior pharyngeal wall when the two surfaces are in apposition, and (c) smaller distance between the velum and the posterior pharyngeal wall when closure is not complete (Iglesias et al., 1980; Lubker, 1968; Moll, 1962). High vowel production also involves greater velopharyngeal sphincter compression (closing force) than low vowel production when velopharyngeal closure is complete (Gotto, 1977; Kuehn & Moon, 1998; Moon, Kuehn, & Huisman, 1994a; Nusbaum, Foly, & Wells, 1935). Velar height differences during sustained vowel productions are relatively strongly correlated with the electrical activity of the *palatal levator* muscles (Bell-Berti, 1976; Fritzell, 1969; Lubker, 1968); less than perfect correlations may relate to partial influences of other muscles involved in trading relationships with the *palatal levator* muscle in velar height adjustments (Fritzell, 1969; Kuehn et al., 1982).

Two possible mechanisms have been proposed to account for the differences observed in velar height between high and low vowel productions. One is that the velum elevates to different degrees because of anatomical constraints imposed through interconnections to structures below (Harrington, 1944; Kaltenborn, 1948; Lubker, 1968; Moll, 1962), with likely candidates being the *glossopalatine* and *pharyngopalatine* muscles. The hypothesis is that the *glossopalatine* muscle, the more important of the two candidates, tethers the velum so that production of low vowels (involving low tongue positions) restricts elevation of the velum and leads to lesser degrees of closure of the velopharyngeal port. The influence of tethering is less for high vowels (involving high tongue positions) because less restriction is placed on velar elevation.

The second proposed mechanism to account for velar height differences between high and low vowel productions has an acoustic-perceptual basis. Specifically, it may be that the velum elevates to different degrees because of acoustic requirements involved in ensuring that the utterance not be perceived as nasal (Curtis, 1968; Lubker, 1968; Moll, 1962). This speculation is based on the results of electrical analog studies of the nasalization of vowels conducted by House and Stevens (1956) and more recently with a computational speech production model by Bunton and Story (2012). Both studies demonstrated that less nasal coupling (velopharyngeal opening) is required to produce the auditory-perceptual judgment of nasal quality for high vowels than for low vowels. Thus, the velar height differences observed for high and low vowels could be purposive adjustments to control the degree of nasalization in the face of different tongue adjustments that influence the flow of acoustic energy through the oral and nasal cavities.

Sustained fricative and nasal consonant productions are accompanied by contrasting velopharyngeal configurations. Sustained fricatives, such as "s" and "z," are accompanied by airtight velopharyngeal closure in children as young as 3 years and adults of all ages (Hoit, Watson, Hixon, McMahon, & Johnson, 1994; Thompson & Hixon, 1979). Airtight closure of the velopharyngeal port is clearly a priority for speech sounds like these that rely on the management of the oral airstream for their production. Such closure has also been found to be accompanied by higher velar elevation and more forward displacement of the posterior pharyngeal wall compared with closure during vowel productions (Iglesias et al., 1980). This difference in velar elevation can be seen by comparing the vowel and fricative images in Figure 4–22.

Sustained nasal consonants are produced with large openings of the velopharyngeal port, as shown in the rightmost image in Figure 4–22. The position of the velum is the same (or slightly higher) for sustained "m" and "n" productions as it is for resting tidal breathing, and *palatal levator* muscle activity is not

---

walls are simply coordinated actions of the *palatal levator* muscles (to elevate the velum) and the *superior constrictor* muscles (to move the lateral pharyngeal walls inward). Those in support of this viewpoint contend that inward movements of the lateral pharyngeal walls occur below the velar eminence associated with insertion of the *palatal levator* muscles into the velum (Shprintzen, McCall, Skolnick, & Lenicone, 1975; Skolnick, 1970; Skolnick et al., 1973) and that the timing of movements of the velum and lateral pharyngeal walls are poorly correlated during speech production in normal individuals (Iglesias et al., 1980). We support this latter viewpoint in our description of velopharyngeal-nasal function and point the interested reader to Moon and Kuehn (2004) for further discussion on this topic.

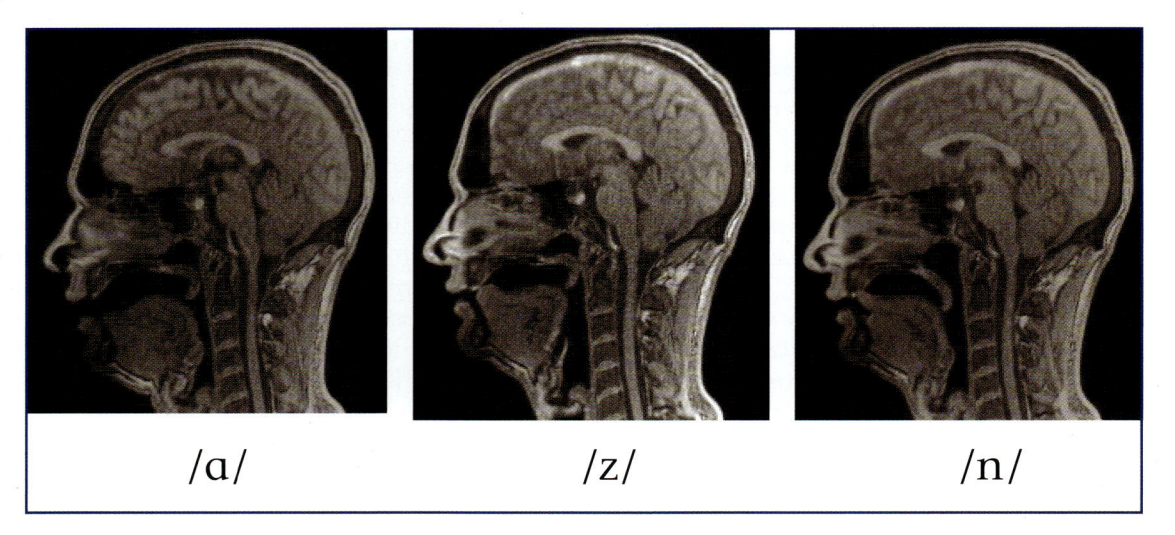

Figure 4-22. Sagittal magnetic resonance images (MRIs) showing different velar elevations associated with production of the vowel "ah," the voiced fricative "z," and the nasal consonant "n" (courtesy of Adam Baker).

discernible (Iglesias et al., 1980; Lubker, 1968). Predictably, sustained nasal consonant productions are accompanied by substantial nasal airflow (Hoit et al., 1994; Thompson & Hixon, 1979).

Running Speech Activities

Running speech activities require rapid adjustments of the velopharyngeal-nasal apparatus. A few minutes spent watching x-ray or real-time magnetic resonance imaging (MRI) recordings of running speech production reveals that velopharyngeal articulation is every bit as fast and intricate as are movements of the mandible, tongue, and lips. In fact, velar elevating and lowering gestures can each occur within a time interval of about a tenth of a second (Kuehn, 1976). The precise pattern of opening and closing and the degree to which the velopharyngeal port is opened or closed relate to the nature of the speech sounds being spoken, the influence of surrounding sounds on the sound being spoken, and the rate at which they are produced (Kent et al., 1974).

When consonants and vowels are combined as they are in running speech activities, primacy of control of the velopharyngeal-nasal apparatus is vested in consonant productions. This is because the production of many consonant elements relies heavily on appropriate management of the airstream. Sacrificing the aeromechanical requirements of these consonants by opening the velopharynx may result in sacrificing the intelligibility of speech. In contrast, sacrificing closure for vowel productions may increase nasalization but has only a minimal effect on speech intelligibility. The consonant elements that rely most on aeromechanical management of the airstream are often referred to as "the pressure consonants" because they are characteristically produced with high oral air pressure and a closed velopharynx. The pressure consonants include stop-plosive, fricative, and affricate speech sounds (see

Playing by Her Own Rule

She was a young woman with a profound bilateral hearing loss. She'd received intensive behavioral therapy for imprecise articulation, but essentially no progress was being made. A puzzled speech-language pathologist made the referral. What was preventing improvement in speech? The answer was found in a recording of nasal airflow. A large burst of airflow was found to accompany each segment of speech that included a voiceless consonant. The young woman had apparently developed a production rule that said, "Only close your velopharynx for speech when your voice is on." It turned out to be a rule that could be changed by displaying nasal airflow for her to monitor on a storage oscilloscope so that she could see her rule in action and adopt a more appropriate one with some guidance. Her velopharynx cooperated and her articulation improved.

Chapter 5 for specific definitions). In contrast, nasal consonants are produced with a low oral air pressure and a relatively wide-open velopharyngeal port.

The control of the velopharyngeal-nasal apparatus during running speech production is not simply a sequencing of separate and independent position and movement patterns for different speech sounds. Rather, the position and movement patterns for two or more speech sounds may occur simultaneously, such that their productions actually overlap and intermingle. Part of this has to do with how the brain prepares in advance for velopharyngeal-nasal adjustments and part has to do with how the mechanical-inertial properties of the velopharyngeal-nasal apparatus influence its behavior. More is said about these principles in Chapter 5.

Underlying the assembling of velopharyngeal-nasal positions and movements is the principle that consonants influence the velopharyngeal-nasal adjustments of all speech sounds (consonants and vowels) within their interval of preparation. The precise influence depends on both the type of consonant and type of vowel. For example, the preparation period for oral consonants results in smaller velopharyngeal port openings (or no opening) for vowels that precede them, whereas the preparation period for nasal consonants results in larger velopharyngeal port openings for vowels that precede them (Warren & DuBois, 1964), as can be seen in Figure 4–23. Furthermore, when a nasal consonant is preceded by two consecutive vowels, the opening of the velopharyngeal port for the nasal consonant is initiated during the production of the first vowel in the sequence (Moll & Daniloff, 1971). Even the presence of a word boundary does not affect this observation, although velar lowering may be delayed somewhat at marked junctural boundaries (McClean, 1973).

Although historically the role of the velopharyngeal apparatus as an "articulatory" structure has been questioned (Moll & Shriner, 1967), the current view is the velopharynx is very much an articulator that receives its commands at the same time as do other articulatory structures (mandible, tongue, and lips). Some have even gone so far as to provide evidence that a portion of the velum—specifically, its lower border—can act as an autonomous oral articulator in the production of selected sounds (e.g., the French uvular fricative; Gick, Francis, Klenin, Mizrahi, & Tom, 2013). Clearly, the function of the velopharynx in speech production is critical to both speech intelligibility (its articulatory role) and voice quality (its acoustic resonance role).

Understandably, the study of velopharyngeal-nasal function for speech production has focused on the expiratory phase of the breathing cycle, the phase of the cycle during which speech is produced. Nevertheless, the velopharyngeal-nasal apparatus also plays an important role during the inspiratory phase of the speech breathing cycle. Running speech breathing usually demands quick inspirations to minimize

Vowel
(closed velopharynx)

Nasalized vowel
(open velopharynx)

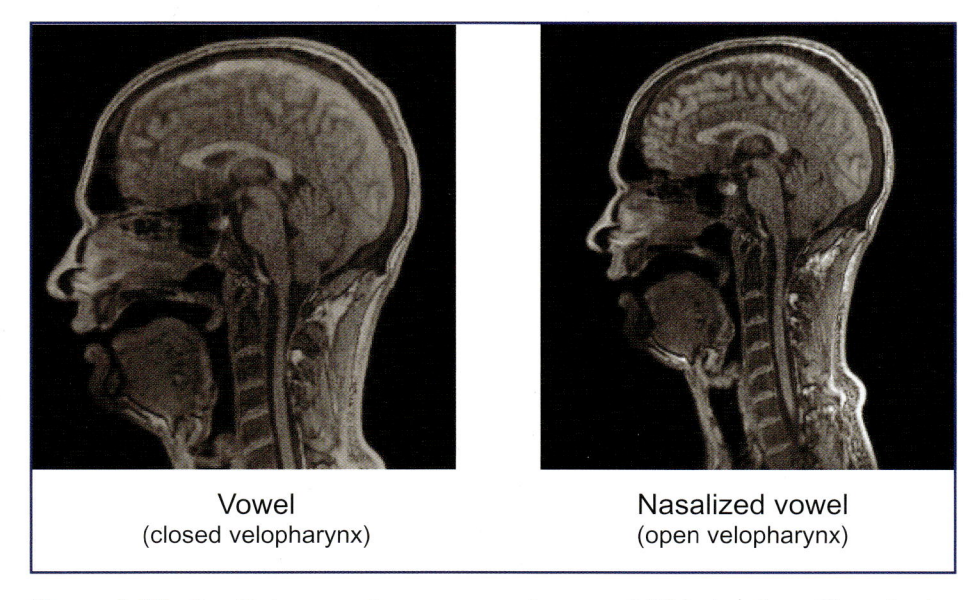

Figure 4–23. Sagittal magnetic resonance images (MRIs) showing different velar elevations for the production of a neutral vowel preceding an oral consonant (*left*) and for the same vowel preceding a nasal consonant (*right*) (courtesy of Adam Baker).

interruptions to the flow of speech, and quick inspirations require a low resistance pathway. The best way to create such a low resistance pathway is to abduct the lips and open the velopharynx simultaneously, and this is, in fact, what people do. Thus, in contrast to resting tidal breathing, during which inspirations are typically routed through the nose exclusively, inspirations are routed through both the mouth and nose during speaking (Lester & Hoit, 2014). This not only allows for quick inspirations, but may also preserve some of the benefits of nasal inspirations, such as air filtration and humidification.

VARIABLES THAT INFLUENCE VELOPHARYNGEAL-NASAL FUNCTION

There are many variables that can influence velopharyngeal-nasal function, some of which have already been mentioned. Three that are covered in this section are body position, age, and sex.

Body Position

Velopharyngeal-nasal function changes with changes in body position, primarily because of the influence of gravity. Each time the velopharyngeal-nasal apparatus is reoriented within a gravity field, alternate mechanical solutions are required to meet the goals for adjusting the velopharyngeal port.

When in an upright position (seated or standing), the pull of gravity tends to lower the velum. In contrast, when in the supine body position, gravity acts to pull the velum toward the posterior pharyngeal wall (Bae, Perry, & Kuehn, 2014; Perry, 2011, Perry, Bae, & Kuehn, 2012). The difference in the resting position of the velum in these two body positions is shown in Figure 4–24.

Movements of the velum away from this rest position, such as those associated with speech production, require different force solutions in the two body positions. In upright, the muscle force required to elevate the velum must overcome the pull of gravity, whereas muscle force required to lower the velum is augmented by this pull. The opposite situation prevails in supine, where the muscle force to move the velum toward the posterior pharyngeal wall is augmented by the pull of gravity, and the muscle force to move the velum away from the posterior pharyngeal wall must overcome the pull of gravity. As might be expected, these different force solutions for upright and supine are accompanied by different muscle activities (Moon & Canady, 1995). Specifically, peak muscle activity (as measured by electromyography) for the *palatal levator* muscle (velar

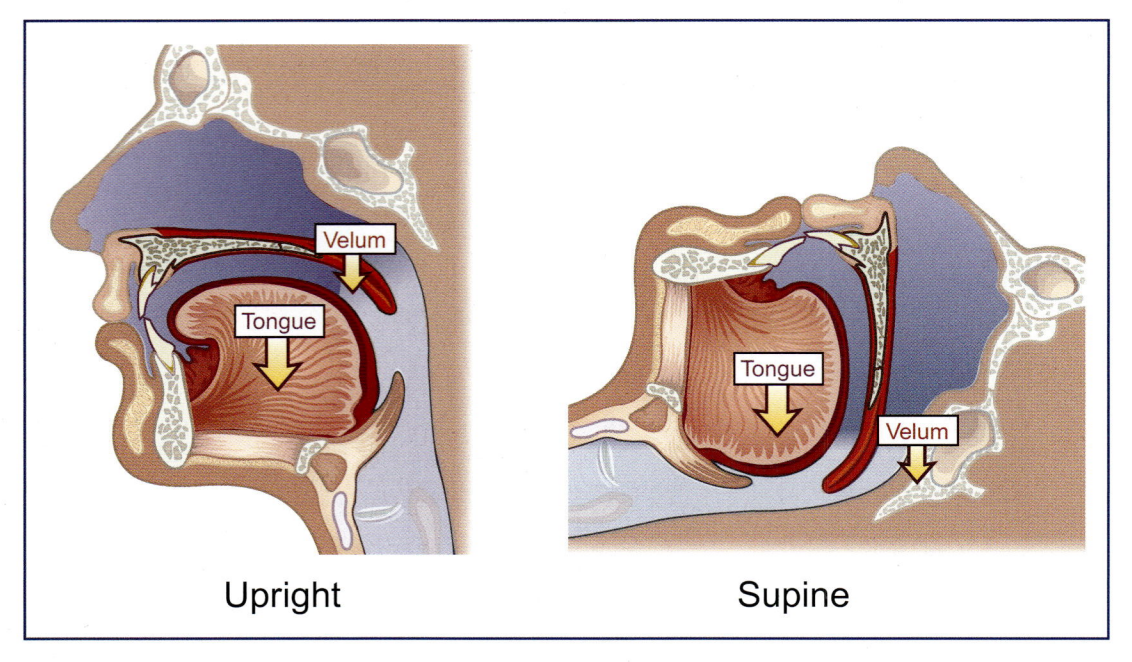

Figure 4–24. The velum at rest in upright and supine body positions. In the upright body position, gravity exerts a downward pull on the velum, whereas in the supine body position gravity pulls the velum toward the posterior pharyngeal wall.

elevator) is lower in the supine body position compared with the upright body position, suggesting that less activation was required when the pull of gravity is in the same direction (toward the posterior pharyngeal wall). Also, the activation level of the *pharyngopalatine* muscle (velar depressor) is usually greater in the supine body position, where the pull of gravity is counter to movement of the velum away from the posterior pharyngeal wall. Interestingly, the position of the velum, though quite similar in the two body positions, tends to be slightly lower in supine (Bae et al., 2014; Perry, 2011), apparently reflecting the lower *palatal levator* muscle activity in that body position.

Reorientation of the velopharyngeal-nasal apparatus in space is not restricted to changes in body position. Reorientation can also mean that the body is maintained in a fixed position and the head is moved about different axes. For example, the head can be pitched about a lateral axis, rolled about a longitudinal axis, and yawed about a vertical axis. Rotation of the head about a lateral axis is an especially common activity (nod your head yes to this statement) that alters the gravitational forces on the velopharyngeal-nasal apparatus, especially the velum. When the head is rotated downward from its usual position (toward a position where the mandible would rest on the rib cage wall), the pull of gravity on the velum is in a direction that tends to pull it away from the posterior pharyngeal wall. In contrast, when the head is rotated upward from its usual position (toward a position where the tip of the nose is maximally elevated), the pull of gravity on the velum is in a direction that tends to pull it toward the posterior pharyngeal wall. Whereas reorientation of the velopharyngeal-nasal apparatus is not noticeable to most people, it may have a profound effect on someone with a neuromotor-based weakness of the *palatal levator* muscles, wherein rotation of the head upward may enhance movement of the velum toward the posterior pharyngeal wall and, thereby, improve velopharyngeal-nasal function for speech production.

Gravitational influences also affect the function of the nasal cavities. For example, nasal patency decreases and nasal airway resistance increases in downright compared with upright body positions (Rudcrantz, 1969). This change in patency appears to relate to vascular changes that cause nasal congestion (Hiyama, Ono, Ishiwata, & Kuroda, 2002).

Age

The structure of the velopharyngeal-nasal apparatus changes across the lifespan as does its function, with the most significant changes occurring during the developmental years. Its function for speech production undergoes maturation during infancy and childhood, but once adulthood is reached, it appears that this function is maintained into senescence. Discussed here are age-related anatomical and physiological changes in the velopharyngeal-nasal apparatus; discussion of other associated upper airway structures is found in Chapter 5.

At birth, the larynx is located high within the neck and the velum and epiglottis are approximated (Kent & Murray, 1982). Around 4 to 6 months of age, the velum and epiglottis separate (Sasaki, Levine, Laitman, & Crelin, 1977) as the larynx moves from the level of the first cervical vertebra to the level of the third cervical vertebra. This downward movement is accomplished primarily by rapid growth of the pharynx in the vertical dimension from about 4 cm in the newborn pharynx (Crelin, 1973) to approximately three times that length in the adult (Sasaki et al., 1977). During that same period, the hard and soft palates grow quickly, with the hard palate growing somewhat more quickly than the soft palate and the growth rate of both becoming more gradual after 2 years of age (Vorperian et al., 2005). As children continue to grow during their first decade, so does the size of the velopharyngeal-nasal structures (Kazlin & Perry, 2016; Vorperian et al., 2009) These developmental changes affect the geometry and mechanical effectiveness of certain muscles. For example, as the palates grow, the orientation of the paired *palatal levator* muscles change in ways that improve their mechanical advantage for elevating the velum (Fletcher, 1973).

Infants are often assumed to be "obligate nasal breathers" because the infant velum and epiglottis are approximated; however, this is not true. The preponderance of evidence indicates that most healthy infants can breathe through the mouth when necessary (e.g., when the anterior nares are occluded) (Miller et al., 1985; Rodenstein, Perlmutter, & Stanescu, 1985). Therefore, the term "preferential nasal breather" is more appropriate to describe the predominant (rather than exclusive) use of the nasal airway for breathing in infants.

The birth cry, the first utterance for most human newborns, is produced with an open velopharynx (Bosma, Truby, & Lind, 1965). Nondistress vocalizations also are often produced with an open velopharynx during the first few months of life (Buhr, 1980; Hsu, Fogel, & Cooper, 2000; Kent & Murray; 1982; Oller, 1986; Thom, Hoit, Hixon, & Smith, 2006). Velopharyngeal closure for nondistress vocalizations (which eventually become speech) increases gradually across the first year and a half of life until it closes for such utterances around 19 months of age (Bunton & Hoit,

2018). A closer look at this developmental trajectory shows that velopharyngeal closure in infants and toddlers is also conditioned by the types of sounds being produced, with sounds that require high oral pressure, such as stops and fricatives, being much more likely to be produced with a closed velopharynx than those that do not require such pressure, such as vowels. Interestingly, other types of utterances do not seem to follow a developmental trajectory and are either closed at all ages (cries, screams, and raspberries) or open at all ages (pre-cry windups, whimpers, and laughs). Children 3 years and older produce imitative speech with a closed velopharynx (Thompson & Hixon, 1979; Zajac, 2000) though certain temporal features of velopharyngeal function during speech production continue to be modified into the teenage years (Leeper, Tissington, & Munhall, 1998; Zajac, 2000; Zajac & Hackett, 2002).

Although speech is produced with airtight velopharyngeal closure by early childhood, the means for achieving this closure may change with development. One example relates to children who have enlarged lymphoid tissue masses in the nasopharyngeal tonsils (adenoids). These tonsils typically grow during the first decade of life and then begin to atrophy (Jaw, Sheu, Liu, & Lin, 1999; Subtelny & Koepp-Baker, 1956) until they are fully atrophied by adulthood. This is illustrated in Figure 4–25. During velopharyngeal closure, children with enlarged nasopharyngeal tonsils typically exhibit velar to adenoid contact and those with larger adenoids show less *palatal levator* muscle contraction (Perry, Kuehn, Sutton, & Fang, 2017). As the nasopharyngeal tonsil tissue recedes with age, velopharyngeal closure must go through a slow reorganization in those children who have been accomplishing closure through abutment of the velum and walls of the pharynx against the enlarged adenoidal tissue. This accommodation is obviously successful given the continuation of airtight velopharyngeal closure during the normal developmental schedule, but it may be interrupted if an adenoidectomy (removal of the adenoids) is performed in a child who is at risk for velopharyngeal problems (Andreassen, Leeper, MacRae, & Nicholson, 1994; Finkelstein, Berger, Nachmani, & Ophir, 1996; Morris, 1975; Siegel-Sadewitz, & Shprintzen, 1986).

Once adulthood is reached, changes in structure and function occur slowly. Like other parts of the body, the velopharyngeal-nasal apparatus changes with age. For example, the pharyngeal muscles weaken and the pharyngeal lumen enlarges (Zaino & Benventano, 1977), sensory innervation declines (Aviv et al., 1994), density of palatal structures change (Tomoda, Morii, Yamashita, & Kumazawa, 1984), and muscle bulk and bone density decrease in this region and elsewhere (Fremont & Hoyland, 2007). Although such changes seem to have the potential to alter velopharyngeal-nasal function for speech production, they do not.

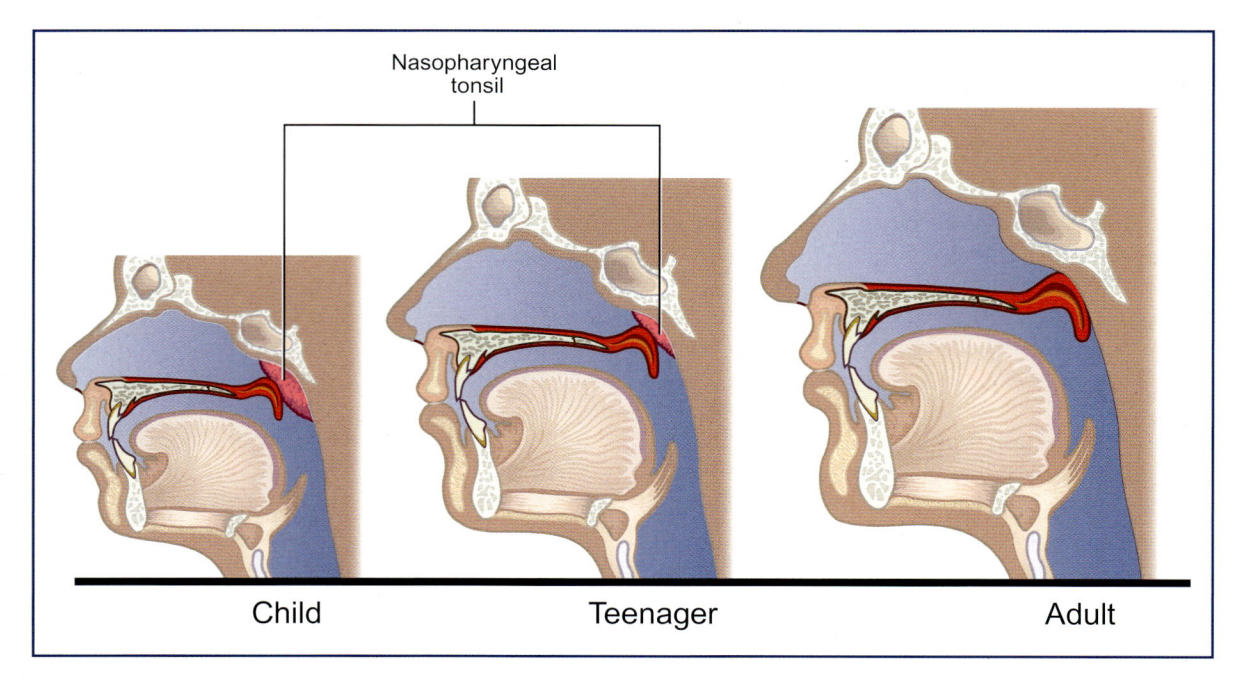

Figure 4–25. Changes in nasopharyngeal tonsil mass during development. The nasopharyngeal tonsil is large in children and atrophies with age. The velopharyngeal structures accommodate to these changes to achieve velopharyngeal closure.

> **When Is a Bad Nose Good and a Good Nose Bad?**
>
> This chapter stresses the functional unity of the normal velopharyngeal-nasal apparatus. This unity is often even better illustrated in an abnormal velopharyngeal-nasal apparatus. Not all speakers with significant velopharyngeal openings during oral consonant productions are destined to exhibit significant speech problems. With the velopharynx and nose being in mechanical series (being in line), an abnormally blocked nose may actually counteract an abnormally opened velopharynx. That is, a bad nose can be a good thing for speech, even if not for breathing. Conversely, a good nose can be a bad thing for speech when there is significant velopharyngeal impairment. The surgeon who attempts to "clean up" a bad nose and does not take into account the status of the velopharynx will sometimes figure this out after the fact when confronted with a child whose speech is worse after nasal surgery.

> **He's an Old Smoothie**
>
> He was a distinguished looking white-haired grandfather. He agreed to serve as a person to be examined by graduate students learning to administer an examination for velopharyngeal-nasal function. Students had been assigned different parts of the examination and told to practice the administration of their part on at least half a dozen people so they could get "calibrated." One student who had dutifully practiced on a group of her peers proceeded to ask the gentleman to open his mouth while she turned on a flashlight and looked in. She methodically looked at structures and made comments to the class as she went along. When she shined the light on the gentleman's hard palate, she paused briefly and said to him, "That's the smoothest hard palate I've ever seen." He smiled back and said, "That's a denture, young lady." And so it was. He took it out and showed it to the class. The moral of this story is don't just practice on your classmates.

The question of whether velopharyngeal function changes with age in adults has been addressed using acoustic and aeromechanical measurements, with somewhat different outcomes. Acoustic studies that used a measure of nasalance (the quotient of nasal sound pressure level to nasal + oral sound pressure level; see Chapter 10) provided ambiguous evidence, with one study showing higher nasalance in older adults compared with younger adults (Hutchinson, Robinson, & Nerbonne, 1978) and another showing little difference (Seaver, Dalston, Leeper, & Adams, 1991). Two later studies that used measures of air pressure and airflow (Hoit et al., 1994; Zajac, 1997) showed no influence of age. This combined acoustic and aeromechanical evidence indicates that velopharyngeal function for speech production does not deteriorate with age, even in the very old. However, it is possible that other variables, such as age-related thinning of bone and tissue and reductions in size of mouth opening, might influence the acoustic speech product.

Sex

Sex makes a difference when it comes to the size of the velopharyngeal-nasal apparatus. For example, men, compared with women, have longer pharynges (Fitch & Giedd, 1999; Jordan et al., 2017; Vorperian et al., 2009), longer *palatal levator* muscles (Bae, Kuehn, Sutton, Conway, & Perry, 2011; Ettema, Kuehn, Perlman, & Alperin, 2002), longer hard palates (Bae et al. 2011), larger and longer soft palates (Jordan et al., 2017; Kuehn & Kahane, 1990; Perry, Kuehn, Sutton, Gamage, & Fang, 2016), and longer noses (Zankl, Eberle, Molinari, & Schinzel, 2002). But do these differences influence velopharyngeal-nasal function for speech production?

There have been many studies comparing velopharyngeal function during speech production in men and women. These include studies that used x-ray techniques to track velar movement (Bzoch, 1968; Iglesias et al., 1980; Kuehn, 1976; McKerns & Bzoch, 1970; Seaver & Kuehn, 1980), electromyography to record velar muscle activity (Seaver & Kuehn, 1980), air pressure and airflow measures to determine velopharyngeal status (open vs. closed) and orifice size (Andreasson, Smith, & Guyette, 1992; Hoit et al., 1994; Thompson & Hixon, 1979; Zajac & Mayo, 1996), and MRI (Jordan et al., 2017). Although the findings revealed some sex-related differences, they were small, idiosyncratic, or contradictory among studies. The only consistent sex-related difference was that the magnitude of airflow during nasal productions is greater in men than women. This is to be expected, given that men have larger airways than women. Therefore, although men and women differ in certain details of velopharyngeal-nasal function in speech production, it is not clear that these differences make a difference functionally or in their application to clinical concerns (McWilliams, Morris, & Shelton, 1990).

REVIEW

The velopharyngeal-nasal apparatus is located within the head and neck and comprises a system of valves and air passages that interconnects the throat and atmosphere through the nose.

The velopharyngeal-nasal apparatus includes the pharynx, velum, nasal cavities, and outer nose.

Forces of the velopharyngeal-nasal apparatus are of two types—passive and active, the former arising from several sources and the latter arising from muscles distributed within different parts of the velopharyngeal-nasal apparatus.

Muscles of the pharynx include the *superior constrictor, middle constrictor, inferior constrictor, salpingopharyngeus, stylopharyngeus,* and *palatopharyngeus*.

Muscles of the velum include the *palatal levator, palatal tensor, uvulus, glossopalatine,* and *pharyngopalatine*.

Muscles of the outer nose include the *levator labii superioris alaeque nasi, anterior nasal dilator, posterior nasal dilator, nasalis,* and *depressor alae nasi*.

Movements of the pharynx enable its lumen to be changed along its length, either by constriction or by dilation at different sites.

Movements of the velum involve shape changes of the structure and are mainly along an upward-backward or downward-forward path.

Movements of the outer nose influence the cross-sections of the anterior nares and are involved in breathing events and the signaling of emotions.

The control variables of velopharyngeal-nasal function include airway resistance offered by the velopharyngeal-nasal apparatus, muscular pressure exerted by the velopharyngeal sphincter to maintain closure, and acoustic impedance in opposition to the flow of sound energy.

Different parts of the nervous system are responsible for the control of different components of the velopharyngeal-nasal apparatus and different activities, with motor and sensory innervation being effected through cranial nerves V, VII, IX, X, and possibly XI.

Functions of the velopharyngeal-nasal apparatus involve changing the degree of coupling between the oral and nasal cavities and between the nasal cavities and atmosphere.

Closure of the velopharyngeal port can be achieved through a variety of movement strategies that involve different actions or combinations of actions of the velum, lateral pharyngeal walls, and posterior pharyngeal wall, strategies that are probably conditioned by velopharyngeal anatomy.

Nasal airflow is modulated by the nasal valve, which consists of external and internal parts, the latter of which is primarily responsible for the governing of nasal patency.

The two sides of the nose go through changes in which their respective nasal concha (turbinates) alternately engorge and constrict in a rhythmical cycle that varies from person to person.

The warming, moistening, and filtering aspects of nasal function are important to health, and nasal breathing prevails until airway resistance becomes excessive, whereupon a switch is made to oral-nasal breathing.

During sustained vowel production, the velum is higher, velar contact with the posterior pharyngeal wall is more extensive, and velopharyngeal sphincter compression is greater for high vowels compared with low vowels.

Sustained fricative consonants are more likely to be produced with airtight velopharyngeal closure than are sustained vowels and sustained nasal consonants are produced with a wide open velopharynx.

Running speech activities involve the combining of consonants and vowels, with primacy of control being vested in consonant productions, especially those that are associated with high oral pressure and little or no opening of the velopharyngeal port.

Position and movement patterns of the velopharyngeal-nasal apparatus may reflect the occurrence of two or more speech sounds simultaneously, such that their productions overlap and intermingle and show evidence of how the brain prepares in advance for velopharyngeal-nasal adjustments and how the mechanical properties of the velopharyngeal-nasal apparatus influence its behavior.

Body position has effects on the velopharyngeal-nasal apparatus due to the influence of gravity.

Velopharyngeal closure for speech production develops gradually during infancy and appears to be relatively stable by 19 months of age with continuing modifications of temporal events during childhood.

Velopharyngeal function for speech production does not change with age during adulthood.

The sex of the speaker does not have a clear influence on velopharyngeal-nasal function for speech production.

REFERENCES

Andreassen, M., Leeper, H., MacRae, D., & Nicholson, I. (1994). Aerodynamic, acoustic, and perceptual changes following adenoidectomy. *Cleft Palate-Craniofacial Journal, 31*, 264–270.

Andreassen, M., Smith, B., & Guyette, T. (1992). Pressure-flow measurements for selected oral and nasal sound segments produced by normal adults. *Cleft Palate-Craniofacial Journal, 29*, 1–9.

Aviv, J., Martin, J., Jones, M., Wee, T., Diamond, B., Keen, M., & Blitzer, A. (1994). Age-related changes in pharyngeal and supraglottic sensation. *Annals of Otology, Rhinology, and Laryngology, 103*, 749–752.

Azzam, N., & Kuehn, D. (1977). The morphology of musculus uvulae. *Cleft Palate Journal, 14*, 78–87.

Bae, Y., Kuehn, D., Sutton, B., Conway, C., & Perry, J. (2011). Three-dimensional magnetic resonance imaging of velopharyngeal structures. *Journal of Speech, Language, and Hearing Research, 54*, 1538–1545.

Bae, Y., Perry, J., & Kuehn, D. (2014). Videofluoroscopic investigation of body position on articulatory positioning. *Journal of Speech, Language, and Hearing Research, 57*, 1135–1147.

Barsoumian, R., Kuehn, D., Moon, J., & Canady, J. (1998). An anatomic study of the tensor veli palatini and dilatator tubae muscles in relation to estachian tube and velar function. *Cleft Palate-Craniofacial Journal, 35*, 101–110.

Bell-Berti, F. (1976). An electromyographic study of velopharyngeal function in speech. *Journal of Speech and Hearing Research, 19*, 225–240.

Bennett, K., & Hoit, J. (2013). Stress velopharyngeal incompetence (SVPI) in collegiate trombone players. *Cleft Palate-Craniofacial Journal, 50*, 388–393.

Boorman, J., & Sommerlad, B. (1985). Levator palati and palatal dimples: Their anatomy, relationship and clinical significance. *British Journal of Plastic Surgery, 38*, 326–332.

Bosma, J., Truby, H., & Lind, J. (1965). Cry motions of the newborn infant. *Acta Paediatrica Scandinavica, 163*, 63–91.

Bridger, G. (1970). Physiology of the nasal valve. *Archives of Otolaryngology, 92*, 543–553.

Buhr, R. (1980). The emergence of vowels in an infant. *Journal of Speech and Hearing Research, 23*, 73–94.

Bunton, K., & Hoit, J. (2018). Development of velopharyngeal closure for vocalization during the first two years of life. *Journal of Speech, Language, and Hearing Research, 61*(3), 549–560.

Bunton, K., & Story, B. (2012). The relation of nasality and nasalance to nasal port area based on a computational model. *Cleft Palate-Craniofacial Journal, 49*, 741–749.

Bzoch, K. (1968). Variations in velar valving: The factor of vowel changes. *Cleft Palate Journal, 5*, 211–218.

Cassell, M., & Ekaldi, H. (1995). Anatomy and physiology of the palate and velopharyngeal apertures. In R. Shprintzen & J. Bardach (Eds.), *Cleft palate speech management: A multidisciplinary approach* (pp. 45–61). St. Louis, MO: Mosby.

Cole, P. (1976). The extrathoracic airways. *Journal of Otolaryngology, 5*, 74–85.

Crelin, E. (1973). *Functional anatomy of the newborn*. New Haven, CT: Yale University Press.

Croft, C., Shprintzen, R., & Rakoff, S. (1981). Patterns of velopharyngeal valving in normal and cleft palate subjects: A multiview videofluoroscopic and nasendoscopic study. *Laryngoscope, 91*, 265–271.

Curtis, J. (1968). Acoustics of speech production and nasalization. In D. Spriestersbach & D. Sherman (Eds.), *Cleft palate and communication* (pp. 27–60). New York, NY: Academic Press.

Dickson, D. (1972). Normal and cleft palate anatomy. *Cleft Palate Journal, 9*, 280–293.

Dickson, D., & Dickson, W. (1972). Velopharyngeal anatomy. *Journal of Speech and Hearing Research, 15*, 372–381.

Drettner, B. (1979). The role of the nose in the functional unity of the respiratory system. *Rhinology, 17*, 3–11.

Ettema, S., Kuehn, D., Perlman, A., & Alperin, N. (2002). Magnetic resonance imaging of the levator veli palatini muscle during speech. *Cleft-Palate-Craniofacial Journal, 39*, 130–144.

Finkelstein, Y., Berger, G., Nachmani, A., & Ophir, D. (1996). The functional role of the adenoids in speech. *International Journal of Pediatric Otorhinolaryngology, 34*, 61–74.

Finkelstein, Y., Shapiro-Feinberg, M., Talmi, Y., Nachmani, A., DeRowe, A., & Ophir, D. (1995). Axial configuration of the velopharyngeal valve and its valving mechanism. *Cleft Palate-Craniofacial Journal, 32*, 299–305.

Fitch, W., & Giedd, J. (1999). Morphology and development of the human vocal tract: A study using magnetic resonance imaging. *Journal of the Acoustical Society of America, 106*, 1511–1522.

Fletcher, S. (1973). Maturation of the speech mechanism. *Folia Phoniatrica, 25*, 161–172.

Foster, T. (1962). Maxillary deformities in repaired clefts of lip and palate. *British Journal of Plastic Surgery, 15*, 182–190.

Fremont, A., & Hoyland, J. (2007). Morphology, mechanisms and pathology of musculoskeletal ageing. *Journal of Pathology, 211*, 252–259.

Fritzell, B. (1963). An electromyographic study of the movements of the soft palate in speech. *Folia Phoniatrica, 15*, 307–311.

Fritzell, B. (1969). The velopharyngeal muscles in speech. *Acta Otolaryngologica, Supplement 250*, 1–81.

Fritzell, B. (1979). Electromyography in the study of the velopharyngeal function—a review. *Folia Phoniatrica, 31*, 93–102.

Gautier, H., Remmers, J., & Bartlett, D. (1973). Control of the duration of expiration. *Respiration Physiology, 18*, 205–221.

Gick, B., Francis, N., Klenin, A., Mizrahi, E., & Tom, D. (2013). The velic transverse: An independent articulator? *Journal of the Acoustical Society of America, 133*, EL208–EL213.

Gotto, T. (1977). Tightness in velopharyngeal closure and its regulatory mechanism. *Journal of the Osaka University Dental Society, 22*, 1–19.

Graber, T., Bzoch, K., & Aoba, T. (1959). A functional study of the palatal and pharyngeal structures. *Angle Orthodontist, 29*, 30–40.

Hairfield, W., Warren, D., Hinton, V., & Seaton, D. (1987). Inspiratory and expiratory effects of nasal breathing. *Cleft Palate Journal, 24,* 183–189.

Harrington, R. (1944). A study of the mechanism of velopharyngeal closure. *Journal of Speech Disorders, 9,* 325–345.

Hiyama, S., Ono, T., Ishiwata, Y., & Kuroda, T. (2002). Effects of mandibular position and body posture on nasal patency in normal awake subjects. *Angle Orthodontist, 72,* 547–553.

Hoit, J., Watson, P., Hixon, K., McMahon, P., & Johnson, C. (1994). Age and velopharyngeal function during speech production. *Journal of Speech and Hearing Research, 37,* 295–302.

Honjo, I., Harada, H., & Kumazasa. T. (1976). Role of the levator veli palatini muscle in movement of the lateral pharyngeal wall. *Archives of Otology, Rhinology, and Laryngology, 212,* 93–98.

House, A., & Stevens, K. (1956). Analog studies of the nasalization of vowels. *Journal of Speech and Hearing Disorders, 21,* 218–232.

Hsu, H., Fogel, A., & Cooper, R. (2000). Infant vocal development during the first 6 months: Speech quality and melodic complexity. *Infant and Child Development, 9,* 1–16.

Huang, Z., Lee, S., & Rajendran, K. (1997). Structure of the musculus uvulae: Functional and surgical implications of an anatomic study. *Cleft Palate-Craniofacial Journal, 34,* 466–474.

Huang, Z., Ong, K., Goh, S., Liew, H., Yeoh, K., & Wang, D. (2003). Assessment of nasal cycle by acoustic rhinometry and rhinomamometry. *Otolaryngology–Head and Neck Surgery, 128,* 510–516.

Hutchinson, J., Robinson, K., & Nerbonne, M. (1978). Patterns of nasalance in a sample of normal gerontologic subjects. *Journal of Communication Disorders, 11,* 469–481.

Iglesias, A., Kuehn, D., & Morris, H. (1980). Simultaneous assessment of pharyngeal wall and velar displacement for selected speech sounds. *Journal of Speech and Hearing Research, 23,* 429–446.

Isshiki, N., Harita, Y., & Kawano, M. (1985). What muscle is responsible for lateral pharyngeal wall movement? *Annals of Plastic Surgery, 14,* 224–227.

Jackson, R. (1976). Nasal-cardiopulmonary reflexes: A role of the larynx. *Annals of Otology, Rhinology, and Laryngology, 85,* 65–70.

Jaw, T., Sheu, R., Liu, G., & Lin, W. (1999). Development of adenoids: A study by measurement with MR images. *Kaohsiung Journal of Medical Sciences, 15,* 12–18.

Jordan, H., Schenck, G., Ellis, C., Rangarathnam, B., Fang, X., & Perry, J. (2017). Examining velopharyngeal closure patterns based on anatomic variables. *Journal of Craniofacial Surgery, 28,* 270–274.

Kaltenborn, A. (1948). *An x-ray study of velopharyngeal closure in nasal and non-nasal speakers* (Master's thesis). Northwestern University, Evanston, IL.

Kazlin, M., & Perry, J. (2016). Relationship between age and diagnosis on volumetric and linear velopharyngeal measures in the cleft and noncleft populations. *Journal of Craniofacial Surgery, 27,* 1340–1345.

Kent, R., Carney, P., & Severeid, L. (1974). Velar movement and timing: Evaluation of a model for binary control. *Journal of Speech and Hearing Research, 17,* 470–488.

Kent, R., & Murray, A. (1982). Acoustic features of infant vocal utterances at 3, 6, and 9 months. *Journal of the Acoustical Society of America, 72,* 353–365.

Koprowski, S., VanLue, M., & McCormick, M. (2018). Treatment of stress velopharyngeal incompetence with injection of hyaluronic acid. *Cleft Palate-Craniofacial Journal, 55,* 615–618. https://doi.org/10.1177/1055665617732788

Kuehn, D. (1976). A cineradiographic investigation of velar movement variables in two normals. *Cleft Palate Journal, 13,* 88–103.

Kuehn, D. (1990). Commentary on Doyle, Casselbrandt, Swarts, and Bluestone (1990): Observations on a role for the tensor veli palatini in intrinsic palatal function. *Cleft Palate Journal, 27,* 318–319.

Kuehn, D., & Azzam, N. (1978). Anatomical characteristics of palatoglossus and the anterior faucial pillar. *Cleft Palate Journal, 15,* 349–359.

Kuehn, D., Folkins, J., & Cutting, C. (1982). Relationships between muscle activity and velar position. *Cleft Palate Journal, 19,* 25–35.

Kuehn, D., Folkins, J., & Linville, R. (1988). An electromyographic study of the musculus uvulae. *Cleft Palate Journal, 25,* 348–355.

Kuehn, D., & Kahane, J. (1990). Histologic study of the normal human adult soft palate. *Cleft Palate Journal, 27,* 26–34.

Kuehn, D., & Moon, J. (1998). Velopharyngeal closure force and levator veli palatini activation levels in varying phonetic contexts. *Journal of Speech, Language, and Hearing Research, 41,* 51–62.

Kuehn, D., & Moon, J. (2005). Histologic study of intravelar structures in normal human adult specimens. *Cleft Palate-Craniofacial Journal, 42,* 481–489.

Kuehn, D., & Perry, J. (2008). Anatomy and physiology of the velopharynx. In J. Losee & R. Kirschner (Eds.), *Comprehensive cleft care.* New York, NY: McGraw-Hill Medical.

Leeper, H., Tissington, M., & Munhall, K. (1998). Temporal aspects of velopharyngeal function in children. *Cleft Palate-Craniofacial Journal, 35,* 215–221.

Lester, R., & Hoit, J. (2014). Nasal and oral inspiration during natural speech breathing. *Journal of Speech, Language, and Hearing Research, 57,* 734–742.

Liss, J., Kuehn, D., & Hinkle, K. (1994). Direct training of velopharyngeal musculature. *Journal of Medical Speech-Language Pathology, 2,* 243–249.

Lubker, J. (1968). An electromyographic-cinefluorographic investigation of velar function during normal speech production. *Cleft Palate Journal, 5,* 1–18.

Malick, D., Moon, J., & Canady, J. (2007). Stress velopharyngeal incompetence: Prevalence, treatment, and management practices. *Cleft Palate Journal, 44,* 424–433.

McClean, M. (1973). Forward coarticulation of velar movement at marked junctural boundaries. *Journal of Speech and Hearing Research, 16,* 286–296.

McKerns, D., & Bzoch, K. (1970). Variations in velopharyngeal valving: The factor of sex. *Cleft Palate Journal, 7,* 652–662.

McWilliams, B., Morris, H., & Shelton, R. (1990). *Cleft palate speech* (2nd ed.). Philadelphia, PA: B. C. Decker.

Miller, M., Martin, R., Waldemar, A., Fouke, J., Strohl, K., & Fanaroff, M. (1985). Oral breathing in newborn infants. *Journal of Pediatrics, 107*, 465–469.

Moll, K. (1962). Velopharyngeal closure on vowels. *Journal of Speech and Hearing Research, 5*, 30–37.

Moll, K., & Daniloff, R. (1971). Investigation of the timing of velar movements during speech. *Journal of Speech and Hearing Research, 50*, 678–684.

Moll, K., & Shriner, T. (1967). Preliminary investigation of a new concept of velar activity during speech. *Cleft Palate Journal, 4*, 58–69.

Moon, J., & Canady, J. (1995). Effects of gravity on velopharyngeal muscle activity during speech. *Cleft Palate-Craniofacial Journal, 32*, 371–375.

Moon, J., & Kuehn, D. (2004). Anatomy and physiology of normal and disordered velopharyngeal function for speech. In K. Bzoch (Ed.), *Communicative disorders related to cleft lip and palate* (5th ed., pp. 67–98). Austin, TX: Pro-Ed.

Moon, J., Kuehn, D., & Huisman, J. (1994a). Measurement of velopharyngeal closure force during vowel production. *Cleft Palate-Craniofacial Journal, 31*, 356–363.

Moon, J., Smith, A., Folkins, J., Lemke, J., & Gartlan, M. (1994b). Coordination of velopharyngeal muscle activity during positioning of the soft palate. *Cleft Palate-Craniofacial Journal, 31*, 45–55.

Morris, H. (1975). The speech pathologist looks at the tonsils and the adenoids. *Annals of Otology, Rhinology, and Laryngology, 84*, 63–66.

Netsell, R. (1990). Commentary. *Cleft Palate Journal, 27*, 58–60.

Niinimaa, V., Cole, P., & Mintz, S. (1981). Oronasal distribution of respiratory airflow. *Respiratory Physiology, 43*, 69–75.

Nusbaum, E., Foly, L., & Wells, C. (1935). Experimental studies of the firmness of the velar-pharyngeal occlusion during the production of the English vowels. *Speech Monographs, 2*, 71–80.

Okada, R., Muro, S., Eguchi, K., Yagi, K., Nasu, H., Yamaguchi, K., . . . Akita, K. (2018). The extended bundle of the tensor veli palatini: Anatomic consideration of the dilating mechanism of the Eustachian tube. *Auris Nasus Larynx, 45*(2), 265–272.

Oller, K. (1986). Metaphonology and infant vocalizations. In B. Lindblom & R. Zetterstrom (Eds.), *Precursors of early speech* (pp. 21–36). New York, NY: Stockton Press.

Perry, J. (2011). Variations in velopharyngeal structures between upright and supine positions using upright magnetic resonance imaging. *Cleft Palate-Craniofacial Journal, 48*, 123–133.

Perry, J., Bae, Y., & Kuehn, D. (2012). Effect of posture on deglutitive biomechanics in healthy individuals. *Dysphagia, 27*, 70–80.

Perry, J., Kuehn, D., Sutton, B., & Fang, X. (2017). Velopharyngeal structural and functional assessment of speech in young children using dynamic magnetic resonance imaging. *The Cleft Palate-Craniofacial Journal, 54*, 408–422.

Perry, J., Kuehn, D., Sutton, B., Gamage, J., & Fang, X. (2016). Anthropometric analysis of the velopharynx and related craniometrics dimensions in three adult populations using MRI. *Cleft Palate-Craniofacial Journal, 53*, e1–e13.

Poppelreuter, S., Engelke, W., & Bruns, T. (2000). Quantitative analysis of the velopharyngeal sphincter function during speech. *Cleft Palate-Craniofacial Journal, 37*, 157–165.

Principato, J., & Ozenberger, J. (1970). Cyclical changes in nasal resistance. *Archives of Otolaryngology, 91*, 71–77.

Proctor, D. (1982). The upper airway. In D. Proctor & I. Andersen (Eds.), *The nose: Upper airway physiology and the atmospheric environment* (pp. 23–44). Amsterdam, Netherlands: Elsevier Biomedical Press.

Rodenstein, D., Perlmutter, N., & Stanescu, D. (1985). Infants are not obligatory nasal breathers. *American Review of Respiratory Disease, 131*, 343–347.

Rudcrantz, H. (1969). Postural variations of nasal patency. *Acta Otolaryngologica, 68*, 435–443.

Ruscello, D. (1982). A selected review of palatal training procedures. *Cleft Palate Journal, 19*, 181–193.

Saibene, F., Mognoni, P., & LaFortuna, C. (1978). Oronasal breathing during exercise. *Pleugers Archives, 378*, 65–69.

Sasaki, C., Levine, P., Laitman, J., & Crelin, E. (1977). Postnatal descent of the epiglottis in man. *Archives of Otolaryngology, 103*, 169–171.

Schwab, B., & Schulze-Florey, A. (2004). Velopharyngeal insufficiency in woodwind and brass players. *Medical Problems of Performing Artists, 19*, 21–25.

Seaver, E., Dalston, R., Leeper, H., & Adams, L. (1991). A study of nasometric values for normal nasal resonance. *Journal of Speech and Hearing Research, 34*, 715–721.

Seaver, E., & Kuehn, D. (1980). A cineradiographic and electromyographic investigation of velar positioning in nonnasal speech. *Cleft Palate Journal, 17*, 216–226.

Shelton, R., Beaumont, K., Trier, W., & Furr, M. (1978). Videopanendoscopic feedback in training velopharyngeal closure. *Cleft Palate Journal, 15*, 6–12.

Shimokawa, T., Yi, S., & Tanaka, S. (2005). Nerve supply to the soft palate muscles with special reference to the distribution of the lesser palatine nerves. *Cleft Palate-Craniofacial Journal, 42*, 495–500.

Shprintzen, R. (1992). Assessment of velopharyngeal function: Nasopharyngoscopy and multiview videofluoroscopy. In L. Brodsky, L. Holt, & D. Ritter-Schmidt (Eds.), *Craniofacial anomalies: An interdisciplinary approach* (pp. 196–207). St. Louis, MO: Mosby.

Shprintzen, R., McCall, G., Skolnick, L., & Lenicone, R. (1975). Selective movement of the lateral aspects of the pharyngeal walls during velopharyngeal closure for speech, blowing, and whistling in normals. *Cleft Palate Journal, 12*, 51–58.

Siegel-Sadewitz, V., & Shprintzen, R. (1986). Changes in velopharyngeal valving with age. *International Journal of Pediatric Otorhinolaryngology, 11*, 171–182.

Skolnick, M. (1970). Videofluoroscopic examination of the velopharyngeal portal during phonation in lateral and base projections—a new technique for studying the mechanics of closure. *Cleft Palate Journal, 7*, 803–816.

Skolnick, M., McCall, G., & Barnes, M. (1973). The sphincteric mechanism of velopharyngeal closure. *Cleft Palate Journal, 10*, 286–305.

Stoksted, P. (1953). Rhinometric measurements for determination of the nasal cycle. *Acta Otolaryngologica, Supplement 109*, 1–159.

Subtelny, J., & Koepp-Baker, H. (1956). The significance of adenoid tissue in velopharyngeal function. *Plastic and Reconstructive Surgery, 12*, 235–250.

Thom, S., Hoit, J., Hixon, T., & Smith, A. (2006). Velopharyngeal function during vocalization in infants. *Cleft Palate-Craniofacial Journal, 43*, 539–546.

Thompson, A., & Hixon, T. (1979). Nasal air flow during normal speech production. *Cleft Palate Journal, 16*, 412–420.

Tomoda, T., Morii, S., Yamashita, T., & Kumazawa, T. (1984). Histology of human eustachian tube muscles: Effect of aging. *Annals of Otology, Rhinology, and Laryngology, 93*, 17–24.

Tucker, L. (1963). *Articulatory variations in normal speakers with changes in vocal pitch and effort* (Master's thesis). University of Iowa, Iowa City.

Vig, P., & Zajac, D. (1993). Age and gender effects on nasal respiratory function in normal subjects. *Cleft Palate-Craniofacial Journal, 30*, 279–284.

Vorperian, H., Kent, R., Lindstrom, M., Kalina, C., Gentry, L., & Yandell, B. (2005). Development of vocal tract length during childhood: A magnetic resonance imaging study. *Journal of the Acoustical Society of America, 117*, 338–350.

Vorperian, H., Wang, S., Chung, M., Schimek, E.M., Durtschi, R., Kent, R., Ziegert, A., & Gentry, L., (2009). Anatomic development of the oral and pharyngeal portions of the vocal tract: An imaging study. *Journal of the Acoustical Society of America, 125*, 1666–1678.

Warren, D., Dalston, R., & Dalston, E. (1990). Maintaining speech pressures in the presence of velopharyngeal impairment. *Cleft Palate Journal, 27*, 53–58.

Warren, D., Drake, A., & Davis, J. (1992). Nasal airway in breathing and speech. *Cleft Palate-Craniofacial Journal, 29*, 511–519.

Warren, D., & DuBois, A. (1964). A pressure-flow technique for measuring velopharyngeal orifice area during continuous speech. *Cleft Palate Journal, 1*, 52–71.

Warren, D., Hairfield, W., & Hinton, V. (1985). The respiratory significance of the nasal grimace. *ASHA, 27*, 82.

Warren, D., Hairfield, W., Seaton, D., & Hinton, V. (1987). The relationship between nasal airway cross-sectional area and nasal resistance. *American Journal of Orthodontics and Dentofacial Orothopedics, 92*, 390–395.

Warren, D., Hairfield, W., Seaton, D., Morr, K., & Smith, L. (1988). The relationship between nasal airway size and nasal-oral breathing. *American Journal of Orthodontics and Dentofacial Orthopedics, 93*, 289–293.

Warren, D., Mayo, R., Zajac, D., & Rochet, A. (1996). Dyspnea following experimentally induced increased nasal airway resistance. *Cleft Palate-Craniofacial Journal, 33*, 231–235.

Zaino, C., & Benventano, T. (1977). Functional, involutional, and degenerative disorders. In C. Zaino & T. Benventano (Eds.), *Radiologic examination of the oropharynx and esophagus* (pp. 141–170). New York, NY: Springer-Verlag.

Zajac, D. (1997). Velopharyngeal function in young and older adult speakers: Evidence from aerodynamic studies. *Journal of the Acoustical Society of America, 102*, 1846–1852.

Zajac, D. (2000). Pressure-flow characteristics of /m/ and /p/ production in speakers without cleft palate: Developmental findings. *Cleft Palate-Craniofacial Journal, 37*, 468–477.

Zajac, D., & Hackett, A. (2002). Temporal characteristics of aerodynamic segments in the speech of children and adults. *Cleft Palate-Craniofacial Journal, 39*, 432–438.

Zajac, D., & Mayo, R. (1996). Aerodynamic and temporal aspects of velopharyngeal function in normal speakers. *Journal of Speech and Hearing Research, 39*, 1199–1207.

Zankl, A., Eberle, L., Molinari, L., & Schinzel, A. (2002). Growth charts for nose length, nasal protrusion, and philtrum length from birth to 97 years. *American Journal of Medical Genetic, 111*, 388–391.

5

Pharyngeal-Oral Function and Speech Production

INTRODUCTION

The pharyngeal-oral apparatus, together with the velopharyngeal-nasal apparatus (discussed in Chapter 4), forms what is called the upper airway. In this book, the term *upper airway* is used in the context of the anatomy and physiology of this region so as to be consistent with terms such as *lower airways, laryngeal airway, velopharyngeal-nasal airway,* and *oral airway*. When referring to the acoustic properties of these regions, different terms are used: the term *vocal tract* is used for the pharyngeal-oral air spaces and the term *nasal tract* is used for the nasal air spaces (see Chapters 8–11).

Although most textbooks consider only the oral component (or the combined oral and velopharyngeal components), this chapter includes the pharynx in its consideration of pharyngeal-oral function. This is because the middle and lower regions of the pharynx function like articulators and acoustic filters in much the same way as do oral structures.

This chapter begins with the anatomy, forces (including muscle forces), and movements of the pharyngeal-oral apparatus. The next sections cover the control variables of the apparatus, its neural control, and its general functions. The final sections are dedicated to articulatory descriptions and processes as well as variables that may influence speech production. Its role during swallowing is discussed in Chapter 16.

ANATOMY OF THE PHARYNGEAL-ORAL APPARATUS

The pharyngeal-oral apparatus is a flexible tube that extends from the larynx to the lips and undergoes an approximate 90-degree bend (like a plumber's elbow joint) at the level of the oropharynx. There, the longer and vertical pharyngeal portion communicates through the oropharyngeal (faucial) isthmus with the shorter and horizontal oral portion. The pharyngeal-oral apparatus is supported by a skeletal structure that provides the framework around which its internal topography is organized.

Skeletal Framework

The full skeletal framework that supports both the velopharyngeal-nasal apparatus and the pharyngeal-oral apparatus is presented and illustrated in Chapter 4. This framework consists of the cervical vertebrae, bones of the skull (see Figure 4–1), and bones of the face (see Figure 4–2). The cervical (neck) segments of the vertebral column lie behind the three subdivisions of the pharynx—laryngopharynx, oropharynx, and nasopharynx—and form part of the substance of their back walls. The skull, made up of several irregularly shaped bones, forms the framework of the head. The facial bones contribute to the formation of the roof, floor, and sides of the oral cavity. The maxilla, mandible, and the temporomandibular joints are particularly prominent pharyngeal-oral structures and are discussed in more detail here.

Maxilla

Figure 5–1 depicts the maxilla. The maxilla forms the upper jaw and most of the hard palate. It consists of two complex bones (one on the left and one on the right) that combine at the midline. The maxilla lends strength to the roof of the oral cavity (as well as to the floor of the nasal cavities) and provides a buttress for

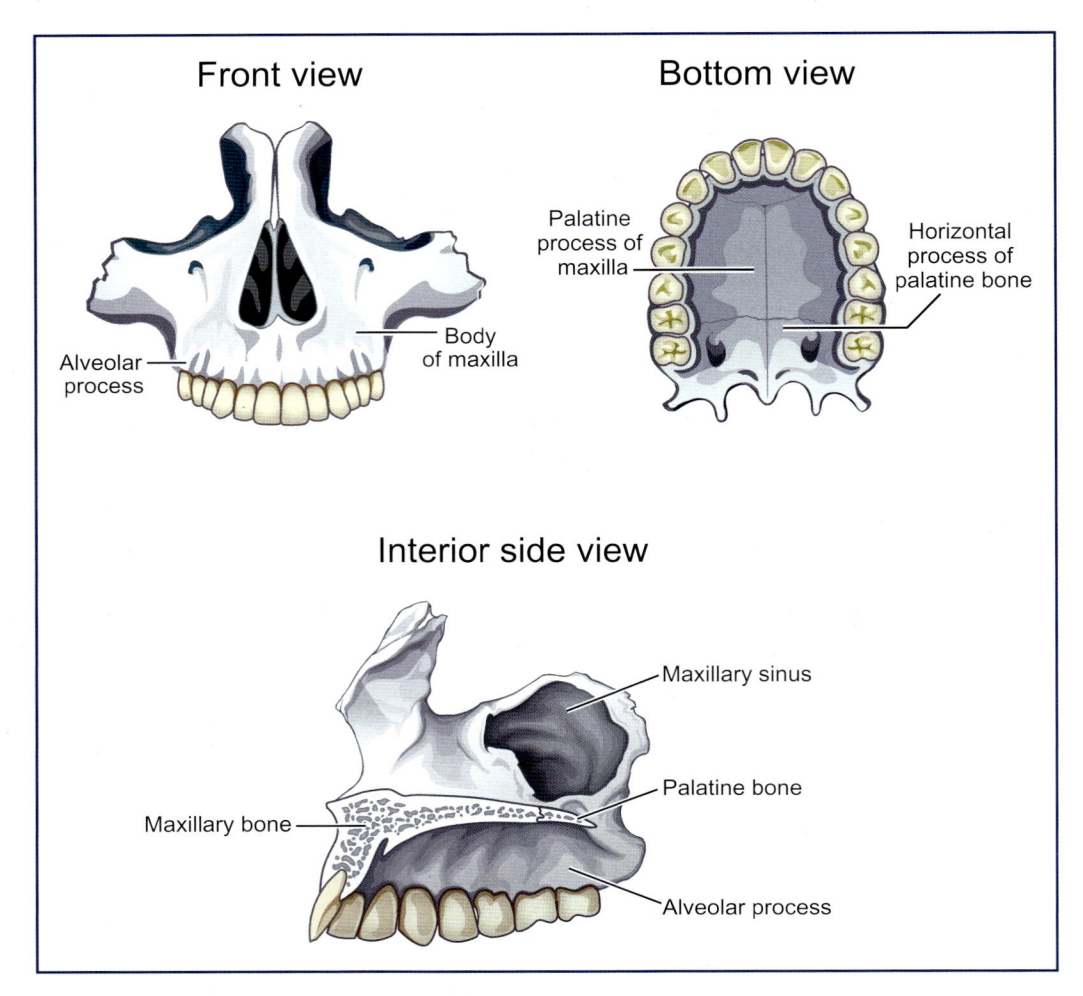

Figure 5–1. Maxilla as shown from front and bottom views.

the facial skeleton. Each bone of the maxilla has a palatine process that extends horizontally to the midline and joins with the palatine process from the opposite side to form the front three-fourths of the hard palate. The back one-fourth of the hard palate is formed by the much smaller palatine bones, which have horizontal processes that extend to the midline from each side to complete that part of the hard palate.

The alveolar process of the maxilla (sometimes called the alveolar arch) is a thick spongy projection that extends downward and houses the upper teeth. This process accommodates 16 permanent teeth (8 on each side). As shown in Figure 5–2, they are the central incisors, lateral incisors, canines (or cuspids), first and second premolars (or bicuspids), first and second molars, and third molar (or wisdom teeth). Infants and young children have only 10 teeth, called deciduous teeth (or baby teeth or milk teeth), which are later replaced by the permanent teeth.

Mandible

Figure 5–3 shows the salient features of the mandible. The mandible (lower jaw) is a large horseshoe-shaped structure when viewed from above or below. Its open end faces toward the back. The front and sides of the mandible together form what is called the body of the structure. The left and right halves of the mandible join at the front through a fibrous symphysis (line of union) that ossifies (turns to bone) during the first year of life. Like the maxilla, the mandible also has an alveolar process that accommodates 16 permanent teeth. These teeth bear the same names as the maxillary teeth.

On each side of the mandible toward the back, there is an upward projection called the ramus (meaning a branch from the body). The location along the bottom of the mandible where each ramus diverges upward is designated as the angle. The upper part of each ramus has two projections, one at the front called the coronoid process and one at the back called the condylar process (also called the condyle). The coronoid process is somewhat rounded, whereas the condylar process has a neck and a prominent head.

Temporomandibular Joints

The mandible articulates with the left and right temporal bones along the sides of the skull to form the temporomandibular joints. As illustrated in Figure 5–4, these joints are located just in front of and below the external auditory meatuses (ear canals). They can be palpated as the mandible is raised and lowered. The temporomandibular joints are enclosed by a fibrous capsule and lubricated by synovial fluid. Each joint is of the condyloid variety in that it consists of an ovoid (egg-shaped) process (the head of the condyle) that fits into an elliptical-shaped cavity within the temporal bone on the corresponding side (Dickson & Maue-Dickson, 1982). The condyle of the mandible (the more rearward of its two processes) is separated from its

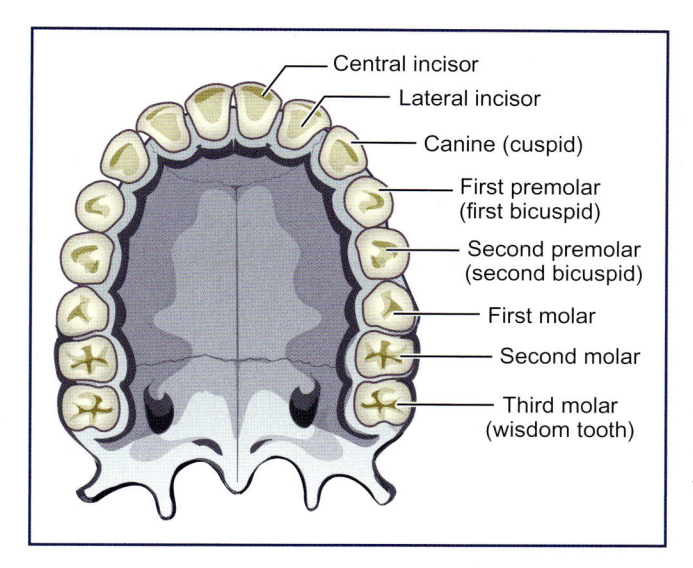

Figure 5-2. The upper teeth. The alveolar process of the maxilla contains 16 permanent teeth (8 on each side) that include incisors, canines, premolars, and molars. Infants and young children have fewer deciduous teeth.

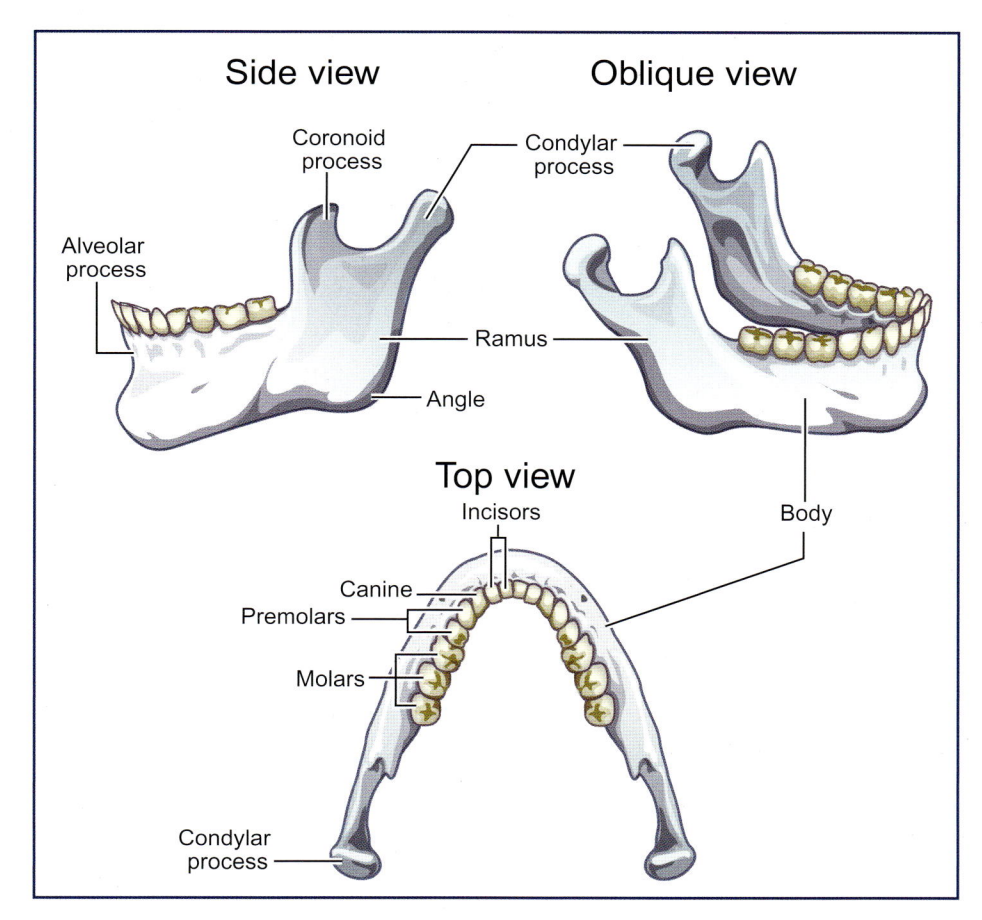

Figure 5-3. Mandible as seen from three different views. The mandibular alveolar process contains 16 teeth that have the same names as their maxillary counterparts.

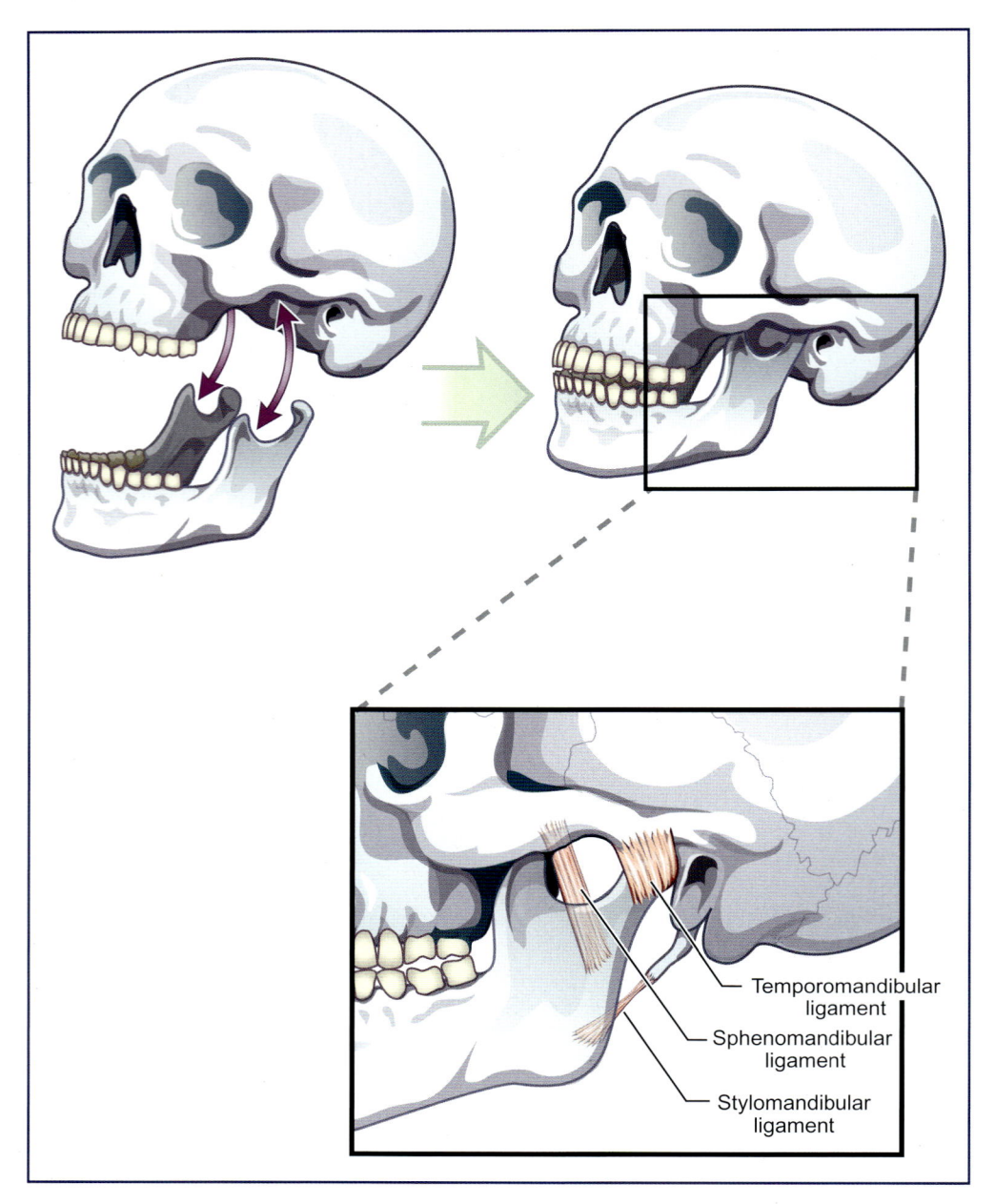

Figure 5–4. Temporomandibular joints and ligaments. The temporomandibular, sphenomandibular, and stylomandibular ligaments limit the motions of the joints in downward, backward, and forward directions.

receiving cavity by a cartilaginous meniscus (crescent) called the articular disk. The surfaces of the condyle and the temporal bone are themselves covered with fibrocartilage (cartilage that contains fibrous bundles of collagen) that is devoid of vascular tissue (Sicher & DuBrul, 1975).

Three ligaments influence the function of each temporomandibular joint (see bottom of Figure 5–4): the temporomandibular ligament, the sphenomandibular ligament, and the stylomandibular ligament. The temporomandibular ligament, which extends between the outer surface of the zygomatic arch and the outer and back surfaces of the neck of the condyle, limits the degree to which the condyle can be displaced downward and backward. The sphenomandibular ligament, which extends between the angular spine of the sphenoid bone and the inner surface of the ramus below the condyle, limits downward and backward displacement of the mandible. The stylomandibular ligament, which extends between the styloid process of the temporal bone to near the angle of the mandible, limits downward and forward displacement of the mandible.

Movements at the temporomandibular joints are conceptualized as movements of the mandible relative to a stabilized skull (although the opposite is possible, such as when the chin is rested on the top of a table and separation of the jaws causes the skull to rotate upward and backward). Movements of the mandible, as mediated through its condyloid processes, has three displacement possibilities: (a) upward and downward, made possible by a hingelike action, (b) forward and backward in a gliding action, and (c) side to side in a gliding action. These displacement possibilities are portrayed individually in Figure 5–5; however, temporomandibular joint movements are often multidimensional and very complex.

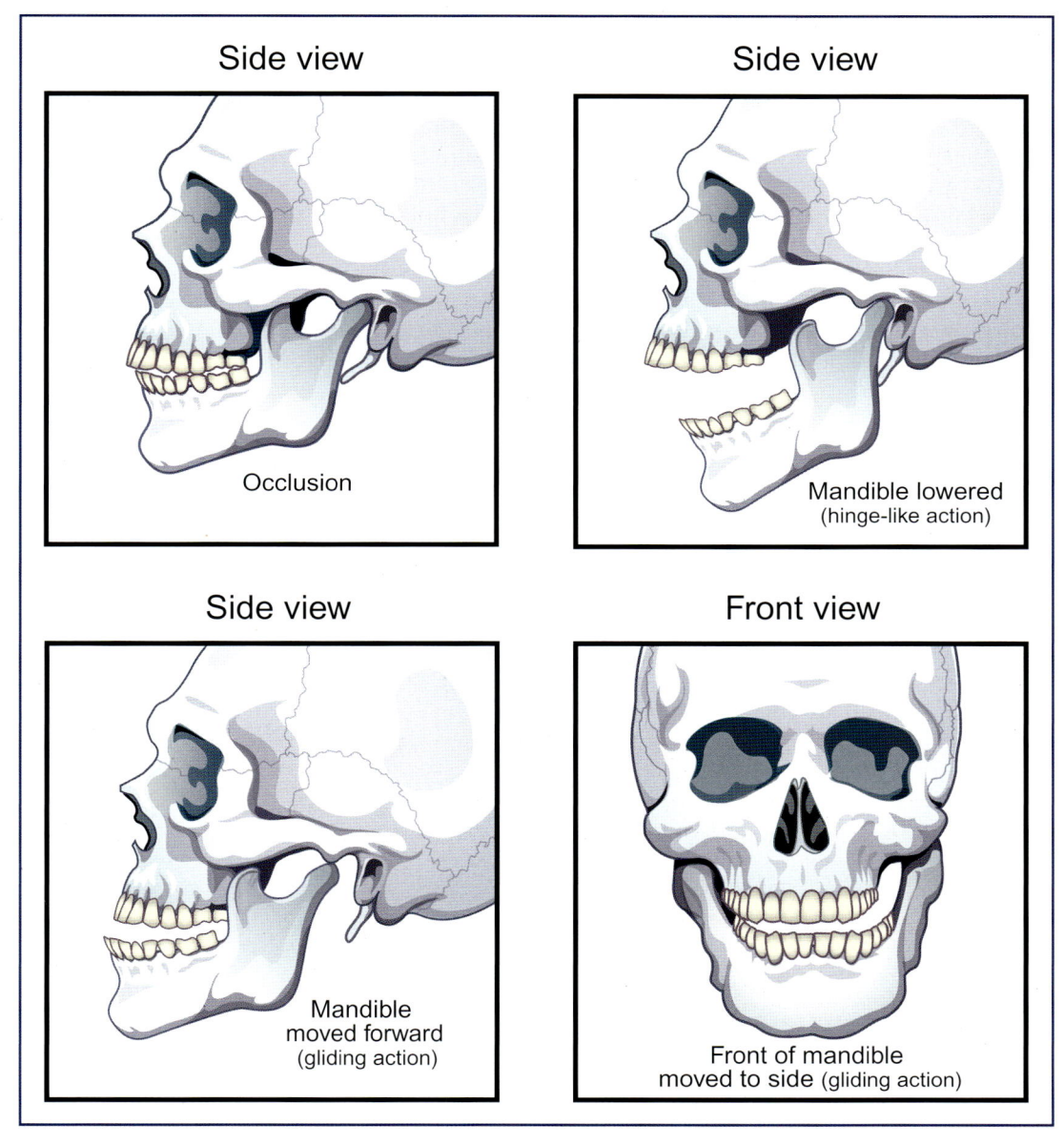

Figure 5–5. Temporomandibular joint movements. These movements include a hinge-like action to lower the mandible, a forward-backward gliding action, and a side-to-side gliding action.

Internal Topography

The internal topography of the pharyngeal-oral apparatus is fashioned around a hollow tube that bends at a right angle at the junction between the pharyngeal and oral portions of the structure. The pharyngeal, oral, and buccal cavities and their mucous lining deserve individual consideration.

Pharyngeal Cavity

Recall from Chapter 4 that the pharynx (throat) is a tube of tendon and muscle that extends from the base of the skull to the larynx. This tube is widest at the top and narrows down its length and is larger side to side than front to back (oval shaped). The lower and middle parts of the pharyngeal tube are designated as the laryngopharynx and oropharynx, respectively, and are the parts of greatest interest in this chapter (see Figure 4–4). The back and sides of the laryngopharynx and oropharynx are ringed by pharyngeal muscles (see Figure 4–10). The lower part of the oropharynx is bounded by the tongue and epiglottis and the upper part of the oropharynx opens into the oral cavity at the front through the anterior faucial pillars (palatoglossal arch). The back wall of the upper part of the oropharynx can be seen when looking back through the faucial isthmus (see Figure 4–5).

Oral Cavity

Figure 5–6 depicts the oral cavity (mouth cavity). The front entryway to the oral cavity is designated as the oral vestibule and is defined to include the lips, cheeks, front teeth, and forwardmost segments of the alveolar processes of the maxilla and mandible. The oral cavity is bounded at the back by the anterior faucial pillars (palatoglossal arch), above by the hard palate and velum, and below by its floor comprising mainly the tongue.

The tongue is a prominent feature of the oral cavity, and its importance in activities such as speaking and singing has long been recognized (Figure 5–7). Although unitary in nature, it is sometimes subdivided into different regions. The subdivisions chosen may have either anatomical or functional bases, depending on their purpose. Anatomical schemes usually recognize a root, pertaining to the vertically oriented back part of the tongue (front wall of the laryngopharynx and oropharynx), and a blade, pertaining to the horizontally oriented part of the tongue (floor of the oral cavity) (Zemlin, 1998). In contrast, functional schemes usually recognize

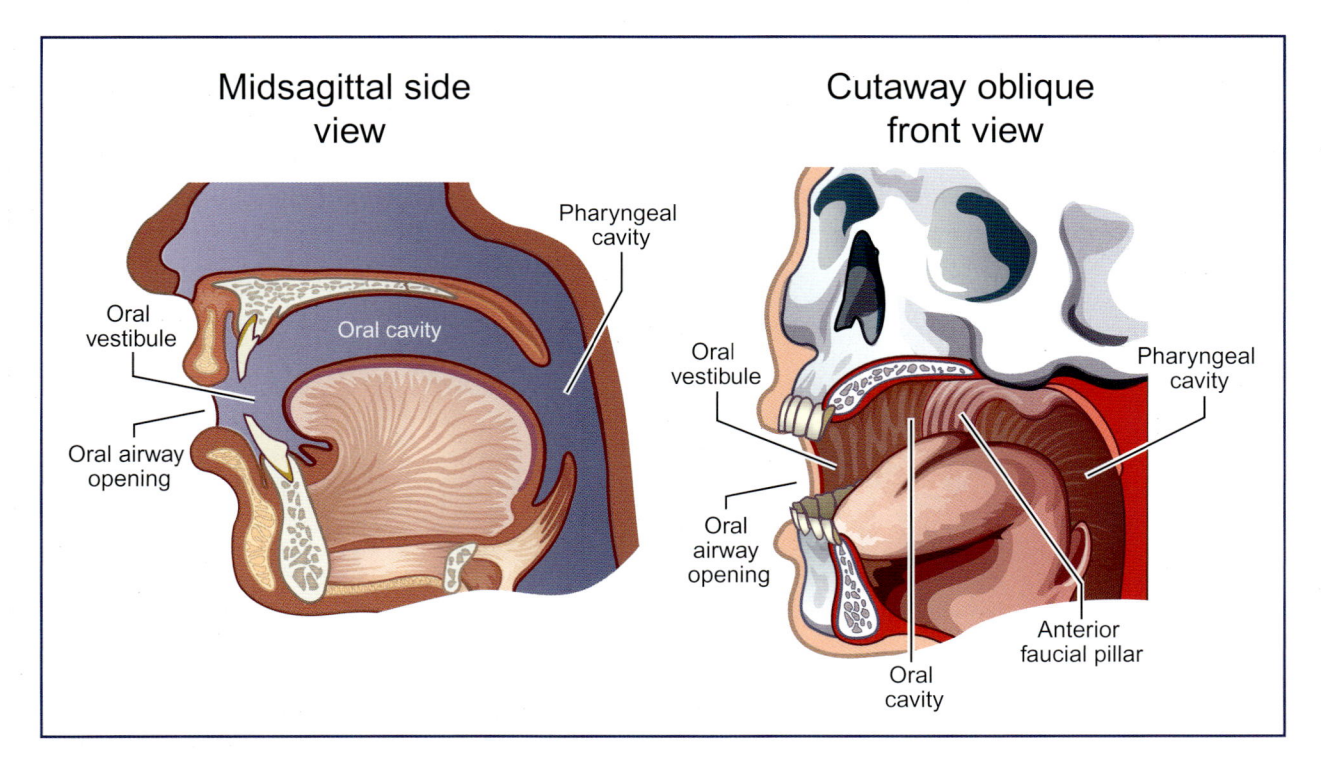

Figure 5–6. Oral cavity. The oral vestibule is the front entryway to the oral cavity and is bounded at the front by the lips and at the back by the front parts of the alveolar processes. The back of the oral cavity is bounded by the anterior faucial pillars.

regions of the tongue that are considered important to the behavior of the structure (Kent, 1997).

Figure 5–8 shows the tongue as consisting of five functional components, called the tip, blade, dorsum, root, and body. The tip of the tongue is the part of its surface nearest the front teeth at rest. The blade is the part of its surface that lies behind the tip and below the alveolar ridge of the maxilla and the front part of the hard palate. The dorsum of the tongue constitutes the surface that lies behind the blade and below the back part of the hard palate and the velum. The root of the tongue designates the part of the surface of the structure that faces the back of the pharynx and the front of the epiglottis. The body of the tongue represents its central mass and underlies the other four surface parts.

Grant Fairbanks (1910–1964)

Fairbanks was a giant in speech science. He also trained others who became distinguished scientists. Fairbanks was a key figure in the development of speech science as a discipline and had a major influence in bringing it to the fore as an integrated science. One of his best-known works was the development of the notion that speech production was controlled in the manner of a servomechanism that relied on sensory feedback. His book titled *Voice and Articulation Drillbook* (Fairbanks, 1960) is a classic and contains the famous *Rainbow Passage* that has been used in more speech research studies than any other reading. Fairbanks died while on a flight between Chicago and San Francisco. The flight was diverted to Denver, where the coroner ruled that he had choked to death while eating. Fairbanks was greatly admired. The three of us are honored to be able to directly trace our professional lineages to him.

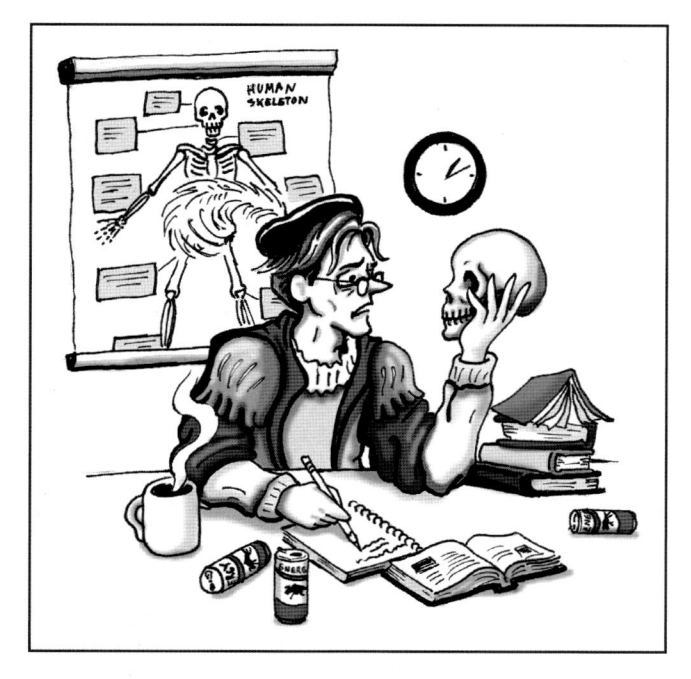

Figure 5–7. "That skull had a tongue in it, and could sing once." Hamlet in *Hamlet*, Act 5, Scene 1, William Shakespeare.

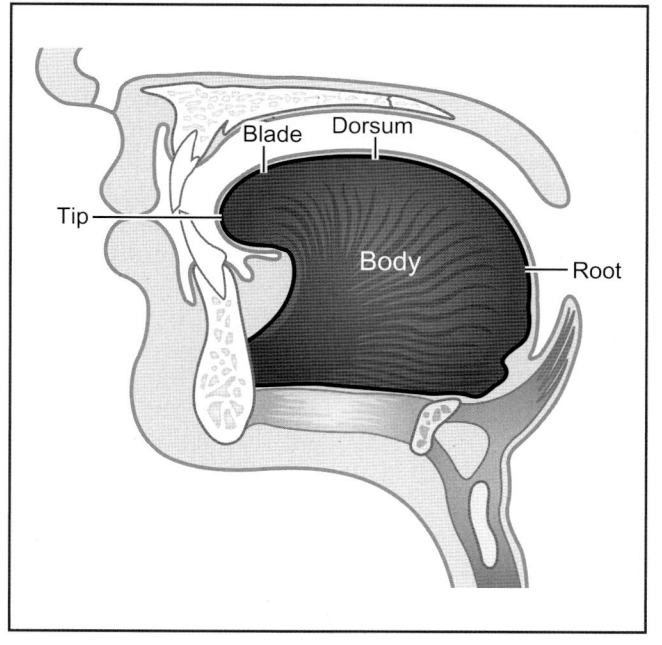

Figure 5–8. Five functional components of the tongue. From front to back, they are the tip, blade, dorsum, and root. The body is the central mass of the tongue that lies below the other four.

Buccal Cavity

The buccal cavity lies to the sides of the oral cavity. This cavity constitutes the small space between the gums (gingivae) and teeth internally and the lips and cheeks (buccae) externally. The buccal cavity connects to the oral cavity through spaces between the teeth and behind the last molars. The status of the lips and cheeks are major determinants of the size of the buccal cavity.

Mucous Lining

The pharyngeal-oral apparatus contains a mucous lining on its internal surfaces. This lining consists of an outer layer of epithelium and an inner layer of connective tissue (lamina propria). The details of this layering differ at different locations within the pharyngeal-oral apparatus, especially the outer layer of epithelium (Dickson & Maue-Dickson, 1982). The most prominent mucosa lining has a shiny appearance and covers all of the soft tissues of the apparatus except the gums, hard palate, and tongue. A so-called masticatory mucosa covers the gums and the hard palate and has a collagen subflooring that causes its epithelium to hold firmly against adjacent bone. The upper surface of the tongue is covered with a specialized mucosa that contains an array of small pockets and crypts that house taste buds.

Dancing in the Moonlight

He was a pleasant young man who was honorably discharged after serving in the military. He had made his way to a large Veterans Administration Medical Center. His only complaint was hearing loss, but the audiologist thought his speech was inconsistent with his hearing test results. The moment he said his name to the speech-language pathologist, there was suspicion that he had impairment of one or both cranial nerves serving the tongue. When asked to open his mouth, the beam of a flashlight revealed a shrunken and wrinkled tongue that seemed to dance around under the surface like a bagful of jumping beans. The signs were classic of lower motor neuron disease and a neurologist reported presumptive bilateral congenital agenesis (failure to develop) of the hypoglossal nerves (motor nerves to the tongue). How had this escaped detection during his physical examination for the military? Perhaps he was only asked to say "ah."

FORCES OF THE PHARYNGEAL-ORAL APPARATUS

Two types of forces are applied to the pharyngeal-oral apparatus: passive and active. Passive force is inherent and always present, but subject to change. The passive force of the pharyngeal-oral apparatus arises from the natural recoil of structures that line its walls, the surface tension between structures in apposition (lips, tongue, gums, hard palate, velum), the pull of gravity, and aeromechanical forces within the pharyngeal and oral portions of the apparatus.

The active force of pharyngeal-oral function comes from the contraction of muscles, some intrinsic (both ends attached within a component) and some extrinsic (one end attached within a component and one end attached outside the component). The function described here for individual muscles assumes that the muscle of interest is engaged in a shortening (concentric) contraction, unless otherwise specified as being involved in a lengthening (eccentric) contraction or a fixed-length (isometric) contraction. The tongue presents a somewhat more complex situation because of its special status as a muscular hydrostat (explained below). Discussed here are muscles of the pharynx, mandible, tongue, and lips.

Muscles of the Pharynx

The muscles of the pharynx are located within the laryngopharynx, oropharynx, and nasopharynx and are discussed in detail in Chapter 4. For the purposes of this chapter, those within the laryngopharynx and oropharynx are of primary interest and are reviewed here briefly.

Muscles of the laryngopharynx and oropharynx can influence the lumen (cavity) of the pharynx (the cross section along its length) in the region that lies behind the tongue, epiglottis, and oral cavity (the back wall of which is easily visualized through the faucial isthmus). The lumen of the pharynx in this region can also be influenced by adjustments of the tongue and epiglottis (see Figure 4–15). Muscles that attach to the laryngopharynx and oropharynx fabric proper (within the posterior and lateral pharyngeal walls) are revisited here. These include the *inferior constrictor* muscle, *middle constrictor* muscle, and *stylopharyngeus* muscle (see Figure 4–10).

The *inferior constrictor* muscle of the pharynx is located toward the bottom of the structure and is sometimes conceptualized as two muscles, the *thyropha-*

ryngeus and *cricopharyngeus* muscles. Its fibers arise from the sides of the thyroid and cricoid cartilages and diverge in a fanlike configuration as they course backward and toward the midline. There they interdigitate with fibers of the paired mate from the opposite side. The middle and upper fibers of the muscle ascend obliquely, whereas the lowermost fibers run horizontally and downward and are continuous with those of the esophagus. When the *inferior constrictor* muscle contracts, it pulls the lower part of the back wall of the pharynx forward and draws the sidewalls of the lower pharynx forward and inward. These actions cause the lumen of the lower pharynx to reduce in cross-section.

The *middle constrictor* muscle of the pharynx is located midway along the length of the pharyngeal tube and is sometimes conceptualized as two muscles, the *chondropharyngeus* and *ceratopharyngeus* muscles. Its fibers arise from the greater and lesser horns of the hyoid bone and the stylohyoid ligament and course backward and toward the midline where they insert into the median raphe (seam) of the pharynx. The uppermost fibers of the *middle constrictor* muscle course obliquely upward and overlap the lower fibers of the *superior constrictor* muscle, whereas the lowermost fibers of the muscle run obliquely downward beneath the fibers of the *inferior constrictor* muscle. Recall that this fiber arrangement is akin to the way in which roof shingles partially overlap. When the *middle constrictor* muscle contracts, it decreases the cross-sectional area of the oropharynx by pulling forward on the posterior pharyngeal wall and forward and inward on the lateral pharyngeal wall. Simultaneous contraction of the left and right *middle constrictor* muscles causes the pharyngeal lumen to constrict regionally in the manner of a sphincter.

The *stylopharyngeus* muscle extends between the styloid process of the temporal bone and the lateral wall of the pharynx near the juncture of the *superior constrictor* and *middle constrictor* muscles of the pharynx. Its fibers run downward, forward, and toward the midline. When the *stylopharyngeus* muscle contracts, it pulls the pharyngeal tube upward and draws the lateral wall of the pharynx toward the side. Together with similar action of its paired mate from the opposite side, it widens the lumen of the pharynx, especially in the region of the oropharynx, but also elsewhere along the length of the pharyngeal tube.

Muscles of the Mandible

Seven muscles provide active forces that operate on the mandible. These muscles are depicted in Figure 5–9 and are responsible for positioning the mandible in accordance with the movements allowed by the temporomandibular joints. Included among these muscles are the *masseter, temporalis, internal pterygoid, external pterygoid, digastric, mylohyoid,* and *geniohyoid*. Their general force vectors are depicted in Figure 5–10.

The *masseter* muscle is a flat, quadrilateral structure that covers much of the outer surface of the ramus of the mandible. Fibers of this muscle are in two layers. An outer layer forms the bulk of the muscle and courses from an aponeurosis along the front two-thirds of the zygomatic arch downward and backward to insert on the angle and nearby outer surface of the ramus of the mandible. An inner layer of fibers courses from the entire length of the zygomatic arch downward and forward to insert into the outer surface of the upper half of the ramus and its coronoid process. Contraction of the outer layer of the *masseter* muscle results in elevation of the mandible and approximation of the mandible and maxilla. The elevation is along a path that is at a right angle to the plane of occlusion of the molars. If the elevation is sufficient, pressure is brought to bear on the molars. Contraction of the inner layer of the muscle also results in elevation of the mandible and additionally exerts a force on the mandible that pulls it backward and aids in approximating the jaws.

The *temporalis* muscle is a broad, fan-shaped structure that covers much of the side of the cranium. Fibers of this muscle originate from the inferior temporal line of the parietal bone and the greater wing of the sphenoid bone. These converge as they course downward under the zygomatic arch and insert on the inner surface and front border of the coronoid process and the front surface of the ramus of the mandible. Fibers toward the front and middle of the muscle course vertically, whereas those toward the back of the muscle have a more horizontal orientation. Contraction of the *temporalis* muscle results in an upward and backward pull on the mandible, with vertically oriented fibers contributing to the upward component and horizontally oriented fibers contributing to the backward component. Activation of the *temporalis* muscle on only one side may result in retraction of the mandible on the same side and movement of the front of the mandible toward the activated side.

The *internal pterygoid* muscle is a quadrilateral structure that follows an orientation that generally parallels that of the *masseter* muscle. Fibers of the *internal pterygoid* muscle originate from the lateral pterygoid plate and the perpendicular plate of the palatine bone. From there, they course downward, backward, and outward to insert on the inner surface of the angle and ramus of the mandible. Contraction of the *internal*

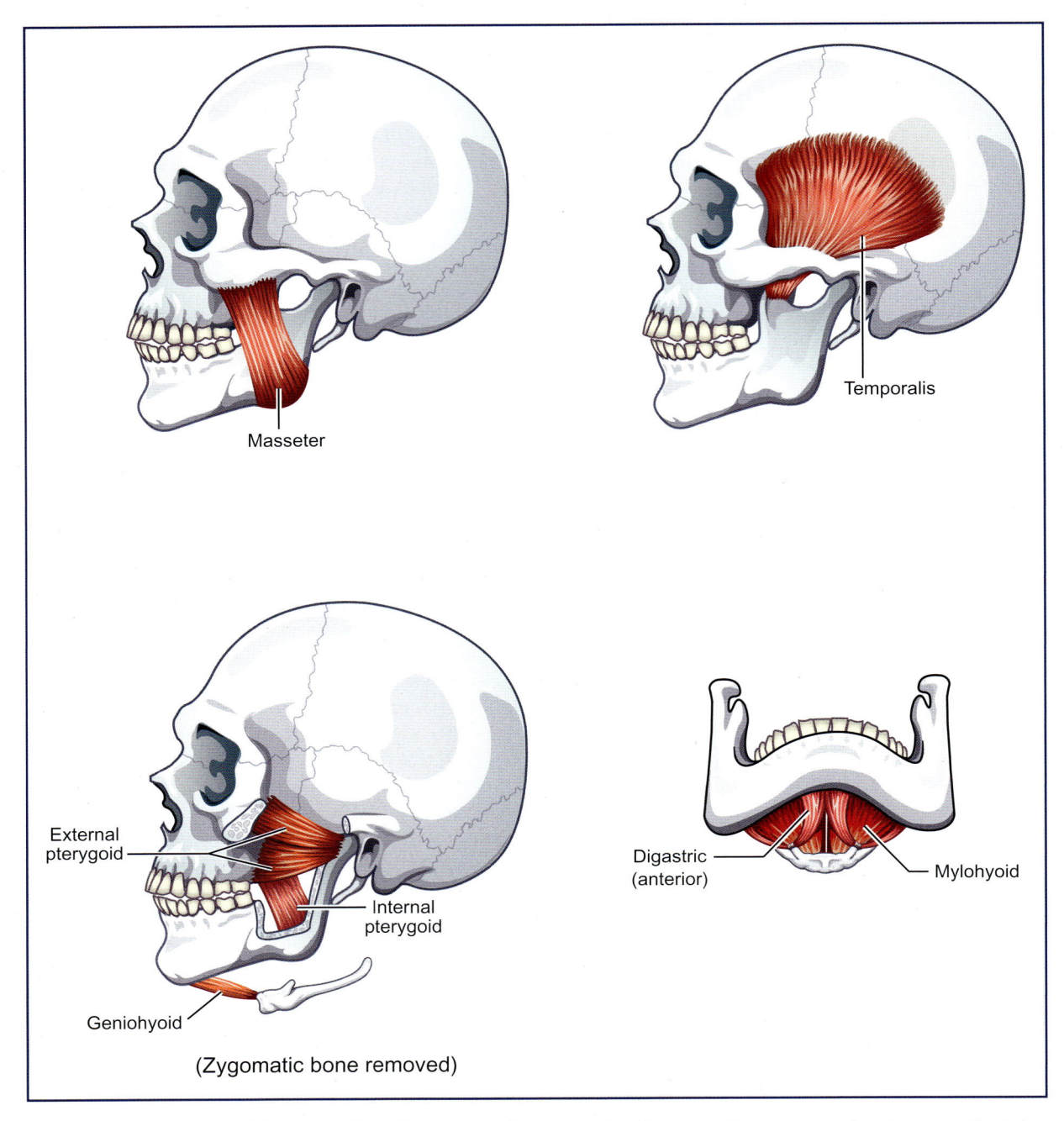

Figure 5-9. Muscles of the mandible. These muscles can raise the mandible (*masseter, temporalis, internal pterygoid*), lower the mandible (*external pterygoid, digastric* [*anterior* belly], *mylohyoid, geniohyoid*), move the mandible laterally (*masseter, temporalis, internal pterygoid, external pterygoid*), move the mandible forward (*external pterygoid*), and move the mandible backward (*masseter, temporalis*).

pterygoid muscle results in elevation of the mandible. Sufficient elevation causes pressure to be placed on the opposing teeth of the mandible and maxilla. Activation of the muscle on only one side may result in slight movement of the corresponding condyle toward the opposite side.

The *internal pterygoid* muscle has a special relationship with the *masseter* muscle. Together these two muscles form a muscular sling that surrounds the angle of the mandible. This anatomical sling holds the angle from above and effectively straps the ramus to the skull. The result is a functional articulation between the man-

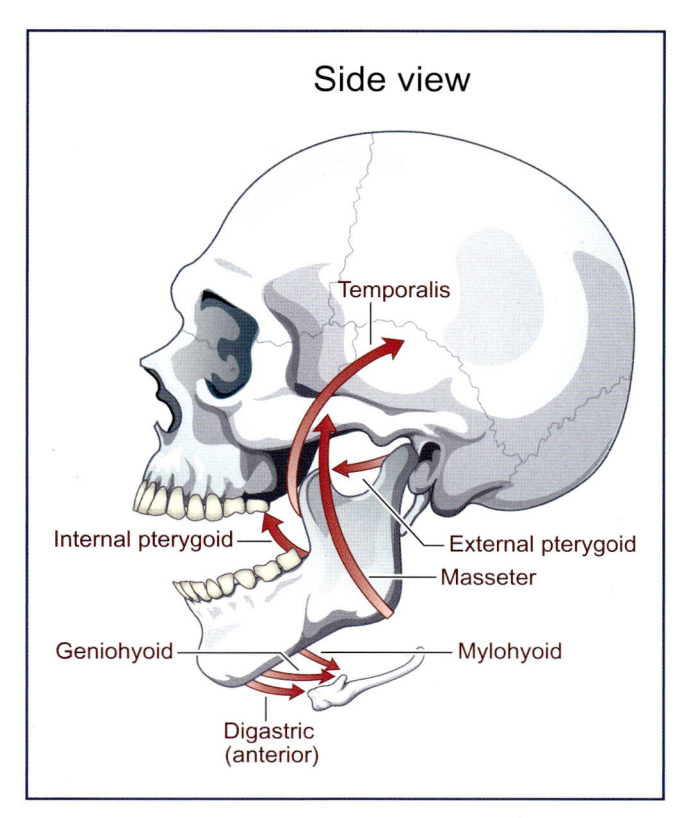

Figure 5–10. Actions of muscles of the mandible. The *masseter* and *temporalis* muscles raise the mandible and pull it backward, the *external pterygoid* muscle slides the mandible downward and forward, and the *internal pterygoid*, *digastric* (*anterior* belly), *mylohyoid*, and *geniohyoid* muscles lower the mandible.

dible and the maxilla, with the temporomandibular joint acting as an enabling guide for movements of the mandible (Zemlin, 1998).

The *external pterygoid* muscle is one of the smaller muscles of the mandible. Fibers of the *external pterygoid* muscle have two origins toward the front, one from the greater wing of the sphenoid bone and one from the lateral pterygoid plate. Fibers from these two points of origin tend to converge as they run generally horizontally backward to insert into the neck of the condyle of the mandible. Contraction of the *external pterygoid* muscle causes the condyle to slide downward and forward. Contraction of the *external pterygoid* muscle on only one side tends to move the front of the mandible toward the opposite side.

Three other muscles have a role in actions of the mandible. These are the *digastric* (*anterior* belly), *mylohyoid*, and *geniohyoid*, all supplementary muscles of the laryngeal apparatus. The structure and function of these muscles are presented in detail in Chapter 3 (and illustrated in Figure 3–24) and are reviewed here only briefly.

The *digastric* is a two-bellied muscle arranged such that it can pull upward on the hyoid bone and/or downward on the mandible. Its action is dependent on the degree to which either or both of these structures are fixed in position by other muscles. With greater relative fixation of the hyoid bone, contraction of the *anterior* belly of the *digastric* muscle results in a lowering of the mandible.

The *mylohyoid* muscle is positioned along the floor of the oral cavity. It is oriented such that its fibers can exert an upward and forward pull on the hyoid bone or a downward pull on the mandible. With greater relative fixation of the hyoid bone, contraction of the *mylohyoid* muscle brings about a lowering of the mandible.

The *geniohyoid* is a cylindrical muscle that lies above the *mylohyoid* muscle. The course of its muscle fibers is essentially parallel to the fiber course of the *anterior digastric* muscle. Orientation of the muscle is such that it can pull upward and forward on the hyoid bone or downward on the mandible. With greater relative fixation of the hyoid bone, contraction of the *geniohyoid* muscle results in a lowering of the mandible.

Muscles of the Tongue

Skeletal support for the overall pharyngeal-oral apparatus comes from vertebrae and bones of the skull and face, but the tongue is endowed with its own "soft skeleton." This personal skeleton is largely connective tissue and serves to both surround and separate different components of the tongue, including its left and right halves (Dickson & Maue-Dickson, 1982). This skeleton also includes a dense felt-like network of fibrous elastic tissue that lies below the epidermis and constitutes an encapsulating structural bag around the tongue (Zemlin, 1998). It is through this special soft skeleton that the eight muscles of the tongue (four intrinsic and four extrinsic) are able to bring about the wide variety of tongue movements that are possible.

The intrinsic muscles of the tongue are the *superior longitudinal*, *inferior longitudinal*, *vertical*, and *transverse* muscles. They are depicted in Figure 5–11.

The *superior longitudinal* is a broad, flat muscle that lies just beneath the expansive upper surface (dorsum) of the tongue. Fibers originate within the root of the tongue from the hyoid bone and course forward in an imbricated pattern (like overlapping fish scales) along the long axis of the tongue. Forward attachments of the muscle are in the region of the front edges of the tongue and the upper surface of the tongue tip. Fibers

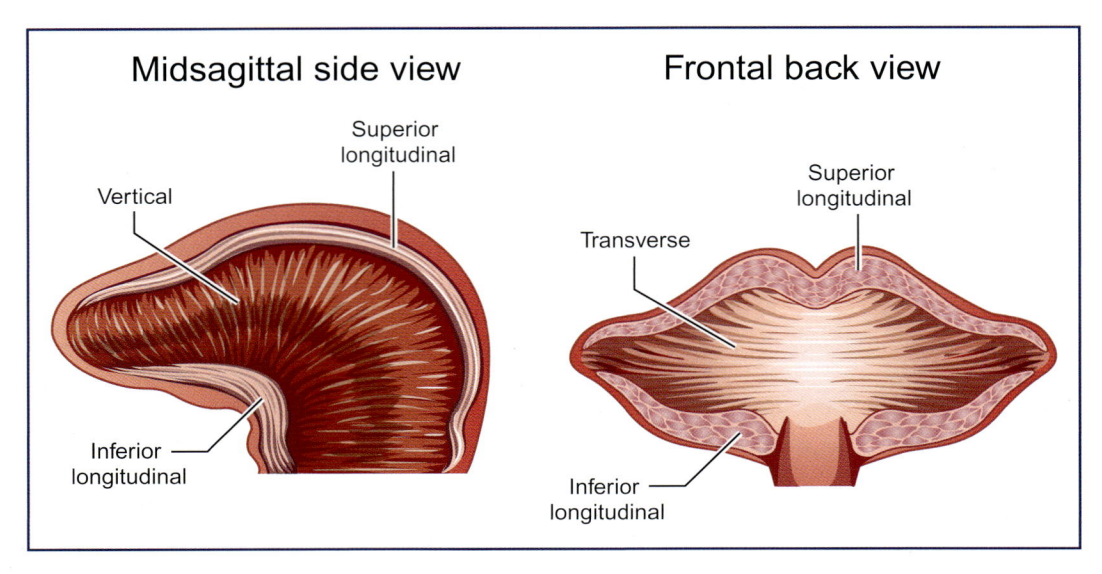

Figure 5–11. Intrinsic muscles of the tongue. These are the **superior longitudinal**, **inferior longitudinal**, **vertical**, and **transverse** muscles.

Gone but Not Forgotten

Arm and leg amputations occurred in large numbers during the Civil War. Amputees from this era reported that pain or other sensations continued to arise from where their missing limbs had been. Some described them as sensory ghosts and many doctors of the time thought that those who reported them had mental problems. Not so. Phantom limb pain or other sensations are now recognized to be common following amputation of any body part and scientists have embraced a number of theories about their origins. Those who have had their tongues amputated (usually surgically and because of cancer) also report tongue pain or other sensations that are analogous to those associated with their better known phantom-limb counterpart. Ghost tongues are most prominent right after surgery and tend to fade away with time, although they are known to abruptly reappear on occasion. All of this is really quite haunting when you think about it.

short imbricated fibers, it can also activate in patterns that differentially affect the regional configuration of the tongue. For example, contraction of fibers toward the front of the tongue can pull the tongue tip upward and toward the side of muscle activation. Simultaneous contractions of comparable fibers in the paired *superior longitudinal* muscles elevate the tongue tip without deviation to either side. For another example, contraction of fibers that insert obliquely into the edges of the tongue can pull the lateral margins of the structure upward to create a longitudinal trough down the center of the tongue toward the front.

The *inferior longitudinal* muscle is positioned near the undersurface of the tongue somewhat toward the side. It arises from the body of the hyoid bone at the root of the tongue and courses forward through the body of the tongue to insert near the lower surface of the tongue tip. Fibers of the *inferior longitudinal* muscle blend with the fibers of different extrinsic muscles of the tongue (discussed below) within the body of the tongue. Contraction of the *inferior longitudinal* muscle shortens the tongue and pulls the tip of the structure downward and toward the same side. Simultaneous contraction of comparable fibers in the paired *inferior longitudinal* muscles pulls the tongue tip downward symmetrically.

The *vertical* muscle originates from just beneath the dorsum of the tongue and courses downward vertically and toward the side through the body of the tongue. Fibers of the *vertical* muscle terminate near the sides of the tongue along its lower surface. There is some suggestion that not all fibers follow a course

near the midline course downward to their attachments, whereas fibers toward the side course obliquely toward the lateral boundary of the tongue. Contraction of the entire *superior longitudinal* muscle can shorten the tongue and increase its convexity from front to back. Because the muscle is composed of a series of through the entire body of the tongue, but rather are found only in the upper half of the tongue (Miyawaki, 1974), or that there is a mixture of short and long fibers, some of which course only through the upper half of the tongue and some of which course all the way to the lower part of the tongue (Abd-El-Malek, 1939). Contraction of the *vertical* muscle results in a flattening of the tongue on the side of action, especially toward its lateral margins. More midline parts of the upper tongue surface may also be lowered on the side of action as a result of pull exerted during the contraction of this muscle.

The *transverse* muscle, as its name implies, courses side to side within the tongue. Fibers of the muscle arise mainly from the median fibrous skeleton of the tongue and course laterally, where they terminate in fibrous tissue along the side of the tongue. Upper fibers fan out in an upward direction, whereas lower fibers fan out in a downward direction. The intermingling of *transverse* muscle fibers with those of other intrinsic and extrinsic tongue muscles is extensive and makes it hard to determine their precise course and location within different parts of the tongue. Some fibers may not extend all the way to the sides of the tongue (Miyawaki, 1974) and the extent to which fibers are located at the back of the tongue is in question (Abd-El-Malek, 1939). The *transverse* muscle is, however, a major constituent in the mass of interwoven muscle fibers that make up the bulk of the tongue. Contraction of the *transverse* muscle results in a narrowing of the tongue from side to side and an elongation of the tongue.

The extrinsic muscles of the tongue include the ***styloglossus, palatoglossus, hyoglossus***, and ***genioglossus*** muscles. These are depicted in Figure 5–12.

The ***styloglossus*** muscle originates from the front and side of the styloid process of the temporal bone and the stylomandibular ligament. Fibers of the muscle course forward, downward, and toward the midline to insert into the sides of the root of the tongue. From there, they run in various directions, but primarily toward the midline and forward within the body of the tongue. Some fibers of the ***styloglossus*** muscle interdigitate with fibers of the ***inferior longitudinal*** muscle, whereas others interdigitate with fibers of the ***hyoglossus*** muscle. Ultimate blending of different fibers makes it difficult to distinguish those of one muscle from another. Contraction of the ***styloglossus*** muscle can have multiple consequences, including that it can: (a) draw the body of the tongue upward and backward, (b) pull the side of the tongue upward to influence the tongue's concavity, (c) shorten the tongue, and (d) pull the tongue tip toward the side.

The ***palatoglossus*** muscle is discussed in Chapter 4 (and illustrated in Figure 4–12) as a part of the velopharyngeal-nasal apparatus. There it is referred to as the ***glossopalatine*** muscle (its origin and insertion

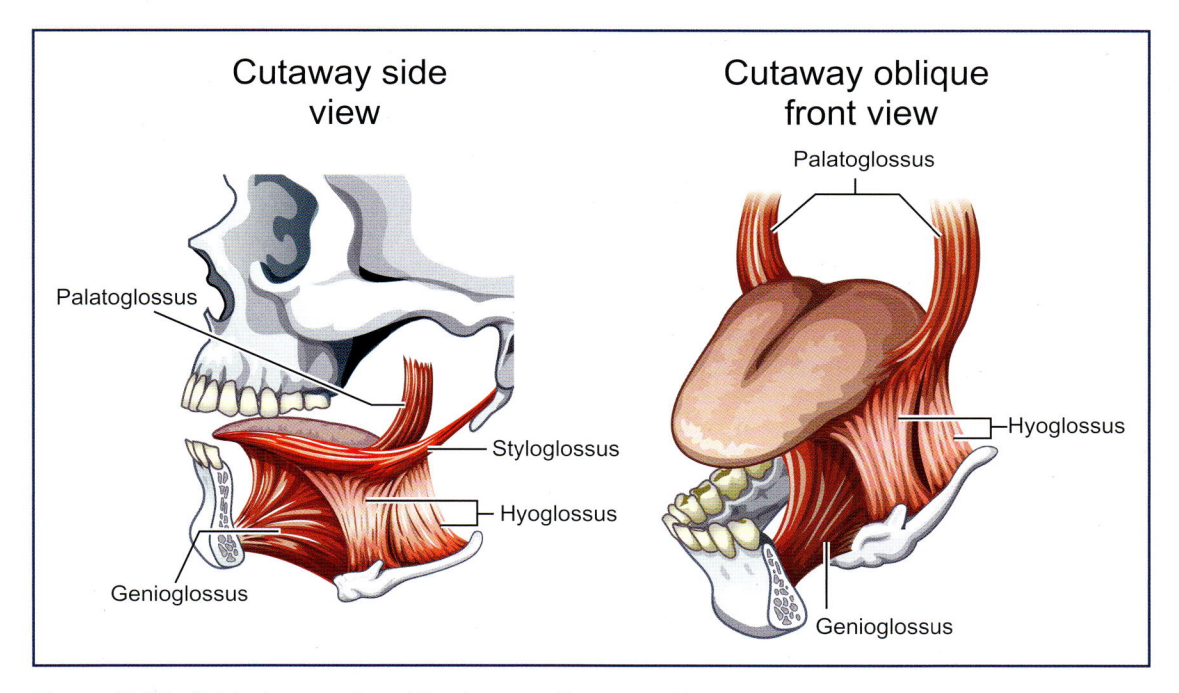

Figure 5–12. Extrinsic muscles of the tongue. These are the ***styloglossus, palatoglossus, hyoglossus***, and ***genioglossus*** muscles.

being reversed in that context). For present purposes, the *palatoglossus* muscle can be thought of as originating from the lower surface of the palatal aponeurosis with its fibers coursing downward, forward, and toward the side (forming the anterior faucial pillar) and inserting into the side of the root of the tongue. There the fibers of the *palatoglossus* muscle blend with those of the *transverse*, *styloglossus*, and *hyoglossus* muscles of the tongue. When the *palatoglossus* muscle contracts, it pulls upward, backward, and inward on the root of the tongue. Through its action, the muscle can displace the tongue mass backward in the oral cavity and increase the concavity of its upper surface. When the left and right *palatoglossus* muscles contract simultaneously, the result is a lengthwise grooving of the upper surface of the tongue.

The *hyoglossus* muscle (see also Chapter 3 and Figure 3–24) is a quadrilateral structure that originates from the upper border of the body and greater cornua of the hyoid bone and extends upward and forward to insert into the side of the tongue toward the rear. Fibers of the *hyoglossus* muscle intermingle with those of the *styloglossus* and *palatoglossus* muscles. Some authors consider one particular bundle of fibers within the *hyoglossus* muscle to be a separate muscle (Zemlin, 1998). This bundle is identified as the *chondroglossus* muscle and has fibers that extend from the hyoid bone farther forward into the tip of the tongue where they intermingle with fibers from intrinsic tongue muscles such as the *inferior longitudinal* muscle. Contraction of the *hyoglossus* (and *chondroglossus*) muscle results in a lowering of the body of the tongue and a backward displacement of its mass. The lowering effect is most pronounced along the sides of the tongue (Dickson & Maue-Dickson, 1982).

The *genioglossus* muscle is complex and makes up a large portion of the tongue. This muscle is fan-shaped and originates as three groups of fibers from the inner surface of the body of the mandible near the midline. The lower fibers course backward to insert into the root of the tongue. The middle fibers course backward and extend upward into the tongue in the region of the juncture between the dorsum and blade of the structure. The upper fibers run vertically and forward to insert into the tip of the tongue (Langdon, Klueber, & Barnwell, 1978), although some authors report that fibers stop short of the tongue tip itself (Doran & Baggett, 1972; Miyawaki, 1974). Collectively, fibers of the *genioglossus* muscle travel through the body of the tongue between layers of muscle fibers formed by the *vertical*, *transverse*, and *superior longitudinal* muscles of the structure (Dickson & Maue-Dickson, 1982). Contraction of the *genioglossus* muscle can have a diverse set of consequences, depending on which particular fibers of the muscle are activated and in what patterns. Possible outcomes are that: (a) the root of the tongue can be moved forward so as to force the tip of the tongue against the teeth or out of the mouth, (b) the front of the tongue can be pulled backward, and (c) the center line of the tongue can be pulled downward so as to form a trough-like depression along the length of the upper surface of the structure.

Figure 5–13 depicts the general force vectors associated with actions of the eight muscles of the tongue. Although discussion of the individual capabilities of the tongue muscles is instructive, it does not do justice to the intricate and interacting forces that can operate on and within the tongue to move it in different ways. Much of this has to do with special properties of the tongue that qualify it as a muscular hydrostat (discussed below under Movements of the Tongue).

Muscles of the Lips

The muscles of the lips are a subset of the muscles of the face. These muscles are more than a dozen in number and are portrayed in Figure 5–14 from different perspectives. The muscles of the lips include one intrinsic (contained within) and many extrinsic (one attachment within) muscles. They are the *orbicularis oris, buccinator, risorius, levator labii superioris, levator labii superioris alaeque nasi, zygomatic major, zygomatic minor, depressor labii inferioris, mentalis, levator anguli oris, depressor anguli oris, incisivus labii superioris, incisivus labii inferioris,* and *platysma*.

Street Talk About Talking

The folk language is filled with indications that the person on the street knows something about pharyngeal-oral function in speech production. Below are some expressions that we generated off the tops of our heads. Look at these and then try to add to the list from your own knowledge of the folk language. Our favorite from the list below is the last one, used during World War II to mean be careful to whom you are talking. Here goes. "That's a real tongue twister." "We were just jawing it." "He's bumping his gums." "They were flapping their cheeks." "She's lying through her teeth." "Don't give me any of your lip." "I don't chew my cabbage twice." "He's running off at the mouth again." "Hold your tongue, young man." "She's a big loudmouth." And our favorite, "Loose lips sink ships."

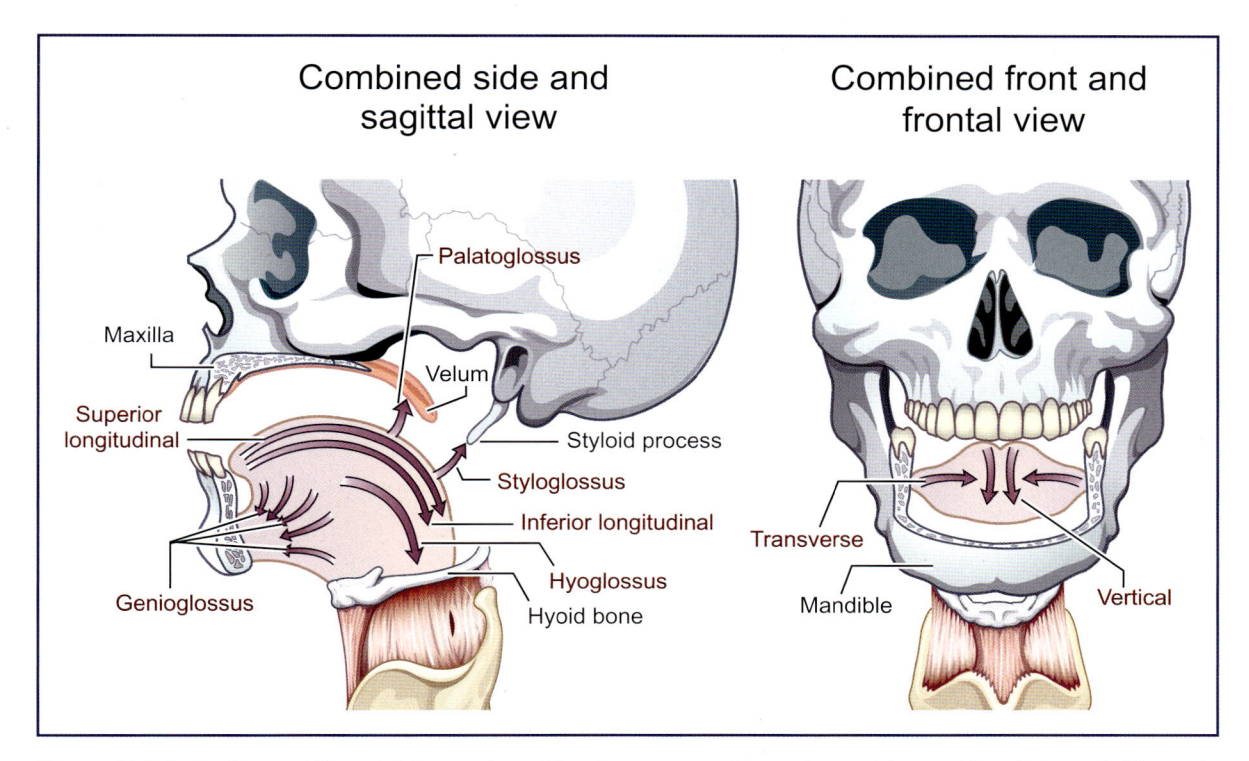

Figure 5–13. Actions of the eight muscles of the tongue as shown from side and front views (with parts cut away). These actions are extremely complex and not easily summarized. Shown here are major actions of each muscle, although other actions are possible.

The *orbicularis oris* is a ring of muscle within the lips that forms a sphincter at the oral end (mouth opening) of the pharyngeal-oral apparatus. This ring of muscle is complex and is constituted of fibers from both intrinsic and extrinsic sources that intertwine to form an airway valve and the most mobile part of the face. Fibers of the *orbicularis oris* muscle that are exclusive to the lips (intrinsic) are arranged in concentric rings around the border of the sphincter. These rings follow the outer contour of the upper and lower lips. The course of the intrinsic fibers of the *orbicularis oris* muscle changes with changes in the angular circumference of the mouth opening. Contraction of the *orbicularis oris* muscle can result in several positional changes of the lips. These include movements of the lips toward one another and forward, which, if extensive enough, can result in closure of the mouth and a forcing together of the lips. The corners of the mouth may also move as a result of activation of the *orbicularis oris* muscle. Such movement can be upward, downward, toward the side, or toward the midline. Action of the *orbicularis oris* muscle may also force the lips and/or corners of the mouth against the teeth.

Those lip muscles that are extrinsic are sometimes subgrouped into sets that follow fiber courses that are transverse (horizontal), angular (oblique to the corners of the mouth), vertical (from above or below), and parallel (adjacent to and alongside the lips). These subsets are considered, in turn, below, and are summarized in Table 5–1. The *platysma*, which is classified as a cervical (neck) muscle, is also discussed because it has extrinsic influences on the lower lip.

The transverse facial muscles that influence the lips are the *buccinator* muscle and the *risorius* muscle. The *buccinator* is sometimes called the bugler's muscle and the *risorius* is often referred to as the laughter muscle.

The *buccinator* muscle is a broad muscle that forms part of the cheek. It originates from the pterygomandibular ligament, the outer surface of the alveolar process of the maxilla, and the mandible from the region of the last molars. Fibers course horizontally forward and toward the midline to insert into the upper and lower lips near the corner of the mouth. Uppermost fibers of the muscle enter the upper lip, whereas lowermost fibers enter the lower lip. Fibers of the central part of the muscle converge near the corner of the mouth and cross such that the lower fibers of that part of the muscle insert into the upper lip and the upper fibers insert into the lower lip. Contraction of the *buccinator*

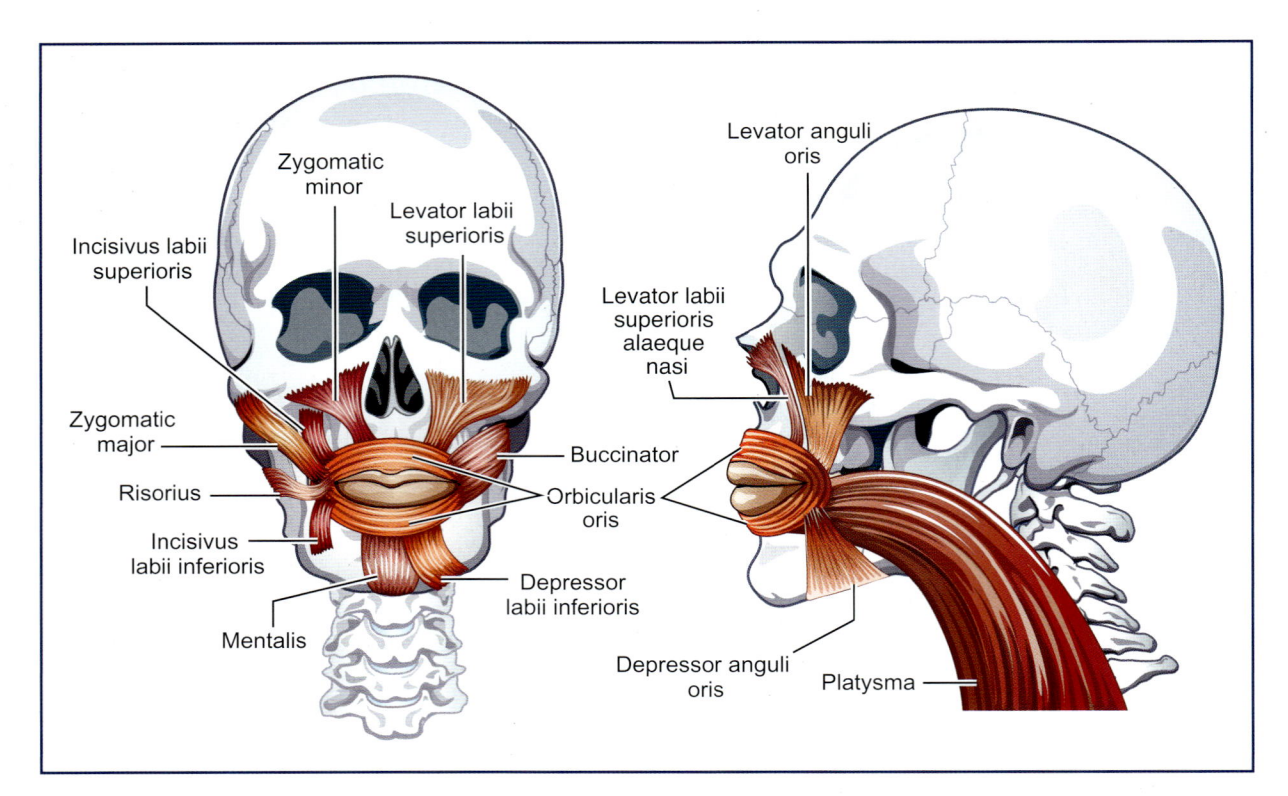

Figure 5-14. Muscles of the lips. All but one of these 14 muscles are extrinsic lip muscles—the exception being a subset of fibers of the **orbicularis oris** muscle. These extrinsic muscles are subgrouped into the transverse (**buccinators** and **risorius**), angular (**levator labii superioris, levator labii superioris alaeque nasi, zygomatic major, zygomatic minor, depressor labii inferioris**), vertical (**mentalis, levator anguli oris, depressor anguli oris**), and parallel (**incisivus labii superioris, incisivus labii inferioris**) muscles. The **platysma** muscle is a neck muscle and is included here because it has extrinsic influences on the lower lip.

Table 5-1. Extrinsic Tongue Muscles Organized According to Their Subgroupings

SUBGROUPS	MUSCLES
Transverse	*Buccinator*
	Risorius
Angular	*Levator labii superioris*
	Levator labii superioris alaeque nasi
	Zygomatic major
	Zygomatic minor
	Depressor labii inferioris
Vertical	*Mentalis*
	Levator anguli oris
	Depressor anguli oris
Parallel	*Incisivus labii superioris*
	Incisivus labii inferioris

muscle can pull the corner of the mouth backward and toward the side. It can also force the lips and cheek against adjacent teeth.

The *risorius* is a small muscle located within the cheek, but closer to the surface than the *buccinator* muscle. It arises from fascia of the *masseter* muscle and courses horizontally forward and toward the midline to insert into the corner of the mouth and the lower lip. Contraction of the *risorius* muscle draws the corner of the mouth backward and toward the side; it may also force the lips against adjacent teeth.

The angular muscle group includes five muscles. These are the *levator labii superioris*, the *levator labii superioris alaeque nasi*, the *zygomatic major*, the *zygomatic minor*, and the *depressor labii inferioris*.

The *levator labii superioris* muscle has a broad origin from below the orbit of the eye, the front of the maxillary bone, and the zygomatic bone. Its fibers course downward and slightly inward and insert into the upper lip. Contraction of the *levator labii supe-*

rioris muscle results in elevation of the upper lip; it may also cause an outward turning (eversion) of the upper lip.

The *levator labii superioris alaeque nasi* muscle originates as a slender slip from the front of the maxilla and courses vertically downward and slightly toward the side. The muscle divides into a nasal segment and a lip segment. Fibers from the lip segment of the muscle insert into the upper lip where they intermingle with fibers of the *orbicularis oris* muscle. Contraction of the lip segment of the *levator labii superioris alaeque nasi* muscle causes elevation of the upper lip. Contraction of the nasal segment of this muscle dilates the anterior naris on the corresponding side, as described in Chapter 4 (and illustrated in Figure 4–14).

The *zygomatic major* muscle has its origin on the side of the zygomatic bone and runs down and toward the midline where it inserts into the corner of the mouth. Fibers associated with its insertion intermingle with those of the *orbicularis oris* muscle. Contraction of the *zygomatic major* muscle pulls backward on the corner of the mouth. At the same time, action of this muscle lifts the corner of the mouth upward and toward the side.

The *zygomatic minor* muscle originates from the inner surface of the zygomatic bone. Its fibers course downward and toward the midline where they insert into the upper lip and interweave with fibers of the *orbicularis oris* muscle. Contraction of the *zygomatic minor* muscle results in elevation of the upper lip. It also pulls the corner of the mouth upward.

The *depressor labii inferioris* is a small, flat muscle located off the midline of the lower lip. Fibers of the muscle originate from the front surface of the mandible and course upward and inward to insert into the lower lip from near the midline to the corner of the mouth. Contraction of the *depressor labii inferioris* muscle pulls the lower lip downward and toward the side. It may also cause the lower lip to turn outward.

The vertical facial muscles are three in number. They include the *mentalis* muscle, *levator anguli oris* muscle, and the *depressor anguli oris* muscle.

The *mentalis* muscle lies on the front of the chin. It is a small muscle that arises from the front and side of the mandible near the midline and inserts into the *orbicularis oris* muscle and the skin overlying the chin. Contraction of the *mentalis* muscle results in upward displacement of the soft tissue of the chin, a forcing of the lower part of the lower lip against the alveolar process of the mandible, and an outward curling of the lower lip. The lower lip may also elevate somewhat during contraction of the *mentalis* muscle. These actions are consistent with the familiar signs of pouting, and, indeed, the *mentalis* muscle is sometimes called the "pouting muscle."

The *levator anguli oris* muscle (also referred to as the *caninus* muscle) originates from the front of the maxilla and courses downward and forward to insert into both the upper lip and the lower lip near the corner of the mouth. There, its fibers intermingle with those of the *orbicularis oris* muscle. Contraction of the *levator anguli oris* muscle draws the corner of the mouth upward and toward the side. Activation of this muscle can also elevate the lower lip against the upper lip and force the lips together.

The *depressor anguli oris* muscle is also sometimes referred to as the *triangularis* muscle. As its alternate name implies, the muscle is roughly triangular in form. This muscle has a broad origin from the outer surface of the mandible. Its fibers course upward and converge before inserting into the *orbicularis oris* muscle at the corner of the mouth and into the upper lip. Contraction of the *depressor anguli oris* muscle pulls the corner of the mouth downward. It also forces the lips together by drawing the upper lip downward against the lower lip.

There are two parallel facial muscles. These are the *incisivus labii superioris* muscle and the *incisivus labii inferioris* muscle.

The *incisivus labii superioris* is a small, narrow muscle that lies beneath the *levator labii superioris* muscle. Fibers of the *incisivus labii superioris* muscle originate from the maxilla in the region of the canine tooth and course parallel to the transverse fibers of the *orbicularis oris* muscle of the upper lip. This muscle inserts near the corner of the mouth where its fibers intermingle with the fibers of other muscles. Contraction of the *incisivus labii superioris* muscle pulls the corner of the mouth upward and toward the midline.

The *incisivus labii inferioris* muscle constitutes the lower lip counterpart of the *incisivus labii superioris* muscle. The *incisivus labii inferioris* muscle lies below the corner of the mouth and underneath the *depressor labii superioris* muscle. It originates on the mandible in the region of the lateral incisor tooth and courses parallel to the transverse fibers of the *orbicularis oris* muscle of the lower lip. The insertion of the *incisivus labii inferioris* muscle is into the region of the corner of the mouth. Contraction of the muscle results in a downward and inward pull on the corner of the mouth. The downward component of this action is antagonistic to the upward pull provided by the *incisivus labii superioris* muscle.

The *platysma* is a very board muscle that covers most of the front and side of the neck and much of the side of the face. The muscle has an extensive origin from a sheet of connective tissue within the neck above the clavicle and may even extend from as far below as the front of the chest wall and regions of the back of the torso. Fibers of the *platysma* muscle run upward and forward to attach to the lower edge of the mandible along the side and interweave with fibers of the opposite side at the front of the mandible. Its fibers have a broad distribution about the face, which includes a blending of fibers associated with different muscles of the lower lip and the corner of the mouth. Contraction of the *platysma* muscle draws the skin of the neck toward the mandible. It may also pull the lower lip and corner of the mouth to the side and downward and/or force the lower lip against the lower teeth and the alveolar process of the mandible.

Figure 5–15 portrays the general force vectors for the 14 muscles of the lips. These vectors summarize the active forces operating on the lips and their consequences on the positioning of the lips and corners of the mouth up and down, side to side, and with regard to compression against the teeth and/or alveolar processes of the maxilla and mandible. When the actions of these muscles are combined, they create a seeming infinite variety of lip adjustments that are intricately involved in human expression.

MOVEMENTS OF THE PHARYNGEAL-ORAL APPARATUS

Movements of the pharyngeal-oral apparatus allow it to perform a variety of functions involved in speech production and swallowing as well as many other activities. Movements of its component parts—the pharynx, mandible, tongue, and lips—are considered individually below.

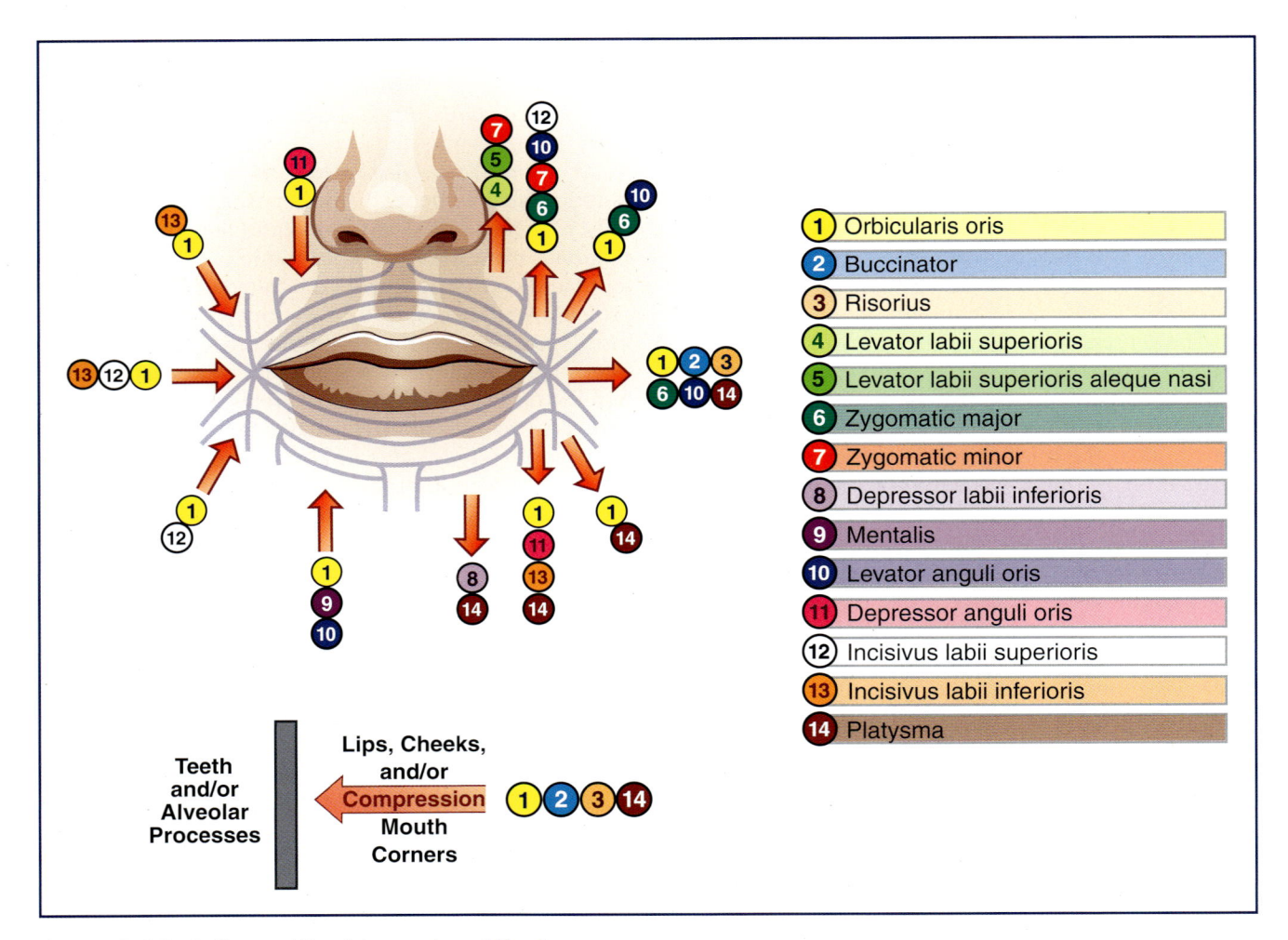

Figure 5–15. Actions of the 14 muscles of the lips.

Movements of the Pharynx

The potential movements of the overall pharynx are discussed in detail in Chapter 4 and illustrated there (see Figure 4–15). Focus here is on potential movements of the laryngopharynx and oropharynx and their roles in changing the regional lumen of the pharynx and the degree of coupling between the oropharynx and the oral cavity through the palatoglossal arch (anterior faucial pillars). These portions of the pharyngeal tube are relatively mobile and present three movement capabilities: (a) inward and outward movement of their sidewalls, (b) forward and backward movement of their back wall, and (c) forward and backward movement of their front wall (tongue and/or epiglottis). These movements enable the lumen of the laryngopharynx and oropharynx to be changed in size and shape.

The pharynx can change in size from a maximally enlarged pharyngeal airway to one that is fully obstructed. In the case of complete obstruction, the walls of the pharynx may not only come in contact, but also undergo forceful compression against one another. Inward movements of the sides of the pharynx are effected mainly through contractions of the *inferior* and *middle constrictor* muscles, and outward movements are effected through contractions of the *stylopharyngeus* muscle. The sides of the pharynx can also be moved inward by lowering of the mandible (thereby creating a smaller and more circular lumen) and moved outward by raising the mandible again (Minifie, Hixon, Kelsey, & Woodhouse, 1970). Inward movements of the back wall can be effected by those same constrictor muscles, and inward movement of the front wall is usually accomplished by the tongue and epiglottis. The position of the upper front wall of the pharyngeal lumen can be changed by the velum and the lower boundary of the lumen is changed when the height of the larynx changes.

The degree of coupling between the pharyngeal cavity and oral cavity can be changed by: (a) upward and downward movements of the tongue, (b) upward and downward movements of the velum, and (c) side-to-side movements of the pillars of the palatoglossal arch (anterior faucial pillars). Maximum coupling is brought about by a combined maximum elevation of the velum and maximum depression of the tongue. Decoupling results when the undersurface of the velum and the upper surface of the tongue are placed in full apposition and the oropharyngeal airway is occluded. When contact between the tongue and the velum occurs, it is also possible to have openings on the left and right sides through which the pharynx and oral cavity are coupled.

Movements of the Mandible

The mandible is capable of a wide range of movements that derive from actions of the temporomandibular joints (see Figure 5–5). Upward and downward movements of the mandible are rotational and take place about a lateral axis that passes through the condyloid processes on the left and right sides of the skull (resembling the swinging of a two-hinged trap door about an axis that extends through the center pins of its hinges). Forward and backward and side to side movements are accomplished through gliding movements of the mandible along the articular facets of the temporomandibular joints. These three movement possibilities (pitching the mandible upward or downward about a lateral axis, rolling it to one side or the other about a longitudinal axis, and yawing it to the left or right about a vertical axis) often combine in activities such as the crushing and grinding associated with chewing.

The mandible can be adjusted in position, but not in shape. Such adjustment is usually considered in relation to the maxilla because it constitutes the opposing jaw for the mandible and is critical to functions that the two structures carry out collaboratively, such as chewing and speech production. Adjustments that lower the mandible result from the action of one or more muscles that include the *external pterygoid*, *digastric* (*anterior*

Early X-Games

This isn't about sports, but about x-rays. Early uses of x-rays to study structures of the upper airway during speech production were quite interesting. A few tidbits should give you an appreciation. A narrow gold chain was often placed down the midline of the tongue to make its longitudinal configuration easy to visualize on single shot lateral head x-rays. Some of the first findings from different laboratories were not in agreement concerning tongue positions during vowel productions. Despite public arguments about linguistic bases for the differences, it turned out that the head had not been fixed in position and variation was related to its rotation from one exposure to another. Then, there were dangers. A pioneer in the use of x-rays for speech research entered old age unable to grow a beard on one side of his face, the side he had frequently bombarded with x-rays to get the view of the speech production apparatus he wanted to study.

belly), *mylohyoid*, and *geniohyoid* muscles. In contrast, adjustments that elevate the mandible result from the action of one or more muscles that include the *masseter*, *temporalis*, and *internal pterygoid* muscles. Side-to-side movements are the domain of the *masseter*, *temporalis*, *internal pterygoid*, and *external pterygoid* muscles. Forward movements are caused by actions of the *external pterygoid* muscle, and backward movements are caused by actions of the *masseter* and *temporalis* muscles.

Movements of the Tongue

The tongue is a fleshy muscular structure that is exceedingly mobile. Its mobility derives from the fact that: (a) it rides with the mandible and goes as a whole where the mandible goes, (b) its position within the oral cavity can be shifted en masse as a body (akin to moving a closed fist around in space), and (c) its shape can be changed markedly and relatively independently of the first two sources of mobility. Movements of the tongue are often segmental and differ along its major and minor axes. Movements of different points on the surface of the structure can be upward and downward, forward and backward, side to side, or different combinations of these. Vertical movements can extend from the trough to the roof of the oral cavity. Front-to-back movements can range from a maximally forward displacement of the tongue out of the mouth to a maximally rearward displacement of the structure against the back wall of the pharynx. Side-to-side movements can range from the stretchable limits of one cheek to the other.

The enormous variety of possible tongue adjustments is truly amazing. The tongue can protrude, retract, lateralize, centralize, curl, point, lick, bulge, groove, flatten, rotate, and do many other things such as "picking between one's teeth." What seems to be a near infinite array of adjustments relates to its special mechanical endowment that allows it to function as a muscular hydrostat (Kier & Smith, 1985; Smith & Kier, 1989). A muscular hydrostat is a pliable structure without bones that has connective tissue that allows it to change shape while maintaining its overall volume. It is a pliable structure that is incompressible and behaves somewhat like a water-filled balloon. Examples of other muscular hydrostats are octopus tentacles and elephant trunks, as depicted in Figure 5–16.

This special property of the tongue, along with its personal soft skeleton that encapsulates it, provides leverages for the eight muscles that give rise to its motive force. Because of its hydrostatic properties, inward displacement of one part of the tongue brings about outward displacement of another part (like squeezing one part of a water-filled balloon and seeing another part bulge outward). Through the selective contraction of different muscle fibers, a relatively rigid but changing support system is created in which the contraction of different muscle fibers can change the location and shape of the tongue.

Although conceptualization of the tongue as a muscular hydrostat has been largely accepted for decades, it has been difficult to study tongue movements from this perspective until recently. New technological advances have allowed the entire tongue volume to be tracked during various activities such as resting tidal breathing (Cheng, Butler, Gandevia, & Bilston, 2008) and speaking (Woo, Xing, Lee, Stone, & Prince, 2016). The challenges to quantification of tongue movement in a 4D landscape (3-dimensional space by time) are still being worked out (e.g., Woo et al., 2017).

Movements of the Lips

The mobility of the face in the region of the lips rivals that of the fine movements of the fingers. Movements of the lips can occur along vertical, side-to-side, and front-to-back dimensions. Each lip can be moved independently of the other or the two lips can be coordinated in their movements. The upper lip is fixed in

> **Take It Away**
>
> The tongue rides with the mandible and goes where it goes. Thus, when trying to interpret changes in the configuration of the tongue surface, it's necessary to determine how much is attributable to adjustment of the tongue and how much is attributable to adjustment of the mandible. Suppose you had a client with a hyperkinetic disease in which both the tongue and mandible went through adventitious involuntary movements. How could you go about parsing them in your evaluation? Not to worry! Have the client speak through clenched teeth or while biting down on a small stack of tongue depressors. Then, the abnormal movements of the tongue are on their own and not confounded by the abnormal movements of the mandible. It's called removing a degree of freedom of performance, and the principle can be applied in many ways when analyzing different speech structures.

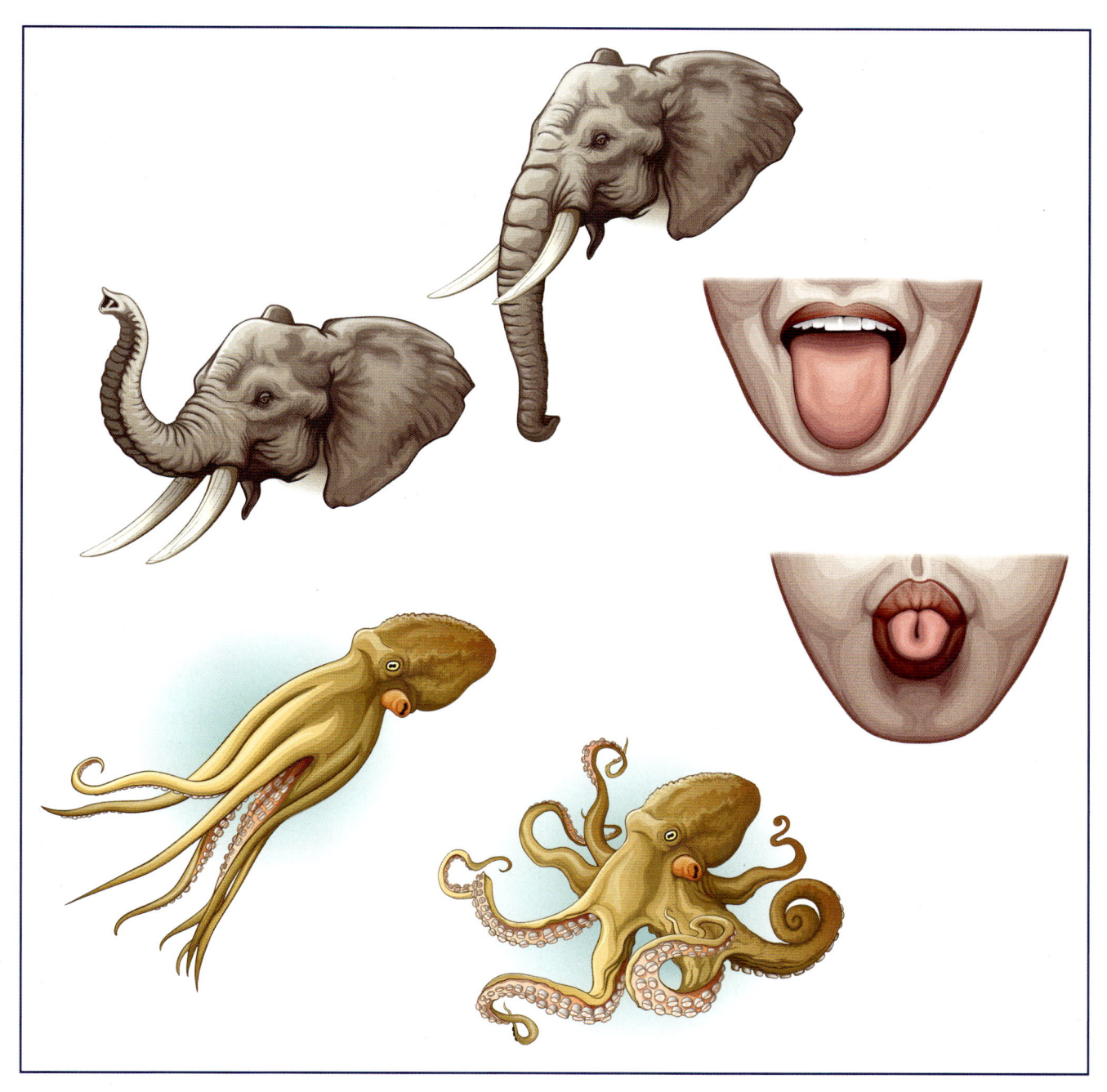

Figure 5–16. Three muscular hydrostats: an octopus arm, an elephant trunk, and a human tongue.

spatial coordinates to the fixed position of the maxilla, whereas the lower lip rides with the mandible so that its movements are dictated, in part, by the prevailing position of the mandible. The lips can be puckered, protruded, retracted, spread, pointed, curled inward and outward, rounded, and plumped and can be associated with a host of facial expressions, such as smiling, smirking, sulking, and sneering. The multitude of possible lip adjustments are effected by different combinations of the more than a dozen muscles that impart forces to the lips. Experimenting with lip movements in front of a mirror gives one an appreciation for the degrees of freedom of lip movement.

Adjustments of the lips can be viewed from a variety of perspectives, such as in relation to influences on: (a) the position and shape of each lip, (b) the position

> **The Cold War**
>
> With prolonged exposure to very cold weather, your face tightens up and your speech slows down. Certain parts of your speech production apparatus actually get stiffer as you chill down. You can live with this because your body, although coping with change at the periphery, is still winning the cold war. Should things get worse, however, such that hypothermia sets in, you'll be in trouble. Hypothermia occurs when your body can't replace heat lost to its surroundings and your core temperature begins to drop. From the usual 98.6°F down to 95°F, your speech will continue to sound normal. Below 95°F down to 90°F, your speech will become slurred and progressively more so as temperature decreases. Once your core temperature passes below 90°F, your speech will be unintelligible. The cooling of the body is simply too much for the nervous system to handle and all remaining resources are devoted to preserving the organism.

and shape of the corners of the mouth, (c) the compression between the lips and/or between one or both lips and the teeth and gums, and (d) the configuration (cross-section and length) of the channel that forms the airway opening. The first two of these are often considered significant contributors to facial expression, whereas compression between the lips is relevant to activities such as drinking through a straw. The configuration of the channel that forms the airway opening is especially critical to the formation of the acoustic speech product. During speaking, this channel is frequently adjusted such that it can be lengthened or shortened, changed in shape, and moved from side to side (consider talking out of one side of the mouth, the so-called sidewinder). The lips may even be in apposition on one side and be parted on the other, as in the dying breed of the smoker who talks with a cigarette hanging from one side of the mouth.

CONTROL VARIABLES OF PHARYNGEAL-ORAL FUNCTION

Several control variables are important in pharyngeal-oral function. Their relative importance depends on the activity being performed, whether it is breathing, speaking, singing, whistling, wind instrument playing, blowing, sucking, chewing, or swallowing. For the purposes of this chapter, discussion is devoted to four control variables: (a) pharyngeal-oral lumen size and configuration, (b) pharyngeal-oral contact pressure, (c) pharyngeal-oral airway resistance, and (d) pharyngeal-oral acoustic impedance.

Pharyngeal-Oral Lumen Size and Configuration

The lumen of the pharyngeal-oral apparatus (its inner open space) can be changed in both size and configuration (shape). Such changes are the result of adjustments in the positions of structures that line the pharyngeal-oral airway.

The open space that constitutes the pharyngeal-oral lumen can be either increased or decreased from the resting configuration. Figure 5–17 summarizes the structures that may contribute individually or in combination to changing the lumen of the airway in the pharyngeal cavity, the oral cavity, and the oral vestibule. Length changes of the pharyngeal-oral lumen can be achieved: (a) within the pharyngeal cavity, by different combinations of adjustments of the velum and larynx, (b) within the oral cavity, by different combinations of adjustments of the tongue and mandible, and (c) within the oral vestibule, by different combinations of adjustments of the lips and mandible. Cross-sectional changes can be achieved: (a) within the pharynx, by different

> **Open Wide**
>
> Your mandible and maxilla are separated by only a small distance when you produce speech. Activities such as calling your dog, yelling at a football game, or singing often get you to open up more. Classical (opera) singing is one activity that gets people to open very wide. One form of classical singing teaches what is referred to as a four-finger jaw position. Try it. Place the four fingers of one hand together and then, with your thumb on that hand pointing upward, insert your fingers vertically at the midline between your upper and lower front teeth. Quite a stretch, isn't it? It comes close to maximum separation between your mandible and maxilla and gives you nearly as large a mouth opening as you can achieve (or tolerate). What a great way to get that beautiful singing voice to radiate outward from the singer to the audience.

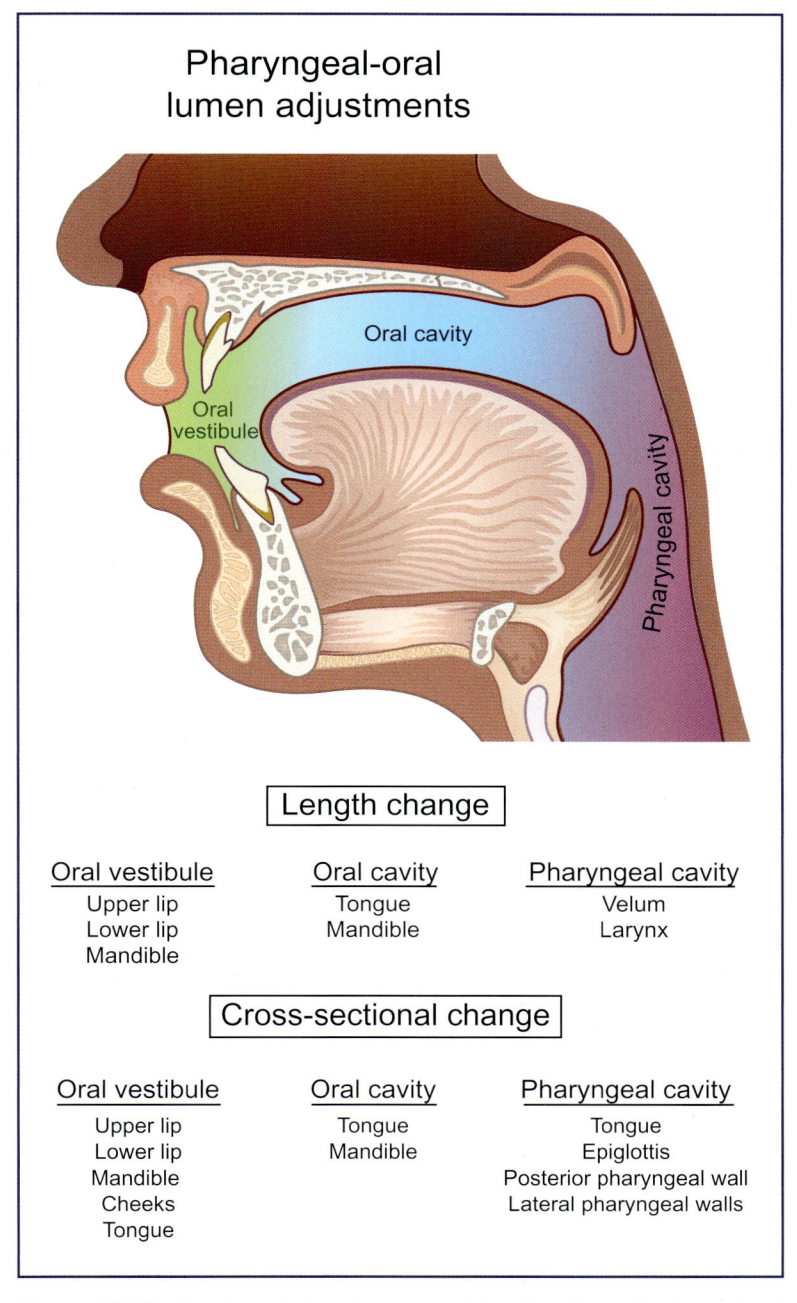

Figure 5-17. Regional structures contributing to adjustments of the pharyngeal-oral lumen. Length changes in the lumen can be achieved by movements of the larynx, velum, tongue, mandible, and lips. Cross-sectional changes in the lumen can be achieved by movements of the pharyngeal walls, epiglottis, tongue, mandible, lips, and cheeks.

combinations of adjustments of the tongue, epiglottis, posterior pharyngeal wall, and lateral pharyngeal walls, (b) within the oral cavity, by different combinations of adjustments of the tongue and mandible, and (c) within the oral vestibule, by different combinations of adjustments of the lips, mandible, cheeks, and tongue.

Given the lengthwise and cross-sectional adjustment possibilities noted, the number of options for luminal changes in the pharyngeal-oral apparatus is exceedingly large. This underpins the fact that the acoustic products that emanate from the pharyngeal-oral apparatus (such as speech and song) can be richly variable.

Pharyngeal-Oral Structural Contact Pressure

Adjustments of the pharyngeal-oral apparatus can result in full obstruction of the pharyngeal-oral lumen at different locations. Full obstruction can be accomplished through structural contact of: (a) the tongue against the pharynx, velum, hard palate, alveolar process of the maxilla, teeth, and lips, and (b) the lips against the teeth and one another. Once two structures are in apposition, the contact pressure between them can be adjusted to meet the needs of the situation. Figure 5–18 portrays structural contact and its resultant compressive force between the tongue and the alveolar process of the maxilla.

Structural contact pressure can be influenced by several factors. These include: (a) muscular pressure exerted by muscular components of the contacting surfaces, (b) surface tension between apposed surfaces that are moist and hold them together, and (c) gravity that weighs down structures and acts on them differently in different body positions. The most significant of these three is the muscular pressure. Contact pressure for an activity may require low-level muscular exertion for soft contact between structures or it may require high contact pressure when it is necessary to fortify the contact in the face of high air pressures in the vicinity.

Pharyngeal-Oral Airway Resistance

Pharyngeal-oral airway resistance is a calculated measure of the opposition provided by the pharyngeal-oral apparatus to mass airflow through it, as portrayed in Figure 5–19. Airway resistance is calculated from the quotient of the pressure drop across any segment of interest and the airflow through that segment. Pharyngeal-oral airway resistance is a property of the airway itself and is airflow dependent. This means that it increases or decreases with increases or decreases in the rate at which air moves, even without changes in the physical dimensions of the pharyngeal-oral airway. However, it is the change in the cross section of the airway that causes the greatest change in pharyngeal-oral airway resistance. By decreasing the cross-sectional

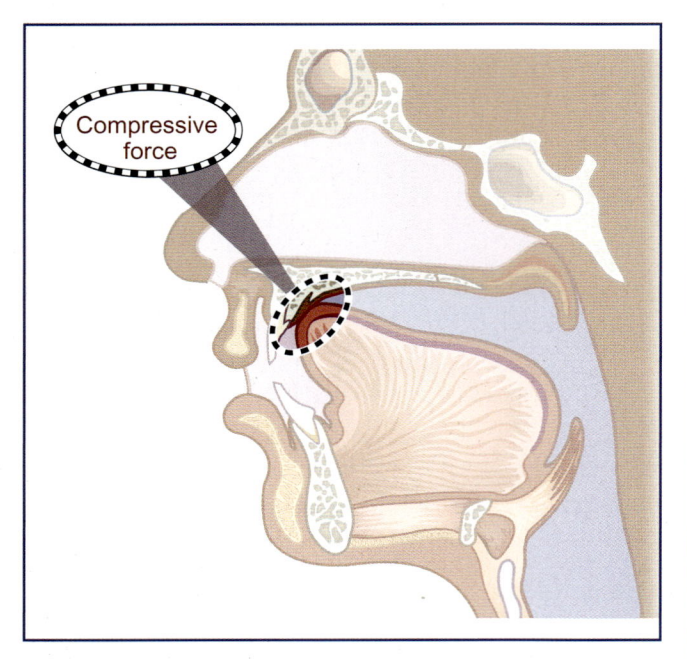

Figure 5–18. Structural contact pressure between the tongue and alveolar process of the maxilla. The magnitude of the contact pressure is determined by the muscular pressure exerted by the different structures, the surface tension between the surfaces, and gravity. Of these three, muscular pressure is by far the most important.

Low Energy Physics

Speech is clearly an energy-producing enterprise. But just how much energy is involved? One scientist has calculated that 300 to 400 ergs of energy is expended in the resultant sound wave when the sentence, "Joe took father's shoe-bench out" is produced at usual loudness (Fletcher, 1953). That's not a sentence that most people run around saying and many readers might not have an appreciation for how 300 to 400 ergs relates to their everyday lives. Perhaps we can help a bit. You and 499 of your closest friends (that's a Boeing-747 aircraft with all the seats filled or an Airbus A380 with a few empty seats) would have to say, "Joe took father's shoe-bench out" together at your usual loudness continuously for a year to produce enough energy to heat a cup of coffee. Holy Starbucks! That's a lot of talking. It would undoubtedly contend for a Guinness World Record, but on nature's energy scale it wouldn't amount to much.

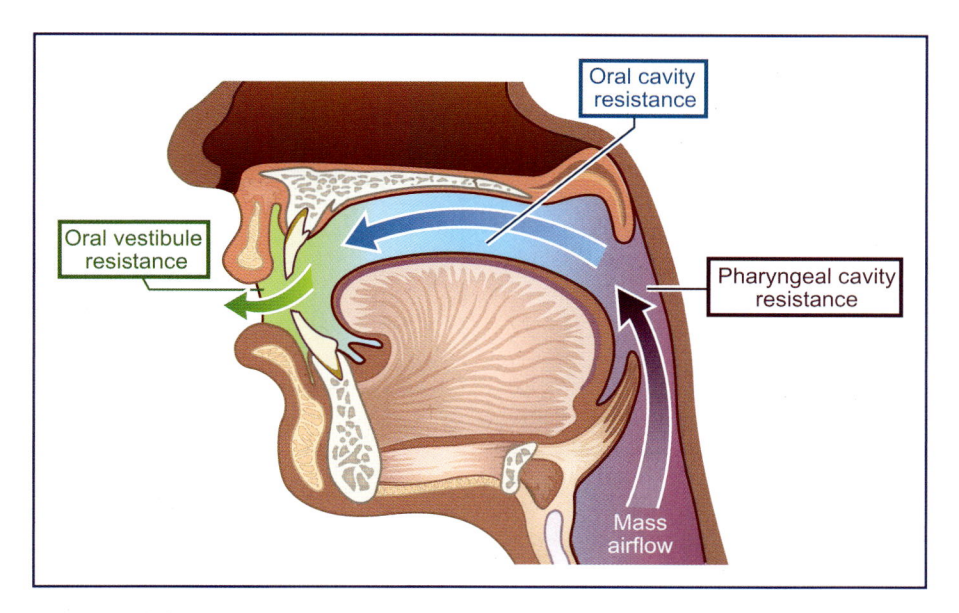

Figure 5–19. Pharyngeal-oral airway resistance is a calculated measure of the opposition of the pharyngeal-oral airway to mass airflow through it. The greatest changes in pharyngeal-oral airway resistance are due to changes in cross-sectional area in the oropharynx, oral cavity, and oral vestibule.

area of the airway anywhere within these regions, the airway resistance will likely increase. Such change can occur anywhere along the length of the pharyngeal-oral apparatus, from larynx to lips, but is most prominently the result of adjustments within the oropharynx, oral cavity, and oral vestibule. The range of potential airway resistance values is from very low (associated with a wide open pharyngeal-oral apparatus) to infinity (associated with a closed pharyngeal-oral apparatus).

Pharyngeal-Oral Acoustic Impedance

The pharyngeal-oral apparatus plays an important role in the control of acoustic impedance, which, like airway resistance, involves opposition to flow. As portrayed in Figure 5–20, this opposition is not to mass airflow, but to the movement of energy in the form of sound waves through the apparatus. These waves function like an alternating current in which adjacent air molecules collide with each other and pass energy on to their neighbors. Acoustic impedance influences how well sound waves propagate through the pharyngeal-oral airway.

Acoustic impedance is determined to a great extent by cross-sectional adjustments of the pharyngeal-oral airway. These adjustments influence the degree of coupling between different segments of the pharyngeal-oral apparatus. When the adjustments increase the

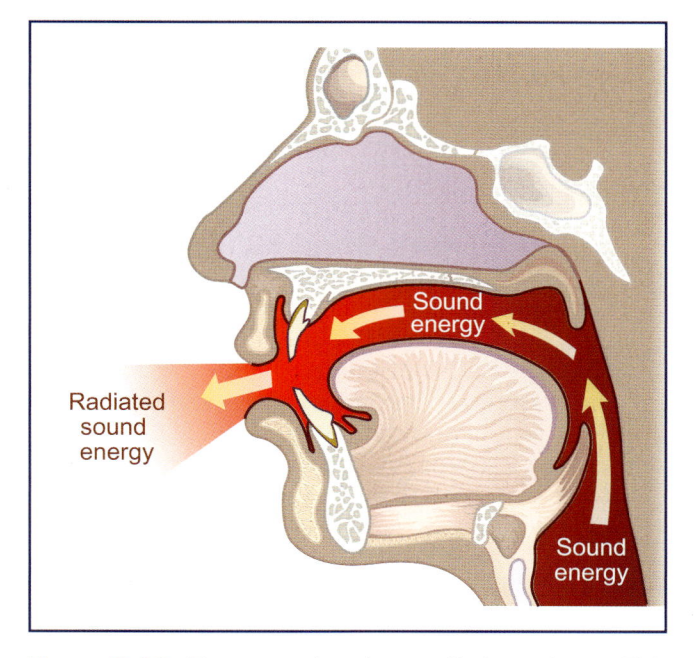

Figure 5–20. Pharyngeal-oral acoustic impedance. This impedance relates to the ease with which sound waves propagate through the pharyngeal-oral airway. The more open the airway, the lower the acoustic impedance. Note that, in this figure, the velopharynx is closed so that velopharyngeal-nasal impedance is near infinite (a small amount of sound energy may be transmitted through the velum via sympathetic vibration).

cross section of the lumen of the pharyngeal-oral airway, sound waves pass relatively freely along the airway. In contrast, when the adjustments decrease the cross section of the lumen of the airway, sound energy does not pass as freely along the airway. Relative decreases in the cross section of the lumen at different locations simultaneously may also influence the degree to which different segments of the pharyngeal-oral airway interact with one another acoustically.

NEURAL SUBSTRATES OF PHARYNGEAL-ORAL CONTROL

Pharyngeal-oral movements are controlled by the nervous system and differ with the activity being performed. Thus, speaking and swallowing, while engaging the same structures of the pharyngeal-oral apparatus, are controlled by different neural substrates and mechanisms.

Although different parts of the central nervous system participate in the control of different pharyngeal-oral activities, the final forms of the control commands are sent through the same set of cranial nerves. These nerves have their origins in the brainstem and course from there to provide motor innervation to the muscles of the pharynx, mandible, tongue, and lips. As shown in Table 5–2, motor innervation of the pharynx is effected through the pharyngeal plexus, which includes fibers from cranial nerves IX (glossopharyngeal), X (vagus), and possibly XI (accessory). Motor innervation to the mandible is effected through cranial nerves V (trigeminal) and the first cervical spinal nerve (C1). Motor innervation of the tongue includes cranial nerves X and XII, whereas motor innervation of the lips is effected through cranial nerve VII (facial).

Sensory innervation to the pharynx is carried by cranial nerves IX and X. Sensory innervation to the mandible is supplied by cranial nerve V. The tongue receives sensory supply from cranial nerves V, VII, and IX, whereas supply to the lips is from cranial nerve V. Neural information traveling along the sensory nerves supplying the pharynx, mandible, tongue, and lips results from the activation of receptors of various types within those structures. These receptors include an array of mechanoreceptors that are differentially distributed (some occurring in certain locations more than others) throughout the tissues of the pharyngeal-oral apparatus. When sound results from pharyngeal-oral activity, mechanoreceptors formed by hair cells within the cochlea (end organ of the auditory system) may be activated. Sensory information from the auditory system is effected via cranial nerve VIII (auditory-vestibular nerve).

The mechanoreceptors within the pharyngeal-oral apparatus are sensitive to a variety of stimuli and are

Table 5–2. Summary of Motor and Sensory Nerve Supply to the Pharynx, Mandible, Tongue, and Lips

COMPONENT	INNERVATION MOTOR	INNERVATION SENSORY
Pharynx	IX[a], X, (XI)[b]	IX, X
Mandible	V, C1[c]	V
Tongue	X[d], XII	V, VII, IX
Lips	VII	V

Note. Peripheral nerves indicated in the table and notes are cranial nerves V (trigeminal), VII (facial), IX (glossopharyngeal), X (vagus), XI (accessory), and XII (hypoglossal) and cervical spinal nerve 1 (C1).
[a]The only pharyngeal muscle innervated by cranial nerve IX is the **stylopharyngeus** muscle.
[b]The branches of cranial nerves IX and X (and possibly XI) that innervate parts of the pharynx are sometimes called the pharyngeal plexus.
[c]The only mandibular muscle innervated by C1 is the **geniohyoid** muscle.
[d]The only tongue muscle innervated by cranial nerve X is the **palatoglossus** muscle.

Ten-Four, Good Buddy

Bell's palsy is a relatively common condition that affects cranial nerve VII, the nerve that innervates the muscles of the face. Upper and lower facial muscles can become weak or paralyzed and speech production can be impaired. Most often the cause is unknown and the problem is on one side. It may involve an autoimmune inflammatory response, a herpes viral infection, or a swelling of the nerve because of allergy. Most people who get Bell's palsy make a full recovery, especially if they're young. Exposure to cold can be a factor in Bell's palsy. Truck drivers who keep the driver's-side window down may contract Bell's palsy. Wind chill for a prolonged period across the side of the face is believed to be a contributing factor to onset of the problem. Which side depends on the country in which you're driving. What's the prevention? Close the window and turn on the air conditioner.

capable of providing the nervous system with many types of information, including information about: (a) muscle length, (b) rate of change in muscle length, (c) muscle tension, (d) joint position, (e) joint movement, (f) touch, (g) surface pressure, (h) deep pressure, (i) surface deformation, (j) temperature, and (k) vibration, among others. Mechanoreceptors within the fabric of the pharyngeal-oral apparatus (and within the auditory system during speech production) provide the central nervous system with information that is used to keep track of the recent status of the pharyngeal-oral apparatus and to guide anticipated actions of the apparatus.

PHARYNGEAL-ORAL FUNCTIONS

The pharyngeal-oral apparatus performs many functions. Those of interest here relate to: (a) degree of coupling between the oral cavity and atmosphere, (b) chewing, (c) swallowing, and (d) sound generation and filtering.

Degree of Coupling Between the Oral Cavity and Atmosphere

Actions of the pharyngeal-oral apparatus determine the degree of coupling between the pharyngeal-oral apparatus and atmosphere. The coupling pathway in this case is through the oral vestibule. When breathing through the pharyngeal-oral apparatus, the oral vestibule is open, whereas when breathing through the velopharyngeal-nasal port, the oral vestibule may be closed. The lips are especially important in changing the degree of coupling between the oral cavity and atmosphere and can influence it not only in cross-section but also by adjusting the length of the channel formed between the oral cavity and the airway opening.

Chewing and Swallowing

Chewing (mastication) is the process of grinding, mashing, gnawing, crushing, and kneading food (nutriment in solid form) with the teeth. This process is aimed at the alteration of food into smaller particle sizes that can be prepared to a swallow-ready consistency. The alignment of the maxilla, mandible, and teeth is important in this process to ensure that proper biting forces can be exerted. Chewing entails extensive movement of the mandible that may have significant vertical, side-to-side, and elliptical components. These depend, in part, on the consistency of the food being manipulated.

> **Myth Conceptions**
>
> The history of speech-language pathology is rich with clinical theories and methods that don't actually involve speech production directly. These have taken many forms. One early one took the point of view that language had its beginnings in chewing and that chewing exercises had a prominent role in the evaluation and management of speech and voice disorders. The originator of this idea said that he conceived the notion when confronted with two Egyptian hieroglyphic scripts that showed a similar sign for eating and speaking. Despite using some of the same pharyngeal-oral structures, chewing and speaking are controlled differently by the nervous system and one is not a precursor or analog of the other. Other forms of nonspeech activities continue to be used even today as if they were somehow beneficial to speech production. We don't subscribe to any of these misconceptions. You shouldn't either.

Actions of the oral cavity and oral vestibule prepare food (by chewing) or liquid for swallowing by positioning the bolus and then propelling it backward into the oropharynx (the velopharynx being closed). Thereafter, muscles of the oropharynx and laryngopharynx act to further propel the prepared substances downward through the pharyngeal tube and into the esophagus. Chapter 16 provides a detailed discussion about the swallowing process that includes consideration of the role played by the pharyngeal-oral apparatus.

Sound Generation and Filtering

Much of the interest in the present chapter is with sound generation and filtering of that sound by the pharyngeal-oral apparatus. Sound generation refers to the creation of an acoustic source, whereas filtering refers to the shaping of the source sound.

Sound generation in the pharyngeal-oral apparatus can be of several types. The two of these that are most important to this book are: (a) transient (popping) sounds, in which the oral airstream is momentarily interrupted and then released, and (b) turbulence (hissing) sounds, in which air is forced through a narrow constriction within the airway.

Sounds such as these that are generated within the pharyngeal-oral apparatus and sounds that are generated in the larynx (by vocal fold vibration, sustained

> **Duck and Cover**
>
> Aeromechanical and acoustic energies come out of your mouth during speech production. Other things also make their way out. One of these is saliva. Your salivary glands might produce up to a quart of liquid in a day. Tiny drops of saliva spew from your mouth when you speak. These are usually invisible and emerge as wet clouds that can hang around an hour or more and settle on nearby listeners. Each word spoken sends about 2.5 droplets of saliva into the atmosphere (Bodanis, 1995). Read this sidetrack aloud and you'll expel about 350 droplets of saliva. Do the same with the Gettysburg Address and the number will reach 700. The United States Constitution would get you about 11,000 droplets. And what would an assembly of 500 people reciting the Pledge of Allegiance get you? Forty thousand droplets dispersed in 500 wet clouds.

noise production such as whisper, or glottal stop production) are filtered (or shaped) by the pharyngeal-oral apparatus. That is, the source frequencies and amplitudes of those frequencies are modified by the sizes and shapes of the different regions of the pharyngeal-oral apparatus (and velopharyngeal-nasal apparatus, if it is coupled to the pharyngeal-oral apparatus). The final acoustic product—that is, the speech heard by a listener or measured in front of the speaker's lips—is determined by the nature of the sound source and how it is filtered as it passes through the various pharyngeal and oral (and nasal, in some cases) cavities. Chapters 7, 8, and 9 contain in-depth coverage of these concepts.

SPEECH PRODUCTION: ARTICULATORY DESCRIPTIONS

The pharyngeal-oral apparatus is a critical player in speech production and is often referred to as the "articulatory" part of the speech mechanism (in this context, an articulator is a movable structure that contributes to the production of speech sounds). In this section, discussion focuses on how speech sounds are described and categorized. In the next major section, discussion turns to articulatory processes and how they play out in real time.

Articulatory descriptions of sound segments are often separated into different types. For each type of speech sound (e.g., vowels), a finer description is made to characterize articulatory differences within the type. These descriptions for the sounds of American English are considered here. For an excellent introduction to articulatory descriptions for virtually all sounds in languages of the world, see https://en.wikipedia.org/wiki/International_Phonetic_Alphabet

The articulatory description presented here considers the broad categories of sonorants and obstruents. Sonorants are sounds produced with a relatively open pharyngeal-oral airway (vocal tract) or nasal airway (nasal tract) which allows air to flow freely from the glottis and through the lips or nose. The sonorants include vowels, diphthongs, and two types of consonants: semivowels and nasals. In American English all sonorants are produced with vocal fold vibration. Obstruents are sounds produced with a constriction or obstruction and include three types of consonants: stops, fricatives, and affricates. In Figures 5–21 and 5–22, sonorants are shown in blue and obstruents are shown in orange.

Vowels

Vowels are usually produced with voicing by the larynx and with velopharyngeal closure (although they can be nasalized, and are in many languages). Figure 5–21 shows how vowels can be described using the three dimensions of *place of major constriction* within the pharyngeal-oral apparatus, *degree of major constriction* within the apparatus, and *degree of lip rounding*. All vowels are sonorants; thus, all of Figure 5–21 is colored blue. Chapter 8 discusses the acoustic counterparts of these three dimensions.

Place of Major Constriction

Place of major constriction specifies the location at which the pharyngeal-oral airway is maximally constricted during vowel production. Three locations are specified for vowels. These include *front*, *central*, and *back*. The term *front* is used to designate constrictions formed between the tongue blade and the alveolar process of the maxilla. The term *central* is used to indicate constrictions formed between the tongue and the hard palate, or when no obvious constriction exists. And the term *back* designates constrictions formed between the tongue and the velum, or between the tongue and the posterior pharyngeal wall. Five vowels fall under the rubric *front* vowels, four are classified as *central* vowels, and five are considered *back* vowels. Changes across the *place of major constriction* dimension can be viewed as shifts in the position of the tongue along the length coordinate of the pharyngeal-oral apparatus.

Place of major oral constriction

Degree of major oral constriction		Front	Central		Back	
						Increasing lip-rounding →
High		i — beat ɪ — bit			u — tooth ʊ — hook	
Mid		e — **capon** ɛ — bet	ɜ˞ — word ʌ — **above**	ɚ — onward ə — **above**	o — boast ɔ — taught	
Low		æ — bat			ɑ — calm	

Figure 5–21. Vowel description. Vowels are sonorants and are categorized for American English in terms of place of major constriction, degree of major constriction, and degree of lip rounding. Vowel symbols are from the International Phonetic Alphabet. Word exemplars are primarily from Fairbanks (1960).

Manner of production

Place of production	Stop-plosive − / +	Fricative − / +	Affricate − / +	Nasal − / +	Semivowel − / +
Labial (lips)	p pole / b bowl			/ m sum	/ w watt
Labiodental (lip–teeth)		f fat / v vat			
Dental (tongue–teeth)		θ thigh / ð thy			
Alveolar (tongue–gum)	t toll / d dole	s seal / z zeal		/ n sun	/ l lot
Palatal (tongue–hard palate)		ʃ ash / ʒ azure	tʃ choke / dʒ joke		/ j,r yacht, rot
Velar (tongue–velum)	k coal / g goal			/ ŋ sung	
Glottal (vocal folds)		h hot /			

Figure 5–22. Consonant description. Consonants can be obstruents (*orange*) or sonorants (*blue*). Consonants for American English are categorized in terms of manner of production, place of production, and voicing. Voiceless and voiced elements are designated by − and + signs, respectively. Consonant symbols are from the International Phonetic Alphabet. Word exemplars are from Fairbanks (1960).

Degree of Major Constriction

Degree of major constriction designates the cross-sectional size of the constricted region of the airway. This dimension typically specifies a *high*, *mid*, or *low* degree of major constriction and corresponds, in most circumstances, to the location of the highest point of the tongue surface in relation to the roof of the mouth. Exceptions occur when the major constriction is formed between the back of the tongue and the posterior pharyngeal wall. *High* degrees of constriction correspond to small cross-sectional areas at the major constriction. *Mid* degrees of constriction are associated with intermediate-size cross-sections. And *low* degrees of constriction involve large cross-sectional areas. The size of the constricted area of the airway is influenced by the height of the jaw, which influences the height of the tongue. For example, low vowels typically have lower mandible positions compared with high vowels.

Lip Rounding

Lip rounding designates the degree to which the lips are protruded and the area between them is reduced. Protrusion often correlates directly with the size of the airway opening at the lips. Thus, an increase in lip rounding signifies a simultaneous lengthening and narrowing of the lip channel along the oral vestibule, whereas a decrease in lip rounding indicates a simultaneous shortening and opening up of the lip channel. This relationship between lip extension and decrease of the airway size is not an anatomical necessity, however, as demonstrated by the fact that some languages have vowel sounds with substantial narrowing of the lip channel without extension of the lips. In American English, lip rounding occurs only on *mid*-constriction and *high*-constriction *back* vowels. For these vowels, lip rounding increases across the *mid* to *high* categories of constriction.

Diphthongs

Diphthongs are sonorant sounds that are vowel-like in nature. The classic phonetic view is that they are transitional hybrids of vowels that are formed by rapidly changing from one vowel adjustment to another. Thus, they are transcribed as pairs of vowels, there being five such pairs in American English—/ɑɪ/ (as in bide), /ɔɪ/ (as in boy), /ɑʊ/ (as in bough), /eɪ/ (as in bait), and /oʊ/ (as in boat)—although diphthongs vary substantially across dialects. In English, each diphthong is formed by a vowel pair in which the first vowel is characterized by a lesser degree of major constriction than the second vowel. Diphthongs may combine vowel pairs that transition: (a) within the same place of major constriction, (b) from back to front places of constriction, and (c) from mid to high degrees of constriction that include increases in lip rounding. Given that diphthongs are transitional hybrids of vowel pairs in the classic phonetic view, their production description may be conceptualized in terms of their vowel beginning and ending points and nearly continuous adjustments in between. This usual phonetic conceptualization of diphthongs is not without controversy. Acoustic studies of diphthong formation have suggested that they have unique features that are different from "pure" vowels and that their transitional components contain defining features that show them to be a different sound class than vowels.

Consonants

Consonants can be classified as obstruents or sonorants, as represented in the color scheme in Figure 5–22. Consonants are described along three dimensions: *manner of production* (five categories), *place of production* (seven categories), and *voicing* (two categories). These three dimensions yield 70 (5 × 7 × 2) unique consonant possibilities. About one-third of these are used in American English.

Raspberries

Raspberries (also called Bronx cheers) are sounds that resemble sustained flatulence (farting). Raspberries are made by blowing air between a protruded tongue and the lips. Adults use raspberries to indicate derision, sarcasm, or silliness. All cultures seem to have a fondness for them. Infants especially like them and use them in their early sound play. Raspberries aren't used as sounds in human languages. Thus, they fade from the repertoire of experimental noises as the infant figures out that they're not an important part of the linguistic code. Nevertheless, the skill acquired is not wasted. They return later on as full-blown Bronx cheers to be used to put someone down, sarcastically cheer a poor sports performance, or be the final gesture after a lost argument. Blow a raspberry the next time you see a primate at a zoo. Most primates make raspberries. You'll either get one back or get a weird look from a resident.

Manner of Production

Manner of production specifies the way in which structures of the laryngeal apparatus, velopharyngeal-nasal apparatus, and pharyngeal-oral apparatus constrict or obstruct the airway during consonant generation. The manner of production dimension includes five categories, referred to as *stop-plosive, fricative, affricate, nasal,* and *semivowel*. Both nasals and semivowels are sonorants but are often described as consonants. They are described here and considered further in Chapter 9.

Stop-plosive consonants begin with occlusion of the oral airway and a buildup of oral air pressure behind the occlusion. The airway is then abruptly opened and a burst of airflow is released. Such actions are generated in association with airtight closure of the velopharynx. Not all stop consonants demonstrate a burst of airflow following occlusion of the oral airway. Some release the pent-up air through a lowering of the velum. This allows air to escape inaudibly through the nasal cavities. This type of stop consonant occurs in American English but is not phonemically distinctive.

Fricative consonants are generated when air is forced at high velocity through a narrowly constricted laryngeal or pharyngeal-oral airway. Such sounds derive their acoustic energy from turbulent airflow near their constrictions and from airflow striking nearby obstacles such as the teeth. Fricative consonants are usually produced with a closed velopharynx, although this is not obligatory if the constriction is upstream of the velopharynx, as in a fricative produced within the larynx (/h/).

Affricate consonants are usually produced with a closed velopharynx. Such consonants start out much like stop-plosive consonants in that the oral airway is occluded and air pressure builds up behind the occlusion. The occlusion for affricate consonants is released less abruptly than for stop-plosive consonants and a burst of airflow. These characteristics of the release phase of affricate consonants are the main features that distinguish their productions from those of stop-plosives.

Nasal consonants are produced with an occluded oral airway and an open velopharyngeal airway. The aeromechanical and acoustic energy associated with their production is transmitted through the nasopharynx and nasal cavities and is emitted from the external nares. They can be described as sonorants because the airway is open via the velopharyngeal airway and to the atmosphere via the nares.

Semivowels are consonant sounds produced with an oral airway that is more constricted than vowels but not as constricted as obstruents. Semivowels are generated with the velopharynx closed and the aeromechanical and acoustic energy associated with their production passing through the pharyngeal-oral airway.

Place of Production

Place of production describes the location of the consonant constriction or occlusion along the laryngeal and pharyngeal-oral airway. This dimension encompasses seven sites: *labial, labiodental, dental, alveolar, palatal, velar,* and *glottal*. In the order listed, these constriction or occlusion sites lie progressively farther inward along the combined pharyngeal-oral and laryngeal airways.

Labial means that only the two lips participate in the primary action having to do with place of production. An exception exists for the semivowel /w/, which is also specified as requiring a high-back tongue configuration. *Labiodental* indicates that the place of production is between the lower lip and the upper teeth. *Dental, alveolar, palatal,* and *velar* places of production designate locations where the tongue contacts or comes very close to contacting the teeth, upper gum ridge (inside the teeth), hard palate, and velum (soft palate and uvula), respectively. The *glottal* place of production entails primary action of the two vocal folds.

Voicing

The *voicing* dimension for stop-plosives, fricatives, and affricates is binary. That is, voice is either on or off for consonant productions, so consonants are categorized as either *voiced* or *voiceless*. Many of the consonants of American English form cognate pairs that differ only on the voicing dimension. Thus, two consonants in a cognate pair match one another in their manner of production and place of production, but differ from one another because one is *voiced* and the other is *voiceless*. In English, cognate pairs exist for the three places of articulation for stop-plosives, the four places for fricatives, and for the single place of articulation for affricates. The nasal and semivowel manners of production are *voiced*.

SPEECH PRODUCTION STREAM: ARTICULATORY PROCESSES

The previous section provides articulatory descriptions related to place/constriction/lip rounding for vowels and place/manner/voicing for consonants. A limitation of these descriptions, however, is that they are timeless. The speech production process is not a linear assemblage of a series of idealized segment characteristics (e.g., place or manner of articulation), nor is it a series of invariant positions and movement sequences strung together like beads on a string (MacNeilage, 1970). Instead, articulatory processes in speech production require discussion of displacements and speeds of articulatory movement, coordination between articulators to produce speech sounds and speech sound sequences, and coarticulation, which is the influence of the articulatory movements of one sound on those of an adjacent sound or even a nonadjacent sound.

Studies of movements of the speech production apparatus, especially of the pharyngeal-oral subsystem, reveal the limitations of a simple articulatory description. X-ray images, obtained from speakers of several different languages, show the mandible, tongue, velum, and lips to undergo continuous movement throughout even the simplest sequence of sounds (Munhall, Vatikiotis-Bateson, & Tohkura, 1995). Such x-ray images reveal the sequencing and coordination of articulatory events to be far more complex than a series of discrete speech sounds abutted to one another. Rather, the speech production stream, as visualized at the level of articulatory movement, appears to be fluid and continuous and to show no obvious boundaries between successive sounds. Moreover, examination of x-ray images suggests that very different movements can be associated with a single speech sound, such as a vowel, depending on the identity of the surrounding consonants. It is no exaggeration to say that the continuous and changeable movements of the articulators correspond poorly with the discrete symbols of phonetic transcription. Speech scientists have spent the last many decades attempting to determine the relationship between articulatory movements and the intuitively appealing idea of speech production being guided by a set of discrete symbols such as phonemes or a phonetic transcription. An important concept that has helped explain certain deviations from the idealized descriptive scheme is that of coarticulation.

Coarticulation

The examination of images of articulatory movements within the pharyngeal-oral apparatus during speech production clearly shows how the articulatory movements for one sound influence the movements for another sound. This mutual influence is most apparent between adjacent sounds, but it can extend across several sounds. For example, in both the words "Sue" [su] and "stew" [stu], the lip rounding that is a part of the phonetic description for /u/ is observed during the [s] part of the articulatory sequence. The same thing happens when the sequence is reversed, as in "twos" [tuz] and "toots" [tuts]. In both cases, lip rounding for the /u/ may extend to the lingua-alveolar fricative /z/ or /s/, even when the fricative is separated from the /u/ by a stop consonant. These are examples of coarticulation, defined as "the influence of one sound on another" (Daniloff & Hammarberg, 1973; Farnetani & Recasens, 2010). These mutual influences of immediately adjacent and nonadjacent sounds on one another explain, in part, why the articulators undergo continuous movement through a sound sequence and why it is so hard to identify clear sound boundaries from records of articulatory movement.

Speech scientists usually agree on two kinds of coarticulation. Forward coarticulation (also called right-to-left coarticulation and anticipatory coarticulation) occurs when the articulatory characteristics of an upcoming sound influence the characteristics of a currently produced sound. The production of lip rounding during the [s] in "Sue" is an example of an upcoming articulatory requirement (the lip rounding for /u/) occurring during the current /s/ articulation. The "forward" and "right-to-left" descriptions are meant to convey the idea that articulatory characteristics ahead in the speech production stream influence currently articulated sounds. Backward coarticulation (also called left-to-right coarticulation and carryover coarticulation) occurs when a currently articulated sound is influenced by the articulatory characteristics of a previous sound in the speech production stream. For example, in the word "toots" [tuts], the articulatory characteristics of the /s/ include some lip rounding because of the previously articulated [u]. The "backward" and "left-to-right" descriptions suggest the idea that the currently articulated sound is being influenced by a preceding articulatory event. A schematic illustration of forward and backward coarticulation is provided in Figure 5–23.

Figure 5–23 contains the terms that pertain to hypothesized mechanisms for the two types of coarticulation. Right-to-left coarticulation has been hypothesized to reflect anticipatory processes (anticipatory coarticulation), and left-to-right coarticulation has been hypothesized to reflect inertial properties of the articulators (carryover coarticulation). These hypothesized mechanisms are associated with what is called the traditional theory of coarticulation. This theory is based on the idea of feature spreading.

Traditional Theory of Coarticulation (Feature Spreading)

Speech sounds are often conceptualized as consisting of a small set of features, consistent with the phonetic [s   u]   [t u t s]

Lip rounding   Lip rounding

Forward coarticulation   Backward coarticulation

Right-to-left coarticulation   Left-to-right coarticulation

Anticipatory coarticulation   *Carryover* coarticulation

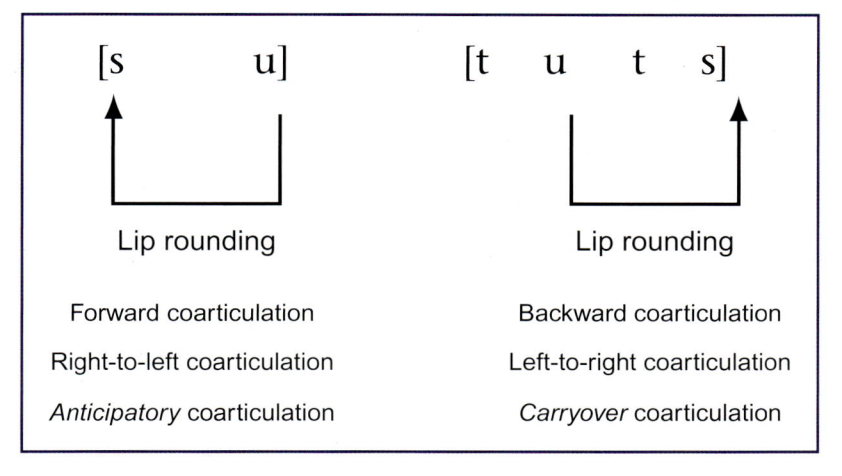

Figure 5–23. Schematic illustration of forward and backward coarticulation. Forward coarticulation (also called right-to-left and anticipatory coarticulation) means that a sound later in a sequence influences the production of an earlier sound in the sequence. Backward coarticulation (also called left-to-right and carryover coarticulation) means that an earlier sound in a sequence influences the production of a later sound. The symbols represent the words "Sue" and "toots."

descriptions discussed above. Many speech scientists combine linguistic theory with the problem of speech motor control by specifying the plan for an articulatory sequence as a string of phonemes, each of which is composed of a "bundle of features" that form the identity of each phoneme. This is very much like the discussion provided above (Figures 5–21 and 5–22) of phonemes described as timeless places of articulation, manners of articulation, and so forth. A small-scale example of this is shown in Figure 5–24, where the words "stew" /stu/, "used" /just/ (as in "used to it"), "bomb" /bɑm/, and "mob" /mɑb/ are shown as phonemic representations specified by a set of features. The features listed in Figure 5–24 are not the complete set for each phoneme, but they suffice to illustrate the concept of feature spreading. Four features are shown, including sonorant, coronal, lip rounding, and nasal. Each of the four features in a phoneme column can be specified as "+," "−," or left blank. A feature specified as "+" means the phoneme is produced with that feature, a specification of "−" indicates the explicit absence of that feature from the phoneme's production, and a blank means that the phoneme is not specified one way or the other for the feature.

Consider the phoneme /s/ as an example of articulatory feature specification (see upper panel of Figure 5–24). /s/ is "−" for sonorant (not produced with an open pharyngeal-oral airway), "+" for coronal (produced by raising the tongue blade to the front of the hard palate), blank (unspecified) for lip rounding, and "−" for nasal (because fricatives are produced with a closed velopharynx). In the traditional theory of coarticulation, the unspecified entries are of great interest because they allow a feature (or features) associated with an upcoming sound to migrate or spread to a currently articulated sound. For example, in the word "stew" /stu/, the unspecified lip rounding feature for /s/ allows the upcoming lip rounding feature for /u/ to be anticipated and produced during the /s/. The same set of conditions applies to the /t/ in "stew." Thus, when the word is articulated, lip rounding occurs on the two sounds prior to /u/. That is, [stu] shows coarticulation in the form of anticipatory lip rounding on the two consonants preceding the vowel for which lip rounding is required. Lip rounding associated with the vowel spreads to the preceding two consonants because it does not compromise their articulatory characteristics. An /s/ or /t/ can be articulated with the lips rounded or spread without changing the phonemic value of the sound. The flip side of this is that conflicting feature specifications cannot be spread through anticipation, because this would compromise the phonemic value of a sound. As an example, the /s/ and /t/ in "stew" are both specified as "−" for sonorant, whereas the vowel /u/ is specified as "+" for this feature. The "+" sonorant specification for /u/ cannot be anticipated for the /s/ and /t/ articulations because it would compromise their articulatory requirement for a

	/s	t	u/	/u	s	t/
Sonorant	−	−	+	+	−	−
Coronal	+	+	−	−	+	+
Lip rounding			+	+		
Nasal	−	−			−	−

	/b	ɑ	m/	/m	ɑ	b/
Sonorant	−	+	+	+	+	−
Coronal	−	−	−	−	−	−
Lip rounding	−	−	−	−	−	−
Nasal	−		+	+		−

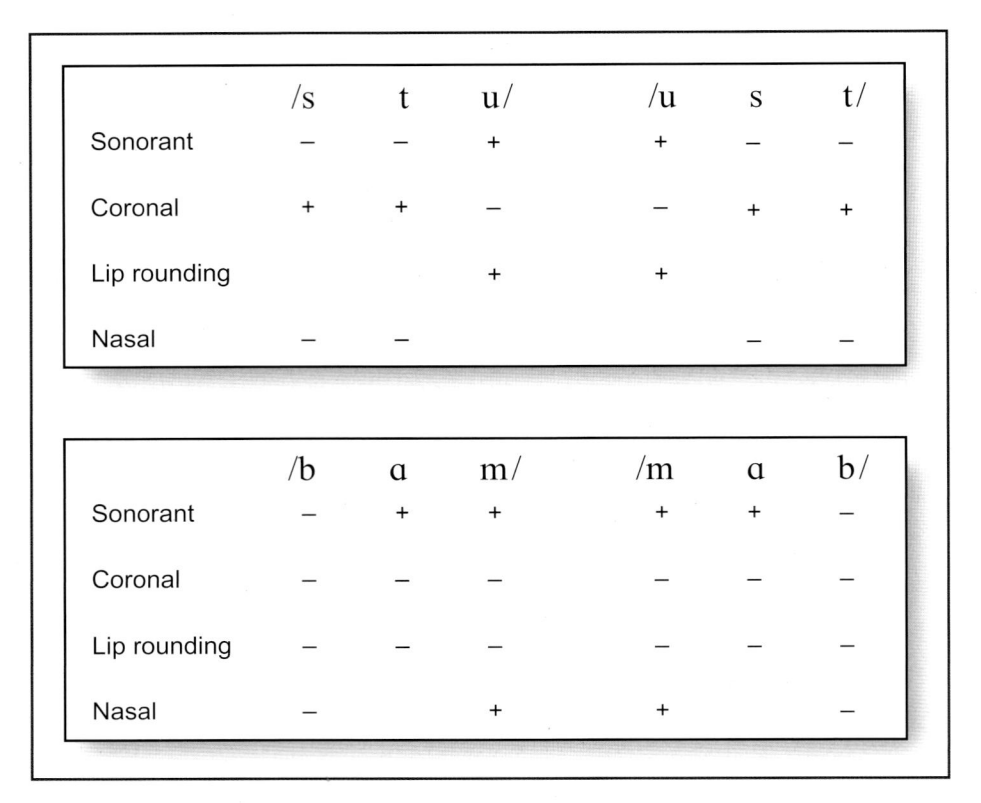

Figure 5–24. Plans for articulatory sequences as strings of phonemes composed of bundles of features, with only selected features represented. Sonorant means that a sound is made with a relatively open pharyngeal-oral airway or free passage through the nasal cavities; coronal refers to consonant sounds made by raising the tongue tip or blade toward the teeth or hard palate; lip rounding refers to vowels or consonants in which rounding of the lips is an integral feature; and nasal means that the sound is made with an open velopharyngeal port. The features are shown as specified (+), absent (−), or not specified (left blank). The symbols represent the words "stew," "used," "bomb," and "mob."

nearly complete constriction (/s/) or obstruction (/t/) of the airway.

A different example of anticipatory (forward) coarticulation is given in the lower left part of Figure 5–24. There, the feature specifications for the phoneme sequence /bɑm/ "bomb" show that all features are specified except the nasal feature for the vowel /ɑ/. The "+" nasal specification for the upcoming /m/ can, therefore, be spread to /ɑ/, resulting in a partially or completely nasalized vowel. In English, nasalization of vowels has no effect on phonemic status, so the feature spreading does not compromise the integrity of the speaker's articulatory intent or the listener's ability to recover the spoken word.

Explanations and mechanisms have been proposed to account for anticipatory coarticulation (Farnetani & Recasens, 2010; Kent, 1976). One explanation is that anticipatory coarticulation constitutes the ability to anticipate articulatory features before they are needed and is one of the ways in which speech production movements are smoothed out and made continuous across a sequence of sounds. This avoids the obviously inefficient situation of having to articulate each phoneme's "bundle of features" in discrete and successive chunks. Thus, the continuous articulation observed in x-ray studies of the movement of the pharyngeal-oral apparatus is an expression of speech motor efficiency.

A proposed mechanism for anticipatory coarticulation is one in which the plan for articulatory behavior is in the form of a sequence of phonemes and their respective feature specifications, such as depicted in Figure 5–24. Quite literally, the phoneme sequence and component features are believed to be represented in the brain. A programming operation, often referred to as a "look-ahead" operator (Daniloff & Hammarberg, 1973; Henke, 1966), scans the phoneme sequence from left to right—the intended output order—and finds features that can be anticipated without compromising the articulatory identity of a sound. In a sense, the look-ahead operator is the mechanism of anticipatory coarticulation and has the task of identifying features that can be spread from a later to an earlier occurring phoneme.

Explanations and mechanisms have also been proposed for carryover (left-to-right or backward) coarticulation. In the traditional view, carryover coarticulation is believed to be the result of articulators being unable to move immediately from one position to the next because they have mass and demonstrate inertia. The right side of Figure 5–24 contains two examples of this. In the upper right sequence, the "+" for the /u/ in "used" specifies rounded lips, which not only occur when the [u] is produced, but remains to some extent during the [s] and possibly even the [t] because the lips cannot move instantaneously from a rounded to an unrounded configuration. Similarly, the example in the lower right part of Figure 5–24 indicates an open velopharyngeal port for the [m] in "mob" which cannot be closed instantaneously for the following [ɑ]. In both cases, an articulatory feature of one sound is carried over to a following sound because the articulators are subject to inertial laws.

Anticipatory and carryover coarticulation are regarded as very different phenomena, even though they both involve feature spreading. Anticipatory coarticulation is thought of as a planning or programming phenomenon, whereas carryover coarticulation is thought to be the result of the physical characteristics of the speech production apparatus. A more general model of speech production, in which the notion of feature spreading is incorporated, is depicted in Figure 5–25. This model shows an input to the speech production apparatus, which, in this case, is the phonemic representation and feature components of the utterance "no seat" (as in "There is no seat in the auditorium"). Figure 5–25 suggests a cognitive representation of a yet to be discovered neural code. As in Figure 5–24, some of the features are specified and some are not. The input is delivered to a programming module, where the look-ahead operator determines the available forward coarticulations. The phonemic input with coarticulatory modifications is translated

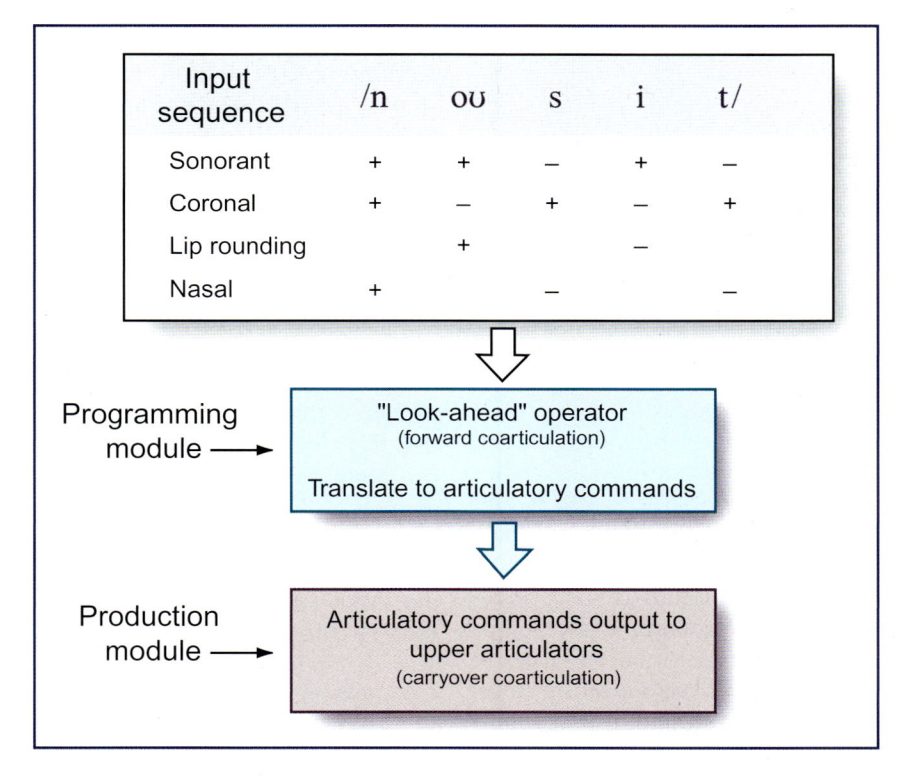

Figure 5–25. General model of speech production in which phonemic representation and feature spreading are operations of the model. The input sequence represents the words "no seat."

into a form suitable for speech production. This translation takes the form of motor commands to the different articulators, including the timing and strength of contraction of the many muscles involved in speech production. These commands are sent to a production module, which implements them in the form of movements of the articulators. Carryover coarticulation occurs at this stage of production, allowing features to spread from left to right as a result of the inertial properties of the articulators.

This view of articulatory production, although greatly simplified, is accepted by most speech-language pathologists. For example, when a client is diagnosed with apraxia of speech, there is an assumption of dysfunction in the programming component of the speech production process. Such programming dysfunction is believed to operate on input units that are very much like the phoneme representations portrayed in Figures 5–24 and 5–25. The details of these units or how they enter into the actual articulatory errors observed in apraxia of speech may vary from explanation to explanation, but the basic structure of the underlying theory is much like the one described in this section. McNeil, Pratt, and Fosset (2004) have provided a detailed account of how errors in apraxia of speech can be accounted for by various speech production models that are all variants of the one depicted in Figure 5–25.

Problems with the Traditional Theory of Coarticulation

Application of the traditional theory of coarticulation to explanations of speech disorders such as apraxia of speech does not mean the theory is universally accepted. In fact, soon after the theory was developed and publicized in the late 1960s and early 1970s, some of its problems became apparent.

One problem with models of coarticulation specified by feature spreading is the assumption (usually implicit) that all sounds may potentially be affected by coarticulation in the same way. This is not the case. The term "coarticulatory resistance" is used to describe the degree to which a vowel or consonant is susceptible to influence from an adjacent consonant or vowel. For example, evidence suggests that the vowel /i/ is more resistant to coarticulation (shows less variation in its production depending on the immediate context) compared with vowels such as /ɑ/ and /u/ (see summary in Chen, Chang, and Iskarous [2015]). Similarly, the fricative /s/ shows a great deal of resistance to coarticulation, whereas the fricative /θ/ is quite variable depending on its context: /s/ therefore shows more coarticulatory resistance than /θ/ (Tabain, 2001). The idea of coarticulatory resistance applies to both vowels and consonants, and may affect speech sound correction strategies when sounds with low versus high coarticulatory resistance are expected to produce more or less variability, respectively, in the production of a sound under treatment.

The main problem with the traditional theory of coarticulation, according to critics, is the requirement of an input representation (phonemes) that may have no reality in the speech production process. Another criticism of the traditional theory is that it requires a mechanism to translate the phonemic representation to articulatory motions, contacts, and configurations. Critics of the traditional theory of coarticulation argue that it is awkward and unnecessary to imagine a speech production process in which a "digital" representation of speech (discrete phonemes) must be translated to an "analog" form (the smooth and continuous movements of the articulators). In other words, the traditional theory lacks a representation of the time element of articulatory behavior. The alternative proposed by these critics is an input to the speech production process that represents articulatory behavior as it unfolds over time.

Articulatory Phonology or Gesture Theory

Theories that reject the ideas of phonemes and their translation to speech motor behavior are variously

---

Raymond D. Kent

Kent has been one of the leading speech scientists in the world for over three decades. He has written extensively on a variety of topics, including speech development, normal speech acoustics, and the acoustics of speech associated with neuromotor speech disorders. His work, along with colleagues, has elucidated much of what is known about speech acoustics and inferred articulatory dynamics in speakers with dysarthria. A distinguishing feature of Kent's work is its multidisciplinary nature. Those who read his articles and books come away with an appreciation for his ability to integrate diverse literatures and bring them to bear on issues in his own discipline. Few can match him and those who know him well affectionately refer to him as "Clark Kent," the character of Superman fame, because of their awe for his powerful influence in speech science. He is retired and lives in Madison, Wisconsin.

called articulatory phonology (Browman & Goldstein, 1992) or gesture theories (Byrd, 1996; Saltzman & Munhall, 1989). The details of these different approaches to the production of articulatory behavior are less important than is a broad understanding of how these theories differ from the traditional theory of coarticulation. Figure 5–26 presents a model of the speech production process in which the focus is entirely on articulatory gestures (movements). The identity and timing of selected gestures are shown for production of the word "sinew" [sɪnju]. Five gestures are listed, including those of the tongue tip, tongue body, velopharyngeal port, lips, and larynx. These gestures unfold in time, from left to right, just as the sounds for the word "sinew" occur in sequence. The time course of each gesture is indicated by the length of its associated rectangle. The onset and offset of the lip rounding gesture are shown to illustrate how the timing of each rectangle should be interpreted.

The primary impression from this display is of the different articulatory gestures occurring at different onsets and offsets throughout the utterance, and of gestures overlapping in time. For example, in addition to the overlap between the open velopharyngeal port gesture and the tongue tip raising gesture for [n], the open port gesture also overlaps with the tongue body gestures for both the preceding [i] and the following [ju]. Thus, the sounds preceding and following the nasal sound are produced with a somewhat open velopharyngeal port. In articulatory phonology or gesture theories, this phenomenon is called coproduction, to indicate that two or more gestures are produced at the same time and overlap to some degree. In the traditional theory, the partial nasalization of [i] is an example of anticipatory coarticulation, and the partial nasalization of [ju] is an example of carryover coarticulation. In the traditional theory both are the result of feature spreading (see Figure 5–24). Articulatory phonology or gesture theorists use the term "coproduction," rather than "coarticulation," to avoid the phoneme representation implications of the traditional theory. The overlap of the open velopharyngeal port gesture with the tongue body gestures for the two flanking vowels is just that—overlap—and does not reflect the operation of an extra programming process (anticipatory coarticulation) or the physical limitation of articulatory movement (carryover coarticulation).

A criticism of the traditional theory of coarticulation is that it does not account for the timing details of articulatory behavior (Kent & Minifie, 1977). For example, x-ray images of articulatory sequences such as occur in the word "bums" [bʌmz] reveal that the

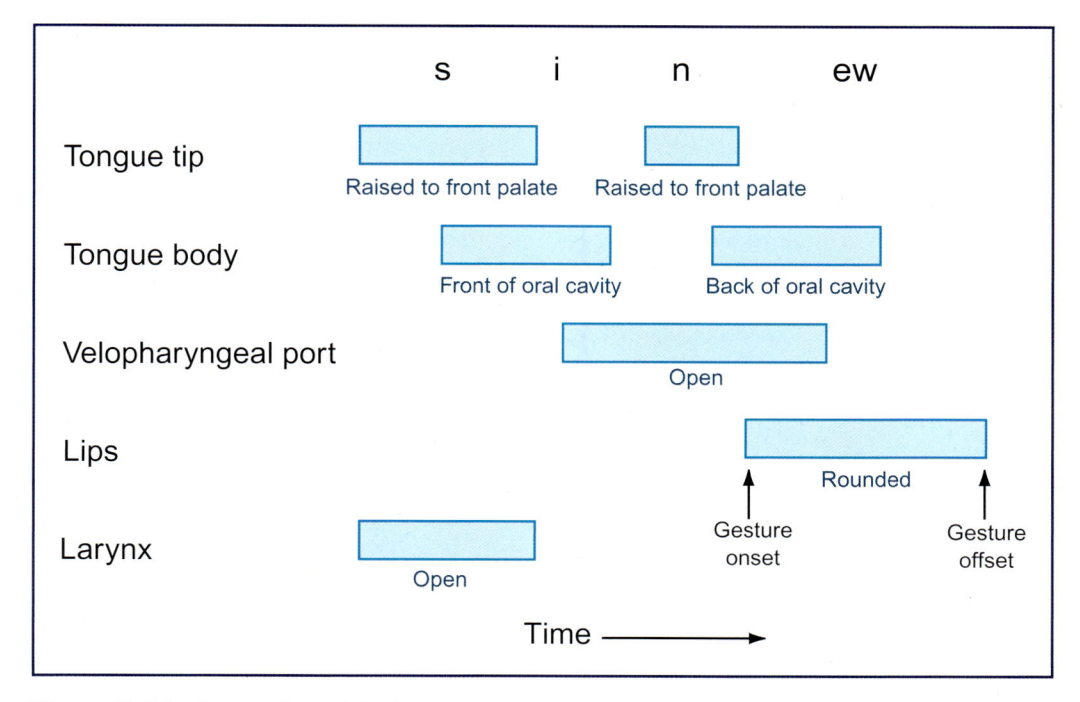

Figure 5–26. General model of speech production in which there is no phonemic representation and focus is on the articulatory gestures (movements). Rectangles delimit the time course of individual gestures of selected articulators. This represents the production of the word "sinew."

velopharyngeal port is actually closing during the lip closure portion of the [m], apparently in anticipation of the fricative requirement of a closed velopharynx. Two questions to be asked are, "How does the traditional theory account for this timing?" and "Why is the nasal '+' specification for [m] contradicted by a *closing* gesture of the velopharyngeal port (like a '−' specification) when the lips are closed for the bilabial nasal?" Articulatory phonology or gesture theories address these two questions by eliminating the plus, minus, or unspecified feature characteristics of sounds and the need for them to have phonemic representation. The closing velopharyngeal port during the lip seal for [m] simply reflects the degree of overlap between gestures of the lips and velopharynx.

In articulatory phonology or gesture theories, it is the sequencing and overlapping of multiple gestures that results in articulatory sequences. An examination of the gestures portrayed in Figure 5–26 suggests that the timing component is complicated. Somehow, the gestures have to be specified for their duration and for their phasing (when one gesture begins relative to another gesture). For example, the first tongue tip gesture (raised to front palate) begins earlier in time than the first tongue body gesture (front of oral cavity). These precise phasings, or timings, of successive articulatory gestures are very important because incorrect phasing can result in poorly formed (and hard to understand) articulatory sequences. An example of this is the larynx gesture (open), which represents the abduction of the vocal folds required for the voiceless fricative [s] at the beginning of the word. If this gesture is phased later relative to the tongue tip gesture and nothing else is changed, a good portion of the vowel [i] may be devoiced and therefore difficult to understand. In articulatory phonology or gesture theories, each gesture can slide in time relative to other gestures. This is a very attractive feature of these theories for certain speech disorders, such as ataxic dysarthria (a speech problem caused by dysfunction of the cerebellum), in which articulatory gestures seem to be pulled apart (not overlapped correctly). The pulling apart of articulatory gestures may be the result of improper phasing or gestures that are allowed to slide too much with respect to each other. The basic structure of articulatory phonology or gesture theories seems to have more potential for application to speech disorders than the traditional theory of coarticulation.

VARIABLES THAT INFLUENCE PHARYNGEAL-ORAL FUNCTION

One need only look at a group of men, women, and children and listen to them speak to know that age and sex have an influence on the structure and function of the pharyngeal-oral apparatus. The effects of age are most apparent during the first couple of decades of life, though they continue on a more gradual time scale throughout the remainder of the lifespan. The influence of sex emerges early in life and is maintained through senescence.

Age

Age brings change and these changes affect the anatomical and physiological substrates that support speaking and swallowing. The pharyngeal-oral apparatus at birth is a far cry from that in adulthood, and the senescent apparatus shows the wear and tear of the aging process when held up against its younger counterpart.

The skeletal framework of the pharyngeal-oral apparatus of the newborn infant differs from that of the adult in both size and configuration, as illustrated in Figure 5–27. At birth, the skull of the newborn is rela-

---

Eye Eye Eye Eye Eye

This title should catch your eye (pun intended). As a clinician you need to develop a good eye for eyes. Eyes can be an eye opener for identifying syndromes that include pharyngeal-oral problems. We can bear eyewitness to this from our own experiences. Consider the physical spacing of the eyes. Most faces are five-eyes wide at eye level. This means that a space the width of one eye should fit between the two eyes and another eye should fit between the outside corner of each eye and the side of the face. Departures from this pattern come in several forms, the most common being that the two eyes are too widely spaced or too narrowly spaced. Any abnormal pattern should catch your eye and immediately cause you to eye the pharyngeal-oral apparatus for frank and subtle abnormalities. Hopefully, we see eye to eye on this. Work on developing your eye for eyes.

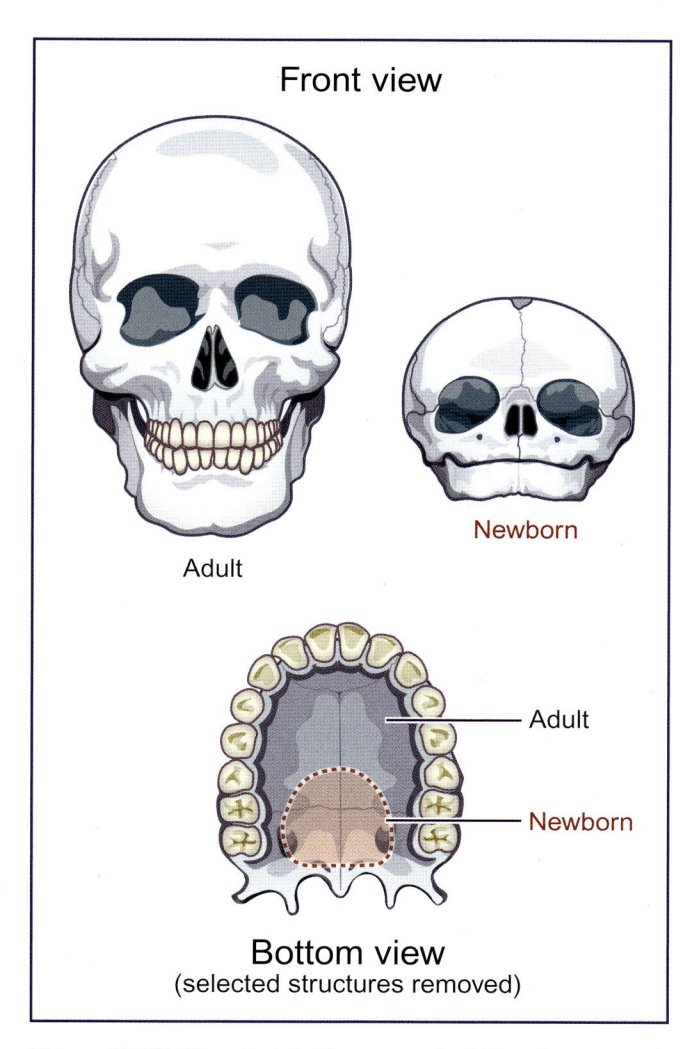

Figure 5–27. The skeletal framework of the pharyngeal-oral apparatus of the newborn infant and the adult.

tively large compared with the body. The facial part of the skull is small, being about one-eighth of the bulk of the cranium of the newborn as opposed to about one-half of the bulk of the cranium in the adult (Zemlin, 1998). After the first year of life, the facial skeleton grows at a much faster rate than the cranial skeleton.

Although the cranium approximates adult size relatively early in childhood, perhaps as early as 6 years of age (Melsen & Melsen, 1982), the facial skeleton continues to grow into adolescence and possibly adulthood (Kent & Vorperian, 1995; Richtsmeier & Cheverud, 1986). During this growth period, the front-to-back depth of the bony palate nearly doubles, whereas the side-to-side expansion of the structure increases significantly less (Zemlin, 1998). The mandible also grows in size and changes in shape during its growth period (Scott, 1976). The body of the mandible increases in length to accommodate the addition of three permanent teeth on each side, and the angle between the ramus and body of the mandible becomes less obtuse (Zemlin, 1998). Growth of the mandible continues until near adulthood and progresses relatively steadily with occasional growth spurts at certain ages (Walker & Kowalski, 1972). Dental development is subject to significant individual variation, its consistent hallmark being the loss of 20 deciduous teeth and their replacement with 32 permanent teeth (Scott, 1976).

Soft structures of the pharyngeal-oral apparatus also undergo nonlinear developmental change during infancy and childhood (Vorperian et al, 2009). In the newborn infant, the pharyngeal cavity is about 4 cm in length and appreciably shorter than the oral cavity (Crelin, 1973). The contour of the junction between the pharyngeal and oral parts of the pharyngeal-oral apparatus is rounded in the newborn infant, assumes an oblique angle at about 5 years of age, and approximates the right-angle configuration of the adult around the time of puberty (Kent & Vorperian, 1995). The predominant feature of pharyngeal development is its vertical enlargement (Vorperian et al., 2005, 2009), with the pharynx tripling in length to become about 12 cm long by adulthood (Tourne, 1991).

The tongue of the newborn infant essentially fills the oral cavity (Crelin, 1976). During the first year of life the structure begins to descend within the neck and continues to do so until about 5 years of age (Laitman & Crelin, 1976). Growth of the tongue is relatively continual throughout childhood and on through puberty, showing occasional growth spurts along the way (Kerr, Kelly, & Geddes, 1991). The patterning of growth of the tongue tends to be in general harmony with the patterning of growth of the mandible (Kent & Vorperian, 1995).

The lips undergo significant developmental change between birth and adulthood. They form a near circular sphincter in the newborn infant, whereas they form a transverse, elliptical sphincter in the adult. Major reconfiguration of the lips occurs during the first 2 years of life (Burke, 1980). Thereafter, lip size changes, with forward growth of the lower lip exceeding that of the upper lip. Rapid growth of the lips is reported to occur between 10 and 17 years of age (Vig & Cohen, 1979). Growth spurts of the lips appear to be correlated with those occurring in the mandible (Walker & Kowalski, 1972).

Along with the anatomical changes described above, various aspects of the nervous system also undergo change. Neural development follows a protracted time course that extends well into adolescence. This development reflects change in cognition, memory, motor control, and other nervous system functions that are relevant to the encoding of movement by the pharyngeal-oral apparatus. Such development is conditioned by nervous system change that involves maturation in synaptic connections, axon diameters, dendrite branching, myelination of motor and sensory pathways, and the establishment of more ingrained neural networks for preferred activities (Benes, Turtle, Khan, & Farol, 1994; Huttenlocher, 1990; Lecours, 1975; Netsell, 1986; Paus et al., 2001).

Characteristic of the development of movement control of the pharyngeal-oral apparatus are sensitive periods in which skill acquisition is continuous but nonlinear and during which incremental increases in performance take what appear to be jumps forward (Netsell, 1986). Certain changes in the development of movement control appear to be governed by factors operating over long periods and involving persistent effects, whereas others occur over shorter periods (Newell, Liu, & Meyer-Kress, 2001). Motor commands to the muscles of the developing pharyngeal-oral apparatus are generated through a background of "neural noise" that may be unrelated to a movement goal (Crossman & Szafran, 1956; Schmidt, Zelaznik, Hawkins, Frank, & Quinn, 1979; Welford, 1956). Such noise influences movement proficiency and is thought to be of major significance but to decrease in importance over the course of development (Jones, Hamilton, & Wolpert, 2002; Smits-Engelsman & Van Galen, 1997; Yan, Thomas, Stelmach, & Thomas, 2000).

Studies of speech production have revealed differences in pharyngeal-oral control in children compared with adults. For example, whereas lip movements during speech production are primarily vertical in adults, they begin as more horizontal (spreading) in infants and develop a more vertical movement component over the first few years of life (Iuzzini-Seigel, Hogen, Rong, & Green, 2015). Nevertheless, the most prominent speech production difference between children and adults is that children speak more slowly (Kent & Forner, 1980; Nittrouer, 1993; Smith & McLean-Muse, 1986; Smith, Sugarman, & Long, 1983; Sturm & Seery, 2007) and with greater variability. Such variability is manifested in amplitude, velocity, timing, and general patterning of pharyngeal-oral movements during speech production (Goffman & Smith, 1999; Green, Moore, Higashikawa, & Steeve, 2000; Green, Moore, & Reilly, 2002; Grigos, 2009; Maner, Smith, & Grayson, 2000; Sharkey & Folkins, 1985; Smith & Goffman, 1998; Smith & McLean-Muse, 1986; Steeve, Moore, Green, Reilly, & McMurtrey, 2008; Watkin & Fromm, 1984).

Transition to faster and more stable speech production continues throughout development. Observations of pharyngeal-oral movements indicate that adult-like performance is not reached until near the end of the teenage years (Smith & Zelaznik, 2004; Walsh & Smith, 2002). Coordinative movement patterns also undergo development across childhood and adolescence in the form of changes in muscle synergies that influence how different structures become functionally coupled to one another during speech performance. An example is how the upper lip, lower lip, and mandible can be variously adjusted to bring about a resultant opening or closing of the lip aperture (Smith & Zelaznik, 2004). While muscle synergies are developing, the diversity of movement routines is also undergoing change. As a child develops, a wider range of movements can be generated, greater variation is possible in the combination of different movements, and the order in which movements can be combined becomes less rigid (Menn, 1983; Nittrouer, 1993). Beyond this, the pace at which speech production skills are acquired and the nature of the developmental trajectory are not uniform across children or structures (Nittrouer, 1993), and may even be manifested in clusters of different developmental profiles (Vick et al., 2012).

Speech production is a motor skill that is functional throughout much of life and is preserved even in the oldest of the old. Once this skill is fully mature, it gives the appearance of involving little effort, proceeding automatically, and being highly ingrained. Most elderly people use this practiced motor skill exceedingly well and produce fully intelligible speech. This does not mean, however, that their speech production is unchanged from what it was decades earlier. As time passes, the structures and processes involved in speech production undergo modification. Although the features of interest are subject to change on different schedules and to different degrees in different parts of the apparatus, the majority of age-related changes manifest after the fifth decade of life (Kahane, 1990). Such changes tend to be gradual and progressive, but the greatest alterations, diminutions, and functional consequences occur during the senescent years.

The structure of the pharyngeal part of the pharyngeal-oral apparatus changes in several ways during adulthood. Overall, it gets larger. In young adults, the lower edge of the cricoid cartilage is positioned at the upper edge of the seventh cervical vertebra. This positioning lowers during adulthood until, by senescence, the lower edge of the cricoid cartilage reaches the bottom of the seventh cervical vertebra and even farther (Wind, 1970). One result of this lowering of the laryngeal framework is that the pharynx lengthens. It also increases in cross-section as the muscles of the pharynx tend to weaken and atrophy and the pharyngeal lumen widens and dilates (Linville & Fisher, 1985; Zaino & Benventano, 1977). The epithelial lining of the pharynx undergoes progressive thinning (Ferreri, 1959), the compliance (relative floppiness) of the pharyngeal tube increases with age (Huang et al., 1998), and the capacity to voluntarily move the pharynx progressively decreases with age (Sonies, Stone, & Shawker, 1984). Sensory innervation in the pharyngeal region decreases and sensory discrimination goes through a significant decline (Aviv et al., 1994; Ferreri, 1959).

The oral part of the pharyngeal-oral apparatus (oral cavity and oral vestibule) also changes in several ways during adulthood. The oral airway undergoes a gradual increase in size with age, probably in both length and cross section, an increase that is believed to continue even into senescence (Israel, 1968, 1973). The oral epithelium thins, loses some of its elasticity, and becomes less firmly attached to adjacent bone and connective tissue (Squire, Johnson, & Hoops, 1976). Salivary production declines and saliva thickens and alters in composition (Baum, 1981; Chauncey, Borkan, Wayler, Feller, & Kapur, 1981), possibly accounting for why the elderly have more oral infections, more oral lesions (sores), and more loose teeth than their younger counterparts (Sonies, 1991).

In those individuals who lose teeth with age, alveolar bone may be resorbed (dissolved), sometimes significantly so (Klein, 1980), although this is less of a problem with current high-quality dental care than in the past (Zemlin, 1998). The bones of the oral cavity and oral vestibule may become more fragile, cartilages may lose some of their resiliency, ligaments may lose some of their elasticity, fat may get redistributed, and muscle bulk and power may wane with aging (Fremont & Hoyland, 2007).

Sensory and motor capabilities of the oral part of the pharyngeal-oral apparatus also decrease with age. For example, oral form, pressure, and touch discrimination are poorer in elderly adults than in young adults (Canetta, 1977). Spatial acuity on the surface of the lips also declines significantly in old age (Bilodeau-Mercure & Tremblay, 2016; Wohlert, 1996b). The tongue may lose strength (Peladeau-Pigeon & Steele, 2017; Vanderwegen, Guns, Van Nuffelen, Elen, & De Bodt, 2013), mobility (Amerman & Parnell, 1982), range of motion (Sonies, Baum, & Shawker, 1984), and sensitivity (Bilodeau-Mercure & Tremblay, 2016) with age. Lip endurance (the ability to exert pressure over time) also declines with age (Bilodeau-Mercure & Tremblay, 2016). Reflex responses of lip muscles are significantly lower in amplitude and longer in latency in elderly compared with young individuals (Wohlert, 1996a).

Some of the age-related changes discussed to this juncture may affect speech production. Three prominently discussed manifestations of aging are changes that affect the resonance properties of the pharyngeal-oral airway, temporal features of speech production, and variability of speech production.

The length and cross-section of the pharyngeal and oral airways increase with age during adulthood and it is reasonable to assume that these changes might influence the resonant properties of the pharyngeal-oral apparatus during speaking. Nevertheless, it is unclear if they do. Although earlier reports have shown older adults to have lower vowel formants (major energy concentrations in the acoustic speech signal) than younger adults (Debruyne & Decoster, 1999; Linville & Fisher, 1985; Linville & Rens, 2001; Scukanec, Petrosino, & Squibb, 1991; Xue & Hao, 2003), others have found no consistent difference with age (Eichhorn, Kent, Austin, & Vorperian, 2017; Sebastian, Babu, Oommen, & Ballraj, 2012). Such contradictory findings are difficult to interpret. Nevertheless, it seems reasonable to speculate that, in those cases where no age effect is apparent, older individuals have made adaptive changes to their speech production to account for any age-related changes in the size and shape of their pharyngeal and oral airways.

Slowing is a hallmark of aging and is viewed as the most pervasive motor characteristic of getting older (Fremont & Hoyland, 2007; Welford, 1982). Slowing in the pharyngeal-oral apparatus is no exception and can be attributed to changes in parts of the nervous system that control the peripheral machinery of the apparatus, as well as to changes in the peripheral machinery itself (Fozard, Vercruyssen, Reynolds, Hancock, & Quilter,

---

Coming and Going

He could feel when it was coming. It would come on slowly, be there for a while, and then go away slowly. When it was gone, the speech sounded normal. But, when it was there, his speech sounded as if he were drunk. We studied him, using him as his own control. What could be better? He perfectly matched himself. The psychiatrist thought the problem was all in his mind. But it turned out otherwise. What made his speech alternately normal and abnormal was a condition called paroxysmal ataxia, an uncontrollable physiological change in the ability to transmit neural signals within the cerebellum. The neurologist who diagnosed the problem was concerned. Paroxysmal ataxia can be a harbinger of another diagnosis to come, multiple sclerosis. The unwanted coming and going of speech signs can mean the ultimate coming of something else unwanted. And so it turned out that this was the fate for this middle-aged man.

1994; Kahane, 1990; Kent & Burkard, 1981; Ulatowska, 1985; Weismer & Liss, 1991). The influence of age on breathing, laryngeal, and velopharyngeal-nasal function (described in Chapters 2, 3, and 4) combine with those of the pharyngeal-oral apparatus to produce a general slowing of speech production with advanced age. This slowing has two bases, one being that articulatory rate slows (longer individual speech segments, syllables, and sentences) and the other being that older speakers pause more often during running speech production (Bilodeau-Mercure & Tremblay, 2016; Bona, 2014; Hartman & Danhauer, 1976; Hoit & Hixon, 1987; Liss, Weismer, & Rosenbek, 1990; Ryan, 1972; Smith, Wasowicz, & Preston, 1987; Wohlert & Smith, 1998).

The variability of movement also undergoes change with age across adulthood. Such variability tends to increase with age and is often considered to be a measure of motor control integrity in general (Nelson, Soderberg, & Urbsheit, 1984; Weismer & Liss, 1991). For example, lip movements during speech production of different rates have been shown to have greater spatiotemporal variability in older adults compared with younger ones (Wohlert & Smith, 1998). Acoustic studies of speech also show greater age-related variability in measures such as sound and syllable durations (Smith et al., 1987; Weismer, 1984; Weismer & Fromm, 1983), and such variability becomes even more pronounced in the oldest of the old (Liss et al., 1990). Speech accuracy has been shown to decline in older individuals, particularly during the production of complex movement and sound sequences (Bilodeau-Mercure et al., 2015).

Sex

Everyone knows that speech usually sounds different when produced by men and women. From discussion in previous chapters, it is clear that sex-related differences in speech production and speech are strongly associated with sex-related differences in laryngeal structure and function, but that structure and function of the breathing apparatus and velopharyngeal-nasal apparatus are only minimally different between the sexes (see Chapters 2, 3, and 4). Here, attention turns to the potential contribution of pharyngeal-oral structure and function to sex-related differences in speech production and speech.

Perhaps the most obvious structural difference between men and women is size. Men tend to be larger than women overall, and this size difference is also reflected in the pharyngeal-oral apparatus. For example, the skull is larger (Zemlin, 1998) and the upper airway (from larynx to lips) is longer in men than women (Fitch & Giedd, 1999). One of the most important sex-related differences for speech production is that the pharynx is longer in men compared with women at rest (Fitch & Giedd, 1999) and during vowel production (Story, Hoffman, & Titze, 1997). Although sex-related size differences emerge strongly at puberty and continue to become more prominent until early adulthood (Fitch & Giedd, 1999; Goldstein, 1980), there are sex-related size differences in selected regions of the pharyngeal-oral apparatus even prior to puberty (Vorperian et al., 2011).

Men tend to be stronger than women. This also holds true for the strength of structures within the pharyngeal-oral apparatus. For example, men produce greater maximum lip forces (Barlow & Rath, 1985) and tongue forces (Youmans & Stierwalt, 2006) than women, though such findings are not universal (Peladeau-Pigeon & Steele, 2017). Also, when maximum tongue force production is normalized to body muscle mass, sex-related differences disappear (Mortimore, Fiddes, Stephens, & Douglas, 1999).

Pharyngeal-oral function during speech production has also been shown to differ somewhat between the sexes. For example, men produce syllable-, word-, and sentence-level utterances (Smith et al., 1987) and repetitions of speech movements (Nicholson & Kimura, 1996) at faster rates than women. Examination of a single structure, the tongue, also shows the same sex-related pattern for speed during diphthong productions and productions of two consecutive vowels, with the posterior tongue moving faster in men than women (Simpson, 2001, 2002). This difference in speed has been attributed to the fact that the male tongue must move a greater distance than the female tongue, particularly in the posterior region of the oral cavity, where the palate is domed and the pharynx is large in men.

Sex-related differences in the size of the pharyngeal-oral apparatus are reflected in speech (the acoustic product) in a number of ways. For example, the frequency spectrum of certain fricative consonants is lower in men than women due to size differences in the resonating cavities (Schwartz, 1968). Perhaps one of the most puzzling differences between the speech of men and women relates to the formant patterns (patterns of energy concentration) associated with vowel production. Although men have lower frequency vowel formants than women across adulthood (Eichhorn et al., 2017), as would be expected from the fact that men are larger than women, the differences in formant values are not what would be expected from size differences alone. Various explanations for this have been offered and include that: (a) women use smaller and longer constrictions than men in their vowel productions and these constrictions contribute to the creation of differ-

> **Faster than a Herd of Turtles**
>
> When you watch someone reading aloud, things are moving all over the place. The mandible, tongue, and lips can all be seen to move from here to there and back and then off again to somewhere else. The coordination among these structures is exquisite and the speech sounds come so fast that they blend together into a beautiful constant stream that flows quickly after the thoughts of the speaker. Running speech production is truly a marvelous thing to watch. The speed of articulatory movements is what impresses many observers. Look at those structures go. But just how fast are they moving? What would you guess? Put it in miles per hour: 500? 250? 125? Or would you guess 65 like a car traveling along a freeway? Well, things aren't always what they seem. The actual speed is less than 1 mile per hour. That's not much faster than a thundering herd of turtles and probably considerably less than your usual walking speed.

ent formant patterns (Fant, 1975); (b) women articulate in ways that create larger acoustic differences among vowels as a means of compensating for the wider distribution of energy across frequency (more widely spaced harmonics) provided by the voice source (Ryalls & Lieberman, 1982), and (c) the relative length of the female pharynx is so much shorter during vowel production (Story et al., 1997).

REVIEW

The pharyngeal-oral apparatus (along with the velopharyngeal-nasal apparatus) forms the upper airway, and is also called the vocal tract when referring to its acoustic properties.

The pharyngeal-oral apparatus is a flexible tube that extends from the larynx to the lips and undergoes an approximate 90-degree forward bend within the oropharynx.

The skeleton of the pharyngeal-oral apparatus consists of the cervical vertebrae and various bones of the skull and especially those of the face.

The maxilla consists of two complexly shaped bones that combine at the midline to form the upper jaw, most of the hard palate, and the alveolar process that houses the upper teeth.

The mandible is a large horseshoe-shaped bone that forms the lower jaw and holds the lower teeth.

The mandible articulates with the left and right temporal bones along the sides of the skull to form the temporomandibular joints, the only freely movable joints of the skull.

Movements of the mandible are conditioned by the mechanical arrangements of the temporomandibular joints, which allow a hinge action of the mandible in relation to the temporal bone, a front-to-back gliding action, and a side-to-side gliding action.

The oropharynx is located midway along the pharyngeal cavity and is the part of the pharynx of greatest importance to function of the pharyngeal-oral apparatus for speech production.

The oral cavity is formed by the teeth, alveolar processes of the maxilla and mandible, hard palate, velum, floor of the mouth (mainly the tongue), and the anterior faucial pillars, and a forward vestibule (entryway) that is formed by the lips, cheeks, teeth, and alveolar processes of the maxilla and mandible.

The buccal (cheek) cavity constitutes the small space between the gums and teeth internally and the lips and cheeks externally and connects to the oral cavity through spaces between the teeth and behind the last molars.

The pharyngeal-oral apparatus contains a mucous lining that consists of epithelium and connective tissues that are different at different locations within the apparatus and includes a general lining mucosa, a masticatory mucosa, and a specialized mucosa.

Passive and active forces act on the pharyngeal-oral apparatus, with active force coming from the contraction of muscles of the pharynx, mandible, tongue, and lips.

Muscles of the pharynx relevant to pharyngeal-oral function are the *middle constrictor, inferior constrictor*, and *stylopharyngeus*.

Muscles of the mandible include the *masseter, temporalis, internal pterygoid, external pterygoid, digastric, mylohyoid*, and *geniohyoid*.

Muscles of the tongue include the *superior longitudinal, inferior longitudinal, vertical, transverse, styloglossus, palatoglossus, hyoglossus*, and *genioglossus*.

Muscles of the lips include the *orbicularis oris, buccinator, risorius, levator labii superioris, levator labii superioris alaeque nasi, zygomatic major, zygomatic minor, depressor labii inferioris, mentalis, levator anguli oris, depressor anguli oris, incisivus labii superioris, incisivus labii inferioris*, and *platysma*.

Movements of the pharynx are vested in its sidewalls, back wall, and front wall and enable the lumen of the pharynx to be adjusted in size and shape, and the degree of coupling between the oropharynx and the oral cavity (through the palatoglossal arch) to be modified.

Movements of the mandible are conditioned by the physical arrangements of the temporomandibular joints and can involve both rotation and translation that combine to provide for vertical, front-to-back, and side-to-side adjustments of the structure.

Movements of the tongue derive from movements of the mandible, shifting of the tongue mass within the oral cavity, and changing of the shape of the tongue in various dimensions, all of which are facilitated by the biomechanical property of the tongue that enables it to function like a liquid-filled, incompressible, and pliable structure (a muscular hydrostat).

Movements of the lips are exceptionally versatile, with each lip being able to move independently or with the two lips coordinated in their movements, and with the range of possible adjustments including puckering, protruding, retracting, spreading, pointing, curling, groping, rounding, and plumping, among others.

The control variables of pharyngeal-oral function include pharyngeal-oral lumen size and configuration, pharyngeal-oral structural contact pressure, pharyngeal-oral airway resistance, and pharyngeal-oral acoustic impedance.

Pharyngeal-oral movements are controlled by the nervous system, with the final forms of control commands sent through cranial nerves to muscles, and with sensory innervation provided through cranial nerves to guide anticipated actions of the pharyngeal-oral apparatus and to keep track of its recent status.

Pharyngeal-oral functions of importance to this text include changing the degree of coupling between the oral cavity and atmosphere, chewing and swallowing, and sound generation and filtering.

The pharyngeal-oral apparatus, well known for its articulatory role in speech production, contributes significantly to the formation of different speech sounds and those sounds that can be described and categorized as sonorants and obstruents and vowels and consonants.

Vowels and diphthongs are sonorants and are produced with voicing by the larynx, exclusion of nasal participation by velopharyngeal closure, and using combinations of structural positions and movements that result in relatively unconstricted configurations of the pharyngeal-oral airway that are classified according to place of major constriction, degree of major constriction, and degree of lip rounding.

Consonant sounds include both obstruents and sonorants and are usually produced with a relatively constricted or obstructed airway, with or without voicing by the larynx, and/or with or without velopharyngeal closure, and using combinations of structural positions and movements that are classified according to manner of production, place of production, and voicing.

The speech production stream is fluid and ongoing and structures of the pharyngeal-oral apparatus move smoothly and nearly continuously from one position to another.

The traditional theory of coarticulation proposes that sounds in the speech production stream influence their neighbors through processes that are anticipatory and scan ahead and processes that are a reflection of the inertial properties of the speech production apparatus.

The traditional theory of coarticulation has been criticized for certain weaknesses and has been replaced by more recent articulatory phonology or gesture theories that propose that sounds in the speech production stream are assembled by the phasing of overlapping movement gestures of different structures and do not require schemes of phoneme representation to account for speech production behavior.

The development of pharyngeal-oral function in speech production involves a transition to faster speech production rates and more stable speech production movements across childhood, along with the development of muscle synergies and movement routines, whereas aging is manifested in changes in the resonances of the pharyngeal-oral airway, a slowing of speech production, and greater variability of performance.

Sex has certain influences on pharyngeal-oral function in speech production and speech that are related to faster utterance rates and movements in men than women and a longer pharyngeal airway in men than women that results in nonuniform differences in formants (resonances) between the sexes.

REFERENCES

Abd-El-Malek, S. (1939). Observations on the morphology of the human tongue. *Journal of Anatomy, 73*, 201–210.

Amerman, J., & Parnell, M. (1982). Oral motor precision in older adults. *Journal of the National Student Speech-Language-Hearing Association, 10*, 55–67.

Aviv, J., Martin, J., Jones, M., Wee, T., Diamond, B., Keen, M., & Blitzer, A. (1994). Age-related changes in pharyngeal and supraglottic sensation. *Annals of Otology, Rhinology, and Laryngology, 103*, 749–752.

Barlow, S., & Rath, E. (1985). Maximum voluntary closing forces in the upper and lower lips of humans. *Journal of Speech and Hearing Research, 28*, 373–376.

Baum, B. (1981). Evaluation of stimulated parotid saliva flow rate in different age groups. *Journal of Dental Research, 60*, 1292–1296.

Benes, F., Turtle, M., Khan, Y., & Farol, P. (1994). Myelination of a key relay zone in the hippocampal formation occurs in the human brain during childhood, adolescence, and adulthood. *Archives of General Psychiatry, 51*, 477–484.

Bilodeau-Mercure, M., Kirouac, V., Langlois, N., Ouellet, C., Gasse, I., & Tremblay, P. (2015). Movement sequencing in normal aging: Speech, oro-facial, and finger movements. *Age, 37*, 1–13.

Bilodeau-Mercure, M., & Tremblay, P. (2016). Age differences in sequential speech production: Articulatory and physiological factors. *Journal of the American Geriatrics Society, 64*, e177–e182.

Bodanis, D. (1995). It's in the air: Skin, stardust, radio waves, vitamins, spider legs. *Smithsonian, 26*, 76–81.

Bona, J. (2014). Temporal characteristics of speech: The effect of age and speech style. *Journal of the Acoustical Society of America, 136*, EL116–EL121.

Browman, C., & Goldstein, L. (1992). Articulatory phonology: An overview. *Phonetica, 49*, 155–180.

Burke, P. (1980). Serial growth changes in the lips. *British Journal of Orthodontics, 7*, 17–30.

Byrd, D. (1996). A phase window framework for articulatory timing. *Phonology, 13*, 139–169.

Canetta, R. (1977). Decline in oral perception from 20 to 70 years. *Perceptual Motor Skills, 45*, 1028–1030.

Chauncey, H., Borkan, G., Wayler, A., Feller, R., & Kapur, K. (1981). Parotid fluid composition in healthy young males. *Advances in Physiological Sciences, 28*, 323–328.

Chen W., Chang, Y., & Iskarous, K. (2015). Vowel coarticulation: Landmark statistics measure vowel aggression. *Journal of the Acoustical Society of America, 138*, 1221–1232.

Cheng, S., Butler, J., Gandevia, S., & Bilston, L. (2008). Movement of the tongue during normal breathing in awake healthy humans. *Journal of Physiology, 586*, 4283–4294.

Crelin, E. (1973). *Functional anatomy of the newborn*. New Haven, CT: Yale University Press.

Crelin, E. (1976). Development of the upper respiratory system. *Clinical Symposia, 28*, 1–30.

Crossman, E., & Szafran, J. (1956). Changes with age in the speed of information-intake and discrimination. *Experientia, 4*, 128–134.

Daniloff, R., & Hammarberg, R. (1973). On defining coarticulation. *Journal of Phonetics, 1*, 239–248.

Debruyne, F., & Decoster, W. (1999). Acoustic differences between sustained vowels perceived as young or old. *Logopedics Phoniatrics Vocology, 24*, 1–5

Dickson, D., & Maue-Dickson, W. (1982). *Anatomical and physiological bases of speech*. Boston, MA: Little, Brown and Company.

Doran, G., & Baggett, H. (1972). The genioglossus muscle: A reassessment of its anatomy in some mammals including man. *Acta Anatomica, 83*, 403–410.

Eichhorn, J., Kent, R., Austin, D., & Vorperian, H. (2017). Effects of aging on vocal fundamental frequency and vowel formants in men and women. *Journal of Voice*. Advance online publication. doi:10.1016/j.jvoice.2017.08.003

Fairbanks, G. (1960). *Voice and articulation drillbook*. New York, NY: Harper & Row.

Fant, G. (1975). Non-uniform vowel normalization. *Speech Transmission Laboratory—Quarterly Progress and Status Report, 2–3*, 1–19.

Farnetani, E., & Recasens, D. (2010). Coarticulation and connected speech processes. In W. J. Hardcastle, F. E. Gibbon, & J. Laver (Eds.), *Handbook of phonetic sciences* (2nd ed., pp. 316–352). Chichester, UK and Malden, MA: Wiley-Blackwell.

Ferreri, G. (1959). Senescence of the larynx. *Italian General Review of Oto-Rhino-Laryngology, 1*, 640–709.

Fitch, W., & Giedd, J. (1999). Morphology and development of the human vocal tract: A study using magnetic resonance imaging. *Journal of the Acoustical Society of America, 106*, 1511–1522.

Fletcher, H. (1953). *Speech and hearing in communication*. New York, NY: Van Nostrand.

Fozard, J., Vercruyssen, M., Reynolds, S., Hancock, P., & Quilter, R. (1994). Age differences and changes in reaction time. *Journal of Gerontology: Psychological Sciences, 49*, 179–189.

Fremont, A., & Hoyland, J. (2007). Morphology, mechanisms and pathology of musculoskeletal ageing. *Journal of Pathology, 211*, 252–259.

Goffman, L., & Smith, A. (1999). Development and differentiation of speech movement patterns. *Human Perception and Performance, 25*, 1–12.

Goldstein, U. (1980). *An articulatory model for the vocal tracts of growing children* (Doctoral dissertation). Massachusetts Institute of Technology, Cambridge, MA.

Green, J., Moore, C., Higashikawa, M., & Steeve, R. (2000). The physiological development of speech motor control: Lip and jaw coordination. *Journal of Speech, Language, and Hearing Research, 43*, 239–255.

Green, J., Moore, C., & Reilly, K. (2002). The sequential development of jaw and lip control for speech. *Journal of Speech, Language, and Hearing Research, 45*, 66–79.

Grigos, M. (2009). Changes in articulator movement variability during phonemic development: A longitudinal study. *Journal of Speech, Language, and Hearing Research, 52*, 164–177.

Hartman, D., & Danhauer, J. (1976). Perceptual features of speech for males in four perceived age categories. *Journal of the Acoustical Society of America, 59*, 713–715.

Henke, W. (1966). *Dynamic articulatory model of speech production using computer simulation* (Doctoral dissertation). Massachusetts Institute of Technology, Cambridge, MA.

Hoit, J., & Hixon, T. (1987). Age and speech breathing. *Journal of Speech and Hearing Research, 30*, 351–366.

Huang, J., Shen, H., Takahashi, M., Fukunaga, T., Toga, H., Takahashi, K., & Ohya, N. (1998). Pharyngeal cross-sectional area and pharyngeal compliance in normal males and females. *Respiration, 65*, 458–468.

Iuzzini-Seigel, J., Hogan, T., Rong, P., & Green, J. (2015). Longitudinal development of speech motor control: Motor and linguistic factors. *Journal of Motor Learning and Development, 3*, 53–68.

Huttenlocher, P. (1990). Morphometric study of human cerebral cortex development. *Neuropsychologia, 28*, 517–527.

Israel, H. (1968). Continuing growth in the human cranial skeleton. *Archives of Oral Biology, 13*, 133–137.

Israel, H. (1973). Age factor and the pattern of change in craniofacial structures. *American Journal of Physical Anthropology, 39*, 111–128.

Jones, K., Hamilton, A., & Wolpert, D. (2002). Sources of signal-dependent noise during isometric force production. *Journal of Neurophysiology, 88*, 1533–1544.

Kahane, J. (1990). Age-related changes in the peripheral speech mechanism: Structural and physiological changes. *ASHA Reports, 19*, 75–87.

Kent, R. (1976). Models of speech production. In N. Lass (Ed.), *Contemporary issues in experimental phonetics* (pp. 79–104). New York, NY: Academic Press.

Kent, R. (1997). *The speech sciences*. San Diego, CA: Singular.

Kent, R., & Burkard, R. (1981). Changes in the acoustic correlates of speech production. In D. Beasley & G. Davis (Eds.), *Aging: Communication processes and disorders* (pp. 47–62). New York, NY: Grune and Stratton.

Kent, R., & Forner, L. (1980). Speech segment durations in sentence recitations by children and adults. *Journal of Phonetics, 8*, 157–168.

Kent, R., & Minifie, F. (1977). Coarticulation in recent speech production models. *Journal of Phonetics, 5*, 115–133.

Kent, R., & Vorperian, H. (1995). Development of the craniofacial-oral-laryngeal anatomy: A review. *Journal of Medical Speech-Language Pathology, 3*, 149–190.

Kerr, W., Kelly, J., & Geddes, D. (1991). The areas of various surfaces in the human mouth from nine years to adulthood. *Journal of Dental Research, 70*, 1528–1530.

Kier, W., & Smith, K. (1985). Tongues, tentacles, and trunks: The biomechanics of movement in muscular hydrostats. *Zoological Journal of the Linnean Society, 83*, 307–324.

Klein, D. (1980). Oral soft tissue changes in geriatric patients. *Bulletin of the New York Academy of Medicine, 56*, 721–727.

Laitman, J., & Crelin, E. (1976). Postnatal development of the basicranium and vocal tract region in man. In J. Bosma (Ed.), *Symposium on the development of the basicranium* (pp. 206–220). Bethesda, MD: Department of Health, Education, and Welfare Publication No. 76–989, Public Health Service, National Institutes of Health.

Langdon, H., Klueber, K., & Barnwell, Y. (1978). The anatomy of m. genioglossus in the 15-week human fetus. *Anatomy and Embryology, 155*, 107–113.

Lecours, A. (1975). Myelogenetic correlates of the development of speech and language. In E. Lenneberg & E. Lenneberg (Eds.), *Foundations of language development: A multidisciplinary approach* (Vol. 1, pp. 121–136). New York, NY: Academic Press.

Linville, S., & Fisher, H. (1985). Acoustic characteristics of women's voices with advanced age. *Journal of Gerontology, 3*, 324–330.

Linville, S., & Rens, R. (2001). Vocal tract resonance analysis of aging voice using long-term average spectra. *Journal of Voice, 15*, 323–330.

Liss, J., Weismer, G., & Rosenbek, J. (1990). Selected acoustic characteristics of speech production in very old males. *Journal of Gerontology, 45*, 35–45.

MacNeilage, P. (1970). Motor control of serial ordering of speech. *Psychological Review, 77*, 182–196.

Maner, K., Smith, A., & Grayson, L. (2000). Influences of utterance length and complexity on speech motor performance in children and adults. *Journal of Speech, Language, and Hearing Research, 43*, 560–573.

McNeil, M., Pratt, S., & Fosset T. (2004). The differential diagnosis of apraxia of speech. In B. Maassen, R. Kent, H. Peters, P. Van Lieshout, & W. Hultstijn (Eds.), *Speech motor control in normal and disordered speech* (pp. 389–413). Oxford, UK: Oxford University Press.

Melsen, B., & Melsen, F. (1982). The postnatal development of the palatomaxillary region studied on human autopsy material. *American Journal of Orthodontics, 82*, 329–342.

Menn, L. (1983). Development of articulatory, phonetic, and phonological capabilities. In B. Butterworth (Ed.), *Language production* (pp. 3–50). Cambridge, UK: Cambridge University Press.

Minifie, F., Hixon, T., Kelsey, C., & Woodhouse, R. (1970). Lateral pharyngeal wall movement during speech production. *Journal of Speech and Hearing Research, 13*, 584–594.

Miyawaki, K. (1974). A study of the musculature of the human tongue. *Bulletin of the Research Institute of Logopedics and Phoniatrics, University of Tokyo, 8*, 23–50.

Mortimore, I., Fiddes, P., Stephens, S., & Douglas, N. (1999). Tongue protrusion force and fatiguability in male and female subjects. *European Respiratory Journal, 14*, 191–195.

Munhall, K., Vatikiotis-Bateson, E., & Tohkura, Y. (1995). X-ray film database for speech research. *Journal of the Acoustical Society of America, 98*, 1222–1224.

Nelson, R., Soderberg, G., & Urbsheit, M. (1984). Alteration of motor-unit discharge characteristics in aged humans. *Physical Therapy, 64*, 29–34.

Netsell, R. (1986). *A neurobiologic view of speech production and the dysarthrias*. San Diego, CA: College-Hill Press.

Newell, K., Liu, Y., & Mayer-Kress, G. (2001). Time scales in learning and development. *Psychological Review, 108*, 57–82.

Nicholson, K., & Kimura, D. (1996). Sex differences for speech and manual skill. *Perceptual and Motor Skills, 82*, 3–13.

Nittrouer, S. (1993). The emergence of mature gestural patterns is not uniform: Evidence from an acoustic study. *Journal of Speech and Hearing Research, 36*, 959–972.

Paus, T., Zijdenbos, A., Worsley, K., Collins, D., Blumenthal, J., Giedd, J., Rapoport, J., & Evans, A. (2001). Structural maturation of neural pathways in children and adolescents: In vivo study. *Science, 19*, 1908–1911.

Peladeau-Pigeon, M., & Steele, C. (2017). Age-related variability in tongue pressure patterns for maximum isometric and saliva swallowing tasks. *Journal of Speech, Language, and Hearing Research, 60*, 3177–3184.

Richtsmeier, J., & Cheverud, J. (1986). Finite element scaling analysis of human craniofacial growth. *Journal of Craniofacial Genetics and Developmental Biology, 6*, 289–323.

Ryalls, J., & Lieberman, P. (1982). Fundamental frequency and vowel perception. *Journal of the Acoustical Society of America, 72*, 1631–1634.

Ryan, W. (1972). Acoustic aspects of the aging voice. *Journal of Gerontology, 27*, 265–268.

Saltzman, E., & Munhall, K. (1989). A dynamical approach to gestural patterning in speech production. *Ecological Psychology, 1*, 333–382.

Schmidt, R., Zelaznik, H., Hawkins, B., Frank, J., & Quinn, J. (1979). Motor-output variability: A theory for the accuracy of rapid motor acts. *Psychological Review, 47*, 415–451.

Schwartz, M. (1968). Identification of speaker sex from isolated, voiceless fricatives. *Journal of the Acoustical Society of America, 43*, 1178–1179.

Scott, J. (1976). *Dentofacial development and growth*. Oxford, UK: Pergamon Press.

Scukanec, G., Petrosino, L., & Squibb, K. (1991). Formant frequency characteristics of children, young adult, and aged female speakers. *Perceptual and Motor Skills, 73*, 203–208.

Sebastian, S., Babu, S., Oommen, N. & Ballraj, A. (2012). Acoustic measurements of geriatric voice. *Journal of Laryngology & Voice, 2*, 81–84.

Sharkey, S., & Folkins, J. (1985). Variability of lip and jaw movements in children and adults: Implications for the development of speech motor control. *Journal of Speech and Hearing Research, 28*, 8–15.

Sicher, H., & DuBrul, E. (1975). *Oral anatomy* (2nd ed.). St Louis, MO: C. V. Mosby.

Simpson, A. (2001). Dynamic consequences of differences in male and female vocal tract dimensions. *Journal of the Acoustical Society of America, 109*, 2153–2164.

Simpson, A. (2002). Gender-specific articulatory-acoustic relations in vowel sequences. *Journal of Phonetics, 30*, 417–435.

Smith, A., & Goffman, L. (1998). Stability and patterning of speech movement sequences in children and adults. *Journal of Speech, Language, and Hearing Research, 41*, 18–30.

Smith, A., & Zelaznik, H. (2004). Development of functional synergies for speech motor coordination in childhood and adolescence. *Developmental Psychobiology, 45*, 22–33.

Smith, B., & McLean-Muse, A. (1986). Articulatory movement characteristics of labial consonant productions by children. *Journal of the Acoustical Society of America, 80*, 1321–1327.

Smith, B., Sugarman, M., & Long, S. (1983). Experimental manipulation of speaking rate for studying temporal variability in children's speech. *Journal of the Acoustical Society of America, 74*, 744–748.

Smith, B., Wasowicz, J., & Preston, J. (1987). Temporal characteristics of the speech of normal elderly adults. *Journal of Speech and Hearing Research, 30*, 522–529.

Smith, K., & Kier, W. (1989). Trunks, tongues, and tentacles: Moving with skeletons of muscle. *American Scientist, 77*, 28–35.

Smits-Engelsman, B., & Van Galen, G. (1997). Dysgraphia in children: Lasting psychomotor deficiency or transient developmental delay? *Journal of Experimental Child Psychology, 67*, 164–184.

Sonies, B. (1991). The aging oropharyngeal system. In D. Ripich (Ed.), *Handbook of geriatric communication disorders* (pp. 187–203). Austin, TX: Pro-Ed.

Sonies, B., Baum, B., & Shawker, T. (1984). Tongue motion in the elderly: Initial in situ observation. *Journal of Gerontology, 39*, 279–283.

Sonies, B., Stone, M., & Shawker, T. (1984). Speech and swallowing in the elderly. *Gerontology, 3*, 279–283.

Squire, C., Johnson, N., & Hoops, R. (1976). *Human oral mucosa*. London, UK: Blackwell Scientific.

Steeve, R., Moore, C., Green, J., Reilly, K., & McMurtrey, J. (2008). Babbling, chewing, and sucking: Oromandibular coordination at 9 months. *Journal of Speech, Language, and Hearing Research, 51*, 1390–1404.

Story, B., Hoffman, E., & Titze, I. (1997, February). Volumetric image-based comparison of male and female vocal tract shapes. *Proceedings of the International Society of Optical Engineering* (pp. 25–37). Bellingham, WA: International Society of Optical Engineering.

Sturm, J., & Seery, C. (2007). Speech and articulatory rates of school-age children in conversation and narrative contexts. *Language, Speech, and Hearing Services in Schools, 38*, 47–59.

Tabain, M. (2001). Variability in fricative production and spectra: implications for the hyper- and hypo- and quantal theories of speech production. *Language & Speech, 44*, 57–94.

Tourne, L. (1991). Growth of the pharynx and its physiologic implications. *American Journal of Orthodontics and Dentofacial Orthopedics, 99*, 129–139.

Ulatowska, H. (1985). *The aging brain: Communication in the elderly*. San Diego, CA: College-Hill Press.

Vanderwegen, J., Guns, C., Van Nuffelen, G., Elen, R., & De Bodt, M. (2013). The influence of age, sex, bulb position, visual feedback, and the order of testing on maximum anterior and posterior tongue strength and endurance in healthy Belgian adults. *Dysphagia, 28*, 159–166.

Vick, J., Campbell, T., Shriberg, L., Green, J., Abdi, H., Rusiewicz, H., Venkatesh, L., & Moore, C. (2012). Distinct developmental profiles in typical speech acquisition. *Journal of Neurophysiology, 107*, 2885–2900.

Vig, P., & Cohen, A. (1979). Vertical growth of the lips: A serial cephalometric study. *American Journal of Orthodontics, 75*, 405–415.

Vorperian, H., Kent, R., Lindstrom, M., Kalina, C., Gentry, L., & Yandell, B. (2005). Development of vocal tract length during early childhood: A magnetic resonance imaging study. *Journal of the Acoustical Society of America, 117*, 338–350.

Vorperian, H., Wang, S., Chung, M., Schimek, E., Durtschi, R., Kent, R., Ziegert, A., & Gentry, L. (2009). Anatomic development of the oral and pharyngeal portions of the vocal tract: An imaging study. *Journal of the Acoustical Society of America, 125*, 1666–1678.

Vorperian, H., Wang, S., Schimek, E., Durtschi, R., Kent, R., Gentry, L., & Chung, M. (2011). Developmental sexual dimorphism of the oral and pharyngeal portions of the vocal tract: An imaging study. *Journal of Speech, Language, and Hearing Research, 54*, 995–1010.

Walker, G., & Kowalski, C. (1972). On the growth of the mandible. *American Journal of Physical Anthropology, 36*, 111–118.

Walsh, B., & Smith, A. (2002). Articulatory movements in adolescents: Evidence for protracted development of speech motor control processes. *Journal of Speech, Language, and Hearing Research, 45,* 1119–1133.

Watkin, K., & Fromm, D. (1984). Labial coordination in children: Preliminary considerations. *Journal of the Acoustical Society of America, 75,* 629–632.

Weismer, G. (1984). Articulatory characteristics of parkinsonian dysarthria: Segmental and phrase-level timing, spirantization, and glottal-supraglottal coordination. In M. McNeil, J. Rosenbek, & A. Aronson (Eds.), *The dysarthrias: Physiology, acoustics, perception, management* (pp. 101–130). San Diego, CA: College-Hill Press.

Weismer, G., & Fromm, D. (1983). Acoustic analysis of geriatric utterances: Segmental and nonsegmental characteristics that relate to laryngeal function. In D. Bless & J. Abbs (Eds.), *Vocal fold physiology: Contemporary research and clinical issues* (pp. 317–322). San Diego, CA: College-Hill Press.

Weismer, G., & Liss, J. (1991). Speech motor control and aging. In D. Ripich (Ed.), *Handbook of geriatric communication disorders* (pp. 205–226). Austin, TX: Pro-Ed.

Welford, A. (1956). Age and learning: Theory and needed research. *Experientia, 4,* 136–144.

Welford, A. (1982). Motor skills and aging. In J. Mortimer, F. Pirozzolo, & G. Maletta (Eds.), *The aging motor system* (pp. 152–187). New York, NY: Preager.

Wind, J. (1970). *On the phylogeny and ontogeny of the human larynx.* Groningen, Netherlands: Wolters-Noordhoff.

Wohlert, A. (1996a). Reflex responses of lip muscles in young and older women. *Journal of Speech and Hearing Research, 39,* 578–589.

Wohlert, A. (1996b). Tactile perception of spatial stimuli on the lip surface by young and older adults. *Journal of Speech and Hearing Research, 39,* 1191–1198.

Wohlert, A., & Smith, A. (1998). Spatiotemporal stability of lip movements in older adult speakers. *Journal of Speech, Language, and Hearing Research, 41,* 41–50.

Woo, J., Xing, F., Lee, J., Stone, M., & Prince, J. (2016). A spatiotemporal atlas and statistical model of the tongue during speech from cine-MRI. *Computer Methods in Biomechanics and Biomedical Engineering: Imaging and Visualization.* doi:10.1080/21681163.2016.1169220

Woo, J., Xing, F., Stone, M., Green, J., Reese, T., Brady, T., . . . El Fakhri, G. (2017). Speech Map: A statistical multimodal atlas of 4D tongue motion during speech from tagged and cine MR images. *Computer Methods in Biomechanics and Biomedical Engineering: Imaging and Visualization.* doi:10.1080/21681163.2017.1382393

Xue, S., & Hao, G. (2003). Changes in the human vocal tract due to aging and the acoustic correlates of speech production: A pilot study. *Journal of Speech, Language, and Hearing Research, 46,* 689–701.

Yan, J., Thomas, J., Stelmach, G., & Thomas, K. (2000). Developmental features of rapid aiming arm movements across the lifespan. *Journal of Motor Behavior, 32,* 121–140.

Youmans, S., & Stierwalt, J. (2006). Measures of tongue function related to normal swallowing. *Dysphagia, 21,* 102–111.

Zaino, C., & Benventano, T. (1977). Functional, involutional, and degenerative disorders. In C. Zaino & T. Benventano (Eds.), *Radiologic examination of the oropharynx and esophagus* (pp. 141–170). New York, NY: Springer-Verlag.

Zemlin, W. (1998). *Speech and hearing science: Anatomy and physiology* (4th ed.). Boston, MA: Allyn & Bacon.

6

Speech Physiology Measurement and Analysis

INTRODUCTION

Much of the knowledge about speech production has been acquired through measurement. This chapter is dedicated to measurement and analysis of speech production physiology as it relates to the function of the breathing apparatus, laryngeal apparatus, velopharyngeal-nasal apparatus, and pharyngeal-oral apparatus. Acoustic measurement and analysis of speech are covered in Chapter 10. This chapter concludes with a section on health care professionals who may use speech physiology measurements in their provision of clinical services.

MEASUREMENT AND ANALYSIS OF BREATHING

Three types of measurements are the focus of this section. They are spirometry (to obtain measures of lung volume and airflow), chest wall surface tracking (to obtain measures of lung volume, airflow, and chest wall shape), and manometry (to obtain measures of pressure). Some of these measurements are made during speech production, but some are not. Those that are included here are commonly encountered in clinical settings and provide information that may be relevant to understanding the nature of a speech breathing disorder.

Spirometry

Spirometry can be used to measure lung volume and airflow. Recall that lung volume is the volume (size) of the air inside the pulmonary apparatus (lungs and lower airways). Lung volume is important for speech production because it has implications for how much speech can be produced on a single breath. Airflow in this context is lung volume change over time and it, too, has implications for how much speech can be produced on a breath.

A wet (or water) spirometer, shown in Figure 6–1, is an old-fashioned instrument that can be used to measure lung volume and airflow. Invented in the 1800s, the wet spirometer includes a chamber containing water and a bell that floats inside the chamber. Air moving into the bell causes it to rise and air moving out of the bell causes it to fall, the height of the bell being directly proportional to the volume of air in the spirometer. A mouthpiece can be used to couple the person to the spirometer (as shown in Figure 6–1), as long as the nose is occluded and the lips are sealed around the mouthpiece; a facemask that covers the mouth and nose is another coupling option. A pen fixed to the bell may provide a record of volume change on paper attached to a drum, or a potentiometer driven by movement of the bell may provide an electrical signal for display on a screen. As long as the spirometer has a drum that rotates at a known speed, the tracing can also be used to calculate airflow (change in volume over time). This tracing is called a spirogram (see also Figure 2–16). Wet spirometers are instructive because their operation is easy to understand. However, they are not in wide used today.

Most of today's spirometers incorporate a pneumotachometer, a device that measures instantaneous airflow (pneumo = relating to the lungs or air; tachometer = instrument that measures speed). A pneumotachometer, such as that illustrated in Figure 6–2, senses airflow in both directions by recording the air pressure difference across a resistive screen (a wire mesh screen, much like a window screen). When air flows across the

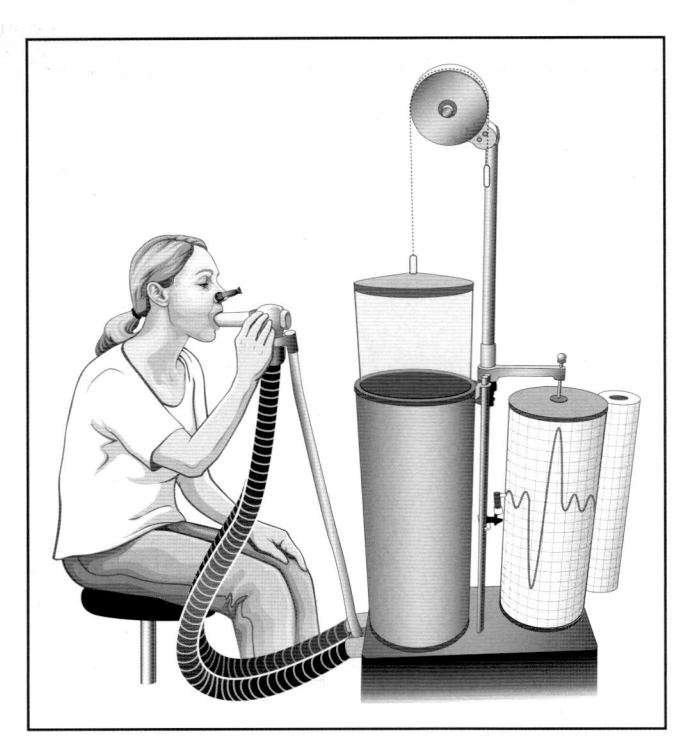

Figure 6-1. Wet spirometer. The tracing on the drum is called a spirogram. This spirogram reflects (*from left to right*) resting tidal breaths followed by an inspiratory capacity (*downward directed tracing*) and a vital capacity (*longest upward directed tracing*) and two more resting tidal breaths. Modified from *Evaluation and management of speech breathing disorders: Principles and methods* (p. 160), by T. Hixon and J. Hoit, 2005, Tucson, AZ: Redington Brown. Copyright 2005 by Thomas J. Hixon and Jeannette D. Hoit. Modified and reproduced with permission.

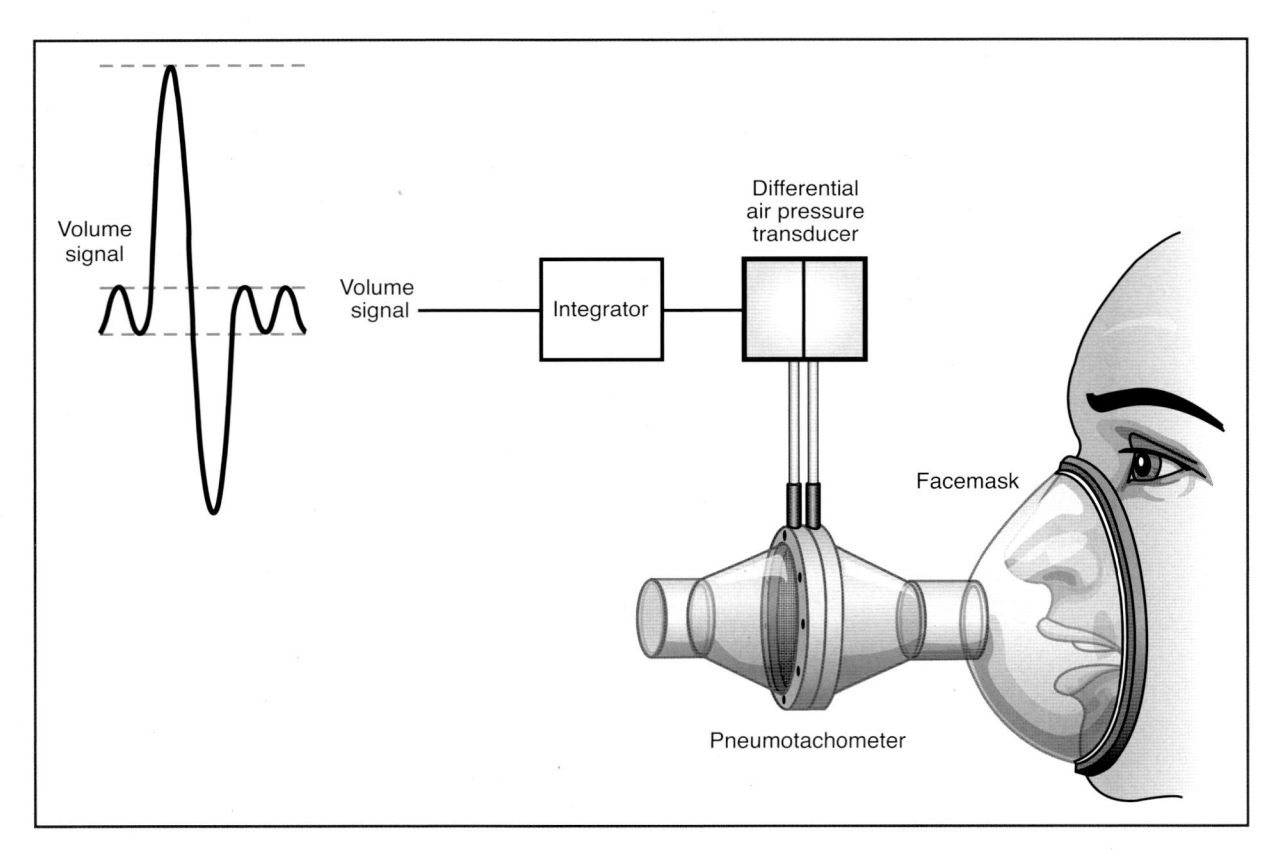

Figure 6-2. A Silverman (or Lilly) type pneumotachometer as a component of a spirometer. The differential pressure transducer senses the pressures on the two sides of the resistive screen and the difference between the two pressures reflects the airflow. This signal can be integrated (summed over time) to create a signal that represents lung volume. From *Evaluation and management of speech breathing disorders: Principles and methods* (p. 162), by T. Hixon and J. Hoit, 2005, Tucson, AZ: Redington Brown. Copyright 2005 by Thomas J. Hixon and Jeannette D. Hoit. Modified and reproduced with permission.

screen, there is a pressure drop from one side (the side of the screen closest to the airflow source) to the other side. The higher the airflow, the greater the pressure drop across the screen. This pressure drop is sensed by a differential air pressure transducer (a transducer that subtracts one pressure from another) and provides an electrical signal proportional to the airflow. This airflow signal can be "added up" over time by a device called an integrator. The integrated (summed) signal provides a measure of volume. An analogy to help understand the difference between measurements of airflow and volume is that an airflow measurement is like reading an automobile's speedometer and a volume measurement (by airflow integration) is like reading the automobile's odometer.

Spirometers can be used to measure most subdivisions of the lung volume, as described in Chapter 2 and illustrated in Figure 2–16. The exceptions are the residual volume and any lung capacities that include the residual volume (functional residual capacity and total lung capacity). This is because, by definition, residual volume cannot be expired voluntarily. (The residual volume can be estimated using indirect measurement approaches, but these are beyond the scope of this book.) One measure not mentioned in Chapter 2, but one often encountered in clinical settings, is the forced vital capacity (FVC). This is like a vital capacity (VC), except that it is obtained by expiring as *quickly* and as fully as possible following a full inspiration. Thus, an FVC differs from a VC only by the speed with which the maneuver is executed. In healthy people, the VC and FVC are comparable. However, the FVC may be much smaller than the VC in someone who has compliant (floppy) airways that collapse in the face of high airflow (thereby trapping much of the air so that it cannot be expired).

Spirometers can also be used to measure ventilation. Recall that ventilation is defined as the movement of air into or out of the pulmonary apparatus and is usually quantified over a given period, such as a minute. In fact, the term *minute ventilation* is commonly used in clinical practice. Minute ventilation is calculated by adding the lung volume inspired (or expired) over the course of a minute.

Sometimes it is of interest to examine the relationship between volume and airflow by generating what are called flow-volume loops. In this case, the pneumotachometer form of spirometer is used to provide direct measures of airflow. A flow-volume loop, such as might be generated by a healthy person, is shown in Figure 6–3. To generate a flow-volume loop, the person is instructed to first breathe out all the air possible, seal the lips around the spirometer mouthpiece, and inspire as quickly and as fully as possible (from residual volume) and then expire as forcefully and as fully as possible (back to residual volume). The trajectory shown in Figure 6–3 indicates that inspiratory flow increases and then decreases during the inspiration phase of the maneuver and that the peak (fastest) expiratory flow occurs at the very beginning of expiration and tapers off from there. The magnitude and shape of the flow-volume loop can be interpreted in ways that help detect and characterize certain disease states.

Spirometers (either wet spirometers or those with pneumotachometers) can be used to measure lung volume and lung volume change (airflow) during speech production; however, the coupling part of the measurement system can be a limiting factor. If a mouthpiece is used (such as that shown in Figure 6–1), measures can only be obtained during productions such as sustained vowels. In contrast, when using a facemask that covers both the mouth and nose, it is possible to produce a wide variety of speech sounds and sound combinations. It is critical that the facemask be sealed airtight around the nose, cheeks, and chin and that the pneumotachometer be sensitive enough to pick up the very high airflows that are produced during running speech production (e.g., during the release of a voiceless stop-plosive). It is also important to recognize that the presence of a facemask may restrict upper airway articulatory movements during speech production.

Chest Wall Surface Tracking

Lung volume and lung volume change (airflow) can be measured in ways other than using a spirometer, one of which involves the use of instrumentation that tracks movement of the chest wall surface. Chest wall surface tracking also provides a way to measure chest wall shape.

Two chest wall surface tracking instruments, respiratory magnetometers and respiratory inductance plethysmographs, are shown in Figure 6–4. Respiratory magnetometers operate on the principle that the rib cage wall and abdominal wall each displace volume as they move and each usually behaves with a single degree of freedom with respect to their movement (meaning that all points on their surface move together). The magnetometers include pairs of electromagnetic coils consisting of generator and sensor (front and back) mates that are used to transduce anteroposterior diameter changes of the rib cage wall and abdominal wall. As the coils move away from each other (as they might during inspiration), the amplitude of the signal "seen" by the sensor coil decreases; as the coils move toward each other (as they might during expiration), the signal amplitude increases. Respiratory

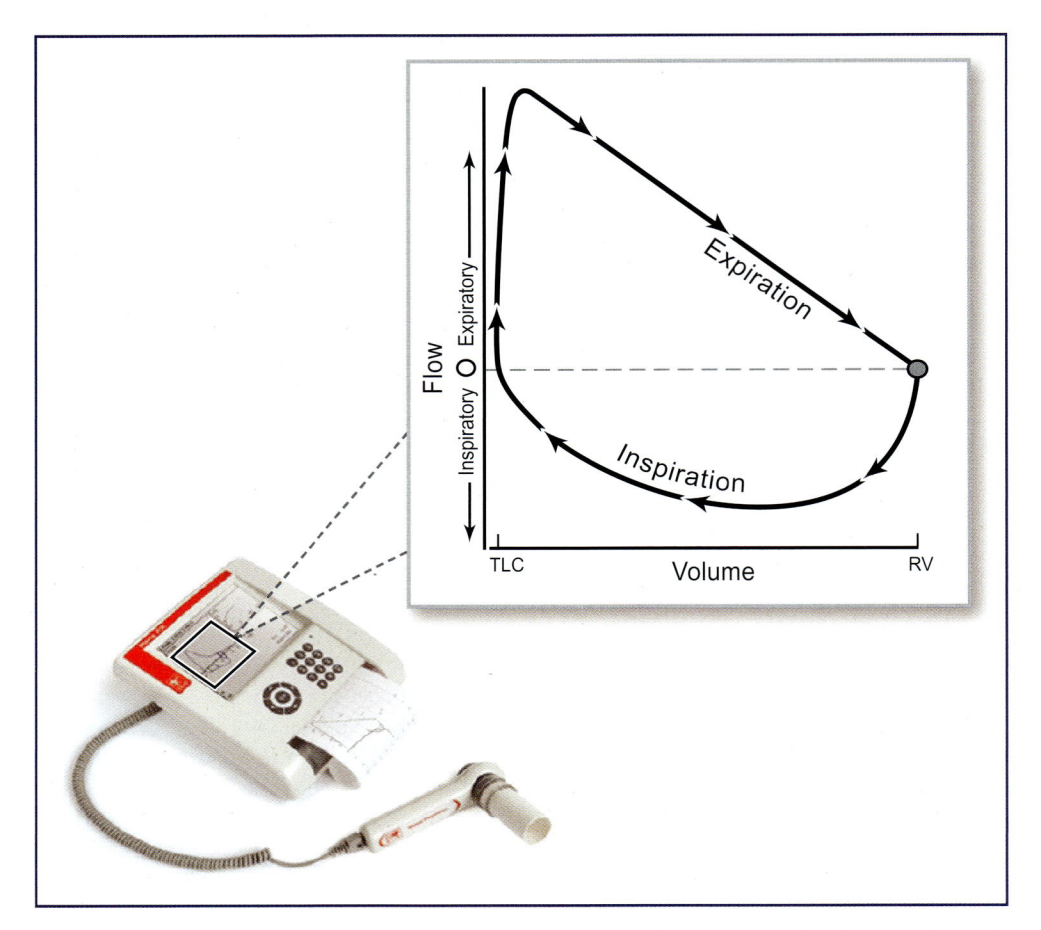

Figure 6–3. Flow-volume loop generated with a hand-held spirometer. Lung volume is shown on the horizontal axis, ranging from residual volume (RV) to total lung capacity (TLC), and flow is shown on the vertical axis, with inspiratory flow increasing downward from zero and expiratory flow increasing upward from zero. As indicated by the arrows, this flow-volume loop was generated by having the person inspire quickly and fully from RV to TLC and then expire quickly and fully back to RV.

inductance plethysmographs operate in a similar manner, except that they include broad elastic bands with embedded electrical wires that sense the average cross-sectional areas of the rib cage wall and abdominal wall. As the bands expand and contract (as they might during inspiration and expiration) the signal outputs change accordingly.

Lung volume and lung volume change can be measured using either respiratory magnetometers or respiratory inductance plethysmographs. To do so, one need merely sum and calibrate the output signals from the electromagnetic coils or the two elastic sensing bands against a known volume (as measured by a spirometer) to obtain a measure of lung volume change from movements of the body surface. The lung volume tracings from summed rib cage and abdominal wall signals look like the tracings found in a spirogram (such as those shown in Figures 2–16 and 6–1).

Chest wall surface tracking may be the best way to measure lung volume, lung volume change, and ventilation during speech production because the speaker's face is unencumbered by a facemask and speech production can proceed relatively naturally. In addition, if the output signals are properly calibrated and monitored, it is possible to determine not just how much volume is being expired, but also exactly where within the vital capacity speech is being produced. As an example, it would be possible to determine that a person was speaking primarily within the inspiratory capacity with occasional encroachments into the expi-

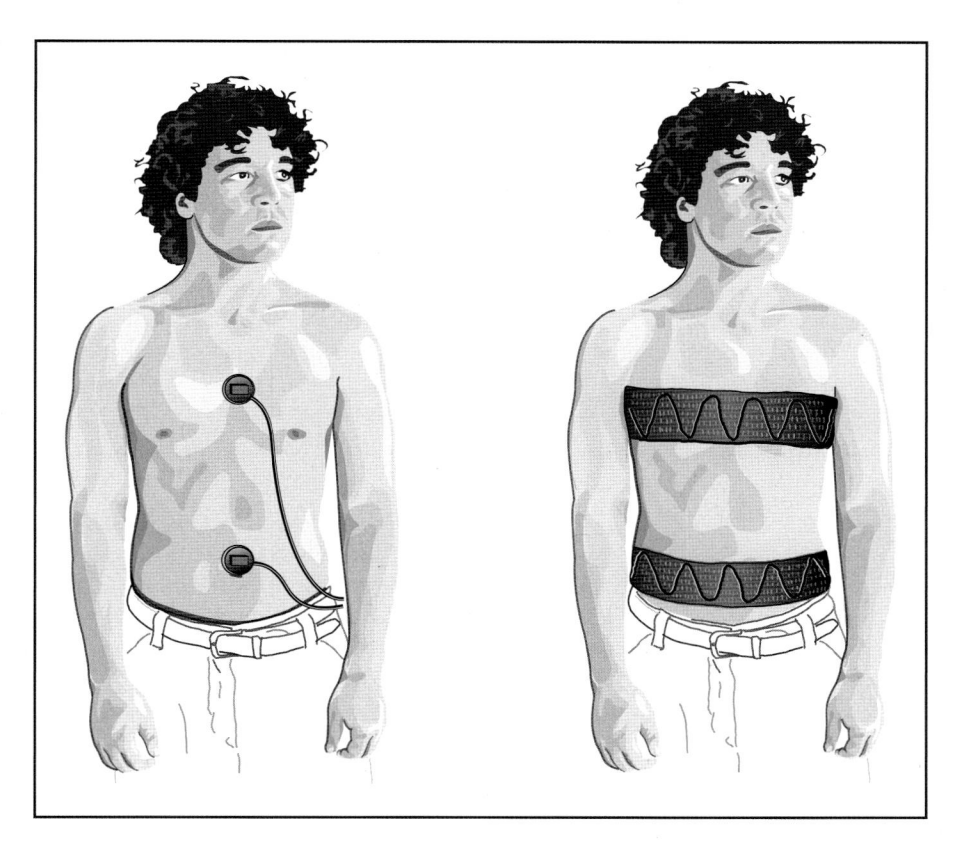

Figure 6–4. Respiratory magnetometers (*left*) and respiratory inductance plethysmographs (*right*). Respiratory magnetometers consist of generator coils, taped to the front of the rib cage wall and abdominal wall, and sensor coil mates, taped to the back at the same axial levels. When the generator and sensor coil mates move closer to one another, the signal amplitude increases, and when they move farther apart, the signal decreases. Respiratory inductance plethysmographs consist of elastic bands embedded with electric wires. When the bands lengthen and shorten (such as when someone inspires and expires), the signals generated by the two bands change accordingly. Signals from respiratory magnetometers and respiratory inductance plethysmographs can be calibrated against a known volume and used to estimate rib cage wall volume, abdominal wall volume, and lung volume. They can also be used to measure chest wall shape. From *Evaluation and management of speech breathing disorders: Principles and methods* (p. 167), by T. Hixon and J. Hoit, 2005, Tucson, AZ: Redington Brown. Copyright 2005 by Thomas J. Hixon and Jeannette D. Hoit. Modified and reproduced with permission.

ratory reserve volume during the production of long breath groups.

Chest wall surface tracking has the additional advantage of allowing for visualization of chest wall shape and changes in shape. This is possible when the rib cage wall signal is displayed against the abdominal wall signal in an *x-y* plot (such as that shown in Figure 2–20). This form of display is very powerful because it allows the examiner to make inferences about potential muscular mechanisms underlying the movements of the chest wall (see Figure 2–22). Chest wall surface tracking has been used to investigate speech breathing in healthy individuals (e.g., Hixon, Goldman, & Mead, 1973) and individuals with speech breathing disorders (e.g., Hoit, Banzett, Brown, & Loring, 1990; Solomon & Hixon, 1993) as well as the effects of behavioral interventions on speech breathing behavior (e.g., Darling-White & Huber, 2017).

Where's the Border?

Borders may or may not be important. Ride your Harley-Davidson motorcycle around the monument at the Four Corners junction from Arizona through New Mexico through Colorado to Utah (for the geographically challenged, this is a continuous left turn) without wearing a helmet and there will be times you're breaking the law and times you're not. You need to know each state's law and identify each border to know your status. But the border between the rib cage wall and the abdominal wall is another story. When the two structures move, it's hard to identify where their two edges meet. The respiratory magnetometers discussed in the text make it so that you don't have to fret such delineation. Magnetometers have the advantage that their coils can be placed at the center of the surfaces being monitored and far away from their edges. Where's the border? Who cares? It's not important to know when using respiratory magnetometers.

Manometry

A pressure-measuring device is called a manometer. Manometers come in many forms and are designed to measure many different types of pressure. The pressure of interest in the present context is alveolar pressure (the pressure inside the alveolar air sacs), a pressure of great relevance to speech production. Alveolar pressure cannot be measured directly in humans; however, it can be estimated from oral pressure under specified conditions. These conditions include that the (a) velopharynx is closed and that the lips are sealed airtight, as any air leak will give a falsely low estimate of alveolar pressure, (b) flow of air between the alveoli and the oral cavity is zero (or nearly zero), and (c) pressure measurement is not influenced by impounding pressure in the oral cavity by adjustments of the cheeks and other oral structures. Three types of manometers that have been used to measure oral pressure are discussed here: U-tube manometers, air-gauge manometers, and pressure transducers (mechanical-electrical manometers).

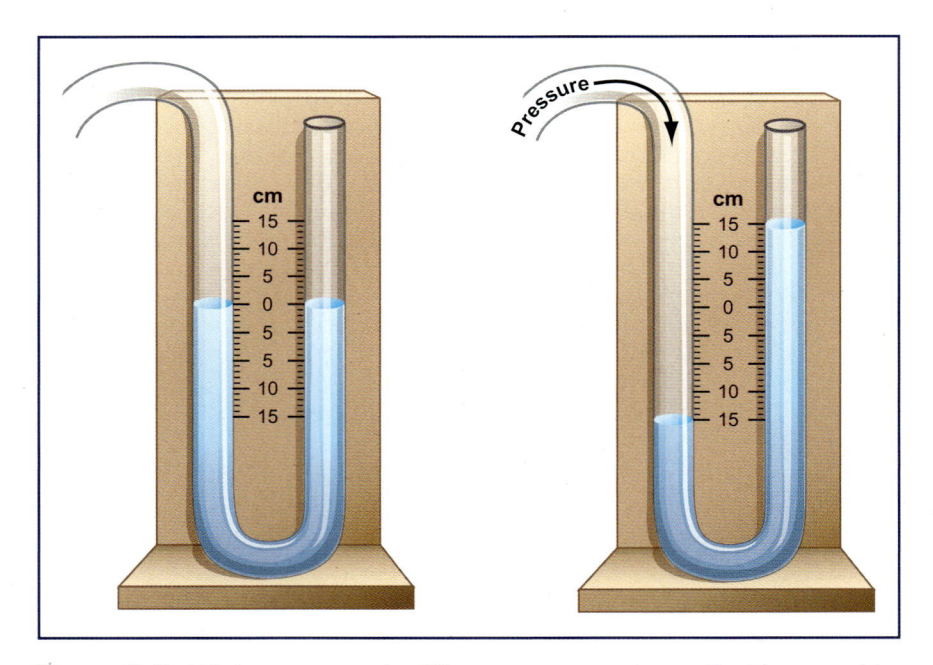

Figure 6–5. U-tube manometer. When a pressure is applied to one side, the water moves within the tube. The distance moved can be measured by a calibration scale marked in centimeters of water (cmH_2O). The U-tube manometer on the right shows a pressure of 30 cmH_2O. The 30 cmH_2O is calculated by measuring the distance (in cm) from where the water column starts on the left side of the manometer (15 cm below 0) to where it ends on the right side (15 cm above 0).

A U-tube manometer is depicted in Figure 6–5. The manometer includes a U-shaped tube containing water, a connecting tube coupled to one arm of the tube, and a calibration scale (in centimeters). To measure pressure, one need only blow into the connecting tube and the water will be displaced by a distance that corresponds to the pressure exerted. In the figure, the manometer shows a 30-centimeter displacement; therefore, the pressure exerted is 30 centimeters of water (cmH$_2$O). U-tube manometers are instructive for understanding the concept of pressure as expressed in "centimeters of water."

Air-gauge manometers, such as the one shown in Figure 6–6, are small and easy to use and are often found in clinical settings. The manometer in the figure has a needle that moves clockwise around the face of the gauge to indicate the pressure being measured. This manometer could be used to measure maximum expiratory pressure (by having the client blow into the tube as forcefully as possible) and maximum inspiratory pressure (by having the client suck from the tube as forcefully as possible). Of course, present-day manometers are often digital rather than analog, like the one shown in the figure.

Pressure transducers can be thought of as mechanical-electrical manometers. The transducer depicted in Figure 6–7 has a metal diaphragm housed within it which deforms when a pressure is applied to one side of it. This deformation is converted into an electrical signal, the amplitude of which varies with the degree of deformation. When the electrical signal is calibrated against a known pressure (by using a U-tube manometer, for example), the transducer provides an accurate measure of the pressure differential across the diaphragm. Of the three types of manometer described here, pressure transducers are by far the best for obtaining measures of oral pressure (as an estimate of alveolar pressure) during speech production.

Measuring oral pressure to estimate alveolar pressure during speech production is somewhat more complicated than measuring oral pressure during nonspeech activities such as blowing. However, it is possible to do when using a pressure transducer system and a particular type of speech sample (Hertegård, Gauffin, & Lindestad, 1995; Netsell & Hixon, 1978). As illustrated in Figure 6–7, a small polyethylene pressure tube is connected to a pressure transducer and the other end of the tube is placed at one corner of the mouth just behind the front teeth so that its end is perpendicular to the flow of air out of the mouth.

The key is to capitalize on a period during speech production when oral pressure and alveolar pressure are essentially equal. This occurs during the closed phase of a voiceless stop-plosive sound (e.g., /p/) when the oral and velopharyngeal valves are sealed airtight and the laryngeal valve is open. At the moment of peak pressure, the pressure recorded in the oral cavity is essentially equal to the pressure in the alveoli. When an utterance sequence includes interspersed voiceless stop-plosives (such as /pipipipipipipi/), the peak oral pressures measured during the consonants can be interconnected to reveal the underlying alveolar pressure contour. This is done by constructing a contour from successive linear interpolations between the peak pressures of adjacent consonants, as illustrated in the lower panel of Figure 6–7.

MEASUREMENT AND ANALYSIS OF LARYNGEAL FUNCTION

Laryngeal physiology can be measured and analyzed using a variety of approaches. This section considers three of them: endoscopy, electroglottography, and aeromechanical observations.

Endoscopy

Visualization of the larynx is one of the most important tools available for determining its status and quantifying its actions. Such visualization entails inserting a viewing device through either the oral or nasal cavities.

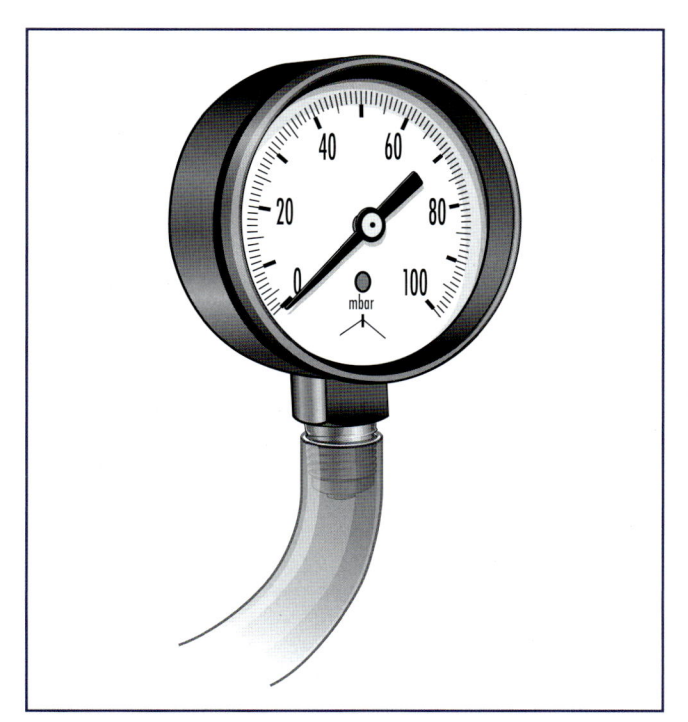

Figure 6-6. Air-gauge manometer. Pressure change is indicated by movement of the needle.

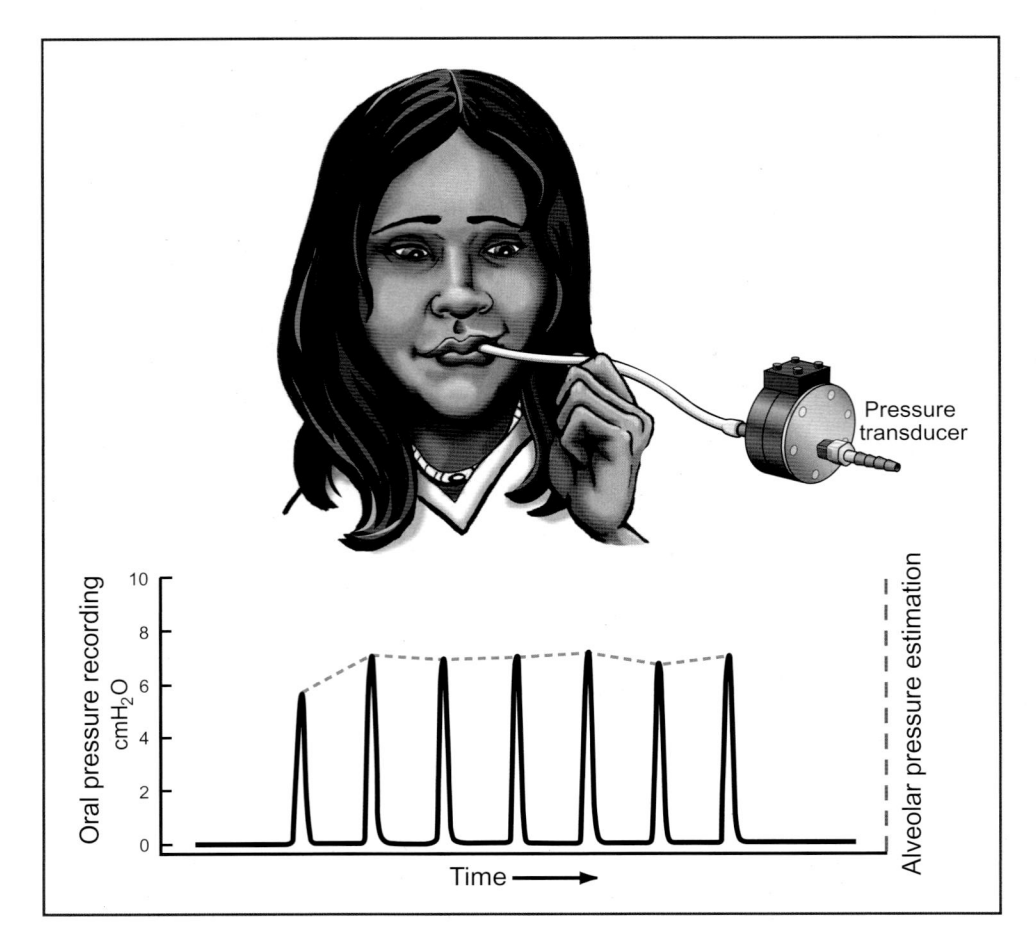

Figure 6–7. Method for estimating alveolar air pressure during speech production. The upper panel shows a person with a small tube inserted between her lips, the other end of which is connected to a pressure transducer. The lower panel depicts the oral pressure tracing associated with the production of "pea-pea-pea-pea-pea-pea-pea." The alveolar pressure is estimated by connecting the peak oral air pressures, as shown by the dashed line. This tracing indicates that most of this utterance was produced with an alveolar pressure of approximately 7 cmH$_2$O.

This method, called endoscopy, includes some form of illumination and some form of optical device that gathers the laryngeal image.

As illustrated in the upper panel of Figure 6–8, visualization via the oral route is most often done with a device called a rigid endoscope that is positioned along the upper surface of the tongue (with the tongue tip pulled forward and out of the way) and into the oropharynx. The image can be viewed through an eyepiece or recorded by one of several different optical recording systems. The rigid endoscope provides an excellent image of the larynx (examples of which are included in Figures 3–26 and 3–27). Nevertheless, it has limitations, one of which is that the client might find the positioning of the device to be uncomfortable and another is that its positioning interferes with movements of pharyngeal-oral structures so that only vowel-like productions can be examined.

As illustrated in the lower panel of Figure 6–8, visualization via the nasal route is accomplished by inserting a flexible endoscope through one side of the nose over the upper surface of the velum and into the pharynx. The flexible endoscope has positional controls so that its distal tip can be oriented to obtain an unobstructed view of the vocal folds. The image can be viewed through an eyepiece or recorded on an optical recording system. A major advantage of the flexible endoscope is that it does not encumber pharyngeal-oral structures so that the behavior of the larynx can be examined during a wide range of speech production activities. Nevertheless, its image is of lower quality than that obtained with the larger rigid endoscope.

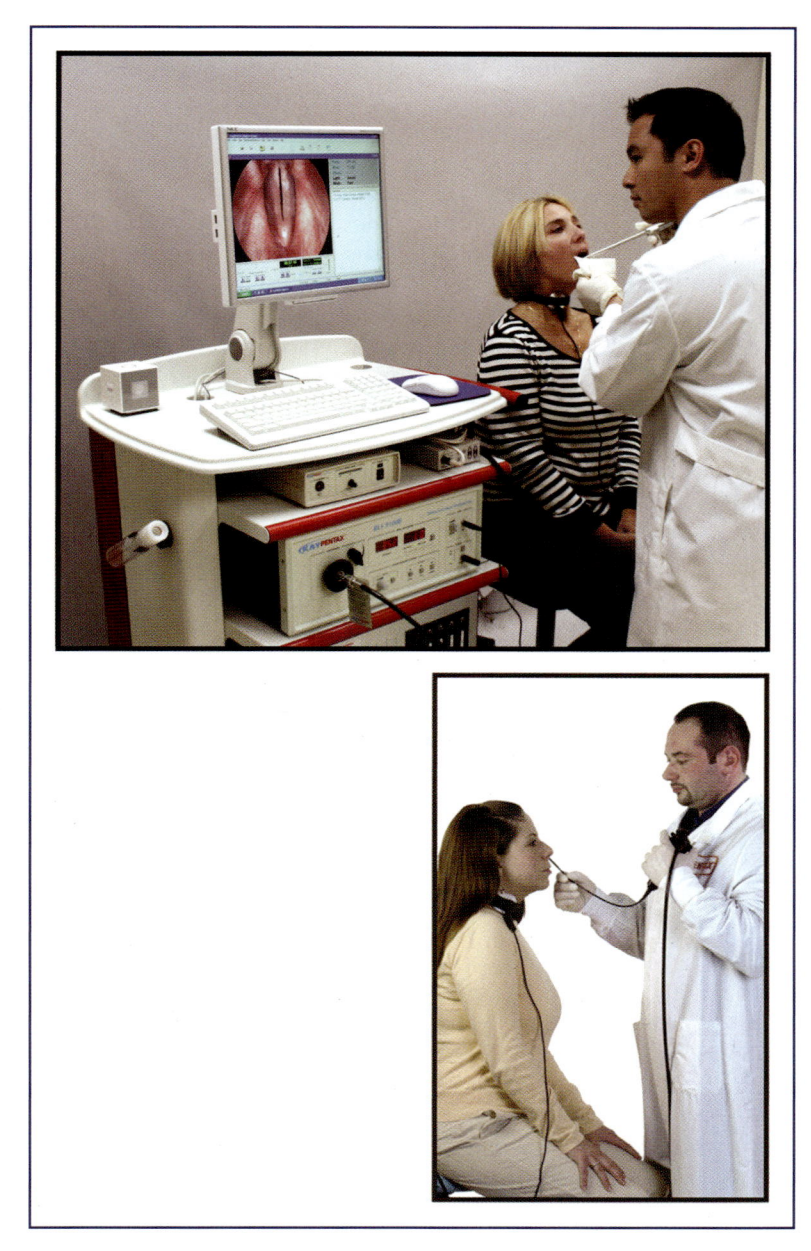

Figure 6–8. Visualization of the larynx via endoscopy. The upper panel illustrates the oral approach with a rigid endoscope. The lower panel illustrates the nasal approach with a flexible endoscope. Images provided courtesy of KayPENTAX, Montvale, NJ. Reproduced with permission.

Endoscopes that use a constant light source are well suited for imaging stationary structures or structures that move relatively slowly. However, the rapid movements of vocal fold vibration cannot be resolved with the naked eye, no matter how good the light source. One way to "slow" these movements is by the optical illusion created with a flashing-light stroboscope. Brief flashes of light illuminate the vocal folds, with each flash being advanced slightly in time with each vibratory cycle such that the phase difference between the vocal fold cycle and the flash cycle progressively increases (Baken & Orlikoff, 2000). This creates the illusion of a slowly moving vocal fold vibration that is actually a composite of the sampling of many successive cycles (Hirano & Bless, 1993). The terms *videoendoscopy* and *videostoboscopy* are sometimes used to differentiate the recording of laryngeal images using a constant light source versus using a stroboscopic light source (Deliyski, Hillman, & Mehta, 2015).

A more recent application of endoscopy is high-speed videoendoscopy, which can record an almost limitless number of images per vocal fold vibratory cycle. A typical rate of 2000 to 8000 frames per second can usually capture at least 20 images per cycle. This means that a fundamental frequency of 200 Hz (with a period—the time between each vocal fold vibration—of 0.005 second or 5 milliseconds) sampled at 2000 frames per second yields an image every 2.5 microseconds. This allows for a detailed analysis of each cycle and offers a more complete picture of vocal fold vibration than does the use of stroboscopy, particularly for clients with voice disorders (Patel, Dailey, & Bless, 2008).

Methods have been developed to quantify the images obtained through the use of videoendoscopy and videostoboscopy and protocols have been proposed to interpret those quantified images in ways that are relevant to clinical practice (Colton & Casper, 1996; Hirano & Bless, 1993; Kendall & Leonard, 2010; Poburka, Patel, & Bless, 2017). Quantification is usually in the form of ratings of structural integrity, nonvibratory movements, and vocal fold vibration (Patel et al., in press). For example, ratings may be obtained for the appearance of the vocal fold edges, extent of vocal fold abduction and adduction, regularity and amplitude of vocal fold vibration, and glottal shape. High-speed videoendoscopy images can also be quantified for clinical applications by using a rating form (Poburka et al., 2017; Yamauchi et al., 2012). However, high-speed videoendoscopy is more frequently used in research applications, with many different automated analyses available to describe specific aspects of vibration. One example involves converting the images into kymographs, tracings that represent movements of a single point at the same transverse level on each of the two vocal folds (Svec & Schutte, 1996).

Electroglottography

Electroglottography is a noninvasive method for estimating the area of contact between the vocal folds (Fourcin, 1974) that capitalizes on the electrical conduction properties of laryngeal tissues. As shown in Figure 6–9, use of an electroglottograph involves the placement of electrodes on both sides of the neck, positioned over the left and right alae of the thyroid cartilage. A weak high-frequency electrical current flows between these two electrodes and a determination is made as to the impedance (opposition) offered to that current flow by laryngeal structures.

Tissues in the vocal folds are good electrical conductors, whereas the air between the vocal folds (when a glottis exists) is an extremely poor electrical conductor. Therefore, the electrical impedance across the larynx rises when the laryngeal airway opens and falls when the vocal folds come into increasingly more extensive contact (Baken & Orlikoff, 2000). Changes in impedance as measured through the use of electroglottography can reflect both slow laryngeal adjustments, such as those associated with abduction and adduction of the vocal folds, and rapid changes in vocal fold contact area, such as those associated with vocal fold vibration (Childers, Hicks, Moore, Eskenazi, & Lalwani, 1990; Childers, Smith, & Moore, 1984; Titze, 1990).

The lower part of Figure 6–9 contains an electroglottographic tracing representing one vocal fold vibratory cycle. This tracing is interpreted to represent the time course of changes in vocal fold contact area over the cycle (Childers & Krishnamurthy, 1985; Colton & Conture, 1990; Lecluse, Brocaar, & Verschuure, 1975; Orlikoff, 1998). Also shown in the figure is a typical analysis procedure applied to electroglottographic data in which the portion of the cycle during which the vocal folds are considered to be approximated (labeled "closed" in the figure) and the portion during which they are not (labeled "open" in the figure) are demarked and measured.

There are other, less commonly used applications of electroglottography. One such application involves the interpretation of certain perturbations in the electroglottographic signal to identify the onset and offset of vocal fold abduction and adduction during speech production (Rothenberg, 2009; Rothenberg & Mahshie, 1988). Another application is to track the vertical position of the larynx within the neck (Rothenberg, 1992), such as during voice therapy (Wistbacka, Sundberg, & Simberg, 2016). This application requires two pairs of electrodes, one pair placed near the lower part of the thyroid cartilage and the other placed near the upper part of the cartilage. Vertical movement of the larynx is reflected in changes in the relative amplitudes of the signals generated by the upper versus lower electrode pairs.

Electroglottography has come to be used by a variety of disciplines concerned with understanding laryngeal behavior during voice production and other activities. The popularity of this method is based on its simplicity and noninvasive nature and because it can be used as both an evaluation tool and a feedback device for management (Baken & Orlikoff, 2000; Kitzing, 1990; Motta, Cesari, Iengo, & Motta; 1990; Smith

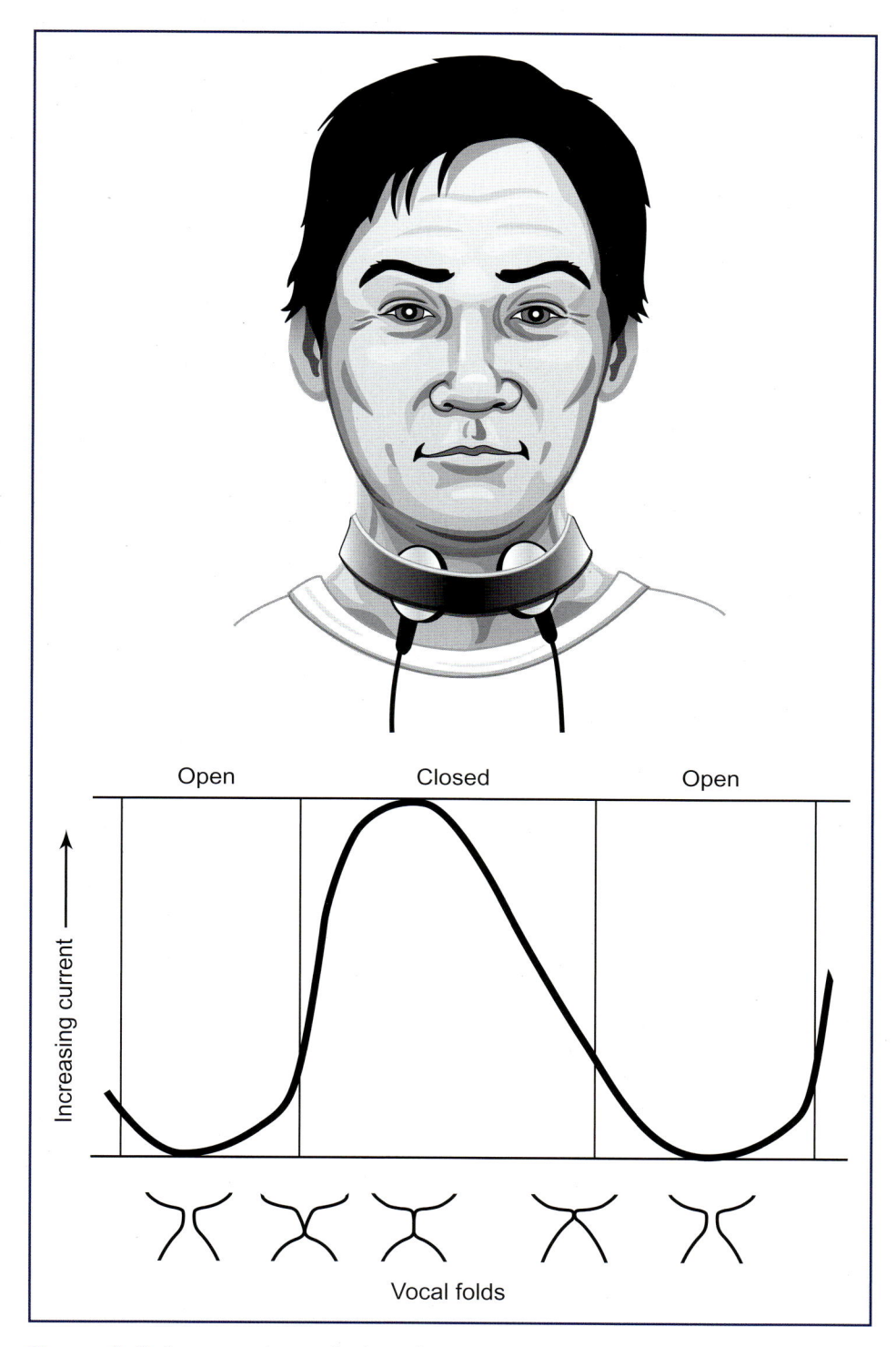

Figure 6-9. Laryngeal monitoring via electroglottography. Two electrodes are placed over the thyroid cartilage and a weak electrical current is passed between them. The resultant tracing reflects the amplitude of current flowing through the larynx. The tracing represents the amplitude of the current signal during one full cycle of vocal fold vibration. When current flow is high, impedance is low; and when current is zero, impedance is infinite. Such tracings are interpreted to indicate when the vocal folds are approximated (in contact) and when they are not, and are labeled as "closed" and "open," respectively, in the tracing.

& Childers, 1983). It can also be used in conjunction with other measurement methods discussed in this section because it does not interfere with the way those methods operate. Although electroglottography is easy to use, there are limitations on what physiological inferences can be made from its signal. For example, discrepancies have been found between the period of presumed vocal fold approximation during the vibratory cycle as determined by electroglottography and the period of approximation as determined from simultaneous endoscopic high-speed videokymographic tracings (e.g., Herbst, Schutte, Bowling, & Svec, 2017).

Aeromechanical Observations

Aeromechanical observations can provide information about the status of the laryngeal airway. Three commonly used aeromechanical observations are airflow through the larynx, calculation of resistance to airflow provided by the larynx, and determination of phonation threshold pressure.

Airflow through the larynx is usually measured with a pneumotachometer, such as that shown in Figure 6–2, located near the airway opening. Under certain conditions, such as during vowel production, the average (mass) airflow through the larynx (translaryngeal airflow) can be estimated at the airway opening because airflow through the larynx is continuous with that at the airway opening. Thus, this average airflow is an indicator of the average openness of the larynx (providing driving pressure does not change) and the extent to which it allows air to pass between the trachea and pharynx (Isshiki & von Leden, 1964). When measuring average airflow, the pneumotachometer system is usually filtered so that only slow (low frequency) airflow events are recorded.

During voice production, the flow of air through the larynx has superimposed on it a rapidly varying component associated with vocal fold vibration. This high-frequency component of the airflow is of interest because of what it reveals about the nature of vocal fold function in generating the sound source for speech (Isshiki, 1985). A common way to acquire a measurement of this cycle-to-cycle airflow waveform is to record airflow changes at the airway opening with a specially designed facemask in which pneumotachometer screens are actually built into its walls. This mask, called a circumferentially vented mask and shown in Figure 6–10, greatly improves the sensitivity of the airflow measuring device and enables the faithful recording of the extremely rapid airflow changes associated with vocal fold vibration. This high-frequency airflow signal, when recorded at the airway opening, is

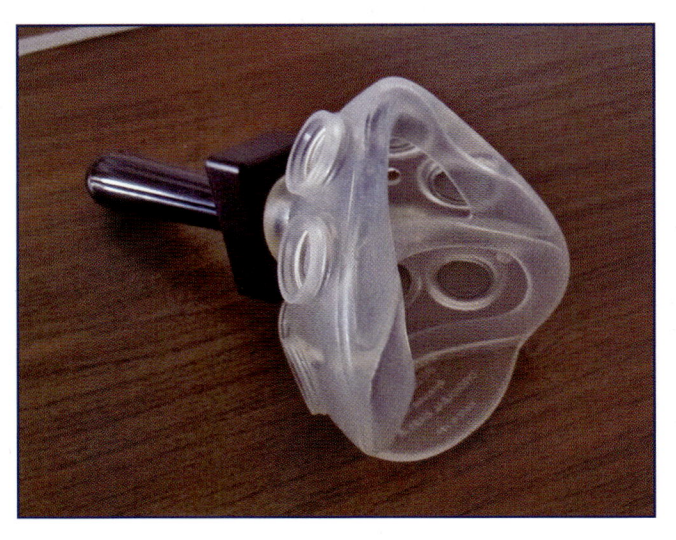

Figure 6–10. A circumferentially vented mask used in measuring fast airflow events (Glottal Enterprises, Inc.). This is a divided mask that allows the user to record oral and nasal flow separately.

not a perfect reflection of the airflow signal generated at the larynx because it has been modified by acoustic effects of the vocal tract (pharyngeal-oral airway). Thus, the airflow signal is subjected to what is called inverse filtering, a filtering algorithm that is designed to minimize the effect of the acoustic properties of the downstream airway on the final airflow waveform (Rothenberg, 1973; also see Chapter 8, Figure 8–3).

Figure 6–11 presents a comparison of average airflow and cycle-to-cycle airflow. Low-pass filtered (average) airflow (red tracings) are superimposed on tracings of fast cycle-to-cycle airflow events associated with voice production (black tracings). The top set of tracings show the full 0.2 second of vocal fold vibration and the bottom set of tracings are zoomed-in images of the last few cycles. The highest peaks in the airflow tracings are responsible for creating the abrupt air pressure changes that become sound.

Airflow through the larynx is influenced not only by the openness of the larynx, but also by the forcefulness with which air is being driven through the airway (D'Antonio, Netsell, & Lotz, 1988). Thus, the best indicator of the general status of the laryngeal airway itself is an estimate of the resistance offered by the larynx to the flow of air through it (van den Berg, Zantema, & Doornenbal, 1957). This requires knowledge of both the air pressure driving the airflow and the resultant airflow.

The most commonly used clinical method for estimating laryngeal airway resistance during voice production is the method of Smitheran and Hixon (1981). This method records oral air pressure and

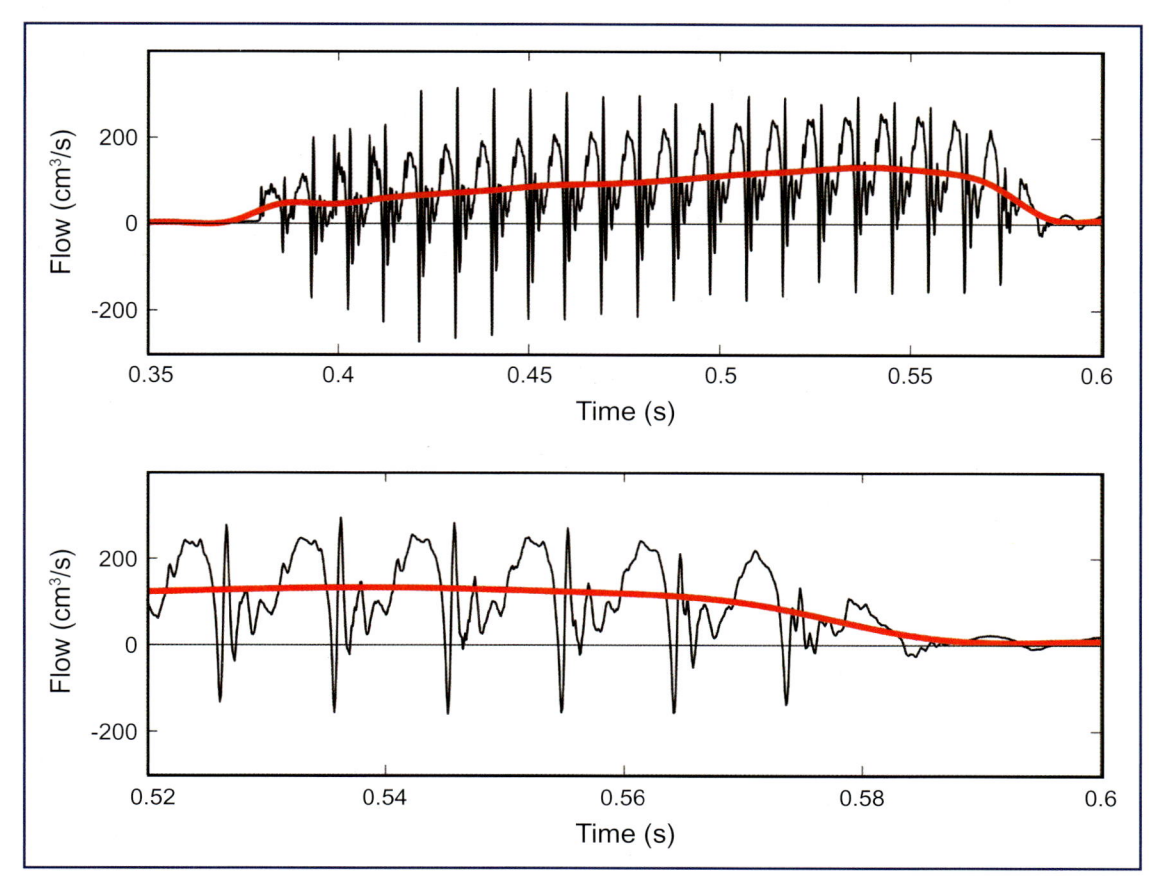

Figure 6–11. Airflow recorded at the airway opening during vowel production. The black tracings show the fast airflow events associated with each cycle of vocal fold vibration. The red tracings represent the average airflow obtained by low-pass filtering the black airflow signal (to filter out high-frequency airflow events). The bottom set of tracings are a zoomed-in image from the upper set of tracings. The fundamental frequency is about 100 Hz (courtesy of Brad Story).

airway-opening airflow to calculate laryngeal airway resistance. As shown in Figure 6–12, measurements are taken at moments that enable estimates to be made of the air pressure difference across the larynx and the airflow through it during vowel productions. Resistance is calculated by dividing the air pressure difference (estimated tracheal air pressure minus estimated pharyngeal air pressure) by the translaryngeal airflow (estimated from the airflow at the airway opening). Resistance values are typically expressed in cmH$_2$O/LPS (centimeters of water/liters per second) and can range from very low (wide open airway) to infinite (airtight closure of the airway). Such resistance values reflect the degree of opening of the laryngeal airway during voice production (Holmberg, Hillman, & Perkell, 1988, 1999; Leeper & Graves, 1984; Smitheran & Hixon, 1981).

Phonation threshold pressure is another aeromechanical measure that can provide information about laryngeal function, or more specifically, vocal fold function. Phonation threshold pressure is defined as the minimum tracheal pressure required to initiate vocal fold vibration and is understood to reflect the status of the vocal folds (viscosity and thickness) and their distance from one another (glottal width) (Titze, 1988). Although there are invasive ways to measure phonation threshold pressure, the most common way to estimate it is by using the noninvasive approach depicted in Figure 6–7, with the client producing the /p/-vowel syllable strings in the quietest voice possible (Verdolini-Marston, Titze, & Druker, 1990). The lower the peak oral pressures during /p/ productions (estimated tracheal pressure), while still maintaining voicing during the vowel segments, the lower the phonation threshold pressure. And the lower the phonation threshold pressure, the healthier vocal fold function is judged to be. Although this measure is relatively easy to obtain, it is not without its limitations. For example, it is common

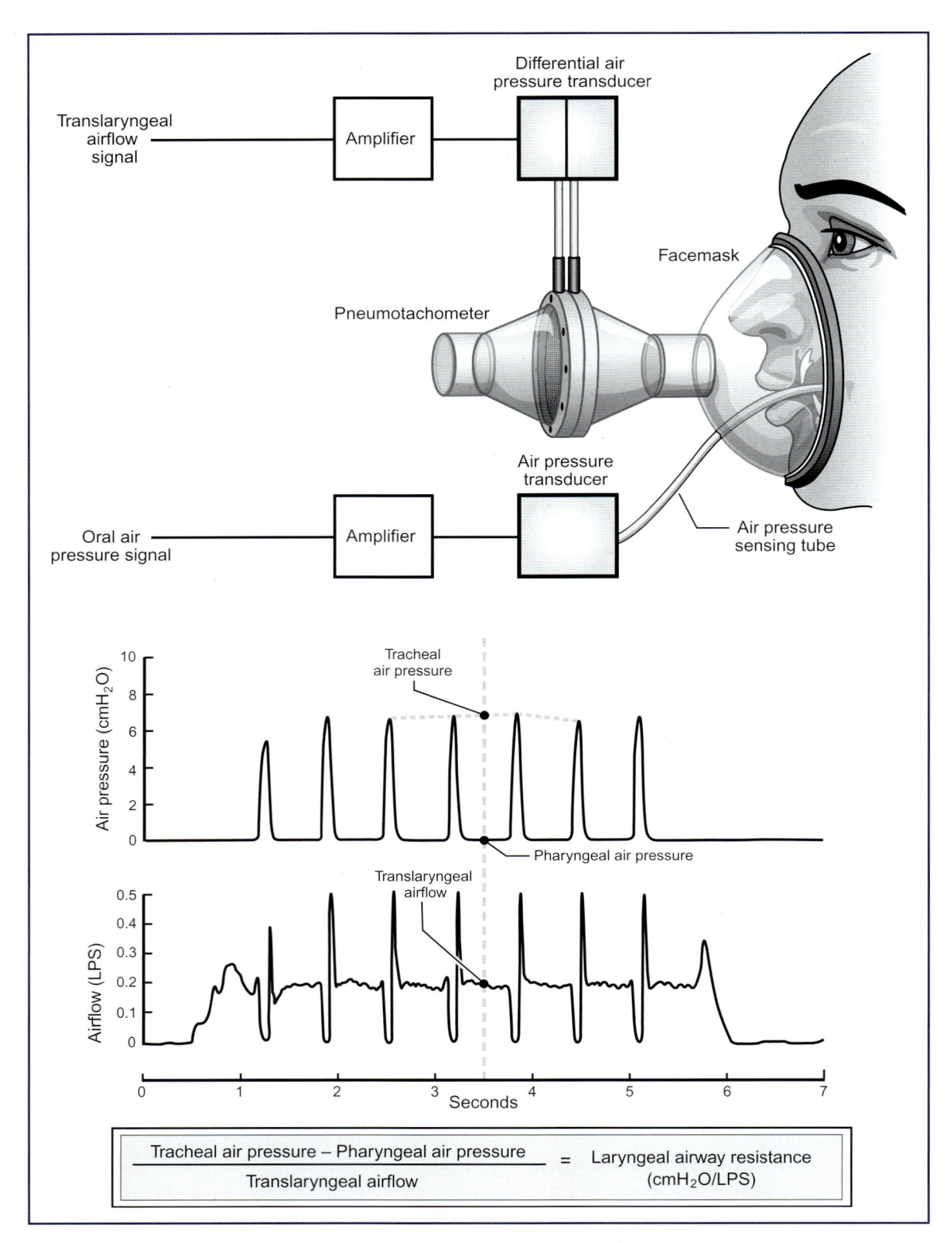

Figure 6-12. Method for determining laryngeal airway resistance during voice production. The upper panel illustrates client-instrumentation interface. The lower panel shows data used for resistance calculation. Laryngeal airway resistance is calculated by subtracting the estimated pharyngeal pressure (oral pressure during vowel production) from the estimated tracheal pressure (peak oral pressure during /p/ productions) divided by the airway-opening flow during the vowel production (in cmH$_2$O/LPS). In this case, the pharyngeal pressure is zero during vowel production, as would be expected with normal resistance being provided by the laryngeal airway. This pressure might be greater than zero in the case of very breathy voice production.

> ### Opposition to Certain Terms of Opposition
>
> Laryngeal airway resistance, discussed in the text, is opposition to the movement of air through the laryngeal airway. This resistance is often mistakenly labeled as vocal fold resistance, glottal resistance, or laryngeal resistance. It's none of these. It's not a measure of the mechanical status of the vocal folds, nor is it a measure of the size of the hole designated as the glottis. Laryngeal airway resistance is a property of the airway itself. To gain a more concrete understanding (pun intended), think of a plaster cast of the inside of a larynx. Nothing in the plaster cast is adjustable. Everything is dead-stiff rigid. Yet, resistance to the flow of air through the cast is airflow dependent. Force air through the cast in either direction and you'll find that laryngeal airway resistance goes up and down as airflow goes up and down. Laryngeal airway resistance isn't something you can look at and measure. It's something you have to calculate.

for the velopharynx to open during soft speech production, which results in a lowering of oral pressure, thereby making it a poor estimate of tracheal pressure (Fisher & Swank, 1997). A useful review of phonation threshold pressure and its potential for clinical application is provided by Plexico, Sandage, and Faver (2012).

MEASUREMENT AND ANALYSIS OF VELOPHARYNGEAL-NASAL FUNCTION

This section considers the instrumental measurement and analysis of the velopharyngeal-nasal apparatus. Two types of measurements are considered here: nasendoscopy and aeromechanical observations. Two other types of instrumental measurements, x-ray imaging and magnetic resonance imaging, are also pertinent to the velopharyngeal part of the apparatus. These are covered in the next section on Measurement and Analysis of Pharyngeal-Oral Function.

Nasendoscopy

Endoscopy (discussed above in the section on Measurement and Analysis of Laryngeal Function) can be used to visualize the velopharyngeal-nasal structures. Although it is possible to visualize the velopharynx from below with a rigid endoscope by turning it "upside down" in the oropharynx (away from the larynx), a flexible endoscope is the most useful instrument for examining the entire velopharyngeal-nasal apparatus (see lower panel in Figure 6–8). When a flexible endoscope is used in this way, the procedure is often referred to as nasendoscopy.

The flexible endoscope inserted through an anterior naris provides an image of the nasal airway as it travels posteriorly until its distal end is positioned above the velum within the nasopharynx. From this perspective (bird's eye view), structures of the nasopharynx and the velopharyngeal port can be examined. The structural part of an examination involves inspecting for any abnormalities such as nasal obstructions or a bifid uvula (cleft in the uvula). The functional part of an examination usually includes making observations while the client breathes quietly and then produces various oral speech samples and some containing nasal sounds.

Nasoendoscopic images can be evaluated both quantitatively and qualitatively. Standard procedures for such evaluations exist (D'Antonio, Marsh, Province, Muntz, & Phillips, 1989; Golding-Kushner et al., 1990) and include measurements and ratings that reflect extent of velar movements, lateral pharyngeal wall (left and right) movements, and posterior pharyngeal wall movements, and the size and shape of the velopharyngeal port. Ratings, rather than physical measures, are more often used in clinical settings—for example, when evaluating change in velopharyngeal function pre- and post-therapy (Pegoraro-Krook, Dutka-Souza, & Marino, 2008).

Aeromechanical Observations

Aeromechanical methods can provide information about the binary status of the velopharyngeal-nasal apparatus (whether it is open or closed), the sizes of different minimum cross-sectional areas of velopharyngeal port, and the magnitudes of opposition to airflow through the apparatus. These methods include measurements of airflow and/or air pressure.

Nasal airflow is a useful index for determining if the velopharyngeal port is open or closed (Thompson & Hixon, 1979). Such airflow is usually sensed with a pneumotachometer attached to a nasal mask, as illustrated in Figure 6–13. The presence of nasal airflow during speech production indicates an open velopharynx, whereas the absence of nasal airflow during speech production indicates a closed velopharynx. It

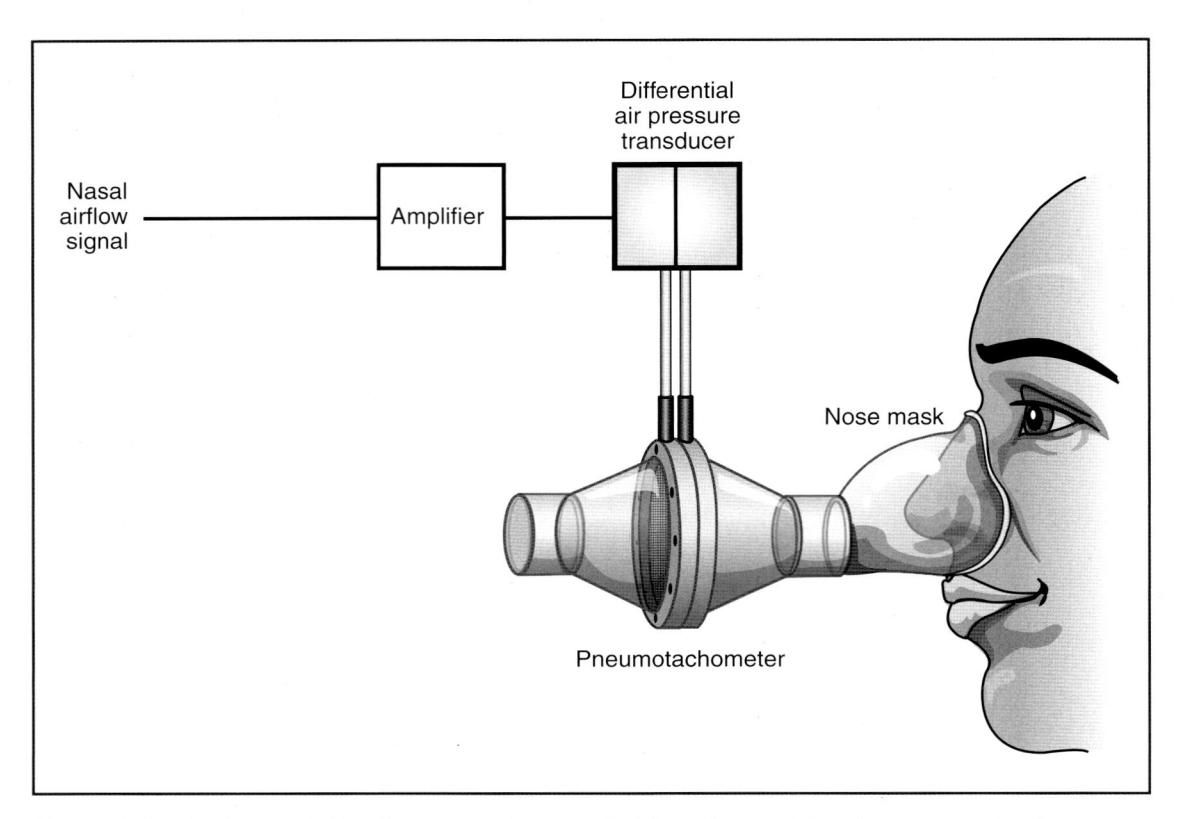

Figure 6–13. Instrumentation for measuring nasal airflow. Nasal airflow is measured with a pneumotachometer system attached to a nasal mask.

Lubker Bumps

Scientists often name phenomena for those who were first to describe them or figure out what they meant. In this regard, the inauguration of the term "Lubker Bumps" seems long overdue. Most who have studied velopharyngeal-nasal function using aeromechanical techniques have encountered very small variations in nasal airflow (usually oscillating around zero airflow) when the velopharynx is closed airtight. These variations, as described by James F. Lubker, result from movements of the velum up and down within a closed velopharynx, acting like a piston in a cylinder to push very small quantities of air in and out of the nasopharynx. The nasal airflow tracings that characterize such piston movements show tiny bumps up and down around zero airflow that reflect true airflows, but ones not generated by the passage of air through the velopharynx. Lubker's reputation deserves to be bumped up a notch for his astute observation.

is important to note that nasal airflow is not the same as nasalance, an acoustic measure that reflects the relative sound pressure level emanating from the nose (described in Chapter 9).

Another simple way to determine whether the velopharynx is open or closed involves monitoring nasal air pressure, an approach first used in a study of velopharyngeal development in infants (Bunton & Hoit, 2018; Thom, Hoit, Hixon, & Smith, 2006) and recently applied to clinical populations (Bunton, Hoit, & Gallagher, 2011; Eshghi, Vallino, Baylis, Preisser, & Zajac, 2017). As shown in Figure 6–14, this approach requires the use of a double-barreled nasal cannula positioned in the anterior nares. This cannula is connected to a sensitive pressure transducer. When the pressure is positive during sound production, this indicates that the velopharynx is open, whereas if the pressure is atmospheric (zero) pressure during sound production, this indicates that the velopharynx is closed.

A pressure-flow technique that is often used to calculate the minimum cross-sectional area of the velopharyngeal port during continuous speech production (Warren & DuBois, 1964) is depicted in Figure 6–15.

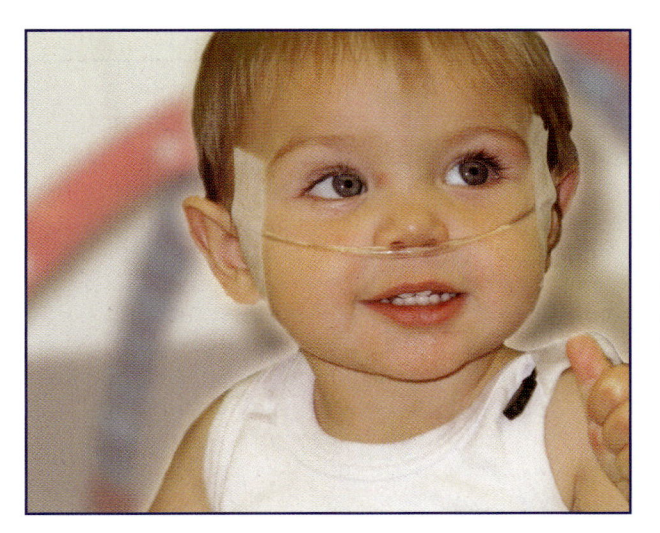

Figure 6-14. Toddler wearing a nasal cannula for monitoring nasal air pressure. The cannula is connected to a sensitive pressure transducer and associated electronics (not shown in the photo).

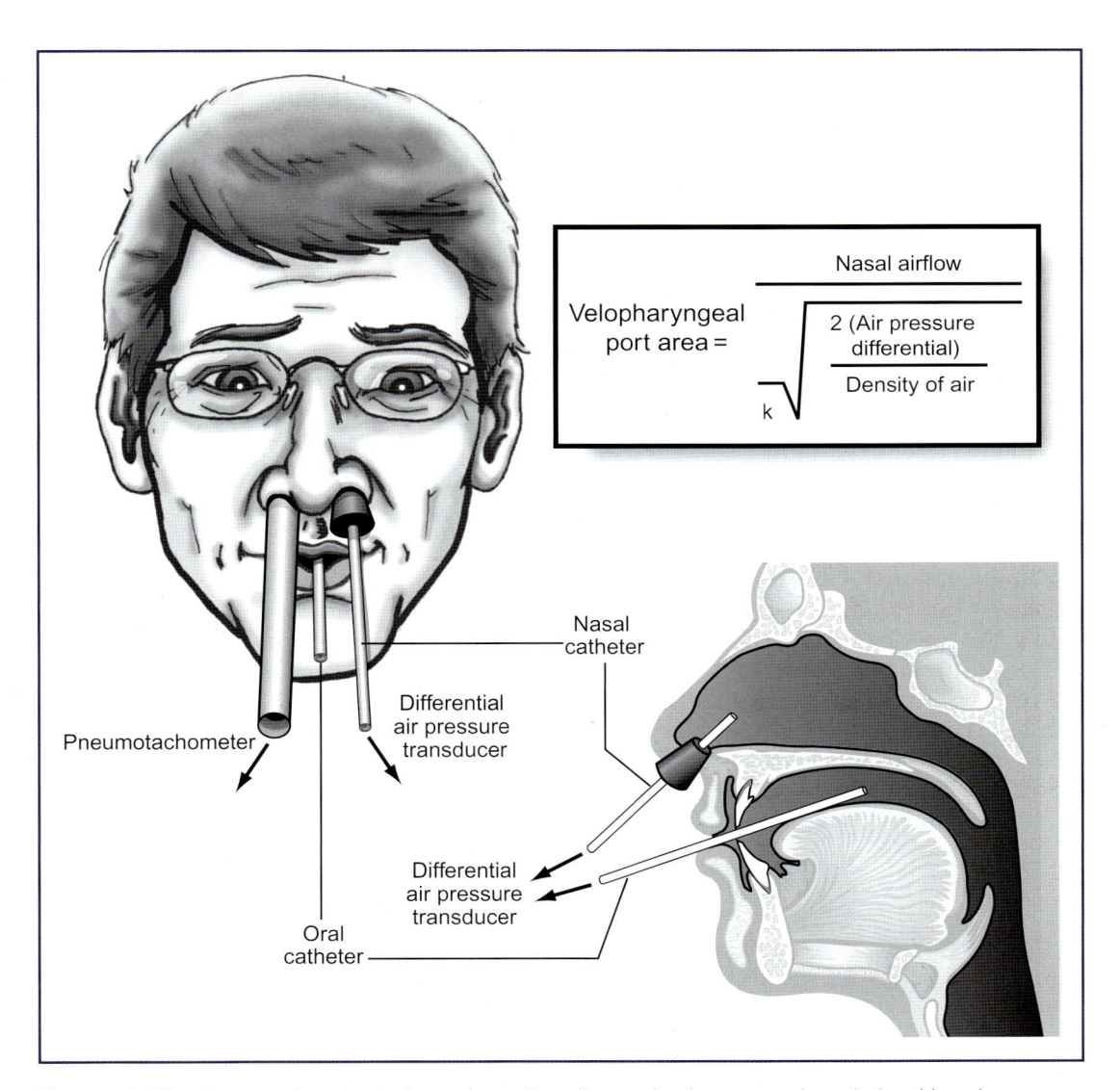

$$\text{Velopharyngeal port area} = \frac{\text{Nasal airflow}}{k\sqrt{\dfrac{2\,(\text{Air pressure differential})}{\text{Density of air}}}}$$

Figure 6-15. Pressure-flow technique for estimating velopharyngeal port size. Nasal pressure and oral pressure are sensed with small tubes connected to pressure transducers, and nasal airflow is sensed by a pneumotachometer. The resultant measures are entered into an equation that calculates the minimum cross-sectional area of the velopharyngeal port.

> **Out Your Nose Like a Garden Hose**
>
> Some think that airflow from the nose is a measure of velopharyngeal port size. It's true that nasal airflow depends on velopharyngeal port size, but it also depends on things like the size of the nostrils and the driving pressure of the breathing apparatus. Observing airflow from the nose is like watching water flow from the end of a garden hose that is being controlled by a friend around a blind corner. Your friend may be adjusting the faucet (changing the driving pressure) or squeezing and releasing the hose (changing its cross-section). We'll exclude the possibility that you're using your thumb to adjust the "nostril" of the hose. Different actions of your friend can make the flow of water change at your end of the hose, but you can't be sure what those actions are. The same is true of airflow from the nose. It can go up or down and you don't know why. It could be because of a single adjustment or a combination of adjustments. Be safe. Don't go with the flow.

Oral and nasal air pressures are recorded along with nasal airflow. The difference in air pressure across the velopharyngeal port and the rate of air movement through it are determined and entered into a working equation that yields the minimum cross-sectional area of the velopharyngeal port at each moment. Although some have proposed that nasal airflow alone is a useful measure of the degree of velopharyngeal opening, this is only true when the size of the velopharyngeal opening is small. As demonstrated by Warren (1967), the relation of nasal airflow to velopharyngeal opening is linear at small velopharyngeal orifice sizes, but the correlation between the two variables decreases as the size of the velopharyngeal orifice increases.

Pressure-flow recordings can also be used to calculate the resistance offered by the airway to the flow of air into and out of the velopharyngeal-nasal apparatus (Warren, Duany, & Fischer, 1969). Resistance across any segment of interest is calculated from the ratio of the air pressure difference across the segment to the rate of air movement through it. Resistance values are airflow dependent, so comparisons of resistance values are usually made at standard airflow values (Allison & Leeper, 1990).

MEASUREMENT AND ANALYSIS OF PHARYNGEAL-ORAL FUNCTION

This section considers instrumental measurement and analysis approaches to evaluating pharyngeal-oral function. The three approaches discussed in this section relate to structural and functional imaging, articulatory tracking, and aeromechanical observations.

Structural and Functional Imaging

Many of the pharyngeal-oral structures that participate in speech production are out of view of the casual observer. Therefore, various forms of imaging are employed to view these structures and their movements. Three types of imaging are of particular interest in the present context: x-ray imaging, magnetic resonance imaging, and ultrasound imaging. The first two of these also provide important means of evaluating velopharyngeal-nasal structures and their movements.

X-Ray Imaging

X-ray imaging is a powerful means of studying the upper airway (pharyngeal-oral apparatus and velopharyngeal-nasal apparatus). Such imaging provided much of the early data on the positions of structures in the form of lateral still x-rays and movements of structures in the form of cinefluorography (motion picture x-rays). Unfortunately, exposure to x-ray poses serious health risks, and regulations are now in place to restrict the amount of exposure allowed.

Lateral still x-rays, like that shown in Figure 6–16, provide a shadow-cast "snapshot" at a moment in time and are useful for examining structures that are stationary. Thus, they can be used to determine the positions of the lips, mandible, tongue, velum, posterior pharyngeal wall, and hyoid bone in relation to one another during sustained speech sounds (such as vowels, nasals, and fricatives) where such structures are relatively fixed in position. x-ray imaging can also be done using frontal views that make it possible to see structures such as the lateral pharyngeal walls (Kuehn & Dolan, 1975) and using multiple views that enable

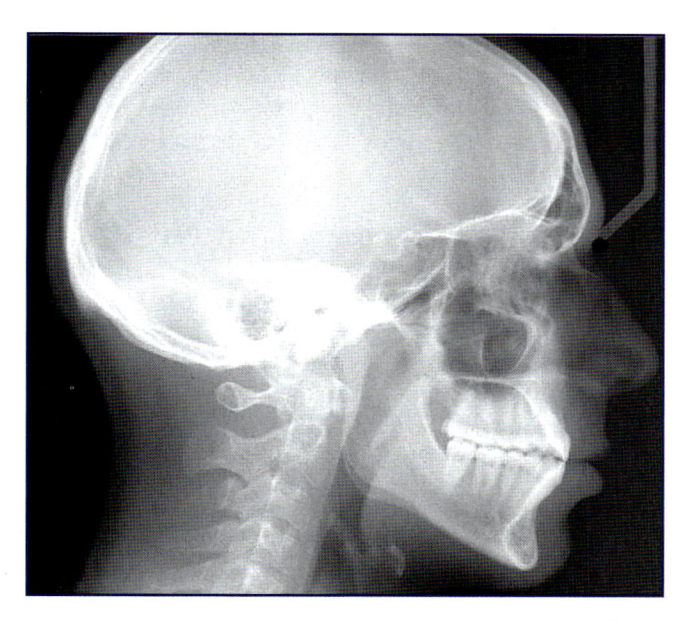

Figure 6–16. Lateral x-ray image of the head and neck. From *Speech and voice science* (p. 266), by A. Behrman, 2007. San Diego, CA: Plural Publishing, Inc. Image provided courtesy of David A. Behrman, DMD, Weill Cornell Medical Center, New York, NY. Reproduced with permission.

imaging of an entire region, such as the velopharynx, in lateral, frontal, and base projections (Skolnick, 1970). Although x-ray imaging offers clear views of bony structures, such as the hard palate, it is often limited in its ability to provide quality images of soft-tissue structures, such as the tongue, unless barium is used to enhance them.

Cinefluorography (or videofluorography) enables the x-ray study of structures in motion (McWilliams & Girdany, 1964; Moll, 1960). A great deal of knowledge about spatial and temporal coordination among structures during speech production (in a two-dimensional coordinate system) has been obtained using this methodology (Kent & Moll, 1975; Magen, Kang, Tiede, & Whalen, 2003; Netsell & Kent, 1976). For certain structures, such as the velopharynx, it is especially revealing to use multiview videofluorography (Golding-Kushner et al., 1990; Lam et al., 2006, Naran, Ford, & Losee, 2017). Speech production data obtained through the use of cinefluorography (or videofluorography) can be analyzed qualitatively or quantitatively. Videofluoroscopy is also used in the evaluation of swallowing and is discussed in Chapter 16.

Magnetic Resonance Imaging

Magnetic resonance imaging (MRI) offers a particularly effective way to observe pharyngeal-oral and velopharyngeal structures and their movements during speech production. MRI is based on the fact that protons (specifically, the nuclei of hydrogen molecules, which are abundant in the body) tend to line up when exposed to a magnetic field (induced by the scanner), and then tend to reorient themselves when hit with radio waves to create a signal of their own. The strength of this signal is proportional to the number of protons in a "slice" of body material, such as tissue, bone, and cartilage. Figure 6–17 shows a static magnetic resonance image of the head and neck in which the pharyngeal-oral structures are clearly visible. Note the clarity of the tongue position and shape compared with that provided in the x-ray image in Figure 6–16.

Technological advances have now made real-time MRI possible wherein high-quality images are captured at a fast sampling rate so that the movements of speech

---

Don't Put Things in Your Ears

Cinefluorographic (motion picture x-ray) studies of speech production require that the head be stabilized. Part of the instrumentation for doing this includes ear rods that fit in the ear canals (like sticking your index fingers in your ears). People aren't eager to try to turn their heads with these in place. We had occasion to see a person fall victim to a sequencing problem when a classroom demonstration about cinefluorography was ending. The lecturer was distracted by a question and stepped on a pedal to lower a hydraulic chair in which this person was sitting before taking out the ear rods (which were bolted to the wall). It was then that the person in the chair discovered a previously unreported reflex called "grab the stabilizer frame, support your weight, and scream at the lecturer." It was do that or be hanged by your ear canals. There are two morals to this story. Don't put things in your ears and don't put things in your ears.

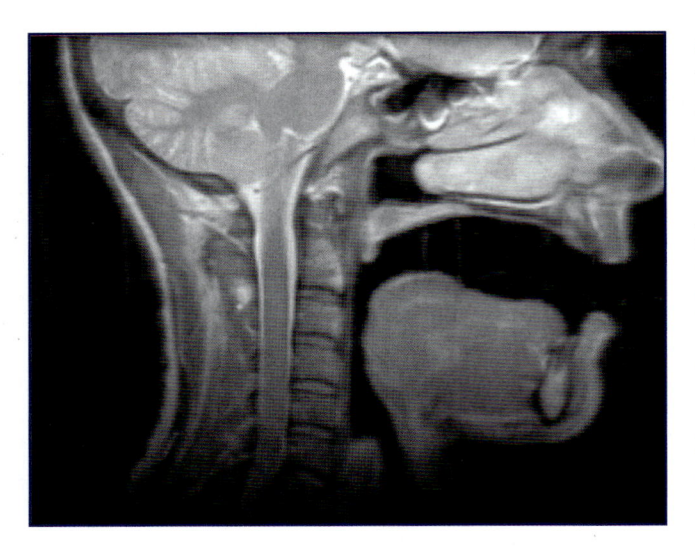

Figure 6–17. Magnetic resonance image of a lateral view of the head and neck (courtesy of Brad Story).

production can be recorded and analyzed (Toutios & Narayanan, 2016). Studies have been conducted using MRI to elucidate articulatory behavior during activities such as normal speaking (e.g., Bae, Kuehn, Conway, & Sutton, 2011), disordered speaking (e.g., Hagedorn et al., 2017; Lander-Portnoy & Goldstein, 2017), singing (Echternach, Burk, Burdumy, Traser, & Richter, 2016), and yodeling (Echternach, Markl, & Richter, 2011).

Ultrasonic Imaging

Ultrasonic methods provide another means for observing pharyngeal-oral function (Kelsey, Minifie, & Hixon, 1969; Stone, 1996). Such methods rely on the use of high-frequency sound waves (above the range that humans can hear) to map the positions and movements of internal structures. A combined sound generator–sound receiver is placed on the outer surface of the pharyngeal-oral apparatus and ultrasonic waves are generated and directed inward through body tissues. These waves propagate until they encounter the internal airway. Because ultrasonic waves do not travel well through air, they are reflected back through the same tissues and are picked up by the receiver. The time it takes for ultrasonic waves to make their round trip provides a measure of how far away the reflecting airway is from the sound generator.

The pharyngeal-oral structures that are most easily imaged with ultrasonic techniques are the dorsal surface of the tongue (Minifie, Kelsey, Zagzebski, & King, 1971; Stone, 2005; Watkin & Rubin, 1989) and the surfaces of the lateral pharyngeal walls (Miller, 2004; Minifie, Hixon, Kelsey, & Woodhouse, 1970; Zagzebski, 1975). When imaging the surface of the tongue, the ultrasonic generator and receiver are positioned below the chin and oriented so that the sound beam can be swept to scan the interface between the airway and the surface of the tongue (Stone, 1996). As shown in Figure 6–18, the tongue can be visualized from different perspectives using midsagittal and frontal scans and its position and configuration can be tracked over time (Davidson, 2005; Stone, Epstein, & Kskarous, 2004). The figure shows the tongue surface facing the hard palate as a white, illuminated band in both planes.

Ultrasonic imaging has been used to investigate aspects of normal speech production (e.g., Stone et al., 2007) and disordered speech production (e.g., Bressman, Radovanovic, Kulkarni, Klaiman, & Fisher, 2011). Ultrasound imaging can also be used in evaluation and management of speech disorders (Preston et al., 2017) and to model visual biofeedback in the management of speech disorders (Fabre, Heuber, Girin, Alameda-Pineda, & Badin, 2017).

Movement of the lateral pharyngeal walls can be monitored by placing the sound generator and sound receiver on the side of the neck corresponding to the lateral pharyngeal wall of interest (Kelsey, Ewanowski, Hixon, & Minifie, 1968). The ultrasonic signal is beamed through the neck and travels until it strikes the pharyngeal airspace and bounces back to the receiver. More than one generator-receiver unit can be placed along the neck to sample different vertical locations along the lateral pharyngeal wall (Miller, 2004; Zagzebski, 1975). Ultrasonic monitoring at the level of the oropharynx has shown that the lateral pharyngeal walls move inward for low vowel productions and outward for stop consonant productions (Minifie et al., 1970).

Articulatory Tracking

The movements of entire structures, such as those seen in x-ray and magnetic resonance imaging, are difficult to measure. One way to simplify the measurement problem is to adhere markers to structures at strategic locations and then track the movements of those markers. This approach, called flesh point tracking, has been used in x-ray microbeam imaging, electromagnetic sensing (articulography), and optoelectronic tracking. A different approach to articulatory tracking is used in electropalatography.

X-Ray Microbeam Imaging

X-ray microbeam technology was developed at the University of Tokyo (Kiritani, Itoh, & Fujimura, 1975) and a microbeam system was installed at the Univer-

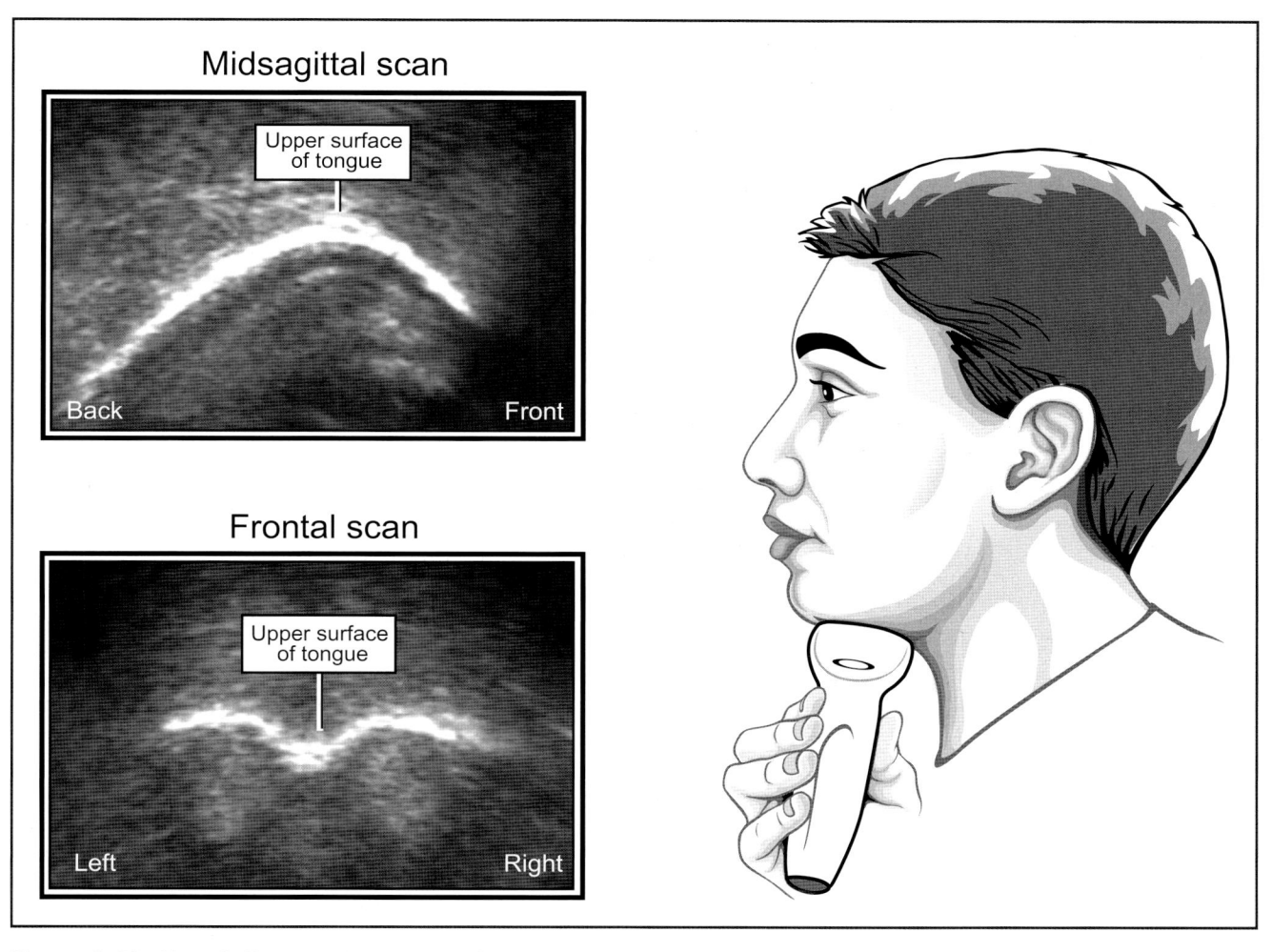

Figure 6-18. Use of ultrasound to image the tongue. A probe containing a generator and receiver is placed under the chin against the skin to obtain images of the tongue's surface. Ultrasonic images of the upper surface of the tongue in midsagittal and frontal perspectives are shown, illustrating lengthwise dorsal configuration and midline grooving, respectively (ultrasound images courtesy of Maureen Stone).

sity of Wisconsin–Madison in a facility supported as a national resource by the National Institutes of Health (NIH) (Westbury, 1991). The x-ray microbeam system was designed to track small pellets adhered to pharyngeal-oral structures using an extremely thin x-ray beam. The beam was focused on the pellets so that surrounding tissue received minimal radiation. Two-dimensional positions of multiple pellets could be tracked simultaneously. For example, multiple pellets could be affixed to the dorsal surface of the tongue to track the movement of different points along its surface. The tracking of specific flesh points removes some of the ambiguities of studying complex gestures, especially those involved in tongue movements (Honda, 2002; Kent, 1972; Wood, 1979). Fortunately, acoustic and perceptual analyses suggest that patterns of tongue movement are not appreciably changed with the pellets in place (Weismer & Bunton, 1999).

Figure 6–19A shows a midsagittal view of the pharyngeal-oral structures with pellets fixed to the outside of the upper and lower lips, on the mandible near the incisors, and at four locations on the dorsal surface of the tongue. Figure 6–19B provides a graphic representation of the movements of the flesh point pellets in two-dimensional space. The graph is oriented to indicate upward movement (toward the palate) when moving vertically along the ordinate and forward movement (toward the lips and beyond) when moving rightward along the abscissa. The tracings were generated with x-ray microbeam data recorded during production of the vowel sequence /iaui/. The movements of the pellets can be "relived" by following the tracings

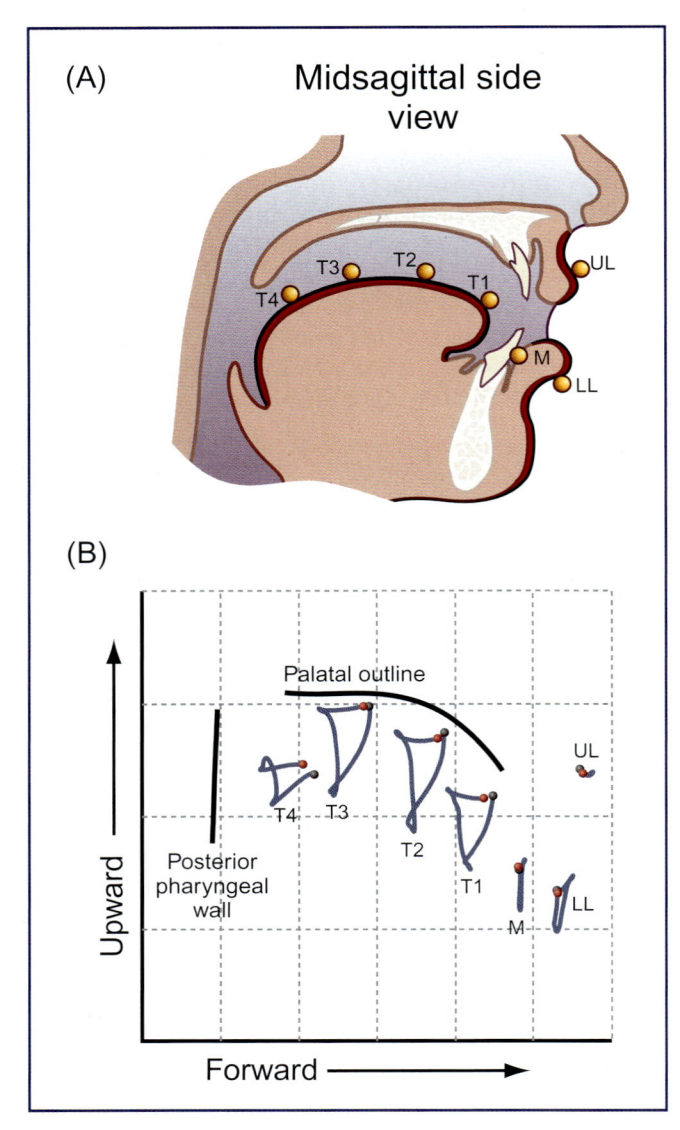

Figure 6–19. Flesh point locations (**A**) and representative tracings (**B**) during the production of the vowel sequence /iaui/. Flesh point locations are shown on the tongue (T), mandible, (M), upper lip (UL), and lower lip (LL). The movement sequence begins at the black dot and ends at the red dot. These locations and tracings apply to x-ray microbeam imaging and electromagnetic sensing (graphic data provided courtesy of Brad Story).

from the black dot (where the production of the first /i/ begins) along the trajectory of the blue line (during the movements associated with /ɑ/ and /u/), to the red dot (the termination of the second /i/). X-ray microbeam data such as these have been exceptionally useful in elucidating kinematic behavior of structures of the pharyngeal-oral apparatus in both individuals with normal speech production (e.g., Green & Wang, 2003; Nittrouer, 1991) and individuals with neuromotor-based speech disorders (e.g., Weismer, Yunusova, & Westbury, 2003; Yunusova, Weismer, & Lindstrom, 2011). Although the x-ray microbeam system was disassembled in 2010, the data that were generated with it continue to undergo analysis.

Electromagnetic Sensing (Articulography)

Electromagnetic sensing also provides a means for tracking the movements of multiple points on pharyngeal-oral structures, but without using x-ray. Electromagnetic sensing, also called articulography, relies on the use of a generator coil (or coils) and several sensor coils. The voltage induced in the receiving coils is inversely proportional to the distance between them and the generating coil(s). Suitable electronic manipulations provide a measure of the position of the receiving coils in one-, two-, or three-dimensional space.

Electromagnetic sensing was first applied to the pharyngeal-oral apparatus in studies of one- and two-dimensional movements of a point on the mandible (Hixon, 1971). Since then, more complex systems have been developed with applications to the study of multiple points on different structures on the inside and outside of the pharyngeal-oral apparatus (Perkell et al., 1992; Schonle et al., 1987; van der Giet, 1977). The most often studied points are on the mandible, lips, and tongue (usually at multiple sites).

Figure 6–20 shows a multiple-coil system called an electromagnetic articulograph (sometimes abbreviated as EMA). This type of system uses a computer algorithm to calculate the distance between generating (transmitting) and receiving coils as the receiving coils move through three-dimensional space over time. The resultant data can be displayed in different ways, including displacement-time plots (showing movement of flesh points over time) or x-y plots (showing the relative movements of flesh points in two-dimensional space, such as that shown in Figure 6–19B). The use of electromagnetic articulography in research and clinical studies is becoming increasingly popular and its measurement continues to be refined (Pattem, Illa, Afshan, & Ghosh, 2018). Articulographic data appear to be driving a more comprehensive understanding of normal and disordered speech production (e.g., Mefferd, 2017; Nip, Arias, Morita, & Richardson, 2017).

Optoelectronic Tracking

Optoelectronic tracking is another technology that can be useful for observing movements of a subset of pharyngeal-oral structures, specifically those structures that are visible externally, such as the lips and

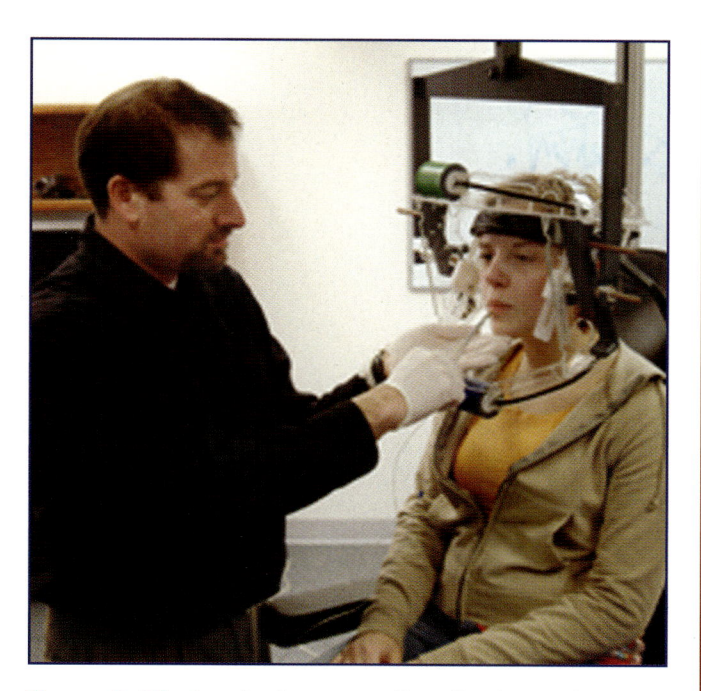

Figure 6–20. An electromagnetic articulograph (EMA) (photograph provided courtesy of Jordan Green).

Cornstarch

Modern systems are available that make it possible to determine the location of tongue contact with the palate. These take advantage of sensors embedded in an acrylic device that is worn like an upper denture. Signals from these sensors are displayed in a computer array that portrays the pattern of contact. The precursor to this electronic means of observation was cornstarch. The roof of the mouth was dusted white with cornstarch and then the articulatory action of interest was executed immediately. A quick look at the roof of the mouth right afterward would reveal where the tongue had made contact with the palate. The resulting pattern could be drawn on paper or photographed from a mirror reflection of the area on the palate where the tongue contact had wiped the cornstarch away. The method was crude in comparison to today's sophisticated techniques, but it worked nonetheless.

jaw. An optoelectronic tracking system requires fixing small markers (either light-emitting or reflective) on the surface of the structures of interest and the positioning of several cameras in different locations. The cameras record the position of the markers and their change in position (movements) in three dimensions. Optoelectronic tracking has been used to investigate lip and jaw movements to address questions related to topics such as normal speech development in children (e.g., Smith & Goffman, 1998; Nip, Green, & Marx, 2011) and speech disorders (e.g., MacPherson & Smith, 2013). An advantage of optoelectronic tracking is that speech can be produced with minimal encumbrance to speech structures. A disadvantage is that only movements of externally visible structures can be tracked.

Electropalatographic Monitoring

Electropalatographic monitoring differs from the other articulatory tracking systems discussed in this section in that it does not use markers to track specific locations and movements of structures. Instead, electropalatography is designed to sense the contact of the tongue against an artificial palate, such as that shown in Figure 6–21A. This form of sensing relies on the construction of an acrylic plate molded to fit against the hard palate of a specific individual. Within the plate are housed dozens of small electrodes, each of which responds (lights up) when the tongue touches it. During speaking, the electrodes are activated in patterns that reflect the contact of the tongue against the artificial palate at each moment, as illustrated in Figure 6–21B. Electropalatography has been used to study the behavior of the tongue during speech production in children and adults (e.g., Gibbon, Lee, & Yuen, 2010; Hardcastle, Barry, & Clark, 1987; Timmins, Hardcastle, Wood, & Cleland, 2011) and in the treatment of articulatory errors in children (Hitchcock, Byun, Swartz, & Lazarus, 2017) and adults (Mauszycki, Wright, Dingus, & Wambaugh, 2016). Nevertheless, it is relevant to note that electropalatography only provides information about tongue contact against the palate and does not provide information about tongue movement per se.

Aeromechanical Observations

Aeromechanical observations provide different insights into the function of the pharyngeal-oral apparatus than do the structural-level observations discussed above. Two common types of aeromechanical observations are oral air pressure and oral airflow.

Oral air pressure is most often measured using a sensing tube attached to an air pressure transducer. One end of the tube is placed in the oral cavity in the region of interest. To measure air pressure behind the lips, the tube might be inserted between the lips and into the oral vestibule (see Figure 6–7). To measure air pressures

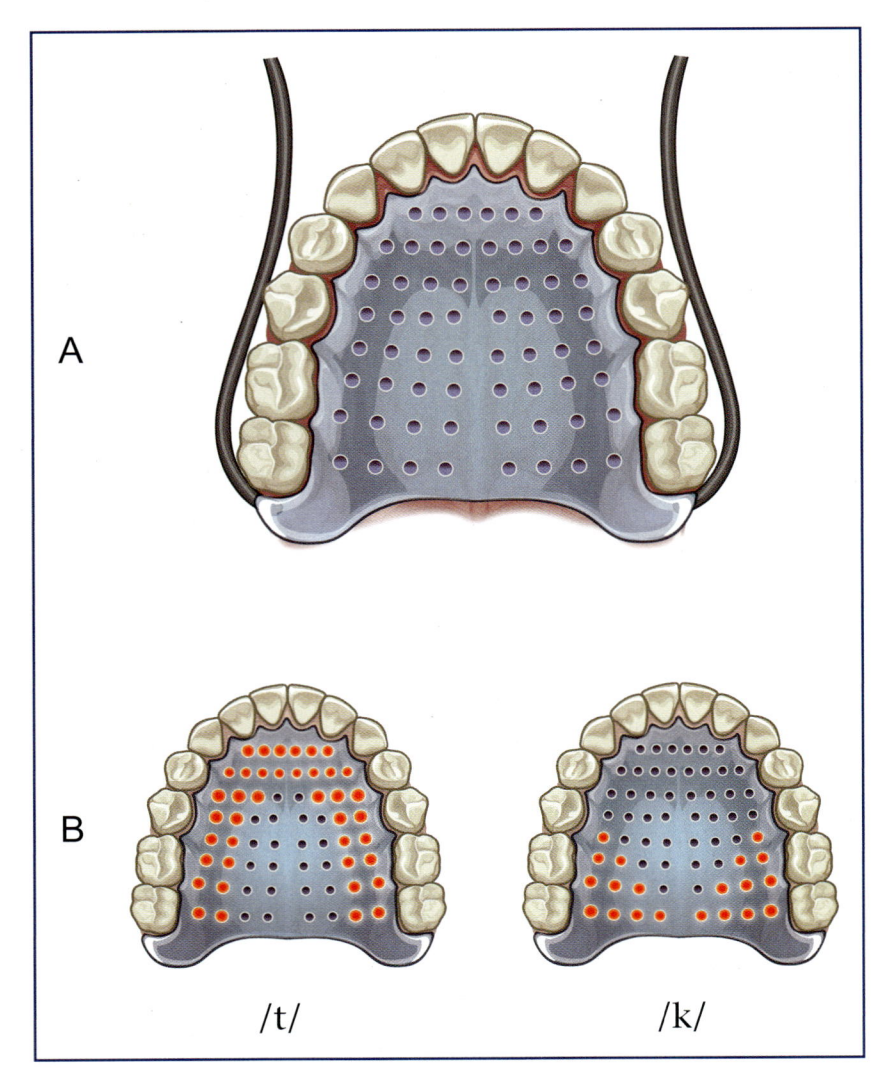

Figure 6–21. Electropalatographic monitoring. The custom-made artificial palate contains many small electrodes (**A**). When the tongue contacts these electrodes, they send a signal that reflects the tongue-palate contact pattern. Examples of typical patterns for the production of /t/ and /k/ are shown (**B**).

behind constrictions formed between the tongue and roof of the oral cavity, the end of the tube is positioned farther back in the oral cavity and might be configured to run between the upper cheek and gum and curve into the airway behind the teeth (Hardy, 1965).

Measures of oral air pressure reflect the force responsible for driving airflow through the pharyngeal-oral airway (Arkebauer, Hixon, & Hardy, 1967). Oral air pressure may differ from the pressure delivered by the breathing apparatus when the velopharynx is open or when the vocal folds offer a significant resistance to airflow. Lower-than-normal oral air pressure may be an indication of poor valving due to slow and/or insufficient movements of structures of the pharyngeal-oral apparatus and may be accompanied by weak-sounding voiceless stop-plosive, fricative, and affricate productions.

Oral airflow is usually measured at the airway opening and is most often channeled through a mouthpiece or facemask to a pneumotachometer, as illustrated in Figure 6–2. Airflow through the pharyngeal-oral apparatus is influenced by the openness of the airway and by the forcefulness with which air is being driven through the airway (Warren, 1996). Higher oral air pressures result in higher oral airflows at the release of stop-plosive consonants or during the formation of a fricative constriction. Measures of oral airflow are instructive regarding the status of the pharyngeal-oral airway (Gilbert, 1973; Isshiki & Ringel, 1964) and, like oral air pressure measures, provide information from which inferences can be made concerning valving adjustments and their integrity (Warren, Hall, & Davis, 1981).

Oral air pressure and oral airflow measures can be combined to calculate airway resistance along different segments of the pharyngeal-oral apparatus. This is done by dividing the air pressure difference between the two ends of a segment by the rate at which air is flowing through the segment, much like the calculation of laryngeal airway resistance described above. For example, this method can be used to determine the resistance offered by an airway constriction used to produce a fricative consonant (Warren, 1996).

Oral air pressure and oral airflow measures can also be combined to calculate the cross-sectional area of the airway at different locations along the pharyngeal-oral apparatus. For example, oral air pressure and oral airflow data can be used to calculate changes in the size of the minimum cross-section (maximum constriction) along the airway during consonant productions (Hixon, 1966; Smith, Allen, Warren, & Hall, 1978; Warren et al., 1981) using an aeromechanical equation similar to the one used to calculate the area of the velopharyngeal port (see Figure 6–15). Figure 6–22 illustrates the change in minimum cross-sectional area within the oral cavity during an /s/ production in a consonant-vowel syllable. As can be seen, the cross-section of the airway decreases significantly during the early part of the /s/, reaches its smallest value coincident with the maximum sound pressure level for the consonant, and then abruptly enlarges as the fricative constriction transitions into the following vowel. Data of this type can be used to define the size of airway constrictions and the precision of their control in both normal individuals and in individuals with structural or neuromotor disorders (Warren et al., 1981).

HEALTH CARE PROFESSIONALS AND CLINICAL MEASUREMENTS

The measurements discussed in this chapter have been instrumental in providing much of the knowledge that informs current understanding of speech physiology and upon which much of the material in Chapters 2 through 5 is based. As such, these measurements have a clear role in research settings where speech scientists strive to uncover the mysteries of speech production. Nevertheless, these measurements also play a role in clinical settings where speech-language pathologists and other professionals may use these measurements in their evaluation (and occasionally management) of their clients with speech disorders. This section offers a brief overview of health care professionals who provide services to clients with speech disorders and who

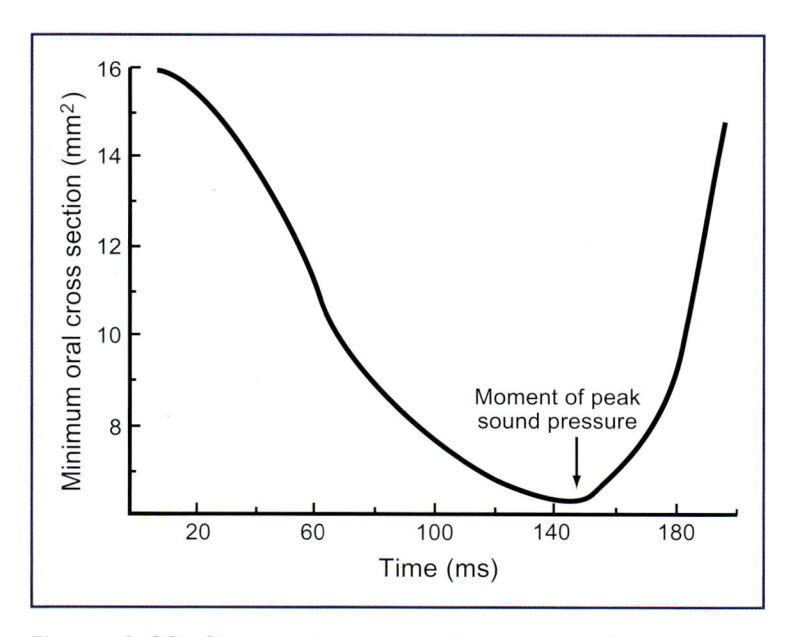

Figure 6–22. Change in cross-sectional area of the oral airway during /s/ production in a syllable context as determined through the use of an aeromechanical equation employing oral air pressure and oral airflow measurements.

use speech physiology measurements such as those described above (as well as other forms of measurement not covered in this chapter). Some of these professionals see a broad range of clients with speech disorders (speech-language pathologists, psychologists, neurologists, and radiologists), whereas others are more apt to provide services to clients with disorders of particular speech subsystems (pulmonologists, respiratory therapists, physical therapists, otorhinolaryngologists, plastic surgeons, dentists, and prosthodontists), as shown in Table 6–1.

The speech-language pathologist is considered the expert in speech disorders. In certain cases, the speech-language pathologist is the only professional to evaluate and manage a person with a speech disorder. A good example of this is an individual with a functional-misuse disorder (with no signs of a physical disorder). A functional-misuse disorder may be manifest in any of the speech subsystems; however, they are most often seen in the form of voice disorders caused by inappropriate use of the laryngeal subsystem, often in conjunction with misuse of the breathing subsystem.

Sally Peterson-Falzone, Clinician-Scientist Extraordinaire

In the adjacent text, we refer to "scientists" and "clinicians" as though they are separate entities. And in many cases they are—the scientist does research and the clinician provides services to clients. But there are also people like Sally Peterson-Falzone, PhD, CCC-SLP, who are both. Sally's contributions have been at the highest levels of science and clinical service, contributions that have changed the lives of children around the world who were born with cleft palates and other craniofacial birth defects. A short list of her contributions includes heading up two long-running NIH grants on craniofacial anomalies, publishing definitive articles and books on the topic, serving as a leader in the American Cleft Palate-Craniofacial Association, and mentoring many others who have stepped into leadership roles. Sally has been described as a "wildly popular" speaker, a "generous and attentive mentor," and a "walking encyclopedia" on how to manage speech in children with clefts of the lip and palate. Although ostensibly retired, Sally continues to perform international humanitarian work and to stir up controversy at international meetings, always with sagacity and wit.

Table 6–1. Health Care Professionals Who May Provide Services to Clients with Disorders Affecting the Four Speech Subsystems (Breathing, Laryngeal, Velopharyngeal-Nasal, and Pharyngeal-Oral)

HEALTH CARE PROFESSIONAL	BREATHING	LARYNGEAL	VELOPHARYNGEAL-NASAL	PHARYNGEAL-ORAL
Speech-language pathologist	X	X	X	X
Psychologist/counselor	X	X	X	X
Neurologist	X	X	X	X
Radiologist	X	X	X	X
Pulmonologist	X			
Respiratory therapist	X			
Physical therapist	X			
Otorhinolaryngologist		X	X	
Plastic surgeon			X	X
Dentist				X
Prosthodontist			X	X

Another example of a speech disorder with no physical basis is "phoneme specific emission" in which a child with an entirely normal speech mechanism has developed the habit of opening the velopharynx on a particular sound, such as an /s/, that should be produced with a closed velopharynx. Evaluation of such cases may include some of the measurements described in this chapter, and management consists of behavioral therapy conducted by the speech-language pathologist alone. In many other types of cases, however, the speech-language pathologist is only one of several professionals involved in a client's care.

The services of a psychologist (or counselor) may be needed when a speech disorder is accompanied by emotional distress. Psychologists have expertise in the psychological bases of behavior and, therefore, can help clients work through psychological issues that may be the basis of a speech disorder, such as in the case of conversion voice disorders (conversion disorders are those that cannot be explained by a medical condition but, rather, result from the conversion of psychic pain or stress into physical symptoms and signs). Psychologists can also help clients and their families cope with the grief and depression that may come with the loss of physical function or the stresses that accompany situations such as having a child with a malformed brain or immature lungs.

A neurologist is a physician with expertise in disorders of the nervous system. Many speech disorders stem from damage or disease of the nervous system and require the oversight of a neurologist. Sometimes a neurologist will refer a client with a known neural disease to a speech-language pathologist for evaluation and management of a concomitant speech and/or swallowing disorder. Other times the speech-language pathologist will be the first professional to see a client who exhibits speech or swallowing signs which are suggestive of an underlying neural impairment. In such cases, it will be the speech-language pathologist who refers the client to the neurologist for a diagnostic evaluation. Examples of the types of individuals who are under the care of a neurologist are those with Parkinson's disease (a degenerative brain disease that causes problems such as slow movement, rigidity, and tremor), cerebral palsy (a nonprogressive disorder of movement and posture due to brain insult occurring in the period of early maturation), and multiple sclerosis (a disease of the myelin that surrounds axons within the central nervous system and causes problems such as muscle weakness and dyscoordination). A neurologist's primary interests in speech physiology measurements are those that provide information about movement speed and accuracy and muscle strength.

A radiologist is a physician who specializes in medical imaging, such as x-ray, computed tomography (CT), and MRI, among others. Such imaging may be used to locate and identify tumors or other abnormalities that might be found in any part of the speech mechanism. The radiologist also oversees radiation treatment of cancerous tumors, such as those that might arise in the lungs, larynx, nasal, or oral parts of the speech mechanism. The role of the radiologist in the diagnosis of swallowing disorders is discussed in Chapter 16.

A pulmonologist is a physician with expertise in breathing disorders. Examples of the types of clients who are under the care of a pulmonologist are those with pulmonary disease, such as cystic fibrosis (a genetic disease that causes excess secretion of mucus and airway obstruction) and those with severe neuromuscular disease, such as muscular dystrophy (a genetic disease that causes weakness and degeneration of muscles). Clients who require ventilator support are always overseen by a pulmonologist. A pulmonologist will often order pulmonary function tests that provide measures of lung volume, airflow, and air pressure that may be of use to the speech-language pathologist. A pulmonologist has the first and last word when it comes to the care of a person with a breathing disorder, because breathing outweighs everything else in importance.

A respiratory therapist carries out specific evaluation and management procedures requested by a pulmonologist, such as performing pulmonary function testing and teaching clients how to clear secretions from their lungs. A speech-language pathologist may work side by side with a respiratory therapist when evaluating or managing clients with certain types of speech breathing disorders, especially those who are supported by ventilators.

A physical therapist has expertise in the evaluation and management of body positioning and movement. Examples of the types of individuals that a physical therapist might evaluate and manage include those with structural deformity, spinal cord or brain injury, and degenerative neural disease, among others. A speech-language pathologist might work together with a physical therapist to determine optimal body positioning for a client with a speech breathing disorder. Measurements of breathing in different body positions are sometimes useful in determining which body position is best for speech production.

An otorhinolaryngologist is a physician who specializes in ear (oto), nose (rhino), and throat (laryngo) disorders (and is, therefore, commonly referred to as an ENT). The otorhinolaryngologist will usually use an endoscope (rigid or flexible, depending on the need) to examine the larynx for possible structural problems (e.g., polyps, nodules, ulcers) or physiological dysfunction (e.g., vocal fold paralysis, tremor, joint ankylosis) or the velopharynx to look for velopharyngeal closure during various activities. Otorhinolaryngologists may perform surgical procedures on clients with craniofacial disorders (such as cleft palate) and neoplastic (tumor) growths in the upper airway and are also the physicians responsible for managing nasal obstructions, auditory (eustachian) tube dysfunction, and middle ear problems. A laryngologist is an otorhinolaryngologist with a subspecialty in diseases of the larynx. Some laryngologists are highly trained in surgical procedures of the larynx that affect voice and are called phonosurgeons. A laryngologist who specializes as a phonosurgeon might be concerned with procedures such as those that influence the mechanical nature of vibration of the vocal fold cover and the enhancement of laryngeal closure through the implantation of different substances into the vocal folds. Endoscopic images provided by the otorhinolaryngologist are of great interest to the speech-language pathologist, and in the best of all circumstances those images are obtained with the speech-language pathologist present to help guide the speech portion of the examination. Measurements of velopharyngeal-nasal and laryngeal function, such as air pressure and airflow, are relevant to both the otorhinolaryngologist and speech-language pathologist for evaluation purposes as well as for documenting the effects of medical and behavioral management.

A plastic surgeon is a physician concerned with surgical repair and/or reconstruction of deformed or destroyed parts of the body as a result of anomalous development, disease, or trauma. Responsibilities of a plastic surgeon might include the repair of clefts of the hard and soft palates in children and any secondary surgical procedure that might be required, such as constructing a surgical flap across the velopharyngeal airway. Responsibilities may also include removal of an invasive tumor from the tongue or jaw and reconstruction of the affected area. In the case of surgery of the outer nose, the plastic surgeon may also perform cosmetic surgery to improve appearance.

The dentist is the specialist responsible for the care and repair of teeth and for surgical procedures associated with the teeth and gums. The dentist plays a prominent role in the management of clients with significant dental problems such as supernumerary (an excess number of) teeth and misaligned teeth. Subspecialists of dentistry include the orthodontist (who corrects tooth irregularities) and the pedodontist (whose focus is dentistry in children). The dentist may also be called on to handle dental problems associated with traumatic injury to craniofacial structures or sequelae to the surgical resection of parts of the mandible and other structures of the facial skeleton. At times, the dentist and the plastic surgeon work closely together in planning a course of management for a client, sometimes with the prosthodontist involved as well.

A prosthodontist is a dentist who specializes in the replacement of missing parts through the fabrication of prostheses. Work of the prosthodontist is concerned with restoring function, appearance, and health to those who have abnormal structures caused by congenital anomaly, disease, trauma, or surgery. Clients who require the services of a prosthodontist include those born with palatal clefts that are exceptionally wide and are managed through the fitting of a palatal obturator, a device that is fixed to the maxillary teeth and occludes the gap between the palatal shelves. Similarly, clients who have large parts of the palate or tongue resected because of cancer may be fitted with a prosthesis as replacement or partial replacement for the excised structure. A prosthodontist may fabricate customized velar-lift prostheses for clients with paresis or paralysis of the velum. A velar-lift prosthesis consists of a plate that extends backward along the roof of the mouth to lift the velum to a horizontal plane and support its weight against the force of gravity. The speech-language pathologist usually works with the prosthodontist to help evaluate the success of different prostheses on velopharyngeal-nasal function during breathing, speaking, and swallowing. Some of the measurements described in this chapter are useful in determining the best prosthesis for the client.

The health care professionals described above represent many, though not all, of those commonly encountered in clinical practice. As should be clear from these descriptions, a team of health care professionals is often required to determine the best strategies for habilitating or rehabilitating clients with speech disorders.

REVIEW

Much of our current understanding of speech production physiology has come from measurement and analysis of the structure and function of the breathing apparatus, laryngeal apparatus, velopharyngeal-nasal apparatus, and pharyngeal-oral apparatus.

Breathing physiology can be measured using spirometry, chest wall surface tracking, and manometry.

Spirometers (wet spirometers and those that include pneumotachometers) can provide measures of lung volume, lung volume change (airflow), and ventilation.

Chest wall surface tracking instruments (respiratory magnetometers and respiratory inductance plethysmographs) can be used to measure lung volume and lung volume change, ventilation, and chest wall shape and shape change.

Manometers are pressure-measuring devices and include U-tube manometers, air-gauge manometers, and pressure transducers (mechanical-electrical manometers), the last of which are the best for measuring oral pressure (from which to estimate alveolar pressure) during speech production.

Laryngeal structure and function can be examined and quantified using endoscopy, electroglottography, and aeromechanical observations.

Laryngeal endoscopy can be performed using a rigid or flexible endoscope, a straight light source or a stroboscopic one, and in some cases, a high-speed imaging system.

Electroglottography is a noninvasive way to track changes in the area of contact between the two vocal folds during speech production.

Aeromechanical measures that provide insight into laryngeal function include airflow (both the slowly changing average airflow and the fast changing cycle-to-cycle airflow associated with vocal fold vibration) and a combination of air pressure and airflow to calculate laryngeal airway resistance during voice production.

Structure and function of the velopharyngeal-nasal apparatus can be examined using nasoendoscopy and aeromechanical observations, as well as certain imaging approaches that are also used to examine the pharyngeal-oral apparatus.

Nasoendoscopy involves the use of a flexible endoscope that is passed posteriorly through the nasal airway and positioned so that the velopharynx can be viewed from above while speech is being produced.

Aeromechanical measurement can provide insight into velopharyngeal-nasal function during speech production and includes measurement of nasal airflow, nasal air pressure, and special methods for combining measures of airflow and air pressure to estimate velopharyngeal-nasal pathway resistance and velopharyngeal port area.

Measurement and analysis of the pharyngeal-oral apparatus includes structural and functional imaging (x-ray imaging, magnetic resonance imaging [MRI], and ultrasound imaging), articulatory tracking (using x-ray microbeam imaging, electromagnetic sensing, and optoelectronic tracking), and aeromechanical observations.

X-ray imaging provided much of the seminal data on upper airway articulatory movements during speech production, whereas real-time MRI and ultrasonic imaging, which carry much less risk than x-ray, continue to refine our understanding of such movements.

Flesh point tracking systems simplify the measurement of articulatory movements by tracking specific points on structures rather than entire structures, something that has been done with an x-ray microbeam system and currently is being done with electromagnetic sensing (articulography) of multiple articulators and optoelectronic tracking of visually accessible articulators.

Electropalatography monitors tongue contact with the palate during speech production with the use of an artificial palate embedded with sensors.

Information about how well the pharyngeal-oral apparatus is valving the airstream during speech production can be obtained by measuring oral pressure and oral airflow.

There are many health care professionals who may participate in obtaining or using these speech physiology measurements, including speech-language pathologists, psychologists (and counselors), neurologists, radiologists, pulmonologists, respiratory therapists, physical therapists, otorhinolaryngologists, plastic surgeons, dentists, and prosthodontists.

REFERENCES

Allison, D., & Leeper, H. (1990). A comparison of noninvasive procedures to assess nasal airway resistance. *Cleft Palate Journal, 27,* 40–44.

Arkebauer, H., Hixon, T., & Hardy, J. (1967). Peak intra-oral air pressure during speech. *Journal of Speech and Hearing Research, 10,* 196–208.

Bae, Y., Kuehn, D., Conway, C., & Sutton, B. (2011). Real-time magnetic resonance imaging of velopharyngeal activities with simultaneous speech recordings. *Cleft-Palate Craniofacial Journal, 48,* 695–707.

Baken, R., & Orlikoff, R. (2000). *Clinical measurement of speech and voice* (2nd ed.). San Diego, CA: Singular.

Behrman, A. (2007). *Speech and voice science.* San Diego, CA: Plural.

Bressmann, T., Radovanovic, B., Kulkarni, G., Klaiman, P., & Fisher, D. (2011). An ultrasonic investigation of cleft-type compensatory articulations of voiceless velar stops. *Clinical Linguistics and Phonetics, 25,* 1028–1033.

Bunton, K., & Hoit, J. (2018). Development of velopharyngeal closure for vocalization during the first two years of life. *Journal of Speech, Language, and Hearing Research, 61*(3), 549–560.

Bunton, K., Hoit, J., & Gallagher, K. (2011). A simple technique for determining velopharyngeal status during speech production. *Seminars in Speech and Language, 32,* 69–80.

Childers, D., Hicks, D., Moore, G., Eskenazi, L., & Lalwani, A. (1990). Electroglottography and vocal fold physiology. *Journal of Speech and Hearing Research, 33,* 245–254.

Childers, D., & Krishnamurthy, A. (1985). A critical review of electroglottography. *Critical Review of Biomedical Engineering, 12,* 131–161.

Childers, D., Smith, A., & Moore, G. (1984). Relationships between electroglottography, speech, and vocal cord contact. *Folia Phoniatrica, 36,* 105–118.

Colton, R., & Casper, J. (1996). *Understanding voice problems: A physiological perspective for diagnosis and treatment* (2nd ed.). Baltimore, MD: Williams & Wilkins.

Colton, R., & Conture, E. (1990). Problems and pitfalls of electroglottography. *Journal of Voice, 4,* 10–24.

D'Antonio, L., Marsh, J., Province, M., Muntz, H., & Phillips, C. (1989). Reliability of flexible fiberoptic nasopharyngoscopy for evaluation of velopharyngeal function in a clinical population. *Cleft Palate Journal, 26,* 217–225.

D'Antonio, L., Netsell, R., & Lotz, W. (1988). Clinical aerodynamics for the evaluation and management of voice disorders. *Ear, Nose, and Throat Journal, 67,* 394–399.

Darling-White, M., & Huber, J. (2017). The impact of expiratory muscle strength training on speech breathing in individuals with Parkinson's disease: A preliminary study. *American Journal of Speech-Language Pathology, 26,* 1159-1166.

Davidson, L. (2005). Addressing phonological questions with ultrasound. *Clinical Linguistics and Phonetics, 19,* 619–633.

Deliyski, D., Hillman, R., & Mehta, D. (2015). Laryngeal high-speed videoendoscopy: Rationale and recommendation for accurate and consistent terminology. *Journal of Speech, Language, and Hearing Research, 58,* 1488-1492.

Echternach, M., Burk, F., Burdumy, M., Traser, L., & Richter, B. (2016). Morphometric differences of vocal tract articulators in different loudness conditions in singing. *PLoS One, 11,* e0153792. doi:10.1371/journal.pone.0153792

Echternach, M., Markl, M., & Richter, B. (2011). Vocal tract configurations in yodelling—prospective comparison of two Swiss yodeller and two non-yodeller subjects. *Logopedics Phoniatrics Vocology, 36,* 109–113.

Eshghi, M., Vallino, L. D., Baylis, A. L., Preisser, J. S., & Zajac, D. J. (2017). Velopharyngeal status of stop consonants and vowels produced by young children with and without repaired cleft palate at 12, 14, and 18 months of age. *Journal of Speech, Language, and Hearing Research, 60,* 1467–1476.

Fabre, D., Heuber, T., Girin, L., Alameda-Pineda, X., & Badin, P. (2017). Automatic animation of an articulatory tongue model from ultrasound images of the vocal tract. *Speech Communication, 93,* 63–75.

Fisher, K., & Swank, P. (1997). Estimating phonation threshold pressure. *Journal of Speech, Language, and Hearing Research, 40,* 1122–1129.

Fourcin, A. (1974). Laryngographic examination of vocal fold vibration. In B. Wyke (Ed.), *Ventilatory and phonatory control systems* (pp. 315–326). London, UK: Oxford University Press.

Gibbon, F., Lee, A., & Yuen, I. (2010) Tongue-palate contact during selected vowels in normal speech. *Cleft Palate-Craniofacial Journal, 47,* 405–412.

Gilbert, H. (1973). Oral airflow during stop consonant production. *Folia Phoniatrica, 25,* 288–301.

Golding-Kushner, K., Argamaso, R., Cotton, R., Grames, L., Henningsson, G., Jones, D., . . . Ysunza, A. (1990). Standardization for the reporting of nasopharyngoscopy and Multiview videofluoroscopy: A report from an International Working Group. *Cleft Palate Journal, 27,* 337–347.

Green, J., & Wang, Y. (2003). Tongue-surface movement patterns during speech and swallowing. *Journal of the Acoustical Society of America, 113,* 2820–2833.

Hagedorn, C., Proctor, M., Goldstein, L., Wilson, S., Miller, B., Gorno-Tempini, M., & Narayanan, S. (2017). Characterizing articulation in apraxic speech using real-time magnetic resonance imaging. *Journal of Speech, Language, and Hearing Research, 60,* 877–891.

Hardcastle, W., Barry, R., & Clark, C. (1987). An instrumental phonetic study of lingual activity in articulation disordered children. *Journal of Speech and Hearing Research, 30,* 171–184.

Hardy, J. (1965). Air flow and air pressure studies. *ASHA Reports, 1,* 141–152.

Herbst, C., Schutte, H., Bowling, D., & Svec, J. (2017). Comparing chalk with cheese—the EGG contact quotient is only a limited surrogate of the closed quotient. *Journal of Voice, 31,* 401–409.

Hertegård, S., Gauffin, J., & Lindestad, P-Å. (1995). A comparison of subglottal and intraoral pressure measurements during phonation. *Journal of Voice, 9,* 149–155.

Hirano, M., & Bless, D. (1993). *Videostroboscopic examination of the larynx.* San Diego, CA: Singular.

Hitchcock, E., Byun, T., Swartz, M., & Lazarus, R. (2017). Efficacy of electropalatography for treating misarticulation of /r/. *American Journal of Speech-Language Pathology, 26,* 1141–1158.

Hixon, T., (1966). Turbulent noise sources for speech. *Folia Phoniatrica, 18,* 168–182.

Hixon, T. (1971). An electromagnetic method for transducing jaw movements during speech. *Journal of the Acoustical Society of America, 49,* 603–606.

Hixon, T., Goldman, M., & Mead, J. (1973). Kinematics of the chest wall during speech production: Volume displacements of the rib cage, abdomen, and lung. *Journal of Speech and Hearing Research, 16,* 78–115.

Hixon, T., & Hoit, J. (2005). *Evaluation and management of speech breathing disorders: Principles and methods.* Tucson, AZ: Redington Brown.

Hoit, J., Banzett, R., Brown, R., & Loring, S. (1990). Speech breathing in individuals with cervical spinal cord injury. *Journal of Speech and Hearing Research, 33,* 798–807.

Holmberg, E., Hillman, R., & Perkell, J. (1988). Glottal airflow and transglottal air pressure measurements for male and female speakers in soft, normal, and loud voice. *Journal of the Acoustical Society of America, 84,* 511–529.

Holmberg, E., Hillman, R., & Perkell, J. (1989). Glottal airflow and transglottal air pressure measurements for male and female speakers in low, normal, and high pitch. *Journal of Voice, 3,* 294–305.

Honda, K. (2002). Evolution of vowel production studies and observation techniques. *Acoustical Science and Technology, 23,* 189–194.

Isshiki, N. (1985). Clinical significance of a vocal efficiency index. In I. Titze & R. Scherer (Eds.), *Vocal fold physiology: Biomechanics, acoustics, and phonatory control* (pp. 230–238). Denver, CO: The Denver Center for the Performing Arts.

Isshiki, N., & Ringel, R. (1964). Air flow during production of selected consonants. *Journal of Speech and Hearing Research, 7,* 233–244.

Isshiki, N., & von Leden, H. (1964). Hoarseness: Aerodynamic studies. *Archives of Otolaryngology, 80*, 206–213.

Kelsey, C., Ewanowski, S., Hixon, T., & Minifie, F. (1968). Determination of lateral pharyngeal wall motion during connected speech by use of pulsed ultrasound. *Science, 161*, 1259–1260.

Kelsey, C., Minifie, F., & Hixon, T. (1969). Applications of ultrasound in speech research. *Journal of Speech and Hearing Research, 12*, 564–575.

Kendall, K., & Leonard, R. (2010). *Laryngeal evaluation: Indirect laryngoscopy to high-speed digital imaging*. New York, NY: Thieme Medical.

Kent, R. (1972). Some considerations in the cineradiographic analysis of tongue movements during speech. *Phonetica, 26*, 293–306.

Kent, R., & Moll, K. (1975). Articulatory timing in selected consonant sequences. *Brain and Language, 2*, 304–323.

Kiritani, S., Itoh, K., & Fujimura, O. (1975). Tongue-pellet tracking by a computer-controlled x-ray microbeam system. *Journal of the Acoustical Society of America, 57*, 1516–1520.

Kitzing, P. (1990). Clinical applications of electroglottography. *Journal of Voice, 4*, 238–249.

Kuehn, D., & Dolan, K. (1975). A tomographic technique of assessing lateral pharyngeal wall displacement. *Cleft Palate Journal, 12*, 200–209.

Lam, D., Starr, J., Perkins, J., Lewis, C., Eblen, L., Dunlap, J., & Sie, K. (2006). A comparison of nasendoscopy and multiview videofluoroscopy in assessing velopharyngeal insufficiency. *Otolaryngology–Head and Neck Surgery, 134*, 394–402.

Lander-Portnoy, M., & Goldstein, L. (2017). Using real time magnetic resonance imaging to measure change in articulatory behavior due to partial glossectomy. *The Journal of the Acoustical Society of America, 142*, doi:10.1121/1.5014684

Lecluse, F., Brocaar, M., & Verschuure, J. (1975). The electroglottography and its relation to glottal activity. *Folia Phoniatrica, 27*, 215–224.

Leeper, H., & Graves, D. (1984). Consistency of laryngeal airway resistance in adult women. *Journal of Communication Disorders, 17*, 153–163.

MacPherson, M., & Smith, A. (2013). Influences of sentence length and syntactic complexity on the speech motor control of children who stutter. *Journal of Speech, Language, and Hearing Research, 56*, 89–102.

Magen, H., Kang, A., Tiede, M., & Whalen, D. (2003). Posterior pharyngeal wall position in the production of speech. *Journal of Speech, Language, and Hearing Research, 46*, 241–251.

Mauszycki, S., Wright, S., Dingus, N., & Wambaugh, J. (2016). The use of electropalatography in the treatment of acquired apraxia of speech. *American Journal of Speech-Language Pathology, 25*, S697–S715.

McWilliams, B., & Girdany, B. (1964). The use of Televex in cleft palate research. *Cleft Palate Journal, 1*, 398–401.

Mefferd, A. (2017). Tongue- and jaw-specific contributions to acoustic vowel contrast changes in the diphthong /ai/ in response to slow, loud, and clear speech. *Journal of Speech, Language, and Hearing Research, 60*, 3144–3158.

Miller, J. (2004). Lateral pharyngeal wall motion during swallowing using real time ultrasound. *Dysphagia, 12*, 125–132.

Minifie, F., Hixon, T., Kelsey, C., & Woodhouse, R. (1970). Lateral pharyngeal wall movement during speech production. *Journal of Speech and Hearing Research, 13*, 584–594.

Minifie, F., Kelsey, C., Zagzebski, J., & King, T. (1971). Ultrasonic scans of the dorsal surface of the tongue. *Journal of the Acoustical Society of America, 49*, 1857–1860.

Moll, K. (1960). Cinefluorographic techniques in speech research. *Journal of Speech and Hearing Research, 3*, 227–241.

Motta, G., Cesari, U., Iengo, G., & Motta, G. (1990). Clinical application of electroglottography. *Folia Phoniatrica, 42*, 111–117.

Naran, S., Ford, M., & Losee, J. (2017). What's new in cleft palate and velopharyngeal dysfunction management? *Plastic and Reconstructive Surgery, 139*, 1343e–1355e.

Netsell, R., & Hixon, T. (1978). A noninvasive method for clinically estimating subglottal air pressure. *Journal of Speech and Hearing Disorders, 43*, 326–330.

Netsell, R., & Kent, R. (1976). Paroxysmal ataxic dysarthria. *Journal of Speech and Hearing Disorders, 41*, 93–109.

Nip, I., Arias, C., Morita, K., & Richardson, H. (2017). Initial observations of lingual movement characteristics of children with cerebral palsy. *Journal of Speech, Language, and Hearing Research, 60*, 1780–1790.

Nip, I., Green, J., & Marx, D. (2011). The co-emergence of cognition, language, and speech motor control in early development: A longitudinal correlational study. *Journal of Communication Disorders, 44*, 149–160.

Nittrouer, S. (1991). Phase relations of jaw and tongue tip movements in the production of VCV utterances. *Journal of the Acoustical Society of America, 90*, 1806–1815.

Orlikoff, R. (1998). Scrambled EGG: The uses and abuses of electroglottography. *Phonoscope, 1*, 37–53.

Patel, R., Barkmeier-Kraemer, J., Awan, S., Courey, M., Deliyski, D., . . . Hillman, R. (in press). Recommended protocols for instrumental assessment of voice: American Speech-Language-Hearing Association Expert Panel to Develop a Protocol for Instrumental Assessment of Vocal Function. *American Journal of Speech-Language Pathology*.

Patel, R., Dailey, S., & Bless, D. (2008). Comparison of high-speed digital imaging with stroboscopy for laryngeal imaging of glottal disorders. *Annals of Otology, Rhinology, and Laryngology, 117*, 413–424.

Pattem, A., Illa, A., Afshan, A., & Ghosh, P. (2018). Optimal sensor placement in electromagnetic articulography recording for speech production study. *Computer Speech & Language, 47*, 157–174.

Pegoraro-Krook, M., Dutka-Souza, J., & Marino, V. (2008). Nasoendoscopy of velopharynx before and during diagnostic therapy. *Journal of Applied Oral Science, 16*, 181–188.

Perkell, J., Cohen, M., Svirsky, M., Matthies, M., Garabieta, I., & Jackson, M. (1992). Electromagnetic midsagittal articulometer systems for transducing speech articulatory movements. *Journal of the Acoustical Society of America, 92*, 3078–3096.

Plexico, L., Sandage, M., & Faver, K. (2012). Assessment of phonation threshold pressure: A critical review and clinical implications. *American Journal of Speech Language Pathology, 20*, 348-366.

Poburka, B., Patel, R., & Bless, D. (2017). Voice-Vibratory Assessment with Laryngeal Imaging (VALI) form: Reliability of rating stroboscopy and high-speed videoendoscopy. *Journal of Voice, 31,* 513.e1–513.e14.

Preston, J., McAllister Byun, T., Boyce, S., Hamilton, S., Tiede, M., Phillips, E., Rivera-Campos, A., & Whalen, D. (2017). Ultrasonic images of the tongue: A tutorial for assessment and remediation of speech sound errors. *Journal of Visualized Experiments, 119,* e55123.

Rothenberg, M. (1973). A new inverse-filtering technique for deriving the glottal air flow waveform during voicing. *Journal of the Acoustical Society of America, 53,* 1632–1645.

Rothenberg, M. (1992). A multichannel electroglottograph. *Journal of Voice, 6,* 36–43.

Rothenberg, M. (2009). Voice onset time versus articulatory modeling for stop consonants. *Logopedics Phoniatrics Vocology, 34,* 171–180.

Rothenberg, M., & Mahshie, J. (1988). Monitoring vocal fold abduction through vocal contact area. *Journal of Speech and Hearing Research, 31,* 338–351.

Schönle, P., Grabe, K., Wenig, P., Hohne, J., Schrader, J., & Conrad, B. (1987). Electromagnetic articulography: Use of alternating magnetic fields for tracking movements of multiple points inside and outside the vocal tract. *Brain and Language, 31,* 26–35.

Skolnick, M. (1970). Videofluoroscopic examination of the velopharyngeal portal during phonation in lateral and base projections—a new technique for studying the mechanics of closure. *Cleft Palate Journal, 7,* 803–816.

Smith, A., & Childers, D. (1983). Laryngeal evaluation using features from speech and the electroglottograph. *IEEE Transactions on Biomedical Engineering, 30,* 755–759.

Smith, A., & Goffman, L. (1998). Stability and patterning of speech movement sequences in children and adults. *Journal of Speech, Language, and Hearing Research, 41,* 18–30.

Smith, H., Allen, G., Warren, D., & Hall, D. (1978). The consistency of the pressure-flow technique for assessing oral port size. *Journal of the Acoustical Society of America, 64,* 1203–1206.

Smitheran, J., & Hixon, T. (1981). A clinical method for estimating laryngeal airway resistance during vowel production. *Journal of Speech and Hearing Disorders, 46,* 138–146.

Solomon, N., & Hixon, T. (1993). Speech breathing in Parkinson's disease. *Journal of Speech and Hearing Research, 36,* 294–310.

Stone, M. (1996). Instrumentation for the study of speech physiology. In N. Lass (Ed.), *Principles of experimental phonetics* (pp. 495–524). St. Louis, MO: Mosby-Year Book.

Stone, M. (2005). A guide to analyzing tongue motion from ultrasound images. *Clinical Linguistics and Phonetics, 19,* 455–501.

Stone, M., Epstein, M., & Kskarous, K. (2004). Functional segments in tongue movement. *Clinical Linguistics and Phonetics, 18,* 507–521.

Stone, M. Stock, G., Bunin, K., Kumar, K., Epstein, M., Kambhamettu, C., . . . Prince, J. (2007). Comparison of speech production in upright and supine position. *Journal of the Acoustical Society of America, 122,* 532–541.

Svec, J., & Schutte, H. (1996). Videokymography: High-speed line scanning of vocal fold vibration. *Journal of Voice, 10,* 201–205.

Thom, S., Hoit, J., Hixon, T., & Smith, A. (2006). Velopharyngeal function during vocalization in infants. *Cleft Palate-Craniofacial Journal, 43,* 539–546.

Thompson, A., & Hixon, T. (1979). Nasal air flow during normal speech production. *Cleft Palate Journal, 16,* 412–420.

Timmins, C., Hardcastle, W., Wood, S., & Cleland, J. (2011). An EPG analysis of /t/ in young people with Down's syndrome. *Clinical Linguistics and Phonetics, 25,* 1022–1027.

Titze, I. (1988). The physics of small-amplitude oscillation of the vocal folds. *Journal of the Acoustical Society of America, 83,* 1536–1552.

Titze, I. (1990). Interpretation of the electroglottographic signal. *Journal of Voice, 4,* 1–9.

Toutios, A., & Narayanan, S. (2016). Advances in real-time magnetic resonance imaging of the vocal tract for speech science and technology research. *Asia Pacific Signal and Information Processing Association (APSIPA) Transactions on Signal Information and Processing, 5.* doi:10.1017/ATSIP.2016.5

van den Berg, J., Zantema, J., & Doornenbal, P. (1957). On the air resistance and the Bernoulli effect of the human larynx. *Journal of the Acoustical Society of America, 29,* 626–631.

van der Giet, G. (1977). Computer controlled method for measuring articulatory activities. *Journal of the Acoustical Society of America, 61,* 1072–1076.

Verdolini-Marston, K., Titze, I., & Druker, D. (1990). Changes in phonation threshold pressure with induced conditions of hydration. *Journal of Voice, 4,* 142–151.

Warren, D. (1967). Nasal emission of air and velopharyngeal function. *Cleft Palate Journal, 4,* 148–156.

Warren, D. (1996). Regulation of speech aerodynamics. In N. Lass (Ed.), *Principles of experimental phonetics* (pp. 46–92). St. Louis, MO: Mosby-Year Book.

Warren, D., Duany, L., & Fischer, N. (1969). Nasal pathway resistance in normal and cleft lip and palate subjects. *Cleft Palate Journal, 6,* 134–140.

Warren, D., & DuBois, A. (1964). A pressure-flow technique for measuring velopharyngeal orifice area during continuous speech. *Cleft Palate Journal, 1,* 52–71.

Warren, D., Hall, D., & Davis, J. (1981). Oral port constriction and pressure-flow relationships during sibilant productions. *Folia Phoniatrica, 33,* 380–394.

Watkin, K., & Rubin, J. (1989). Pseudo-three-dimensional reconstruction of ultrasound images of the tongue. *Journal of the Acoustical Society of America, 85,* 496–499.

Weismer, G., & Bunton, K. (1999). Influences of pellet markers on speech production behavior: Acoustical and perceptual measures. *Journal of the Acoustical Society of America, 105,* 2882–2894.

Weismer, G., Yunusova, Y., & Westbury, J. (2003). Interarticulator coordination in dysarthria: An x-ray microbeam study. *Journal of Speech, Language, and Hearing Research, 46,* 1247–1261.

Westbury, J. (1991). The significance and measurement of head position during speech production experiments using the x-ray microbeam system. *Journal of the Acoustical Society of America, 89*, 1782–1791.

Wistbacka, G., Sundberg, J., & Simberg, S. (2016). Vertical laryngeal position and oral pressure variations during resonance phonation in water and in air: A pilot study. *Logopedics, Phoniatrics, Vocology, 41*, 117–123.

Wood, S. (1979). A radiographic analysis of constriction locations for vowels. *Journal of Phonetics, 7*, 25–43.

Yamauchi, A., Imagawa, H., Yokonishi, H., Nito, T., Yamasoba, T., Goto, T., . . . Tayama, N. (2012). Evaluation of vocal fold vibration with an assessment form for high-speed digital imaging: Comparative study between healthy young and elderly subjects. *Journal of Voice, 26*, 742–750.

Yunusova, Y., Weismer, G., & Lindstrom, M. (2011). Classifications of vocalic segments from articulatory kinematics: Healthy controls and speakers with dysarthria. *Journal of Speech, Language, and Hearing Research, 54*, 1302–1311.

Zagzebski, J. (1975). Ultrasonic measurement of lateral pharyngeal wall motion at two levels in the vocal tract. *Journal of Speech and Hearing Research, 18*, 308–318.

7

Acoustics

INTRODUCTION

Physical acoustics encompasses a huge range of topics, many of which are not covered in this text. The information presented here is selected to serve as a foundation for the study of speech acoustics (Chapters 8–11), auditory anatomy and physiology (Chapter 13), and auditory psychophysics (Chapter 14). Readers interested in a full, technical treatment of acoustics should consult the classic textbook by Beranek (1986, originally published in 1954). Entertaining histories of acoustics as a scientific discipline have been published by Hunt (1978) and Beyer (1999).

Acoustics has been studied for centuries (Hunt, 1978). Over these many years a rich foundation of knowledge has evolved that is not specific to individual, contemporary studies in the scientific literature. This chapter does not cite a large or even modest number of publications, but rather derives its presentation from a composite of textbook material written by Beranek (1986), Blackstock (2000), and Kinsler, Frey, Coppens, and Sanders (2000).

This chapter addresses a series of questions. Answers to these questions provide a foundational understanding of speech acoustics and audition. The questions are as follows:

1. What are pressure (sound) waves, and how can they be measured?
2. What is sinusoidal motion, and which measurements are relevant to its description?
3. What are complex acoustic events, and how are they related to sinusoids?
4. What is the phenomenon of resonance, and how is resonant frequency determined in mechanical and acoustical systems?
5. What does it mean to say that a resonator "shapes" an input?
6. What is the difference between a resonator and a filter?

Secret Acoustical Society?

The leading acoustics organization in the world is the Acoustical Society of America (ASA), founded in 1929. Roughly 35 scientists attended the initial 1929 meeting of the Society (that's the number counted in a photograph taken of the attendees at the meeting). Today, ASA has over 7,000 members, who study all aspects of acoustics. The Society encourages open exchange of ideas and education in acoustics. It wasn't always so. The science of acoustics goes way back to the Ionian philosopher Pythagoras (ca. 575–495 BC), the same fellow after whom a famous geometry theorem is named. Pythagoras enjoyed a sort of guru status, and his followers decided that their investigations should be kept secret to protect their intellectual sanctity. We know the Pythagoreans made numerous observations about acoustical events, but alas, we only learned about these through indirect sources—leaks in the system. So, the first Acoustical Society was really a Secret Acoustical Society.

PRESSURE WAVES

This section considers the nature of pressure waves. It discusses the forces that govern such waves, how local changes in air pressure occur, how pressure waves propagate through space, and how such waves can be measured and represented.

The Motions of Vibrating Air Molecules Are Governed by Simple Forces

Sound can be defined as the propagation of a pressure wave—a *sound wave*—in space and time. Clarification of this definition requires a precise definition of exactly what is meant by the term *pressure wave*.

Sound is always propagated through some medium. The various media that conduct sound waves (e.g., water, steel, air) are composed of molecules that are compressible, the degree of compressibility depending on the medium. In other words, molecules of these media may, under the influence of a force, be displaced away from their rest positions (where "rest positions" refers to the positions when no forces are applied to the medium) and moved closer to nearby molecules. The resulting "bunching up" of molecules, relative to their distribution at rest, shows that the medium is compressible.

The molecules of all sound-conducting media share the characteristics of *elasticity* and *mass*. Elastic objects oppose displacement, and do so with greater magnitude as they are moved farther from their rest positions. A common example of this is a rubber band. When the rubber band is completely collapsed, it is in its rest position. As the rubber band is stretched, it becomes stiffer. Increasing the stretch on a rubber band not only increases its stiffness, but makes it more difficult to stretch. Massive objects oppose being accelerated and decelerated (that is, they have *inertia*: "a body in motion tends to stay in motion"), and do so with greater magnitude as they become more massive. The effect of mass on motion is easily appreciated by the speeding automobile that does not stop instantly when the brakes are applied.

Opposition to displacement (elasticity) and acceleration/deceleration (inertia) result in energy storage. This stored energy can be expressed as motion of the object even in the absence of an external force. This topic is taken up in greater detail below.

The sound-conducting medium of interest for speech is, at least in most cases, air. The number of molecules in a cubic inch of air, referred to as the density of air and symbolized with the Greek letter *rho* (ρ), is approximately 4×10^{23}. The density of molecules in water is about four times greater than that in air, and in steel about eleven times greater than air.

With air as the medium, a schematic drawing[1] can be used to illustrate the concepts mentioned above. Imagine, as shown in Figure 7–1, four columns of air molecules (labeled 1, 2, 3, 4) extending across some distance. Five rows, labeled A, B, C, D, E, show the state of these molecules at successive moments in time. Row A (hereafter, time A) shows the molecules at rest, with no external forces applied to them. This rest position is indicated across all times by the dashed lines extending downward throughout the four columns of molecules. Note the even spacing between the molecules across time A.

Molecules at rest are still in motion (this small motion is referred to as *Brownian* motion), but the average spacing between any pair of molecules will be roughly equivalent, as shown in Figure 7–1, time A. Because the molecules at time A are not being displaced from their rest positions and thus not being accelerated, they store no elastic or inertial energy (other than the negligible energies stored due to Brownian motion). At time B, the molecule in column 1 is subjected to a *force* (indicated by the rightward directed arrow) that moves it rightward, away from its rest position and in the direction of the molecule at position 2. For present purposes, a *force* can be thought of as any push or pull applied to an object. As the molecule moves farther from its rest position, it opposes increasing displacement by generating an increasing *recoil force*, which is exerted in the direction of the rest position, or the direction opposite to its current motion. Stated in a different way, the original force of the rightward push is transferred to the air molecule, whose rightward displacement is increasingly opposed by the tendency of the molecule to recoil back to its rest position. The current motion continues away from the rest position because the original force of the push still exceeds the recoil force. The recoil force is the stored energy resulting from the displacement of the molecule from its rest position. Recoil is a hallmark of all elastic objects.

At position 2, time B, several things happen. First, the spacing between molecules 1 and 2 is now minimal compared with their spacing at rest (time A). At position 2, time B, the molecules are bunched up, and molecule 1 bumps molecule 2, just as the push originally bumped molecule 1 to get this process under way. Second, the molecule that was originally pushed to start the process and is now displaced relatively far from its rest position generates a strong recoil force to return to its rest position. At some point, the recoil force equals and then exceeds the original force and thus stops its rightward motion and begins to move leftward, back toward the rest position. Assume that the bump of molecule 2 by molecule 1 occurs at the same time as the recoil force of molecule 1 becomes greater than the original force on it. Molecule 1 therefore imparts a displacing force on molecule 2 and generates its own force to return to its rest position.

---

[1] A *schematic* drawing is basically a graphical model that attempts to capture the important aspects of a phenomenon while reducing or eliminating other information. For example, a stick person is a schematic of the human form, and a road sign indicating a curve is a schematic of the actual layout of a curving roadway.

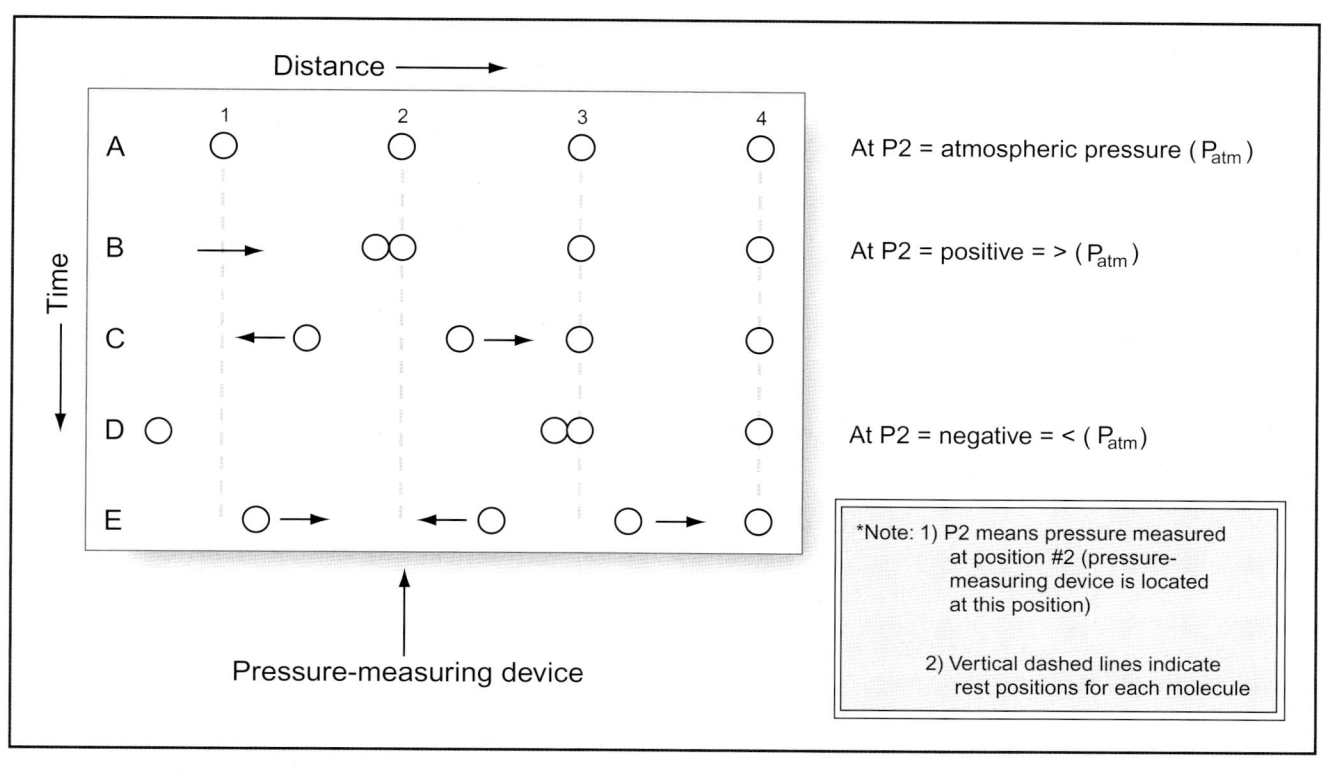

Figure 7-1. Schematic drawing of the vibration of air molecules around their rest positions. Rest positions of four molecules are shown at time "A" at positions 1, 2, 3, and 4. Time is indicated by the rows A, B, C, D, and E. A pressure-measuring device is located at the rest position of molecule 2. See text for details.

At time C, the molecule from position 1 is headed back toward the rest position (leftward-directed arrow). The molecule from position 2, having been bumped by the position 1 molecule, now moves away from its rest position and in the direction of the molecule at position 3 (rightward-directed arrow). At time D, the molecule from position 2 is bumping into the molecule at position 3, and is also about to reverse its direction—just like the situation discussed above for time B, position 2. The molecule from position 1, however, has gone *through* its rest position, and is displaced far to the left—note at time D the wide separation of the molecules from positions 1 and 2. Clearly, the elastic recoil forces caused the molecule from position 1 to move back toward the rest position at time E, but why doesn't the motion stop at the rest position—why has it passed the rest position at point 1? The answer is that inertial forces do not allow the molecule to "stop on a dime" at the rest position, but drive the molecule through rest and to the rightward extreme. The molecule, which has mass and opposes acceleration and deceleration, does not decelerate instantly to stop at the rest position, but rather continues its motion through that point in space. As the molecule passes through the rest position and continues to move away from it, it is once again stretched and develops recoil force. The molecule continues this motion until the recoil forces again overcome the forces driving the molecule away from its rest position (primarily inertial). Once again, the motion is reversed, and the molecule heads back in the direction of the rest position. And once again, the motion does not stop at the rest position because of inertial forces; the molecule continues to move back and forth around the rest position.

It is important to understand that the forces maintaining the back and forth motion of the molecule around the rest position are a product of the motion itself: recoil and inertial forces result from the motion of the molecule. These forces are intrinsic to the motion of the molecule, rather than imposed from an outside source (as was the case with the bumping force that initiated the motion).

After the original application of the force at position 1, therefore, the back and forth motion is maintained by energy stored by the molecule itself. If the molecules were vibrating in a *frictionless* medium, in which no energy was lost because of heat generation, the back and forth motion would continue indefinitely. Realistically, heat loss due to air molecules rubbing against each other and other surfaces eventually cause the back and forth motion to die out if external forces are not continuously reapplied to the air molecules. However, the principles of recoil and inertia forces still apply to a dying-out motion. The frictional forces compete with the recoil and inertial forces and, in the absence of external forces (such as another bump), eventually dominate the latter two and end the motion.

The Motions of Vibrating Air Molecules Change the Local Densities of Air

The motion of air molecules and the forces that control that motion have been described. How can this description lead to an understanding of pressure waves? Assume that a device for measuring air pressure is placed at position 2 in Figure 7–1. *Pressure* can be defined as the force exerted over a unit area (P = F/A) and is proportional to the density of air. When air molecules are more densely packed in some unit volume, they collide with each other more frequently and generate more force and more pressure within that volume. Conversely, when air molecules are less densely packed, the collisions are less frequent and the pressures are relatively lower. At time A in Figure 7–1, there are no external forces applied to the air molecules and the density of air is that associated with air at rest (recall the 4×10^{23} figure given above). The pressure measured at time A, position 2 (or at any other position at time A, because the density of air at rest is the same at any spatial location) is referred to as *atmospheric pressure*. The actual value of atmospheric pressure is not important to the current discussion,[2] but the *reference function* of this pressure is important. In the following discussion, atmospheric pressure (symbolized hereafter as Patm) is considered as zero (0) pressure. At time B, the schematic drawing shows two molecules close together at position 2, indicating a relatively denser packing of air molecules at that position compared with time A. The pressure measuring device at time B, position 2 measures a higher pressure than at time A because the denser packing of molecules involves more frequent collisions and higher forces. Any time a pressure is above the reference pressure Patm, it is referred to as *positive pressure*. The more tightly packed the molecules, the more positive the pressure.

At time D, position 2, the first and second molecules are widely separated in space. This represents a case where the density of air is less than it is at Patm. The pressure-measuring device records a value below Patm, which is a *negative pressure*. The less tightly packed the molecules, the more negative the pressure.

These positive and negative pressures are not positive or negative in any absolute sense. They are only positive (above) or negative (below) with respect to the reference pressure Patm. Figure 7–2 shows the result of the continuous bunching up and spreading apart of the air molecules schematized in Figure 7–1.

The three rows labeled A, B, D in Figure 7–2 correspond to the same rows in Figure 7–1 (rows C and E from Figure 7–1 have been omitted from Figure 7–2), indicating three different times in the evolving history of air molecule movement. At time A, each of the multiple dots represents an air molecule, and the collection of these molecules is shown evenly distributed across space, as expected if the medium is not affected by an external force. The pressure at any point throughout the distribution, measured at any location in space from the left to the right edge of the dot display, is Patm.

At time B, this distribution has been changed to one in which regions of low and high density alternate across space. The heavily shaded areas represent high densities (as when two molecules are immediately adjacent, Figure 7–1, time B, position 2), and the lightly shaded areas represent low densities (Figure 7–1, time D, position 2). At time D, regions of high and low densities again alternate across space, but their locations have been reversed from those at time B. In other words, for a given point in space (such as position 2), what was a high-density and high-pressure area at time B is a low-density, low-pressure area at time D. Areas of high density and high pressure are called areas of *compression* or *condensation*[3]; areas of low density and low pressures are called areas of *rarefaction*.

Pressure Waves, Not Individual Molecules, Propagate Through Space and Vary as a Function of Both Space and Time

Recall what was said earlier about the motion of individual air molecules. They move around a rest position, the movement resulting from inherent elastic and inertial forces. The molecules themselves, however, do not *propagate* across space. What moves across space

---

[2] Atmospheric pressure at sea level is 101, 325 pascal (Pa) (or 101.3 kPa), 14.7 pounds per square inch (an alternative unit of pressure), or 1013 *millibars* (another alternative unit of pressure).
[3] Condensation is the result of compression. For purposes of this text, compression and condensation are used interchangeably.

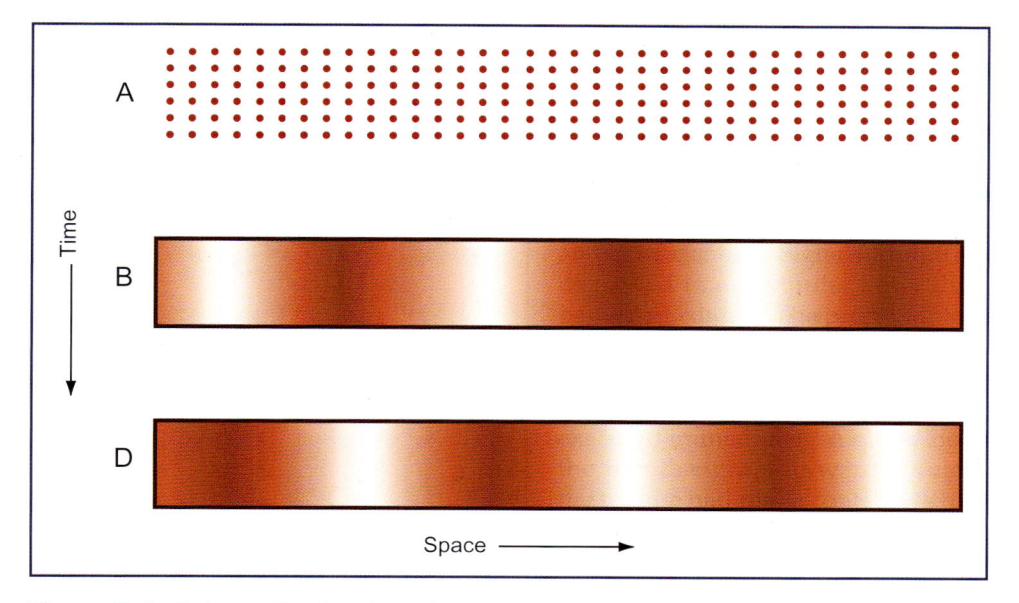

Figure 7–2. Schematic drawing of pressure waves, distributed in space and time. A, B, and D correspond to discrete times depicted in Figure 7–1. At a given point in space, pressure changes over time.

is the *pressure wave*, shown in Figure 7–2 from left to right as the sequence of high and low densities (pressures), or the sequence of compression (condensation) and rarefaction areas. Because these alternating regions of high and low pressures are the result of the back and forth movement of air molecules, which alternately bunches them up and spreads them apart, a given point in space sometimes has high pressure (such as time B, position 2 in Figure 7–1), and sometimes has low pressure (time D, position 2 in Figure 7–1). Thus, a pressure wave extends across space at a specific instant in time (examine Figure 7–2, across time B or D) and varies in time at a specific point in space (Figure 7–2, compare times B and D at any point in space).

When a pressure wave moves away from the *source* of the sound waves (the origin of the forces that initiated the displacement of air molecules), the alternating regions of high and low pressures often project more or less in a straight line, as shown from left to right in Figure 7–2. These kinds of sound waves are called *plane waves*, because the sequence of high and low pressures can be thought of as a series of pressure "slices," or planes, extending away from the source. The pathway followed by plane waves may vary as a function of frequency, as discussed below. For the present discussion, only plane waves are considered, but other kinds of pressure waves are possible (for example, those moving sideways from a source, rather than in a straight line away from the source: see comment on this in Chapter 11).

The Variation of a Pressure Wave in Time and Space Can Be Measured

There are specific measures of the temporal (time) and spatial (space) variation of pressure waves. A firm grasp of these measures is essential to understanding important aspects of the acoustic theory of vowel production, covered in Chapter 8.

Temporal Measures

Figure 7–3A redraws a portion of the molecule motion shown in Figure 7–1. Of interest is the motion of the first molecule, shown in Figure 7–3A as a shaded circle. As in Figure 7–1, space (distance) is shown from left to right, and time from top to bottom (times A, B, C, D, E, occurring in succession). The numbers 1, 2, 3, 4, and 5 above the filled circles show the position of the first molecule at five discrete points in time, starting from the molecule at the rest position "1" and ending back at the rest position "5." At time B (molecule labeled "2"), the molecule is immediately adjacent to the next molecule, which creates a region of compression, or high pressure, at the point in space indicated by the upward-pointing arrow. The pressure at this point in space becomes somewhat negative at time C (molecule labeled "3"), more negative yet at time D (molecule labeled "4"), and returns to Patm at time E (molecule labeled "5").

The motion of the filled-circle molecule is shown as a function of time in Figure 7–3B. When any magnitude

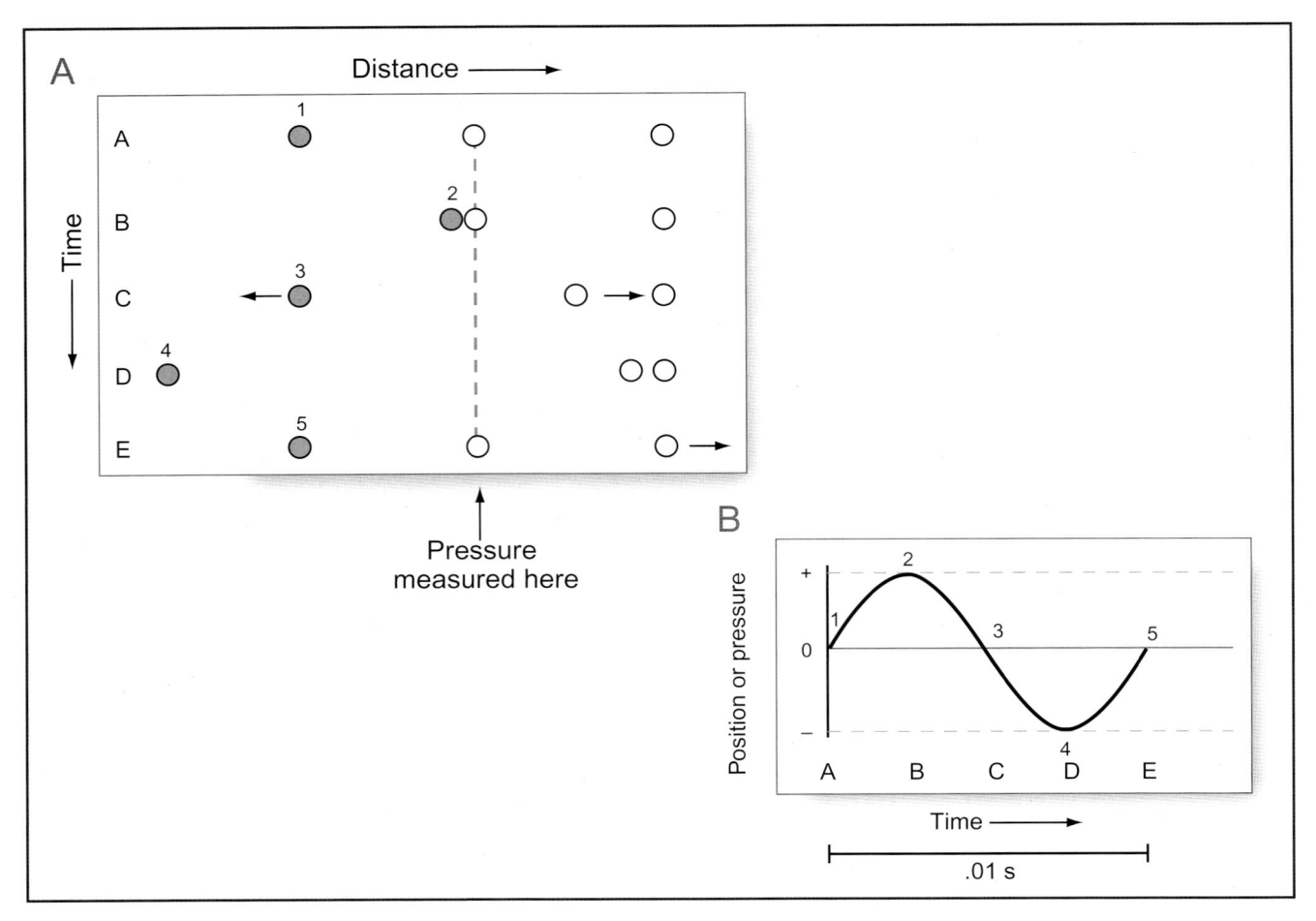

Figure 7–3. A. Schematic drawing of the vibration of an air molecule (*filled circles*) around its rest position. Numbers above the molecule indicate five successive points in time throughout its vibratory cycle. **B.** Plot of the position of the filled-circle molecule and the pressure measured at the location of the second molecule during one vibratory cycle.

(such as displacement, pressure, speed, and so forth) is shown as a function of time, the plot is called a *waveform*. This waveform shows the position of the molecule from rest position (1), to the rightward extreme (2), the return through the rest position (3), at the leftward extreme (4), and finally back at the rest position (5). The discrete positions are connected to illustrate the continuous motion of the molecule throughout the vibratory cycle. This waveform shows one complete *cycle of motion* of the molecule. If the molecule continues to move after point 5, it repeats the 1 through 5 sequence of motions and produces another cycle with the same characteristics.

The y-axis of the waveform in Figure 7–3B is also labeled pressure because it is easy to show that air pressure (measured at position 2) and position of the first molecule change in the same way over time. The rightmost extreme of molecule movement ("2" in Figure 7–3A) is also the time when air compression is maximum at the pressure measurement point, the leftmost extreme ("4") will occur at the same time as a rarefaction at the pressure measurement point, and the rest positions ("1" and "5") will be associated with Patm. Positions between these discrete times will have pressures somewhere between compressions and Patm or rarefactions and Patm. Thus, the waveform in Figure 7–3B shows the temporal variation of the pressure wave. The period (T) is the time taken to complete one full cycle of motion; T is given by the formula: $T = 1/f$, where f = frequency. The filled-circle molecule is plotted as *a continuous function of time* as shown in Figure 7–3B. Figure 7–3A only indicates 5 discrete points in time, but Figure 7–3B shows every possible position of the molecule from time A through E, and how those positions change over time. Time is shown on the x-axis and molecule position (or air pressure) is shown on the y-axis. The horizontal line separating the upper and lower halves of the waveform indicates the rest position of the molecule, that is, when pressure = Patm. The numbers 1, 2, 3, 4, and 5 given in Figure 7–3A are indicated on the time plot in their appropriate locations. According to the time scale shown on the waveform in Figure 7–3B, it takes .01 second to complete one cycle of molecule motion. For this waveform $T = .01$ second (s) or $T = 10$ milliseconds (ms).

In this example, .01 s and 10 ms are the same value, but expressed in different units. In speech and hearing applications, it is typical to express time units in ms. For reference purposes, 1 s = 1000 ms, 0.1 s = 100 ms, 0.01 s = 10 ms, and 0.001 s = 1 ms. In some hearing applications (see Chapters 13 and 14), time may be expressed in units as small as microseconds (μs; 1 μs = 0.000001 s).

The time variation of a repeating, cyclic motion, like the one shown in Figure 7–3B, can also be expressed in terms of *frequency*, symbolized with an *f*. Frequency (*f*) is the inverse of period (*T*):

$$f = 1/T \qquad (1).$$

The units for frequency are *hertz*, abbreviated as Hz, which stands for "cycles per second." The number resulting from the formula indicates how many complete cycles of vibration occur in one second. When formula (1) is applied to the 10-ms period in Figure 7–3B, the result is $f = 1/10$ ms or $f = 1/.01 = 100$ Hz.

Because frequency (*f*) is the inverse of period (*T*), as one variable (e.g., *f*) increases, the other (e.g., *T*) decreases. Longer periods are associated with lower frequencies, and shorter periods are associated with higher frequencies. Figure 7–4 shows the relationship between frequency and period ranging from 1.0 ms to 10.0 ms. For this graph, period is plotted on the *x*-axis, and is changed in steps of 0.5 ms (i.e., 1.0 ms, 1.5 ms, 2.0 ms, 2.5 ms . . . 10.0 ms). The corresponding frequency values, computed by $f = 1/T$, are plotted on the *y*-axis. The inverse relationship between the two expressions of cyclic variation is clearly seen in the way the plotted points descend on the *y*-axis as the value on the *x*-axis increases. Note also that the relationship between *T* and *f* is not *linear*. In a perfectly linear relationship between two variables, equal-sized change in one variable is accompanied by equal-sized change in the other variable. If the relationship between *T* and *f* were perfectly linear, each 0.5-ms step in *T* would be accompanied by a constant change in *f*. In Figure 7–4, however, the frequency changes (*y*-axis) accompanying the 0.5-ms steps in the region of 10 ms (*x*-axis) are much smaller than the frequency changes accompanying 0.5-ms steps in the region of 1.0 ms. This is an example of a curvilinear relationship between two variables. For instance, the 0.5-ms change between 9.0 and 9.5 ms on the *x*-axis produces a change in *f* of approximately 6 Hz, but the same 0.5-ms change between 2.5 and 3.0 ms produces a change in *f* of more than 65 Hz.

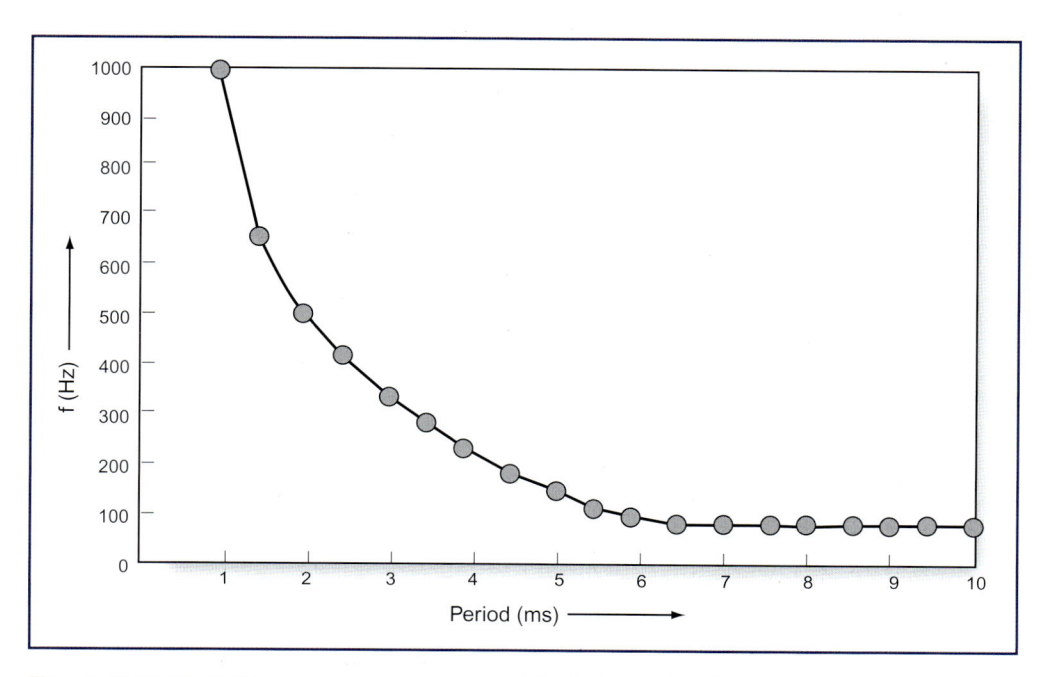

Figure 7–4. Plot of frequency versus period that shows the inverse and nonlinear relationship between the two variables.

Spatial Measures

In Figure 7–2, pressure waves were depicted as alternating regions of high and low pressures extending across space. Portions of two pressure waves are shown in Figure 7–5, one corresponding to a frequency of 100 Hz, the other corresponding to a frequency of 1000 Hz. The *x*-axis is labeled as distance and is scaled from 0 to 500 centimeters (cm) (equivalent to roughly 0 to 195 inches). The portions of the pressure waves for both frequencies shown in Figure 7–5 consist of sequences of high- and low-pressure regions. The high-pressure regions are shown as the more heavily shaded areas, indicating relatively dense packing of air molecules, and the low-pressure areas are shown as lightly shaded, indicating the relatively sparse packing of molecules. It is immediately apparent that one complete variation across space between high and low pressures associated with the 100-Hz sound covers a greater distance than the corresponding variation across space for the 1000-Hz sound. The measurement of spatial variation of a pressure wave is called the *wavelength*, which is the distance covered by a high-pressure region and its succeeding low-pressure region (or by a low-pressure region and its succeeding high-pressure region). Wavelength is symbolized by the Greek letter *lambda* (λ), and is shown for both pressure waves in Figure 7–5 as extending from the leading edge of the first high-pressure region (i.e., the position in space where the pressure first becomes positive relative to Patm) to the leading edge of the next high-pressure region. In accord with the definition given immediately above, wavelength includes the distance covered by the first high-pressure region and its succeeding low-pressure region.

Wavelength has an inverse relationship to frequency. The higher the frequency, the shorter the wavelength. This acoustic law is illustrated in Figure 7–5 where the 1000-Hz sound has a much shorter wavelength than the 100-Hz sound. The formula for wavelength is:

$$\lambda = c/f \text{ or } f = c/\lambda \tag{2}$$

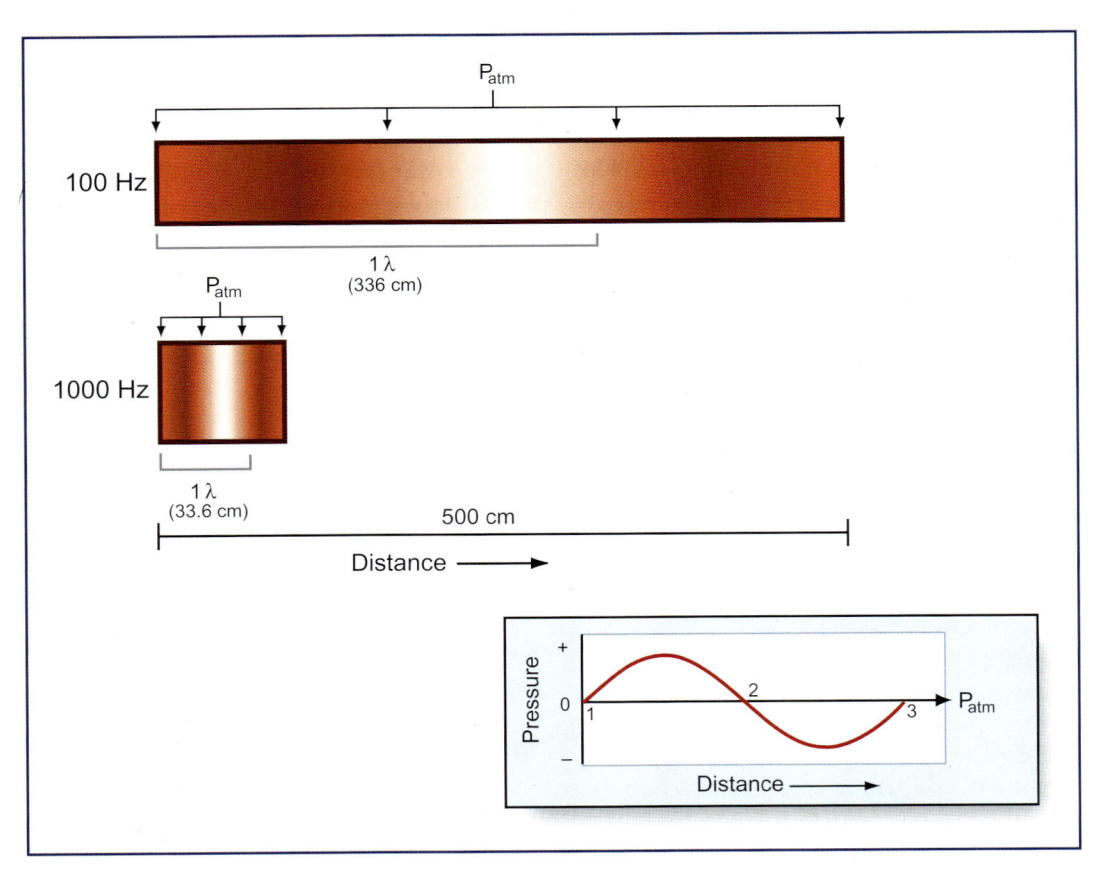

Figure 7–5. Illustration of the measurement of wavelength. Wavelength is the distance covered by a cycle of pressure variation. This distance is marked as 1λ on the 100-Hz and 1000-Hz signals. Wavelength is longer for the 100-Hz signal. The bottom right inset shows pressure variation plotted as a function of distance.

where f = frequency and c = the speed of sound in air, which is a constant and has a value of approximately 33,600 cm/s (roughly 1100 ft/s). If the values of the frequencies shown in Figure 7–5 are plugged into the formula along with the value for the constant c, the wavelengths for 100 Hz and 1000 Hz are approximately 336 cm (100 Hz) and 33.6 cm (1000 Hz), respectively.

Note also that the "boundaries" of the low- and high-pressure regions in Figure 7–5 are marked as Patm. As described above, this indicates that as the pressure varies across space, there are points where the pressure is equal to Patm. The pressure varies across space by going above Patm, below it, above it, and so on. The changes in pressure across space are gradual. The graded nature of these pressure changes is illustrated in Figure 7–5 by the continuous changes in the shadings of the compression and rarefaction regions, with the heaviest shading occurring at the most positive pressure and the lightest shading at the most negative pressure.

The continuous changes in pressure across a single wavelength are also shown in the inset to Figure 7–5, where pressure (y-axis) is shown as a function of distance (x-axis). The horizontal line in this inset is Patm, the reference pressure. Pressure increases relative to Patm ("1" in the inset) until it reaches a positive peak, then decreases and passes through Patm ("2" in the inset) as it goes to the negative peak, then reverses again to return to Patm ("3" in the inset). This is a different way to plot the pressure waves shown in the main part of the figure.

The concept of wavelength is critical to understanding why different configurations of the vocal tract (the "tube" of air shaped by the articulators, extending from vocal folds to the lips) result in different spectra for different vowels (see Chapter 8). Wavelength is also an important concept in understanding the variation of auditory sensitivity as a function of frequency, which is explained in large part by the resonance of the ear canal which is an air-filled tube closed at one end (see Chapter 13).

Wavelength and Direction of Sound

Pressure waves that are primarily plane waves move in a straight line away from their source. When sound waves encounter an object along their path, however, straight-line propagation may change. In general, frequencies with very long wavelengths may bend around objects in their path, whereas frequencies with very short wavelengths do not bend and may strike the object. The short wavelengths cause pressure variations to reflect off the object. These pressure reflections interact with the original pressure wave as well as with the multiple reflections.

The relationship between wavelength and objects within the path of a pressure wave is more precisely related to the respective magnitude of the wavelength and the size of the object in its path. If the wavelength of a pressure wave (or of components of a pressure wave with many frequencies; see below) is substantially greater than the size of the object—say, the diameter of a human head—the wave will bend around the object. The same pressure wave, with the same wavelength, may not bend around a massive building.

As discussed in Chapter 14, the issue of wavelength and objects within the path of a pressure wave is relevant to the acoustic information used by humans to localize a sound source in space. If the typical head diameter of the adult female head is roughly 56 cm, wavelengths associated with frequencies of 500 Hz and below can bend around the head ($\lambda = c/f$; 33,600/500 = 67.2 cm).

Pressure Waves: A Summary and Introduction to Sinusoids

The motions of air molecules can produce pressure waves, which are the basis of sound. Pressure waves vary across space and time, and both variations can be described and measured using simple mathematics.

To this point, the examples and explanations of these events have been *schematic*, or simplified to some degree. For example, very little has been said about the causes, or *sources*, of air molecule motions and resulting pressure waves. Moreover, the motions discussed so far have been very simple, whereas many acoustic events—such as speech—involve complex vibrations of air molecules caused by the motions of complex sources. Even the most complex vibrations, however, can be broken down into a set or group of the simple vibrations described above. It is also the case that a complex vibration can be generated by taking a set of these simple motions and adding them together; complex acoustic events can be created by combining many individual simple acoustic events. The understanding of simple vibrations is the basis for understanding the more complex vibrations observed in most acoustic events.

The simple motions and resulting pressure waves discussed above are called *sinusoidal* motions and waves. Sinusoidal motions are the simplest form of vibration. More complex vibrations can be broken down ("decomposed") into a set of individual sinusoids. The inverse of this decomposition is that complex acoustic events occur when a group of sinusoids are combined together. A formal description of sinusoidal motion is presented next, along with the idea that complex sounds are the sum of their component sinusoids.

> ### Sound Speed
>
> Speed of sound in air varies as a function of air temperature, and to a lesser degree as a function of humidity and altitude. The higher the temperature, the faster the propagation of sound waves. Students will find slightly different values used in different texts. Thirty-three thousand six hundred centimeters per second is roughly the value that is measured at 0 degrees Celsius (32 degrees F). Speed of sound in air increases as temperature rises because molecules move faster at higher, compared with lower, temperatures. Speed of sound also varies with the nature of the conducting medium. Sound propagation is about 4 times faster in water compared with air, and about 11 times faster in steel compared with air (everyone knows the trick of putting an ear to a railroad track to "hear" an oncoming train that is far away from your ear). The general rule is: the denser the medium, the faster the sound conduction.

SINUSOIDAL MOTION

In the foregoing discussion of pressure waves, the motion of air molecules was described as governed by simple laws of elasticity and inertia. The effects of recoil and inertial forces produce the oscillation of the molecule around a rest position. This sinusoidal motion (also called *simple harmonic motion*) has a simple conceptual and mathematical basis.

Sinusoidal Motion (Simple Harmonic Motion) Is Derived from the Linear Projection of Uniform Circular Speed

Imagine, as shown in Figure 7–6A, a circle of some arbitrary radius with its four right angles defined by the radius lines AB, BC, CD, and DA. The filled dot at point A indicates an object that rotates continuously around the circumference of the circle, in a counterclockwise direction. When the object rotates around the circle, it does so with *uniform circular speed* (UCS). In UCS, the rotating object crosses equal angles in equal amounts of time. In the example shown in Figure 7–6A, this means that the time it takes the rotating point (*filled dot*) to travel from point A to B will equal the time it takes to travel from point B to C, point C to D, and point D back to A. This is consistent with the definition of uniform circular motion given above, because the angles defined by lines AB, BC, CD, and DA all equal 90 degrees and each 90-degree angle (or each 45-degree angle, or 30-degree angle, and so forth) is traversed in an equal amount of time.

Sinusoidal motion can now be defined as the *linear projection of uniform circular speed*. This is illustrated in Figure 7–6B, where one-half of the circle has been partitioned into four angles of 45 degrees each. Alongside the circle is a vertical line, the top and bottom of which have the same location as the top and bottom of the circle (point C is located at the top of the circle). At each point along this half-circle motion, a horizontal dashed line has been drawn to intersect the vertical line. The horizontal lines *project* the labeled points (points A through E) along the circle to the vertical line—hence the expression "linear projection of UCS." Remember that each of the 45-degree angles shown in Figure 7–6B is traversed by the rotating object in equal amounts of time.

The result of the linear projection of UCS can be best appreciated by comparing the points on the vertical line to the corresponding points on the circle. The projection of point A on the circle results in point A' on the line, which divides the line into upper and lower segments of equal length. Point B on the circle projects to point B' on the line, and point C on the circle projects to point C' on the line. The interesting comparison here is the length of the linear segment A'-B' to B'-C'. Clearly the segment A'-B' is longer than the segment B'-C', yet these two segments result from the projection of points spanning *equivalent arcs*. In other words, when the circular motion involves equal distances (that is, motion covering equal angles), the linear projection of the points defining those angles does not yield equal linear distances.

As the point moves from point C to point E, its linear projection is superimposed on the same line segment (A'-C') originally covered when the point rotated from A to C. The result of this projection is now from C' to A', which is the reverse of the original projection. As the rotating point moves from E to F, the linear projection extends from A' to F', and the projection of the rotation from F to A is superimposed on the A'-F' line segment, but now in the opposite direction.

Discrete angles on the circle illustrate the linear projection of UCS, but as the point rotates about the circle, the angles change continuously as they are projected to the line segment. The linear projection of a complete rotation around the circle looks very much like the motion of the air molecule in Figures

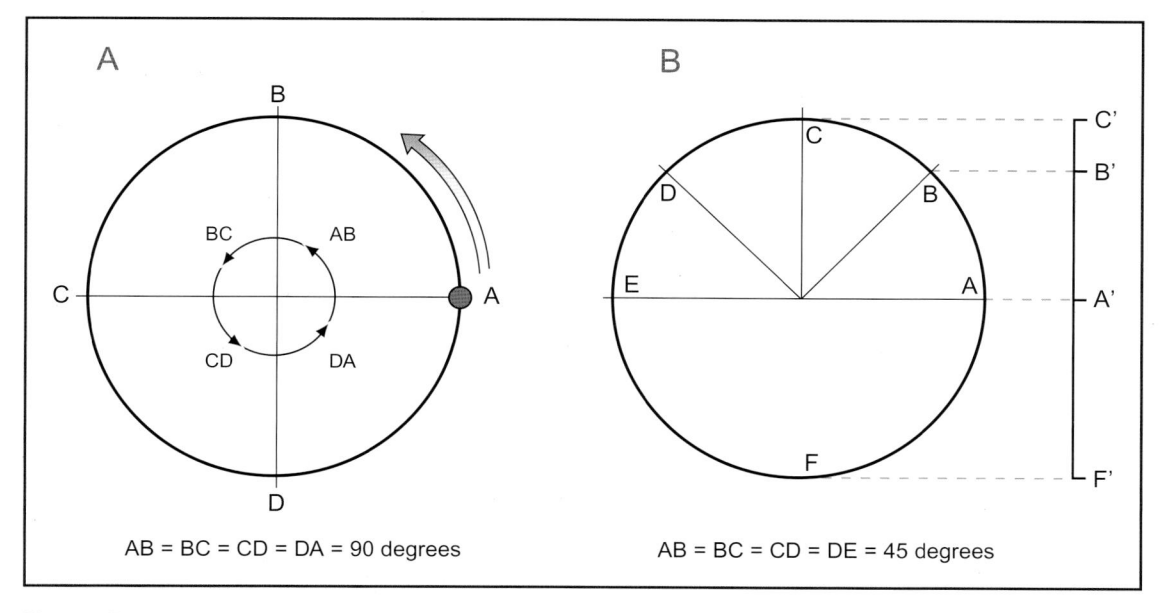

Figure 7-6. Derivation of sinusoidal motion from the linear projection of uniform circular speed. **A.** Filled dot moving around larger circle at uniform circular speed which means it crosses equal angles in equal time intervals. **B.** Projection of points along the circumference of the larger circle to a line segment, showing how projection from equal angles does not result in equal linear segments. See text for details.

How Sound Points

Acoustic wavelengths are not only longer for low frequencies and shorter for highs, but straighter for highs and more bendy for lows. If you wanted to "aim" a sound wave with great accuracy, a high frequency is a good choice because it tends to move in a relatively straight line. Wavelengths of low frequencies, on the other hand, can wrap around objects and, in general, be a curvy aural nuisance. The directional properties of sound waves are one of the many important variables engineers consider when they design warning sirens, such as those used on emergency vehicles or weather alert systems. The text has some additional information on the consequences of relatively long versus short wavelengths.

7–1 and 7–3. A' on the linear segment is the rest position, whereas C' and F' are the extremes of the linear displacement. One complete cycle involves motion from the rest position A' to the one extreme (C'), back through the rest position to the other extreme (F'), and then back to the rest position. In fact, if the line segment in Figure 7–6B is turned on its side with C' to the right and F' to the left, the motion described by the linear projection of the rotating point is the same as the motion of air molecules described above.

When the Linear Projection of Uniform Circular Speed Is Stretched Out in Time, the Result Is a Sine Wave

Imagine now that the rotating object in Figure 7–6A is a small ring through which a pencil is inserted and that the motion described by UCS is marked on paper beneath the circle. If the circle is moved from left to right across the paper at a constant speed and without disturbing the UCS of the rotating ring, the pencil line draws the motion as a function of time. The resulting waveform would look like the one on the right in Figure 7–7 (and the ones in Figures 7–3 and 7–5) and is called a *sine wave*. This is displacement shown as a function of time. If the time scale is known, the period (and its inverse, frequency) can be determined using the simple computation of Formula (1)—$f = 1/T$. Note also the corresponding positions on the circle and resulting waveform (given by A, B, C, D in Figure 7–7).

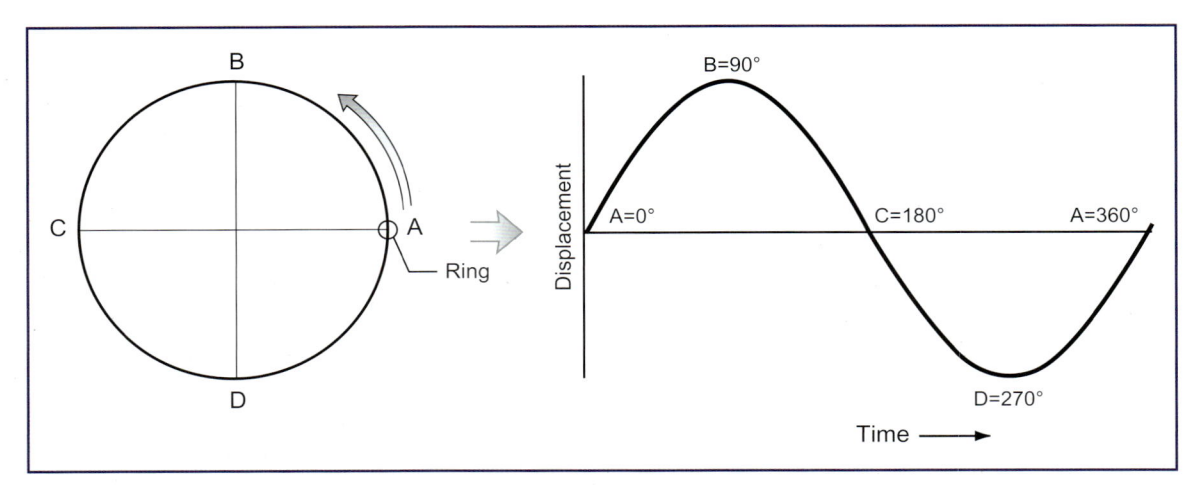

Figure 7–7. Linear projection of uniform circular speed, shown as a function of time. If a pencil is inserted through the ring at A on the large circle (*left side of figure*) during uniform circular speed, and the motion is traced as the pencil is moved from left to right, the result is the sinusoidal waveform on the right side of the figure. Angular notation on the waveform at the right corresponds to angles crossed during motion around the circle on the left.

Sinusoidal Motion Can Be Described by a Simple Formula and Has Three Important Characteristics: Frequency, Amplitude, and Phase

Sinusoidal motion can be described by three characteristics, or *parameters*. The first of these parameters is frequency, which has been defined above as the number of full cycles occurring in a 1-s interval. If one complete rotation about a circle is equivalent to one cycle of vibration, it is easy to see how a faster speed of rotation results in a higher frequency. A faster speed of rotation reduces the amount of time required to complete one full revolution around the circle. This is equivalent to saying that the period, T, is reduced with faster circular speeds. As Formula (1), $f = 1/T$, and Figure 7–4 indicate, a reduction in T is associated with an increase in f.

The second parameter is amplitude, symbolized as A. Amplitude can be thought of in terms of displacement of an air molecule from the rest position. The circle in Figure 7–6 provides a simple illustration of variations in A. The vertical line onto which points are projected from the circular motion corresponds in length to the size (diameter) of the circle. The extremes of the linearly projected motion are, therefore, defined by the diameter of the circle. If the circle is made larger or smaller, the extremes of the linearly projected motion are greater or smaller, respectively. Amplitude of vibration (for the current purposes, the same as molecule displacement) is directly related to the size of the circle from which sinusoidal motion is derived.

The third parameter, phase, symbolized by the Greek letter φ (*phi*), describes the position of the sinusoidal motion relative to some arbitrary reference position. For example, in Figure 7–7, assume that position A is the reference point. Using the circular basis of sinusoidal motion, the location or *phase* of point B can be described as 90 degrees relative to point A, because the radii extending to points A and B form a 90-degree angle. Similarly, the phase of points C and D are 180 degrees and 270 degrees, respectively, relative to the reference point A. This phase angle description applies to the waveform in Figure 7–7 as well, because points along the waveform are simply points around the circle, extended in time. With A as the waveform reference point, a time corresponding to a *lag* of 90 degrees is equivalent to a quarter of a complete cycle, 180 degrees would be a half cycle, and so forth.

These examples use phase to compare points within a single waveform, but phase can also be used to compare points across two waveforms of identical or different frequencies. Phase relations between two or more sinusoids of different frequencies are discussed below in the section dealing with complex waveforms.

A simple formula describes sinusoidal motion as a function of time. This *sinusoidal function* is used to determine the displacement of an object (i.e., an air molecule) at any instant in time, and is computed as follows:

$$D = A \sin(2\pi ft + \varphi) \tag{3}$$

where D = the displacement of the object at a given instant, A = the maximum displacement of the object from the rest position, f = the frequency of the motion, t = the specific time at which the displacement D is being computed, and φ = the starting phase of the motion (like the reference point described above). The constant 2π (equaling 360 degrees, or one full revolution around the circle) reflects the circular origin of sinusoidal motion and when multiplied by "ft" converts the expression in parentheses to angular notation. The *sine* is a trigonometric function, the sinusoid function that converts angles to real numbers.

Tables of sine values for angles between 0 and 360 degrees are available in any basic trigonometry text or on the Internet. Sine values vary between 0 and +1.00 for angles ranging from 0 to 90 degrees, and between +1.00 and 0 for angles ranging from 91 to 180 degrees. Between 180 and 360 degrees, these values have mirror-image negative values, ranging from 0 to –1.00 (270 degrees) and then back to 0 (360 degrees).

If the starting phase (φ) in Formula (3) is assumed to be zero (that is, if we are not concerned about the absolute starting phase of the waveform), the formula for sinusoidal motion can be simplified to:

$$D = A (\sin \theta) \qquad (4)$$

where D = displacement, A = maximum displacement, as above, and θ = the angle formed between the reference radius (i.e., the radii projected to point A in Figures 7–6 and 7–7) and the radius projected to any other point along the circle. For the sequence of angles formed as an object rotates around the circle (that is, 0 to 360 degrees), application of this formula yields a sine wave.

Sinusoidal Motion: A Summary

A sine wave is a waveform that results from the linear projection of UCS. A sine wave is *periodic*, because multiple rotations around the circle produce a sequence of multiple waveforms having the same period. Because the period is the same for all cycles of the vibration, sinusoids by definition and derivation have only a single frequency. A sinusoidal waveform can be described by a simple formula in which period, amplitude, and phase are the parameters.

Because a sinusoid involves only a single frequency, it is the simplest type of acoustic event. Sinusoids are the "building blocks" of acoustic events containing many frequencies. Acoustic events that contain many frequencies have *complex waveforms*, which may or may not repeat over time. The next section describes complex acoustic events.

COMPLEX ACOUSTIC EVENTS

Two types of complex events are considered: (a) those in which the waveform pattern repeats over time, and (b) those in which no repeating pattern can be identified. When an acoustic event contains more than one frequency and has a waveform with a repeating pattern, it is called a *complex periodic* event. An acoustic event with more than one frequency and no repeating pattern is called a *complex aperiodic* event.

Complex Periodic Events Have Waveforms That Repeat Their Patterns Over Time and Are Composed of Harmonically Related Frequency Components

Figure 7–8 shows two different complex periodic waveforms and associated spectra. Both waveforms, shown above their respective spectra, share the property of a repeating pattern over time and have the same period of roughly 8 ms and hence a *fundamental frequency* of around 125 Hz ($f = 1/8$ ms $= 1/.008$ s $= 125$ Hz). The fundamental frequency is determined by the rate of repetition of the major waveform pattern, as indicated by the marked periods on the two waveforms. Even though the fundamental frequency is nearly identical for the two waveforms, the appearance of the waveforms is clearly different. The frequencies in addition to the fundamental frequency, and their amplitudes and phase relations, give the waveforms their unique appearance.

Waveform displays are said to show an acoustic event in the *time domain*, because the event is shown as a function of time. This is a useful way to display an acoustic event, but if one is interested in the frequencies and their amplitudes that give waveforms their unique appearance, a different type of display is required. When an acoustic event is examined in the *frequency domain*, the individual frequencies and amplitudes that contribute to a complex acoustic event are displayed. The frequency domain of an acoustic event is shown by a *spectrum*, which can be defined as a plot of *relative amplitude* (y-axis) as a function of frequency (x-axis). Spectra are shown immediately below the two waveforms in Figure 7–8; the two spectra are quite different.

The spectrum of the waveform in Figure 7–8A shows frequency components at odd number multiples

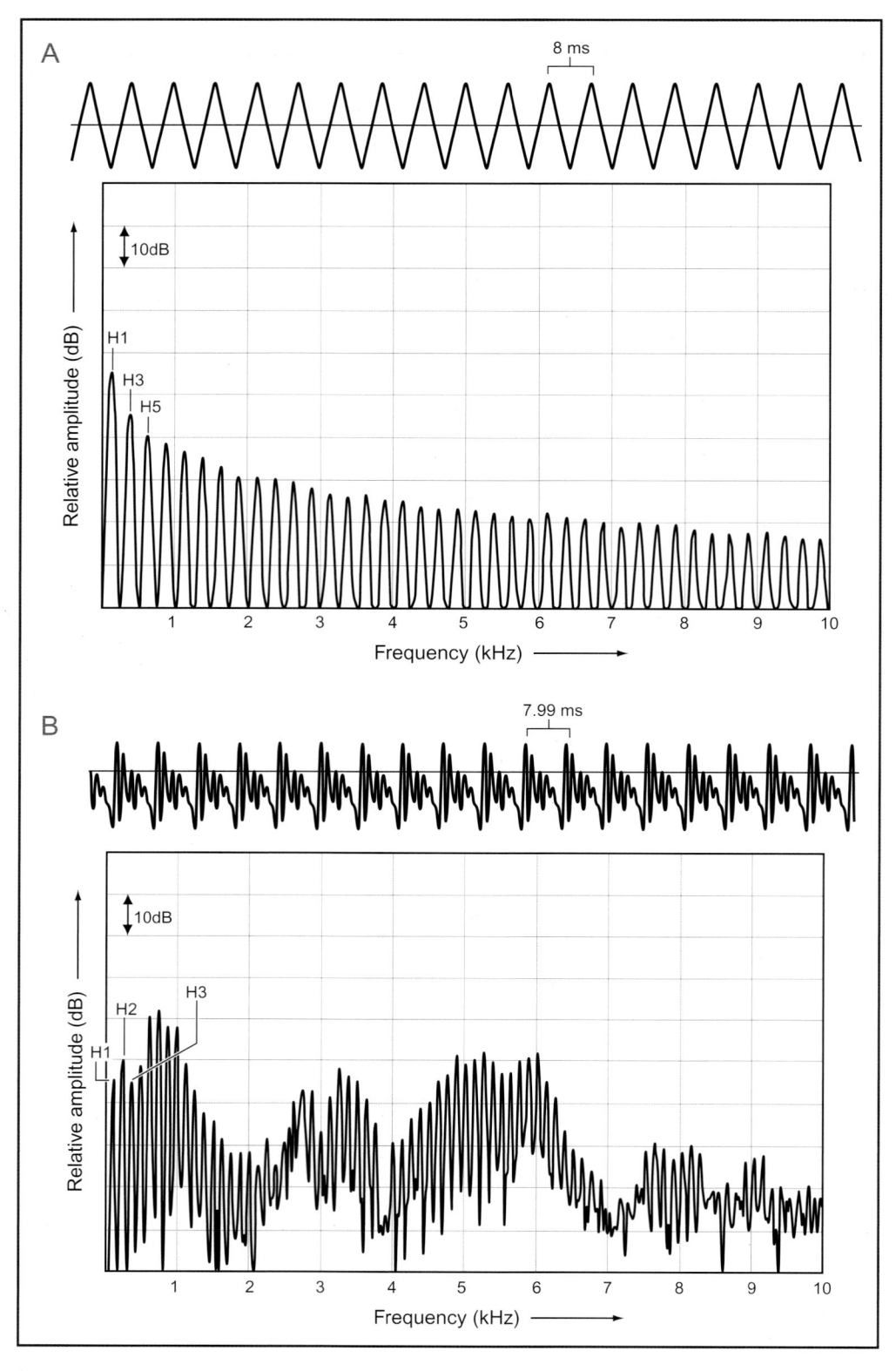

Figure 7-8. Two complex periodic waveforms and their spectra. **A.** Waveform and spectrum of a 125-Hz triangular wave. The period of one cycle (8 ms) is marked on the waveform, and the first (H1), third (H3), and fifth (H5) harmonics are marked on the spectrum. **B.** Waveform and spectrum of the vowel /a/ produced by an adult male. The period of one cycle (7.99 ms) is marked on the waveform, and the first (H1), second (H2), and third (H3) harmonics are marked on the spectrum.

(1, 3, 5, 7, 9 ... n) of the fundamental frequency (125 Hz). This spectrum contains frequency components at 125 Hz: the fundamental frequency, or first harmonic (H1), 375 Hz (H3), 625 Hz (H5) ... 125 × (2n − 1) Hz, where n is the number of harmonic components in the spectrum. The relative amplitudes of the frequencies, represented by the heights of the harmonic components (i.e., the magnitude on the y-axis), decrease consistently as frequency increases. In this spectrum, therefore, a higher frequency (e.g., 625 Hz, the fifth harmonic of 125 Hz) always has less energy than a lower frequency (e.g., 375 Hz, the third harmonic).[4] Waveform (A) is a common test signal used in electronics shops and laboratories, and is called a *triangular wave*. A triangular wave is said to have an odd-integer series of harmonics.

The waveform in Figure 7–8B is the time-domain representation of the vowel /ɑ/ spoken by an adult male. The marked period of the waveform is 7.99 ms, almost identical to the 8-ms period of the triangular wave in Figure 7–8A. The periods of the two waveforms are not perfectly identical because it is difficult, even for someone with training in voice and articulation, to produce a vowel with an exact frequency (the triangular wave was produced with a computer program capable of synthesizing exactly a period of 8 ms). The frequency domain representation (i.e., the spectrum) shows why the /ɑ/ waveform is different from the triangular waveform in Figure 7–8A. First, the /ɑ/ spectrum contains harmonics at whole-number multiples of the fundamental frequency (that is, 125 Hz × 1, 2, 3, 4, 5, 6, 7, 8, 9 ... n), not just odd-number multiples. An easy way to verify this difference is to compare the two spectra for the number of harmonics between 0 and 1000 Hz. The triangular wave shows four harmonics from 0 to 1000 Hz, whereas the vowel /ɑ/ shows eight. The vowel spectrum is harmonically denser than the triangular wave spectrum. A second difference between the two spectra is the pattern of amplitudes as a function of harmonic frequency. Unlike the spectrum of the triangular wave, the relative amplitudes of the frequency components do not decrease systematically with increasing frequency. Rather, the relative amplitudes fluctuate as frequency increases (moving rightward on the x-axis), sometimes increasing and sometimes decreasing. For example, note in the vowel spectrum the greater relative amplitude of the fifth and sixth harmonics (roughly from 600–750 Hz) compared with the amplitude of the second harmonic (around 250 Hz). The different harmonic densities, the different variation of amplitude as a function of frequency, plus different phase relations among the frequencies (not discussed here) all contribute to the different appearance of triangular wave and vowel waveforms. Both, however, are clearly periodic and different in shape from a sinusoidal (single-frequency) waveform.

A Complex Periodic Waveform Can Be Considered as the Sum of the Individual Sinusoids at the Harmonic Frequencies

Complex periodic waveforms have spectra with multiple, harmonically related frequencies. Energy at these frequencies is *discrete*, which means that between the harmonic frequencies (e.g., at 250 Hz in Figure 7–8A, which is between the first and third harmonics of the triangular wave spectrum) there is little or no energy. The multiple harmonic frequencies occur at the same time, and it is their combination that produces the complex waveforms seen in Figure 7–8. Earlier in this chapter, the idea was advanced that understanding sinusoidal vibration was important because even the most complex acoustic events can be broken down into their component sinusoids.

The spectral representations shown in Figure 7–8 provide a snapshot, averaged across an interval of time, of the component sinusoids of a complex acoustic event. In a sense, the spectrum shows the acoustic event with the individual frequency components "pulled apart" and displayed with their individual, relative amplitudes. The formal analysis required to produce a spectrum of a waveform is called *Fourier analysis*, a mathematical tool that decomposes a complex time-domain function (e.g., a complex periodic waveform) into the set of its simple functions (i.e., sinusoids). In this text, the mathematical details of Fourier analysis are not discussed, but the conceptual basis of the process, the ability to break down a complex acoustic event into its simple components, is important. Fourier analysis is implemented in almost every speech analysis computer program. For example, the spectra in Figure 7–8 were constructed using TF32 (Milenkovic, 2001), a computer program written by Professor Paul Milenkovic of the University of Wisconsin–Madison. Using mouse-controlled cursors, the user selects the portion of the waveform to be analyzed (in Figure 7–8, the waveform portions shown were the ones subjected to Fourier analysis) and selects a function that instructs the program to perform a Fourier analysis. The Fourier

---

[4] A formal discussion of sound intensity level and sound pressure level (two ways to describe the energy in an acoustic event) is provided in Appendix 7–A of this chapter. For the present discussion, the term "relative amplitude" is used to describe the energy relations between two or more frequency components in a spectrum. These energy relations are expressed in decibels (dB).

analysis function automatically displays spectra like those shown in Figure 7–8.

The conceptual basis of Fourier analysis can be "stood on its head" to show that a group of simple functions (sinusoids) add together to produce a complex acoustic event. For example, if a computer program synthesizes a sinusoid at 125 Hz, the result is a simple waveform with a period of $T = 8$ ms. If the program synthesizes another sinusoid at 375 Hz which is added to the 125 Hz waveform, the new waveform is not sinusoidal but retains the original period of 8 ms. The new waveform is a complex periodic event, with two frequency components. If this process is repeated for a large series of odd-integer harmonics, whose synthesized amplitudes decrease as a function of frequency, the waveform eventually becomes triangular. The progression from a sinusoidal to a triangular waveform reflects the addition of all odd-integer harmonics whose amplitudes decrease across frequency in a specific way. The period of the triangular waveform, however, equals the period of the lowest frequency component, which in this case is 8 ms (that is, the period of 125 Hz). This is the Fourier concept stood on its head. Instead of decomposing a complex acoustic event into its component sinusoids, a complex acoustic event is synthesized, or constructed, from the addition of many different sinusoids. In a complex periodic waveform, the period is always that of the lowest frequency component (the fundamental frequency, or first harmonic) in the spectrum.

The idea that a complex acoustic event can be "built up" from the waveforms of individual component sinusoids is associated with the *superposition principle*. When the waveforms of different sinusoidal frequencies are viewed on the same time scale, at any point in time the amplitude of the complex waveform is the sum of the amplitudes of each of the component sinusoids, at that point in time. It is as if the sinusoids are superimposed on each other to create a complex waveform whose shape over time reflects the amplitude contributions of each of the component sinusoids.

A special and interesting demonstration of the superposition principle is the phenomenon called *beats*, illustrated in Figure 7–9. At the top of the figure, two sinusoids are shown on a common time scale, which is marked by the calibration line of 100 ms at the bottom of the figure. The sinusoid drawn in brown has a period of .002 ms, and therefore a frequency of 500 Hz. The sinusoid drawn in blue has a period of .00198 ms, corresponding to a frequency of 503 Hz. The left horizontal bar above the sinusoids shows one cycle of the waveform with $f = 503$ Hz, and the right horizontal bar shows one cycle of the waveform with $f = 500$ Hz. The time difference between the duration of these cycles—that is, the difference in the periods—is subtle but can be seen on close inspection. The two sinusoids in this example have the same maximum amplitude. The superposition principle is demonstrated by the complex waveform at the bottom of the figure (in black) that shows how the fluctuations in its amplitude are the result of the sum of the amplitudes of the individual components at the top of the figure. The amplitude variations of the complex waveform are the result of the slowly changing phase relations between the two component sinusoids.

With the lower frequency of 500 Hz considered the reference waveform, over time the peak amplitude of the sinusoidal waveform for $f = 503$ Hz seems to "catch up" and then fall behind the waveform for $f = 500$ Hz. Three cycles into the displayed waveforms, the peak amplitudes of the two component sinusoids are nearly in phase, adding their maximum amplitudes and resulting in the maximum amplitude of the complex waveform (extend the downward-pointing arrow labeled "in phase" to the complex waveform to verify the statement). A little more than two cycles later, the two component waveforms are nearly out of phase by 180 degrees, with the blue waveform at peak positive amplitude, the brown waveform at peak negative amplitude. At this point in time the amplitudes of the two waveforms nearly cancel each other; extending the "out of phase" arrow to the complex waveform reveals a very low amplitude, as expected from the superposition principle. The superposition principle applies to any number of component sinusoids that contribute to a complex waveform: at any point in time, add the amplitudes of the components to determine the amplitude of the complex waveform.

Beats are the perceptual result of two similar sinusoids slowly and systematically going in and out of phase. The completely "in phase" moment in time and "out of phase" moment repeat at a rate equal to the difference between the component frequencies. In the example shown in the figure, the in-phase/out-of-phase repetition is three times per second, and when these two sinusoids are played together, a listener should hear a periodic loudness variation occurring at a rate of three times per second; the relatively slow, repeating loudness variations are the beats. Guitar players know this phenomenon well when they tune the instrument using harmonics of different strings but the same note. Tuning is achieved by turning the tuning pegs until the beats are eliminated (that is, when the harmonics of the two strings are the same frequency). Beats may also be used to tune other stringed instruments, including the piano.

In phase   Out of phase

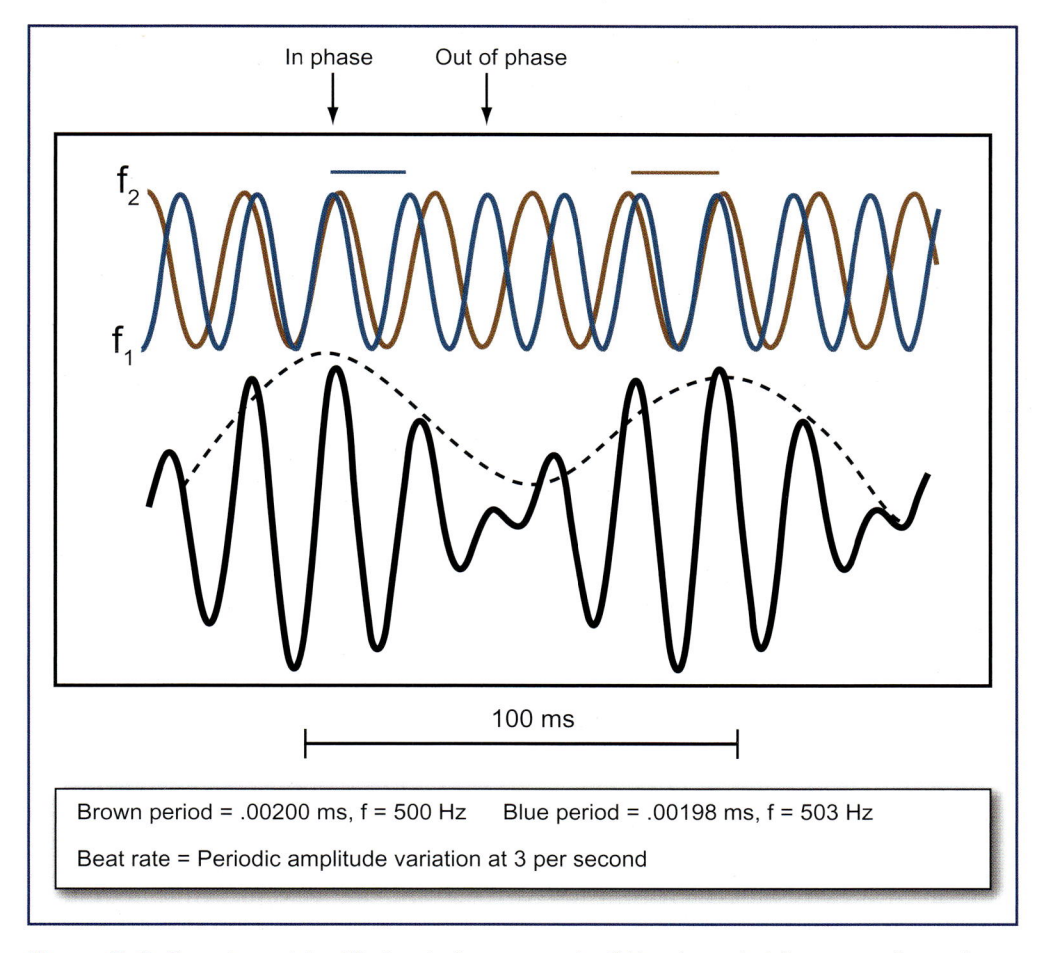

f₂

f₁

100 ms

Brown period = .00200 ms, f = 500 Hz   Blue period = .00198 ms, f = 503 Hz

Beat rate = Periodic amplitude variation at 3 per second

Figure 7-9. Two sinusoids differing in frequency by 3 Hz, played at the same time, showing how the slowly changing phase relationships between the two waves produce a phenomenon called beats. When the two waves are in phase their combined amplitude is at maximum, when the two waves are 180 degrees out of phase their combined amplitude is at minimum. The result is a sound that varies slowly in loudness, at a rate equal to the difference in frequency between the two waveforms.

When two or more sinusoids are related to each other by a whole number multiple, they are said to be in a harmonic relationship. Moreover, when the individual sinusoidal components of an acoustic event are harmonically related, the complex event will be periodic (see section below on complex aperiodic events). In the case of the spectrum shown in Figure 7–8A, the 375 Hz harmonic component is three times the fundamental frequency of 125 Hz and is, therefore, called the third harmonic of the fundamental frequency. In the triangular wave spectrum, there is no second harmonic (which would be 250 Hz for a 125-Hz fundamental frequency). The component at 625 Hz is the fifth harmonic (5 × 125 Hz), the component at 875 Hz the seventh harmonic (7 × 125 Hz), and so on. In the vowel spectrum,

Pending Further Notice

Ever wonder about the connection between words such as "pendant," "pending," "pendulous," "pendulum"? They all derive from a seventeenth-century Latin word meaning "hanging down," which in turn probably derives from a thirteenth-century Scandinavian word meaning "wag" or "fluctuate." A pendulum does wag back and forth—it varies in position as a function of time. It does so with simple harmonic motion and obeys the same principles discussed here for the simple motions of air molecules.

which has a consecutive integer series of harmonics, there is a second (250 Hz), third (375 Hz), and fourth (500 Hz) harmonic (and so on). Later in this text, the spectrum associated with the acoustic result of vocal fold vibration is discussed, and the role of harmonics generated by this vibration is shown to be important to the acoustic theory of speech production.

Complex Aperiodic Events Have Waveforms in Which No Repetitive Pattern Can Be Discerned, and Frequency Components That Are Not Harmonically Related

Figure 7–10 shows two pairs of waveform-spectrum displays for two different complex aperiodic acoustic events. These waveforms are composed of multiple frequencies, but in contrast to the waveforms in Figure 7–8, neither shows a repetitive pattern over time. The lack of a repetitive pattern reflects the lack of periodicity, hence the term "complex *a*periodic acoustic event." Because there is no repetitive pattern, it is not possible to compute a period for these waveforms. Complex aperiodic waveforms, therefore, do not have a fundamental frequency.

The frequency composition of complex aperiodic acoustic events cannot be inferred with much accuracy from their waveforms, but rather must be obtained from direct examination of the spectrum (remember that in a complex periodic waveform, the ability to compute the period and hence the fundamental frequency from a waveform allows at least a partial identification of other frequency components because of their harmonic relationship to the fundamental). The spectra shown in Figure 7–10 were obtained by Fourier analysis, just as they were for the complex periodic events shown in Figure 7–8. The decomposition of complex waveforms into their component sinusoids follows the same general principles for both periodic and aperiodic events. Figure 7–10A shows the waveform and spectrum of a brief time interval of white noise. White noise is a type of complex aperiodic acoustic event that contains, in theory, energy at all frequencies (from 1 Hz to infinity); the amplitudes of each of these frequencies vary randomly over time. In theory, white noise has equal average energy at all frequencies. Stated otherwise, the spectrum of a "perfect" white noise is flat.

The white noise waveform shown in Figure 7–10A has a total duration of 150 ms, and the spectrum was computed for this interval. The spectrum, which displays frequencies from 1 to 10.0 kHz, is not perfectly flat but shows a continuous and slow increase in energy from low to high frequencies. This white noise was obtained from free software on the Internet, so perhaps the algorithm for generating the noise was not accurate or something about the way the signal was processed resulted in the deviation from a perfectly flat spectrum. Nevertheless, because of the absence of harmonics in this spectrum it is much more difficult to identify discrete frequency components such as those seen in the spectra of Figure 7–8. Rather, the energy appears to vary in a random and continuous fashion.[5] The use of a truly flat-spectrum white noise as a test signal is important in the upcoming discussion of resonance and resonators (see Figure 7–19 and accompanying text). Figure 7–10B presents the waveform and spectrum of a sustained /ʃ/, a voiceless fricative (as in the first sound of "ship") produced by grooving the blade of the tongue against the hard palate. Like the white noise waveform, there is no repeating pattern, and like the white noise spectrum, it is difficult to identify discrete frequency components because of the absence of harmonics. This spectrum shows an increase of energy from very low frequencies to higher frequencies, but the peak energy in the /ʃ/ spectrum occurs around 5000 Hz. Above 5000 Hz, the energy declines gradually, giving the overall *spectral shape* an appearance of symmetry, with low amplitudes below 3000 Hz and above 7000 Hz, and higher amplitudes between 3000 and 7000 Hz. The characteristics of this spectrum are consistent with /ʃ/ spectra reported in the literature and described in Chapters 10 and 11.

Complex Acoustic Events: A Summary

Complex acoustic events are composed of more than one frequency, and may be periodic or aperiodic. Complex periodic events have a repetitive waveform pattern and, therefore, a fundamental frequency. The higher-frequency components are harmonically related to this fundamental frequency. Complex aperiodic events do not have a fundamental frequency because the waveform pattern is nonrepetitive. The frequencies in the spectrum do not stand in a harmonic relationship to one another.

Complex acoustic events can be displayed in either the time or frequency domain. When Fourier analysis is applied to a time-domain representation a com-

---

[5]The actual shape of a computed spectrum depends on the way in which the acoustic signal has been processed (e.g., including such variables as the type of microphone and possibly tape recorder used, the specifications of the computer program used to perform the analysis, and so forth). In the spectra presented in this text, it is safe to assume that frequencies between 100 Hz and 9000 Hz are minimally affected by these variables.

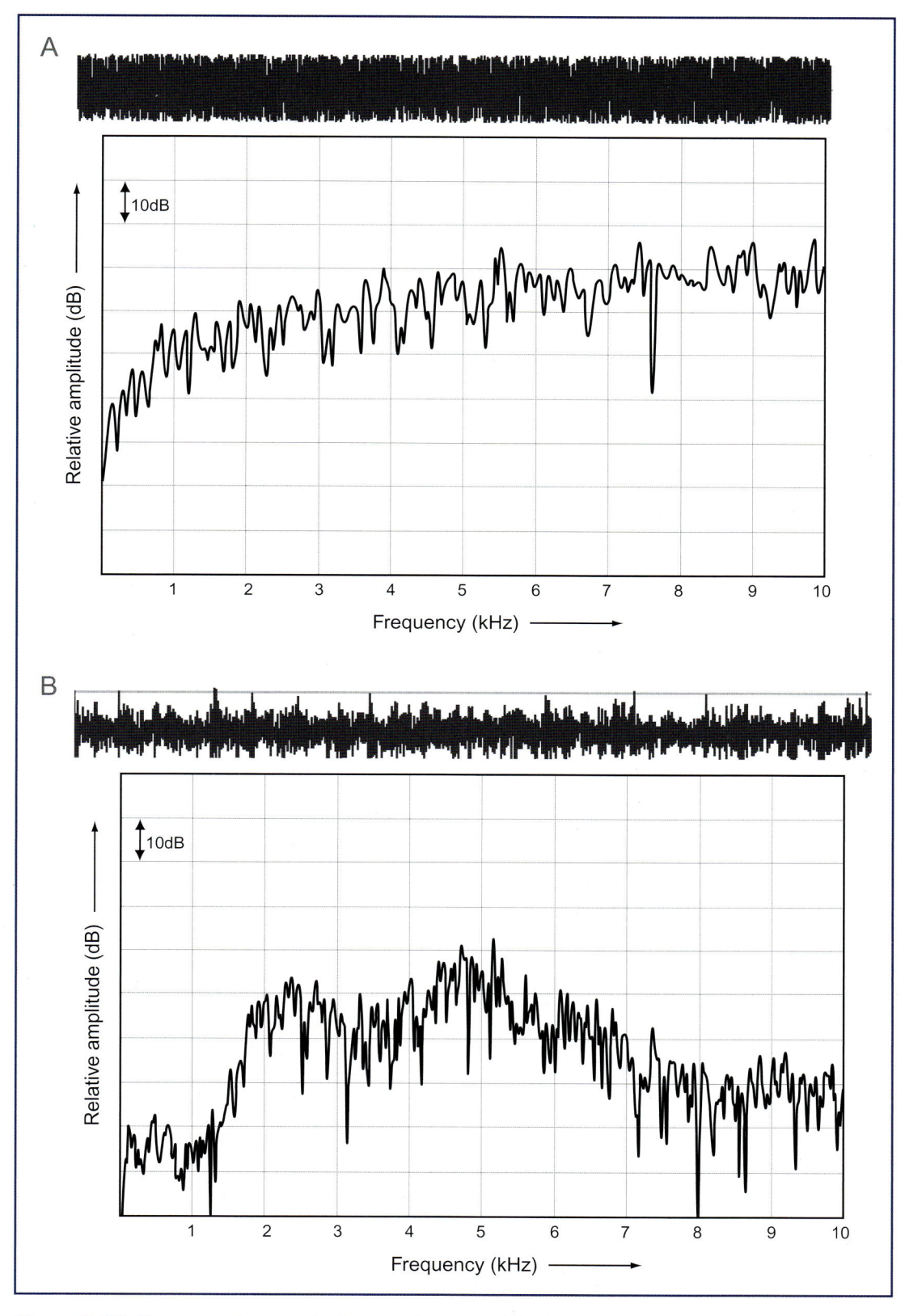

Figure 7–10. Two complex aperiodic waveforms and their spectra. **A.** Waveform and spectrum of a white noise produced by freeware on the Internet. **B.** Waveform and spectrum of a sustained /ʃ/ produced by an adult male. The two waveforms do not have periods, and discrete harmonics do not appear in their spectra.

plex waveform is decomposed into its simple, sinusoidal functions. This process identifies the component frequencies and their amplitudes. This frequency-domain representation of an acoustic event is called a spectrum.

The time and frequency domains are two alternative representations of acoustic events. The two domains do not show different events, just different ways of looking at the same event. The simplest example of this was provided earlier, when the period and frequency of a sinusoid were defined as the inverse of each other ($f = 1/T$, or $T = 1/f$). The period is derived from the time-domain representation, and the frequency, of course, is derived from the frequency domain. One of the major advances in acoustic phonetics occurred when an instrument was developed that combined the time and frequency domain representations into a single display. This instrument, the *sound spectrograph*, is discussed in Chapter 10.

To this point, the discussion of complex acoustic events has been restricted to cases where the sound can be related strictly to the vibration of one object. For example, when a tuning fork is struck, the vibrating tines of the fork displace the surrounding air molecules and are, therefore, the source of the pressure waves heard as sound. Similarly, the vibrating diaphragm (a woofer or tweeter) in one of the loudspeakers connected to an amplifier serves as the source of pressure waves heard as music. Many acoustic events, including the production of speech sounds and the sounds of most musical instruments, involve an interaction between a source of sound, like the ones discussed above, and a resonator (or resonators). A resonator is part of an acoustic system that emphasizes certain frequencies in a source vibration and rejects certain other frequencies. Attention is now turned to a detailed consideration of resonance.

RESONANCE

Resonance is the phenomenon whereby an object vibrates with maximum energy at a particular frequency or range of frequencies. Sometimes the term "natural frequency" is used synonymously with the term "resonance." To say that an object has a natural frequency, or that it resonates at a particular frequency, does not mean that the object vibrates at only one frequency. It simply means that there is a frequency that "naturally" produces a vibration of greatest amplitude, even while other frequencies produce vibrations of lesser amplitude. The reasons why objects have "natural frequencies" are the focus of this section.

Vibratory objects include almost anything in the world. The main vibratory object of concern in this book is, of course, air; but the phenomenon of resonance extends to other objects, sometimes with startling outcomes. For example, most people know about the ability of some vocalists to shatter a wine glass with a loudly sung note, or the comedic scene in films where an opera singer hits a note of extremely high frequency and intensity, causing mirrors, windows, vases, eyeglasses, and other assorted objects to break apart. These are all examples of vibratory energy in air, emerging from a singer's vocal tract and being transferred to a mechanical object and causing it to vibrate. If a frequency produced by the singer coincides with the natural or resonant frequency of the solid object and the energy transfer from air to solid is sufficient, the solid may begin to vibrate. If the energy transfer from air to solid is very efficient at the natural frequency of the solid, its vibration may become violent enough to cause the solid to break apart. Perhaps one of the most startling examples of resonance is when a bridge is set into vibration by the rhythmic marching of soldiers. If the synchronized marching frequency is the same as the resonant frequency of the bridge, it is transferred very efficiently to the bridge, which responds with large-amplitude swaying (vibrations) that can endanger its structural integrity.

The concept of resonance is introduced here by describing a simple mechanical model. Then, because energy can be transferred from vibrating objects to volumes of air, acoustic resonance is discussed in detail. The discussion shows how concepts from mechanical systems are directly applicable to acoustical systems.

Fourier Analysis Was Hot in the Nineteenth Century

Sometimes the most important aspects of one scientific discipline have their origins in a different scientific area. Fourier analysis was "invented" by one Baron J. B. J. Fourier (1768–1830), who wrote a famous textbook whose French title can be translated as "Analytic Theory of Heat." This text had nothing to do with acoustics, but did take up the problem of periodic variations in heat. Fourier designed his analysis to decompose these complex variations into their simple harmonic components, and in the middle of the nineteenth century a German physicist named Georg Ohm (1789–1854) argued for the application of Fourier analysis to the decomposition of complex tones into simple ones.

Mechanical Resonance

Mechanical systems can be used to understand acoustical systems. This is illustrated using a spring-mass model to describe the phenomenon of resonance and to explain how mass and elasticity determine resonant frequencies.

A Spring-Mass Model of Resonance

Figure 7–11A shows a simple mechanism consisting of a mass (e.g., a small block of wood) labeled M, a spring labeled K, and a fixed surface to which the spring-mass assembly is attached. The spring-mass model in Figure 7–11A is not under the influence of any external forces (i.e., it is not being pushed or pulled) and is, therefore, at rest. Not surprisingly, if the mass is pulled away from the fixed surface (that is, the spring is stretched) and then released (Figure 7–11B), the result is a back-and-forth motion around the original rest position (rest position indicated by the vertical dashed line at the right of the figure). As the spring-mass assembly vibrates, the spring is alternately stretched (Figure 7–11B) and compressed (Figure 7–11C) relative to its rest length (Figure 7–11A or 7–11D). Figure 7–11D shows the spring-mass model as it passes through the

---

Calm Yourself with Dissonance

Everyone is familiar with the peculiar sound evoked from a partially filled wine glass by rotating a finger around the lip of the glass. This party trick is rooted in the ancient practice of meditating with the assistance of Tibetan Singing Bowls. In ancient times, these bowls were constructed from a mixture of several different metals such as gold, copper, silver, and iron. The different proportions of metals used to craft the bowls determined their unique resonant properties, elicited by stroking the bowl's edge with a leather mallet. Here is what is interesting about these resonant characteristics: the peaks in the spectrum of a vibrating Tibetan Singing Bowl often produce a highly dissonant musical chord, unlike the nicely balanced chords we typically associate with soothing music. The multiple resonances of a Tibetan Singing Bowl sound vaguely like outer space sounds from a 1950s science fiction movie. Yet these sounds are considered well matched to the calming practice of meditation.

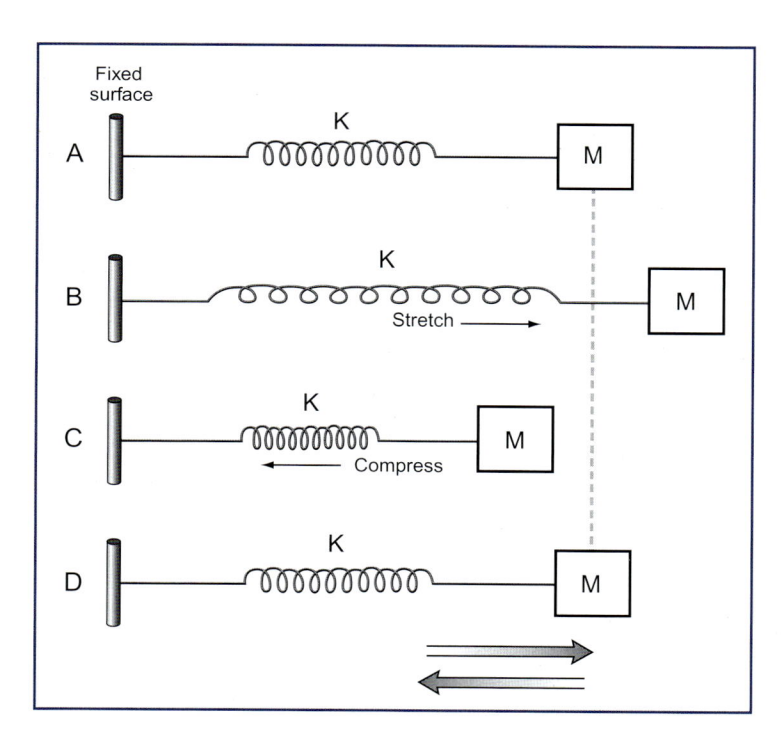

Figure 7–11. Spring-mass model that illustrates the concept of mechanical resonance. K = stiffness and M = mass. **A.** Model at rest. **B.** Model stretched from its rest position. **C.** Model compressed relative to its rest position. **D.** Model passing through its rest position during vibration.

rest position, either in the direction of stretching (right-pointing arrow) or compression (left-pointing arrow). The difference between Figures 7–11A and 7–11D is that Figure 7–11A shows the model at rest (no forces applied), whereas 7–11D shows a single moment in time during vibration when the spring-mass model is at a length corresponding to the length at rest.

The period of the vibration is equal to the amount of time required to complete one full cycle of motion (from rest, to maximum stretch of the spring, back through rest to maximum compression of the spring, and then back to rest). Alternatively, one could measure the frequency simply by counting the number of complete vibrations occurring in some unit of time and then converting to Hz, the number of complete cycles in 1 s. The motion of this spring-mass model is exactly like the one described above for the motion of air molecules (see Figures 7–1 and 7–3). The relevant question here is, What determines the frequency of a spring-mass model after it has been set into motion by a manual stretch?

The Relative Values of Mass (M) and Elasticity (K) Determine the Frequency of Vibration of the Spring-Mass Model

As described earlier, the mass and elasticity properties of an air molecule play a critical role in maintaining the motion of the molecule. This idea is pursued here, but now with reference to the specific properties of M and K that determine vibratory frequency of the spring-mass model.

Mass. The mass of an object is defined as its weight divided by a constant, which is the value of acceleration due to gravity. Formally,

$$M = \text{weight}/g_o \qquad (5)$$

where weight can be measured in pounds or grams and g_o is the symbol used to denote acceleration due to gravity, the value of which is 9.8 m/s². Because g_o is a constant, mass is considered for the remainder of this discussion as directly proportional to weight.

Objects with mass have the property of inertia, meaning that they offer opposition to being accelerated and decelerated. This property explains why, when an air molecule recoils from a stretched or compressed position back toward the rest position, it does not stop at the rest position. The inertial forces inherent in the air molecule oppose deceleration as the molecule approaches rest position, causing the motion to continue past rest and toward the other extreme position. Similarly, when recoil forces overcome inertial forces and reverse the direction of movement back toward the rest position, the molecule does not reach full speed immediately because the inertial forces oppose acceleration. These same inertial forces apply to the vibration of the spring-mass model. The explanation of mass and inertia provides the clues to how mass affects the frequency of vibration. Keep in mind, both recoil and inertial forces are acting at the same time during the vibration, with one or the other dominating depending on the position of the vibratory object.

Imagine that the mass in Figure 7–11 is replaced with a heavier one. Because the new mass is greater than the old one, it demonstrates greater inertial forces. The new mass therefore opposes being accelerated and decelerated to a greater degree than the old mass. How does this affect the motion of the spring-mass model? If the new spring-mass model opposes acceleration and deceleration more than the old one, it takes more time for the model to move through one complete cycle. This is the result of the greater time required to initiate movement at points in the cycle where the direction of motion is reversed (as at the end of a maximum displacement) or to slow down the movement as the spring-mass model goes through the rest position and moves to the other displacement extreme. Thus, the effect of adding mass to the spring-mass model is to increase the period of vibration, which is the same as decreasing the frequency. All other things being equal, an increase in mass decreases the resonant frequency of a vibratory object.

Stiffness. The elasticity of an object is defined by the amount of force required to displace the object some distance. Elasticity is typically measured in terms of *stiffness*, which can be expressed formally as:

$$K = \text{force}/\text{meters} \qquad (6)$$

where K is the symbol for the quantity *stiffness*, force is measured in units called *newtons*, and *meters* indicates a linear distance. Stiffness is typically schematized by a spring, as shown in Figure 7–11 and several upcoming figures.

Force can be described in terms of an equivalent weight (mass) required to displace an object some distance. For example, 1 newton is roughly equivalent to the application of 0.224 pounds (or 98.7 grams; 1 pound = 454 grams) of force to an object. If there were a scale sensitive enough to register accurately fractions of a pound, and enough force were applied manually to make the scale register 0.224 pounds, 1 newton of force would have been applied to the scale.

The elasticity formula shown above suggests that stiffer objects require greater force to displace them over some standard distance. This concept is illustrated in Figure 7–12, which shows two spring-mass models mounted on either side of a measuring rule marked off in centimeters. For this demonstration, the two masses (M1 and M2) are assumed to be equal, but the springs, labeled K1 and K2, have some unknown difference in stiffness. The difference in the stiffness of K1 and K2 can be determined as follows. First, both spring-mass models are resting at "0" on the centimeter rule, so 1 cm can be designated as a standard displacement for both models. Next, a wire is attached to the mass of each model, and this wire is connected to a scale which registers the amount of weight applied to the spring-mass model to cause a displacement of 1 cm. The stiffer spring, according to Formula (6), is the one requiring more weight (greater force) to produce a displacement of 1 cm. As shown in Figure 7–12, if K2 is greater than K1, then F2 (where *F* = force) must be greater than F1 to produce the standard displacement of 1 cm.

In the discussion of air molecule motion, it was noted that as a molecule is displaced from its rest position, a recoil force is developed and exerted in the direction of the rest position. When any spring is stretched or compressed away from its rest position, it stores these recoil forces, which become greater with increasing displacement from the rest position. When the two springs in Figure 7–12 are stretched 1 cm away from their rest positions, it follows that the stiffer spring—K2—will generate a greater recoil force to return to the rest position because it required a greater force to displace it the standard distance of 1 cm. If the two springs are suddenly let go after their extension to 1 cm, they both spring back toward the rest position, but K2's movement is faster because its recoil forces are greater than those of K1 at equivalent displacements. In other words, greater recoil forces are associated with greater rates of movement when the forces are permitted to produce motion (as in the case of "letting the spring go").

Now assume that the original spring in Figure 7–11 is replaced with one having greater stiffness. The greater recoil forces, and thus recoil speeds, of the new spring will decrease the time required for the model to complete a full cycle of vibration. Stated in another way, if the motion of the spring-mass model is faster because of a stiffer spring, it will take less time to move back and forth. Thus, the effect of increasing stiffness is to decrease the period, which is the same as increasing the frequency. All other things being equal, an increase in stiffness increases the resonant frequency of a vibratory object.

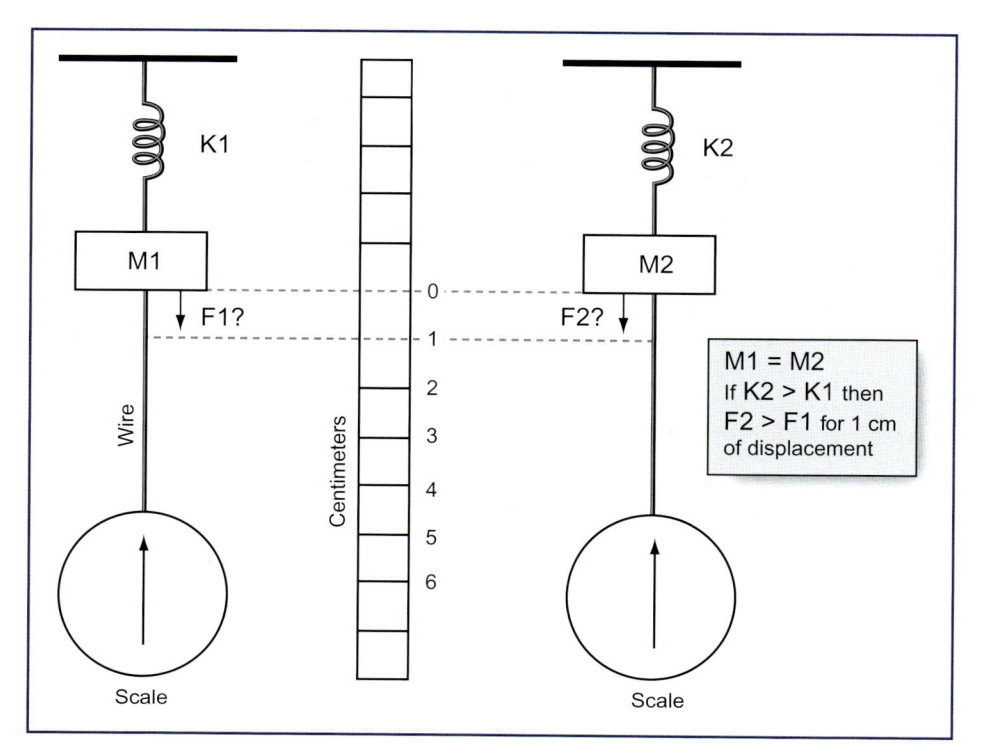

Figure 7-12. Measurement of stiffness. If the spring on the right (K2) is stiffer than the spring on the left (K1), all else being equal, a greater force is required to displace the K2-M2 spring-mass model a 1-cm unit of length.

The Effects of Mass and Stiffness (Elasticity) on a Resonant System: A Summary

The foregoing discussion of the factors that determine the resonant frequency of a spring-mass model can be summarized by the following formula:

$$fr = 1/2\pi \times \sqrt{K/M} \qquad (7)$$

where fr = resonant frequency, K = stiffness, and M = mass; $1/2\pi$ is a constant related to the circular origin of sinusoidal motion. According to the formula, an increase in the numerator K increases the resonant frequency fr, whereas an increase in the denominator M decreases fr. The formula and preceding discussion also show that a decrease in fr can be accomplished either by a decrease in stiffness or an increase in mass. Similarly, an increase in fr can be accomplished either by an increase in stiffness or a decrease in mass. In more complicated resonant systems, both stiffness and mass vary independently, and their combination (more precisely, their ratio) determines the resonant, or natural, frequency of the system.

Tacoma Narrows Bridge

A spectacular episode of apparent wind-induced resonance occurred in 1940, when the half-mile-long Tacoma Narrows Bridge in Washington State responded to high winds with vibrations of increasingly large amplitude and eventually collapsed into the Puget Sound (see Petroski, 1992 for an interesting account of bridge structures and the potential dangers of resonance). There has been some controversy over the years about the exact cause of the bridge's collapse, but one factor seems to be that the wind "forced" the bridge to resonate and twist rhythmically until it broke apart and collapsed. Search "Tacoma Narrows Bridge" on the Internet to see photographs and a brief movie of the bridge as it responded to the winds and collapsed.

Acoustic Resonance: Helmholtz Resonators

The concepts just developed in the discussion of mechanical resonance are directly applicable to a model of acoustic resonance called *Helmholtz resonance*. Helmholtz resonance is named in honor of Hermann von Helmholtz, a German scientist who lived in the late nineteenth century, constructed acoustic resonators, and studied the laws governing their vibratory behaviors. A discussion of Helmholtz resonance shows how concepts of mechanical resonance are not only equally valid in an acoustical system, but also directly applicable to certain aspects of vowel production, as discussed in Chapter 8.

Figure 7–13A shows a drawing of a Helmholtz resonator. The resonator consists of a neck having some length l, a circular opening with radius a, and a bowl having radius R. The air contained within this resonator can be separated into two functional components corresponding to the resonator neck and bowl, respectively.

The Neck of the Helmholtz Resonator Contains a Column, or Plug of Air, That Behaves Like a Mass When a Force Is Applied to It

The air within the neck can be thought of as a plug of air having some mass. When a force is applied to this plug of air, or *acoustic mass*, it offers opposition to being accelerated and, once set in motion, offers opposition to being decelerated. This acoustic mass, symbolized as Ma and alternately called an *inertance* to highlight the analogy to inertial forces offered by mechanical masses, behaves just like the masses described above in the discussion of spring-mass models.[6]

To continue the analogy from mechanical resonators, an increase in Ma decreases the resonant frequency (fr) of a Helmholtz resonator. Ma can be increased in a Helmholtz resonator by one of two physical modifications to the neck section. First, the neck can be lengthened (greater l in Figure 7–13A). A longer neck increases the number of air molecules within the plug, adding the mass of the newly included molecules to the ones in the original plug. This is a straightforward analogy to the mechanical case of increasing the weight

---

[6]Technically, a "perfect" acoustic mass is a plug of air that can be accelerated, but not compressed. What this means is that when a force is applied to one end of a plug of air, the air molecules in the plug move (accelerate) as a unit without changes in air density (that is, pressure). In other words, the air molecules within the plug are not forced closer together because of the application of the force. The analogy to a mechanical mass is direct. When a force is applied to a solid mass, the laws of inertia dictate completely the movement of the mass provided there is no compression (e.g., bending, twisting, splitting) of the molecules making up the solid. See Footnote 7 for a similar explanation of a "perfect" acoustic compliance.

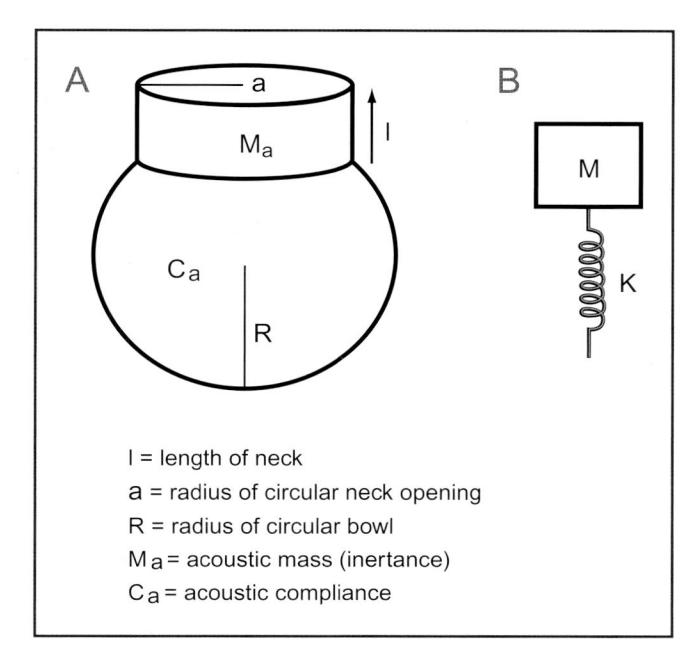

Figure 7–13. **A.** Helmholtz resonator and dimensions that determine its resonant frequency. **B.** Spring-mass model that is analogous to the Helmholtz resonator.

l = length of neck
a = radius of circular neck opening
R = radius of circular bowl
M_a = acoustic mass (inertance)
C_a = acoustic compliance

acceleration must be to these higher speeds and deceleration must be from the higher speeds. The narrower plug, therefore, offers greater functional opposition to acceleration and deceleration than the wider plug. These greater acceleration and deceleration effects will add to the period, and, therefore, decrease frequency. All other things being equal, a narrower neck opening reduces resonant frequency compared with a wider neck opening, because the narrower opening is associated with greater Ma.

The Bowl of a Resonator Contains a Volume of Air That Behaves Like a Spring When a Force Is Applied to It

The second functional component of the Helmholtz resonator is the bowl. When a force is applied to the air in the bowl, the molecules are compressed or expanded, just like the spring in the spring-mass model. When the air is compressed, the molecules exert a recoil force to "spring back" to their rest positions. When the air is expanded, the molecules exert a force to "'spring back" to their rest position. These recoil forces, summed over all the air molecules within the bowl, are expressed as pressures above or below Patm. Compressions create positive pressures (>Patm), and expansions create negative pressures (<Patm). The term *acoustic compliance* (C_a) is used to denote the stiffness properties of the volume of air within the resonator bowl. Compliance is the inverse of stiffness, so a stiffer volume of air is said to be *less* compliant, and vice versa.[7]

Following the analogy from mechanical resonators, an increase in Ca (i.e., a decrease in the stiffness) decreases the *fr* of a Helmholtz resonator. Ca can be varied in a Helmholtz resonator by changing the size of the bowl: larger bowls (those with larger internal radii, R in Figure 7–13) are more compliant, smaller bowls less compliant. For a given applied force, molecules in a larger bowl have more room to be displaced from their rest positions and are therefore more compliant (i.e., less stiff). Molecules in a smaller bowl have less room to be displaced, and therefore are less compliant (i.e., stiffer). The analogy to a spring is straightforward. Imagine two springs of the same material and the same

of a solid mass. The second way to increase Ma is to decrease the size of the neck opening (decreasing a in Figure 7–13A), even with a constant neck length. At first glance, this seems counterintuitive, because a decrease in the size of the neck opening, making it more narrow, should decrease the number of molecules in the air plug, and, therefore, make it less, rather than more, massive. Functionally, however, the effect of narrowing the neck size and hence the air plug is to cause the molecules within the plug to move at a greater speed during vibration, and hence require longer acceleration and deceleration times to and from the higher speed. When air molecules are flowing and encounter a constriction, they tend to speed up. The narrower the constriction, the greater the speed of the molecules. Thus, given two air plugs of the same length but differing degrees of narrowness, the narrower air plug responds to an applied force in a more mass-like way because

---

[7]In theory, a "perfect" compliance is a volume of air that can be compressed (or expanded), but not accelerated (this is the opposite of the definition of a perfect inertance, given in Footnote 6). This means that the molecules within the volume are all displaced from their rest positions by compression or expansion, but not accelerated to new rest positions (for example, 3 cm away from their old rest positions). Under this definition, the compressing or expanding force is expressed equally throughout the air volume in the form of increased or decreased pressures. If some of the molecules are accelerated and thus moved from their original rest positions, the pressure changes are not uniform throughout the volume. Another way to say this is that some of the applied compression or expansion force is "lost" in the acceleration of air molecules. Imagine a mechanical spring to which a compression force is applied. If the spring changes position in addition to being compressed, meaning its position has been accelerated to some degree, some of the applied force is "lost" to the movement of the spring, and the recoil force does not equal the applied force.

number of coils per unit length, but of different absolute lengths (say, 5 and 15 cm). If each of these springs is compressed the same distance (say, 1 cm), the shorter spring develops a greater recoil force than the longer spring. The small versus large air volume effect on acoustic compliance, where small bowls have low Ca (more stiff), and large bowls have high Ca (less stiff), can be explained in the same way.

A mechanical model of a Helmholtz resonator looks just like a spring-mass model. The correspondence between the two systems is captured by the orientation of the spring-mass model to the right of the Helmholtz resonator in Figure 7–13B. In both systems, an increase in mass lowers the resonant frequency and an increase in stiffness (a decrease in compliance [Ca] in an acoustic system) raises the resonant frequency. An increase in mass lengthens the period (because of increased inertial effects) and an increase in stiffness shortens the period (because of increased recoil forces and, hence, recoil speeds).

Another way to demonstrate the analogies between the mechanical and acoustical resonant systems is to show what happens when the air in the Helmholtz resonator is made to vibrate. Figure 7–14 shows four "snapshots" of a Helmholtz resonator at different points in a vibratory cycle. In all four snapshots, the colored plug or cylinder in the vicinity of the neck represents Ma, and the "cloud" of dots within the bowl represents Ca. The movement of the air plug relative to the volume of air within the bowl can be likened to a piston moving in and out of a volume of air or, of course, to a mass alternately compressing and expanding a spring. In snapshot A, the plug (Ma) and volume (Ca) of air are essentially at their rest positions. The pressure measured inside the bowl is "0" (Patm), because the air molecules are not stretched or compressed relative to their rest positions. Snapshot B shows the air plug displaced into the bowl, which compresses the volume of air and raises the pressure, as indicated by the denser cloud of dots. The compressed air molecules generate recoil forces in the outward direction, which eventually overcome the inertial force of the inward moving plug and drive it back toward the neck opening. The plug is driven outward, passes through its rest position because of its own inertial forces, and extends past the neck opening, as shown in snapshot C. At snapshot C, the molecules in the bowl are stretched relative to their rest positions and the pressure is negative, as indicated by the sparser cloud of dots. The stretched molecules generate an inward recoil force that ultimately overcomes the inertial force of the outward-going air plug and pulls it back through the rest position (snapshot D).

The analogy between mechanical and acoustical resonant systems can be summarized by means of the formula for the resonant frequency of a Helmholtz resonator. One version of the formula is the same as that given for the spring-mass model, namely,

$$fr = 1/2\pi \times \sqrt{K/M} \quad (7)$$

but it is desirable for the expression to have direct relevance to the case of a Helmholtz resonator. The resonant frequency of a Helmholtz resonator is given by:

$$fr = c/2\pi \times \sqrt{S/Vl}. \quad (8)$$

In this formula, the constant "$c/2\pi$" differs from the mechanical case ($1/2\pi$) only by the inclusion of the constant c = speed of sound in air. S = the surface area of the opening of the neck. The inclusion of S in the

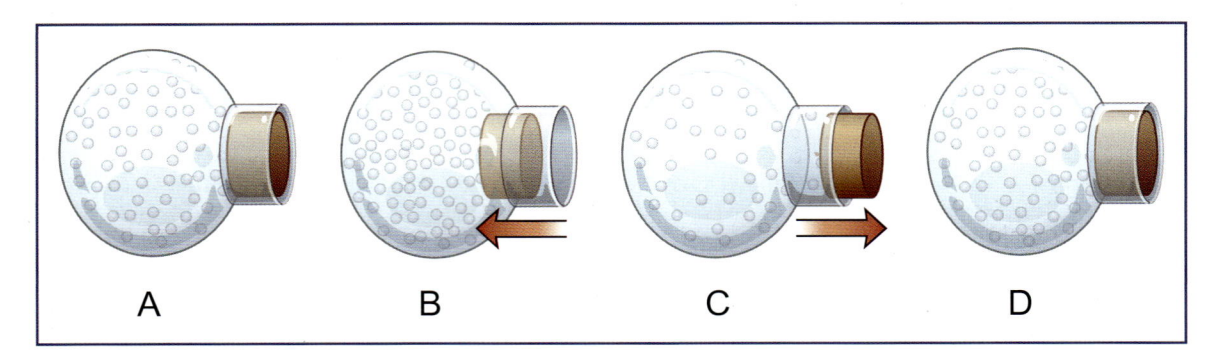

Figure 7–14. Four "snapshots" of the air in a Helmholtz resonator during vibration at resonance. The plug of air in the neck of the resonator is depicted by the shaded cylinder. The volume of air within the bowl of the resonator is depicted by the cluster of dots. Snapshots A, B, C, and D show four different moments in time during a vibratory cycle. **A.** Rest position. **B.** Plug of air displaced into the resonator bowl, causing compression of air within the bowl. **C.** Plug of air extending out of the resonator bowl and neck, causing expansion of air within the bowl. **D.** Plug of air passing through the rest position.

numerator indicates that as the surface area increases (as the neck becomes wider) the resonant frequency increases. This is consistent with the statement given above that wider necks are associated with smaller Ma. V = the volume of the resonator bowl, which when larger increases the Ca and thus lowers the resonant frequency (hence its placement in the denominator). And finally, l = length of the neck, is in the denominator because longer resonator necks are associated with greater Ma and, therefore, a lower resonant frequency.

Acoustic Resonance: Tube Resonators

Not all acoustic resonators are shaped like a Helmholtz resonator, in which the neck and bowl are physically and functionally distinct. *Tubes* are a class of resonators with substantial relevance to speech acoustics as well as other sonic events such as music. A critical concept in the understanding of tube resonance is that of *wavelength*, discussed earlier in this chapter (see Figure 7–5 and accompanying text). First consider what happens when a tube of *uniform cross-sectional area* (i.e., a tube having no constrictions), with both ends open to atmosphere, is exposed to sound energy.

Figure 7–15 pictures a tube open at both ends and a loudspeaker that produces sound energy at one end. If the loudspeaker is producing a complex acoustic event with many different frequencies, the tube is exposed to pressure waves that have a wide variety of wavelengths (recall that frequency and wavelength, related by the formula $\lambda = c/f$, are inverse functions of one another). Many of the pressure fluctuations associated with these varying frequencies propagate through the tube only weakly, but a small group of frequencies produce very strong pressure fluctuations within the tube. These frequencies have wavelengths—distributions of sound pressure in space—that match the pressure conditions at the open ends of the tube.

What are the pressure conditions at the two open ends of the tube in Figure 7–15? Under normal conditions, the pressure at both ends is Patm. Therefore, there must be frequencies whose wavelengths distribute pressure over space in such a way to have Patm at the two ends of the tube. Immediately below the tube in Figure 7–15, a wavelength (pressure as a function of

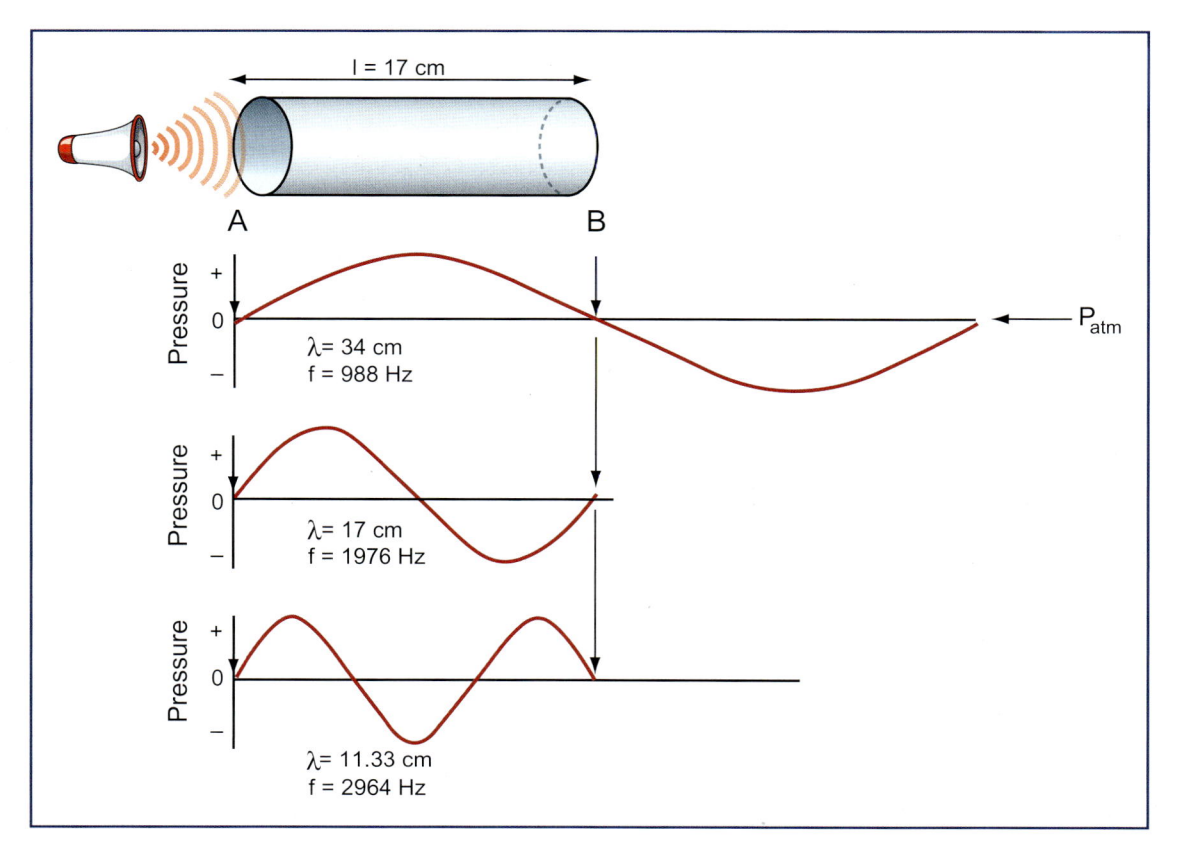

Figure 7–15. A tube 17 cm in length and open at both ends. The pressure distributions are shown for the first three resonant frequencies.

> **Three Shakers and Movers**
>
> The human body is subject to vibration and has an overall resonant frequency as well as different resonant frequencies for different parts. For example, the breathing apparatus has its own resonant frequency. One way to determine this resonant frequency is to seal the body inside a chamber below the shoulders. Powerful loudspeakers attached to the chamber are used to create large sinusoidal pressure variations at the surface of the breathing apparatus (the torso), while airflow from the mouth is monitored. The frequency of pressure swings is changed up and down while the magnitude of the airflow is recorded. The greatest peak-to-peak airflow will occur at the resonant frequency of the breathing apparatus. Your authors have such resonant frequencies of about 4, 5, and 6 Hz. Thus, each of us has a breathing apparatus that shakes best at a different frequency. Maybe you can guess something about our body sizes from these numbers.

distance; review the inset of Figure 7–5) is shown along the same distance spanned by the tube. As described earlier, a wavelength is composed of the full range of pressure variations between the maximum positive and maximum negative pressures. In Figure 7–15, the complete wavelength immediately below the tube is shown beginning at Patm, going to the maximum positive pressure, then passing through Patm and going to maximum negative pressure, and then back again to Patm. Note that the pressures at the beginning (point A) and at half of this wavelength (point B) match the pressure at the open ends of the tube. The downward-pointing arrows in Figure 7–15 indicate the first two points along this wavelength where the pressure = Patm. Those points correspond in space with the open ends of the tube. When this half-wavelength matches the pressure conditions at the open ends of the tube, the pressure fluctuation within the tube is very strong and the tube resonates at the frequency corresponding to the full wavelength.

The concept of resonance, wherein an object vibrates with maximum amplitude at one frequency (or multiple frequencies, as in the case of a tube), applies to tubes by virtue of *standing waves*. Recall that at a given point in space, the pressure associated with a periodic acoustic event varies over time from atmospheric, to maximally positive, to atmospheric, to maximally negative, and then back to atmospheric. In a continuing vibration, this pressure variation at one point in space repeats over and over. A standing wave occurs when the vibrating air molecules within a tube produce the same pressure variations at the *same location* within the tube, and these pressures reinforce each other and build up to their maximum value. These are called standing waves because even though the pressures at the one point within the tube vary over time, the reinforcing of the pressures at the same locations within the tube produces what appears to be a "frozen" distribution of pressure. At some point along this "frozen" distribution of pressure, a pressure maximum is located, and this maximum has a higher pressure than the pressures associated with other frequencies. The frequency associated with the wavelength that produces these maximum pressures vibrates with maximum amplitude, compared with many other frequencies of the complex acoustic events. According to the definition of resonance provided above, this frequency is a resonance of the tube.

Unlike Helmholtz resonators, which have a single resonant frequency, tubes open at both ends have multiple resonant frequencies because multiple frequencies have wavelengths that match the requirement of Patm at the ends of the tube. Standing waves occur at all these resonant frequencies, because the pressures at the ends of the tube reflect off the walls of a closed end (see below), or have a functional "reflection" at an open end. At an open end of a tube, where P= Patm, the molecules are passing through the rest position and therefore have the greatest speed and capability of producing high-pressure regions within the tube during vibration (recall that as a molecule passes through its rest position it does so at top speed). The reflected wave adds to the pressure distribution(s) of the resonances until the "frozen" wave is built up by the reflections. The pressure distributions shown in Figure 7–15 that "fit" the tube length are examples of such "frozen," maximum-amplitude pressure distributions. In the case of a tube open at both ends, maximum pressure(s) always occur somewhere within the tube, but never at the ends where the pressure must be Patm to produce a standing wave.

There is a simple formula for calculating the resonant frequencies of a tube open at both ends. The discussion above implies that if the length of the tube is known, one must double it to get another wavelength, and thus another frequency, that produces the desired pressure match at the ends of the tube (and another standing wave). Because half the wavelength "fits" the pressure conditions at the ends of the tube for the lowest resonance, the formula is called the *half-wavelength rule* and is expressed as:

$$fr = n \times c/2l \qquad (9)$$

where fr = resonant frequency, c = the constant, speed of sound in air, l = the length of the tube, and n = a multiplier that can be any integer 1, 2, 3 ... n. For the 17 cm tube length in Figure 7–15, the computation of resonant frequency for $n = 1$ is $fr = 1 \times 33{,}600 / 2 \times 17 = 988$ Hz.

This is the lowest resonant frequency of the tube, but as implied by the multiplier n in the formula, not the only resonant frequency. Tube resonators have multiple resonances because, as mentioned above, there are other frequencies whose wavelengths meet the requirement of Patm at both ends of the tube. For example, a frequency of 1976 Hz has a wavelength of 17 cm, exactly the length of the tube. Application of the formula produces a second resonant frequency of 1976 Hz, as predicted ($\lambda = c/f$; $17 = 33{,}600/f$; and inverting the formula, $f = c/\lambda$, so $f = 33{,}600/17 = 1976$ Hz). The spatial distribution of pressure for 1976 Hz has Patm at both ends of the tube, as shown in the middle pressure distribution in Figure 7–15. Similarly, a frequency of 2964 Hz has a wavelength of 11.33 cm, with 1½ of these wavelengths equaling 17 cm, the length of the tube. As shown in Figure 7–15, one-and-one-half wavelength is associated with a frequency of 2964 Hz, the third resonant frequency of the tube. The pressure distribution for 1½ wavelength "fits" into a tube open at both ends so that Patm is matched to the ends of the tube. In theory, an infinite number of wavelengths "fit" the tube according to the pressure requirement of Patm at the open ends. A tube resonator open at both ends, therefore, has an infinite number of resonant frequencies, at whole number multiples (1, 2, 3, ... n) of the lowest resonant frequency.

Another important class of tube resonators are those with one end closed, as seen in Figure 7–16 where the right-hand side of the tube is closed. As in the case of the tube open at both ends, a loudspeaker generates a wide variety of frequencies at one end of the tube (the open end), but the tube generates large-amplitude pressure fluctuations for only a selected few of these frequencies. These selected frequencies (i.e., the resonant frequencies) are determined by wavelengths whose pressure distributions match the pressures at the ends of the tube. The pressure condition at the open end of the tube in Figure 7–16 is already known—it is Patm. But what is the pressure condition at the closed end of the tube? Recall from the earlier discussion of sound waves that pressures are proportional to the number of air molecule collisions per unit time. At the closed end of the tube, the number of collisions per unit time is higher than at any other location within the tube, and

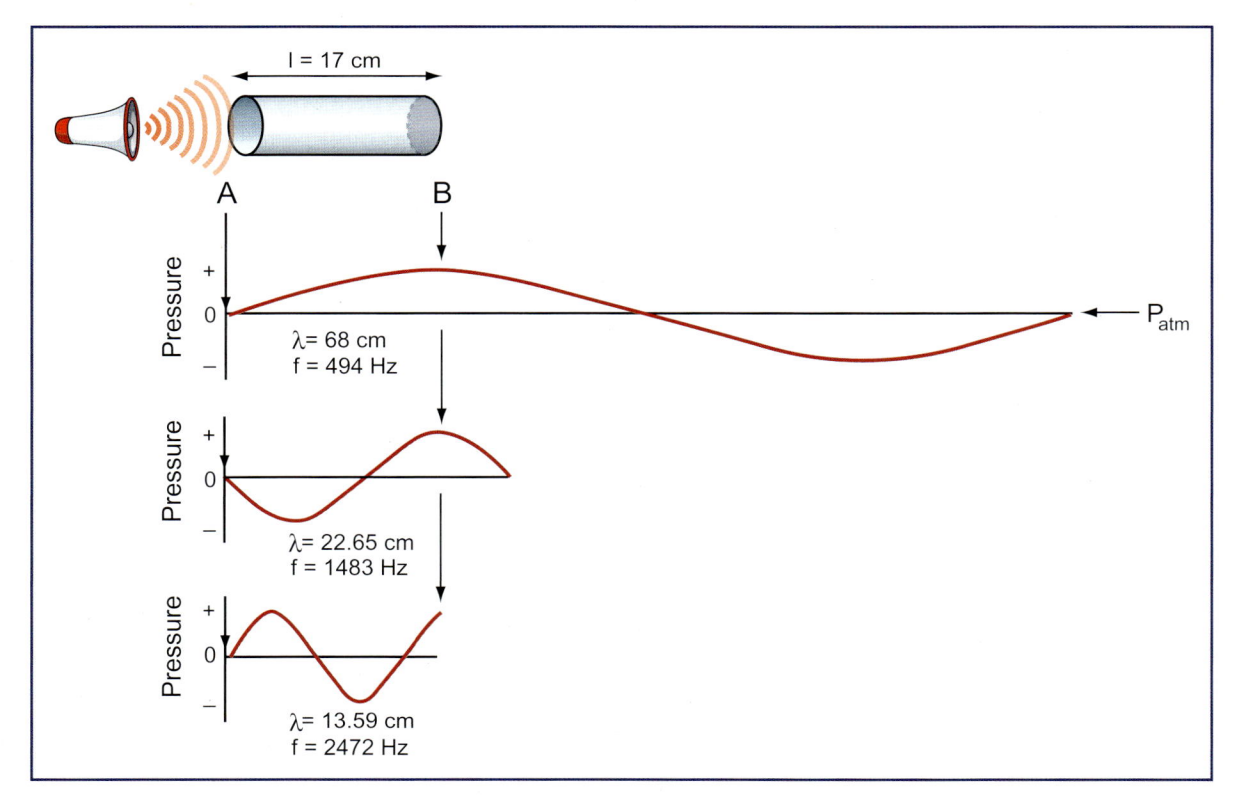

Figure 7–16. A tube 17 cm in length and closed at one end (*right*). The pressure distributions are shown for the first three resonant frequencies.

certainly much higher than at the open end of the tube. This is because the closed end serves as a barrier to the motion of air molecules, which move around and are deflected into other molecules immediately adjacent to the barrier. This results in the largest number of air molecule collisions per unit time within the tube, and hence the highest pressure within the tube. The correct "matching" pressure at the closed end of the tube is the greatest pressure along the wavelength. Pressure should be "0" at the open end (Patm), and maximum at the closed end. When the pressures along a wavelength match these conditions, a standing wave results where the "frozen" pattern is associated with a resonant frequency of the tube.

A complete wavelength contains two maximum pressures, one on the positive side of Patm and one on the negative side (see Figure 7–5, inset). In Figure 7–16, the wavelength immediately below the tube is lined up in space with the tube so that 0 pressure is at the open end of the tube, and the first maximum pressure, which happens to be the positive maximum that occurs one-quarter of the way along the full wavelength, is at the closed end. One-quarter of a wavelength "fits" the pressure requirements for resonance of this tube. The resonance pattern of a tube closed at one end is expressed by the *quarter-wavelength rule*, written as follows:

$$fr = (2n - 1) \times c/4l \qquad (10)$$

where fr = resonant frequency, c = the constant, speed of sound in air, l = the length of the tube, and $2n - 1$ is a multiplier that specifies the pattern of higher resonances. For a tube 17 cm in length and $n = 1$ (the lowest resonant frequency), the computation is $fr = ((2 \times 1) - 1) \times 33,600/68 = 494$ Hz.

Just as in the case of a tube open at both ends, other wavelengths meet the pressure requirements of a tube closed at one end. In Figure 7–16, the next shorter wavelength (i.e., the next higher frequency) that meets the pressure requirements is one that fits three-quarters of its length into the tube. If 0 pressure is located at the open end of the tube, at three-quarters of the wavelength, the pressure is at the positive maximum, which meets the pressure requirement of the closed end. The next shorter wavelength fits five-quarters (a full wavelength plus one quarter) into the tube, the next one seven-quarters, and so forth. In each case, the next shorter wavelength—and thus the next highest frequency—has a pressure distribution that meets the requirements of the tube. Note that the series of wavelengths increases by odd integers, that is, 1/4, 3/4, 5/4, 7/4 ... $(2n - 1)/4$. This explains the resonant frequency multiplier in the quarter-wavelength formula.

Resonance in Tubes: A Summary

An important aspect of a tube is that it resonates at multiple frequencies. This is because wavelengths of multiple frequencies—not just a single frequency—have pressure distributions for resonance that meet the pressure requirements at the ends of the tube. Examples of the multiple wavelengths that meet the pressure requirements of tubes open at both ends or closed at one end are shown in Figure 7–15 (*open at both ends*) and Figure 7–16 (*closed at one end*). It is important to understand that when a tube resonates, the wavelengths of the multiple resonant frequencies are all producing their unique pressure distributions within the tube at the same time. If a snapshot could be taken of the pressure distribution within a tube closed at one end, the standing waves for *each* of the resonant frequencies would be visible. Figure 7–17 shows a hypothetical example of this for the first three resonant frequencies of a tube closed at one end. The snapshot shows the expected maximum pressure at the closed end for all three standing waves corresponding to the first three resonant frequencies, but also additional maximum pressures (e.g., see arrows) near the middle and toward the open end of the tube. These other maximum pressures are from the standing waves of the higher resonant frequencies, and all are present when the tube resonates. The pressure distributions are superimposed on each other when the air in the tube is vibrating.

A fair amount of attention has been devoted to the resonant patterns of tubes because the physical principles are directly applicable to speech acoustics. In fact, a good model of the vocal tract as an acoustic resonator

Beer and Flutes

"Aeroacoustics" is the study of how air interacts with or influences mechanical structures. When you blow across the edge of that half-filled beer bottle in your hand, the air from your mouth is like a jet (a narrow "beam" of air) that exerts a force on the volume of air within the bottle; a resonant tone results. Typically, the less air in the bottle, the higher the tone. The air in the bottle and within the neck is like a Helmholtz resonator, and the air jet across the top is a force applied to the air in the bottle. The interaction of these two factors produces the tone through a very complex set of resonance and air-jet phenomena. In a general sense, flutes produce tones by this kind of aeroacoustic interaction.

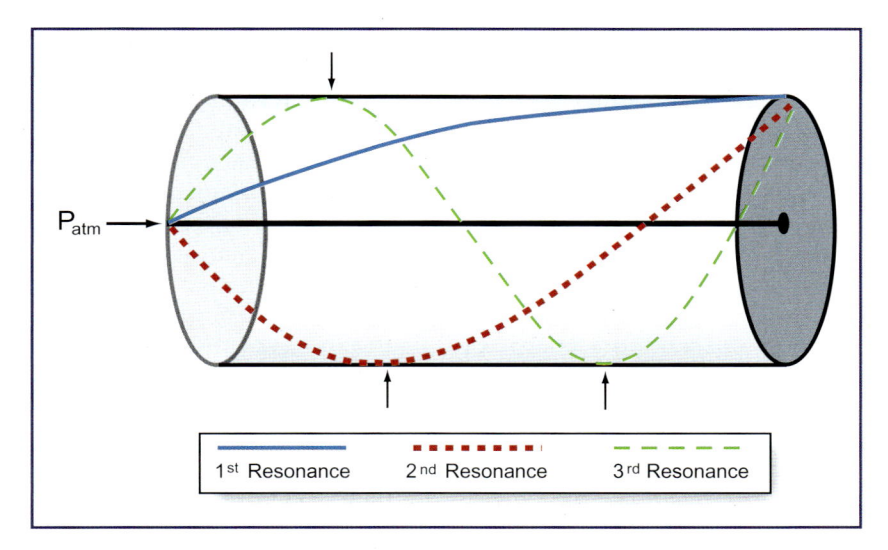

Figure 7–17. Simultaneous pressure distributions for the first three resonant frequencies within a tube closed at one end (*right*). Pressure distributions for all three resonant frequencies occur simultaneously in the vibrating tube (i.e., they are superimposed on one another). The thick horizontal line depicts atmospheric pressure as a reference point within the tube, in relation to the pressure distributions of the three resonances.

is a tube closed at one end. And if the pressure distributions within a vibrating tube are understood, as described above, the relationship of the configuration of the vocal tract to the acoustic output of the vocal tract can be easily understood. Chapter 8 presents these ideas in specific detail.

Resonance Curves, Damping, and Bandwidth

The examples of vibration discussed so far have not included considerations of energy loss. Natural vibratory phenomena are characterized by loss of energy over time. The effect of this loss of energy is to reduce the amplitude of vibration over time, and eventually to terminate the vibration. Thus, a spring-mass model, when set into sinusoidal motion, has increasingly smaller displacements over time as energy is lost. The spring-mass model ultimately ceases moving when the forces responsible for the loss of energy overcome recoil and inertial forces. This applies equally to acoustic systems such as Helmholtz resonators and tubes, where the displacement of air molecules responsible for propagation of a pressure wave gradually diminishes to zero if the source of sound (such as the loudspeaker in Figures 7–15 and 7–16) is removed from the vicinity of the resonator. A mechanical or acoustical resonator with no energy loss factors would, in theory, continue to vibrate forever after being set into vibration.

This introductory comment concerning the impact of energy loss in resonant systems refers exclusively to time-domain phenomena. Because time-domain and frequency-domain phenomena have an inverse relationship to one another, energy loss affects vibratory frequencies as well as waveforms (times). After a brief review of factors responsible for energy loss in vibratory systems, the relationship between the time and frequency aspects of vibrations affected by energy loss factors is discussed. The term *damping* is used to describe energy loss in vibratory systems. *Lightly damped* systems have minimal energy loss and *heavily damped* systems have substantial energy loss.

Energy Loss (Damping) in Vibratory Systems Can Be Attributed to Four Factors

The factors causing energy loss in vibrating systems include friction, absorption, radiation, and gravity.

Friction is a substantial source of energy loss in vibratory systems and is produced when objects rub against each other or against other structures, producing heat. In a mechanical system such as a spring-mass model, the mechanical parts (the mass and spring) rub against air molecules as they move and generate heat. If the mass is mounted in a wooden track, additional heat is generated as the mass slides along the track.

In acoustic systems, air molecules rub against each other and against the walls of the resonator (such as the soft tissues of the vocal tract), generating heat and expending energy. When frictional factors are present, some portion of the vibratory energy is dissipated (lost) in the form of heat. This dissipated energy cannot be recovered and, therefore, degrades the vibration.

Absorption of vibratory energy occurs when the vibrating object transfers (and thus loses) some of its energy to another structure. If a spring-mass model is mounted on a wall, some of the vibratory energy of the model is transferred to the wall and lost by absorption. Air molecules vibrating within the vocal tract are absorbed by vocal tract tissues, causing the latter to vibrate. In this case, the transfer of vibratory energy may result in an effective vibration of (for example) the cheeks, but the energy is lost from the vibrating air.

Radiation of sound is a form of energy loss typically associated with acoustic resonators. When air is vibrating within a resonator, some of the sound energy escapes, or radiates, from the tube and is lost. The obvious application of radiation loss in the vocal tract is the escape of sound energy from the mouth and nose.

Gravity is the force that attracts any mass to the earth. Gravity can cause energy loss in any vibrating object by exerting a force on the object that opposes the forces inherent to the vibration (such as recoil and inertia). This is not a major consideration in energy loss in acoustic vibratory systems. An example of energy loss due to gravity is the degradation of pendulum motion. The attraction of the mass (technically, the pendulum) at the end of the "arm" (called a leader) to the earth results in degradation of the pendulum motion.

Time- and Frequency-Domain Representations of Damping in Acoustic Vibratory Systems

The top of Figure 7–18 shows a Helmholtz resonator of unknown resonant frequency. Obviously, the frequency can be determined with Formula (8) by making the appropriate physical measurements, such as the length and radius of the neck and the volume of the bowl, but the resonator characteristics can also be determined by performing an experiment. The small outlet at the bottom right of the resonator bowl serves as an output through which acoustic energy is radiated and measured. Assume a microphone is mounted directly over this hole and attached to a computer that can record acoustic waveforms and compute spectra by Fourier analysis. The time- and frequency-domain characteristics at the output can be related to the same characteristics at the input.

A small-scale experiment performed with this setup demonstrates the effect of damping on the time- and frequency-domain representations of Helmholtz resonance. For this experiment, the air within the resonator must be excited using a very brief *input* stimulus. For example, the air within the resonator can be excited by a single tap on the outside of the resonator, perhaps using a small hammer as shown in Figure 7–18. The tap is an *impulse-like* event, designed to have an extremely brief duration that will not interfere with the *response* of the resonator (i.e., the vibration of the air within the resonator). The hammer tap provides a source of vibration to the resonator—turning it on, so to speak—but the source is withdrawn immediately and the subsequent response is observed. Now imagine that the experiment is performed twice, once with the resonator having minimal energy loss factors (lightly damped) and the second time with increased energy loss factors (more heavily damped).

The damping factors can be increased for the second experiment by (for example) placing more of the resonator bowl in contact with some absorptive material or decreasing the ease with which air molecules move within the resonator by increasing the roughness of the interior surface (thus increasing friction). For both experiments, the brief input energy—the tap—must be identical so that differences in the acoustic measurements at the output can be attributed to the differences in damping, and not differences in the characteristics of the input.

Figure 7–18A shows a waveform (left) and spectrum (right) of the acoustic energy associated with the resonator response in the condition of light damping. Two notable observations about the waveform are: (a) the amplitude is relatively large immediately following the input and then decreases over time until it is zero; and (b) the waveform is periodic but does not appear to be strictly sinusoidal, which suggests that the acoustic event is characterized by more than one frequency component.

The response of the lightly damped resonator in the frequency domain is seen in the spectrum to the right of the waveform. The relative amplitude scale has been arbitrarily marked 0 dB at the point of maximum energy in the resonator response, and the negative numbers indicate sound levels (in dB) less than this maximum energy point. The function shown in the spectrum is called a *resonance curve*, which displays the measurement of sound levels at all frequencies of interest (i.e., it is a frequency-domain representation of the resonator response). Because resonance is defined as the frequency at which an object (in this case the air within the resonator) vibrates with maximum energy, this resonance curve shows a natural or resonant frequency of 500 Hz. The frequency at which peak sound energy occurs along the resonance curve defines the resonant frequency.

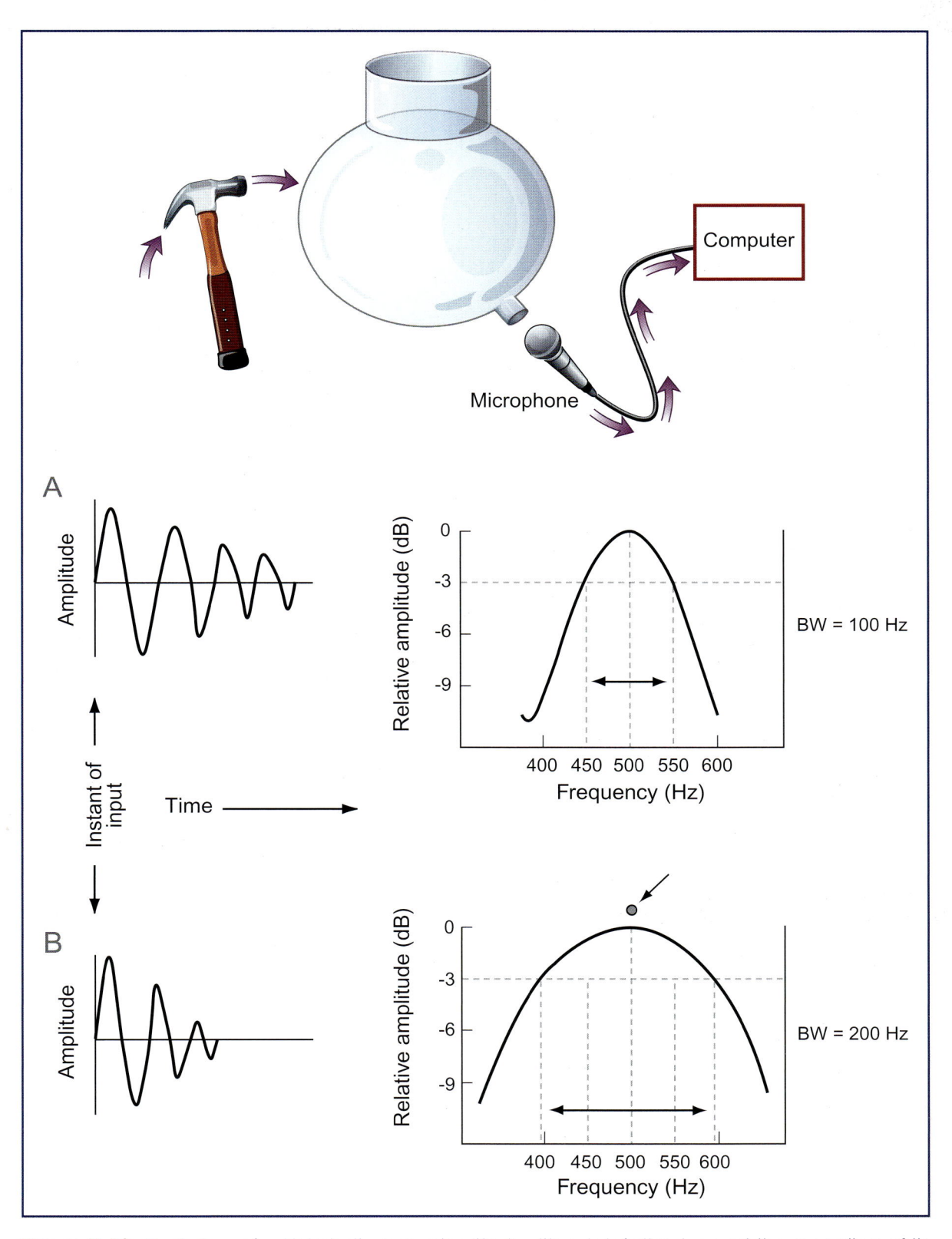

Figure 7-18. Excitation of a Helmholtz resonator (*top*) with a brief stimulus and the recording of its response (*bottom*). Time- (*waveforms at left*) and frequency-domain (*spectra at right*) displays resulting from excitation are shown on the left and right, respectively, in both **A** and **B**. The resonator is more lightly damped in **A** than in **B**.

279

The other frequencies along the resonance curve—those not associated with peak energy, but clearly showing some vibratory energy—reflect energy loss factors affecting the vibration of air within the resonator. If there were no energy loss factors in this Helmholtz resonator, the spectrum would show a single line at 500 Hz, indicating vibratory energy at a single frequency. Such a resonator is said to be *perfectly tuned*. Damping factors in a resonator change this tuning and produce energy at frequencies other than the natural frequency. The frequency-domain index of this tuning, and thus of damping, is called the *bandwidth* of the resonator. Bandwidth is defined as the range of frequencies between the two *3-dB-down points* on either side of the peak energy. In Figure 7–18A, a horizontal dashed line has been extended from the −3 dB level on the y-axis to intersect the resonance curve on either side of the peak (500 Hz). From each of these intersecting points a vertical line has been dropped to the x-axis (frequency). The vertical lines show the frequencies where the energy is 3 dB less than the energy at the resonant frequency of 500 Hz. These frequencies are 450 Hz to the left and 550 Hz to the right of the peak at 500 Hz. The bandwidth of this resonance, shown on the spectrum by the horizontal line terminated in arrows, is 100 Hz.

In Figure 7–18B, the time- and frequency-domain results are shown for the same resonator with greater damping. Here the waveform clearly decays faster over time and the bandwidth is wider than in Figure 7–18A. The spectrum in Figure 7–18B has been drawn to show an important feature of the effect of increased damping on the resonance curve: the single dot in the middle of the spectrum (arrow in Figure 7–18B) is the location of peak energy for the lightly damped resonator in 7–18A, and the peak of the more heavily damped resonance is shown at 0 dB, as in Figure 7–18A. The more heavily damped resonance of Figure 7–18B clearly does not produce the same amount of energy at the resonant frequency as the more lightly damped resonance of 7–18A, but the resonant frequency is the same for both resonators.

Peak energy in Figure 7–18B is still at 500 Hz, even though it is weaker than the peak energy in 7–18A. The most notable difference between parts A and B is the bandwidth, which is wider in B (200 Hz, indicated by the horizontal line ending in arrows).

Why is bandwidth defined in terms of the 3-dB-down points on the resonance curve? The energy in a sound wave performs *work* (such as causing an effective displacement of the human eardrum, and thus having an important effect in the perception of sound), and there is a range of sound levels below the peak that is still effective in doing this work. The term *power* is typically used by scientists to designate the work capability of energy, and it can be shown that half of the peak sound power is equivalent to 3 dB below the peak sound level. The concept of the *half-power points* designating the lower limit of effective sound energy is the origin of the use of 3-dB-down points to determine bandwidth. Note that the half-power (3-dB-down) points are used by agreement of the community of individuals interested in sound, and do not necessarily reflect any inherent truths about the effective nature of sound energy. This kind of *operational definition* is very common in all sciences, and serves the purpose of allowing scientists to communicate with one another and share research experiences and terminology within a common measurement framework.

An Extension of the Resonance Curve Concept: The Shaping of a Source by the Acoustic Characteristics of a Resonator

In Figure 7–18 a brief input (the hammer tap) was used to show the relationship between the speed of decay of the resonant waveform and the bandwidth of the resulting spectrum derived from a resonance curve. This impulse approach to the excitation of the resonator is useful in showing that damping can be defined in the time or frequency domains. This idea is now extended by demonstrating how a resonator shapes the energy of an input signal.

Figure 7–19 shows an experimental arrangement like that in Figure 7–18, except now a continuous white noise serves as the input signal to a Helmholtz resonator (Figure 7–19A) and a tube resonator (Figure 7–19B). A continuous, perfect white noise is an excellent input

---

Organic Music-Making: Hats Off to Tube Resonators

Everyone is familiar with pipe organs, the massive array of different-lengthed tubes rising above a keyboard, the heart-thumping sound of a truly great keyboard instrument. Obviously, a pipe organ can generate tones over a wide range of resonant frequencies by having pipes of different length. But it also achieves frequency variation with *individual* pipes by providing the organist with controls for "capping" one end of the tube, or leaving both ends open. The different resonant frequencies are heard as different pitches and sound qualities (see Chapter 14 on Psychoacoustics). Really, pipe organs are ear candy in disguise as resonating tubes.

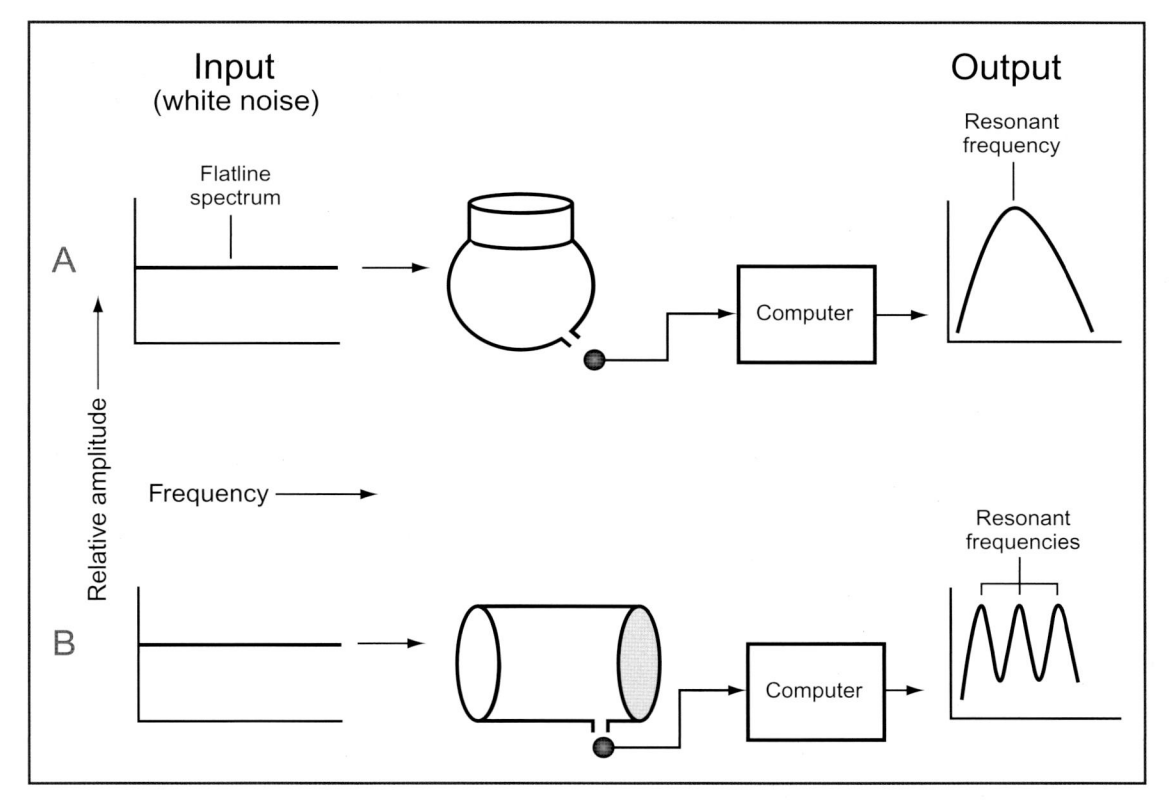

Figure 7–19. Input-output relations for a Helmholtz resonator (**A**) and a tube resonator (**B**), using white noise with a perfectly flat spectrum as the input signal. In both cases, the resonator "shapes" the input signal, as shown by the output spectra to the far right in the two panels.

signal for evaluating the characteristics of a resonator, because the average sound level at any frequency is equivalent to the average sound level at any other frequency. This is shown in Figure 7–19 by the flatline spectrum for the input signals. Because the average sound level in the input signal is equivalent at all frequencies, any modification of the spectrum at the output of the resonator must be due to characteristics of the resonator. Stated otherwise, any difference between the input and output spectra must be due to the resonator only, because the energy in the input spectrum is constant as a function of frequency.

Figure 7–19A shows how the Helmholtz resonator *shapes the input spectrum*. The air in the resonator vibrates with maximum energy at one frequency—the resonant frequency—and with less energy at other frequencies. The resonance curve is like the one shown in Figure 7–18, its shape being the result of both the physical dimensions of the resonator (which determine the resonant frequency) and the energy loss factors. The difference between the input and output spectra in Figure 7–19A is solely a result of the resonator characteristics.

Figure 7–19B shows the *input-output function* for a tube closed at one end. The tube shapes the flat input spectrum by resonating at multiple frequencies (only three are shown in Figure 7–19). Each peak in this output spectrum is a resonant frequency, and the bandwidth around each peak is determined by energy loss factors which may differ as a function of frequency (see Chapters 8 and 9).

The concept of resonators shaping an input to produce an output is a crucial one for understanding the acoustic theory of speech production. A flat input spectrum has been used to illustrate this concept, but the shaping idea applies to any situation where an input is applied to a resonator. Another way to think about the effect of a resonator on a sound source is to consider the former a *filter*. A filter is any device that passes certain inputs (i.e., allows those inputs to get through) and rejects others (i.e., stops them from getting through). Acoustic filters such as Helmholtz or tube resonators pass certain frequencies (especially the resonant frequencies) and reject others to varying degrees. In the case of speech production, the vocal tract can be considered as a filter that passes or rejects frequencies generated by different sources (such as the source energy generated by the vibrating vocal folds).

Filters take many forms, and digital techniques allow scientists to program a wide range of filter types and shapes. The most common filters used in speech and hearing research are low-pass filters, which pass low frequencies while rejecting high frequencies; high-pass filters, which pass high frequencies while rejecting low frequencies; and bandpass filters, which pass a range of frequencies while rejecting both low and high frequencies on either side of the band. Each of these filter types has a cutoff frequency (or frequencies) where frequency begins to be blocked. For example, a low-pass filter may pass frequencies between 1 Hz and 1000 Hz, blocking frequencies above 1000 Hz. In this case, the cutoff frequency is 1000 Hz. The cutoff frequency for a high-pass filter is the frequency at the low end of the filter where frequencies first begin to be blocked. This cutoff frequency can be manipulated like the cutoff frequency of low-pass filters. Digital filters can be programmed to have any cutoff frequency.

The shape of these filters typically does not include an instantaneous blocking of frequencies above (low-pass) or below (high-pass) the cutoff. Rather, the filter has a "roll off" (also called a "rejection rate") from the cutoff frequency so that frequencies above or below the passband do not decline too rapidly. As one example, a filter may have a rejection rate of 24 dB per octave, which means that the ability of the filter to pass rejected frequencies below (or above) the cutoff decreases as frequency moves away from the cutoff frequency. For most applications, "brick wall" filter cutoffs, in which no energy is allowed to pass in the rejection band (imagine a filter with no roll-off from the cutoff frequency) have undesirable effects on the signal processed by the filter.

Bandpass filters have two cutoff frequencies, one on the lower end of the filter, the other on the high end. A narrowband filter with a low-frequency cutoff of 950 Hz and a high-frequency cutoff of 1050 Hz passes frequencies from 950 to 1050 while rejecting frequencies below 950 Hz and above 1050 Hz. These cutoff frequencies can be manipulated to achieve any width, making the filter either wider (passing a greater range of frequencies) or narrower (passing a smaller range of frequencies).

These filter types have been used, and continue to be used, in speech and hearing research. For example, narrow-band noises have been used extensively in hearing research to determine the signal processing characteristics of the cochlea and auditory nerve. Low-pass, high-pass, and bandpass filters have been used to discover the frequency ranges that are necessary to transmit intelligible speech. This is important for landline and cell phone transmission, where wider bandwidths are more expensive and companies research the narrowest band (usually in the form of a bandpass filter) that transmits intelligible speech.

Resonance, Damping, Bandwidth, Filters: A Summary

The vibratory patterns of air in resonators are not only characterized by the resonant frequency (the frequency with maximum vibratory energy), but by energy loss factors that determine the shape of the curve around the peak. The energy loss factors, or damping of a resonance, can be described in either the time or frequency domain. Greater energy loss is associated with more rapid decay of vibratory amplitude over time and with wider bandwidths. For a given resonator, variations in damping have no effect on the resonant frequencies (i.e., the locations of peaks in the spectrum), but may reduce the energy at the resonances. A simple way to determine the acoustic characteristics of a resonator is to perform an input-output experiment, wherein the input is a signal having the same energy at all frequencies. When this input signal is used to excite the resonator, any differences between the input and output spectra must reflect the characteristics of the resonator. Resonators are said to shape, or filter, inputs, and in so doing produce an output that reflects the combination of the input and resonator characteristics. There are many different filter shapes that can be applied to research in speech and hearing sciences.

REVIEW

Pressure waves can be understood by examining the motions of air molecules during vibration.

These motions are governed by various forces, including those due to the elasticity and inertial properties of air molecules.

Sinusoids are the simplest type of acoustic vibration and can be considered as the elementary components of more complex vibrations.

A mathematical technique, Fourier analysis, allows a decomposition of a complex acoustic event into its component sinusoids.

When a computer program is used to construct a spectrum for a portion of a waveform, the program applies the Fourier technique to decompose the complexities in the time domain (the waveform) into the component sinusoids, and displays the components in the frequency domain (a spectrum).

Fourier analysis is valid for acoustic events that repeat in time (complex periodic sounds) and for those that do not repeat in time (complex aperiodic sounds).

A complex periodic acoustic event has frequency components at whole-number multiples of the lowest component, which is called the fundamental frequency; the multiples are called harmonics.

A complex aperiodic acoustic event is composed of many frequencies which are not in harmonic relationships to one another; there is no fundamental frequency in a complex aperiodic event.

Beats are a special case of a complex periodic waveform, in which two sinusoids differing in frequency by only a few Hz move in and out of phase at regular intervals and therefore produce a waveform with a periodic amplitude variation equal to the frequency difference between the two sinusoids.

Resonance is the phenomenon in which an object vibrates at a single frequency, or multiple frequencies, with maximal amplitude.

Two types of resonators—Helmholtz and tubes—were considered in detail.

The frequencies at which Helmholtz and tube resonators vibrate are governed by specific laws.

A Helmholtz resonator has a single resonant frequency, whereas tube resonators have multiple resonant frequencies.

Resonators shape, or filter, the acoustic energy in a sound source.

Factors that contribute to energy loss determine how long a vibration continues and the bandwidth of the output spectrum.

Filters can be low-pass, high-pass, or bandpass, and may have multiple bandpass locations (as in the case of tube resonators).

The shaping of a source by a resonator is critical to the understanding of the acoustic theory of speech production.

REFERENCES

Beranek, L. (1986). *Acoustics*. New York, NY: American Institute of Physics.
Beyer, R. (1999). *Sounds of our times*. New York, NY: Springer-Verlag.
Blackstock, D. T. (2000). *Fundamentals of physical acoustics*. New York, NY: John Wiley and Sons.
Hunt, F. (1978). *Origins in acoustics*. New Haven, CT: Yale University Press.
Kinsler, L. E., Frey, A. R., Coppens, A. B., & Sanders, J. V. (2000). *Fundamentals of acoustics* (4th ed.). New York, NY: John Wiley and Sons
Milenkovic, P. (2001). *TF32. User's manual*. Madison, WI: University of Wisconsin.
Petroski, R. (1992). *To engineer is human: The role of failure in successful design*. New York, NY: Vintage.

APPENDIX 7–A

The Decibel Scale

Humans can hear an enormous range of sound energy because the auditory mechanism can process such a great range of sound pressures. The numbers associated with this huge range of pressures are more manageable for clinical and scientific purposes by expressing sound levels as the logarithm of pressure ratios multiplied by a constant value. The sound levels resulting from this computation are expressed as decibels in sound pressure level (dB SPL). This appendix is a brief description of the dB scale. First, the dB scale for intensity level (IL) is described. Then, the relationship between intensity and pressure ratios is defined, followed by a description of pressure ratios to express the magnitude of sound energy in dB SPL.

INTENSITY LEVEL

The term "intensity" refers to the magnitude of sound energy. Sound intensity has a specific, technical definition. To understand the concept of sound intensity, it is necessary to define the terms *power* and *watt*. Power is the rate of doing work, which can also be described as the amount of energy consumed per unit time. The unit of power is the *watt*, and the unit time over which watts are expressed is 1 second.

$$\text{Power} = \text{watts/sec.} \quad (1)$$

Recall that sound waves propagate away from a source longitudinally, as a series of planes of varying density of air molecules. Sound intensity is defined as power distributed over the area of any one of these planes. The standard unit area over which watts are distributed is the square meter (m^2).

$$\text{Sound intensity} = \text{watts}/m^2. \quad (2)$$

When applied to human hearing, the ratio of sound intensities ranging from barely audible (threshold of hearing; see Chapter 14) to a maximum sound intensity that causes auditory pain (and perhaps pain in other areas of the body) is 100 trillion to 1 (100,000,000,000,000:1). Scientists recognized that expressing sound intensity on a scale with such an enormous range of numbers was cumbersome. To solve this problem, they transformed sound intensity ratios with base-10 logarithms. The scale resulting from the logarithmic transformation is called the bel scale. The bel is computed as:

$$\text{bel} = \log_{10}(I/I_o). \quad (3)$$

In this expression I_o is a reference intensity. The standard reference intensity is defined as the sound intensity associated with the auditory threshold (i.e., the lowest sound intensity that can be heard); obtained from normal-hearing young adult listeners. This reference is 1 picowatt/m^2 (a picowatt = 10^{-12} watts, or .000000000001 watts). Intensities higher or lower than the reference intensity can be expressed in bels after logarithmic transformation. There are many free $\log_{10}$ calculators on the Internet (e.g., https://www.rapidtables.com/calc/math/Log_Calculator.html).

The logarithm of 1 = 0. This means that when a measured intensity is identical to the reference intensity ($I = I_o$), bels = 0. Following the logic above, 0 bels corresponds to the average intensity at the threshold of hearing. An increase in the value of the numerator by one order of magnitude (I multiplied by 10) gives a ratio of 10:1, and the logarithm of 10 is 1. The logarithm of a ratio of 100:1 = 2, the logarithm of a ratio of 1000:1 = 3, and so on. Therefore, a 10:1 intensity ratio = 1 bel, a 100:1 intensity ratio = 2 bels, a 1000:1 intensity ratio = 3 bels, and so on. Table 7A–1 shows intensity ratios from 1:1 to 10,000,000,000:1, their logarithms, and associated bel values.

As can be seen by comparing the first and third columns of Table 7A–1, each successive whole-number increment along the bel scale corresponds to large, and increasingly larger, increments in intensity. For example, the difference between 3 and 4 bels is an intensity increment of 1,000 to 10,000 watts/m^2 and the difference between 4 and 5 bels is an intensity increment of 10,000 to 100,000 watts/m^2. The scale can also be used to reflect intensity ratios between whole-number increments that are not simply order of magnitude changes. For example, the logarithm of an intensity ratio of 1500:1 is 3.176. With rounding, this is equivalent to 3.18 bels above the reference intensity.

Table 7A-1. Intensity Ratios, Their Logarithms, and Associated Bel and Decibel Values

INTENSITY RATIO	LOGARITHM	BELS	dB
1	0	0	0
10	1	1	10
100	2	2	20
1,000	3	3	30
10,000	4	4	40
100,000	5	5	50
1,000,000	6	6	60
10,000,000	7	7	70
100,000,000	8	8	80
1,000,000,000	9	9	90
10,000,000,000	10	10	100

The bel scale is further refined by eliminating decimals. This is accomplished by a partition into 10 equal steps of the difference between each 10-fold increment in bels. This decibel (dB) scale has whole number increments (e.g., 31, 32, 33, 34, 35, 36 dB). The formula for the dB scale for sound intensity level is:

$$dB = 10 \log_{10} (I/I_o). \quad (4)$$

In the example above, an intensity ratio of 1500:1 gives:

$$dB = 10 \log_{10} (1500/1) = 10 \times (3.176) = 31.76 \text{ dB IL}$$

With rounding, an intensity ratio of 1500:1 is 32 dB above (greater than) the reference intensity. Recall that I_o, the reference intensity, is 1 picowatt/m², or 10^{-12} watts/m². In the example immediately above, the proper way to express the intensity level is 32 dB re: 1 picowatt/m². The value of 32 dB IL re: 1 picowatt/m² is the same as 3.2 bels IL re: 1 picowatt/m².

The measurement of sound intensity poses several problems. The most formidable problem is the need to have accurate measures of air particle velocity to obtain accurate measures of power. Microphones can be built to measure these velocities, but they are very expensive and difficult to calibrate. Calibration of a microphone uses a known input to a microphone (such as a known air molecule velocity), which is compared with the output of the microphone; in the best-case scenario, the output is an exact match to the known input. This exercise is difficult to complete for direct measurements of intensity. Fortunately, there is a relationship between intensity and pressure that allows sound energy to be expressed as dB sound pressure level (SPL). Moreover, microphones sensitive to pressure are reliable, easily calibrated, and reasonable in cost.

SOUND PRESSURE LEVEL

The relationship between intensity and pressure is straightforward: intensity is proportional to the square of pressure (p).

$$I \sim p^2. \quad (5)$$

It follows that a *ratio* of intensities is proportional to a *ratio* of pressures squared:

$$I/I_o \sim (p^2/p^2_o). \quad (6)$$

As in the dB scale for intensity, the subscript "o" in the denominator of the pressure ratio denotes a reference pressure, defined in the same way as the reference intensity: that is, the reference pressure for the computation of SPL is the sound pressure associated with the average threshold among normal-hearing young adults.

The reference pressure (force/area) for measurement of SPL is 20 µPa/m², where µ is the symbol for "micro" and Pa stands for pascal (a unit of force); 20 µPa = .000020 Pa. The force part of the ratio is expressed in newtons (units of force), and the area is standardized to 1 m² (1 newton is the force required to accelerate a mass of one kilogram at an acceleration of 1 m/sec²).

The proportionality between sound intensity and sound pressure allows the dB formula to be expressed as:

$$dB \text{ IL} = 10 \log (I/I_o) \sim dB \text{ SPL} = 10 \log (p^2/p^2). \quad (7)$$

A basic property of logarithms is that $\log (x^n) = n * \log (x)$. The expression given above for dB SPL = 10 log (p^2/p^2) can therefore be expressed without the exponents as:

$$dB \text{ SPL} = 2 * 10 \log (p/p_o) = 20 \log (p/p_o). \quad (8)$$

The exponent is removed by multiplying its value by 10. Thus, dB SPL = 20 log (p/p_o). As pointed out years ago by Beranek (1954), among the advantages of measuring sound levels in pressure units, rather than intensity units, is the fact that the human ear responds to pressure variations over time.

The reference pressure for SPL—20 µPa—is substantially smaller than atmospheric pressure, which is 101,325 Pa. Why can people hear such small pressure variations when atmospheric pressure is so much higher? The answer is that atmospheric pressure is more or less static, and when it changes it does so on a very slow time scale. In contrast, *sound* pressures vary at a much faster rate.. The tympanic membrane (eardrum) vibrates in response to these sound pressure variations, setting into motion the structures of the middle and inner ears (Chapter 13).

Table 7A–2 shows the relationship between sound pressure ratios, their associated logarithms, and decibels in SPL. Table 7A–2 covers the same dB range shown in the intensity table presented above.

Using Table 7A–2, it is possible to determine that a pressure ratio of 100, plugged into the SPL formula, is 20 * log (100) = 40 dB SPL. The logarithm of 100 is 2, thus 20 × 2 = 40. Like intensity, each 10-fold pressure increment is partitioned into 10 dB steps, allowing expression of a continuous range of dB SPL re: 20 µPa. As in the example given for intensity, a pressure ratio of 1500:1, whose logarithm is 3.176, is expressed in SPL as 20 log (3.176) = 64 dB SPL (value rounded up one half-step from 63.652).

equivalent sound intensity and sound pressure levels requires some calculation.

Consider the following example of a sound pressure ratio of 1500:1 which is associated with an SPL value of 64 dB re: 20 µPa. With $I \sim p^2$, the square of the pressure ratio of 1500:1 must be obtained to get the corresponding intensity ratio. The square of 1500 is 2,250,000, and the log of this value is is 6.35.. Plugging this log into the intensity level formula 10 log (I/I_o) results in an intensity level of 64 dB re: 1 picowatt/m^2 (10*6.352) = 64 dB). Equivalent dB values expressed in intensity level and sound pressure level are the result of converting a pressure ratio to an intensity ratio.

The doubling of intensity level and of sound pressure level has different outcomes. On the sound pressure level scale, a doubling is associated with a change of 6 dB; that is, for a 2:1 change in pressure, the log of 2 = .301, 20 log (.301) = 6 dB SPL. In contrast, a 2:1 change in intensity yields 10 log (.301) = 3 dB IL. These different dB changes for the same ratio do not mean that the sound *energy* changes are different for intensity and sound pressure levels. The 2:1 ratio applied to both sound intensity level and sound pressure level must account for $I \sim p^2$, so the ratio of 2:1 in pressure terms is equivalent to a ratio 4:1 in intensity terms. The logarithm of 4 = .602, and 10 log (.602) = 6 dB IL.

INTENSITY LEVEL AND SOUND PRESSURE LEVEL

There is often confusion about the similarities and differences between intensity level and sound pressure level. Both are expressed on dB scales and both have standard reference values which reflect the same magnitude of sound energy but in different units, as described above. Both also have reference levels that are based on the threshold of hearing, but to express

Table 7A–2. Sound Pressure Ratios, Their Associated Logarithms, and Decibels in SPL

PRESSURE RATIO	LOGARITHM	dB
1	0	0
10	1	20
100	2	40
1,000	3	60
10,000	4	80
100,000	5	100

SOUND LEVELS AND DISTANCE FROM THE SOUND SOURCE

Intensity levels and sound pressure levels should always be reported with information on the distance of the listener (or recording device) from the sound source. For plane waves, sound energy decreases as the inverse of distance from a source. The measured sound pressure level for a sound source that emits a constant sound pressure level is greater at 5 than at 10 feet distance from the source. Distance from the source is not an issue when sound signals are delivered under headphones; there is a standard practice for calibrating headphones that does not require the specification of distance from the source.

REFERENCE PRESSURE AND THE MEANING OF 0 dB

Zero dB SPL does not indicate the absence of sound energy. This is because the reference pressure is based on the average hearing thresholds of a group of young adults with normal hearing. Some young adults can detect sound pressure levels that are the same or even less than the reference value. This means that negative dB values occur when the measured sound pressure level at an individual's threshold is less than the standard reference value. For example, with 20 µPa as the reference pressure, a sound pressure of 10 µPa has an SPL of −6 dB:

$$dB\ SPL = 20 \log (p/p_o)$$

$$dB\ SPL = 20 \log (10\ \mu Pa/20\ \mu Pa)$$

$$\log 0.5 = (-0.301)$$

$$SPL = 20 * (-0.301) = -6\ dB\ SPL\ re{:}\ 20\ \mu Pa$$

The sound pressure level decibel scale can be used with any reference pressure, even if the scale is most often used with the reference values described above. In certain circumstances, a clinician or researcher may be interested in dB differences from an SPL above the standard reference pressure. For example, audiologists are often interested in the dB level required to understand speech in persons with hearing loss. In this case the reference is the sound pressure level corresponding to the person's elevated threshold (i.e., hearing losses have thresholds greater than the sound pressure that corresponds to the threshold for normal hearing). The point here is that a unit change in dB—1 dB, for example—is the same at any location on the full scale. The computation of sound pressure level uses the same formula for any sound pressure reference.

8

Acoustic Theory of Vowel Production

INTRODUCTION

Speech scientists and speech-language pathologists are indebted to Gunnar Fant, a Swedish speech scientist, and Kenneth Stevens, a Canadian speech scientist who spent his career at the Massachusetts Institute of Technology in Boston, for the development of the theoretical basis of speech acoustics. Fant worked on the theory in the 1940s and 1950s, and published his classic book, titled *Acoustic Theory of Speech Production*, in 1960. Stevens began publishing his work in the 1950s and in 1998 published a text titled *Acoustic Phonetics*. Previously, two Japanese scientists (Chiba & Kajiyama, 1941) developed a mathematical theory of vocal tract acoustics like Fant's, but this work was essentially unknown in Western hemisphere countries until well after World War II. Fant, Stevens, and several other scientists continued to develop and refine the theory in the 1950s, 1960s, and 1970s. Indeed, the theoretical development continues today. In particular, a text published by Flanagan (1972) and more recent work (e.g., Lammert & Narayanan, 2015; Story, 2005; Story & Bunton, 2017) are excellent sources for the advancement of speech acoustic theory. Much of the information in this and the following chapter is drawn from these sources.

The acoustic theory of vowel production can be stated in very broad terms, as follows: for vowel production, the vocal tract resonates like a tube closed at one end, and shapes an input signal generated by the vibrating vocal folds. The two major concepts suggested in this broad statement of the theory—the resonance patterns of a tube closed at one end, and the shaping of an input by a resonator—are covered in Chapter 7. For this chapter, the broad statement of the theory refers only to vowel production. The theory is

---

Fathers of Speech Acoustics

Professor Gunnar Fant (1919–2009) was a famous speech acoustician and is widely regarded as one of the fathers of speech acoustics. Fant was born in Sweden in 1919 and spent most of his career in the Department of Speech, Hearing, and Music at the Royal Institute of Technology (KTH) in Stockholm. Fant founded this department in 1951 as the Speech Transmission Laboratory, after spending 1949 and 1950 at the Massachusetts Institute of Technology working with another giant in the field, Professor Kenneth Stevens (1924–2013). Over the years, Fant's department generated a wealth of valuable research, all of which was reported in a famous, recurring publication called the *KTH Speech Transmission Laboratory Quarterly Progress Report*. Fant's 1960 book, *Acoustic Theory of Speech Production*, is one of a very few knowledge touchstones for the serious speech scientist. The student who reads and comprehends Fant's text, as well as Professor Stevens' (a second intellectual father) magnificent 1998 text *Acoustic Phonetics*, which can be considered a successor to, and enlarger of, Fant's classic book, can claim to be well informed about the many aspects of speech acoustics.

most precise for the case of vowels, primarily because its mathematical basis works best for the resonant frequencies of vowels (compared with many consonants). The theory also addresses consonant acoustics, which is covered in Chapter 9. To explore the acoustic theory of vowel production in greater depth, this chapter addresses the following set of questions:

1. What is the precise nature of the input signal generated by the vibrating vocal folds?
2. Why should the vocal tract be conceptualized as a tube *closed* at one end (compared with open at both ends)?
3. How are the acoustic properties of the vocal tract determined?
4. How does the vocal tract shape the input signal?
5. What happens to the resonant frequencies of the vocal tract when the tube is constricted at a given location?
6. How is the acoustic theory of vowel production confirmed?

WHAT IS THE PRECISE NATURE OF THE INPUT SIGNAL GENERATED BY THE VIBRATING VOCAL FOLDS?

The periodic vibration of the vocal folds provides the input signal for vowels to the vocal tract resonator. This periodic vibration is referred to as the *source* for vowel acoustics. As discussed in Chapter 7, any signal can be studied in both the time and frequency domains. Much of what follows is a condensation of work done by Fant (1979, 1982, 1986) as refinement of the theory first published in 1960.

The Time Domain

The time-domain characteristics of the signal produced by vocal fold vibration are complex. The larynx, a structure of cartilage, membrane, ligament, and muscle (Chapter 3), is not easily accessible for direct measurement of vocal fold behavior. When a microphone is placed directly in front of a speaker's lips while he or she phonates a vowel, the recorded acoustic event will reflect the *combination* of source (vocal fold) and resonator (vocal tract) acoustics. There is no simple way to look at the waveform (time domain) of a vowel recorded in this way (such as that shown in Figure 7–8B) and identify the time or frequency characteristics due only to vocal fold vibration. Some other approach must be found to separate the waveform of a recorded vowel into the parts contributed by (a) the vibrating vocal folds and (b) the resonating vocal tract.

One of the earliest attempts to understand the details of vocal fold vibration was described by Farnsworth (1940), who took high-speed motion pictures of the vibrating vocal folds by filming images of the folds as reflected in a laryngeal mirror. When played back in slow motion, these films allowed Farnsworth to view, on a frame-by-frame basis, movements of the vocal folds and the changing configuration of the glottis (the space between the vocal folds) throughout individual cycles of vocal fold vibration. A sequence of images of one vocal fold cycle, like those examined by Farnsworth but collected with a contemporary device, is shown in Figure 8–1. The cycle begins with the vocal folds fully approximated (image 1). The folds separate gradually to a maximum width of the glottis (image 5), then begin to move back to the midline until they are once again fully approximated (images 6–10). Scientists examined images such as these and for each frame of a vocal fold cycle measured the width and length of the glottis. These measurements allowed them to derive the glottal area, based on the width and length measures, on an image-by-image basis. Glottal area as a function of time was plotted for a complete cycle of vocal fold vibration.

A typical *glottal area function*, symbolized as A_g, is shown in Figure 8–2A for two cycles of vocal fold vibration. The baseline in this plot represents full approximation of the vocal folds (i.e., $A_g \sim 0$), and upward movement of the function indicates increasingly greater separation of the vocal folds (i.e., increasing A_g). One cycle of vocal fold vibration is defined as the interval between successive separations of the vocal folds, as marked in Figure 8–2. Note that the vocal folds are fully approximated for a substantial portion of each cycle (nearly 40% of each cycle). The moment immediately before the vocal folds separate has been chosen arbitrarily as the initiation of each cycle. The duration of these cycles of vocal fold vibration may range from as little as 1 ms or less (for some opera or pop singers who can produce extremely high-pitched notes) to the more typical 5 ms (adult women, as shown in Figure 8–2) or 8 ms (adult men).

The A_g function shown in Figure 8–2 is not an acoustic signal, but rather reflects a pattern of vibration that produces an acoustic signal. How does one obtain the acoustic signal associated with vocal fold vibration—separate from the influence of the cavities in the vocal tract—and how is this signal related to the A_g function just described?

Imagine that it was possible to suspend, immediately above the vocal folds, a device that measures the magnitude of airflow streaming through the glottis as a

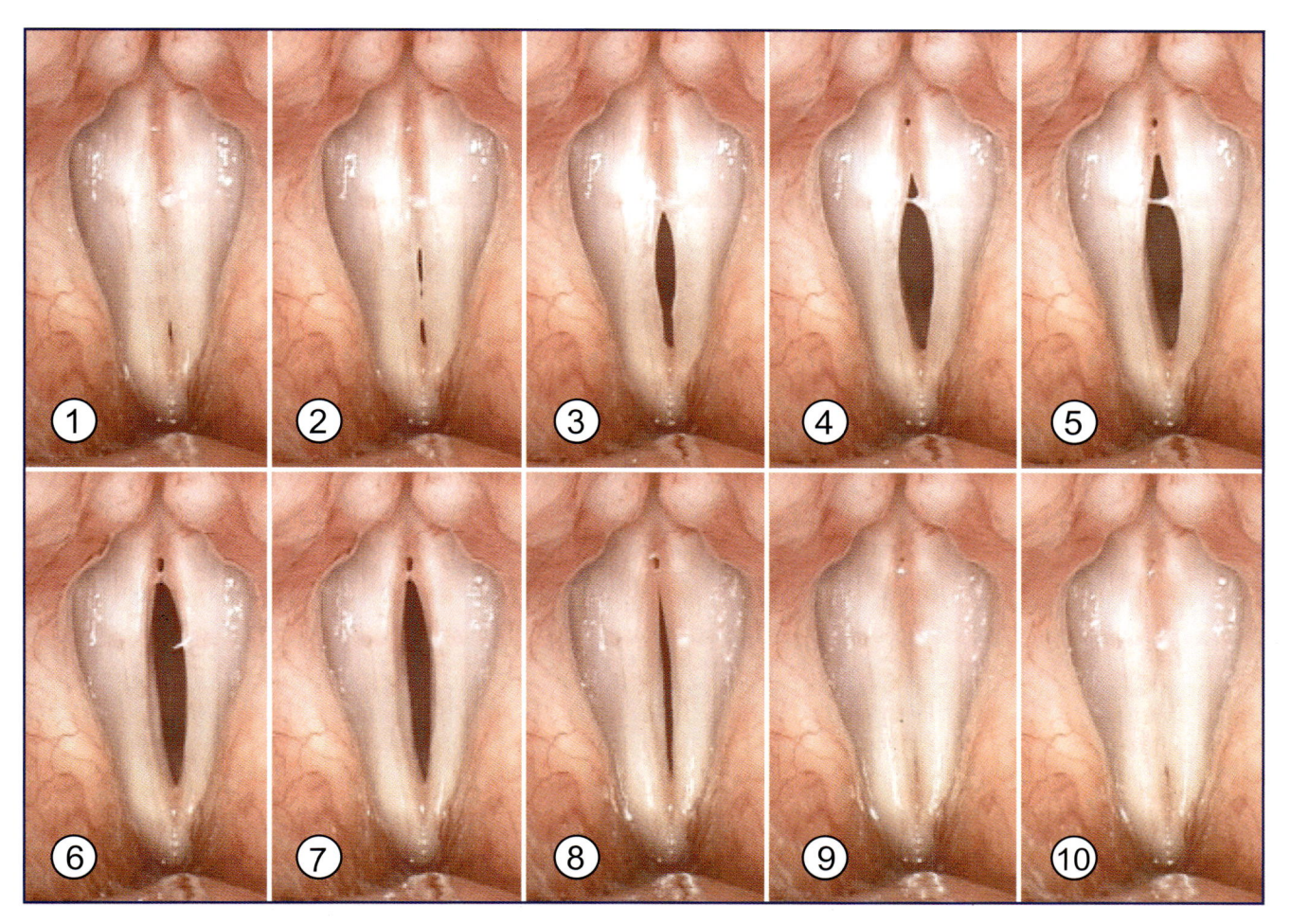

Figure 8–1. Successive images from one complete cycle of vocal fold vibration recorded via videostroboscopy (see Chapter 6). The cycle begins in the upper left frame (image 1) with the vocal folds approximated. The folds begin to separate in image 2 and reach maximum separation in image 5. Closing of the vocal folds takes place in images 6 through 10. Images provided courtesy of KayPENTAX, Montvale, NJ. Reproduced with permission.

function of time. When the vocal folds separate during a vibratory cycle (e.g., during phonation of a vowel) airflow through the glottis is expected because speech is produced with tracheal pressures greater than those in front of the lips (i.e., Patm), and air always flows from regions of higher pressure to regions of lower pressure (Chapter 3). Intuitively, the magnitude of this airflow should be zero when the vocal folds are fully approximated, and maximum when the vocal folds are widest apart (when Ag is the largest). In other words, the airflow coming through the glottis should increase as Ag increases, and decrease as Ag decreases. A plot of the magnitude of airflow coming through the glottis as a function of time (Figure 8–2B) looks a lot like the Ag function shown in Figure 8–2A. The time-domain plot of airflow through the glottis is a *glottal flow* function, symbolized as V̇g. Because the V̇g reflects movement of air molecules, which results in sound pressure waves (see Chapter 7), V̇g is the proper signal to study as the acoustics of the source—vocal fold vibration—in vowel production.

The V̇g function shown in Figure 8–2B looks very much like the Ag function (the detailed differences between the two types of waveforms will not be discussed in this text). Nevertheless, as noted above, actual measurement of the flow coming through the glottis in a phonating human is extremely difficult, if not impossible. Instead, scientists obtain V̇g signals using an indirect approach.

Imagine a situation in which the input signal is the vibration of the vocal folds and the filter is a resonance curve associated with a specific shape of the vocal tract. From the discussion of tube resonators in Chapter 7, and introductory comments concerning the vocal tract

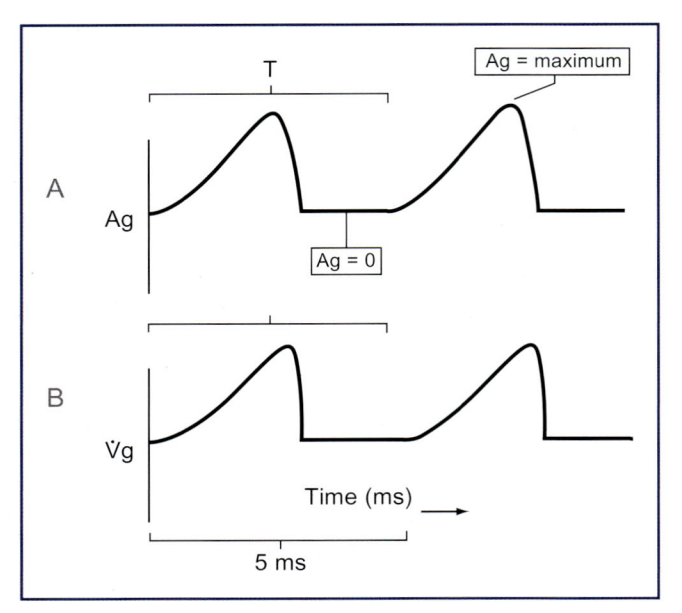

Figure 8–2. **A.** Glottal area function (Ag) for two cycles of vocal fold vibration. Upward displacements represent increasingly larger glottal areas, which are proportional to glottal widths measured from images like those in Figure 8–1. **B.** Glottal airflow function (V̇g) obtained by inverse filtering (see text). Upward displacement indicates increasing magnitude of airflow passing through the glottis.

resonating like a tube closed at one end, multiple peaks are expected in the resonance curve. The input signal plus a resonance curve for the vocal tract tube resonator are shown in the upper part of Figure 8–3. When the input signal—here labeled "glottal source signal"—is applied to the vocal tract filter, the resulting waveform is the output labeled "speech signal" (Figure 8–3, upper right panel). That speech signal represents the blending of the input and filter characteristics. Because of this blending, the output signal cannot reveal the exact characteristics of the input (source) signal unless the output signal is separated into its source and filter parts.

A technique to recover the source signal from the blended signal is called "inverse filtering" as demonstrated in the lower part of Figure 8–3. On the left is the speech signal, the same one as in the upper right-hand panel of the figure. This is the "blended" signal reflecting the influence of both the source and vocal tract filter. The blended signal serves as input to a resonance curve that is "flipped" like a mirror image of the vocal tract filter shown in the top of the figure. In the flipped, or inverse, filter, there are valleys at the precise locations of the peaks in the upper filter function. If the inverse filter is constructed correctly, when the "blended" input signal is run through it, the resonances are subtracted from the signal, and what remains at the output of the filter is the glottal source signal. This is shown in the lower right panel as "recovered glottal source signal." In essence, the sequence of the bottom panel reverses that of the top panels, with the special adjustment of flipping the filter function.

Technical details of inverse filtering are not important here, and the technique is more complicated (and often trickier) than implied by the straightforward logic of Figure 8–3. For current purposes, the ability to recover a glottal source signal—such as the V̇g signal—is the central issue. There are three important features of the V̇g signal shown in Figure 8–2B.

First, as noted above for the Ag signal, the V̇g signal is periodic, meaning that its characteristic shape repeats over time. The rate at which it repeats over time is the fundamental frequency (F0) of vocal fold vibration, or how many times per second the vocal folds go through complete cycles of vibration. In adult women, a typical F0 is around 190 to 200 Hz, in men around 115 to 125 Hz, and in 5-year-old children around 250 to 300 Hz (Kent, 1997; Lee, Potamianos, & Narayanan, 1999). As shown in Figure 8–2 the period (T) of this time-domain signal is easily measured, and the inverse of the period is the F0 (see Chapter 7 for a discussion of $f = 1/T$).

The second important feature of the V̇g signal produced by most people in ordinary conversation is the shape of the opening and closing portions of each cycle. The slope of the opening phase is shallower than the slope of the closing phase, making each cycle appear as if it is "leaning to the right." This shape feature is seen clearly in the V̇g signal of Figure 8–2B. The steepness of the closing phase is important because it reflects how rapidly the vocal folds come together at the end of each cycle. The more rapidly the vocal folds come together, the steeper the closing part of the V̇g signal. This has great importance to the frequency-domain characteristics of the source, as discussed in the next section.

The third important feature is that the V̇g signal shows some portions where the vocal folds are apart (i.e., where airflow is coming through the glottis), and some portions where the vocal folds are approximated. The ratio of open time to closed time for each cycle, which in normal voices is typically around 1.2:2 (i.e., the vocal folds are open approximately 60% of each cycle), may be an important determinant of how much of the source signal is periodic and how much is aperiodic. This is important when considering the physiological and acoustical basis of pathological voice quality.

Figure 8–2 shows that the V̇g signal does not have a sinusoidal shape, but is periodic. Material covered in

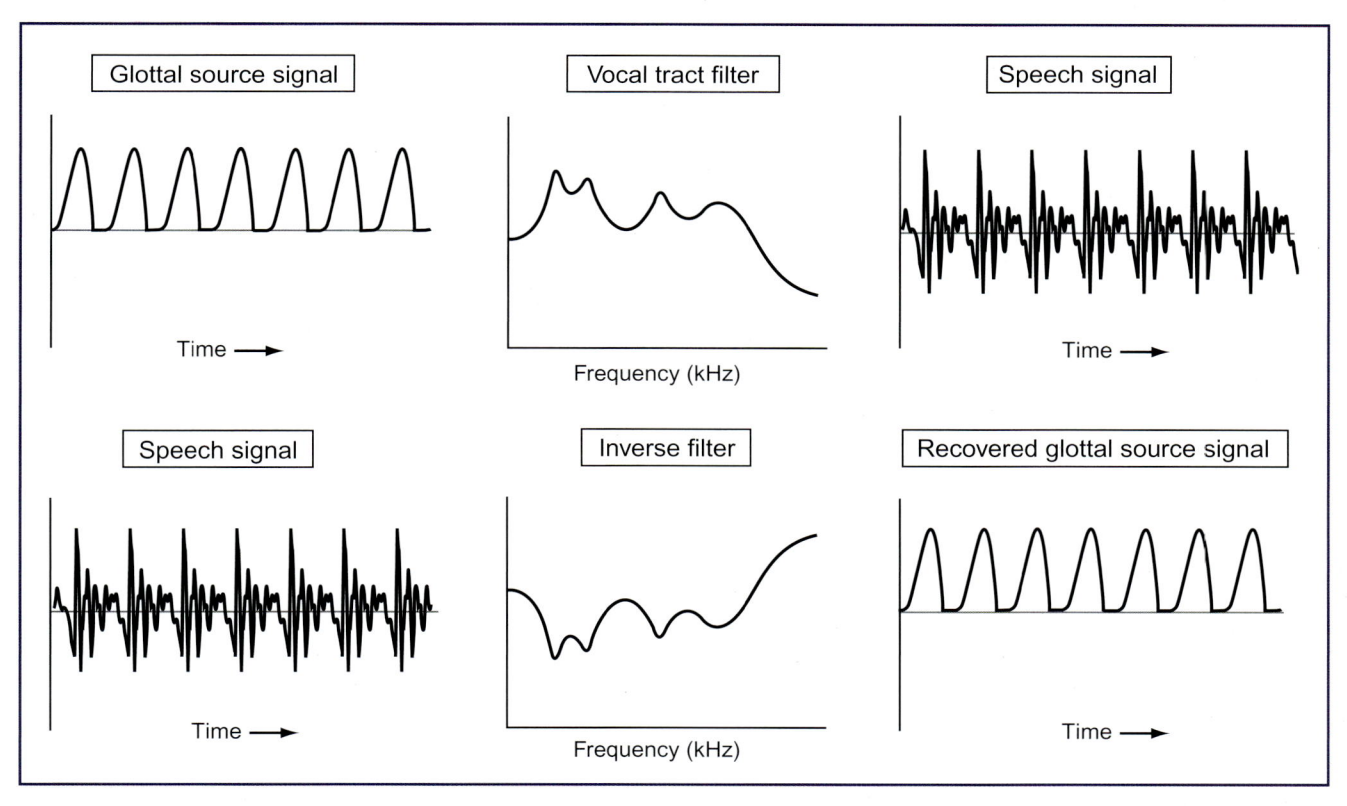

Figure 8–3. Schematic representation of steps in the inverse filtering process. *Top row of panels:* Glottal source signal serves as input to a multipeaked filter function associated with a vocal tract configuration and results in an output which is the speech signal recorded at the lips. This speech signal is a blend of the source signal and the filter characteristics. The three-panel sequence summarizes the source-filter theory of vowel acoustics. *Bottom row of panels:* The output signal shown in the top right waveform now serves as the input to an "inverse filter," which is the "flipped" or mirror image of the filter function in the middle of the top row of panels. The inverse filter inverts the peaks shown in the top filter function and subtracts the resonances from the input signal. The result of the process is the recovered glottal source signal shown in the bottom right panel. Figure provided courtesy of James Hillenbrand, PhD, Western Michigan University, Kalamazoo, Michigan. Reproduced with permission.

Chapter 7 suggests that the signal is a complex periodic waveform. Determination of the frequency components of a complex periodic waveform requires analysis of source acoustics in the frequency domain.

The Frequency Domain

The $\dot{V}g$ signal shown in Figure 8–4A can be submitted to Fourier analysis to identify the frequency components contributing to this source waveform. A typical spectrum resulting from Fourier analysis is shown in Figure 8–4B. The important features of this spectrum are: (a) the series of frequency components at consecutive-integer multiples of the lowest-frequency component; and (b) the relative amplitudes of the frequency components that decrease systematically as frequency increases. This is the *glottal source spectrum*.

The lowest frequency of the glottal source spectrum is the fundamental frequency (F0), which corresponds to the rate of vibration of the vocal folds. The F0 is also called the *first harmonic* (H1) of the source spectrum. The other frequency components in the glottal source spectrum are whole-number multiples of the F0. There is a component at two times the F0 (the second harmonic, H2), three times the F0 (the third harmonic, H3), four times the F0 (the fourth harmonic, H4), and so on. In theory the number of harmonics in the glottal source spectrum is infinite, but the progressive reduction in relative amplitude with increasing frequency greatly limits the significance of very high frequency harmonics.

The reduction of energy (relative amplitude) in the harmonic components of the glottal source spectrum as frequency increases is clearly seen in Figure 8–4B. Moving from left (lower frequency) to right (higher frequency) on the *x*-axis, the vertical lines showing the

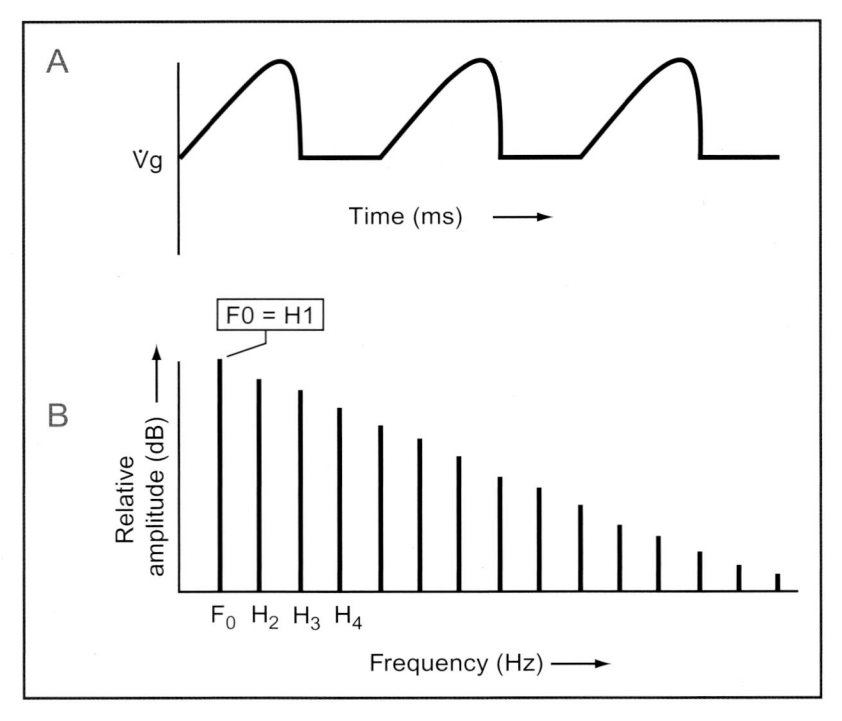

Figure 8–4. Time-domain (**A**) and frequency-domain (**B**) representations of acoustics resulting from vocal fold vibration. The time domain is represented by the glottal airflow waveform ($\dot{V}g$). The frequency domain is represented by the glottal spectrum resulting from vocal fold vibration and indicates F0, the fundamental frequency (first harmonic), and H2, H3, and H4 (the second, third, and fourth harmonics, respectively). The harmonics above H4 (arbitrarily chosen as the last-labeled harmonic on the graph) continue to be whole-number multiples of the F0.

amplitude of the components become progressively shorter. This energy reduction is systematic, with the relative amplitude decreasing 6 to 12 dB for each octave increase in frequency. This gives the typical glottal spectrum a distinctly "tilted" appearance. As discussed below, changes in the mode of vocal fold vibration affect the extent to which the glottal spectrum is "tilted."

In the summary of the time-domain characteristics of the glottal source, three major characteristics were identified, including: (a) the periodic nature of the waveform, (b) the shape of the waveform, and (c) the ratio of open to closed time. Discussion turns now to how each of these features affects the glottal source spectrum.

The Periodic Nature of the Waveform

The $\dot{V}g$ waveform repeats over time, is not sinusoidal, and is, therefore, a complex periodic event. The repetition of the $\dot{V}g$ waveform is not perfectly periodic, but rather has very small variations in the periods of successive glottal cycles. Vocal fold vibration is therefore referred to as *quasi-periodic*. Throughout this discussion, the term "period" refers to the average period—the small, period-to-period variations are not considered further here. The period of the glottal waveform depends on the rate of vibration of the vocal folds, which varies according to a number of factors, including sex and age (see Chapter 3). Figure 8–5 shows two $\dot{V}g$ waveforms (left part of figure) having different periods, and their associated glottal spectra (right part of figure). Note that both waveforms show the $\dot{V}g$ over a 40-ms interval. The top waveform has a period of 8 ms (typical of many adult males), the inverse of which is an F0 of 125 Hz. This 125 Hz F0 is shown as the lowest-frequency component in the glottal spectrum to the right of the waveform. The bottom waveform has a period of 5 ms (typical of many adult females), the inverse of which is an F0 of 200 Hz. This F0 is shown as the lowest-frequency component in the corresponding glottal spectrum. The harmonics of the female glottal spectrum (bottom) are more widely separated than the harmonics of the male glottal spectrum (top). This

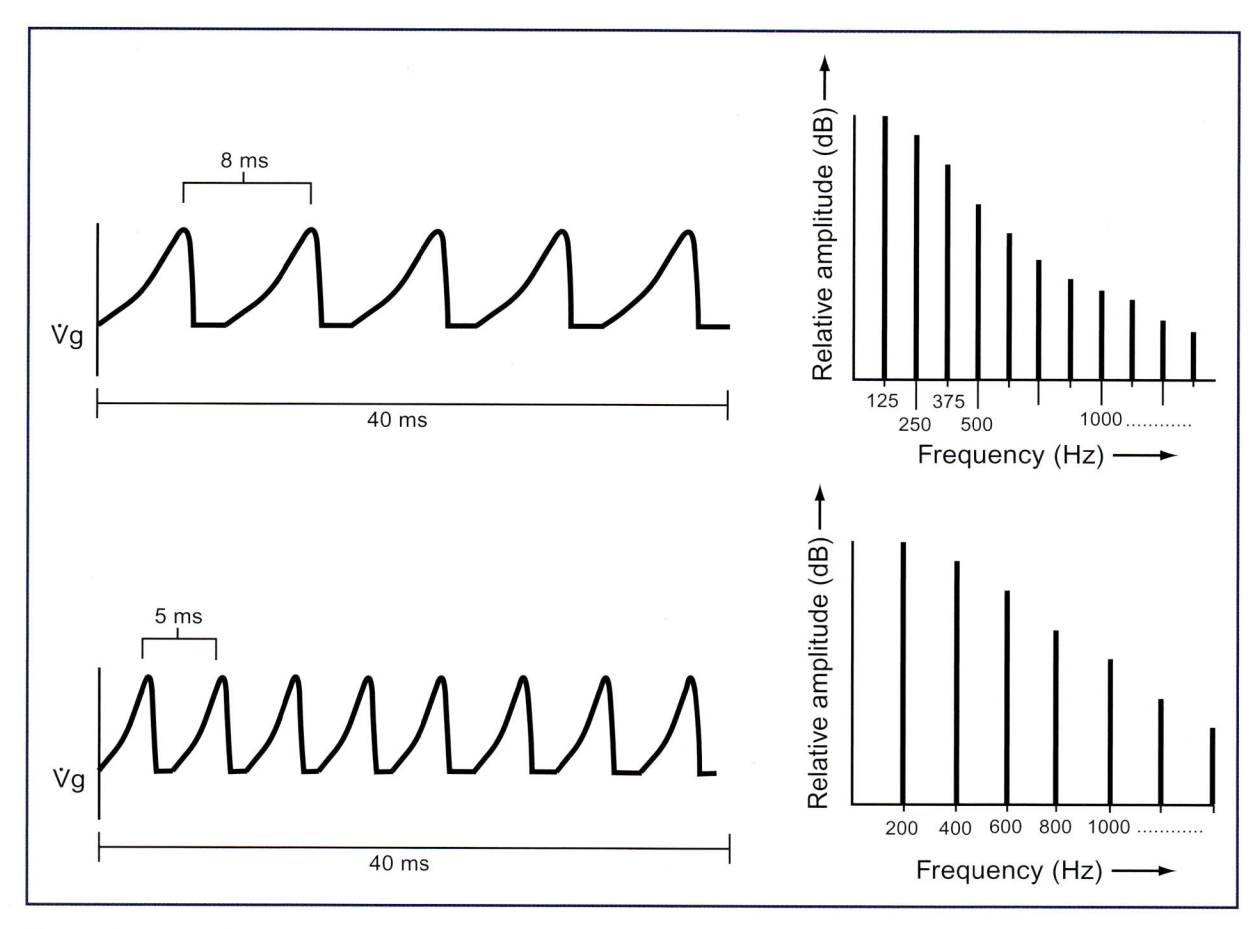

Figure 8–5. Two V̇g waveforms having different periods, and their associated glottal spectra. *Top:* period = 8 ms, F0 = 125 Hz. *Bottom:* period = 5 ms, F0 = 200 Hz. Both waveforms show V̇g over a 40-ms interval. Note the greater number of cycles within this interval for the F0 = 200-Hz waveform (*lower waveform*), compared with the F0 = 125-Hz waveform (*upper*). Note wider spacing of harmonics in the glottal spectrum where F0 = 200 Hz (*bottom*) compared with F0 = 125 Hz (*top*).

follows from the fact that the glottal spectrum consists of a consecutive integer series of harmonics: higher F0s yield greater spacing between successive harmonics compared with lower F0s. The glottal spectra of speakers with low F0s are more densely packed with harmonics compared with the glottal spectra of speakers with high F0s. This difference between the glottal spectra of low versus high F0s explains, in part, why spectrographic analysis of vowels produced by adult males tends to be easier than spectrographic analysis of vowels produced by adult females and children (see Chapter 10).

The Shape of the Waveform

The opening and closing parts of the V̇g waveform create a shape that appears to be "leaning to the right," and the steepness of the closing slope reflects how rapidly the vocal folds return to the midline for each cycle. There is a systematic relationship between this closing slope and the "tilt" of the glottal spectrum: the steeper the closing slope in the V̇g waveform (the faster the vocal folds return to the midline on each cycle), the less tilted the glottal spectrum. This relationship is exemplified in Figure 8–6, where the V̇g waveform on the left has a steeper closing slope than the V̇g waveform on the right (see arrows indicating slopes on the closing part of the waveforms). *CP* in Figure 8–6 is the closed phase of the glottal cycle, or the portion of each cycle when the vocal folds are fully approximated, whereas *OP* stands for open phase. Note the spectra associated with these two glottal waveforms. The glottal spectrum for the waveform with the relatively steep closing slope shows progressive reduction in relative amplitude with increasing frequency, but not nearly as dramatically as the glottal spectrum for the waveform with the shal-

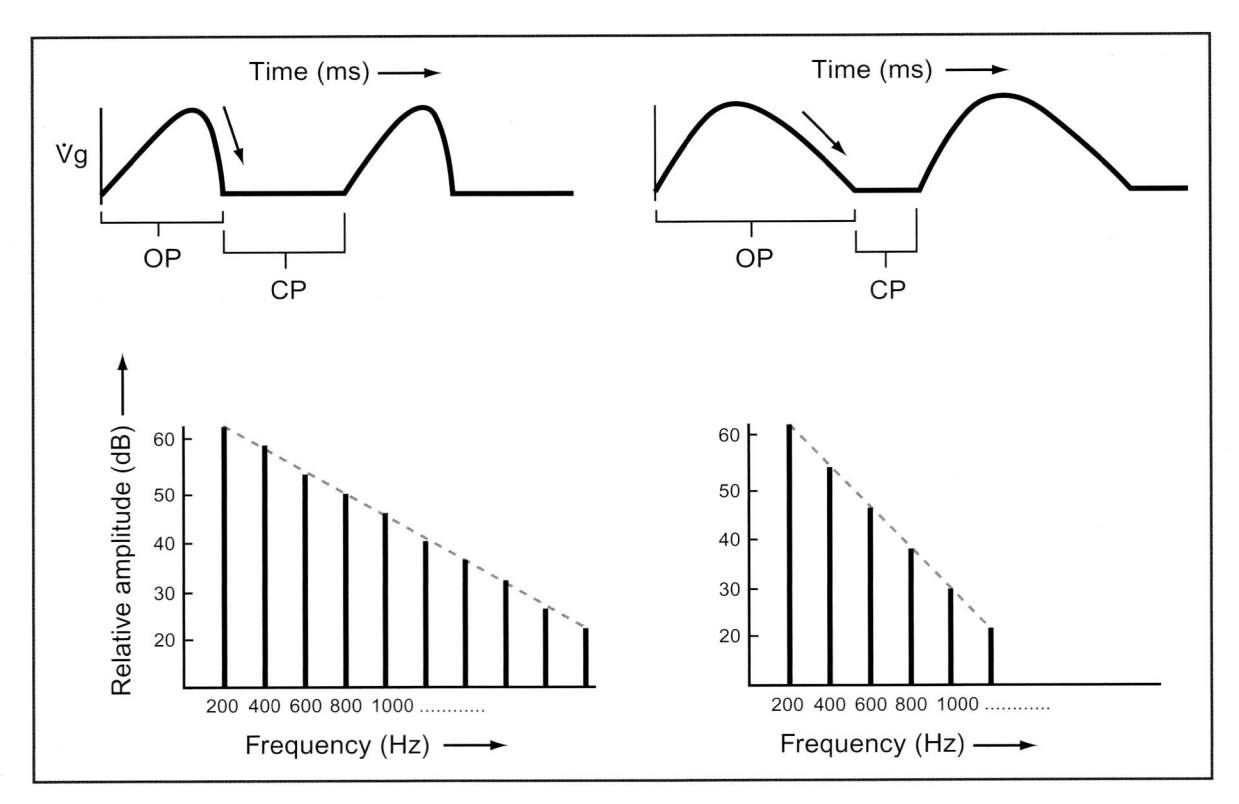

Figure 8-6. Schematic illustration of the speed of vocal fold closing and tilt of the glottal spectrum. The two upper panels show V̇g waveforms, one with relatively rapid closing of the vocal folds (*left*), and one with relatively slow closing of the vocal folds (*right*). Relative speeds of closure are portrayed by the slope of the arrows alongside the closing phase of the functions. The glottal spectra immediately below the two waveforms demonstrate how speed of closure affects the tilt of the spectrum. CP = closed phase (time). OP = open phase (time).

lower closing slope. The dashed line connecting the tops of the vertical lines in the two spectra shows the rapid reduction in energy across frequency when the closing slope in the time domain is shallow (right-hand part of figure) compared with when it is steep (left-hand part of figure). The spectrum with the dramatic reduction in harmonic energy is more tilted than the spectrum with the more gradual reduction in energy. In theory, a glottal spectrum with "no tilt" would be one in which the relative amplitudes of all harmonic components were equal (the dashed line connecting the tops of the vertical lines would be strictly horizontal), and a glottal spectrum with "infinite tilt" would be one in which there was energy at the first harmonic (F0), but at no other frequencies.

Another way to express the concept of tilt of the glottal spectrum is to have a reference value of 8 dB per octave (midway in the range of 6–12 dB per octave given above) as the typical reduction in harmonic amplitude across frequency. V̇g waveforms with very steep closing slopes (e.g., Figure 8–6, left panel) have a smaller dB change per octave (<8 dB per octave), and those with very shallow closing slopes have a larger dB change per octave (>8 dB per octave).

These concepts are important in understanding the physiological and acoustical bases of *hyperfunctional* and *hypofunctional* voice disorders. In hyperfunctional voice disorders, the vocal folds move together too rapidly and forcefully on each closing phase of vocal fold vibration, resulting in a glottal spectrum with less than normal tilt, or too much energy in the higher-frequency harmonics. Listeners interpret the voice quality associated with reduced tilt of the glottal spectrum as abnormal, sometimes using the term *pressed voice* to describe what they hear. A pressed voice sounds overly effortful or strained. In hypofunctional voice disorders, the vocal folds move together more slowly and less forcefully, the result being a highly tilted glottal spectrum because there is so little energy in the higher-frequency harmonics. The quality of a voice with greater than normal tilt is often heard by listeners as weak, breathy, and thin.

> ### Imperfect Perfection
>
> The quasi-periodic nature of vocal fold vibration is largely a result of subtle aeromechanical imperfections. Vocal fold vibration is driven by aerodynamic forces and sustained by mechanical ones. These forces do not repeat themselves across successive cycles with absolute precision. If the forces do not repeat themselves exactly, the thing they are forcing—vibration of the vocal folds—does not either. In early versions of talking computers (speech synthesizers), scientists used a perfectly periodic, complex tone to simulate the source for vowels. Listeners didn't like it. It sounded mechanical, robotic, unfriendly. The solution was to take this complex periodic waveform and introduce into it a small amount of "jitter," or very minimal variation in the cycle-to-cycle period. Listeners found this much more pleasing. More human, you could say.

The Ratio of Open Time to Closed Time

For each cycle in a typical $\dot{V}g$ waveform, the vocal folds are apart about 60% of the time, and approximated about 40% of the time. The two waveforms in Figure 8–6 show that a waveform with a shallower (slower) closing phase is also likely to have more open time throughout a complete cycle. Similarly, a waveform with a steeper (faster) closing phase is likely to have less open time and, therefore, a longer closed phase throughout a complete cycle. Because the speed of closing is often correlated with the open time or closed time (greater speed, less open time; less speed, more open time), less open time is generally associated with a less tilted glottal spectrum, and more open time with a more tilted glottal spectrum. The closing speed and ratio of open phase to closed phase (OP/CP) are somewhat redundant descriptions of $\dot{V}g$ waveforms (and spectral characteristics).

Nature of the Input Signal: A Summary

To answer the first question posed at the outset of this chapter, the input signal generated by the vibrating vocal folds is a complex periodic waveform whose spectrum consists of a consecutive integer series of harmonics at whole-number multiples of the F0. The harmonics in the glottal spectrum systematically decrease in relative amplitude with increasing frequency. These harmonics serve as input to the vocal tract resonator, which shapes that input according to its resonant characteristics. Consideration turns now to the vocal tract resonator.

WHY SHOULD THE VOCAL TRACT BE CONCEPTUALIZED AS A TUBE CLOSED AT ONE END?

The vocal tract is an acoustic resonator. In Chapter 7, two general classes of acoustic resonators—Helmholtz and tube—are described. For the present discussion, accept on faith that the vocal tract is a tube resonator (The bend in the vocal tract is not acoustically relevant). It is easy to provide the proof of the tube-resonance characteristics of the vocal tract, as shown in a later section of this chapter. One obvious proof is the relationship between tube length and tube resonances: shorter tubes have higher resonant frequencies than longer tubes. This is consistent with the higher resonant frequencies of children's vocal tracts compared with longer vocal tracts and lower resonant frequencies of either men or women. For the same reason, women have higher resonant frequencies than men. Comparison of vowel resonant frequencies for men, women, and children is presented in Chapter 11.

If the vocal tract is regarded as a tube resonator, the question must be asked, "Does it resonate as a tube open at both ends, or closed at one end?" The answer to this question requires a brief reconsideration of the vibrating vocal folds, and how this vibration influences the acoustic output of the vocal tract.

Figure 8–7 shows two signals in the time domain, collected synchronously during phonation of a vowel. The upper signal is $\dot{V}g$, discussed above at some length. The upper-pointing arrows mark the instant in time at which the vocal folds snap together during each cycle of vibration. At these instants, when the airflow through the glottis is suddenly blocked by closure of the airway, the air immediately above the vocal folds becomes compressed and initiates a pressure wave through the vocal tract. Now, consider the situation just described. At the vocal fold boundary of the vocal tract, there is, for an instant, no airflow and the air molecules become compressed, whereas at the open, oral boundary of the vocal tract air molecules move freely between the lips. This appears very much like the aeromechanical conditions found in a resonating tube closed at one end, where pressure is maximum at the closed end and flow is maximum at the open end (see Chapter 7). Each time the vocal folds snap together, a pressure wave is set up in the vocal tract and obeys the rules of resonance in a tube closed at one end. Another way to say this is

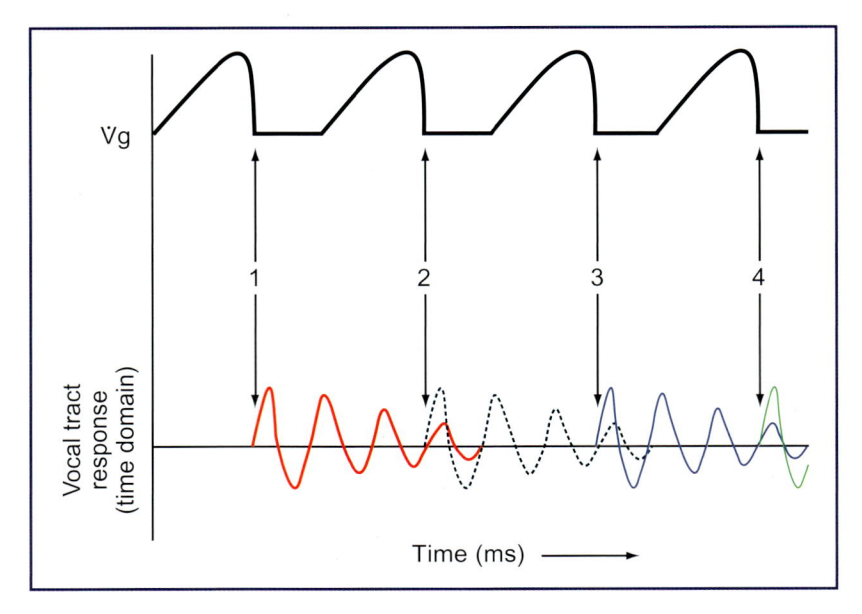

Figure 8–7. Schematic waveforms showing excitation of a vocal tract resonance (*bottom waveform*) by the vibrating vocal folds (*top waveform*). The top waveform, V̇g, shows four periods, with the instant of closing for each cycle marked by an upward-pointing arrow. The waveform of the vocal tract response shows a damped vibration at a resonant frequency of 500 Hz. This vibration is initiated each time the vocal folds snap shut, as indicated by the downward-pointing arrows. The amplitude of the damped vocal tract resonance decays over time. The damped resonator vibration from one vocal fold excitation overlaps with each new excitation of the resonance. The overlap of damped resonator vibration from each excitation causes the resonator response to sum, consistent with the superposition principle described in Chapter 7. All vocal tract resonances, according to the quarter-wavelength rule, are excited by the closing of the vocal folds, but only a single resonance waveform (for 500 Hz) is shown for the sake of clarity.

that the vocal tract resonances are *excited* each time the vibrating vocal folds snap together. Because the excitation occurs when the folds approximate and the oral end of the vocal tract is open for vowel production, the vocal tract resonates like a tube closed at one end.

In Chapter 7, a model of resonance was described in which a hammer tapped a resonator, thus exciting the resonant frequency (Helmholtz resonator) or frequencies (tube resonator). Imagine the hammer being controlled by a periodic motor, rotating it toward the resonator and striking it, then pulling back away, rotating it back toward the resonator and striking it again, and so forth. The continuous motion of the hammer back and forth, toward and away from the resonator, is important to producing the excitation of the resonator, but the actual *instant* of excitation of the resonator corresponds to the point in time when the hammer strikes the resonator. The analogy to excitation of the vocal tract resonances is fairly direct. The motion of the vibrating vocal folds (the swing of the hammer) is important to the resonance of the vocal tract, but the actual excitation of the resonances occurs only at the instant in time of vocal fold approximation.[1]

The Response of the Vocal Tract to Excitation

What does it mean to say that the vocal tract resonances are *excited* each time the vibrating vocal folds snap together? The answer is found in the bottom trace of Figure 8–7, where a waveform is initiated each time

---

[1] This is a simplified description of vocal tract excitation by the vibrating vocal folds. Other, weaker sound sources may be associated with different phases of each vocal fold cycle, and may provide excitation of the vocal tract resonances.

> ### Of Beer Bottles and Vocal Tracts
>
> When the vocal tract is excited by the sudden "snapping shut" of the vocal folds, the source excitation has the form of a glottal spectrum. A series of such excitations, such as the 190 or so per second expected for an adult female, gives the excitation spectrum its "nice" form of discrete harmonics. This harmonic spectrum is shaped by the vocal tract filter. A historical footnote in speech acoustics was the idea that the excitation of the vocal tract was like the edge tones described in the Chapter 7 sidetrack titled "Beer and Flutes." In this view, the resonant chambers of the vocal tract are excited by the individual puffs of air coming through the vocal folds during each cycle of vibration. The air puffs "force" air in the vocal tract into resonance, much like blowing across the opening of a beer bottle forces the air inside the bottle to produce a tone. This was called the "inharmonic theory" of vocal tract acoustics; it is not correct. The correct view is called the "harmonic theory," for obvious reasons. The vocal tract shapes an acoustic source spectrum according to its resonant properties, rather than having its resonant frequencies "forced" into vibration by an aerodynamic event such as the air puff.

the vocal folds snap together. For purposes of simplification, a waveform for only a single resonant frequency is shown in the bottom signal of Figure 8–7, but waveforms are initiated for each resonant frequency of the tube. Think of the vocal tract response waveform shown in Figure 8–7 as corresponding to the first resonance of the tube, with a frequency of 500 Hz. The period of that waveform is 2 ms (500 = 1/T, T = .002 s or 2 ms). Note how the resonance waveform responding to the first excitation is initiated with relatively great amplitude, which declines over each successive cycle until the vibration dies out completely (red waveform). In the example of Figure 8–7 note also that the resonance is *re*-excited before the previous waveform dies out completely (compare the amplitudes of the vocal tract response from excitation 1 (red waveform) and excitation 2 (black, dashed-line waveform). The large, 500-Hz vocal tract vibration at excitation 2 overlaps the small (decaying) vibration from excitation 1. Similar "re-excitations" are shown at excitations 3 (blue waveform) and 4 (green waveform). If Figure 8–7 showed the waveforms of all the excited and re-excited resonances, the vocal tract response signal would be visually too "busy" to illustrate the main point of this discussion, which is that the vocal tract responds to excitation with damped oscillations at each of its resonant frequencies. The oscillations are damped because there is energy loss in the vocal tract due to the factors discussed in Chapter 7 (friction, absorption, and radiation).

To this point, emphasis has been placed on the time-domain characteristics of the source signal and the response of the vocal tract. The focus now turns to the question of how the vocal tract resonances shape the input signal to produce an acoustic output at the lips. Stated more simply: "What is the acoustic basis of the events known as vowel sounds?" The best approach to this problem is to consider the source signal and vocal tract resonances in frequency-domain terms.

How Are the Acoustic Properties of the Vocal Tract Determined?

As discussed in Chapter 7, acoustic resonators can be described in the frequency domain by a resonance curve (see Figure 7–18). The peak of the resonance curve defines the resonant frequency of the resonator, and the width of the curve between the 3-dB-down points—the bandwidth—provides an index of the amount of energy loss in the vibration. Assume, for this discussion, a vocal tract shape associated with schwa (/ə/), a shape very much like a tube having uniform cross-sectional area from the glottis to the lips. This shape is like that of the straight tubes considered in Chapter 7, for which there are no constrictions, or narrowings, along the length of the tube. With knowledge of the length of the tube and its one closed end, the quarter-wavelength rule can be applied to obtain the multiple peaks of the resonance curve—that is, the resonant frequencies of the tube. The shapes of the resonance curves (determined by the bandwidths) are also important, so some additional calculations are necessary to arrive at a full resonance curve for the vocal tract tube.

If the mathematical tools are available to determine the bandwidths of the multiple resonances, the resonance curve for a vocal tract tube 15 cm in length and shaped for the vowel schwa looks something like the one shown in Figure 8–8. As expected, the lowest (first) resonant frequency is at $c/4l$ = 560 Hz (where c = 33,600 cm/s and l = 15 cm), the second resonance at 1680 Hz (3 × 560), and the third at 2800 Hz (5 × 560). Although the vocal tract tube has, like any other tube, an infinite number of resonances, only the first three are shown for the sake of clarity (as well as for other reasons that will become apparent as this discussion proceeds).

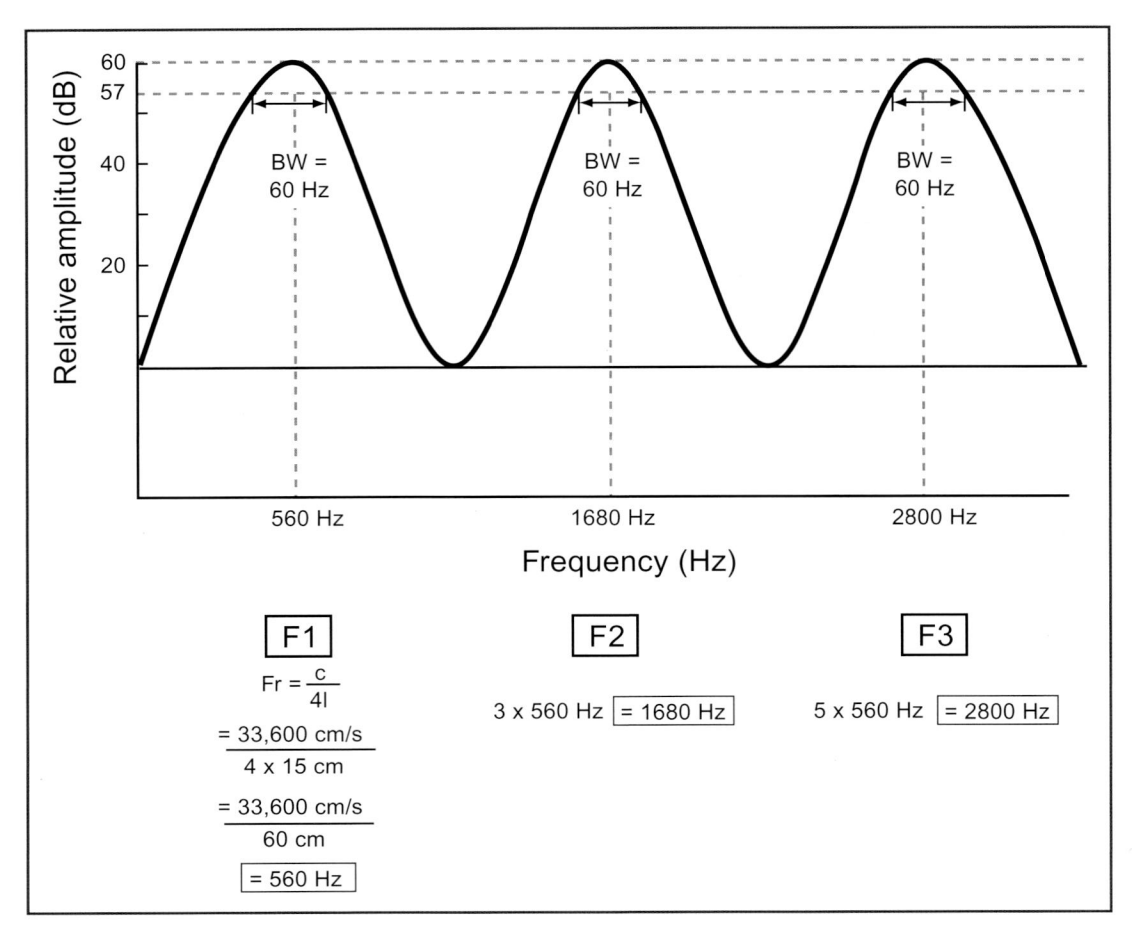

Figure 8–8. Resonance curve for a vocal tract tube in the shape of the schwa /ə/ and having a length of 15 cm. The resonant frequencies along the curve are computed by the quarter-wavelength rule, and the bandwidth of each resonance is assumed to be 60 Hz. Only the first three resonances of the tube are shown.

The bandwidths are indicated for each peak of the resonance curve by the range of frequencies between the 3-dB-down points. For the present discussion, the bandwidths for each of the three resonances have been set to 60 Hz.

The example in Figure 8–8 was generated using simple principles established in Chapter 7 (the quarter-wavelength rule), as well as an "on faith" assumption about bandwidths. Fant (1960) needed a more comprehensive theory, however, because for most vowels the vocal tract tube does not have a uniform cross-sectional area from the glottis to the lips. Rather, *vocal tract configurations* typically involve constrictions along the path from glottis to lips, some of which are relatively tight.

Fant approached the problem of drawing the resonance curves for different vocal tract shapes in the following way. He took sagittal x-ray pictures of an adult male speaker's productions of a variety of Russian and Swedish vowels. The soft and hard tissues of the speaker's vocal tract (tongue, lips, hard palate, velum, part of the pharynx) were coated with barium paste, which allowed easier identification of the outlines of structures in the developed film. Figure 8–9 shows a magnetic resonance image (MRI) of a speaker producing a high back rounded vowel, with the boundaries of the air tube outlined and the air tube itself slightly shaded (note the constriction produced by the tongue, as well as by the rounded lips). The outlined, shaded tube includes boundaries defined by the walls of the larynx superior to the vocal folds, the pharynx, hard palate, velum, tongue, lips, and other surfaces. Although Figure 8–9 is an image type much more advanced than the standard x-ray images used by Fant, his approach can be explained just as effectively using the MRI example. Fant used the x-rays he obtained for many different vowels to outline the varied vocal tract shapes. When

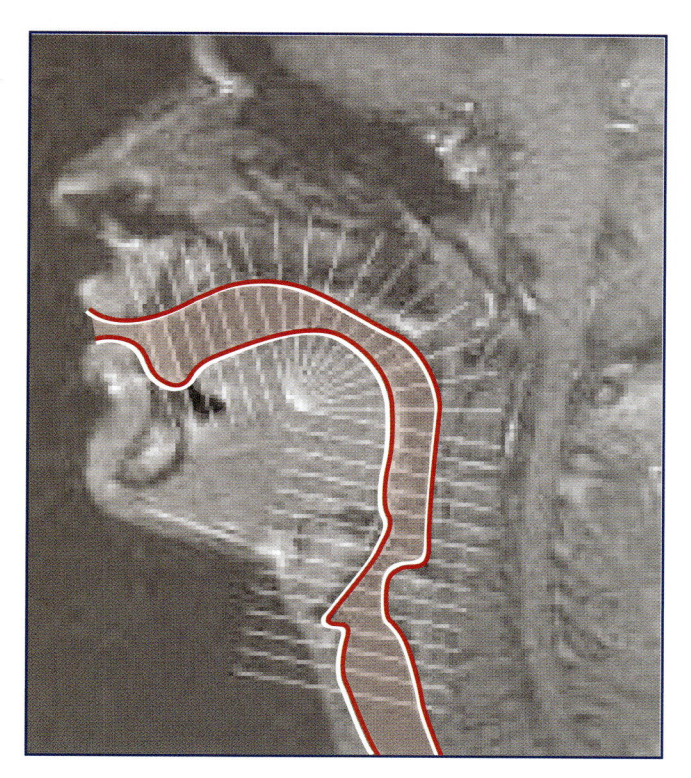

Figure 8–9. Sagittal magnetic resonance image (MRI) of a male speaker producing a vocal tract configuration for the vowel /u/. Boundaries of the vocal tract are outlined to show the shape of the vocal tract tube and how its dimensions vary from glottis to lips. Background image obtained from the Audiovisual-to-articulatory SPeech Inversion (ASPI) project. Retrieved September 2, 2012, from http://aspi.loria.fr. Reproduced with permission.

the structures are outlined in this way, the column of air extending from the glottis to the lips can be conceptualized as a tube of varying cross-sectional area.

The vocal tract length of the speaker studied by Fant (1960) was approximately 17.5 cm. Fant plotted the varying cross-sectional area of the vocal tract by estimating the area of the air tube at 0.5-cm increments from glottis to lips. This "sectioning off" of the vocal tract is shown in Figure 8–9 by the sequence of straight lines drawn through the vocal tract tube. If a line is imagined running straight forward from the glottis to the lips, along the long axis of the vocal tract, each of the straight lines seen in Figure 8–9 intersects this long axis line at a right angle. The length of the intersecting line within the vocal tract—between the red outline in Figure 8–9—defines the "size" of the vocal tract tube at that location. The distance between adjacent lines defines a small section, or "tubelette" within the vocal tract (Story, 2005), for which width measurements can be made. For example, the tubelettes are quite narrow toward the back of the oral cavity, where the tongue is raised toward the boundary of the hard and soft palates. The tubelettes are much wider toward the front of the vocal tract. Fant sectioned his vocal tract images into 35 "pieces" (2 measurements per cm of vocal tract, 2 × 17.5 = 35). The width of each of these section lines was measured and entered into a simple formula to compute the area for that slice of the vocal tract. What emerged from this exercise was an *area function of the vocal tract*.

Area Function of the Vocal Tract

An area function of the vocal tract is a plot of cross-sectional area as a function of distance along the vocal tract from glottis to lips. This distance is described by the succession of the measurement "slices" shown in Figure 8–9. Figure 8–10 shows an area function for the vowel /i/. Area, in cm^2, is plotted on the y-axis and section (slice) number (i.e., distance) is plotted on the x-axis. The low section numbers are near the glottis (i.e., section 1 is immediately above the glottis), and the measurement of section areas moves toward the lips from left to right. Each section number has an area value, so the function is actually a sequence of discrete points. For illustration purposes, the discrete points have been connected and the area function is represented in Figure 8–10 as a continuous line. This is justified because the measurements of successive slices were sufficiently close (in 0.5-cm increments) to minimize the likelihood of major changes in cross-sectional vocal tract area between the measurement steps.

The area function in Figure 8–10 shows relatively large cross-sectional areas in the lower and upper pharyngeal regions (the left side of the x-axis), with relatively smaller areas toward the front of the vocal tract. Tight constrictions—that is, small cross-sectional areas—are present between sections 22 and 27. The entire area function is intuitively consistent with phonetic descriptions of the vowel /i/ as a high-front vowel, for which the major constriction is in the front of the vocal tract.[2] Area functions were measured by Fant for many different vowels.

Area functions are the link between the configuration of the vocal tract tube, as shaped by the oral and

---

[2]The relatively large areas in the back portion of the vocal tract may not be intuitive from a standard phonetic perspective, which typically classifies vowels according to: (a) the degree of tongue advancement, (b) the height of the tongue, and (c) the degree of lip rounding. There is evidence that pharyngeal dimensions, especially above the laryngeal vestibule, are predictable from the height and advancement of the tongue.

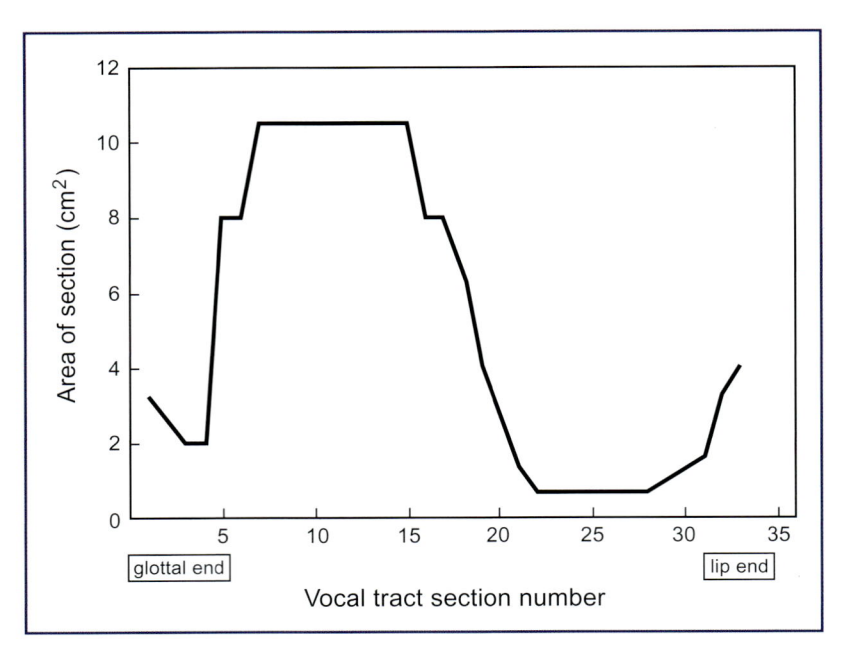

Figure 8-10. Area function for the vowel /i/ plotted from data reported by Fant (1960, p. 115). Vocal tract section number (from 1 to 35, with sections extending from the glottis to the lips) is plotted on the x-axis. Cross-sectional area (in cm²) is plotted on the y-axis.

pharyngeal structures, and the resonant frequencies of that tube. Fant (1960) developed a mathematical technique for estimating the tube resonances from the area function. The specifics of the mathematical technique are not covered here, but the conceptual link between the area function and estimation of vocal tract resonant frequencies is straightforward, and makes use of information developed in Chapter 7.

Chapter 7 described the role of mass and compliance in determining the resonant frequency of an acoustical resonator. Imagine that the air contained within the boundaries of any two adjacent measurement points in the vocal tract (that is, within a tubelette corresponding to the small air column between two measurement lines) has certain mass and compliance properties. If these properties are specified for each of the 35 sections of air, nearly all information relevant to the resonant frequencies of the vocal tract is available. Fant's mathematical theory allowed him to estimate mass and compliance properties from the area measurement for each section, or tubelette. Based on the mass and compliance estimates from *all* 35 sections, the theory produced an estimate of the resonant pattern for the entire vocal tract. When mathematical information concerning energy loss factors was included, Fant was able to draw the complete resonance curve (resonant frequencies and bandwidths as in Figure 8–8) for a given vocal tract configuration.

The conceptual basis of Fant's (1960) theory is, therefore, fairly simple. If the mass and compliance characteristics of the vocal tract tube can be determined, the resonance curve for the tube can be constructed. Because the vocal tract resonates like a tube, there are multiple peaks (i.e., resonances) along the resonance curve, each with its own bandwidth.

At this point in the development of Fant's (1960) theory, it is important to recognize that the vocal tract resonance curve is computed from the measured area function. The resonant peaks are determined mathematically, rather than measured by analyzing the spectrum of a produced vowel. For this reason the computed resonance curve is called a *theoretical spectrum*, or a *filter function*. This filter function shows where the resonances for this a given vocal tract configuration should be. The term *filter function* is particularly interesting, because it implies that the vocal tract acts like a filter, allowing energy to pass only at certain frequencies. It also implies that the filter function shows the frequencies at which energy does not pass. The regions of the spectrum where energy passes through, of course, are those regions at and in the immediate vicinity of the resonant peaks. The next section discusses the way in which the source spectrum and filter function (theoretical spectrum) are combined to produce an output spectrum—a measured spectrum, as for a phonated vowel. This discussion shows why the theoretical spectrum (the filter function) is not always precisely the same as the output spectrum (the spectrum of a produced vowel).

HOW DOES THE VOCAL TRACT SHAPE THE INPUT SIGNAL? (HOW IS THE SOURCE SPECTRUM COMBINED WITH THE THEORETICAL VOCAL TRACT SPECTRUM TO PRODUCE A VOCAL TRACT OUTPUT?)

The two questions heading this section are variants of the same problem, which is to determine how the acoustic characteristics of the source and vocal tract combine to produce a vocal tract output for a vowel. The frequency-domain representation of the vocal tract output is called an *output spectrum*. This is the spectrum measured, with appropriate instruments, from an actual vowel produced by a talker.

Figure 8–11 presents a simple graphic answer to the question posed above. The input (source) spectrum, as described in a preceding section, is shown at the left of the figure. The filter function is shown in the middle of the figure as a resonance curve with three peaks, corresponding to the first three resonances of a vocal tract tube in an /i/ shape. Note the multiplication sign between the input spectrum and filter function. To determine the output of the vocal tract (the right panel in Figure 8–11), the energy in the input spectrum is multiplied by the energy in the filter function.[3] To be a little more explicit about what this process of multiplication means, the axes of both the input (source) spectrum and the filter function are the same—frequency on the x-axis, relative amplitude on the y-axis (i.e., they are both spectra). The input spectrum shows the relative amplitude of discrete frequency components, and the filter function shows the frequencies at which energy applied to it will be "amplified" (the resonances) or "de-emphasized" (the valleys of the resonance curve, between the resonances). The multiplication described here is simply another way to understand the shaping of the input (source) spectrum by the filter function. The harmonics in the input (source) spectrum are shaped by the form of the filter function. At resonant frequencies of the filter function, energy in the input (source) spectrum is strongly multiplied, and appears in the output spectrum as prominent energy components. At valleys in the filter function, energy in the input (source) spectrum is multiplied weakly or not at

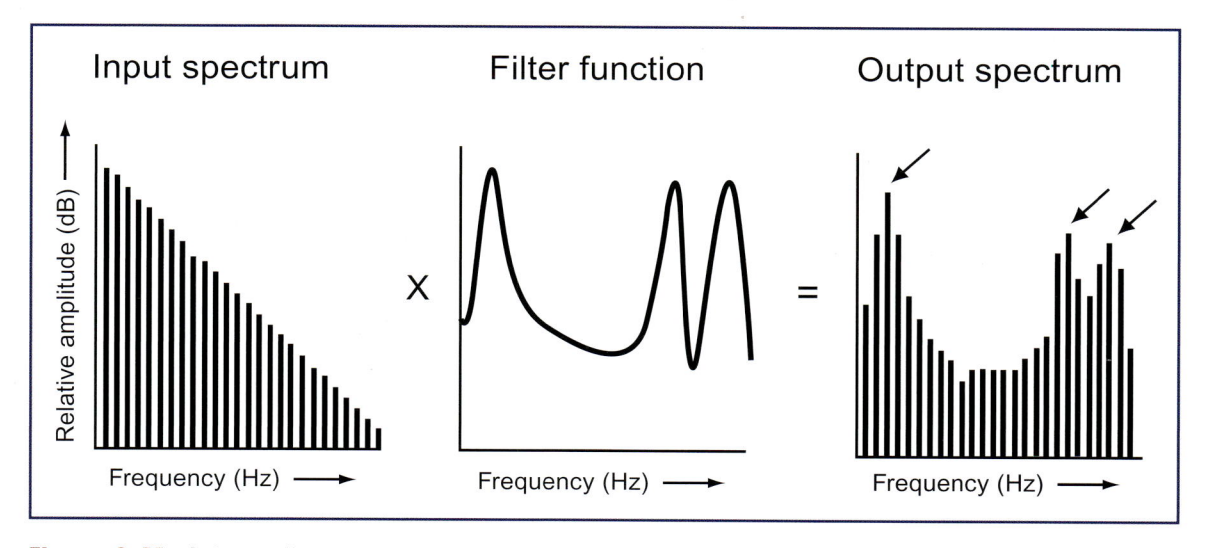

Figure 8–11. Schematic representation of how the source or input spectrum and filter function are combined to produce a vocal tract output. The left panel depicts the input spectrum, the middle panel the filter function for a vocal tract in an /i/ configuration, and the right panel the output spectrum. The output spectrum shows which harmonics are and are not emphasized by combining the input and filter functions. The peaks in the output spectrum are formants (F1, F2, F3) representing the first three resonant frequencies of the vocal tract.

---

[3] The idea of the source being multiplied by the energy in the filter function is somewhat of a simplification, but one that does not violate the essentials of the theory. In precise mathematical terms, the output of the vocal tract is determined by the convolution of source and filter energy. It is like a "blending" of the source and filter functions.

all, and does not appear (or appears only weakly) in the output spectrum.

The result of the multiplication of the input (source) spectrum by the filter function (equivalently, the shaping of the input [source] spectrum by the filter function) is indicated by the "=" sign shown in the output spectrum of Figure 8–11. The output spectrum shows the harmonics, now reshaped from their form in the input (source) spectrum. An important feature of the glottal source spectrum is the systematic decrease in harmonic amplitude as frequency increases, but in this output spectrum some of the higher-frequency harmonics have greater relative amplitude than some of the lower-frequency harmonics. This is because the shaping of the input (source) spectrum by the filter function emphasizes some higher-frequency harmonics while de-emphasizing some lower-frequency harmonics. The rise and fall of the harmonic amplitudes in the output spectrum of Figure 8–11 follow closely the locations of the resonances in the filter function. However, all peaks in the filter function were computed as having roughly equal amplitudes, but in the output spectrum the higher-frequency "peaks" (see arrows) have less amplitude than the lower-frequency peaks (note the decline in peak amplitude across the three peaks in the output spectrum). This is because the energy available in the input (source) spectrum decreases with increasing frequency, meaning there is less energy to multiply by the roughly equivalent peaks in the filter function. An output spectrum may show a general decrease in harmonic energy with increasing frequency, but in some cases higher-frequency harmonics have greater amplitude than lower-frequency harmonics.

The distinction between harmonics in the source (input) spectrum and peaks in the output spectrum can be confusing, so it is useful to pursue this description a little further. In the output spectrum of Figure 8–11, there is a series of harmonics whose amplitudes rise and fall according to peaks and valleys of the filter function. But there is no systematic relationship between the frequency locations of the harmonics in the source (input) spectrum and the peak frequencies of the filter function. The frequencies (harmonics) in the source (input) spectrum are determined by the rate of vibration of the vocal folds (the F0), and the frequencies of the peaks in the filter function are determined by the configuration of the vocal tract. In the acoustic theory of vowel production the source and filter are independent.[4] Two simple examples of the independence of the source and filter in the theory are as follows: (a) for a given speaker, the same vowel (produced by a single filter function) can be produced with many different F0s and, therefore, many different source spectra; and (b) for a given speaker, many different vowels can be produced with the same F0. Either the source or the filter can be adjusted without affecting characteristics of the other component.

A graphic example (Figure 8–12) illustrates the independence of the source and filter in the acoustic theory of vowel production. The example also highlights a distinction in the theory between *computed* (theoretical) *and measured* resonances. Figure 8–12 shows two graphs, both of which have a computed filter function with resonances at 300 Hz (0.3 kHz), 2300 Hz (2.3 kHz), and 3000 Hz (3.0 kHz). This filter function is a reasonable set of formant frequencies for an adult male production of /i/. Because the source spectrum and filter function are shown as spectra, they can be superimposed. The F0s of the two source spectra are slightly different (by 20 Hz) and so are the frequencies of the consecutive-integer series of harmonics. For example, for the F0 of 100 Hz there is a 3rd harmonic at 300 Hz, a 23rd harmonic at 2300 Hz, and a 30th harmonic at 3000 Hz. In this case, there is harmonic energy *exactly* at the location of the computed resonances of the filter function, as well as harmonic energy 100 Hz above and below these frequencies. The harmonic energy around

---

Hardheaded Speech Acoustics

First (Chapter 7) we used a hammer analogy for the excitation of resonators, then in the previous sidetrack we said that wasn't exactly the way the vocal tract was excited for speech; now we're going to say that the vocal tract *can* be excited "inharmonically," if you care to do so. Vowel-like vocal tract sounds can be produced by banging the skull (usually toward the front of the head, in the middle, with your knuckles) with the vocal tract open (flicking the neck with your fingers can produce roughly the same effect). Try this with your vocal tract in the shape of the vowel in "oh" and then "ee." You'll probably hear the difference, and most certainly a listener will. This is simply the case of the vocal tract being excited by a source different from the harmonic glottal spectrum. The vocal tract responds to these head thumps or finger flicks with damped oscillation of the resonant frequencies.

---

[4]This statement is true for the purposes of this textbook; it can be shown that there are some effects of the filter on the source under certain conditions, but these are beyond the scope of this text.

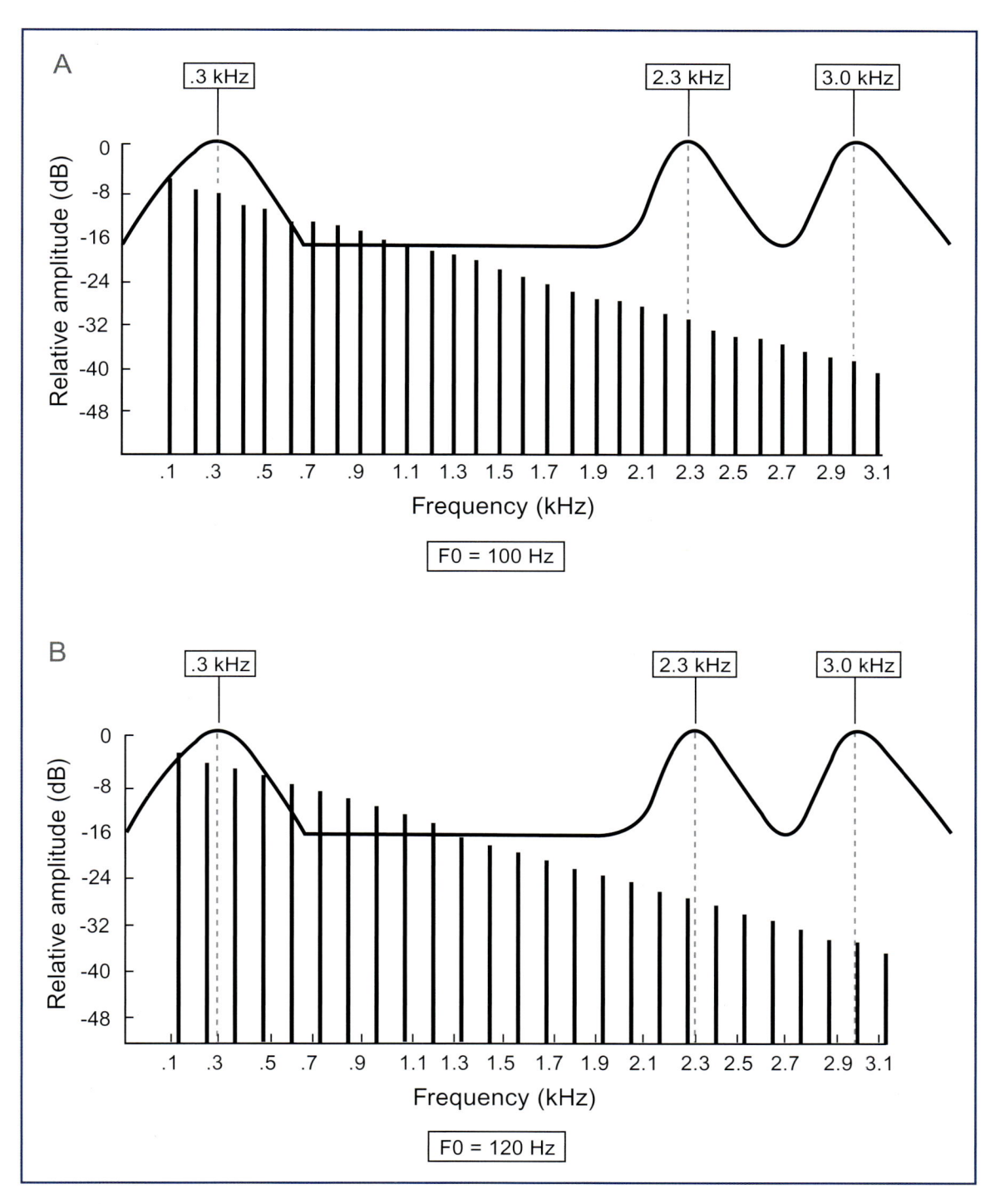

Figure 8-12. A single filter function (appropriate for the vowel /i/) superimposed on two source spectra having different fundamental frequencies and, therefore, different spacing between harmonics. In panels **A** and **B**, the filter function is superimposed on a source spectrum having an F0 = 100 Hz and 120 Hz, respectively. When F0 = 100 Hz, frequencies of the harmonics match the frequencies of the computed (theoretical) resonances of 300 Hz, 2300 Hz, and 3000 Hz. When F0 = 120 Hz, frequencies of the harmonics do not match the first and second resonances, but do match the third resonance (120 × 25 = 3000 Hz).

the peaks in this filter function, but especially exactly at the peaks, will contribute to emphasizing energy in the output spectrum in the immediate region of the computed peaks.

In fact, when the energy in this source spectrum is multiplied by the values along the filter functions, the peaks in the output spectrum are likely to coincide exactly with the computed (theoretical) peaks because there is harmonic energy precisely at the location of the computed peaks. This is the case for the superimposed source and filter characteristics in Figure 8–12A.

Now consider the case of the source spectrum and filter function in Figure 8–12B. Here the F0 of 120 Hz does *not* produce harmonics coinciding exactly with the computed peaks at 300 Hz and 2300 Hz, but the 25th harmonic matches the theoretical resonance at 3000 Hz. The 2nd and 3rd harmonics in this source spectrum are located at 240 and 360 Hz, values in the general neighborhood of the computed first resonance at 300 Hz, but not exactly so as in Figure 8–12A. Similarly, the 19th and 20th harmonics of 120 Hz are located at 2280 and 2400 Hz, values that do not coincide exactly with the computed second resonance of 2300 Hz. When the energy at these harmonic frequencies is multiplied by the values along the filter function, the general region around the first and second computed resonances is emphasized in the output spectrum, but the location of these peaks in the output spectrum may not coincide exactly with the theoretical peaks in the filter function.

Harmonics in the source spectrum are not *purposely* matched with the locations of the computed (theoretical) peaks of the filter function. They do not have to be matched in this manner, because the general region of resonance given by a computed peak is emphasized in either case (i.e., whether or not a harmonic is exactly located at a peak in the filter function). This discussion explains why the output peaks in the measured spectrum may not coincide exactly with the computed (theoretical) peaks in the filter function. A computed (filter function) and measured (output spectrum) peak are exactly the same only when a harmonic in the source spectrum has the same frequency as a *computed* resonance.

The general regions of resonance in the output spectrum have been emphasized in this discussion, rather than specific values of harmonics. In the output spectra—the kinds of spectra typically measured in the laboratory—these regions of high energy are called *formants*. Because the individual harmonics are not of great importance in vowel output spectra, vowel spectra are typically shown as smooth curves that trace an *envelope* along the varying harmonic amplitudes that result from the shaping of the source spectrum by the filter function. Figure 8–13 presents output spectra for the isolated vowels /i/ (top spectrum), /ɑ/ (middle spectrum), and /u/ (bottom spectrum), spoken by an adult male. These spectra show how a *spectral envelope* can be drawn by connecting the tops of the harmonic lines with a smooth curve. The harmonic spectra in

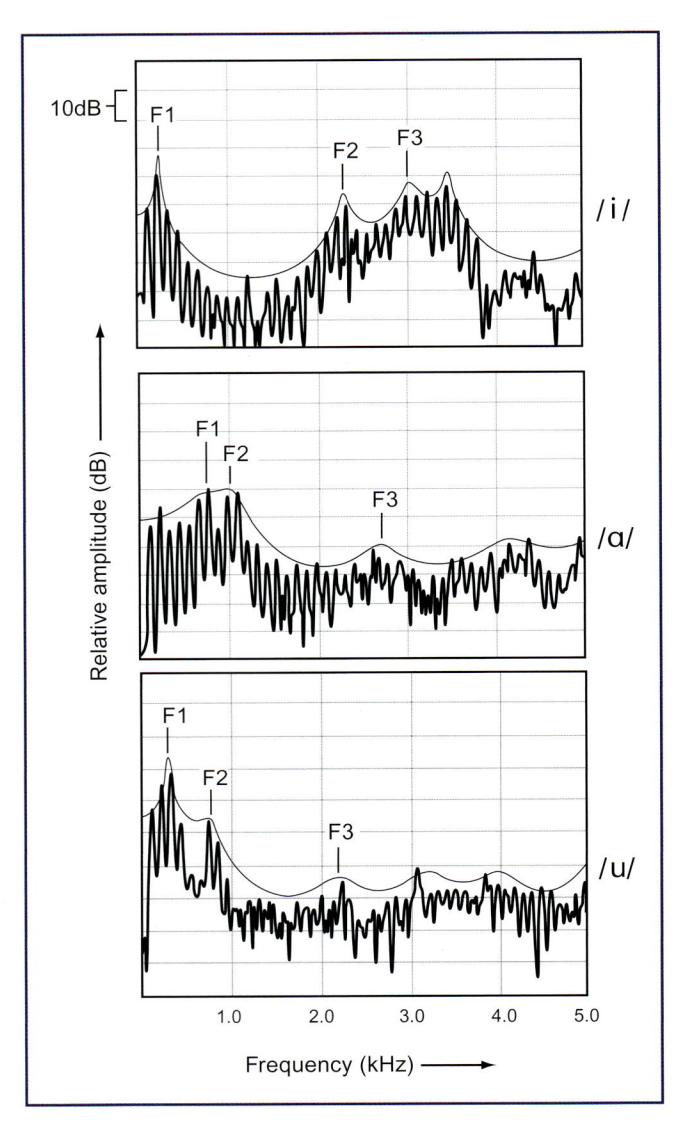

Figure 8–13. Output spectra for the vowels /i/ (*top panel*), /ɑ/ (*middle panel*), and /u/ (*bottom panel*), showing how the tops of the harmonics computed by Fourier analysis can be connected to draw a smooth curve, or spectral envelope, computed by linear predictive code (LPC) analysis. The peaks in the envelope are the formant frequencies, marked F1, F2, and F3 in each spectrum. Spectra are shown for the 0- to 5-kHz range. Each vertical division (*y*-axis, relative amplitude) is equal to 10 dB.

Figure 8–13 were generated with Fourier analysis, whereas the smooth, spectral envelopes superimposed on the tops of the harmonics were generated by linear predictive code (LPC) analysis, a digital algorithm that locates formant frequencies (discussed more fully in Chapter 10). Each spectral envelope shows three peaks, labeled *F1*, *F2*, and *F3* (F1 = first formant, F2 = second formant, F3 = third formant). The higher-frequency peaks typically have lower amplitude than the lower-frequency peaks, primarily because the energy in the source spectrum decreases with increasing frequency (see above). The relative amplitudes of peaks in the output spectrum do not seem to be particularly important for either the acoustic or perceptual specification of vowels, at least in natural speech (Kiefte & Kluender, 2005; but see Kiefte, Enright, & Marshall, 2010) so the frequency locations of the measured peaks—the formant frequencies—dominate the discussion of vowels.

A great deal of research reviewed in Chapter 11 demonstrates that the first three peaks in a vowel spectrum have great importance for the acoustic and perceptual specification of vowel identity. The frequency locations of these first three peaks is sometimes referred to as the *F-pattern* of a vowel. For example, the F-patterns of the vowels shown in Figure 8–13 are F1 = 237, F2 = 2283, and F3 = 3058 Hz for /i/, F1 = 775, F2 = 1012, F3 = 2713 Hz for /ɑ/, and F1 = 280, F2 = 732, and F3 = 2218 Hz for /u/ (measurements made by author GW). Although the F-pattern of a vowel is always stated in terms of these three frequencies, the exact frequency value attached to each of the formants does not mean that other frequencies in the vowel spectrum are unimportant in the acoustic and perceptual specification of vowels. It is better to think of these numbers as *center frequencies* denoting a region of *spectral prominence*. In the region of spectral prominence for each formant, there is a small range of frequencies that reflects the resonance characteristics of the vocal tract (recall the discussion of bandwidth in Chapter 7). The F-pattern is always stated with respect to the frequencies measured at the highest peaks in the output spectrum.

Formant Bandwidths

Chapter 7 presented a brief discussion of the factors responsible for energy loss in acoustic systems. These factors, which include friction, absorption, and radiation, are all operative in the vocal tract and contribute to the shape of the resonances (formants) in the output spectrum.

When air molecules vibrate within the vocal tract, they rub against each other and against soft and hard tissues. This friction generates heat, which dissipates a small amount of the vibratory energy. The vibration of the air molecules may also be taken up by nearby structures whose own resonant frequencies are close to the frequencies propagated through the vocal tract. For example, the cheeks and possibly the tongue appear to have resonant frequencies around 200 Hz, close to the typical first formant frequencies of several vowels (Fujimura & Lindquist, 1971). When a formant frequency is close to the resonant frequency of a structure such as the cheek, the tissue will absorb some of the energy and transform it into its own vibratory event. This absorption of acoustic energy by vocal tract structures is another form of energy loss and contributes to the damping of vocal tract resonances. Under certain conditions, such as when the nasal cavities are connected to the oral cavity because the velopharyngeal port is open, or the oral cavity is connected to the subglottal cavities (e.g., the trachea) because the vocal folds are abducted, the amount of energy loss may be greatly increased partly because there is more tissue to absorb sound energy. Thus, nasalized vowels tend to have greater formant bandwidths than non-nasalized vowels, and the bandwidth of the first formant is greater when a vowel is produced with breathy, compared with typical, phonation. Finally, the radiation of sound from the mouth results in some loss of energy as the sound changes environment from an enclosed tube (the vocal tract) to the open atmosphere. Megaphones are effective in transmitting sound over a great distance

---

All /i/'s and /u/'s Are Not Created Equal

As Fant proposed, formant frequencies completely specify vowels, but the more you look into the relationship between formant values and vowel identity, the more you realize this statement requires qualification. One such qualification has emerged from the recent trend in speech acoustics research comparing acoustic phonetic data between different languages. Although many different languages "share" certain vowels, such as /i/ and /u/, the formant frequencies often differ across the languages. How is it that the same vowel—at least one transcribed with the same phonetic symbol—has a different F-pattern in different languages? Think about it. We'll tell you more in Chapter 11.

partly because their gradually flared design decreases the radiation loss from the vocal tract to the atmosphere. The flare of the megaphone provides a gradual transition from the vocal tract shape to the "shape" of the atmosphere, reducing the amount of energy loss in the propagation of sound from the vocal tract to the atmosphere.

Table 8–1 (data from Fujimura & Lindqvist, 1971) contains some estimates of formant bandwidths and provides a rough range of the formant values associated with the bandwidths. The formant values are provided to support the statement that vowel resonances are relatively *sharply tuned*. In other words, the resonances in the spectrum have narrow bandwidths compared with the frequencies of those resonances. For example, bandwidths of 45 to 90 Hz are relatively narrow compared with typical F1 values, which range between 250 and 800 Hz, depending on the vowel. The bandwidths obtained by Fujimura and Lindqvist (1971) are very similar to recent formant bandwidth values of 50 to 90 Hz for each of the first three formants (Hanna, Smith, & Wolf, 2016).

How does bandwidth affect the acoustic categorization and perception of vowel sounds? Earlier it was noted that the F-pattern (the first three formant frequencies) seemed to be sufficient as an acoustic index of vowels. Information on formant amplitudes and bandwidths does not seem to be particularly useful for the acoustic categorization of vowels. When speech synthesizers systematically increase the bandwidth of vowel formants while maintaining constant formant frequencies, listeners do not hear a change in vowel category. Rather, vowels are perceived as increasingly "muffled" as bandwidths are increased. This "muffling" effect is sometimes heard in the speech of children and adults with craniofacial deficits and associated velopharyngeal insufficiency or incompetence. The perception of muffled vowels in these speakers may be explained, in part, by the increased bandwidths resulting from the undesired coupling of the oral and nasal cavities. Even though the increased "muffling" of vowel quality may not affect the perception of vowel categories, there may be an effect on general speech intelligibility and naturalness.

Acoustic Theory of Vowel Production: A Summary

Information presented to this point can be summarized as follows. First, the input, or source, for vowel production is the acoustic result of vocal fold vibration. This acoustic event can be described in the frequency domain as a series of consecutive integer harmonics whose energy decreases systematically with increasing frequency. The exact shape of the glottal spectrum depends on how rapidly the vocal folds snap together on each cycle of vibration. When the vocal folds snap together very quickly, the harmonic energy decreases relatively slowly with increasing frequency (less tilted spectrum). When the vocal folds move together slowly, the harmonic energy decreases relatively rapidly with frequency (more tilted spectrum).

The resonator in vowel acoustics is the vocal tract, which extends from the top margin of the vocal folds to the lips. The vocal tract resonates like a tube closed at one end, the closed end being the vocal folds, the open end being the lips. Vocal tract resonances are excited at the instant of closure for each cycle of vocal fold vibration. This excitation causes the vocal tract to respond with an infinite series of damped resonances.

A theory developed by Fant (1960) relates the area function of the vocal tract to the specific resonant frequencies of the tube. The area function is a plot of the cross-sectional area of the vocal tract from glottis to lips. The area function is a description of the shape of the air column formed by the articulators and the more or less fixed structures of the vocal tract (such as the posterior pharyngeal wall and hard palate). Using this shape to estimate the mass and compliance of consecutive sections of the air column, Fant calculated the resonant frequencies of differently shaped tubes (i.e., air columns). For current purposes, calculation of only the lowest three resonances is important. The resonance curve that results from these calculations shows the peaks at resonant frequencies, the bandwidths of those peaks, and the valleys between the peaks. This curve is called the filter function. At any frequency, the filter function shows how the energy at the corresponding frequency in the glottal spectrum is transferred by the vocal tract. At frequencies where there are peaks in the filter function, energy transfer is maximum, meaning that the energy appears prominently in the

Table 8–1. Approximate Bandwidths of the First (F1), Second (F2), and Third (F3) Formants of Vowels Frequency Ranges Over Which the Bandwidths Apply.

	F1	F2	F3
Bandwidth	45–90	40–90	40–150
Formant frequency ranges	250–800	500–2500	2400–3300

Note. All values are in Hz and include data for men and women.
Source: These data were taken from graphs published by Fujimura and Lindqvist (1971).

output spectrum. At frequencies where there are valleys in the filter function, the energy at corresponding frequencies in the glottal spectrum does not appear prominently in the output spectrum.

The actual acoustic event that emerges from the lips—a vowel sound—is the product of the acoustic characteristics of the glottal spectrum (the amplitudes of the harmonic frequencies) and the varying amplitudes along the filter function. The output spectrum shows which frequencies are prominent and which are not. Peaks in the output spectrum, where energy transfer is maximal, are called formants. The first three formant frequencies of a vowel are referred to as the F-pattern of that vowel. The F-pattern is vitally important to understanding speech acoustics and perception.

The acoustic model of the vocal tract as a tube closed at one end is a central concept in the development of this theory. The tubes studied in Chapter 7 all had uniform cross-sectional area, like a straight pipe having no constrictions along its length. The articulation of the schwa may be performed with a vocal tract shape somewhat like a straight tube or pipe, but other vowels clearly require tube shapes of varying cross-sectional area from glottis to lips. Is there a straightforward way to understand how constrictions along the vocal tract tube cause changes in the resonant frequencies of a straight tube with one end closed? With no constrictions in a tube closed at one end, the quarter-wavelength rule accounts for the resonant frequencies, provided the length of the tube is known. What happens to these resonant frequencies when a constriction is introduced somewhere in the tube? Fortunately, the mathematical details of Fant's (1960) theory do not need to be studied to understand why the resonances change with constrictions in a tube. There is a simple conceptual basis for these changes, and the background for the concepts has already been established in Chapter 7. Discussion now turns to constrictions in the vocal tract tube, and their effect on formant frequencies.

WHAT HAPPENS TO THE RESONANT FREQUENCIES OF THE VOCAL TRACT WHEN THE TUBE IS CONSTRICTED AT A GIVEN LOCATION?

At the end of the discussion of tube resonances in Chapter 7, a graph (Figure 7–16) is shown of the pressure distributions for the first three resonances of a tube open at one end. This graph is reproduced in Figure 8–14A. The pressure distributions for the first three resonances correspond to one-quarter of the wave-

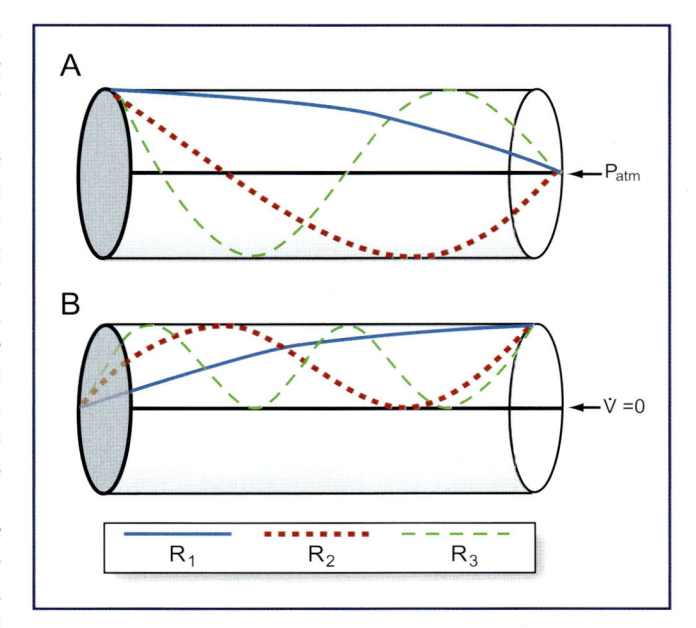

Figure 8–14. **A.** Reproduction of Figure 7–17 showing the pressure distributions corresponding to the first three resonances of a tube closed at one end. Pressure distributions follow the quarter-wavelength rule. **B.** Velocity distributions for the first three resonances of the tube shown in A. Velocities at any point in the tube are the mirror image of the pressure distributions. Thus, when pressure is maximum, velocity is zero, and vice versa. The center horizontal line in A represents Patm, whereas the center horizontal line in B represents zero velocity.

length for the first resonance (solid blue curve), three-quarters for the second resonance (short-dashed red curve), and five-fourths for the third resonance (long-dashed green curve). (In these graphs "maximum pressure" can mean either maximum positive or maximum negative pressure. The sign of maximum pressure is not important for the discussion that follows.) As stated in Chapter 7, there are many other pressure distributions in this tube corresponding to the higher resonances. They are not shown here partly for reasons of clarity, but also because the first three resonances are of chief concern in vowel acoustics as they relate to vowel categories.

Figure 8–14 shows the three pressure distributions superimposed on one another. The expected maximum pressures at the closed end of the tube can be seen for all three distributions, as well as other locations of maximum and zero (atmospheric) pressure that are associated with different wavelengths. For example, the first resonance has maximum pressure at the closed end, which falls to Patm at the open end. The second resonance has maximum pressure at the closed end, which

> **The Unknown Vocal Tract**
>
> Type in the words "voice disguise acoustics" on a search engine and you will be directed to all sorts of sites for electronic devices that guarantee to change your voice so people can't recognize it. With so many millions of voices in the world, it is remarkable that people can make fantastically accurate identifications based on a relatively brief voice sample. No wonder, then, that voice disguise is big business (we won't dwell on why you would want to disguise your voice). In the old days, some would-be voice disguisers spoke through the cardboard tube inside a roll of toilet paper, effectively lengthening their vocal tracts and lowering all formant frequencies. Others (this one turns up in old movies) put a handkerchief over the telephone receiver to "muffle" their voices, increasing sound absorption and, therefore, widening formant bandwidths. These antique maneuvers are easily reversed by signal processing tricks that "take away" the suspected cover-up. Modern electronic devices make it much harder to undo the disguise and recover the real voice behind the deception.

decreases to Patm one-quarter of the way toward the open end, decreases to maximum (negative) pressure three-quarters of the way to the open end, and returns to Patm at the opening. Examination of the pressure pattern for the third resonance reveals two regions of maximum pressure in addition to the maximum pressure at the closed end. Thus, along the length of the tube there are multiple regions of maximum pressure derived from the superimposed pressure patterns for the three lowest resonances.

Regions of high pressure result when molecules are packed together and in a relatively motionless state (i.e., at one of the extremes of the simple harmonic motion). It follows that if a measurement is made of the velocity of air molecules at the regions of high pressure in the tube, the value would be zero (i.e., no displacement as a function of time = zero velocity). Patm is indicated in Figure 8–14 by a horizontal, solid black line running through the center of the tube. When the wavelengths associated with the different resonances cross this line, meaning that their pressure value is equal to Patm, the air molecules are minimally packed together and move at their maximum velocity. Note the inverse relationship between pressure and velocity in the tube. When pressure is maximum, velocity of air molecules is zero, and when pressure is zero (= Patm), velocity is maximum. In fact, when the distributions for air molecule velocity are drawn for the first three resonances, they are mirror images of the distributions of pressure shown in Figure 8–14A. Those velocity distributions are shown in Figure 8–14B. The velocity pattern for the first resonance is shown by the solid blue line, for the second resonance by the short-dashed red line, and by the third resonance by the long-dashed green line. The figure shows the mirror image relationship between pressure and velocity distributions within the tube. This concept of pressure and velocity distributions within the tube is critical to understanding why and how resonances of the tube change when a constriction occurs at a specific location.

Imagine a constriction placed in the tube, exactly at a location of maximum pressure (and, therefore, zero velocity of air molecule movement). This situation is schematized in Figure 8–15A, which shows the three-quarters wavelength distribution of pressure associated with the second resonance. The constriction is shown as a blue hump that narrows the tube, at a location of maximum pressure. What is the effect, if any, of this constriction on the air vibrating within the tube? The constriction in the region of maximum pressure compresses the air molecules even more, forcing them closer together and farther from their rest positions. As air molecules (or any elastic object) are displaced farther from their rest positions, they become stiffer. Thus, a constriction in a region of maximum pressure increases the stiffness of the air molecules for that wavelength. Increased stiffness in a vibratory system results in a higher resonant frequency, which is exactly what happens in this example. The second resonance of the tube in Figure 8–15A, with a constriction placed at a maximum pressure region along its wavelength, increases in frequency relative to the case when the tube has no constrictions. Stated otherwise, if the length of a tube with no constrictions is known, the second resonance (symbolized here as $fr2$) of this unconstructed tube can be computed as $fr2 = (3) \times c/4l$. When a constriction is placed at a region of maximum pressure, the second resonance increases relative to the value computed for the unconstricted tube. The resonances of the unconstricted tube are reference frequencies, and the frequencies of constricted tubes can be regarded as deviations from these reference values.

What happens if the constriction is moved back in the tube to a location of zero pressure (Patm), where velocity is maximum (Figure 8–15B)? In the region of the tube where velocity is maximum, the air molecules are moving at top speed. To attain that top speed, the molecules must undergo substantial acceleration. As described in Chapter 7, objects with mass (like air)

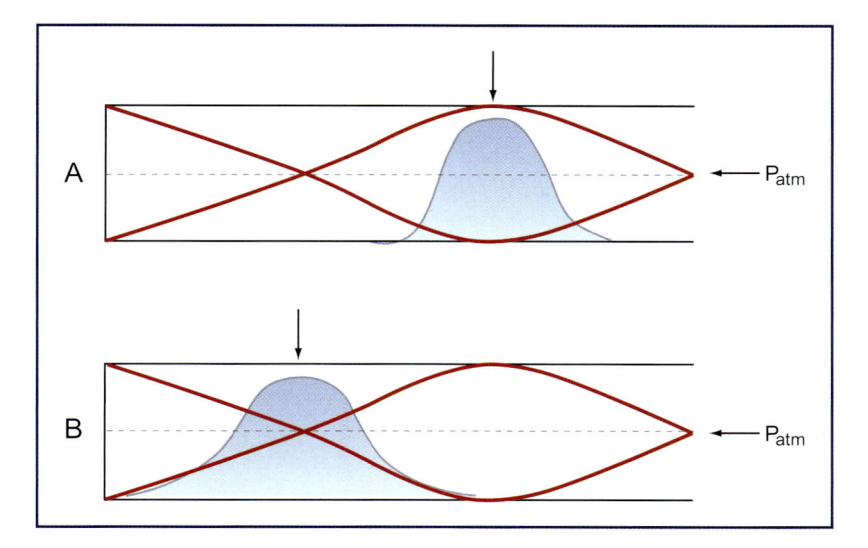

Figure 8–15. A. Tube closed at one end showing the three-quarter-wavelength distribution of pressure associated with the second resonance. A constriction (shown as a blue hump that narrows the area of the tube) is placed in the tube at the pressure maximum (*arrow*), about three-quarters of the way toward the open end. **B.** Same tube and pressure distribution as in A, but with the constriction positioned farther back in the tube, at a location where pressure = 0 and velocity is maximum. Pressure distributions are shown as both positive and negative, emphasizing the maximum pressure locations regardless of sign.

demonstrate inertia, which is an opposition to acceleration and deceleration. When air molecules are flowing through a tube and encounter a constriction, they speed up, increasing their effective mass at the point of constriction. The increase in effective mass means that the molecules demonstrate increased inertia, with increased time required to accelerate to maximum velocity. The narrower the constriction, the higher the velocities of the air molecules and hence the greater the inertial effects. This is the explanation for the increased acoustic mass of Helmholtz resonators with narrower necks. Logic suggests that when a constriction is placed at a location of maximum velocity (zero pressure), the tube resonance in question decreases relative to the case when the tube is not constricted. This is because a constriction in the region of a velocity maximum has the effect of increasing the acoustic mass (due to narrowing of the passageway in which air molecules are vibrating), which will lower the resonant frequency of a vibratory system. Thus, the second resonance of the tube in Figure 8–15B shows a decreased frequency, relative to the reference tube (a straight tube), when the constriction is placed at a velocity maximum.

The examples given in Figure 8–15 make use of the pressure (or its mirror image, velocity) distribution only for the second resonance of a tube closed at one end, but the principles generalize to the pressure (or velocity) distributions of all tube resonances. The principles, and some subprinciples, are as follows:

1. The resonances of a tube closed at one end, with no constrictions, are the reference resonances for tubes with constrictions.
2. A constriction located at a pressure maximum raises the frequency of the resonance whose wavelength "carries" the pressure maximum. This is because the constriction increases the stiffness of the air molecules along that wavelength.
   - The greater the degree of the constriction at a pressure maximum, the stiffer the air molecules become and, therefore, the greater the increase in the resonant frequency (tighter constrictions at pressure maxima result in greater increases in the resonant frequency).
3. A constriction located at a velocity maximum lowers the frequency of the resonance whose wavelength "carries" the velocity maximum. This is because the constriction increases the acoustic mass of the air molecules along that wavelength.
   - The greater the degree of the constriction at a velocity maximum, the more inertive are the moving air molecules and, therefore, the greater

the decrease in the resonant frequency (tighter constrictions at velocity maxima will result in greater decreases in the resonant frequency).

4. A constriction between a pressure or velocity maximum changes the frequency of the relevant resonance according to the relative magnitudes of the pressure and velocity at the point of constriction. Thus, a constriction at a point where the pressure is above Patm, but not maximum, may increase or decrease the resonant frequency, depending on the actual magnitudes of the pressures and velocities at that point in the tube. The effects of constrictions on resonant frequencies are continuous (i.e., they do not apply only at pressure or velocity maxima).

In principles 1 and 2, the phrase "whose wavelength *carries* the pressure (velocity) maximum . . ." is important, because the constrictions shown in Figure 8–15 affect only the second resonance (because it is that resonance's pressure and/or velocity maxima that are being constricted). The effects of the constrictions are always specific to the pressure (or velocity) regions of a particular resonance. But the point has been made that the pressure (or velocity) distributions for *all* resonances are "superimposed" on each other as the tube vibrates. A reasonable question is: "What happens when a constriction occurs on these superimposed distributions?"

Figure 8–16 displays a midsagittal view of a vocal tract, below which are three tubes closed at one end. The vocal tract drawing is lined up with the tubes such that the glottal end matches the closed (right) end of the tubes, and the lip opening matches the open (left) end of the tubes. It is useful to think of the tubes as straightened out versions of the vocal tract, in which the right-angle bend of the pharyngeal-oral airway has been eliminated. The top tube shows the pressure distribution for the first resonance, the middle tube the pressure distribution for the second resonance, and the bottom tube the distribution for the third resonance. These superimposed pressure distributions are shown separately here for the sake of clarity. For this discussion, assume a tube length of 15 centimeters (like the length of an adult female vocal tract), which in the case of no constrictions would yield the first three resonances at $c/4 \times 15 = 560$ Hz, 1680 Hz (3×560), and 2800 Hz (5×560) (where $c = 33{,}600$ cm/s).

Imagine a constriction placed toward the front of the vocal tract, at the location indicated by the number "1" in Figure 8–16. This constriction location is like that expected for the high-front vowel /i/. The corresponding location of this constriction along the three pressure distributions is shown by the vertical, dotted

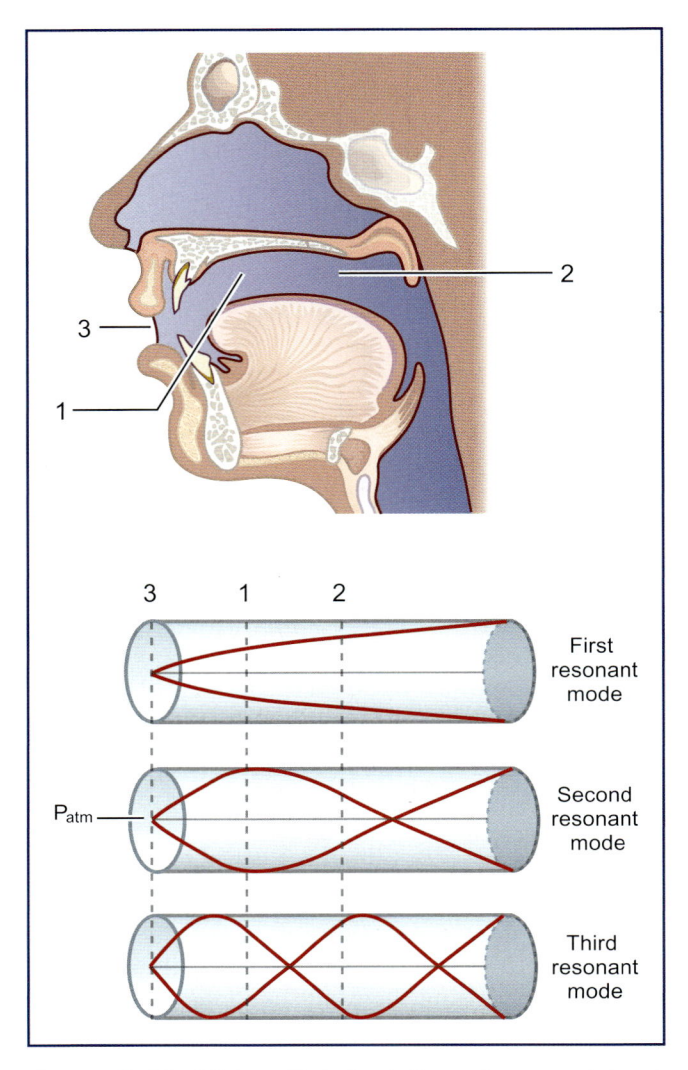

Figure 8–16. Midsagittal depiction of a vocal tract, below which are three tubes showing the pressure distributions for the first three resonances. The closed (*right*) end of the tube is analogous to the glottal end of the vocal tract, whereas the open (*left*) end of the tube is analogous to the lips. The numbers 1, 2, and 3 show locations of hypothetical constrictions within the vocal tract and their corresponding locations relative to the pressure distributions within the tube. High pressures within the tubes are indicated when the wavelength pressure distribution is against the edges of the tube. Sign of the pressure is not relevant. The thin horizontal line within each tube indicates atmospheric pressure.

line extending down from the number "1." The constriction falls at a region of relatively low pressure (i.e., relatively high velocity) for the first resonance, maximum pressure for the second resonance, and between zero and maximum pressure for the third resonance, perhaps closer to maximum than zero pressure. The effect of this constriction on the first resonance is to lower its frequency somewhat relative to the resonance when the tube is unconstricted (i.e., 560 Hz), because it occurs at a region of relatively high velocity, toward the front of the tube. The constriction increases the acoustic mass, which produces a lower resonant frequency relative to the first resonance of the unconstricted reference tube. The same constriction occurs at a maximum pressure region for the second resonance. The constriction, therefore, increases the second resonant frequency relative to the second resonance of the reference tube, because the molecules along this wavelength become stiffer as the region of high pressure is compressed. Finally, the constriction occurs between zero and maximum pressure for the third resonance, but closer to the maximum pressure. The third resonance has a slightly higher frequency compared with the third resonance of the reference tube. In this case, the constriction slightly increases the acoustic stiffness for this resonance.

It is important to recognize that a single constriction causes different effects for the different resonances, depending on the location of the constriction and the distributions of pressure (or velocity) along the tube. The effects of the constriction are all simultaneous, but may cause changes in resonant frequencies in different directions relative to the resonance of the reference tube. Constriction "1," for example, causes a decrease in the first resonance, a large increase in the second resonance, and a somewhat smaller increase in the third resonance.

Example 2 in Figure 8–16 shows a more posterior constriction in the vocal tract, one consistent with the production of the high-back vowel /u/. The dotted line extending through the tubes from the number "2" shows a constriction at a mid-pressure (mid-velocity) location for the first resonance, close to a velocity maximum for the second resonance, and close to a pressure maximum for the third resonance. Compared with constriction "1", constriction "2" results in a somewhat higher first resonant frequency, a much lower second resonant frequency (because constriction "2" occurs close to a velocity maximum for the second resonance, whereas constriction "1" occurs at a pressure maximum), and perhaps a higher third resonance.

Example 3 in Figure 8–16 is like a constriction at the lip opening of the vocal tract. This is an interesting case because the constriction occurs at a region of zero pressure (maximum velocity) for all three resonances. This constriction should lower all three resonant frequencies, because it increases the acoustic mass for all resonant modes. In fact, lip rounding, which produces a constriction at the open end of the tube, has the effect of lowering all resonant frequencies of the vocal tract. In addition, note that the tongue-constriction effects described above for constriction "2," as in the vowel /u/, may be changed if lip rounding (constriction "3") is combined with the tongue constriction. For example, the slight raising of the third resonance produced by tongue constriction "2" (close to a pressure maximum—see Figure 8–16) may be offset by the effect of lip constriction, which lowers the resonant frequency.

In summary, any constriction in the vocal tract affects all resonant frequencies of the tube. Because the pressure (or velocity) distributions for all resonances are superimposed on each other when the air in the tube vibrates, any constriction affects the pressure (or velocity) distributions for every resonance. The concepts of stiffness and mass explain why a constriction in the region of a pressure maximum raises a resonant frequency, and why a constriction in the region of a velocity maximum lowers a resonant frequency. A given resonance may be affected by two simultaneous constrictions, for example by the tongue and lips, but the stiffness and mass rules described here still explain what happens to the resonance when a previously straight tube is constricted at two locations.

Vowel articulation is the creation of vocal tract tubes with different area functions. The area functions are modified by the kinds of constrictions described above, which result in different resonant frequencies for different vowels. There is a lawful connection between articulatory configuration and vocal tract resonant (formant) frequencies.

The theory of tube resonance presented above is referred to as *perturbation theory*. It is called perturbation theory because it explains how the resonances of a tube are changed when the cross-sectional dimensions of the tube are perturbed, or constricted. The theory explains why constrictions in a tube modify the resonant characteristics of the tube. Because the ultimate interest is in the relationship between articulatory configurations and vocal tract resonances, it is convenient to have a small set of articulatory rules that account for changes in vocal tract resonant frequency with changes in vocal tract shape. This would be much simpler than asking exactly where a constriction is located relative to the pressure (velocity) distributions of the resonant modes. Stevens and House (1955) studied this problem, and developed a *three-parameter model of vowel articulation* to account for the relationships between vowel articulations and vocal tract resonances. It is useful to describe this model in some detail because it illustrates one way in which the acoustic theory of vowel production was tested.

> ### A Chance Encounter
>
> A professional speech acoustician, on vacation in the city of Odense, Denmark, spends a July day in 2004 visiting several museums. At the end of the day he is tired, but still has the Funen Art Museum on his list of visits. On the second floor he discovers the work of Martin Riches (http://martinriches.de). Riches' art is the creation of what he calls "machines," two of which are arty speech synthesizers! Riches is not a speech acoustician, but he read Fant's book and created a piece he calls "The Talking Machine." Riches studied Fant's area functions and based on them carved vocal tract shapes out of wood blocks for all sounds, then fitted them with a reed as a source and powered each reed/block with an air supply. The vocal tract blocks are mounted within a frame and the machine talks when the operator enters a word on a keyboard (visit https://www.youtube.com/watch?v=WClZcQo9l6Q) The synthesized speech is very intelligible. Not a bad demonstration of the "truth" of area functions, and pleasing art as well.

The Three-Parameter Model of Stevens and House

Fant (1960) developed his theory by marking sagittal tracings of the vocal tract into 35 half-centimeter sections from glottis to lips. Based on the cross-sectional area of each of these sections, Fant estimated their effective acoustic mass and stiffness. If the acoustic mass and stiffness are known for each of the 35 vocal tract sections, then it is known for the entire vocal tract, and the full set of vocal tract resonances can be computed.

Stevens and House (1955) created an analog model of Fant's theory by using their knowledge of the resonant properties of electrical circuits. The model can be explained by describing several simple characteristics of electrical circuits and components (prior knowledge of electrical circuit theory is not necessary to follow this discussion). The term *analog model* indicates that the electrical model is studied as an analogy of the acoustic properties of the vocal tract.

A simple electrical circuit is shown in the lower right-hand part of Figure 8–17. The circle labeled "S" represents a source of energy that supplies a flow of electrons to the circuit. This flow of electrons is called *current*, and the two long curved arrows around the bottom of the circuit show it flowing both from the negative side of the source to the positive side, and vice versa. This current source generates a sinusoidal signal, depicted in the upper left-hand part of Figure 8–17, with the speed of electron movement varying between zero (e.g., at the peaks of the sinusoid, when the direction changes from upward to downward, or vice versa) and a maximum value (e.g., when the sinusoid is passing through the "rest" position as shown in the waveform in the upper left part of figure). The sinusoidal variation of the current also accounts for the alternating movement of the electrons (i.e., from negative to positive, and positive to negative) indicated by the two curved arrows around the bottom of the circuit.

The circuit in Figure 8–17 contains three components. The component labeled R is a *resistor*, whose primary characteristic is to offer *frictional opposition* to the passage of electrons through the circuit. Friction, as discussed in Chapter 7, is a form of energy loss in which molecules rubbing against one another produce heat and, therefore, dissipate energy. Stevens and House (1955) used resistors in their model to simulate a component of energy loss in the vocal tract and thus the bandwidth characteristics of the formants.

The resonances (formants) of the vocal tract were simulated by Stevens and House (1955) with the components labeled L and C. L stands for an *inductor*, an electrical component that opposes the acceleration and deceleration of moving electrons. If electrons are moving around a circuit with changing velocities, the accelerations are sometimes very high, and other times very low and even zero. Acceleration is defined as the change in velocity over time, so at those times during sinusoidal motion when the velocity is approaching zero—when velocities have to change rapidly from very high to near zero—there will be very high accelerations (or decelerations). One example of a high acceleration and deceleration is the part of the waveform in Figure 8–17 where velocity is changing rapidly over time to reduce to zero, just before the waveform changes directions from up to down. The inductor opposes these high accelerations and decelerations, which are greater for high compared with low frequencies. Not only do the changes from high to low velocities (and, therefore, high accelerations) occur more rapidly for high compared with low frequencies, but there are more such changes per unit time for high frequencies. The discussion of the role of acoustic mass in determining resonant frequencies is based on the concept of inertia, the tendency for objects to oppose being accelerated and decelerated. The inductor opposes acceleration of electrons in the way that objects having mass oppose accel-

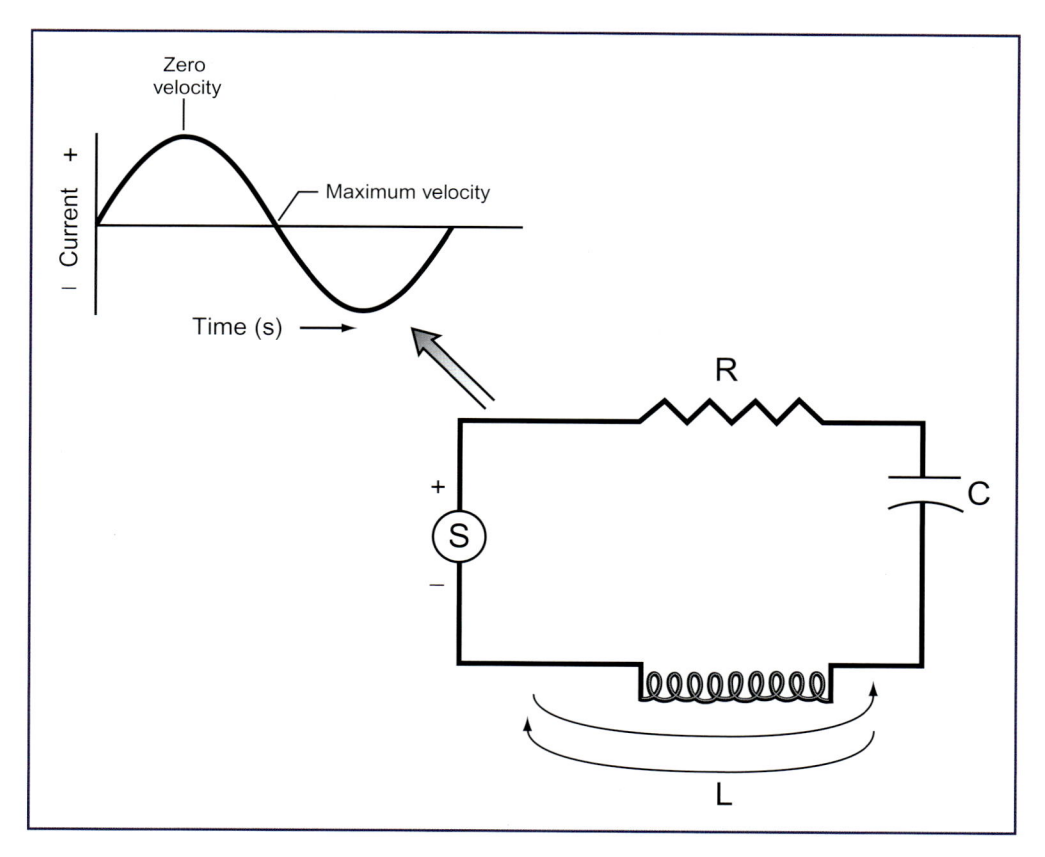

Figure 8–17. Schematic portrayal of a simple RLC electrical circuit (*bottom right*). *S* indicates a source of energy that produces current in the circuit. Current varies sinusoidally, as shown in the waveform inset (*top left*) of the figure. *R* = resistor. *L* = inductor. *C* = capacitor. When current flows through the circuit, *R* dissipates some of the energy in the form of heat, whereas *L* and *C* react to the current, as explained in the text. The waveform inset in the upper left part of the figure shows how current varies as a function of time.

eration and deceleration. The inductor can, therefore, be used in an electrical circuit to simulate an acoustic mass in the vocal tract.

The C in the circuit stands for a *capacitor*, an electrical component that stores electrons and offers opposition to the flow of current in proportion to how many electrons it has stored. The capacitor can be thought of as a closed container through which electrons try to flow. As electrons enter this container, they sometimes get stuck inside, and the capacitor gradually "fills up" with more and more electrons. The fuller the capacitor, the harder it is to get more electrons inside, which results in a reduction of current in the circuit. The current is reduced because the electron flow in the overall circuit is partially blocked by the nearly full capacitor. Imagine a closed volume of air, as in the bowl of a Helmholtz resonator (e.g., see Figure 7–13). If a plunger is placed in the neck of the resonator and moved into the bowl at an *intended* constant velocity, the air inside the bowl becomes increasingly stiff with increasing displacement of the plunger. Because the increasing stiffness develops a recoil force in proportion to the displacement of the air molecules (i.e., the displacement of the plunger), the *intended*, constant velocity of the plunger is opposed by the increasingly stiff air molecules. Thus, even though the plunger velocity was intended to be constant, the developing and increasing recoil force slows down the plunger movement. This is a fancy way to explain the fact that, with any spring (i.e., any volume of air), the more it is displaced from its rest position, the more difficult it is to move in the direction of the compression. Note the direct analogy to the electrical capacitor. The fuller the capacitor (the more the air molecules are compressed), the more opposition (an increasing recoil force) it offers to current flow. The capacitor is, therefore, an electrical version of an acoustical compliance (the inverse of stiffness), and can be used in an electrical circuit to simulate an acoustical compliance in the vocal tract.

Inductors and capacitors come in different sizes, much like masses and springs come in different weights and stiffness, respectively. Like Fant (1960), Stevens and House (1955) estimated the cross-sectional area, and hence the acoustic mass and compliance, of each one of 35 sections of the vocal tract. They used rules (not discussed here) to select the proper inductor and capacitor to simulate the acoustic mass and compliance of each section. They developed a device having 35 connected "RLC circuits" (circuits with a resistor [R], inductor [L], and capacitor [C]). The selection of the LC components was a simulation of the vocal tract area function, which depends on articulatory configuration. The LC settings of the whole 35-section device was an electrical model of articulatory configuration for vowels.

This last point, that the model can be interpreted in terms of articulatory configuration, is especially important. Ideally, it is useful to know the precise acoustic output for every possible vocal tract configuration (assuming a constant source spectrum). For any number of reasons, it is impossible to command a human to produce all these different configurations (but they can give it a try: see Ladefoged & Bladon, 1982). An electrical simulation of vocal tract (articulatory) configuration, however, allows small and precise changes in the configuration and observations of the resulting output. This is exactly what Stevens and House (1955) did. They changed the model's L and C characteristics in small steps to generate a complete "map" of the transform of vocal tract configuration to vocal tract acoustic output. By using an appropriate, electronically generated wave to simulate the source waveform, and an instrument to measure peaks in the output spectrum of the 35-section model, they measured the "formants" of the model for all possible articulatory configurations.

Based on these manipulations of the model, Stevens and House (1955) offered the following conclusions. The mapping between vocal tract configuration and vocal tract output for the first three formants did not need to be specified for each possible articulatory configuration. Instead, the mapping was well described with just three parameters.[5] More importantly, the three parameters make sense in terms of traditional phonetic descriptions of vowel articulation. The parameters include (a) *tongue height*, (b) *tongue advancement*, and (c) *configuration of the lips*.

Tongue Height

In traditional phonetic description, vowel tongue height describes the relative height of the tongue at the location of the major vocal tract constriction. For American English vowels made in the front of the vocal tract, the tongue height series from lowest (most open vocal tract) to highest (most closed vocal tract) is /æ,ɛ,e,ɪ,i/. The corresponding series for American English back vowels is /ɑ,ɔ,o,ʊ,u/. When Stevens and House (1955) simulated changes in tongue height (or equivalently, mouth opening), the main acoustic effect was on the first formant frequency (F1). Specifically, F1 decreased with increases in tongue height (as vowels went from low to high). This effect was more pronounced for the front vowel series compared with the back vowel series (see section on perturbation theory above).

Figure 8–18 illustrates the tongue height-F1 relationship by plotting tongue height on the *x*-axis and F1 on the *y*-axis. High tongue heights (short distances between the highest point on the tongue and the palate), as in vowels like /i/ and /u/, are indicated by low numbers on the *x*-axis ("0" represents complete closure of the vocal tract, as in a stop consonant). Moving from left to right on the *x*-axis represents high to low tongue heights. The tongue height-F1 relationship is plotted separately for front (filled circles connected by a solid line) and back (unfilled circles connected by a dotted line) vowels. For front vowels, the graph shows that F1 changes from about 250 Hz to slightly below 500 Hz as the tongue moves from a high to low position. For back vowels, there is only a small change with adjustments of tongue height, but it is in the same direction as the change for front vowels.

Tongue Advancement

Tongue advancement refers to the position of the major constriction for a vowel along the anterior-posterior (front-back) dimension of the vocal tract. In American English, the major constrictions for vowels such as /æ,ɛ,e,ɪ,i/ are toward the front of the vocal tract, whereas the major constrictions for /ɑ,ɔ,o,ʊ,u/

---

[5]Scientists typically deal with very complex phenomena, with many variables, but do not like to summarize their observations by describing each phenomenon and every variable. They are always looking to reduce the complexity of the real system to a few manageable parameters. If these few parameters capture the major performance characteristics of the system, this type of complexity reduction is deemed appropriate. Stevens and House's (1955) three-parameter model does not work perfectly, but it provides a good approximation to the relation of vocal tract configuration to vocal tract output.

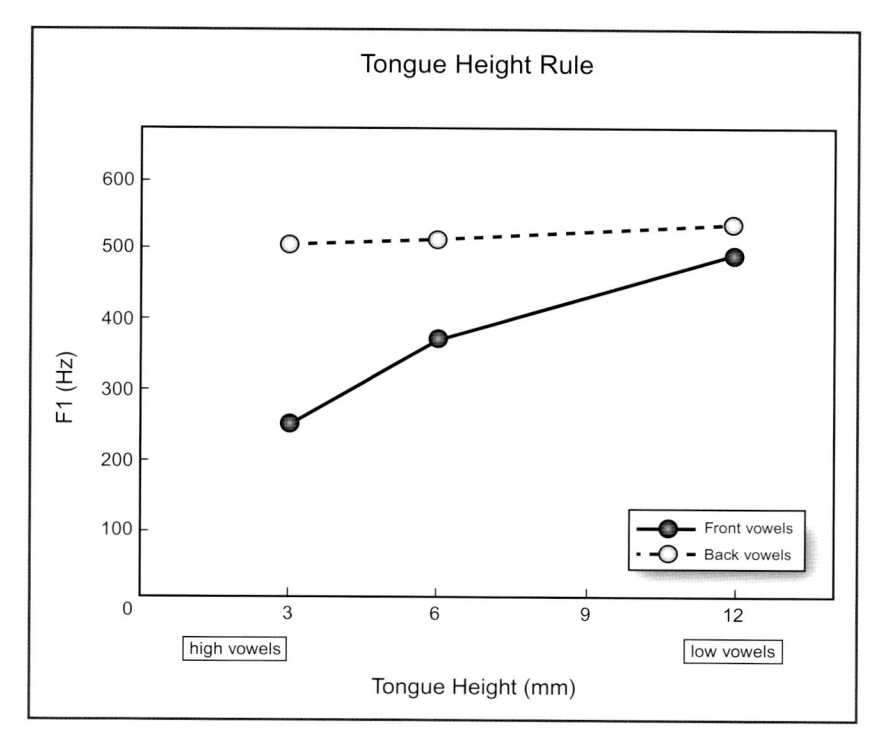

Figure 8–18. Graph illustrating the effect of changes in tongue height on the first formant frequency (F1). Tongue height is plotted on the x-axis as the distance between the highest point of the tongue and the palate. Higher numbers indicate lower tongue heights (that is, a more open vocal tract). Frequency of F1 is plotted on the y-axis. Filled circles, connected by solid lines, plot the effect for front vowels. Unfilled circles, connected by dashed lines, plot the effect for back vowels. Data extrapolated from Stevens and House (1955).

are toward the back of the vocal tract. There are also a few vowels in American English whose constrictions are in a relatively central location in the vocal tract (between front and back vowels). These would include /ɛ,ə,ʌ,ɝ,ɚ/ (note that /ɛ/ is considered as both front and central, depending on textbook, dialect, and so forth). When Stevens and House (1955) held all other factors constant as they simulated constrictions from the back to front of the vocal tract, two clear effects were observed. First, as the constriction moved from back to front, the frequency of F2 increased dramatically. This effect was more dramatic when the model was set for high tongue heights (as in moving from an /u/ to /i/ configuration) compared with low tongue heights (as in moving from an /ɑ/ to /æ/ configuration). Second, back-to-front movements also resulted in a decrease in the frequency of F1.

A summary of these findings is that increases in tongue advancement result in an increasing F2 and a decreasing F1. The effect of tongue advancement on F2 is shown in Figure 8–19. Tongue advancement, plotted on the x-axis, is measured as the distance of the major vowel constriction from the glottis. Small distances (to the left of the x-axis) represent relatively back constrictions, and large distances relatively front constrictions. To simplify the presentation, F2 values are plotted only for a constriction at 4 cm above the glottis (a back constriction) and at 13 cm above the glottis (a front constriction). Filled circles connected by solid lines plot F2 values for a relatively high tongue height (shown in Figure 8–19 by $r = 0.4$ mm indicating the radius of the constriction between the highest point on the tongue and the palate), and unfilled circles connected by dotted lines plot F2 values for a relatively low tongue height and relatively wider constriction (indicated by $r = 0.8$ mm). For high tongue positions (filled circles), moving the tongue from back to front results in an F2 change from about 1000 Hz to 2250 Hz. For low tongue positions (unfilled circles) the same increase in tongue advancement changes the F2 from roughly 1300 Hz to 1800 Hz. These effects are shown as linear changes (straight lines connecting the two measurement points)

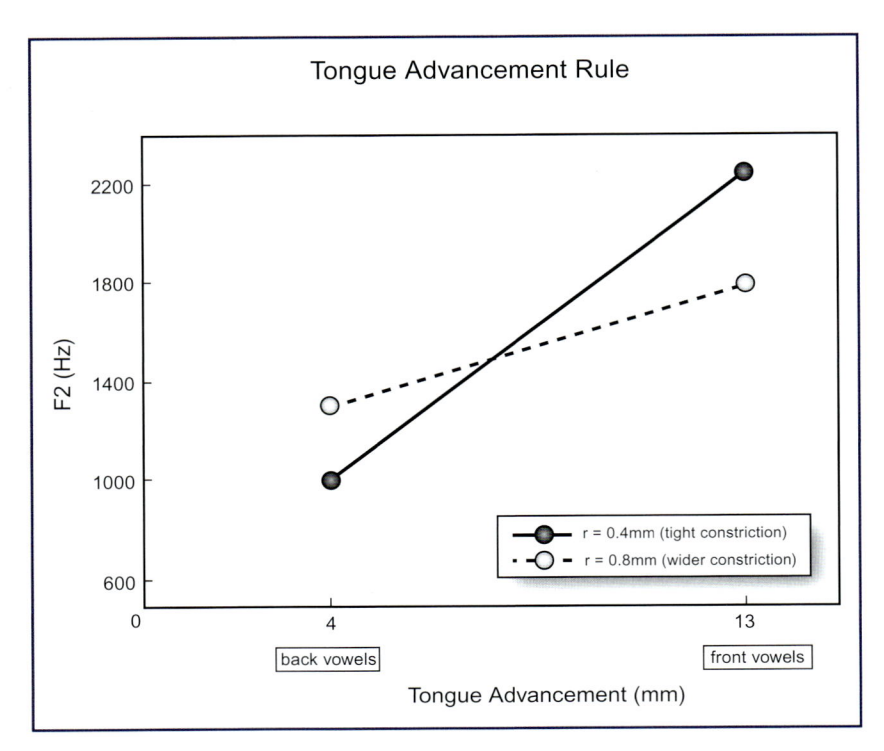

Figure 8-19. Graph illustrating the effect of changes in tongue advancement on the second formant frequency (F2). Tongue advancement is plotted on the x-axis as the distance of the major vocal tract constriction from the glottis. Higher numbers indicate constrictions made more forward (toward the front) of the vocal tract. Frequency of F2 is plotted on the y-axis. Filled circles, connected by a solid line, plot the effect for relatively small constriction radii (relatively high tongue heights). Unfilled circles, connected by a dashed line, plot the effect for relatively large constriction radii (relatively low tongue heights). Data extrapolated from Stevens and House (1955).

for the sake of simplicity, but articulatory-to-acoustic transformations are, in many cases, not linear. Readers interested in more details of the complex nature of articulatory-to-acoustic transformations are encouraged to consult Stevens and House (1955) and Stevens (1989).

Configuration of the Lips

Some vowels of American English are produced with rounded lips. These vowels include /u,ʊ,o,ɔ/. American English does not have a vowel contrast that depends on rounded versus unrounded lips. For example, the high-back-rounded vowel /u/ does not have a high-back unrounded counterpart. Many languages of the world, however, do have vowels distinguished by lip rounding. For example, Swedish has a rounded and unrounded high-front vowel (/i/ versus /y/), and Japanese has a rounded and unrounded high-back vowel (/u/ versus /ɯ/).[6] Stevens and House recognized the importance of lip rounding in languages of the world by systematically varying lip configuration in their model and observing the effects on formant frequencies. They conceptualized the lip section of the vocal tract as a separate "compartment," whose dimensions could be measured by calculating: (a) the area enclosed by the open lips, and (b) the length of the "compartment," measured as the distance between the front of the teeth and the most forward edge of the lips.

---

[6]Rounded vowels are disappearing in many dialects of American English. The vowel /u/ is losing rounding and may also be losing its back vowel characteristics, with a tendency toward fronting (Fridland, 2008). Both phonetic trends are not surprising. There is no high vowel between /i/ and /u/ in English (as there is in, for example, Russian), and no contrast between rounded and unrounded vowels. This is discussed more fully in Chapter 11.

Imagine a speaker's face when he or she is producing an exaggerated /u/, with lips rounded. If one looked at the speaker from the front, the rounding of the lips produces a very small mouth opening (i.e., the opening between the lips having a small area). If one looks from the side and knows roughly where the speaker's teeth are, the lips extend well in front of the teeth, creating a long lip "compartment." The opposite occurs when the lips are spread, as in the vowel /i/. For /i/ there is a relatively large area between the spread lips, which are pulled close to the teeth making the distance between the teeth and lips relatively small. Stevens and House used the ratio of the area of the opening enclosed by the lips (*A*) to the length of the lip compartment (*l*) as an index of lip rounding, with smaller values of the ratio *A*/*l* (smaller area, longer length) indicating more rounded lips. They applied the same principles of electrical-to-acoustic modeling used for tongue height and tongue advancement, and observed the effects of different degrees of lip rounding on formant frequencies. By varying lip rounding at different settings for tongue height and tongue advancement, Stevens and House identified a comprehensive range of acoustic effects due to lip rounding.

The general effect of lip rounding is as follows: as the lips become more rounded, *all* formant frequencies decrease. In a general sense, this makes sense because rounding of the lips is analogous to extending the length of the vocal tract, and longer vocal tracts have lower formant frequencies. In addition, lip rounding decreases the area enclosed by the inside border of the lips, creating a narrower resonator neck which decreases the resonant frequencies of the vocal tract (see section in Chapter 7 on Helmholtz resonators). The vocal tract is typically not a tube with uniform cross-sectional area, however, so lip rounding does not affect all resonances equally. The greatest decreases in formant frequencies with lip rounding are seen in F2, with somewhat lesser (but roughly equal) effects on F1 and F3. Moreover, the influence of lip rounding on F2 depends substantially on tongue height: the higher the tongue, the more lip rounding causes F2 to decrease.

The effects of lip rounding on F2 are illustrated in Figure 8–20. Two degrees of lip rounding are plotted on the *x*-axis, but the range of *A*/*l* values is potentially continuous between the two values in the plot. An *A*/*l* ratio of 0.4 represents a highly rounded condition and a ratio of 6.7 a highly spread (unrounded) condition. For each rounding condition, there are four plotted points. High-back vowels are shown by filled circles connected by a heavy solid line, low-back vowels by unfilled circles connected by a heavy dashed line, high-front vowels by lightly shaded diamonds connected by a thin solid line, and low-back vowels by unfilled diamonds connected by a thin dashed line. Consistent with Stevens and House's (1955) general findings concerning the effects of lip rounding on vowel formants, all points at the 0.4 *A*/*l* value have lower F2 values than corresponding points at the 6.7 value. If the amount of F2 change from the 0.4 to 6.7 value is studied for each vowel type, there are greater effects of lip rounding on the F2s of high compared with low vowels.

Importance of the Stevens and House Rules: A Summary

The findings of Stevens and House (1955) are often stated in the form of simple rules for relating changes in articulatory configuration to changes in formant frequencies. A clear statement of these rules is a good way to summarize the preceding discussion.

Rule 1. F1 varies inversely with tongue height. The higher the tongue, the lower the F1. The rule applies more dramatically to front as compared with back vowels.

Rule 2. F2 increases, and F1 decreases, with increasing tongue advancement. The rule applies dramatically for high vowels, and less so for low vowels.

Rule 3. All formant frequencies decrease with increased rounding of the lips, but the major effect is on F2. The rule applies more dramatically to high as compared with low vowels.

Dynamic Analogies

In the text, mechanical, aerodynamic, acoustic, and electrical systems have been introduced. In several cases, a single physical principle has been shown to be relevant to all systems. Take inertia, for example. Inertia is a property of things having mass, such as a block of wood. In an aerodynamic system, a plug of air has mass, called an inertance, which has relevance to acoustic resonance. Inertance, in turn, can be simulated with the electrical component called an inductor. The representation of a single physical concept in several different systems is referred to as a *dynamic analogy*. The term is used particularly for the representation in electrical circuits of mechanical and acoustic concepts, as in the Stevens and House model. Dynamic analogies have been exploited to create electrical models of the auditory system, as well.

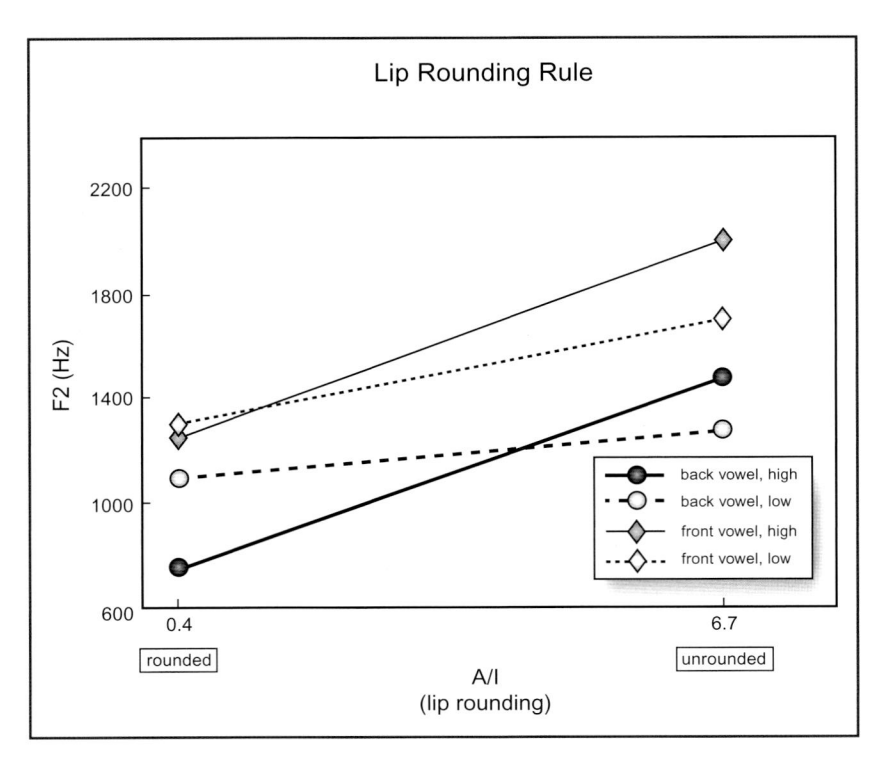

Figure 8–20. Data showing the effect of changes in lip rounding on the second formant frequency (F2). Lip rounding is plotted on the x-axis as the ratio of the area of the lip section to the length of the lip section (A/l). Higher numbers indicate more spread lips (less lip rounding). Frequency of F2 is plotted on the y-axis. Filled circles, connected by a thick solid line, show the effect for back, high vowels. Unfilled circles, connected by a thick dashed line, show the effect for back, low vowels. Filled diamonds, connected by a thin solid line, show the effect for front, high vowels. And unfilled diamonds, connected by a thin dashed line, show the effect for front, low vowels. Data extrapolated from Stevens and House (1955).

An additional aspect of Stevens and House's (1955) modeling experiment is worthy of mention. The behavior of the third formant was not as easily related to changes in articulatory dimensions (tongue height, tongue advancement, configuration of the lips) as were F1 and F2. The changes in F3 that were observed tended to be rather small, regardless of the articulatory change. The only rule relevant to F3, therefore, is the one concerning lip rounding. The fact that the Stevens and House rules are reliable is supported by data showing that articulatory parameters for vowels, such as location and degree of constriction, can be inferred from formant frequencies and their amplitudes (Iskarous, 2010).

The Connection Between the Stevens and House Rules and Perturbation Theory

The Stevens and House (1955) rules can be thought of as articulatory summaries of the resonance rules described in perturbation theory. In perturbation theory, constrictions in the region of high velocities produce a decrease in the resonant frequency. According to Rule 1, F1 varies inversely with tongue height. Figure 8–21A summarizes this articulatory rule within the framework of perturbation theory. There the pressure distribution is shown for the first tube resonance, and articulatory constriction locations are indicated for back and front vowels. The location for the front vowel constriction corresponds to a relatively low pressure, and, therefore, high velocity, along this wavelength. Constrictions at the front vowel location will decrease the frequency of the first resonance (i.e., the first formant), with greater constrictions producing greater frequency decreases. The same degrees of constriction for back vowels will not produce such dramatic decreases in the first resonant frequency because at this location the velocity is not as high. This parallels the behavior of F1 with changes in tongue height. The effect on F1 of increasing the constriction is much greater for front compared with back vowels, as summarized in Figure 8–18.

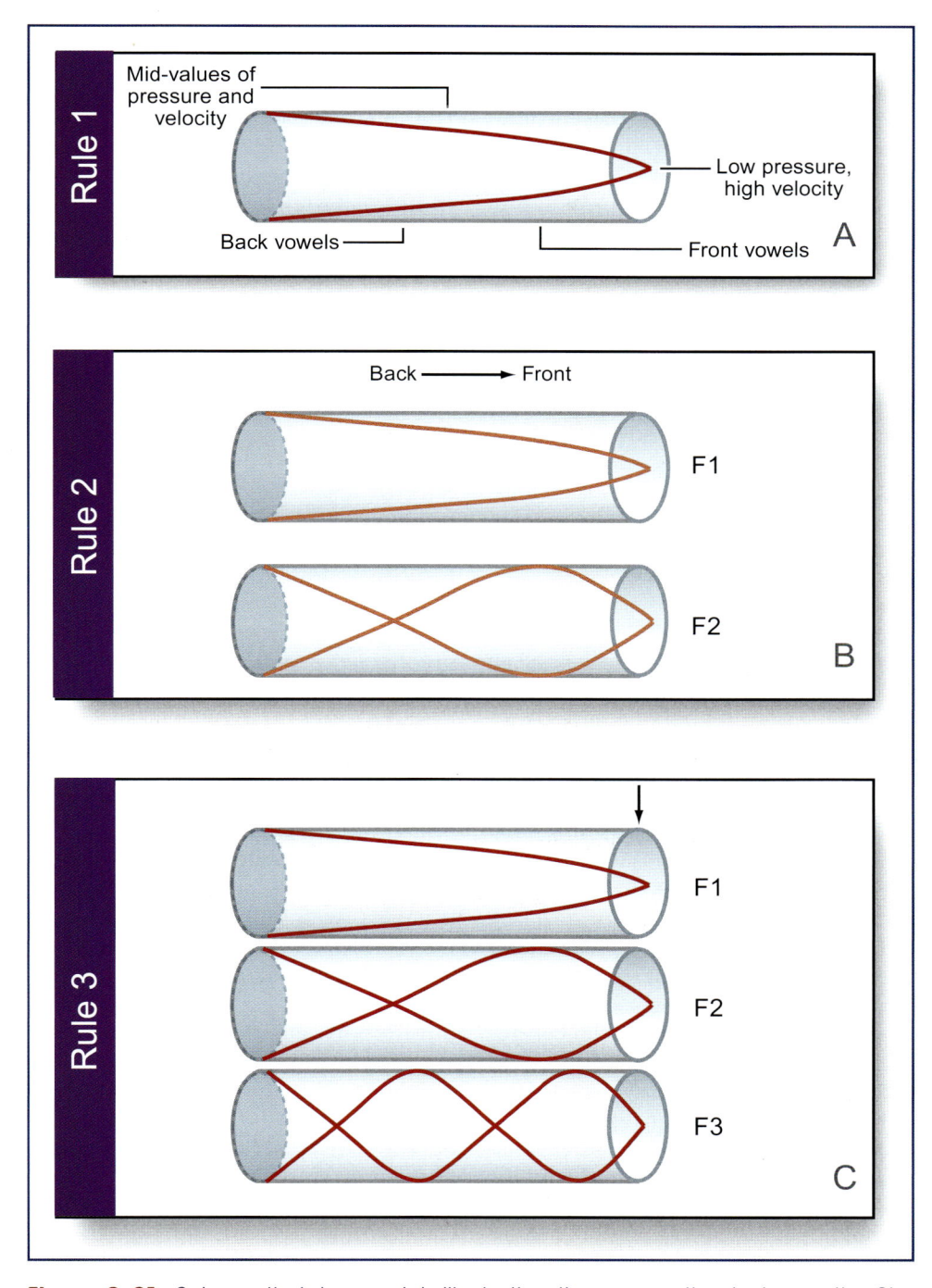

Figure 8–21. Schematic tube models illustrating the connection between the Stevens and House (1955) rules and perturbation theory. **A.** Pressure distribution for F1, showing how perturbation theory is related to the tongue height rule. **B.** Pressure distributions for F1 and F2, showing how perturbation theory is related to the tongue advancement rule. **C.** Pressure distributions of F1, F2, and F3, showing how perturbation theory is related to the lip rounding rule.

Figure 8–21B shows how Rule 2 relates to perturbation theory. The effect of tongue advancement on F2 is illustrated by the lower tube, which shows the pressure distribution for the second resonance (i.e., a three-quarter-wavelength distribution of pressure). The location marked "back" is approximately at the constriction location for /u/, where the pressure is near zero and the velocity is, therefore, near maximum. As the constriction moves forward, the pressure increases to a maximum in the region of the vocal tract constriction for /i/ ("front" in Figure 8–21B). Tongue advancement from an /u/ constriction to an /i/ constriction moves from a region of low to high pressure (high to low velocity). According to perturbation theory, this movement is associated with increasing F2. In addition, because the effect of constrictions on resonant frequencies is greatest for very tight constrictions, the effect on F2 will be greater for higher compared with lower vowels, as summarized in Figure 8–19. The upper tube in Figure 8–21B reproduces the distribution of pressure for the first resonance, and shows why tongue advancement results in a lowering of F1. As the tongue moves forward, the pressure for the first resonance is increasingly lower and the velocities increasingly greater. A more frontal constriction is located at higher velocities, and results in lower resonant frequencies.

Finally, Figure 8–21C illustrates the relationship between perturbation theory and Rule 3, which states that rounding the lips reduces the frequencies of all formants. The downward-pointing arrow indicates a constriction at the open end of the tube, which shows the pressure distributions for the first three resonances. For each distribution, the pressure is zero at the open end, and the velocity is maximum. A constriction at the open end of the tube, therefore, lowers all formant frequencies (see Figure 8–20).

Importantly, Stevens and House's (1955) complete mapping of the relation of vocal tract configuration (articulatory configuration) to formant frequencies resulted in the interesting discovery that more than one vocal tract configuration produced the same formant frequencies. This finding introduced a special consideration in the articulatory interpretation of formant frequency measures. If each set of formant frequencies is associated with a unique vocal tract configuration, acoustic analysis allows a straightforward interpretation of the vocal tract configuration that produced the formant frequencies. As Stevens and House showed, however, this did not appear to be the case. The inference of vocal tract configuration from the F-pattern is ambiguous in certain cases. The inability to specify a precise articulatory configuration from formant frequencies is referred to as the *nonuniqueness problem*, because there is not a unique (i.e., a single) vocal tract configuration that produces a given F-pattern. In many cases, though, the F-pattern provides enough information to make fairly accurate guesses about vocal tract configurations (Iskarous, 2010). This leads to a consideration of the importance of the Stevens and House findings.

Why Are the Stevens and House Rules Important?

The systematic study of articulatory behavior in speech production has a relatively brief history. Interest in phonetics has a solid historical basis, but concentrated study of the physiological and acoustic behavior of the vocal tract did not begin until well after the beginning of the twentieth century. The relative youth of the science of speech production can be explained on the basis of technical limitations. Before the twentieth century, instruments for direct visualization of some of the "hidden" articulators (such as the tongue, velum, and larynx) were not available, nor was it possible to make acoustic recordings and perform spectral analyses of vocal tract output.

The seeds for the explosive growth in communication sciences as a vibrant academic discipline were sown in the 1950s and 1960s, a period during which Fant developed and elaborated his acoustic theory. This period also saw the first systematic collection and analysis of data concerning tongue behavior during speech. x-ray motion pictures, a technology originally developed for medical diagnoses of gastrointestinal function (upper and lower GI studies), were adapted to the study of speech production. A participant's tongue and other articulators were coated with barium paste to make the soft tissue more visible in the developed films. The films were analyzed by hand tracing the outlines of articulatory structures on a frame-by-frame basis. In later variations on this technique, small pellets were fixed to the tongue, lips, and velum and the movements of these points were measured by hand from the x-ray films. This approach eliminated the need to trace articulators frame-by-frame, using sometimes poorly imaged vocal tract structures, but still required an intensive effort on the part of an investigator or clinician. The latest development of this technology involves computerized tracking of the movements of small coils placed on the tongue and other articulators, using electromagnetic fields (Berry, 2011; Hoole & Zierdt, 2010; Perkell, Cohen, Svirsky, Matthies, Garabieta, & Jackson, 1992; see Chapter 6). The automated collection/storage of the moving pellets greatly reduces the amount of time required to collect data on articulatory movement during speech.

This brief digression on techniques for visualizing hidden articulators highlights the challenge of obtaining information on the articulatory function of structures such as the tongue. Most of these techniques involve a substantial amount of subject preparation (e.g., fixing pellets, or magnetic coils, to the tongue), and the instruments are not readily available to practitioners (see below). Moreover, any x-ray technique carries with it some health hazard (there are no currently known health hazards associated with electromagnetic techniques), and the cost of and expertise required to use any of these techniques limit their broad application.

This is where the importance of the Stevens and House rules enters the picture. These rules allow a practitioner to examine an acoustic record of an utterance, locate the formant frequencies, and *infer* the likely vocal tract configuration(s) that produced those formants. Because of the nonuniqueness problem, there may be some ambiguity in these inferences, but for the most part, the formant frequencies provide good information on articulatory positions and time histories (changes in position over time). This can be accomplished by making recordings of a person's speech and submitting the recordings to proper analyses.

Who are the practitioners referred to above? They include researchers and clinicians, both of whom are interested in having access to techniques that allow them to draw objective, cost-effective, and *noninvasive* conclusions about a speaker's articulatory behavior. A noninvasive technique is one in which instruments do not have to be introduced into the body (e.g., into the mouth) to obtain diagnostic and prognostic information, or one that does not create a potential health risk to the participant or client. X-ray procedures are invasive, and the electromagnetic technologies mentioned above are partially invasive and not cost- or time-effective in a clinical setting. The use of acoustic analysis to draw reasonable inferences about articulatory behavior is the most likely technique to upgrade the ability of speech-language clinicians to account for their diagnostic and management observations concerning speech production abnormalities. There is a high level of skill required to make these inferences, but it is the purpose of texts such as this one, and appropriate university-level coursework, to supply the foundation for these skills.

Another Take on the Relationship Between Vocal Tract Configuration and Vocal Tract Resonances

The formant frequencies of the vocal tract tube can be understood using the rules for calculating the resonant frequencies of a tube with a uniform cross-sectional area, and knowing how and why those resonances are modified when the tube is perturbed by a constriction. The shape of the vocal tract tube yields the area function, which is really another way to express the articulatory configuration for a given vowel. The continuous area function from glottis to lips, and its effect on formant frequencies, can be reduced to three variables whose changes affect formant frequencies in systematic ways. This is what Stevens and House (1955) accomplished: the expression of tube acoustics in terms of variables relevant to a phonetician—tongue height, tongue advancement, and lip rounding.

Another approach to understanding the effects of articulatory configuration on vowel acoustics is based on a simple resonator model. This approach deserves mention because it has been used in educational settings in which students are taught vocal tract acoustics. The *Connected Tube Model* (Arai, 2012) represents the vocal tract as a sequence of connected but discrete tubes, as represented in Figure 8–22. Tube models are shown for the vowels /i/, /e/, /ɑ/, /o/, and /u/, with the glottal end of the vocal tract at the left and the lip end on the right. In the tube model for /i/, the large-diameter back tube is seen separated from the equally large-diameter but much shorter front cavity by a long tube of very narrow diameter. The large back tube represents the cavity behind the front constriction for /i/, and the large front tube represents the short open cavity in front of the /i/ constriction. The /i/ constriction is represented by the narrow-diameter connecting tube between the two larger tubes.

What is interesting about this model is that the simple mathematical rules discussed in Chapter 7 for determining the resonant frequencies of tubes and Helmholtz resonators can be applied to this rather crude model to determine the first three formant frequencies of a vowel. For example, in the case of the three-tube model for /i/ at the top of Figure 8–22, the back cavity can be regarded as a tube open at both ends, the front cavity as a tube closed at one end (where the closed end is the beginning of the narrow constriction and the open end is at the mouth), and the back cavity attached to the narrow passageway formed by

---

The Idiomatic Toolbox: Speech Phrases

"Don't give me any lip," "Flapping your gums," "Jawboning," and "Gave him a real tongue lashing" are all well-known phrases that refer to speech acts. To make their point, these phrases refer to part of the speech production apparatus that can be seen more or less easily. It is probably not an accident that potential phrases referring to "hidden" articulators, such as, "Oh, raise your velum, please!" to ask someone to stop whining and "Slow down your vocal folds!" to calm someone, are not in the idiomatic toolbox.

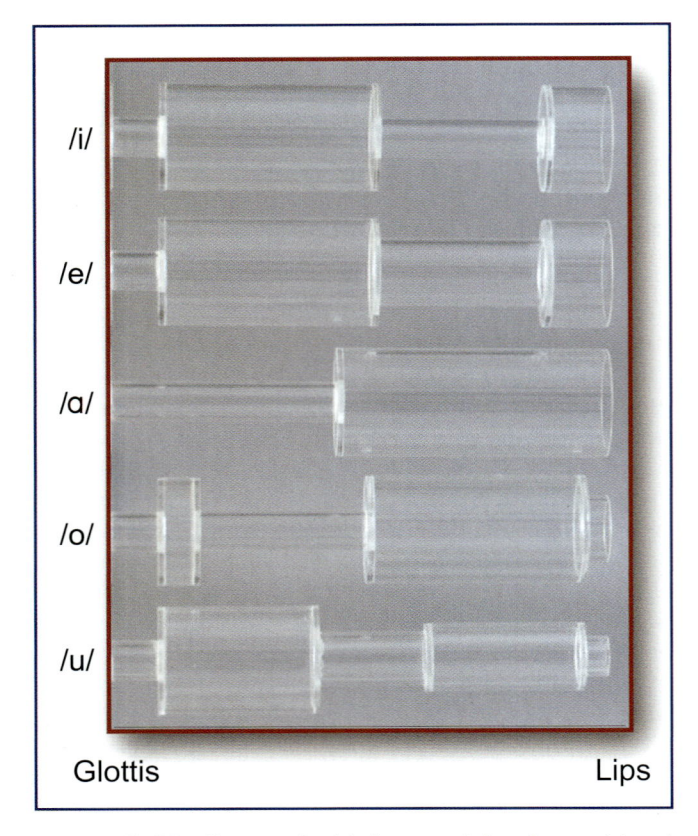

Figure 8–22. Connected tube models of vocal tract configurations for the vowels /i/, /e/, /a/, /o/, and /u/, from top to bottom. The glottis end of the vocal tract is to the left, and the lip end to the right. Photograph from Arai (2012), reproduced with modifications by permission.

the constriction as a Helmholtz resonator (the neck is formed by the narrow-diameter constriction, the bowl by the large-diameter back cavity). If the appropriate tube lengths and bowl radii (in the case of the back cavity when functioning as a Helmholtz resonator) are measured and the values plugged into the formulas given in Chapter 7 for tubes either open at both ends (half-wavelength rule) or closed at one end (quarter-wavelength rule), or for a Helmholtz resonator, an interesting result emerges from the computations. The Helmholtz formula produces a resonant frequency similar to the F1 for /i/, the half-wavelength formula a resonant frequency similar to F2 for /i/, and the quarter-wavelength formula a resonant frequency similar to F3 for /i/ (Arai, 2012, see his Figure 7 and 8). Resonator computations on the crude tube models shown in Figure 8–22 for /e/, /a/, /o/, and /u/ also produce F1, F2, and F3 values similar to those observed for the natural adult productions of these vowels. Note in Figure 8–22 the differences among the connected tube models for the five vowels.

On the one hand, this may seem like a trivial demonstration. After all, a brief examination of the five connected tube models in Figure 8–22 shows precisely the sort of vocal tract configuration differences expected in a comparison between any two of these vowels. For example, the primary difference between the tube models for /i/ and /e/ is the larger-diameter "constriction tube" for /e/ compared with /i/, which in phonetic terms is the same as saying the tongue forms a constriction for both /i/ and /e/ in the front part of the vocal tract, but the constriction is not quite as tight for /e/. Another comparison example is that the tube model for /a/ is distinguished from the other tube models by the long, large-diameter tube in the front of the model and the long, narrow-diameter tube in the back of the model. This is expected for a vowel typically described as having a substantial constriction between the tongue and the pharynx and a wide-open front cavity (that is, a low-back vowel). What is surprising, perhaps, is how well the simple-resonator model computations of formant frequencies match with actual formant frequencies measured from persons producing these vowels. Keep in mind that these matches occur even though real area functions change *continuously* (smoothly) from glottis to lips. In contrast, the resonator models of Figure 8–22 show connections between adjacent resonators characterized by large, sudden changes in resonator diameter. In the /i/-tube model, for example, the two larger cavities do not blend smoothly into the constriction cavity, but appear to be "glued" to the smaller constriction cavity with no gradual connection. This suggests a certain degree of inexactness in the transformation from vocal tract configuration to formant frequencies; stated more simply, in certain cases it appears "precise" articulation is not required to achieve a target vowel output.

There are limitations to the connected tube model. It works best for vowels that separate the vocal tract into easily recognizable cavities in front of and behind well-defined constrictions. For vowels with "straighter" tubes but some constriction, such as /æ/ and /ɛ/, a connected tube model may not be effective for predicting actual formant frequencies. As it turns out, however, the vowels for which the connected tube model is effective—the ones shown in Figure 8–22—are among the most frequently occurring vowels in languages of the world.

CONFIRMATION OF THE ACOUSTIC THEORY OF VOWEL PRODUCTION

Theories serve as proposed explanations of how and why something happens. Fant's (1960) theory is designed to explain how vowel sounds happen, but like all theories it may be false, either completely or, perhaps, just in parts. The confirmation of the acoustic theory of vowel production has taken several forms, including analog experiments and human experiments.

Analog Experiments

The experiments of Stevens and House (1955) were based on an electrical model of the acoustic characteristics of the vocal tract. Stevens and House made their model sound like human vowels (albeit crudely) when they selected electrical components to simulate the area functions of the vocal tract. For example, because the model sounded like an /i/ when the components mimicked an /i/ area function, this was compelling evidence in favor of the theory. If the vocal tract did not resonate like a tube closed at one end and respond acoustically to constrictions according to the principles of perturbation theory, it is hard to see why the electrical model worked so well. Many scientists believed that the electrical analog experiments served as strong confirmation of Fant's (1960) theory.

Human Experiments

A powerful way to test the correctness of Fant's (1960) theory is to compare formant patterns predicted from the area functions with those actually measured when people produce vowels. The formant patterns predicted from area functions depend on the "goodness" of various aspects of the theory. If the calculated (theoretical) formants match the measured formants, the theory can be broadly confirmed.

A comparison of theoretical and human formant frequencies is shown in Figure 8–23, in the form of F1-F2 (left) and F2-F3 (right) plots. These are very popular plots, wherein the values of two formant frequencies are plotted as coordinates in a simple scatterplot (in theory, a plot could be made of three or more simultaneous formant frequencies, as a set of coordinate points in three-space, or n-space for more than three formants). In the left plot, F1 is on the x-axis, and F2 is on the y-axis. In the right plot F2 is on the x-axis and F3 is on the y-axis.

In both plots, the filled circles (labeled "electrical analog") show theoretical locations of F1-F2 or F2-F3 coordinates as generated by an electrical analog of the vocal tract constructed by Fant, based on the area functions obtained from his x-rays of the vocal tract. Fant's analog was very much like the one studied by Stevens and House (1955). These points are theoretical in the sense that they are based on the ability to use the area function to estimate the inertances (acoustic masses) and compliances (the inverse of acoustic stiffness) of small sections of the vocal tract and to represent those with inductors and capacitors in an electrical model that can generate sound. The unfilled circles (labeled "human") are actual formant frequencies measured by Fant (1960, p. 109), from sustained vowels produced by the speaker whose vocal tract was x-rayed for the study. Data are shown for three vowels, /i/, /ɑ/, and /u/.

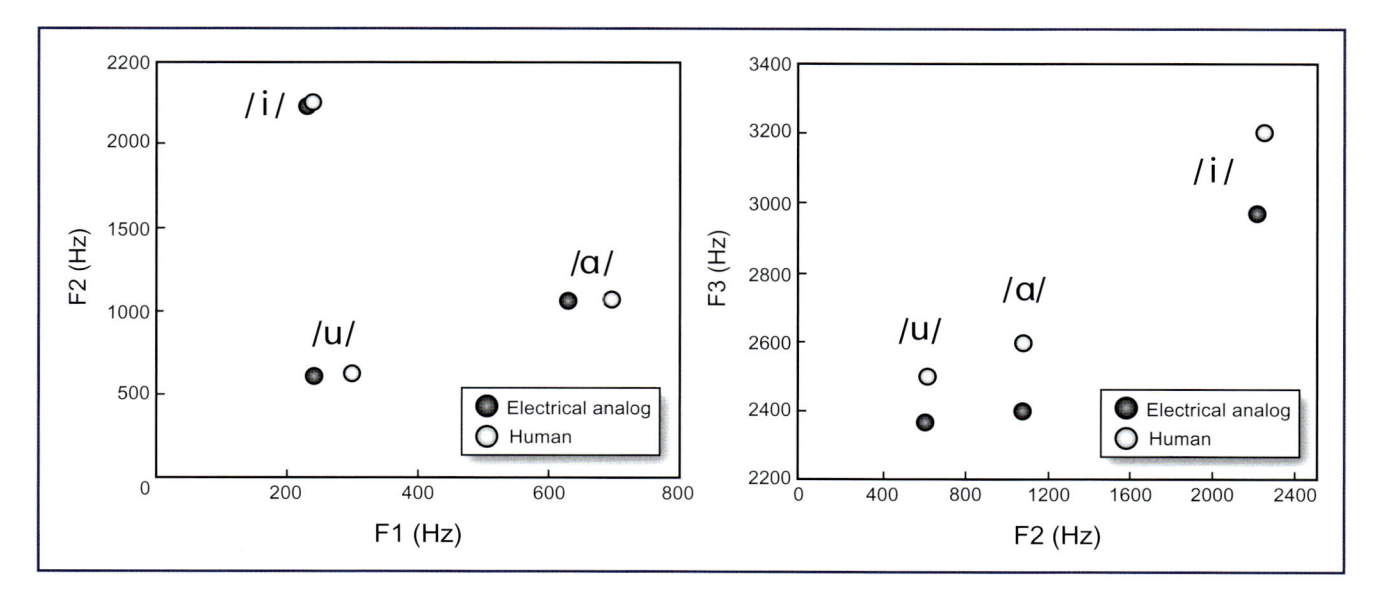

Figure 8–23. F1-F2 (*left*) and F2-F3 (*right*) plots for the vowels /i/, /u/, and /ɑ/ produced by an electrical analog based on Fant's (1960) theory (*filled circles*) and by a human producing the vowels during an x-ray filming procedure (*unfilled circles*). Agreement between the theoretical and human data suggests that the acoustic theory of vowel production is generally correct. Data plotted from Fant's (1960) Table 2.31-1 on p. 109.

One test of the goodness of the theory is the extent to which the theoretical (electrical analog) points agree with the human points. Examination of the two plots in Figure 8–23 suggests that the agreement is impressive, especially for F2. Even in cases where there are differences between the theoretical and human measurements (as in F1 for /u/ and /ɑ/, and in F3 for all three vowels), the differences are relatively small. These data suggest that Fant's (1960) theory predicts human formant frequency data with a high degree of accuracy.

It should also be noted that the electrical analog generates formant measures from the area functions for /i/, /u/, and /ɑ/ that are consistent with the Stevens and House (1955) rules listed and explained above. For example, /i/ is the highest and most front vowel in the phonetic working space and, therefore, has a very high F2 and very low F1. The opposite case is seen for the back and low vowel /ɑ/, which has a low F2 and high F1. This is yet another piece of evidence in favor of the theory's goodness.

Why don't the human and electrical analog formant frequencies match exactly? There are several ways to answer this question, but the general answer is, "The lack of exact matches between the theoretical and human formant frequency coordinates does not invalidate the theory." First, it is very rare for a theory to be confirmed by exact, quantitative matches to theoretical predictions (at least in speech acoustics). Scientists always expect some error between their predicted (theoretical) and obtained measurements. There may be some error in estimating the area functions, perhaps deriving from certain inexact measures of the x-ray images. Alternatively, the measures of formant frequencies, whether done by hand or by computer, are subject to error. Second, and perhaps most importantly, a theory can be correct in many ways but subject to refinement in its details. This is certainly the case for the acoustic theory of vowel production. It is correct, for example, to claim that the area function predicts the locations of formant frequencies, but the precision of those predictions—how close the actual, measured values are to the theoretical values—may depend on details that have yet to be discovered, or ultimately, may be unknowable.

REVIEW

The acoustic theory of vowel production includes a source, or input (the vibrating vocal folds which produce a glottal spectrum), and a filter (the vocal tract resonator), which combine to produce an acoustic output measured directly in front of the lips.

The source produces a complex periodic waveform whose spectrum consists of a consecutive-integer series of harmonics.

The vocal tract filter, or resonator, can be modeled as a tube closed at one end.

When the source and filter combine to produce an output spectrum, the peaks in this spectrum are referred to as formants.

The formants are essentially the resonances of the vocal tract, which change according to changes in the shape of the vocal tract tube.

The vocal tract configuration for a schwa is most like the case of a tube closed at one end and having uniform cross-sectional area (i.e., no constrictions) from one end to the other; this tube has a set of formant frequencies predicted from the quarter-wavelength rule.

When constrictions are introduced into the tube—when articulatory configuration changes from schwa to other vowels—the formant frequencies change according to rules.

These rules can be stated in terms of the location of a constriction relative to pressure and velocity distributions within the tube so that constrictions near a pressure maximum will increase the formant frequency, whereas constrictions near a velocity (flow) maximum will decrease the formant frequency.

The explanation of formant frequency changes based on constriction locations relative to pressure and flow distributions within a tube is called perturbation theory.

Alternatively, the rules can be stated in articulatory terms as described by Stevens and House (1955), which include: (a) tongue height, (b) tongue advancement, and (c) configuration of the lips.

Increases in tongue height (higher tongue heights) result in decreases in F1, increases in tongue advancement (moving the tongue from back to front) result in increases in F2 and decreases in F1, and increased lip rounding decreases all formant frequencies but most notably F2.

The lawfulness of the relations between articulatory configuration for vowels and the formant frequencies of the vocal tract acoustic output make it possible to infer articulatory behavior from the acoustic analysis, without need for direct examination of articulators such as the tongue.

REFERENCES

Arai, T. (2012). Education in acoustics and speech science using vocal-tract models. *Journal of the Acoustical Society of America*, 131, 2444–2454.

Berry, J. J. (2011). Accuracy of the NDI wave speech research system. *Journal of Speech, Language, and Hearing Research, 54*, 1295–1301.

Carré, R. (2004). From an acoustic tube to speech production. *Speech Communication, 42*, 227–240.

Chiba, T., & Kajiyama, M. (1941). *The vowel: Its nature and structure*. Tokyo, Japan: Tokyo-Kaiseikan.

Fant, G. (1960). *Acoustic theory of speech production*. The Hague, Netherlands: Mouton.

Fant, G. (1979). Glottal source and excitation analysis. *Speech Transmission Laboratory—Quarterly Progress and Status Report, 1*, 85–107.

Fant, G. (1982). Preliminaries to the analysis of the human voice source. *Speech Transmission Laboratory—Quarterly Progress and Status Report, 4*, 1–27.

Fant, G. (1986). Glottal flow: Models and interactions. *Journal of Phonetics, 14*, 393–399.

Farnsworth, D. (1940). High speed motion pictures of the human vocal cords. *Bell Laboratories Record, 18*, 203–208.

Flanagan, J. (1972). *Speech analysis, synthesis, and perception*. Berlin, Germany: Springer-Verlag.

Fridland, V. (2008). Patterns of /uw/, /ʊ/, and /ow/ fronting in Reno, Nevada. *American Speech, 83*, 432–454.

Fujimura, O., & Lindqvist, J. (1971). Sweep-tone measurements of vocal tract characteristics. *Journal of the Acoustical Society of America, 49*, 541–558.

Hanna, N., Smith, J., & Wolf, J. (2016), Frequencies, bandwidths, and magnitudes of vocal tract and surrounding tissue resonances, measured through the lips during phonation. *Journal of the Acoustical Society of America, 139*, 2924–2936.

Hoole, P., & Zierdt, A. (2010). Five-dimensional articulography. In B. Maasaen & P. van Lieshout (Eds.), *Speech motor control: New developments in basic and applied research* (pp. 331–349). Oxford, UK: Oxford University Press.

Iskarous, K. (2010). Vowel constrictions are recoverable from formants. *Journal of Phonetics, 38*, 375–387.

Kent, R. (1997). *The speech sciences*. San Diego, CA: Singular.

Kiefte, M., Enright, T., & Marshall, L. (2010). The role of formant amplitude in the perception of /i/ and /u/. *Journal of the Acoustical Society of America, 127*, 2611–2621.

Kiefte M., & Kluender, K. R. (2005). The relative importance of spectral tilt in monophthongs and diphthongs. *Journal of the Acoustical Society of America, 117*, 1395–1404.

Ladefoged, P., & Bladon, A. (1982). Attempts by human speakers to reproduce Fant's nomograms. *Speech Communication, 1*, 185–198.

Lammert, A. C., & Narayanan, S. S. (2015). On short-term estimation of vocal tract length from formant frequencies. *PLoS One, 10*, https://doi.org/10.1371/journal.pone.0132193

Lee, S., Potamianos, A., & Narayanan, S. (1999). Acoustics of children's speech: Developmental changes of temporal and spectral parameters. *Journal of the Acoustical Society of America, 105*, 1455–1468.

Perkell, J. S., Cohen, M. H., Svirsky, M. A., Matthies, M. L., Garabieta, I., & Jackson, M. T. (1992). Electromagnetic midsagittal articulometer systems for transducing speech articulatory movements. *Journal of the Acoustical Society of America, 92*, 3078–3096.

Stevens, K. (1989). On the quantal nature of speech. *Journal of Phonetics, 17*, 3–46.

Stevens, K. (1998). *Acoustic phonetics*. Cambridge, MA: MIT Press.

Stevens, K., & House, A. (1955). Development of a quantitative description of vowel articulation. *Journal of the Acoustical Society of America, 27*, 484–493.

Story, B. (2005). A parametric model of the vocal tract area function for vowel and consonant simulation. *Journal of the Acoustical Society of America, 117*, 3231–3254.

Story, B. H., & Bunton, K. (2017). An acoustically-driven vocal tract model for stop consonant production. *Speech Communication, 87*, 1–17.

9

Theory of Consonant Acoustics

INTRODUCTION

Chapter 8 showed how concepts from basic acoustics (Chapter 7) are used to construct a theory of vowel acoustics. The theory can be viewed as a combination of the following concepts: (a) input signals, (b) resonance and resonators, and (c) output signals. As stated in Chapter 8, the basic theory was presented for the case of vowels because the theory is most precise and accurate for this class of sounds. There is, however, an acoustic theory of *speech* production, not just vowel production. The purpose of this chapter is to establish the theoretical basis for the vocal tract acoustics of non-vowel sounds. Many of the concepts developed for the vowel theory are applicable in this chapter, but some new concepts, specific to the acoustics of consonants, are introduced. The following questions are addressed:

1. Why is the acoustic theory of speech production more accurate for vowels compared with consonants?
2. What are the acoustics of coupled resonators, and how do they apply to consonant acoustics?
3. What is the theory of fricative acoustics?
4. What is the theory of stop acoustics?
5. What is the theory of affricate acoustics?
6. What kinds of acoustic distinctions are associated with the voicing contrast for obstruents (stops, fricatives, and affricates)?

WHY IS THE ACOUSTIC THEORY OF SPEECH PRODUCTION MOST ACCURATE AND STRAIGHTFORWARD FOR VOWELS?

Table 9–1 lists several reasons why the acoustics of sound classes such as obstruents, nasals, and at least one semivowel require some elaboration of the theory outlined for vowels. First, the theory of vowel acoustics is relatively simple because the resonators can be described as extending from the source to lips within a single tube. The single tube, in this case, is the vocal tract, and the source is the vibrating vocal folds. There are sound classes, however, for which the single tube model is not adequate. For example, production of the nasal sounds /m/, /n/, and /ŋ/ involves two major

Table 9–1. Reasons Why the Acoustics of Obstruents, Nasals, and Some Semivowels Are Not Completely Covered by the Theory of Vowel Production Presented in Chapter 8

> 1. The production of nasals, laterals, and obstruents includes *coupled* resonator tubes, rather than the single-tube resonators of vowels. The acoustics of coupled, or *shunt*, resonators are different from the acoustics of single-tube resonators.
>
> 2. The important acoustic energy in vowels is located at frequencies below 4000 Hz, for which the wavelengths exceed the cross-sectional dimensions of the vocal tract. In this case, only plane waves propagate in the vocal tract, and the acoustics are easily related to the area function. Obstruent sounds have important energy at frequencies above 4000 Hz, where wavelengths are less than the cross-sectional dimensions of the vocal tract. In this case, the sound waves are more complex than planar and the area function does not completely describe the tube acoustics.
>
> 3. Vowels have a complex periodic source produced by vocal fold vibration, this source being located at one end of the single-tube resonator. Obstruents have aperiodic sources produced by air flowing through and against vocal tract structures. These sources may be located between resonant cavities of the vocal tract.

tubes—the pharyngeal-oral and nasal—which communicate with each other.[1] This arrangement, wherein a "shunt" or "sidebranch" resonator is attached to a main resonating tube, produces certain acoustic effects different from those associated with vowels.

Second, the important frequencies for vowels, which are below about 4000 Hz, have wavelengths considerably longer than the cross-sectional dimensions of the vocal tract. To make this statement more concrete, consider the cross-sectional areas of the vowel /i/ along the length of the vocal tract. In measurements reported by Fant (1960, p. 115), the cross-sectional areas of the vocal tract for /i/ ranged between 0.65 cm^2 (at the site of the front constriction) and 10.5 cm^2 (in the region of the relatively open pharynx). The F-pattern for /i/ reported by Fant (1960, p. 109) for a representative speaker is F1 = 240 Hz, F2 = 2250 Hz, and F3 = 3200 Hz. By applying the wavelength formula ($\lambda = c/f$) to these frequencies and assuming the speed of sound in air (c) to be 33,600 cm/s, $\lambda 1$ (wavelength for F1) = 140 cm, $\lambda 2$ = 14.9 cm, and $\lambda 3$ = 10.3 cm. Because the range of cross-sectional areas given above are far greater than the simple distances (i.e., radii) used to compute the areas, the wavelengths computed for the first three formants are clearly greater than the cross-sectional dimensions of the vocal tract for the vowel /i/. The importance of this fact is that, in the case of vowels, *sound waves travel through the vocal tract primarily as plane waves*. In other words, when the wavelengths of frequencies are greater than the cross-sectional dimensions of a tube such as the vocal tract, the pressure waves propagate along the long axis of the tube (from one end to the other), but not in other dimensions (such as from the center to the sides of the tube). When pressure waves are propagated mostly as plane waves, the area function of the tube can be used with great accuracy to predict the resonant frequencies of the tube.

At frequencies above 4000 Hz, many wavelengths are shorter than the cross-sectional dimensions of the vocal tract, and pressure wave propagation in the vocal tract is more complex. Correspondingly, the mathematics underlying the theory for cases in which wavelengths are smaller than the cross-sectional dimensions of the vocal tract are also more complex, and more prone to error. Many consonants—especially obstruents, which include stops, fricatives, and affricates—have substantial amounts of energy above 4000 Hz, so the theory is not as accurate for this class of sounds compared with vowels.

Finally, the theory of vowel acoustics includes a complex periodic source, described in Chapter 8. The spectrum of the voicing source is related in a straightforward way to the complex, periodic motions of the vocal folds. In obstruent consonants, however, many sources are aperiodic and depend on complex interactions between airflow and structures within the vocal tract. In addition, some sources for obstruents are located *between* resonant chambers of the vocal tract, rather than at one end of the vocal tract as in the case of vowels.

The first section of this chapter presents theoretical concepts required to understand coupled or "shunt" resonators. The next section discusses vocal tract aeromechanics in obstruent production, and their relationship to concepts from vowel acoustics. Subsequent sections cover points 2 and 3 in Table 9–1 and show how the acoustics of stops, fricatives, and affricates are logical consequences of aeromechanical events associated with the articulatory positions, configurations, and movements in obstruent production.

THE ACOUSTICS OF COUPLED (SHUNT) RESONATORS AND THEIR APPLICATION TO CONSONANT ACOUSTICS

The English nasals /m/, /n/, and /ŋ/ are produced with oral airway closure and an open velopharyngeal port. Because the oral closure involves a complete obstruction to airflow through the vocal tract, /m/, /n/, and /ŋ/ are sometimes called "nasal stop consonants." In fact, the place of complete closure for the three nasals is the same as the place of closure for the stops /b/, /d/, and /g/ (and cognates /p/, /t/, and /k/). Nasals are, therefore, like stop consonants produced with an open, rather than closed, velopharyngeal port. The interval during which the oral closure coincides with an open velopharyngeal port is referred to as the *nasal murmur*. This term is used to distinguish the acoustics of nasals produced with complete oral closure (the nasal murmur) from the acoustics of vowels produced with a somewhat open velopharyngeal port—that is, nasalized vowels. The theory of nasal murmurs is discussed first, followed by the more complex case of *nasalization*, the term used to describe the acoustic effect of coupled resonators with an open oral tract.

Nasal Murmurs

Figure 9–1 shows a schematic tube model of the vocal and nasal tracts during production of an /m/. The

---

[1]Chapter 4 contains detailed discussion of the double-barreled nature of the nasal cavities and its functional significance. Nevertheless, because the double-barreled nature is relatively inconsequential to the acoustic product, it is treated as a single tube in the present context.

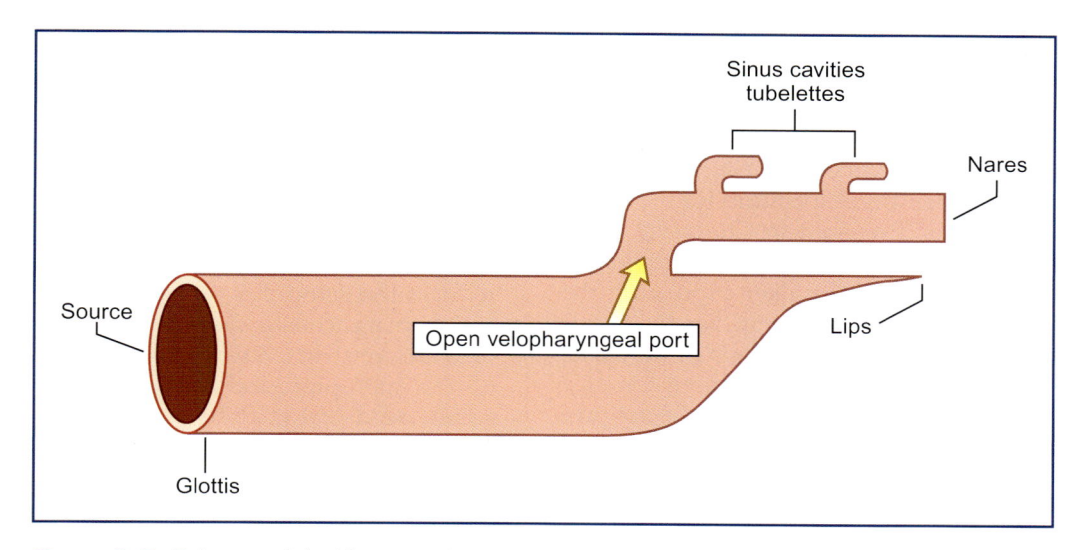

Figure 9–1. Tube model of the vocal tract with coupled resonators. The open velopharyngeal port couples the nasal and pharyngeal-oral cavities, and the sinus cavities are coupled to the nasal cavities. The front end of the tube, where the lips are located, is closed.

nasal tract part of this model is highly simplified and schematic for the purposes of this discussion; for beautiful computerized tomography (CT) and magnetic resonance images (MRI) of a human nasal tract, see Serrurier and Badin (2008), their Figure 6.

Several features of the model in Figure 9–1 are different from the vowel tube model discussed in Chapter 8. First, the lip end of the pharyngeal-oral tube is closed, consistent with labial closure for /m/. The rest of the pharyngeal-oral tube has been constricted roughly in the shape appropriate for the vowel /i/ (tight constriction in the front of the vocal tract, more open tube in the back). Second, the velopharyngeal port is open, also consistent with the production of /m/ or any other nasal sound. As shown in Figure 9–1, the open velopharyngeal port couples the pharyngeal-oral and nasal tracts. Tubes coupled in this way are referred to as *shunt resonators*, one of the resonators being a shunt, or diverging tube, relative to the other resonator. Third, additional shunt resonators are coupled to the nasal tract, shown as tubelettes communicating with the nasal cavities. These tubelettes represent the sinuses, which contribute in important ways to the acoustics of nasal sounds (Dang & Honda, 1996; Dang, Honda, & Suzuki, 1994). The source is located at the glottal end of the tube and has a harmonic spectrum produced by the vibrating vocal folds, just as in the production of vowels. All English nasals are produced as voiced sounds.

As in the case of vowels, the resonators shown in Figure 9–1 shape the spectrum of the source. When shaping the source spectrum for vowels, there are frequency regions at which sound transmission through the vocal tract is maximum. Those regions appear in both the theoretical (i.e., computed from the mathematical theory) and measured spectra as peaks, otherwise known as resonances or formants. The frequency regions between these spectral peaks, or spectral valleys, have substantially less energy than the resonances because the vocal tract shape does not emphasize energy in these regions. Although the reasoning in this last statement may sound circular, it serves to highlight the primary difference between theoretical and measured spectra of vowels on the one hand, and nasals on the other. In the case of the coupled (shunt) resonators shown in Figure 9–1, there are frequency regions where sound energy hits a kind of acoustic dead end, and is "trapped," thus producing *antiresonances*. For example, the closed oral tube shown in Figure 9–1 shapes a frequency region of the source spectrum, but that energy is "trapped" in the closed resonator. Energy may also be trapped in the smaller sinus resonators shown in Figure 9–1, because the sinus cavities are closed resonators. These regions of antiresonance, where energy is trapped because two or more tubes are coupled together and one or more of the tubes has a dead end, can be calculated based on resonator type and size, just as in the vowel theory. An antiresonance affects a measured spectrum in several ways, most notably by eliminating or reducing energy in its vicinity.

Because the nose is an acoustic tube open to the atmosphere at the nares, nasal murmurs have resonances (formants) related to the shape and size of the nasal passages. Antiresonances originate in the sinus cavities and the closed oral cavity. The nasal cavities extend from just behind the nasal septum to the outlet of the nasal cavities at the nares (Pruthi, Espy-Wilson,

& Story, 2007). Nasal sounds, therefore, have spectra consisting of a mix of resonances and antiresonances. The concept of an antiresonance is illustrated in Figure 9–2, which shows theoretical speech-sound spectra from Fant (1960) for a vowel (/ɑ/) and two nasals (/m/ and /n/). The theoretical spectrum for the vowel /ɑ/ was computed, as discussed in Chapter 8, from the estimated area function derived from a midsagittal x-ray tracing of a single speaker producing the sustained vowel. The theoretical spectra for the nasals were also estimated from area functions of the nasal cavities, but the process was somewhat more complex than the case for vowels. Sagittal x-rays could not produce a satisfactory image for the computation of nasal area functions, so Fant used a plastic model of the nasal cavities obtained from a cadaver, and adjusted this model to fit the dimensions of the single (live) speaker. The nasal area functions derived from this model were submitted to the mathematical theory that generated the nasal resonances and antiresonances resulting from the coupling of the nasal and pharyngeal-oral cavities. It should be noted that modern imaging techniques allow very accurate reconstructions of nasal and sinus cavity dimensions and, therefore, estimates of nasal cavity area functions (Dang & Honda, 1996; Dang et al., 1994; Serrurier & Badin, 2008).

The first three peaks in the theoretical vowel spectrum are shown clearly in Figure 9–2A. These peaks correspond to the first three formants of the vowel /ɑ/. Note how the peaks in this spectrum are *sharply tuned*, with relatively narrow bandwidths. Of special interest are the valleys of the computed resonance curve. The arrow on the vowel spectrum indicates a valley around 1800 Hz where the energy is nearly 40 dB less than the energy of the first peak. This is a substantial energy difference between the highest peak in the spectrum and the valley, but note that the valley develops between the second and third peaks in a relatively gradual way. Stated otherwise, the vowel spectrum does not show a sharply tuned, "upside-down" peak along its resonance curve. The valley in the vowel spectrum is partly the result of the decreasing energy in the source spectrum with increasing frequency (see Chapter 8), and partly the result of the close spacing of F1 and F2 for this vowel (see Fant, 1973, Chapter 1, for information on formant frequency spacing and formant intensity).

> **Of Mufflers, Heating Systems, and Nasals**
>
> The concept of shunt resonators is well known to engineers interested in noise reduction in cars, motorcycles, and heating systems. A shunt resonator traps energy at certain frequencies and reduces the amount of energy radiating (coming out) from an acoustic system. This is why car mufflers are constructed with multiple side branches off the main pipe, and heating ducts often have small, dead-end chambers off their main path. Although nasals don't "require" sound reduction, listeners seem to take advantage of it and use it as one cue that a nasal has been produced.

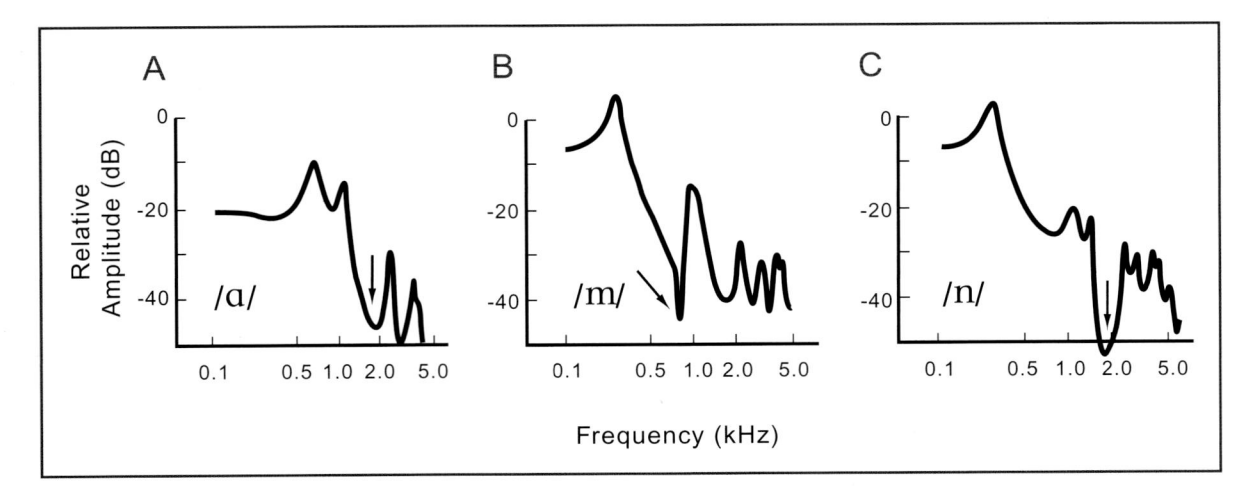

Figure 9–2. Computed spectra based on area functions, showing resonances for /ɑ/ (*panel A*) and resonances and antiresonances for two nasal murmur spectra /m/ (*panel B*) and /n/ (*panel C*). From *Acoustic Theory of Speech Production* (pp. 144, 153), by G. Fant, 1960, The Hague: Mouton. Copyright 1960 by Mouton de Gruyter. Modified and reproduced with permission.

> ### The Sinuses Are Helmholtz Resonators, Part I
>
> In a beautifully done experiment, Dang and Honda (1996) used MRI to measure the structural characteristics of the sphenoid, maxillary, and frontal sinuses in three participants. These characteristics included the volume of each sinus, as well as the dimensions of the small anatomical "tube" connecting the sinus cavity to the main nasal pathways. For each sinus volume, Dang and Honda computed a value for compliance, and for each connecting tube a value for inertance. They entered these values into the formula for Helmholtz resonators (see Chapter 7) and obtained the theoretical location of antiresonance frequencies for each sinus (remember: the sinuses are closed cavities). Then they compared the calculated antiresonance frequencies with actual measurements of antiresonances during the participants' production of nasals. The calculated and measured antiresonance frequencies matched within 10% of each other!

The theoretical spectrum for /m/ shows peaks, much like the vowel spectrum, but it also shows a reverse, or upside-down, peak. This sharply tuned reverse peak, which is indicated in Figure 9–2B by an arrow, occurs around 800 Hz and is the antiresonance that results from trapped acoustic energy in the closed pharyngeal-oral cavity. The antiresonance peak shows relatively sharp tuning, which distinguishes it from the broader valleys seen in vowel spectra. Fant (1960) showed that the frequency of this antiresonance is related to the size of the pharyngeal-oral cavity in which the acoustic energy is trapped. In other words, the frequency location of these reverse (negative) peaks is based on the same resonator rules as the frequency location of the positive peaks referred to as formants. Larger cavities yield antiresonances with lower frequencies; smaller cavities yield antiresonances with higher frequencies.

This latter point is made clear by examination of the theoretical spectrum for /n/ shown in Figure 9–2C. The reverse peak in this spectrum—the antiresonance—is located just below 2000 Hz (see arrow), which is substantially higher than the 800 Hz antiresonance for /m/. Based on the relation of resonator size to frequency, the different frequency locations for the antiresonances of /m/ versus /n/ make sense. The cavity in which acoustic energy is trapped for /m/ is substantially larger than the cavity in which energy is trapped for /n/. The reasoning extends to the case of the velar nasal /ŋ/, for which the point of constriction may result in an extremely small cavity behind the constriction made by the tongue dorsum against the posterior end of the hard palate or anterior end of the soft palate. When the coupled cavity is extremely small, the antiresonance associated with the oral cavity is located at a relatively high frequency, probably well above 3000 Hz. The absence of a coupled cavity, and hence a cavity in which acoustic energy can be trapped, occurs if the point of constriction for the velar nasal is sufficiently posterior in the vocal tract so that the pharyngeal and nasal cavities appear as a single tube with no side branches. In this case, there may be no oral antiresonance, but a pattern of resonances determined by the configuration of the continuous pharyngeal-nasal tube.[2] Midsagittal tracings of vocal tract configurations for /m/, /n/, and relatively anterior and posterior constrictions for /ŋ/, adapted from Fant (1960), are shown in Figure 9–3 to summarize these concepts of sidebranch resonance and coupled cavity size. Dashed outlines show the size of the closed pharyngeal-oral cavity in which energy is trapped. The absence of a cavity indicated by a dashed outline, in the right-hand vocal tract of Figure 9–3, is the case of an extremely posterior point of constriction for /ŋ/.

Although this discussion has focused on the antiresonance feature of the nasal murmur spectra shown in Figure 9–2, nasal murmurs have prominent resonances. In Figures 9–2B and 9–2C, the first peak in the nasal murmur spectra for both /m/ and /n/ occurs roughly between 250 Hz and 300 Hz and has a relatively high amplitude. According to Fant (1960), the first resonance of the velar nasal /ŋ/ also occurs in this frequency region. This relatively high-amplitude, low-frequency (250–300 Hz) formant can be considered a constant feature of all nasals. The high amplitude of the first nasal resonance is greater than the amplitudes of higher-frequency nasal resonances, but typically of lesser amplitude compared with formant amplitudes of vowels preceding or following a nasal murmur, as in a vowel-consonant-vowel (VCV) sequence in which C is a nasal murmur (see Chapter 11). The constancy across nasals of the first nasal

---

[2]Even with an /ŋ/ constriction that is sufficiently posterior to eliminate any coupling between the oral and nasal cavities, there may be antiresonances in the spectrum because of the sinuses, which function like resonators coupled to the nasal cavities (i.e., sidebranch resonators to the nasal cavities). Dang and Honda (1996) have made direct measurements of the frequencies of the sinus antiresonances. Their results suggest that the sinuses contribute antiresonances within the 500 to 1000 Hz region.

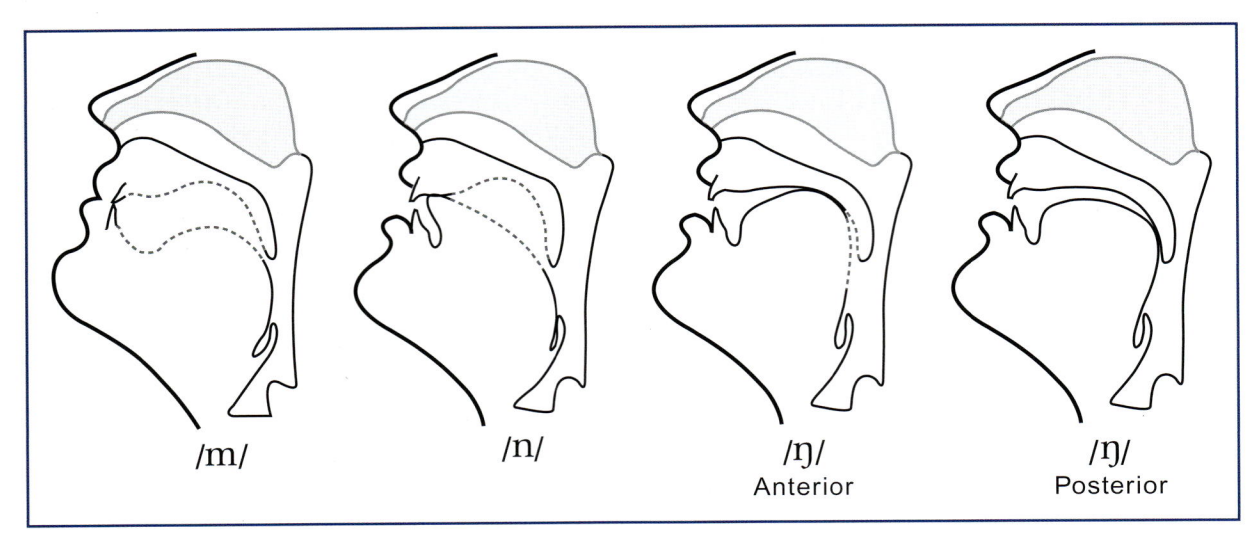

Figure 9-3. Midsagittal tracings of the vocal tract for /m/, /n/, and /ŋ/. The two right-hand vocal tracts show a relatively anterior and a relatively posterior constriction for /ŋ/, respectively. The size of the coupled oral cavity in the first three vocal tracts is enclosed by the dashed lines. The size of this cavity is largest for /m/, somewhat smaller for /n/, and very small for /ŋ/ when the constriction is anterior. There is no dashed line in the rightmost vocal tract because the extreme posterior point of constriction does not permit coupling between the oral and nasal cavities. In this case, the pharynx and nasal cavities act as a continuous, single-tube resonator. From *Acoustic Theory of Speech Production* (p. 140), by G. Fant, 1960, The Hague: Mouton. Copyright 1960 by Mouton de Gruyter. Modified and reproduced with permission.

resonance, or F1 of the nasal murmur, suggests that it originates in cavities of the same size for all murmurs. The combined pharyngeal and nasal cavities are the constant resonators across nasal murmurs. In people with a structurally intact speech production apparatus, there are typically no time-varying constrictions of the nasal cavities—the nasal tract does not change shape during speech production, as does the oral tract. Similarly, the shape of the pharyngeal section of the vocal tract is fairly constant across different places of articulation for nasal murmurs. The effect of this constant tube shape of the pharyngeal-nasal cavities is the production of a low-frequency formant that is an acoustic "signature" of a nasal murmur. In addition to this low F1, nasal murmurs have a series of higher formants occurring roughly at 1000 Hz (nasal F2), 2000 Hz (nasal F3), 3000 Hz (nasal F4), and so on. These upper formants of the nasal murmur, however, tend to be quite sensitive to surrounding phonetic context and are variable across speakers (Fujimura, 1962).

Energy Loss in the Nasal Cavities, Antiresonances, and the Relative Amplitude of Nasal Murmurs

The resonances generated by the nasal tract tend to have greater bandwidths than the resonances of a typical vowel spectrum. In Chapter 8, the factors of absorption, friction, radiation, and gravity were identified as sources of energy loss in the transmission of sound through the vocal tract and into the atmosphere. The wider bandwidths of nasal resonances are largely accounted for by high absorption factors in the nasal cavities. These high absorption factors are related to the extensive surface area within the nasal cavities, which contain many complicated folds and recesses. There is more tissue to absorb sound in the nasal cavities than there is in the vocal tract. Because of this, the damping of nasal resonances, as revealed by the bandwidths of nasal formants, tends to be greater than the damping of oral (vowel) resonances.

The combined effects of an antiresonance and the relatively greater damping of nasal resonances tend to make nasal murmurs weak in relative amplitude compared with vowels (Pruthi & Espy-Wilson, 2004). Antiresonances not only eliminate energy at the exact frequency location of their "reversed peaks," but also reduce energy at surrounding frequencies. Increased damping results in less intense resonant peaks. Because the overall amplitude of a sound can be thought of as the sum of all energy along the resonance curve (i.e., the sum of all amplitudes at all frequencies in a spectrum), speech sounds with antiresonances and increased damping, such as nasals, naturally have less overall amplitude than sounds such as vowels that do not have antiresonances and have minimal damping.

Nasal Murmurs: A Summary

A *nasal murmur* is defined as the sound produced when the velopharyngeal port is open and there is a complete obstruction to the oral airstream. This description encompasses the sound class of English nasal consonants transcribed as /m/, /n/, and /ŋ/. In the production of nasal murmurs, two major tubes are coupled: the nasal tube, which is open to the atmosphere, and the oral tube, which is completely sealed from the atmosphere by articulatory closure. The sealed oral tube shapes the source spectrum according to its resonator size, but the energy shaped by that tube is trapped because its outlet to the atmosphere is closed. This results in an antiresonance, or a reverse peak in the spectrum. The sinus cavities coupled to the nasal tract also function as closed resonators and contribute antiresonances to the spectrum of a nasal murmur. Antiresonances affect a measured spectrum by reducing or eliminating energy at and around the frequency of the reversed peak. The energy in the spectrum of a nasal murmur is also reduced because of the relatively high damping of nasal formants that results from absorption of sound by the extensive tissue surface area in the nasal cavities. Whereas antiresonances are an important characteristic of nasal murmurs, there are also resonances of the nasal cavities, the most important of which is a low-frequency formant between 250 and 300 Hz. This formant frequency is relatively constant for the three nasals of English, because the pharyngeal and nasal cavities responsible for the formant do not change shape across different places of articulation. Higher formants for nasal murmurs can be measured as well, with F2 at approximately 1000 Hz, and upper nasal formants (F3, F4, etc.) at 1000 Hz intervals (F2 = 2000 Hz, F3 = 3000 Hz, and so forth). These formants reflect resonances of the nasal cavities.

Nasalization

The acoustic theory of nasalization has many similarities to the theory of nasal murmurs but is somewhat more complicated. As in nasal murmurs, the pharyngeal-oral and nasal airways are coupled, but in the case of nasalization both tracts are open to atmosphere. The overall output of the vocal tract for nasalized vowels represents a mixture of the resonant characteristics of the nasal and pharyngeal-oral cavities, as well as the effects of their coupling.

When the nasal and pharyngeal-oral airways are coupled, with both open to atmosphere, sound waves propagate through both airways and radiate from the mouth and nares. Each of these tracts has resonant characteristics dependent on the size of the cavities (and, hence, the inertance and compliance of the air in those cavities). The oral resonances are roughly, but not exactly (see below), the same as when the nasal cavities are not coupled to the pharyngeal-oral cavities. Thus, one major effect of coupling the nasal to the pharyngeal-oral cavity during vowel production is the addition of resonances from the nasal cavities to resonances of the vocal tract.

Another effect of coupling the oral and nasal cavities is the addition of antiresonances into the spectrum. In nasalized vowels, antiresonances are the result of energy trapped in the paranasal sinuses (Dang et al., 1994; Havel, Hoffman, Mürbe, & Sundberg, 2014; Stevens, Fant, & Hawkins, 1987). The main antiresonance in nasalized vowels occurs at a relatively low frequency, between 300 Hz and 1000 Hz. Interestingly, the primary *resonance* of the nasal cavities also occurs in this frequency region, as does the first formant (F1) of most non-nasal vowels. Nasalized vowels, therefore, contain a low-frequency spectrum (~300–1000 Hz) having a nasal resonance, an antiresonance, and a pharyngeal-oral resonance (the F1 of the oral vowel). For several writers (Hawkins & Stevens, 1985; Stevens et al., 1987), this resonance-antiresonance-resonance pattern in the region around F1 of the oral vowel is the defining acoustic feature of nasalization.

The low-frequency spectra of four nasalized and non-nasalized vowels are shown in Figure 9–4. Each panel shows the energy level, in relative amplitude (dB), across a frequency range of 0 Hz to 1300 Hz. The "zero" point on the dB scale is arbitrary. The blue curve in each panel shows the spectrum for the non-nasalized vowel and the red curve shows the spectrum for the nasalized version of the vowel. The articulatory difference between non-nasalized and nasalized vowels is the configuration of the velopharyngeal port. For non-nasalized vowels, the port is closed, whereas for nasalized vowels, the port is open.[3] For the vowel /ɑ/ in Figure 9–4 there are peaks in the non-nasalized spectrum (blue curve) at roughly 680 Hz and 1100 Hz, and

---

[3]This statement may or may not be absolutely true. It is possible that the shape of the vocal tract is slightly different for the same vowel produced with the velopharyngeal port open (nasalized vowel) versus closed. The relevant research has not (as far as the authors know) been done (but see the computer modeling work by Pruthi, Espy-Wilson, & Story, 2007; and Rong & Kuehn, 2010).

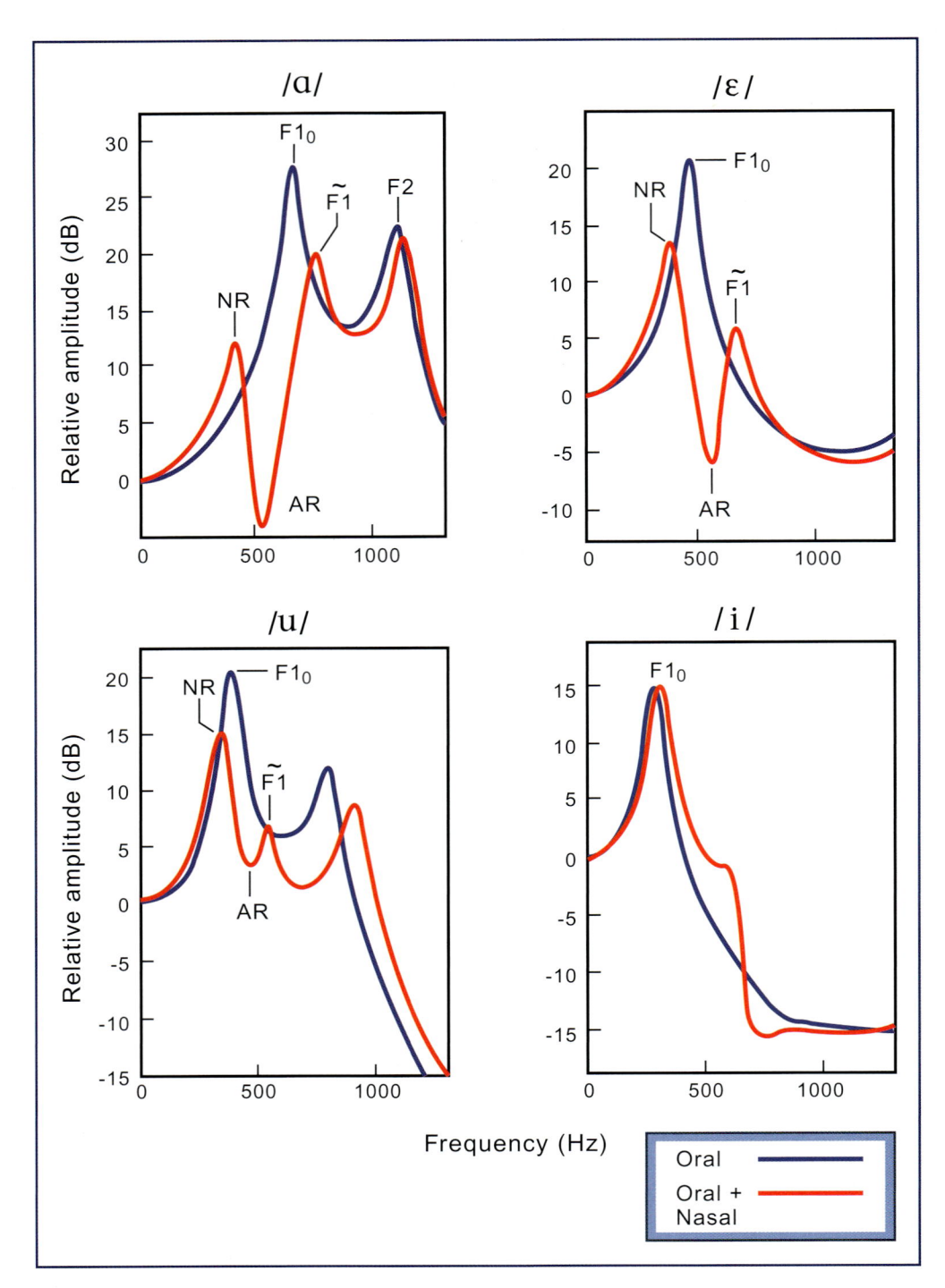

Figure 9–4. Spectra for the vowels /ɑ/, /ɛ/, /u/, and /i/ for non-nasalized (*blue curves*) and nasalized (*red curves*) productions. Frequency is plotted between 0 and 1300 Hz on the x-axis and relative amplitude, in dB, is plotted on the ordinate. NR = nasal resonance. AR = antiresonance. $F1_o$ = F1 of non-nasalized vowel. $\tilde{F1}$ = F1 of nasalized vowel. For each vowel except /i/, there is a nasal resonance-antiresonance-F1 pattern in the nasalized spectra. In the case of /i/, the nasal resonance is canceled by the antiresonance because of the small coupling (small velopharyngeal port opening) between the oral and nasal cavities. From "Some acoustical and perceptual correlates of nasal vowels," by K. Stevens, G. Fant, and S. Hawkins in *In Honor of Ilse Lehiste* (p. 246), edited by R. Channon and L. Shockey, 1987, Dordrecht, Netherlands: Foris. Copyright 1987 by Foris. Modified and reproduced with permission.

the absence of sharply tuned reversed peaks (antiresonances). The frequency location of the peaks is consistent with the typical F1 and F2 values observed in /ɑ/ spectra of adult males. The label F1$_o$ indicates the first oral resonance (i.e., the first formant) of the non-nasalized vowel. The spectrum for the nasalized /ɑ/ (that is, /ɑ̃/: red curve) shows oral peaks in roughly the same location as the F1$_o$ and F2 peaks of the non-nasalized spectrum, but the nasalized peaks are at somewhat higher frequencies than the non-nasalized peaks; this is especially the case for $\widetilde{F1}$ compared with F1$_o$. Note the label $\widetilde{F1}$ indicating the location of the first oral resonance for /ɑ̃/.

The /ɑ̃/ spectrum is different from the /ɑ/ (non-nasalized) spectrum in several ways. First, $\widetilde{F1}$ has lower amplitude than F1$_o$. There is also an amplitude difference for the two F2 peaks (around 1100 Hz), but not of the same magnitude. Second, there is an antiresonance, labeled AR on the graph, just above 500 Hz in the /ɑ̃/ spectrum. This antiresonance is a result of the coupling of the sinus cavities to the pharyngeal-oral and nasal cavities. The antiresonance also accounts for the relatively low amplitude of $\widetilde{F1}$ compared with F1$_o$. Recall that antiresonances reduce energy at and around their frequency locations. The location of the antiresonance, just above 500 Hz, is close enough to the F1 of /ɑ̃/ to have a substantial effect on its amplitude. Third, there is a low-amplitude peak in the nasalized spectrum, around 400 Hz, that is not present in the non-nasalized spectrum. This is the primary resonance of the nasal tract, labeled NR. This nasal resonance mixes with the oral resonances and is seen clearly in the output spectrum of a nasalized vowel.

The resonance-antiresonance-resonance pattern in /ɑ̃/, therefore, consists of the nasal tract resonance (NR) around 400 Hz, the antiresonance (AR) just above 500 Hz, and the F1 around 700 Hz. This general pattern is seen for other nasalized vowels, with variations that depend on vowel identity. Note for the vowels /ɑ̃/, /ɛ̃/, and /ũ/ how $\widetilde{F1}$ is shifted up in frequency relative to F1$_o$, as well as the lower amplitude of $\widetilde{F1}$ compared with F1$_o$. In each of these cases, the antiresonance resulting from the coupling of sinus cavities to the pharyngeal-oral and nasal cavities reduces the amplitude of the first oral resonance. Also noteworthy is the consistent frequency of the nasal resonance (NR) for the vowels /ɑ̃/, /ɛ̃/, and /ũ/. This consistency has the same explanation as the consistent nasal resonance in nasal murmurs. The area function of the pharyngo-nasal tract does not change substantially during speech production, and therefore neither do its resonances.

The non-nasalized and nasalized spectra shown in Figure 9–4 for /i/ seem to violate these acoustic principles of nasalization. No antiresonance (AR) is indicated, nor is there a nasal resonance (NR). The absence of the resonance-antiresonance-resonance pattern in the /ĩ/ spectrum can be attributed to the small amount of coupling between the pharyngeal-oral and nasal cavities for this vowel. It is well known that the size of the velopharyngeal port in nasalized vowels is greater for low and mid-vowels (such as /ɑ/ and /ɛ/) than it is for the high vowel /i/ (Bell-Berti, 1993). Stated in acoustic terms, the coupling between the pharyngeal-oral and nasal cavities is greater for low and mid-vowels than it is for high vowels such as /i/. When the coupling between the pharyngeal-oral and nasal cavities is small, the nasal resonance (NR) and the antiresonance (AR) have essentially the same frequency. A resonance and antiresonance associated with the same cavity and therefore the same resonant

---

The Sinuses Are Helmholtz Resonators, Part II

Yes, the locations and shapes of the sinus cavities are fixed inside your head and yes, they are relatively far from the action where articulatory changes modify the area function of the vocal tract. The sinuses are even relatively far from the ever-changing area of the velopharyngeal port. It might be assumed, then, that for a given person the (anti)resonant frequencies of these sinus resonators contribute in a fixed way to the spectrum of a nasalized vowel: their acoustic consequences would seem to be above the fray of the acoustic consequences of moving the tongue, jaw, velum, and so forth. Not so, according to Pruthi, Espy-Wilson, and Story (2007), who combined MRI measurements of the vocal and nasal tracts with electrical modeling analysis to show that for nasalized vowels, the precise frequencies of antiresonances originating in the sinus cavities change with changes in the vocal tract area function, as well as with the degree of openness at the velopharyngeal port! Interestingly, sinus (anti)resonant frequencies are not affected by different places of articulation for nasal murmurs—they are constant. But the hypernasality of dissatisfaction is basically a vowel thing, so the next time you are asked to stop complaining, nod knowingly and state that whining is acoustically complex, as are you.

> ### More to Vowels Than Meets the Ear
>
> How are vowels distinguished in a language? Well, according to tongue height, tongue advancement, and lip configuration, right? Actually, a more precise answer is yes but not absolutely. In their 1996 book, *The Sounds of the World's Languages*, the great phoneticians Peter Ladefoged (1925–2006) and Ian Maddieson described and discussed "minor features of vowel quality," meaning vowel differences involving contrasts of (for example) voice quality and nasalization. Among the several "minor" contrasts in vowel quality discussed by Ladefoged and Maddieson, the opposition between an oral vowel and its nasalized counterpart (/i/ vs. /ĩ/, for example, as in French or Portuguese) is said to be the most common among languages of the world.

frequency but with different signs cancel each other and their effects are not seen in the output spectrum. The absence of a nasal resonance and antiresonance in the /ĩ/ spectrum is a result of this cancellation. The lack of effect of an antiresonance on F1 for /ĩ/ is apparent in the nearly identical amplitudes of $F1_o$ and $\tilde{F1}$.

The specific acoustic characteristics of nasalized vowels depend very much on precisely which vowel is nasalized. In a study employing a computer-implemented, electrical model of the vocal and nasal tracts plus the sinuses, "equivalent" coupling of the oral and nasal tracts for high and low vowels (that is, the same area of opening of the velopharyngeal port for high and low vowels) produced very different changes in the low-frequency spectrum of the respective vowels (Rong & Kuehn, 2010). This indicates an acoustic interaction between the size of the velopharyngeal port and vocal tract configuration for a vowel. An appropriate response to the question of how an open velopharyngeal port changes the formant and antiresonance characteristics of the nasalized vowel spectrum requires a question in return: Which vowel are you asking about? (A similar result was reported by Pruthi, Espy-Wilson, & Story, 2007.)

Nasalization: A Summary

Nasalization is the term used to describe the production of vowels with an open velopharyngeal port. The acoustic theory of nasalization differs from the theory of nasal murmurs because in the former the oral airway is open, whereas in the latter the oral airway is closed. The primary acoustic effects of nasalization are seen in the frequency range between 0 and 1000 Hz and include: (a) the introduction of an "extra" resonance from the nasal tract, usually in the 300 to 500 Hz region; (b) an antiresonance located at a slightly higher frequency than the nasal tract resonance, probably due to trapping of energy in the paranasal sinus cavities, which act as sidebranch resonators to the main nasal cavities; and (c) a first oral resonance ($\tilde{F1}$), which may be slightly higher in frequency and of lesser amplitude than the non-nasalized F1 ($F1_o$). The reduction of $\tilde{F1}$ amplitude is due to the nearby antiresonance. Because of the reduction in $\tilde{F1}$ amplitude, nasalized vowels typically have less overall amplitude than corresponding non-nasalized vowels.

The Importance of Understanding Nasalization

Why is nasalization important? (see Stevens et al., 1987). First, when English vowels are articulated either before or after nasals, some portion of the vowel is produced with an open velopharyngeal port. Even though the vowels of English are described as non-nasal and, therefore, are specified as having a closed velopharyngeal port, the open velopharyngeal port required for the nasal consonant will "spread" an acoustic effect to adjacent vowels. This spreading of articulatory (and, therefore, acoustic) characteristics from one segment to another is called *coarticulation*, as discussed in Chapter 5. The open velopharyngeal port for the nasal murmur cannot be closed instantaneously for the articulation of a following vowel. Thus, a vowel following a nasal consonant is nasalized for a brief time, during which the output of the vocal tract reflects the effects of combined oral and nasal acoustics. Similarly, a vowel preceding a nasal consonant is nasalized for a certain interval when the velopharyngeal port is opened prior to the oral articulation of the nasal murmur. This opening of the velopharyngeal port during the vowel is often thought to reflect anticipation of the articulatory requirements of the nasal murmur. Even though there is no contrast in English between nasalized and non-nasalized vowels, these coarticulatory effects may serve as important cues to the phonetic perception of an upcoming nasal consonant.

The second reason for understanding nasalization is suggested by the closing statement of the preceding paragraph. Whereas English does not have a *phonemic* opposition for nasalized and non-nasalized vowels, such contrasts are phonemic in languages such as French and Hindi (a language spoken in northern India). A comprehensive theory of speech acoustics should be able to explain the acoustic basis of sound systems for many (if not all) languages of the world (see Sidetrack, "More to Vowels Than Meets the Ear").

A third reason for considering an acoustic theory of nasalization is the more practical one of children and adults with structural or neurological disorders that prevent the decoupling of the pharyngeal-oral and nasal cavities in speech production. Craniofacial anomalies, seen in many different syndromes, often involve structural deficits of the velopharyngeal port area which make velopharyngeal closure inadequate or impossible. Many neurological diseases cause *dysarthria*, which affects the ability of muscles of the speech apparatus to function properly. A typical sign in many cases of dysarthria is chronic or intermittent hypernasality, sometimes similar to that seen in craniofacial anomalies. Regardless of the cause of inadequate or absent velopharyngeal closure, the effect is the same: the chronic or intermittent nasalization of vowels (as well as additional effects on consonant production and acoustics). Speech-language pathologists should know the theory of nasalization as part of their basic scientific knowledge and as a foundation for diagnostic, prognostic, and management plans and statements. A speech-language pathologist who understands the acoustics of nasalization is able to provide a coherent account to other health care professionals, such as physicians, as to why the speech of a child with a repaired cleft palate but lingering velopharyngeal inadequacy produces "muffled" and soft speech. As a further example of how speech acoustics theory can inform clinical practice, recent theoretical work of Rong and Kuehn (2010) has shown how the acoustic results of nasalizing a vowel may be compensated by adjustments of the oral cavity. Rong and Kuehn (2010) used modeling techniques—very similar to the techniques used by Stevens and House, described in Chapter 8, except with the electrical circuits implemented by computer software—to show that nasal formants and antiresonances may be minimized or even eliminated by proper adjustments of the oral articulators. Rong and Kuehn's work suggests the possibility of speech-language pathologists teaching a child to modify oral postures to offset chronic or intermittent nasalization effects.

Coupled (Shunt) Resonators in the Production of Lateral Sounds

Figure 9–5A shows a tracing from a midsagittal x-ray of a speaker producing an /l/. Note the contact of the tongue apex at the alveolar ridge (arrow). Behind this contact, MRI data have shown the front part of the tongue to be somewhat grooved and the tongue dorsum raised very close to the soft palate. This tongue configuration has two parallel air passageways, one on either side of the midline of the vocal tract (Narayanan, Alwan, & Haker, 1997). This type of /l/ production is referred to as a *lateral* manner of articulation, to denote the articulatory configuration just described and hence the propagation of sound waves through the lateral passageways.[4] The cavity immediately behind the apical closure, however, traps sound energy at frequencies determined by the size of the closed resonator and therefore introduces an antiresonance into the /l/ spectrum. The cavity behind the apical closure can be considered a shunt resonator, in much the same way as described above for nasals.

The antiresonance in lateralized /l/ spectra derives from the cavity extending from the apical closure to the uvula, as indicated in the x-ray tracing of Figure 9–5A by the horizontal line ending in short vertical bars. Figure 9–5B shows the computed (theoretical) and measured spectra for an articulatory configuration like that shown in Figure 9–5A. If the spectra shown by the solid (theoretical) and dashed (measured) lines are compared, both show roughly the same frequency location of the antiresonance (*AR*), or reverse peak. This antiresonance occurs between 1800 and 2000 Hz and produces a substantial "dip" in the spectrum between the second and third formants. The antiresonance probably has the greatest effect on the amplitude of F3, which is quite low in both the theoretical and measured /l/ spectra in Figure 9–5B.

Coupled (Shunt) Resonators in the Production of Obstruent Sounds

Shunt resonators also occur in obstruent production. For all sounds considered so far (vowels, nasals, laterals), the theory involves a voicing source located at the back (glottis) end of the vocal tract tube. The production of obstruents, however, involves a source of sound located *between* two resonating cavities. For example, in the production of /ʃ/ there is a noise (aperiodic) source generated near the supraglottal constriction. An MRI of a speaker producing an /ʃ/ is shown in Figure 9–6. The lips are to the right of the image and the air-filled cavities are shown as illuminated passageways. The /ʃ/ constriction is indicated by an arrow, and in and

---

[4]The articulatory configurations for /l/ may not conform to the lateral description given here. For example, word-final /l/ (as in the words *bowl* and *heel*) is often produced with a retracted tongue and no contact with the alveolar ridge (the "dark /l/" discussed in many phonetics textbooks). Some dialects use the lateralized version of /l/ more often than do other dialects.

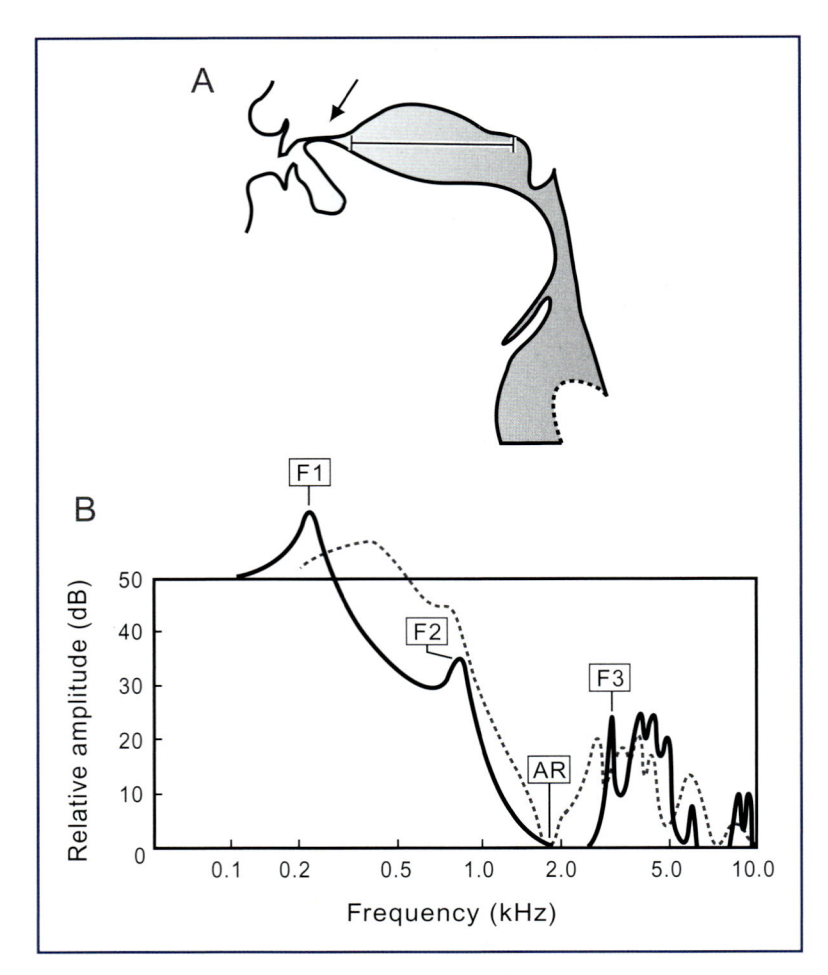

Figure 9–5. A. Midsagittal x-ray tracing of a lateral /l/ production. The contact of the tongue apex to the alveolar ridge is indicated by an arrow. The cavity where energy is trapped, thus introducing an antiresonance into the /l/ spectrum, is indicated by the horizontal line ending in short vertical bars. **B.** Theoretical (*solid line*) and measured (*dotted line*) spectra for lateralized /l/. Note the antiresonance (AR) in the region 1800 to 2000 Hz in both the theoretical and measured spectra. F1, F2, and F3 are indicated on the theoretical spectrum. From *Acoustic Theory of Speech Production* (pp. 163, 165), by G. Fant, The Hague: Mouton. Copyright 1960 by Mouton de Gruyter. Modified and reproduced with permission.

near this constriction a source of frication energy is generated (see below for more details on frication sources). Just as the vibrating vocal folds produce a spectrum shaped by the vocal tract resonators, the /ʃ/ noise source has its spectrum shaped by the vocal tract. Even though the /ʃ/ noise source sits roughly between two resonators—the cavity in front of the constriction (Figure 9–6, "front cavity") and the cavity behind the constriction (Figure 9–6, "back cavity")—both cavities contribute to the vocal tract output because sound waves propagate away from the source in both directions (forward and backward). Because the back cavity is effectively closed, it traps energy at frequencies determined by its size and generates an antiresonance. The back cavity acts as a coupled or shunt resonator in the production of /ʃ/, and its antiresonance has an influence on the shape of the output spectrum. These kinds of coupled or shunt resonators are seen in the production of fricatives, stops, and affricates, as discussed more fully in the next section.

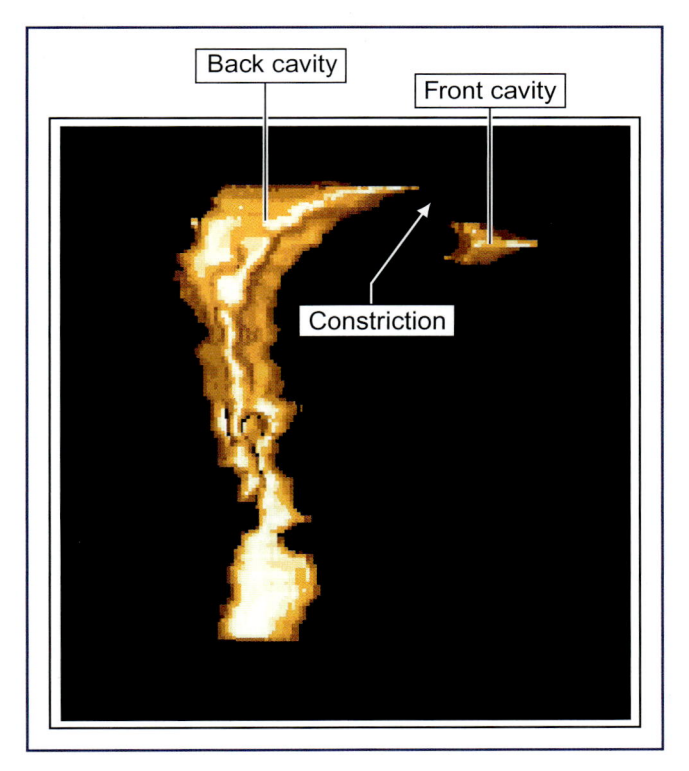

Figure 9–6. Midsagittal MRI of a speaker's vocal tract in the articulatory configuration for /ʃ/. The arrow indicates the /ʃ/ constriction, which is one location of the noise source whose spectrum is shaped by the front and back cavities. The back cavity is effectively a closed resonator and is a coupled, or shunt, resonator, contributing an antiresonance to the /ʃ/ spectrum. Image provided courtesy of Brad Story, PhD, University of Arizona, Tucson. Reproduced with permission.

WHAT IS THE THEORY OF FRICATIVE ACOUSTICS?

Special features of fricatives make the theory of fricative acoustics different from those of the sounds discussed thus far. These features can be understood by considering the general nature of fluid flow in pipes, and how different conditions within a pipe may change the nature of the flow and its acoustic results.

Fluid Flow in Pipes and Source Types

As mentioned above, obstruents are produced with a noise source, usually located in the vicinity of the major constriction or at the point where an obstacle (e.g., the teeth) interrupts airflow within the vocal tract. These noise sources are aperiodic (unlike the periodic voicing source) and can be related to patterns of airflow in the vicinity of the major constrictions or obstacles. In cases where the obstruent is voiced (such as a /b/, /z/, or /dʒ/), the voicing source may occur simultaneously with the vocal tract noise source. This case of *mixed sources* is discussed more fully in a later section of this chapter.

An understanding of aperiodic noise sources requires some background information on how patterns of airflow in tubes are modified at constrictions along the path of flow. Figure 9–7 shows a tube in which air molecules are flowing, as indicated by the parallel arrows. The arrowheads show the direction of the flow. Air is flowing through the tube because there is a *pressure differential* between the two ends of the tube. Air flows from regions of higher pressure to regions of lower pressure, so the movement of air molecules from left to right implies that $P1$ is greater than Pr (where r means "reference," in the present case atmospheric pressure). The pressure differential $P1 - Pr$ is assumed to be constant for the remainder of this discussion.

When air molecules flow through a tube in parallel streams, as shown in Figure 9–7, the flow is referred to as *laminar*. If the air flowing within the tube is not compressed as it moves from one end of the tube to the other, the air volume flowing past any one point in the tube per unit of time must be equivalent to the air volume flowing past any other point in the tube in the same unit of time. "Volume" can be interpreted as an amount, such as one might place in a container. It is typically measured in liters (L) (like milk, soda, or any other fluid, air being a fluid).

Consider the tube shown in Figure 9–7 and imagine two volume-measuring instruments, one placed at a wide section of the tube (M1) and the other at a narrow section (M2). According to the law stated above, the volume of air moving past M1 in 1 s must equal the volume moving past M2 in the same time interval. Although the measurement instruments are shown at single points along the tube, the volume is measured by "accumulating" the flow past the points over a fixed time period (in the current example, 1 sec). The only way to get the same volume per unit time through a narrow section of the tube (at M2) as through a wide section of the tube (at M1) is for the speed of the air molecules to be greater through M2. Thus, air molecules flowing through a tube speed up as they move through a constriction.

Figure 9–8 reproduces the essential features of Figure 9–7 and adds two new phenomena with direct relevance to obstruent production, including the immediate case of fricatives. First, the flowing air molecules

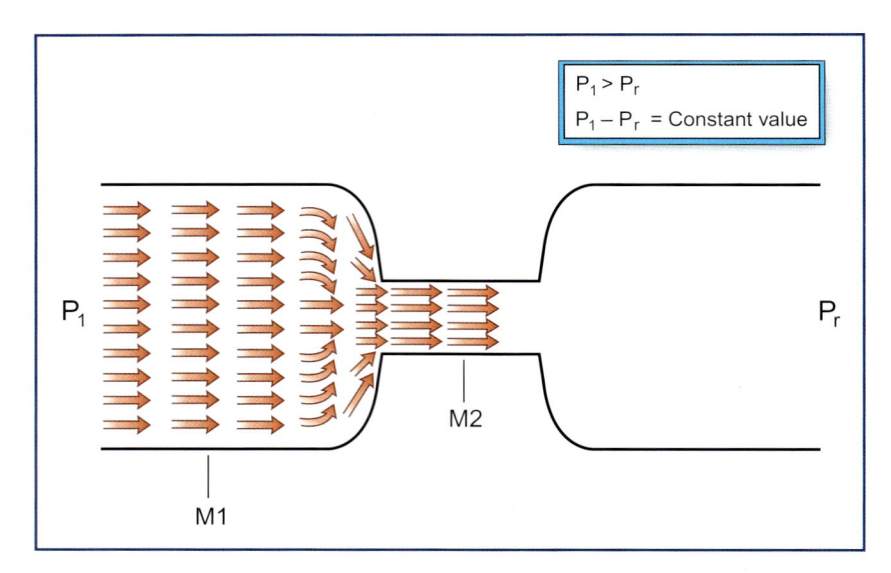

Figure 9–7. Laminar airflow within a tube. Laminar airflow is indicated by the parallel lines ending in arrowheads. Because pressure at the left of the tube (P_1) is greater than pressure at the right of the tube (P_r), air flows from left to right, toward the lower pressure. M1 indicates a measuring device placed at a relatively wide part of the tube and M2 indicates a measuring device placed at a relatively constricted part of the tube.

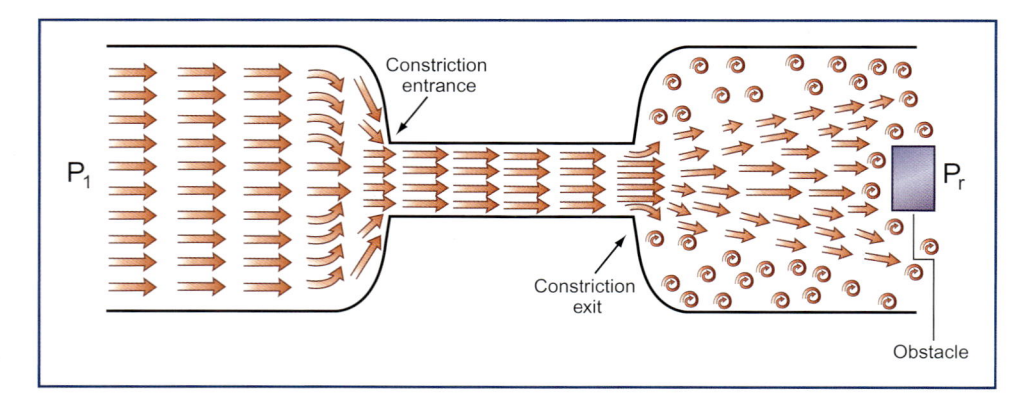

Figure 9–8. Air flowing in a tube, as in Figure 9–7. This tube has a very narrow constriction through which air is forced by a pressure differential across the two ends of the tube. Parallel lines indicate laminar airflow. Laminar airflow emerges from the constriction as a narrow jet, at the edges of which are rotating, erratically moving air molecules called turbulent flow. An obstacle is in front of the constriction and in the path of the airflow. When the laminar jet strikes the obstacle, air molecules move erratically and create additional turbulent airflow.

are shown both entering and exiting the constriction. Second, the flowing air molecules are shown striking a small rectangular obstacle, near the right-hand end of the tube.

As the air molecules enter the constriction they undergo an increase in speed. These fast-moving molecules "shoot out" of the constriction exit in the form of a narrow stream or *jet* which expands as it moves downstream, toward the end of the tube. The jet of air emerges from the constriction as a group of narrowly focused parallel lines. Figure 9–8 shows circular motions of air molecules along the edges of the jet. This circular flow pattern, which is different from the parallel streaming of laminar flow, is called *turbulent flow*, or *turbulence*. When a constriction is narrow enough and the flow through it is sufficiently rapid, turbulent flow is produced in the manner shown in Figure 9–8. Because the temporal and spatial characteristics of these rotating air molecules are random (i.e., they are not periodic), their acoustic correlate is aperiodic. The complex aperiodic acoustic event resulting from turbulent flow provides a sound source for fricatives, which have the narrow constrictions and high flows discussed in conjunction with Figure 9–8. In fricative production, the turbulence generated at the exit of the supralaryngeal (above the larynx and within the vocal tract) constrictions results in a *frication source*. This frication source is shaped by the resonant characteristics of the vocal tract, just as the vocal tract shapes the glottal source spectrum in vowel production.

The obstacle shown in Figure 9–8 produces a similar effect on the streaming air molecules. When molecules strike the obstacle, they rotate and move erratically if certain conditions are met, producing a significant amount of turbulent flow. The turbulence in the region of the obstacle functions as a frication source, just like the turbulence in the region of the constriction exit. When there is a sufficiently narrow constriction and a flow of sufficient magnitude (the conditions necessary to generate turbulent flow), plus an obstacle in the path of the expanding air jet "shooting out" from the constriction, multiple frication sound sources may exist. For example, one source might be located near the constriction exit and the other at the "downstream" obstacle. In addition, air molecules moving along the walls of the vocal tract may generate rotational patterns of airflow that result in aperiodic acoustic energy, also a potential sound source for fricatives. These "wall sources" are typically of weak intensity and associated with fricative articulations toward the back of the vocal tract (as in the voiceless velar fricative /x/ or voiceless pharyngeal fricative /ħ/).

What is the difference in the acoustic characteristics of a frication sound source with and without an obstacle like the one shown in Figure 9–8? Imagine an experiment in which the frication source characteristics generated by air rushing through a constriction is first measured without the obstacle in place, followed by an experiment in which the obstacle is placed in the path of the air jet. The primary difference in the source spectrum is a greater amount of overall energy in the "constriction + obstacle" case compared with the "constriction only" case. In fact, if the linear distance between a constriction and a downstream obstacle is not too great, the frication source at the obstacle is powerful enough to dominate the overall amplitude of the acoustic event.

The tube model shown in Figure 9–8 is a good representation of the aeromechanic and acoustic conditions generated in actual fricative productions. Fricatives are associated with narrow constrictions and relatively high airflows. Lingual fricatives such as /s/, /z/, /ʃ/, and /ʒ/ have obstacles in the form of teeth that contribute significantly to turbulent flow and aperiodic noise sources.

An estimate of the source spectrum for fricatives is presented in Figure 9–9. Just as in the case of the voicing source for vowels, direct measurement of the spectral characteristics of frication sources are nearly impossible, but must be inferred from the study of mechanical and computer models as well as acoustical theory (Shadle, 1985, 1990). The spectrum shown in Figure 9–9 is not precisely correct but is likely to be a close approximation to the aperiodic source spectrum for fricatives. Stevens (1998), based on his own work and that of Shadle (1985, 1990), argued that a source spectrum like the one shown in Figure 9–9 is applicable to *all* fricatives. This "prototype" fricative source spectrum has slowly declining energy over the 0 to 10 kHz frequency range, with a roughly 20 dB difference between the highest-amplitude low-frequency energy and the lowest-amplitude high-frequency energy. In the 0 to 5 kHz range, the spectral energy changes only a little—the source spectrum is nearly flat. There are fricative-specific modifications of this prototype fricative source, the most prominent one being the relative amplitude of the whole spectrum. Fricatives with greater source energy—those with obstacles (teeth) relatively close to the constriction—move the spectrum up the relative amplitude scale but leave the basic spectral shape unchanged (Stevens, 1998). Fricatives produced in the front of the vocal tract, near its exit to the atmosphere, have a source spectrum of the prototype shape but moved down on the relative amplitude scale. These fricative-specific changes in the overall level of the "prototype" source spectrum are indicated in Figure 9–9 by arrows pointing up for /sʃzʒ/ and down for /fθvð/. In addition, because voiceless fricatives have greater oral pressure (P_o, see below) and hence greater airflow through the constriction compared with their voiced cognates, the "prototype" fricative source spectrum is of greater amplitude for voiceless compared with voiced fricatives.

Actual fricative source spectra may deviate from the prototype shown in Figure 9–9 for several reasons. As demonstrated by Shadle (1985, 1990), the shape and degree of the fricative constriction, the magnitude of airflow through the constriction, the angle at which

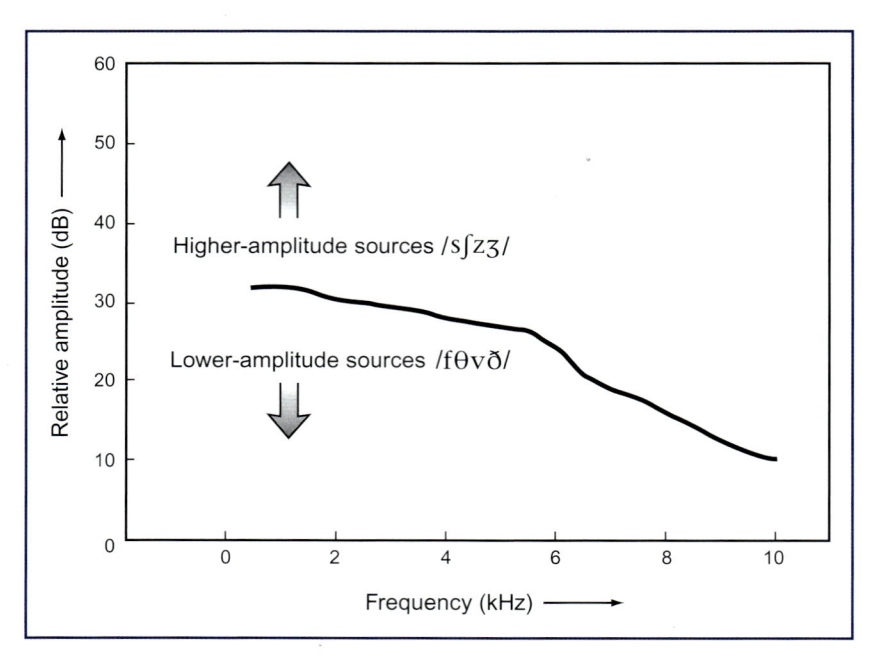

Figure 9–9. "Prototype" source spectrum for fricatives, modeled after data described by Stevens (2000) and the work of Shadle (1985, 1990). The entire prototype spectrum is moved up the relative amplitude scale for fricatives in which an obstacle in the path of airflow contributes heavily to the source energy (/sʃzʒ/) and down the scale for fricatives in which obstacles play only a minor role or no role at all (/fθvð/).

airflow strikes an obstacle, and the distance of the constriction from an obstacle are all factors that adjust details of the fricative source spectrum shape. These factors vary across individuals as a result of varying anatomy of the vocal tract as well as differences across individuals in pressures used to drive air through constrictions. These variations, however, do not change the general description of an aperiodic source spectrum that gradually declines in energy from low to high frequency and is flat from 0 to 5 kHz.

Aeromechanic/Acoustic Effects in Fricatives: A Summary

The source of sound in fricatives represents a transformation of aeromechanical energy (in the form of turbulent flows) to acoustic energy (in the form of aperiodic waveforms and their spectra). The tube model of Figure 9–8 shows how air flowing through a constriction leads to the formation of a jet, around which turbulent flow is generated. This air jet may strike obstacles in its path and generate additional turbulent sound sources, which in some cases are the primary (dominant) source of acoustic energy. Air flows through a constriction because there is a pressure differential across it. In fricative production, pressure is higher in back of the constriction than in front of it. If the size of the constriction stays constant and the pressure differential across the constriction varies, what happens to the source spectrum? This is a reasonable and relevant question, because the same fricative may be

---

Good Dental Health = Nice Fricatives

Even before Shadle's (1985) experiments on how obstacles influence the aperiodic source for fricatives such as /s/ and /ʃ/, the University of Michigan phonetician J. C. Catford (1917–2009) had described a relevant little experiment in his 1977 text *Fundamental Problems in Phonetics*. He located two people with full dentures and asked them to produce /s/ and /ʃ/ with their dentures in and with them out. Catford compared the teeth-in with teeth-out fricative spectra and found a dramatic difference in spectral intensity. The more intense fricative spectra occurred for the teeth-in productions, of course.

produced with very different pressures depending on factors such as the stress, speaking style, and position of the fricative in a word. For example, fricatives occurring in the word-initial position (e.g., the /s/ in *sake* [/seɪk/]) are produced with greater pressure than fricatives in word-final position (e.g., the /s/ in *case* [/keɪs/]). If the pressure differential is greater in the word-initial position, the magnitude of flow through the constriction is greater as well. With all other factors constant, an increase in the pressure differential results in increased airflow through and out of the constriction.

Fortunately, the answer to the question concerning the source spectrum is not complicated. When the pressure differential and, therefore, airflow through a fricative constriction increases, the major effect appears to be an overall increase in the sound amplitude of the source. There do not appear to be major effects of increased airflow on the *shape* of the spectrum. So, if the probable source spectrum shown in Figure 9–9 is adjusted for changes in the pressure differential across the constriction and the resulting magnitude of airflow through the constriction, the significant spectral adjustment is an up or down movement along the relative amplitude axis.

A Typical Fricative Waveform and Its Aeromechanical Correlates

An acoustic waveform for the sequence /æsæ/ is shown at the top of Figure 9–10. Note the contrast between the periodic glottal pulsing of the surrounding vowels with the aperiodic amplitude variations in the fricative waveform. The fricative waveform is a *noise waveform* because of the absence of periodic variations.

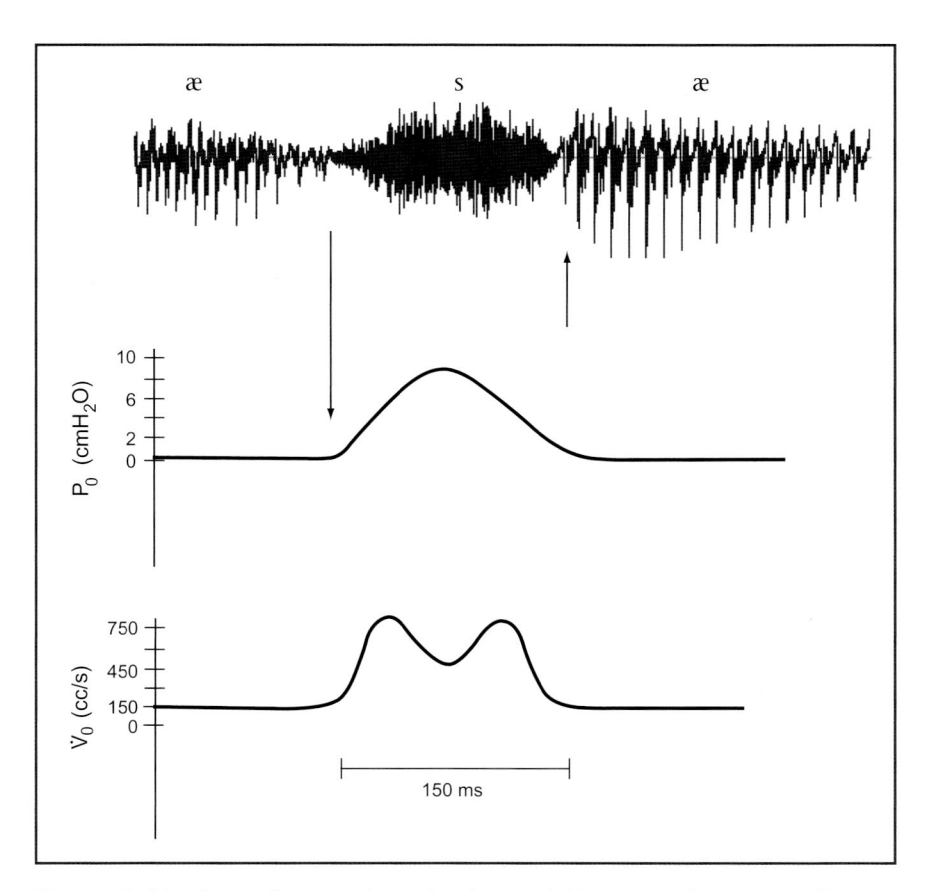

Figure 9–10. Acoustic waveform for /æsæ/ (*top panel*), shown with synchronized oral pressure (*middle panel*) and oral airflow (*bottom panel*) records. Oral pressure, P_o, is near zero during the first vowel and begins to rise at the onset of aperiodic energy in the waveform. Pressure returns to near zero for the second vowel. Oral airflow, $\dot{V}_o$, is 150 cc/s for the first vowel, increases during the /s/, and shows two peaks during the fricative before returning to 150 cc/s for the second vowel.

Immediately below the acoustic waveform are two additional waveforms, one showing the time history[5] of air pressure in the vocal tract, the other the time history of air flowing through the vocal tract. The oral pressure (P_o) is measured *behind* the point of constriction (e.g., for /s/, behind the location where the apex and anterior blade of the tongue form a groove in the vicinity of the alveolar ridge and anterior palate). Airflow is measured as it emerges from the mouth. The air pressure and airflow histories are synchronized in time with the acoustic waveform. The air pressure measured within the vocal tract, called *oral pressure* (P_o), is nearly zero during the first vowel and begins to increase (become positive) at the instant when the acoustic signal changes from periodic to aperiodic (downward arrow pointing to P_o trace). The P_o reaches a maximum value of about 8 centimeters of water (cmH_2O) in the middle of the aperiodic /s/ waveform and then begins to fall back toward zero, toward the end of the fricative and onset of glottal pulsing for the second vowel (see upward arrow pointing to the acoustic waveform, Figure 9–10). P_o is nearly zero during the vowels because the vocal tract is open to atmosphere; pressure inside and outside the vocal tract is nearly the same.[6] The airflow during the fricative is relatively high, about five times the magnitude of flow during the vowels. The fricative flow has a "double-peaked" appearance very common for fricative production (Klatt, Stevens, & Mead, 1968). These double peaks probably reflect the time-varying tightness of the fricative constriction throughout the fricative duration. For present purposes, the relatively high airflow is of primary interest because of its capacity to produce turbulence when it shoots through the fricative constriction and/or strikes an obstacle.

Mixed Sources in Fricative Production

The production of the English fricatives /v/, /ð/, /z/, and /ʒ/ involves turbulence, but may also be accompanied by vibration of the vocal folds. These voiced fricatives are produced with two types of sources—one associated with the aperiodic, turbulent flow generated in the vocal tract and the other with periodic vibration of the vocal folds. This is a case of a mixed source (Fant, 1960), in which two sources are active in the production of a sound. When there is a mixed source, both source spectra are shaped by the resonant characteristics of the vocal tract. It is as if the two sources are superimposed on each other, and the vocal tract resonators act on them (i.e., shape their spectra) simultaneously.

Shaping of Fricative Sources by Vocal Tract Resonators

The foundation for understanding resonances in fricative production has been prepared by: (a) the discussion of resonator size and resonant frequency (Chapter 7) and (b) the discussion above of antiresonances in cases where sources are located between two resonant cavities.

The narrow vocal tract constriction required for fricatives divides the vocal tract into a front and back cavity. The source energy, located close to the constriction or in front of the constriction (e.g., at the teeth), is propagated in both directions along the long axis of the vocal tract, and possibly in other directions as well. Both the front and back cavities shape the source spectrum. However, the back cavity behaves as if it is "closed" and traps energy at frequencies determined by its size (i.e., just as open cavities—cavities that radiate sound to the atmosphere—amplify energy at frequencies determined by their size). The back cavity shapes the source spectrum by introducing antiresonances into the fricative output spectrum. The front cavity, being open to the atmosphere, shapes the source spectrum by emphasizing a frequency region of the spectrum. The emphasized frequencies appear in the output spec-

---

[5]"Time history" is a term used to describe the variation of a signal over time. The acoustic waveform shows the time history of amplitude variations. Time histories have been shown for other signals, including pressures, flows, movements of the articulators, voltages associated with muscle contraction (electromyograms, or EMGs), and formant frequencies, to name a few measurable phenomena relevant to speech production.

[6]Material from Chapter 8 may appear to contradict the discussion in this chapter. The text states that the pressure inside the vocal tract is zero during vowels because there are no substantial supralaryngeal constrictions, yet the discussion of perturbation theory in Chapter 8 included description of pressure variations along the wavelengths associated with vocal tract resonances. At the maximum pressure peaks of these wavelengths the pressure is clearly above Patm. How can the statements made in this chapter about P_o being nearly zero during vowel production be reconciled with the clearly positive pressures at certain points along the wavelengths of the resonant (formant) frequencies of vowels? The answer is, the positive pressures along the wavelengths are at local points only (at a given cross-sectional slice of the vocal tract), and reflect relatively high-frequency pressure fluctuations (typically above 300 Hz). These are *acoustic* pressures in the sense that they are a characteristic of sound waves, as described in Chapter 7. P_o, an aeromechanical phenomenon, is a measure of the low-frequency (slow) compressibility of the *entire air volume in the vocal tract*, rather than at a single cross-sectional slice of the tube. It is low frequency because the rise and fall of the pressure occurs over a period of roughly 0.06 to 0.12 s (60–120 ms), close to the duration of stop closure intervals and fricative noise intervals (see Figure 9–10 and Figure 9–16). The aeromechanical pressure symbolized by P_o is, therefore, a whole-volume, slowly varying event, whereas the acoustic pressures along the resonant wavelengths within the vocal tract tube are local (single-slice), rapidly varying events. This explains why the apparent contradiction is, happily, only apparent, and illustrates the difference between the acoustic and aeromechanical levels of observation introduced in Chapter 7.

trum as high-amplitude regions, or broad peaks across a range of frequencies.

A simplified rule for the way in which these cavities shape fricative spectra is as follows. As the cavity in front of the constriction gets smaller, the resonances of the frication spectra move to higher frequencies. This is consistent with the idea that air volumes in smaller resonating cavities are stiffer than air volumes in larger cavities. As the cavity behind the constriction gets smaller, the resonant frequency of the antiresonances increases for the same reason.

Fricative spectra contain peaks, but they are not as easy to identify as they are in vowel spectra. The peaks in fricative spectra are often broad, extending over a large frequency region. This is unlike vowel spectra in which the peaks are relatively narrow, with bandwidths in the 40 to 70 Hz range. Figure 9–11 presents examples of fricative spectra for /f/, /θ/, /s/, and /ʃ/. The fricatives were spoken in an /æCæ/ frame, where C = fricative; the spectra were computed from the middle 50 ms of the frication noises. These spectra have a frequency range of 0 to 10 kHz (x-axis) and relative amplitude marked off in 10 dB steps (y-axis). Each fricative was recorded under exactly the same conditions, so relative amplitudes can be compared directly across the four spectra.

The /f/ and /θ/ spectra are both relatively weak compared with the /s/ and /ʃ/ spectra. The peak amplitudes in the /s/ and /ʃ/ spectra are approximately 20 dB greater than the peak amplitudes for /f/ and /θ/. The /f/ spectrum is relatively flat, whereas the /θ/ spectrum has increasing amplitude up to 5.0 kHz and relatively flat or slightly decreasing energy above 5.0 kHz. There is either a very small or nonexistent cavity in front of the constrictions for /f/ and /θ/, so their spectra are likely to have an extremely high resonance

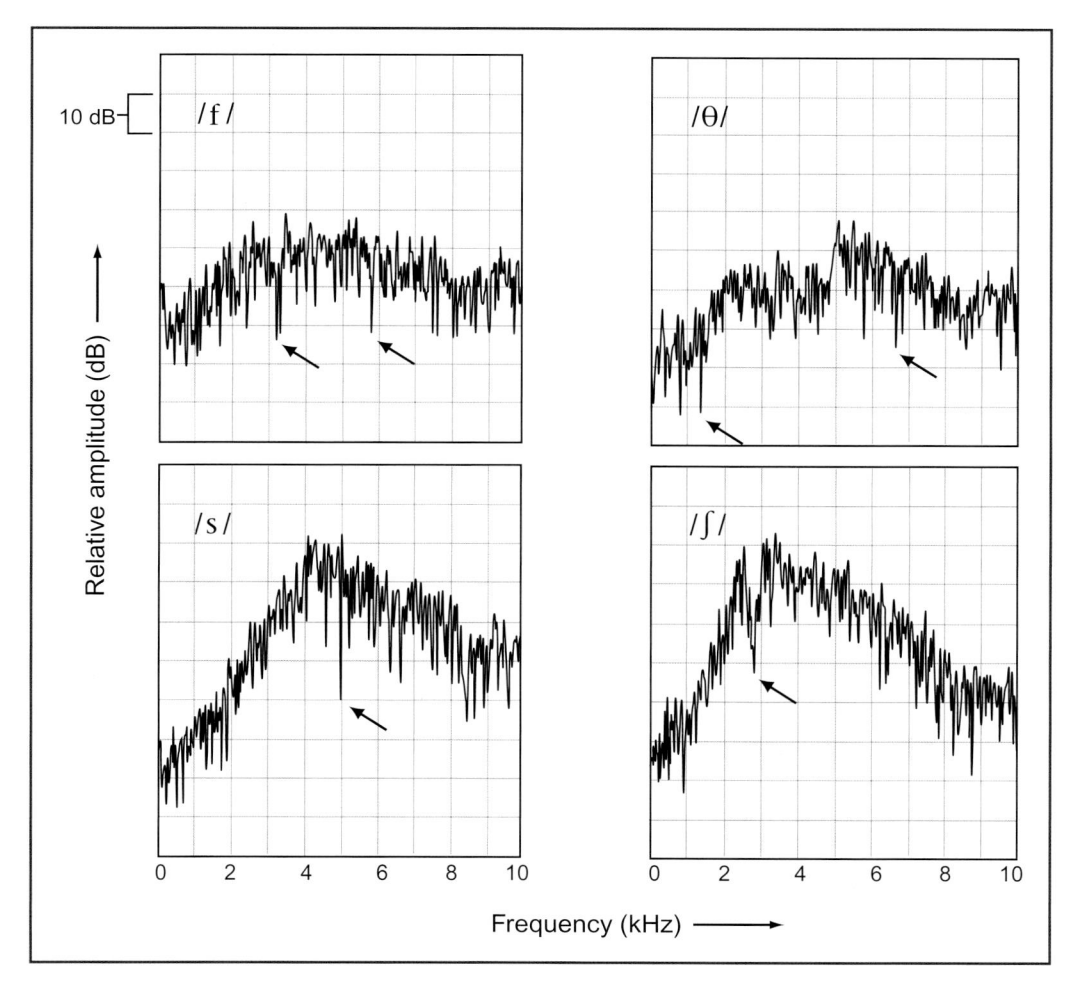

Figure 9–11. Output spectra for /f/ (*upper left*), /θ/ (*upper right*), /s/ (*lower left*), and /ʃ/ (*lower right*), produced by a 57-year-old adult male with complete dentition. The fricative spectra were computed from 50 ms intervals extracted from the middle of the frication noises in an /æCæ/ frame, where C = fricative. Arrows indicate probable antiresonances.

> ### Sound Change
>
> Speech sounds are subject to evolutionary selection. Linguists call this diachronic sound change, where the sound system of a language changes over time. One reason for these changes is that a sound must be sufficiently distinct from other sounds so that it can function phonemically. When two phonemes in a language have very similar acoustic characteristics, their effectiveness as separate phonemes may be compromised. In the language of evolution, the sound system is subject to selection pressure: if two acoustically similar sounds are not doing the phonemic job, they merge. When the merger is complete, the two sounds function as allophones of one phoneme. A sound change seems to be happening for /f/ and /θ/ in African American English. These two fricatives are interchangeable in certain word positions. The low-amplitude, very similar spectra for /f/ and /θ/ make them ideal candidates for this kind of sound change—well known in the history of many languages.

Figure 9–12 summarizes the relation of constriction location to the frequency location of major resonances. The sequence of spectra is associated with a vocal tract maneuver in which one of the authors (GW) moved his tongue continuously from an /x/ to an /s/

frequency, or perhaps no clear region of resonance. In the case of an extremely small resonating cavity, the resonance may be above the frequency limit of the spectra in Figure 9–11 (10 kHz) and, therefore, not visible in these plots. If the constriction is sufficiently anterior in the vocal tract and there is no effective front resonating cavity, the spectra may look like unfiltered versions of the source spectrum. Compare, for example, the shape of the prototype fricative source spectrum shown in Figure 9–9 to the /f/ output spectrum shown in Figure 9–11. With the exception of the low frequencies, the two spectra are quite similar. The /f/ and /θ/ spectra of Figure 9–11 also reflect the influence of antiresonances, as indicated by the upward-pointing arrows aimed at sharp "dips" in the spectra.

A comparison of the /s/ and /ʃ/ spectra in Figure 9–11 illustrates nicely the principle of cavity size and resonant frequency. The constriction location for /s/ is more forward in the vocal tract than it is for /ʃ/, resulting in a smaller front cavity for /s/. Higher frequency peaks should, therefore, be observed for /s/ compared with /ʃ/. Examination of the /s/ and /ʃ/ spectra in Figure 9–11 confirms this, showing a prominent, broad peak between 4.0 and 5.0 kHz for /s/ compared with the peak in the /ʃ/ spectrum located between 2.5 and 3.5 kHz. The probable locations of antiresonances in the /s/ and /ʃ/ spectra are indicated by upward-pointing arrows.

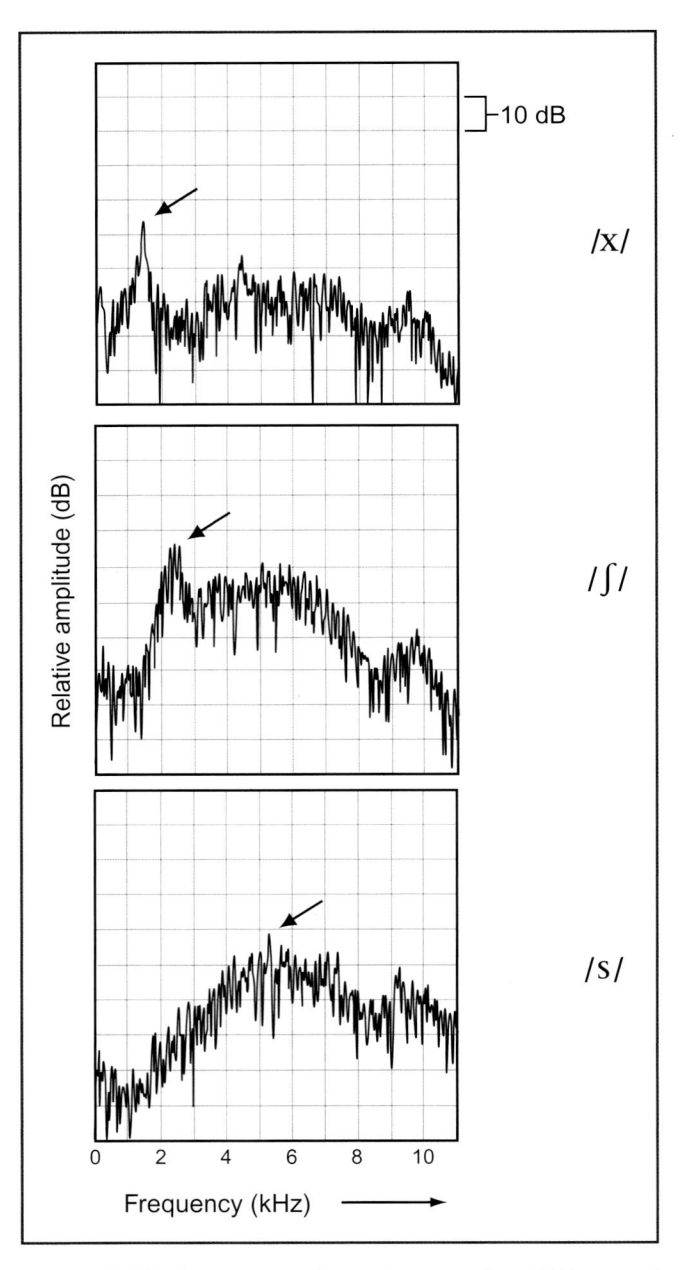

Figure 9-12. Sequence of spectra as author GW moved his tongue continuously forward from an /x/ to /s/ position while generating frication noise. Each spectrum is a "slice in time" from the continuous back-to-front gesture. The change in frequency emphasis as the tongue moves forward is related to the increasingly smaller front cavity. Arrows indicate peaks in the spectra.

position, sliding it forward while generating frication noise. The /x/ sound is a fricative heard in languages such as German and Yiddish (as in German "ach" /ɑx/ and Yiddish "chutzpah" /xʊtspə/). The three spectra were computed at "slices" in time from the beginning (top spectrum), middle (middle spectrum), and end (bottom spectrum) of the tongue-sliding gesture. The major concentration of spectral energy moves from a lower to a higher frequency region as the constriction is moved forward. The peak energy in the /x/, /ʃ/, and /s/-like positions of the tongue, indicated by arrows, are located at 1.5, 2.4, and 5.3 kHz, respectively. These increasing frequencies are consistent with the increasingly small front cavity as the constriction is moved from back to front in the vocal tract.

Measurement of Fricative Acoustics

Both spectral and temporal measures are important in the description of fricative acoustics. The measures reviewed below are used frequently in scientific and clinical applications, but do not exhaust the possible measures that could be used to describe fricative acoustics.

Spectral Measurements

In the acoustic theory of vowel production, the measurement of formant frequencies is an important way to capture the essential acoustic characteristics of vowels. The F-pattern (the frequencies of the first three formants) is an accepted way to represent the acoustic characteristics of vowels. Unfortunately, there is no standard way to measure and summarize fricative spectra. The goal of a measurement strategy for fricative spectra is to obtain a number, or a small set of numbers, that reliably distinguishes between fricatives having different places of articulation, and possibly even between fricatives having the same place of articulation but different voicing characteristics.

Figure 9–13 shows two different approaches to the measurement of fricative spectra, using /f/ (top) and /s/ (bottom) spectra as examples. These fricative spectra are smoothed versions of the ones shown in Figure 9–11. "Smoothed" means that the general shape of the spectrum is shown as a curve connecting the peaks of the Fourier spectrum. The smoothing technique is discussed further in Chapter 10. The arrows in each spectrum point to the primary peak, or the frequency associated with the greatest amplitude. This measurement is called the *peak frequency* of a fricative spectrum. This approach to the measurement of fricative spectra is conceptually similar to the measurement of peaks

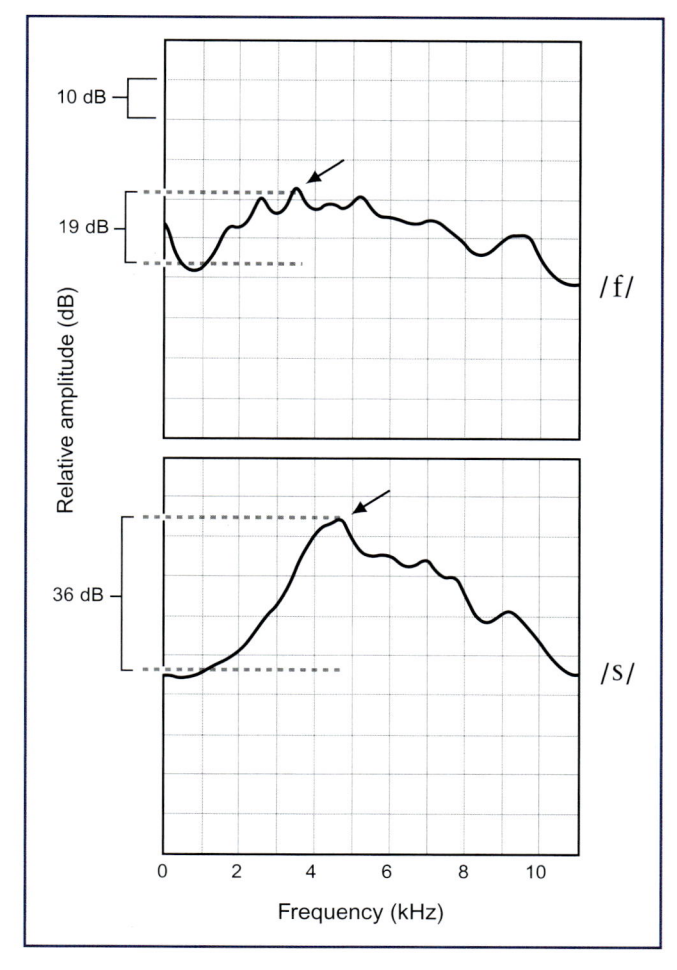

Figure 9–13. An /f/ (*upper panel*) and /s/ (*lower panel*) spectrum, showing two different ways to quantify spectral characteristics. Peak frequencies in both spectra are shown by downward-pointing arrows. Dynamic range of each spectrum is indicated by the distance between the upper and lower dashed lines.

(formants) in vowel spectra. Because the primary resonance of fricatives depends on the size of the front cavity, the peak frequency is, in many cases, correlated with the place of articulation. Higher peak frequencies are expected for fricatives with smaller front cavities (such as /s/), and lower peak frequencies for fricatives with larger front cavities (such as /x/ or /ʃ/). In Figure 9–13 the /f/ peak frequency of 3.5 kHz is clearly different from the /s/ peak at 4.6 kHz.

Although there has been some success classifying fricative place of articulation with peak frequency measurements (Jongman, Wayland, & Wong, 2000), the measures are not as reliable in separating fricatives as formant frequency measures are for separating vowels. Fricative spectra usually have multiple peaks of relatively similar amplitude, making the use of a single peak frequency relatively unreliable in distinguishing among different places of fricative articulation. This is illustrated in Figure 9–13 by the /f/ spectrum, which has three peaks—at 2.6, 3.5 (highest amplitude peak), and 5.2 kHz, all having very similar amplitudes. What if measurements were made of the frequencies of the two or three highest peaks in a fricative spectrum? This increases the *dimensionality* of the measurement (as in vowels, where three peaks are used) and may lead to better acoustic discrimination of fricative place of articulation. Unfortunately, the peaks in fricative spectra are often not as well defined (sharply tuned) as in vowel spectra and can be difficult to identify. This has led scientists to explore other types of measurements, possibly in combination with the measurement of peak frequency(ies).

One such measurement is the *dynamic range* of a fricative spectrum. Figure 9–13 shows, for the two spectra, the range of amplitudes between the highest and lowest energies along the smoothed curves. This range is indicated on each spectrum by the two horizontal, dashed lines. The range value in decibels is shown to the left of each spectrum. In this example, the dynamic range measurement has been limited to the frequency range 1.0 to 10.0 kHz to avoid low energies at the extremes of the spectrum. The substantially larger dynamic range of 36 dB for /s/ compared with 19 dB for /f/ is a quantitative approach to capture the subjective visual impression of the relative flatness of the /f/ spectrum compared with the /s/ spectrum. Although dynamic range measurements have not been explored in detail for fricative spectra (see Shadle, 1985), the combination of such a measure with peak frequencies may result in better ability to distinguish between the acoustic characteristics of fricatives like /s/ and /ʃ/, or /f/ and /θ/ (or their voiced cognates).

Fricative spectra can also be quantified by treating the spectrum as a distribution of numbers and computing parameters that describe the central tendency, dispersion, tilt, and "peakiness" of the set of numbers. One of the first lessons of basic statistics concerns the characteristics of a *normal distribution*. Using the normal distribution as a reference, any distribution can be described by: (a) an average, or *mean* of all the numbers (i.e., the central tendency); (b) a *variance*, which is the tendency of the numbers to spread more or less around the mean (dispersion); (c) a *skewness*, an index of how much the distribution curve deviates from symmetry and leans left or right (tilt); and (d) a *kurtosis*, an index of how much the distribution deviates from "normal" peakiness (either more "peaky" or more flat). These four measures are called the first four *moments* of a distribution, and when applied to acoustic spectra

> **Parsing Parsimony**
>
> The term "reducing the dimensionality" of a measurement problem is well known in all branches of science, including speech acoustics. How many numbers does it take to represent the fricative /ʃ/ so that it is completely distinguishable from other fricatives? Is it sufficient to measure the peak frequency at the halfway point of a fricative waveform, or do you need additional numbers (such as secondary and tertiary peak frequencies, fricative amplitude, and so forth)? Scientists typically prefer the simplest measurement possible, so they spend a lot of time determining the smallest set of numbers required to capture the essence of a physical phenomenon. The concept of *parsimony*—achieving adequate description or explanation using the simplest measures—is deeply entrenched in the souls of scientists.

they are called *spectral moments*. It is easy to see how the spectra in Figures 9–11, 9–12, and 9–13 look like distributions of numbers that deviate from the typical "bell shape" of the normal distribution.

Computer programs are available to compute spectral moments. These programs provide a four-number index (mean, variance, skewness, and kurtosis) of a fricative spectrum, or of any speech sound spectrum. The measures are obtained automatically and rapidly, and certain fricatives can be distinguished from each other quite well using this approach (Forrest, Weismer, Milenkovic, & Dougall, 1988). The articulatory interpretation of spectral moments, however, is sometimes not straightforward, which may limit their application in clinical settings. Spectral moments are discussed in greater detail in Chapter 11.

Temporal Measurements

The waveform in Figure 9–10 illustrates the different appearance of vowel (periodic) and fricative (aperiodic) energy. Even in the case of voiced fricatives, for which the acoustic result of vocal fold vibration may be mixed with frication noise, vowels and fricatives look quite different in a waveform display. The different appearance of vowels and fricatives permits *segmentation* of the waveform into pieces that correspond to vowels, and pieces that correspond to fricatives. The "pieces" correspond to *segment durations* (defined along the *x*-axis of the waveform), where "segment" refers to a sound category (vowel or fricative). Specific rules for the temporal segmentation of speech waveforms and *spectrograms* are given in Chapter 10. Segment durations (see Chapter 11) have been used frequently to describe and classify different types of speech disorders.

The Acoustic Theory of Fricatives: A Summary

The acoustic theory of fricatives shares with the acoustic theory of vowels the concepts of source and filter. In fricative production there is a source generated supralaryngeally, as a result of turbulent airflow: (a) in the vicinity of the constriction, (b) at an obstacle in the path of airflow, or (c) along the walls of the vocal tract. Turbulent noise sources may be generated at any combination of these three sites. Turbulent sources are aperiodic and have a spectrum that is nearly flat, or in some cases slightly falling, as a function of frequency. When airflow strikes an obstacle directly, as in the case of /s/ and /ʃ/ where the obstacle is the teeth, the frication source has relatively great amplitude. When airflow strikes other surfaces in a more indirect manner, as in the case of /f/ and /θ/ where airflow may glance off the teeth and/or lips, or when the airflow moves along the vocal tract walls or encounters no obstacles in its pathway, the frication source is relatively weak. These differences in source amplitude are largely responsible for the pronounced, overall amplitude differences between English fricatives with constrictions in the vocal tract (/s/, /z/, /ʃ/, /ʒ/) versus those with constrictions at the outlet of the vocal tract (/f/, /θ/, /v/, /ð/).

The filter in fricative production is the vocal tract, as it is for vowels. Because the source propagates in both directions along the long axis of the vocal tract, and even from side to side in the tube, all cavities contribute to the shaping of the source spectrum. This is true even though the source location may be well in front of the cavity behind the constriction. The primary resonances in fricative spectra originate in the cavity in front of the constriction. As this cavity decreases in size, as when a fricative constriction is moved from the back to front of the vocal tract, the primary resonances increase in frequency. Fricative spectra also contain antiresonances, which are due primarily to the back cavity and its behavior as a closed resonator that traps acoustic energy.

There is no standard approach to the measurement of fricative spectra, as there is in the case of vowels. However, three candidate measurements—peak frequencies, dynamic range, and spectral moments—appear to be useful. Future research should show which of these (or other) measures does the best job of distinguishing between the fricatives, and which can be most easily interpreted in articulatory terms.

WHAT IS THE THEORY OF STOP ACOUSTICS?

Figure 9–14 shows a tube model like the one shown for fricative aeromechanics (see Figure 9–8). Unlike the tube in Figure 9–8, which contains a narrow constriction through which air flows, the tube in Figure 9–14 has a complete constriction (at the downward-pointing arrow). The complete constriction is like a closed valve blocking the flow of air. When a pressure differential exists between the two ends of the tube, with P_1 greater than P_r, air flows from the left end of the tube to the right end, as shown by the arrows in Figure 9–14. The airflow is blocked by the complete constriction, causing compression of the air molecules behind the place of articulation. Compression of air molecules results in increasing pressure that rises until the constriction is released (i.e.,

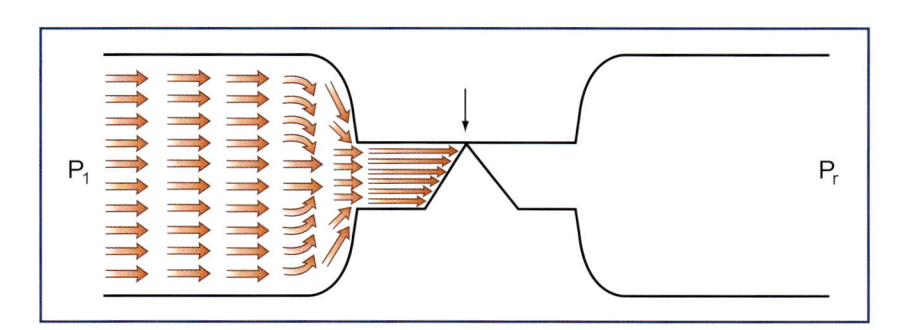

Figure 9–14. Airflow in a tube like that in Figures 9–7 and 9–8, except that a complete constriction in the tube (*arrow*) prevents air from passing through to the right side. Pressure builds up behind the constriction, as is the case for stop consonants. P_1 is the pressure behind the constriction and P_r is the reference pressure (atmospheric pressure).

the valve is opened) or the air volume becomes maximally stiff and cannot be compressed further.

During speech production, completely closed tubes such as the one shown in Figure 9–14 occur for the articulation of stop consonants. The complete blockage of airflow for stops may be formed at several places throughout the vocal tract (at the lips, between the tongue and various locations along the hard and soft palates and pharynx [as in Arabic], and at the glottis). In connected speech these complete blockages last no longer than about 100 ms (1/10 of a second). When air flowing through the vocal tract is blocked by a stop constriction, molecules within the volume behind the constriction are compressed simultaneously and uniformly. For example, in the production of a voiceless stop consonant, the vocal folds are separated and the volume behind a vocal tract constriction includes the air spaces of the trachea and lungs (in addition to those of the vocal tract). The nasal cavities are excluded from this volume because the velopharyngeal port is closed for production of stops (as it is for all obstruents in English). The complete blockage of airflow takes place during the closure (constriction) interval. When the vocal folds are open as in voiceless stops, pressure is uniform throughout the cavities behind the constriction.

This condition is illustrated in the schematic speech production apparatus of Figure 9–15A, where a complete lingua-alveolar constriction is shown for the voiceless stop /t/, and the volume behind the constriction is indicated by the shaded area. Three pressures are indicated within this volume. *Oral air pressure* is symbolized by P_o, which is the pressure measured within the vocal tract. P_t is *tracheal air pressure*, measured immediately below the vocal folds. P_{alv} is *alveolar air pressure*, or the pressure inside the lungs. When air is compressed behind a complete vocal tract constriction for a voiceless stop, the peak (highest) value of P_o is equivalent to the peak values of P_t and P_{alv} because the vocal folds are abducted. In

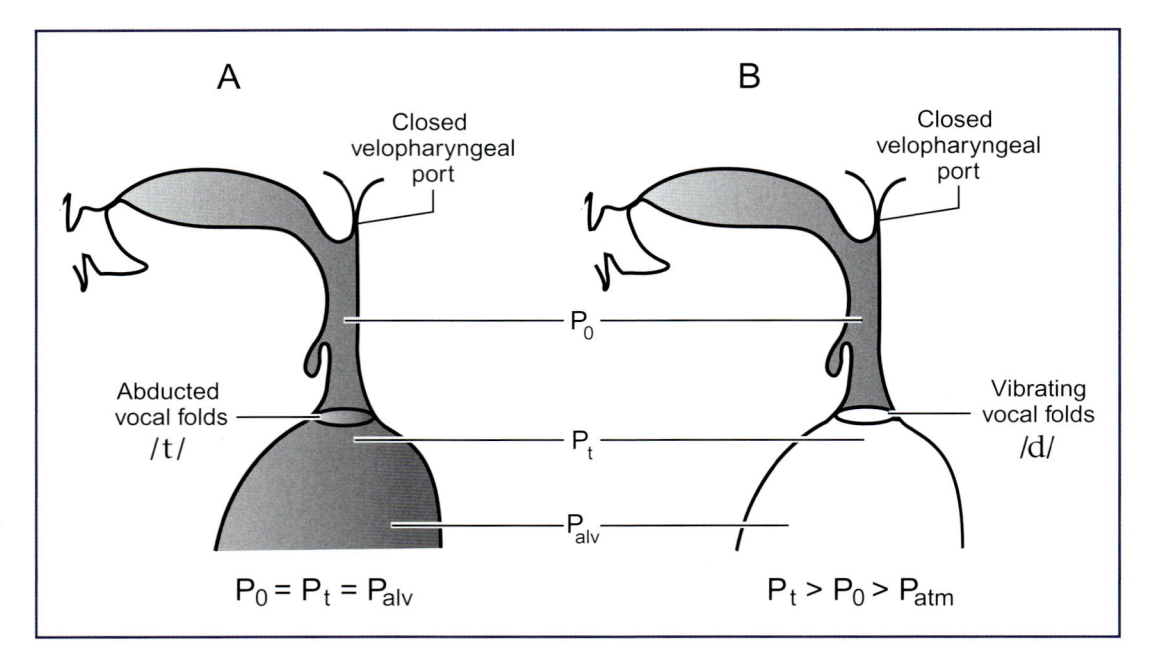

Figure 9–15. **A.** Schematic drawing of the speech production apparatus, showing a complete constriction immediately behind the alveolar ridge for the voiceless stop /t/. The volume of air that is compressed during the stop closure interval is indicated by the shaded parts of the drawing and includes the vocal tract spaces behind the constriction as well as the spaces within the trachea and lungs. Oral, tracheal, and alveolar air pressures are equal during the stop closure interval. **B.** Schematic drawing of the speech production apparatus, showing a complete constriction immediately behind the lingua-alveolar ridge for the voiced stop /d/. The volume of air that is compressed during the stop closure interval is indicated by the shaded parts of the drawing and includes only the spaces between the stop constriction and the larynx. Tracheal air pressure is greater than oral air pressure and both are greater than atmospheric air pressure. The unshaded oval at the level of the glottis indicates laryngeal closure during the closed phase of the vibratory cycle.

an utterance such as /ata/, P_o is nearly zero (Patm) during the first vowel, begins to rise when the constriction is made for /t/ until a magnitude of 5 to 10 cmH$_2$O is reached, and drops rapidly back to zero when the constriction is released into the following vowel. During vowel production, P_t and P_{alv} are above zero (around 5–10 cmH$_2$O) so that air can flow from the trachea and through the vocal folds, setting the latter into vibration for the vowel.

In the case of voiced stop consonants, the aeromechanical situation is somewhat different because the vibrating vocal folds separate the tracheal and pulmonary air volumes from the vocal tract air volume. In this case, the peak value of P_o does not equal P_t and P_{alv} because as air flows through the vibrating vocal folds there is some loss of pressure, resulting in P_o values that are generally lower than the pressures in the trachea and lungs. In Figure 9–15B the shaded area behind the lingua-alveolar constriction shows the compressible volume associated with P_o for voiced stops. This volume extends only between the constriction and the vocal folds, the latter shown as an unshaded oval to indicate the closed phase during each vibratory cycle. When P_t is greater than P_o by a critical amount (usually about 2 cmH$_2$O) the vocal folds continue to vibrate during the voiced stop closure interval, because air flows from the higher (tracheal) to lower (vocal tract) pressure region.[7]

Values of P_o for voiced stops, ranging between about 3.5 and 8.0 cmH$_2$O, are typically about 1.5 cmH$_2$O less than values for voiceless stops. The duration of the closure interval for voiced stops is about the same as that for voiceless stops, usually not exceeding 100 ms.

Both voiceless and voiced stops, therefore, have a buildup of P_o during their closure intervals. The vocal tract is "sealed" by the stop articulation (e.g., between the lips, or between the tongue and palate) as well as by closure of the velopharyngeal port. The seal briefly prevents air from escaping the vocal tract and nasal tract to the atmosphere and results in the P_o buildup. The next step is to link these aeromechanical events with the acoustic characteristics of stop consonants.

Intervals of Stop Consonant Articulation: Aeromechanics and Acoustics

Stop consonant articulation has several successive components. These include the closure, release (burst), frication, and aspiration intervals (the latter only occurring for voiceless stops). Voice-onset time (VOT) includes the burst, frication, and aspiration intervals in the case of voiceless stops, and the burst and frication intervals for voiced stops.

Closure (Silent) Interval

In an articulatory sequence such as /ata/ the vocal tract is open for the first vowel and then closed for the /t/ by contact of the tongue tip with the alveolar ridge. The closure interval of the stop is also called the *silent interval*, during which the vocal tract radiates little or no acoustic energy. Closure intervals of voiceless stops are typically completely silent, but the closure intervals of voiced stops may show evidence of weak periodic energy due to vibration of the vocal folds. This weak periodic energy is not the result of a pressure wave emerging from the mouth or nose, because the vocal tract is completely sealed. Rather, vocal fold vibration during a closure interval causes the walls of the vocal tract to vibrate. These tissue vibrations are transferred to the air surrounding the head and neck in the form of low-energy pressure waves which may be sensed by the ear or by a microphone.

Figure 9–16 shows two speech waveforms to illustrate the closure interval for the stops in /ata/ (left) and /ada/ (right). P_o and $\dot{V}_o$ (oral air pressure and airflow) traces are shown below and synchronized in time with each acoustic waveform. The vowels surrounding the closure intervals are easily identified by their large amplitude, periodic energy. For the /ata/ traces, a pointer marked "onset of /t/ closure" indicates the final glottal pulse of the first vowel, after which there is minimal or no acoustic energy for a period of about 70 ms. This is the closure interval of the voiceless stop consonant. The onset of the /d/ closure is also indicated

---

[7]There are cases in which P_o rises to the same magnitude as P_t during the closure interval of a voiced stop. When this occurs, there is no pressure differential across the glottis, and hence no airflow and no vocal fold vibration. This set of conditions might even be more common if it were not for an articulatory gesture that seems to be specific to voiced stops. In several studies (Bell-Berti, 1975; Kent & Moll, 1969), it has been shown that the volume of the cavity behind the vocal tract constriction and above the glottis *enlarges* during the closure interval of voiced stops (the same pharyngeal enlargement occurs for voiced English *fricatives*, suggesting the enlargement is associated with obstruent voicing in general, and not just stop voicing; see Proctor, Shadle, & Iskarous, 2010). The enlargement is accomplished by muscular mechanisms that widen the pharynx, lower the larynx, and raise the velum. In a closed volume, the product of pressure and volume is a constant; this aeromechanical characteristic of closed volumes is known as *Boyle's law*. Thus, if the volume behind the constriction and above the vocal folds is enlarged during the closure interval, the pressure within that volume is reduced, consistent with Boyle's law. The reduced pressure tends to keep P_o below P_t, and allows vocal fold vibration throughout much or all of the closure interval. This enlargement of the vocal tract volume behind the constriction does not occur for voiceless stops because there is no need to maintain a pressure difference across the glottis (i.e., there is no need to maintain vocal fold vibration, which requires a pressure difference across the glottis).

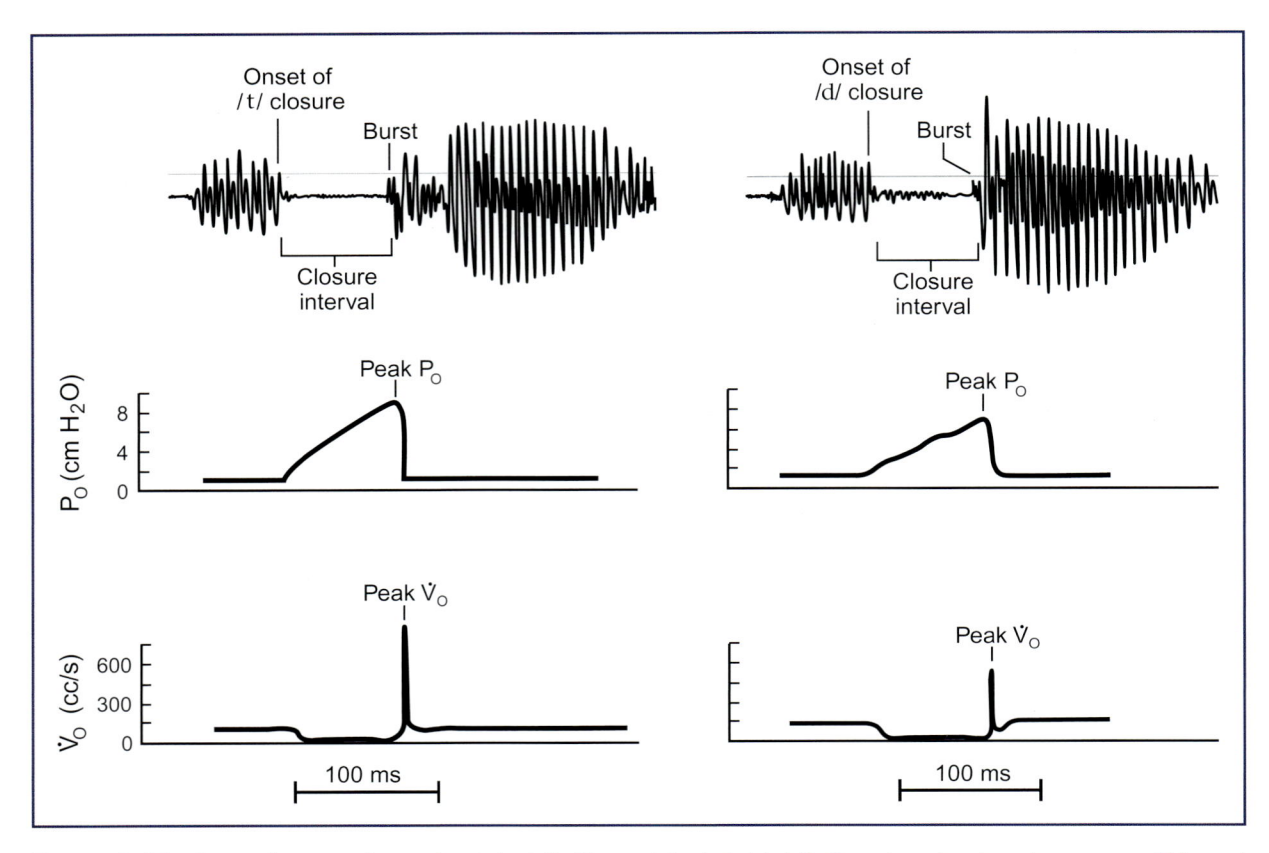

Figure 9–16. Acoustic waveforms for /ɑtɑ/ (*left*) and /ɑdɑ/ (*right*). Synchronized oral pressure (P_o) and oral airflow ($\dot{V}_o$) signals are shown below each acoustic waveform. See text for details.

by a pointer, but in this case the following closure interval contains weak, periodic energy, as shown by the low-amplitude glottal pulses that terminate shortly before the burst. This is the energy from vocal fold vibration, transmitted to the microphone via vibration of orofacial tissue such as the neck and cheeks.

The airflow coming through the mouth ($\dot{V}_o$) is approximately 130 cc per s during the first vowel, and decreases rapidly to zero at the onset of the closure interval. For both waveforms, P_o is nearly zero (Patm) during the vowels and begins to rise at the onset of the closure interval. The P_o continues to rise until it is released by the release of the constriction, marked on the waveforms as "burst" (see next section). At the instant of release of the stop closure there is very high airflow (peak $\dot{V}_o$). The stop constriction is opened suddenly and the high P_o developed during the closure interval decreases to nearly Patm over an interval of just a few ms. The relationship between the aeromechanical and acoustical events shown in Figure 9–16 for /ɑtɑ/ and /ɑdɑ/ is elaborated in the following descriptions of the burst, frication, and aspiration intervals.

Release (Burst) Interval

The sudden drop of P_o at the instant of stop closure release creates an acoustic source of energy, originally referred to by Fant (1960) as *shock excitation*. Shock excitation sources have very brief durations (perhaps no longer than 2 ms) and relatively flat spectra. As in the case of turbulent noise sources for fricatives, shock excitation sources for stops are located in the vicinity of the constriction and their spectra are shaped mainly by the cavity in front of the constriction. In Figure 9–16, the acoustic result of the sudden release of P_o is shown as the sudden "spike" or burst at the end of the closure interval. Bursts are distinctive acoustic characteristics of both voiceless and voiced stops, although they are not always present for stop production in casual speech or out-loud reading of sentences and paragraphs (see Byrd, 1993, and Chapter 11). The greater P_o for voiceless compared with voiced stops (compare peak P_o for voiceless and voiced stops in Figure 9–16) results in greater amplitude for voiceless stop bursts (Stevens, 1998).

Good Things Come in Small Packages

Stop bursts have extremely short life spans—typically less than 0.002 s in duration—and often have low amplitudes, at least when compared with vowels. Yet despite their seemingly small physical attributes, they have played a large role in theories of speech production and perception. A small experiment using speech analysis software can demonstrate the power of this little acoustic event: on the hard disk of the computer, record a speaker saying /pɑ/, /tɑ/, and /kɑ/, and use any speech analysis program to isolate a 4 to 5 ms "piece" of each stop, beginning from the onset of the burst. Play each of the three very brief "pieces" to listeners and ask them if they hear a /p/, /t/, or /k/. From these tiny bits of information, most listeners will hear the "correct" stop.

Frication and Aspiration Intervals

When the constriction is released, the pressure differential between the cavity behind the constriction (P_o) and the cavity in front of the constriction (Patm) generates an airflow of relatively great magnitude. This event is shown in Figure 9–16 by the sudden, high airflows and especially the peak $\dot{V}_o$ which marks the release of the stop constriction.

The passage of flow through narrow constrictions in the vocal tract and at the glottis explains the final two phases of stop consonant acoustics. In the discussion of the aeromechanical basis of the acoustic characteristics of fricatives (see Figure 9–8), turbulence occurs when a flow of sufficient magnitude passes through a sufficiently narrow constriction. Turbulent airflow produces the aperiodic acoustic energy of fricatives, as shown in the waveform of Figure 9–10. In the production of stop consonants there is a brief interval during which conditions are met for the generation of turbulent airflow, and hence fricative-like aperiodic energy. In /ɑtɑ/, for example, as the tongue breaks the stop constriction and moves toward an open vocal tract configuration for the following vowel there is a brief interval when a very narrow constriction is formed between the tongue and alveolar ridge. The airflow "spike" shown in Figure 9–16 moves through this narrow constriction and, as in the case of fricatives, generates turbulence at the outlet of the constriction and perhaps at the teeth as well.

The acoustic time-domain result of the turbulent flow is illustrated in the waveform shown in Figure 9–17. This waveform is like a zoom-lens view of the intervals from the burst to the following vowel. The burst in Figure 9–17 is clearly followed by an interval of aperiodic energy, labeled the *frication interval*. This acoustic interval, which typically lasts for roughly 30 to 50 ms, reflects the time during which the conditions

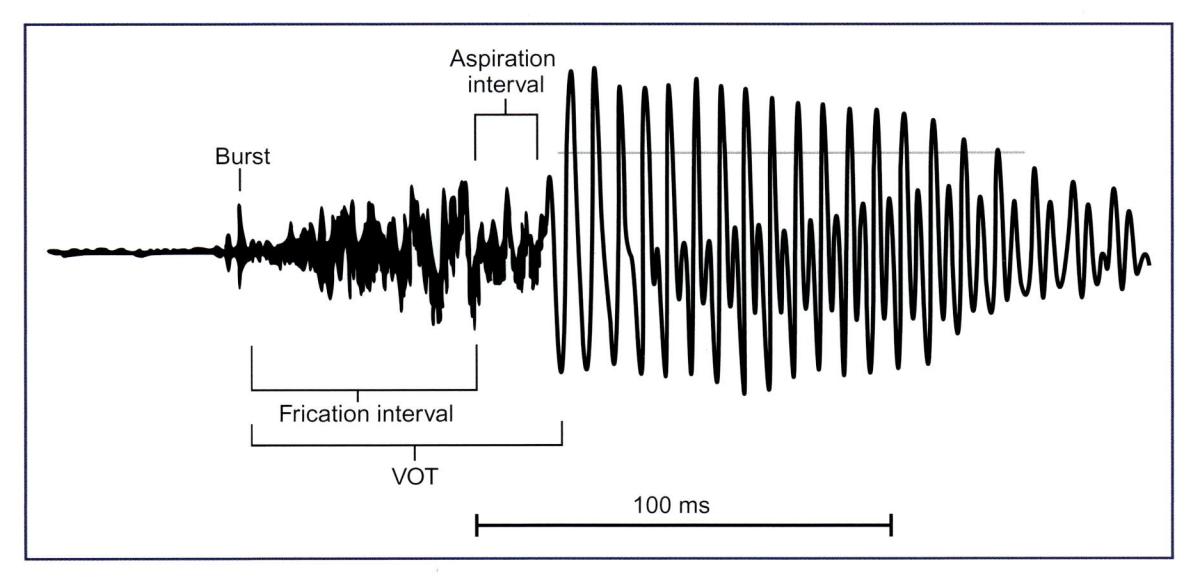

Figure 9–17. A "zoom" picture of a speech waveform showing the burst, frication, and aspiration intervals of a voiceless stop consonant. The sum of the time intervals for the burst, frication, and aspiration intervals is the voice-onset time (VOT).

for turbulent flow are met at the stop constriction as it expands into the configuration for the following vowel. The frication interval of stops lasts only a brief time because as the tongue continues to move away from the alveolar ridge, the size of the constriction increases and quickly becomes too large to sustain turbulent flow. In addition, the flow decreases rapidly from its peak and becomes too low to generate turbulence.

Figure 9–17 also shows a brief *aspiration interval* following the frication interval. Like the frication interval, the aspiration interval is the acoustic product of turbulent airflow. In this case, however, turbulence is produced at the glottis rather than at or around a constriction formed by the upper articulators. In the case of voiceless stops between two vowels, the vocal folds vibrate for the first vowel but must be separated to prevent vocal fold vibration during the closure interval. The separation of the vocal folds is followed by their return to midline for the phonation requirements of the following vowel. As the vocal folds are moving together, there is a brief interval, immediately before complete approximation, during which there is a very narrow glottal constriction. The airflow through this narrow constriction produces turbulent airflow, the acoustic result of which is the aspiration interval shown in Figure 9–17. A typical aspiration interval has a duration of 10 to 30 ms. In stop consonant production, the aspiration interval is only found for voiceless stops. This is because in voiceless stops the vocal folds are brought together for resumption of vibration much more slowly than they are in each cycle of vocal fold vibration, and the airflow through the glottis is greater when the vocal folds are brought together slowly compared with the very brief closing durations of the folds when they vibrate. In other words, the conditions for turbulent flow at the glottis (sufficiently narrow constriction, high airflow) are present for voiceless but not voiced stops.

Both the frication and aspiration intervals are the result of turbulent airflow. Fant (1960) proposed the terms *frication noise* and *aspiration noise* to designate the location of the turbulent flow. Frication noise is the acoustic result of turbulence generated in the vocal tract (at or around a constriction formed by the upper articulators) and aspiration noise is turbulence generated at the glottis. Note in Figure 9–17 the much lower amplitude of the aperiodic energy during the aspiration, compared with the frication, interval. Aspiration noise is typically quite weak, but a clear amplitude distinction like that seen in Figure 9–17 between the frication and aspiration noise is not always so obvious.

Voice-Onset Time

The interval from the stop burst to the first glottal pulse of the following vowel is called *voice-onset time* (VOT). The VOT of voiceless stops includes the burst, frication, and aspiration intervals, as marked in Figure 9–17. The VOT for voiceless stops is usually somewhere between 40 to 80 ms, but may vary according to several factors which are discussed more fully in Chapter 11. VOT for voiced stops is generally less than 20 ms, and voicing may precede the stop burst (see Chapter 11).

Shaping of Stop Sources by Vocal Tract Resonators

As in vowels and fricatives, the acoustic output of the vocal tract for stops is the result of source spectra

---

Phonatory Turbulence

Turbulent flow in the vicinity of the vocal fold edges and structures immediately above the glottis—the ventricular folds and epiglottis, for example—does not occur in "normal" phonation, or is so weak that it is inaudible. But what is "normal" phonation? We all know people with breathy voices, who have no laryngeal pathology, and whose voices are not regarded as "abnormal." Listening to such a voice, you hear a tonal quality (due to vibration of the vocal folds) plus a noisy quality (due to turbulence). How is this possible? Weak closing phases during vocal fold vibration allow high flows through the glottis which can emerge from the glottal constriction as a jet, with randomly rotating molecules at the borders of the jet. As described in this chapter, these rotating molecules just outside the laminar jet are turbulent flows, which generate aspiration noise. In addition, high flows through the glottis may strike the ventricular folds and sides of the epiglottis, causing air molecules to spin and generate aspiration noise. The ventricular folds and epiglottis are obstacles in the path of the high airflow through the glottis. Try changing your voice quality in small steps from the one you use regularly to a little breathy, a lot breathy, and then to a whisper: a big part of what you are doing through this sequence of voice qualities is adding more aspiration noise into the mix.

shaped by vocal tract resonators. Stop sources are considered first, followed by a discussion of how those sources are shaped by the resonators.

The Nature of Stop Sources

The silent, burst, frication, and aspiration intervals of stop consonant production are each produced with different sources. An alternate way to say this is that stops are produced with a *succession* of changing sources. The silent interval of a voiceless stop has no source, whereas the silent interval of a voiced stop has a vocal fold vibration source. However, this voiced source is not shaped by a vocal tract filter in the same way as vowels, nasals, other vocalic sounds such as diphthongs and semivowels. Because the vocal tract is closed during a stop interval, the filtering of vocal fold vibration is, as noted above, the vibration of the vocal tract walls and tissues of the neck, which only pass very low frequencies.

The burst has a shock excitation source, which gives way to two turbulent noise sources in the case of voiceless stops (frication and aspiration) or a single turbulent noise source in voiced stops (frication). Just as in the case of fricatives, it is difficult to state the precise spectral characteristics of the sources for stop consonants. Estimates of stop source spectra are available in the acoustic phonetics literature.

The shock excitation source of the burst is a brief event, lasting only as long as the time required for the peak P_o developed during the closure interval to decline to Patm, following release of the stop (see Figure 9–16). This interval lasts only a few milliseconds, and may be as brief as 0.5 ms (Stevens, 1998). Shock excitation qualifies as an *impulse-like event*, or one that is characterized by a large change in amplitude (in this case, pressure) over a very brief interval. Impulse-like events spread acoustic energy across a wide range of frequencies, producing a spectrum with roughly equal energy at all frequencies. The source spectrum of shock excitation is consistent with that of an impulse-like event; like the frication source spectrum, the shock excitation spectrum decreases in energy as frequency increases. For the purposes of this text it can be assumed that the source spectrum of shock excitation is like that shown for fricatives in Figure 9–9. The different places of articulation for stop consonants have only a slight effect on the shock excitation source spectrum. Fant (1960) suggested that the source spectrum for /t/ shock excitation is flatter (shows a shallower decrease in energy across frequency) than the source spectra for /p/ and /k/. This description of shock excitation source spectra also applies to the voiced cognates (/b,d,g/).

Source spectra for the frication interval are essentially the same as source spectra for fricatives shown

---

Counteracting Pop

Vocalists are notorious for "chewing the microphone" as they sing. This is one way to control variations in voice intensity that result from changing the distance between the mouth and microphone. If the singer is lip-to-foam or lip-to-metal, the only variations in voice intensity heard by the crowd are those with artistic intent—that is, changed by the singer as she or he delivers the song. The "foam" to which the singer's lips are applied is called a wind- or pop-screen (you've seen a version of these in videos of artists recording vocals in the studio). Pop screens are designed specifically to disperse the bursts produced for /p/s and /b/s. When the intraoral pressure is released for bilabial stops, the sudden spike of airflow has the potential to overdrive the microphone, producing acoustic distortion. Some pop screens are better described as digital filters or compression algorithms; these eliminate the need for the screens. Pop screens or their digital versions scatter bilabial airflow spikes and prevent them from creating aural unpleasantries.

---

in Figure 9–9. The aeromechanical phenomena that produce sources for fricatives, and sources for the stop frication intervals, are identical. Figure 9–9 shows some place-of-articulation differences in the source spectra for fricatives, and these apply to the frication intervals of /p,b/ versus /t,d/ and /k,g/. The frication source for bilabials typically has weaker energy than the frication sources for lingua-alveolar and dorsal stop consonants, consistent with the place-related differences in frication source energy shown in Figure 9–9.

The source spectrum for the aspiration interval of voiceless stops has energy concentrated in the mid-frequencies (1.0–4.0 kHz), with less energy in the lower and higher frequencies. A single aspiration source spectrum applies to all three places of articulation of stops, because variation in place of articulation does not affect the acoustic result of turbulence at the glottis. This source spectrum is somewhat different from the relatively flat source spectra of the shock excitation and frication intervals.

The Shaping of Stop Sources

The acoustic shaping of the shock excitation and frication sources in stop articulation is consistent with the shaping of fricative sources. Shock excitation and frication sources are typically located within the vocal tract, between two resonators. As in the case of fricatives, the cavity in front of the stop source provides the primary emphasis of energy (resonance) in the output spectrum, and the cavity behind the source contributes one or more antiresonances to the output spectrum.

Figure 9–18 presents typical spectra for the three stop places of articulation, measured over a 10=ms interval beginning at the burst. The spectra have been smoothed in the same way as the fricative spectra in Figure 9–13. These spectra were derived from voiceless stops, but the description provided here can be applied to their voiced cognates as well. The shapes of these three burst spectra are consistent with the ideas developed above in the section on fricative spectra. For example, the bilabial stop /p/ does not have a vocal tract cavity in front of the constriction. A relatively flat output spectrum for the /p/ burst is expected because there is no front cavity to emphasize a particular region of the shock excitation source spectrum. The /p/ burst spectrum shown in Figure 9–18 (left spectrum) is, in fact, relatively flat between roughly 0 Hz and 7000 Hz (compare this with the description of the /f/ output spectrum and Figure 9–11). Note the slight tilt of the /p/ burst spectrum, indicating a gradual decrease in energy with increasing frequency. This flat or gradually declining spectrum is considered a classic characteristic of bilabial stops. As in fricatives, the cavity behind the shock excitation source contributes antiresonances to the spectrum.

The effect of the size of the cavity in front of the constriction is illustrated by comparing the burst spectra for /t/ (Figure 9–18, middle spectrum) with that for /k/ (Figure 9–18, right spectrum). The energy in the /t/ burst spectrum rises sharply from 0 Hz to 4.5 kHz, with a clear spectral emphasis (the location of greatest energy) between 4.0 and 5.0 kHz. The /k/ burst spectrum, on the other hand, shows a prominent peak at 1.5 kHz, in addition to peaks around 4.0 kHz. The emphasis at higher frequencies in the /t/ burst spectrum makes sense because the cavity in front of the constriction is smaller than in the case of /k/. As the cavity in front of the stop constriction becomes smaller, the emphasis in the spectrum moves to higher frequencies. The general *spectral shapes* of stop bursts are related to articulatory configurations in the same way as discussed above for fricatives. Chapter 11 contains a detailed discussion of spectral shapes for stop bursts.

Stop burst spectra contain antiresonances. The same rules relating cavity size to location of frequency peaks (or reverse peaks) apply to the locations of antiresonances as well as to resonances: Large cavities yield low-frequency resonances or antiresonances, and small cavities yield high-frequency resonances or antiresonances. The spectra in Figure 9–18 do not show antiresonances because the smoothing of the spectra ignores the locations where large "dips" occur.

Measurement of Stop Acoustics

Both spectral and temporal measurements have been used to quantify the acoustic characteristics of stops. As in the case outlined earlier for fricatives, the discussion below is not exhaustive but rather describes frequently made measurements.

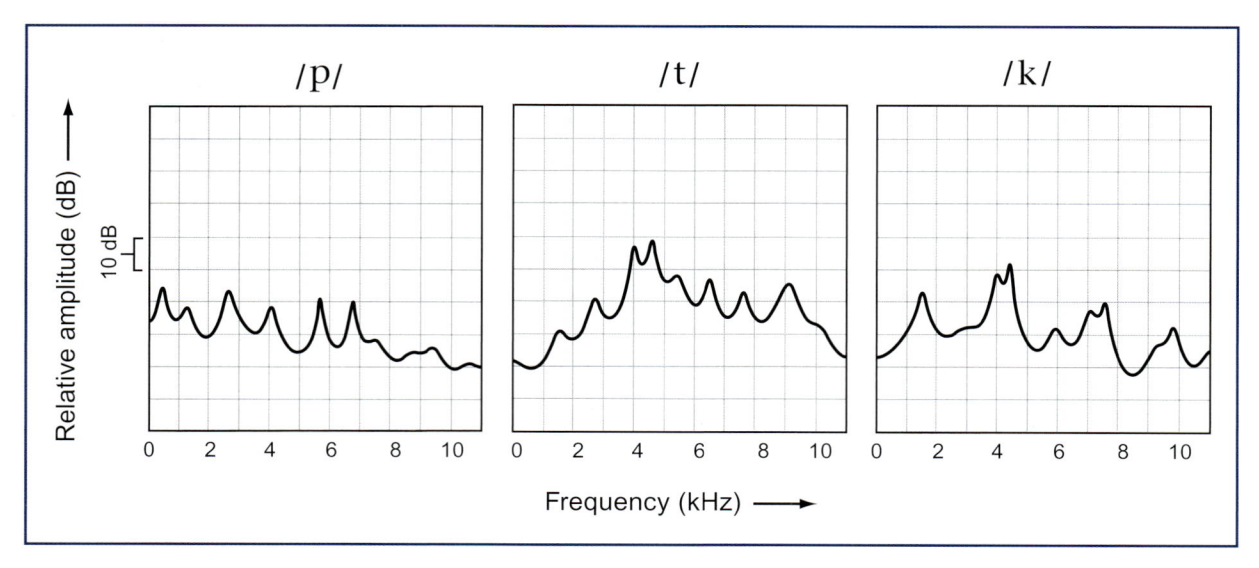

Figure 9–18. Sample output spectra (smoothed) for the burst interval of voiceless stop consonants. Each spectrum is computed from a 10-ms interval starting at the burst. The spectra for voiced stop consonants are similar, but may show less overall energy and some additional low-frequency energy.

Spectral Measurements

Surprisingly, even though stop burst spectra have played a prominent role in theories of speech production and perception, there has not been much agreement concerning their measurement. As in the case of fricatives, there is much discussion (and not much agreement) concerning the proper way to measure stop spectra.

Similar to fricative spectra, the goal of a measurement strategy for stop burst spectra is to obtain a small set of numbers that distinguishes among the three places of articulation. Stop burst spectra have numerous peaks and valleys, as is evident in the three spectra shown in Figure 9–18. These spectra are similar to fricative spectra (compare spectra in Figure 9–18 with those in Figure 9–11). Thus, peak frequencies can be measured for stop burst spectra but have the same problems as those discussed for fricatives. Similarly, dynamic range can be measured for burst spectra, but laboratory experience suggests that this does not provide a useful way to distinguish stop place of articulation.

Many researchers have focused their attention on the shape of the stop burst spectrum. Earlier, spectral moments were described as one means to obtain a numerical index of the shape of fricative spectra. When spectral moments are applied to stop burst spectra, they do a good job of distinguishing place of articulation (Forrest et al., 1988; see additional discussion in Chapter 11). A non-numerical, *prototype* approach to the classification of place of articulation for stop consonants involves the use of *spectral shape templates*. These templates, developed originally by Blumstein and Stevens (1979), provide a prototype, or template burst spectrum, for each place of articulation and an allowable range of variability for a "real" stop burst spectrum to fit one of the prototypes. For example, if a stop burst spectrum fits within an allowable range of variability for the bilabial prototype, or template, it is classified as a bilabial stop.

Blumstein and Stevens (1979) constructed the templates based on careful examination of many burst spectra computed over the 0 to 5000 Hz frequency range, and using the templates quantified the number of spectra from naturally spoken stops that were correctly classified. They had relatively good success in this exercise, classifying place of articulation correctly about 85% of the time. This success makes the template approach attractive because it offers a relatively simple procedure for classifying acoustic events (burst spectra) according to phoneme category (i.e., place contrasts). For example, the spectral templates can be stored digitally for comparison to real burst spectra for the purpose of identifying place of articulation. In a clinical setting, this may serve as a simple approach to objective evaluation of a client's articulatory capabilities for stop consonants. The procedure has certain limitations, however, which have to be worked out prior to widespread clinical or research use. The classification accuracy of the original templates was evaluated by Blumstein and Stevens using a small number of speakers (three) who articulated simple syllables in a very careful way. It is not known if the same template approach can be used for child speakers, older speakers, or any speaker using a more casual form of articulation. Also, it is not clear how to interpret an "unclassifiable" burst spectrum. In Blumstein and Stevens' study, some spectra did not fit *any* of the templates; how should these be classified? Persons with speech disorders often produce stops that sound as if they are "in between" the normal places of articulation. The template system must be expanded to capture these important articulatory events. These are areas in need of careful research if the objective measures are to have an impact in the clinic (see Chapter 11 for more material on spectral templates for stop consonant place of articulation).

Spectral measurements can also be made of frication and aspiration intervals following the stop release. The measurement issues for these spectra are the same as discussed above for the burst. The details of frication interval spectra for the different places of articulation are similar to the details of burst spectra. Spectra of aspiration intervals of voiceless stops have not been studied extensively, but generally show a pattern similar to the formant pattern of the following vowel. This is because the aspiration source, located at the glottis, excites the resonances of the vocal tract as it is opening following the stop release.

Temporal Measurements

As in the case of fricatives, temporal segmentation of stop consonant waveforms is relatively straightforward. The waveforms in Figures 9–16 and 9–17 show the closure interval and VOT segments clearly. In real speech waveforms, it is often more difficult to find the dividing lines between the burst, frication, and aspiration intervals. Many measurements of closure intervals and VOTs have been reported in the literature and applied to clinical populations.

Stop Consonants: A Summary

Stops are produced when there is a constriction in the vocal tract that completely blocks the airstream for a brief interval. During the closure interval the pressure behind the constriction (P_o) builds up and is suddenly released when the articulators break the constriction. The sudden drop in pressure serves as an acoustic source called shock excitation, the spectrum of which is shaped by the vocal tract cavities. Typically, the cavity in front of the stop constriction provides the major resonance that shapes the shock excitation source, whereas the cavity in back of the constriction contributes antiresonances to the output spectrum.

Following the closure interval, there is a sequence of acoustic events associated with stops. For voiceless stops, the sequence is the burst, frication interval, and aspiration interval. The burst is associated with the release of P_o, the frication interval with high airflow rushing past the narrow vocal tract constriction immediately following the release, and aspiration interval with high airflow rushing past the vocal folds as they move together in anticipation of phonation for the following vowel. The aeromechanical basis of the frication and aspiration intervals is turbulent airflow, the acoustic counterpart of which is aperiodic energy (i.e., noise). Voiced stops have burst and frication intervals, but lack an aspiration interval because the vocal folds are not separated from the midline during the closure interval, as they are for voiceless stops.

The spectra of the burst and frication intervals are unique for each of the three stop places of articulation. The uniqueness of these spectra can be traced largely to the size of the cavity in front of the constriction. In bilabial stops, the cavity is infinitely large (i.e., there is no vocal tract cavity), so the output spectrum tends to be flat. In lingua-alveolar stops, the cavity is very small, which results in a high-frequency emphasis in the output spectrum. In dorsal stops, the cavity is relatively large, resulting in a concentration of energy in the midfrequencies of the output spectrum.

The output spectra of voiced and voiceless stops at the same place of articulation are essentially the same, with greater overall amplitude for the voiceless stop spectra. Voiced and voiceless stops may be distinguished from each other by: (a) the appearance of glottal pulses during the closure interval of voiced but not voiceless stops and (b) longer VOTs for voiceless compared with voiced stops.

WHAT IS THE THEORY OF AFFRICATE ACOUSTICS?

Affricates combine features of stop consonants and fricatives. Like stops, affricates have a closure interval during which P_o rises and is released when the articulatory constriction is broken. This results in a burst similar to a stop burst. A relatively long interval of frication energy generated by turbulent airflow follows the burst, again just as in the case of stops. What seems to distinguish affricates from stops is the long interval of this frication noise. In stops, the frication has a duration between 30 and 50 ms, whereas in affricates this interval may have a duration of 60 to 80 ms. As described above, frication noise occurs when the conditions for turbulent airflow exist, these conditions being: (a) a flow of sufficient magnitude and (b) a sufficiently narrow constriction. The longer frication interval in affricates compared with stops suggests that immediately after the release of an affricate the conditions for turbulence exist for a greater amount of time. This is why affricates have been described as "slowly released stops." The affricates of American English, which include /tʃ/ and /dʒ/, may also have a place of articulation that is different (slightly posterior) from the lingua-alveolar place of /t/ and /d/. Affricates are discussed more fully in Chapter 11.

ACOUSTIC CONTRASTS ASSOCIATED WITH THE VOICING DISTINCTION IN OBSTRUENTS

Four intervals for stop consonants have been defined and discussed. The first three (closure interval, burst, and frication interval) apply to both voiceless and voiced stops, whereas the aspiration interval is only found for voiceless stops. VOTs of voiceless stops are typically longer than those of voiced stops, partly because of the aspiration interval in the former case. Typical VOTs for voiced stops are between 0 and 20 ms, whereas VOTs for voiceless stops are typically between 40 and 80 ms. A VOT of zero means that glottal pulsing begins at the same time as the release of the stop (i.e., the burst). The difference in VOTs for voiceless and voiced stops is shown in Figure 9–16 by comparing the top two waveforms.

The relatively short VOTs of voiced stops not only are due to the absence of the aspiration interval, but also reflect burst and frication intervals that are somewhat shorter than those found in voiceless stops. The shorter burst and frication intervals are probably the result of the lower P_o in voiced compared with voiceless stops. In addition, the vocal folds begin vibrating almost immediately after release of the vocal tract closure for voiced stops. This is because, during the stop closure, the vocal folds are held near or at the midline, and if the pressure difference across the folds is sufficient they vibrate to produce voicing, as shown in the closure interval of Figure 9–16 (right). At the release of a voiced stop, the vocal folds are in position to begin vibration for the following vowel.

The activity at the level of the larynx for voiceless stops and other voiceless obstruents is substantially

> ### Slowly Released Slops
>
> Affricates combine stop (closure and burst) and fricative features (a relatively long period of frication noise). This phonetic double identity is represented in the transcription symbols for English affricates, /tʃ/ and /dʒ/. But are affricates really two sound classes—stops and fricatives—in rapid succession, or should they be accorded their own unique sound class? The famous linguist/phonetician Leigh Lisker (1918–2006) called affricates "slowly released stops," by which he meant they were neither stops nor fricatives, but something different. Another form of evidence for the unique status of affricates is what happens when the sound class is involved in a spoonerism, or as the linguists like the call them, "metathetic errors." "Flipping the channel" becomes "chipping the flannel"; the /tʃ/ in "channel" does not separate into a stop and fricative component, with either one moving independently (nor does the /fl/ cluster separate for this switch: chipping the flannel—that's another story). Here is another one that makes the same point for /dʒ/, spoken by actor Peter Sellers in the Pink Panther classic *A Shot in the Dark* (1964): "killed him in a rit of fealous jage." Linguists such as Stephanie Shattuck Hufnagel (Massachusetts Institute of Technology), Victoria Fromkin (1923–2000, UCLA), and Gary Dell (University of Illinois) have studied these errors to shed light on the sound systems of languages.

different than in the case of voiced stops. This activity receives detailed consideration in Chapter 11, where acoustic data and physiological interpretations are presented on the voicing distinction for stops, fricatives, and affricates.

REVIEW

A theory of consonant acoustics was presented, with special emphasis on the acoustic basis of antiresonances and the aeromechanical basis of noise sources.

A theory of consonants is similar in some respects to the theory of vowel acoustics, but also differs from the latter in important ways.

Antiresonances occur when two resonators are coupled, as in the case of nasals and laterals, or when a source sits in-between two vocal tract resonators, as in the case of stops, fricatives, and affricates.

Nasal murmur and nasalization spectra include antiresonances as well as resonances; the antiresonances have the effect of reducing or eliminating the amplitude of resonances in the output signal.

Lateral /l/ has an antiresonance originating in the closed cavity between the tongue tip contact with the alveolar ridge and the tongue dorsum contact (or near contact) with the soft palate.

The primary resonator in obstruent production is determined by the size of the resonator in front of the constriction.

The relationship of aeromechanical phenomena to speech acoustic phenomena is critical in consideration of fricative, stop, and affricate acoustics.

Turbulent airflow is generated when a sufficiently high airflow is forced through a sufficiently narrow constriction.

The acoustic correlate of turbulence is noise, which accounts for frication and aspiration sources in the speech production apparatus.

Stop consonants have a shock excitation source, which is the acoustic result of sudden release of the positive oral pressure developed during the silent interval.

The measurement of consonant spectra is complicated, but several alternative approaches are discussed.

VOT, the duration between a stop consonant burst and the first glottal pulse of a following vowel, is a well-studied temporal measurement of stop consonants.

Affricates are best understood as slowly released stop consonants.

Data from several studies in which stop, fricative, and nasal spectra have been measured are presented in Chapter 11.

REFERENCES

A shot in the dark [Motion picture]. (1964). B. Edwards (Director). United States: MGM Entertainment.
Bell-Berti, F. (1975). Control of pharyngeal cavity size for voiced and voiceless stops. *Journal of the Acoustical Society of America, 57,* 456–461.
Bell-Berti, F. (1993). Understanding velic motor control: Studies of segmental context. In M. Huffman & R. Krakow (Eds.), *Phonetics and phonology: Nasals, nasalization, and the velum* (pp. 63–85). New York, NY: Academic Press.
Blumstein, S., & Steven, K. (1979). Acoustic invariance in speech production: Evidence from measurements of the

spectral characteristics of stop consonants. *Journal of the Acoustical Society of America, 66,* 1001–1017.

Byrd, D. (1993). 54,000 American stops. *UCLA Working Papers in Phonetics, 83,* 97–116.

Catford, J. (1977). *Fundamental problems in phonetics.* Bloomington, IN: Indiana University Press.

Dang, J., & Honda, K. (1996). Acoustic characteristics of the paranasal sinuses derived from transmission characteristic measurement and morphological observation. *Journal of the Acoustical Society of America, 100,* 3374–3383.

Dang, J., Honda, K., & Suzuki, H. (1994). Morphological and acoustical analysis of the nasal and paranasal cavities. *Journal of the Acoustical Society of America, 96,* 2088–2100.

Fant, G. (1960). *Acoustic theory of speech production.* The Hague, Netherlands: Mouton.

Fant, G. (1973). *Speech sounds and features.* Cambridge, MA: MIT Press.

Forrest, K., Weismer, G., Milenkovic, P., & Dougall, R. (1988). Statistical analysis of word-initial voiceless obstruents: Preliminary data. *Journal of the Acoustical Society of America, 84,* 115–124.

Fujimura, O. (1962). Analysis of nasal consonants. *Journal of the Acoustical Society of America, 34,* 1865–1875.

Havel, M., Hoffman, G., Mürbe, D. & Sundberg, J. (2014). Contribution of paranasal sinuses to the acoustic properties of the nasal tract. *Folia Phoniatrica et Logopaedica, 66,* 109–114.

Hawkins, S., & Stevens, K. (1985). Acoustic and perceptual correlates of the non-nasal-nasal distinction for vowels. *Journal of the Acoustical Society of America, 77,* 1560–1575.

Jongman, A., Wayland, R., & Wong, S. (2000). Acoustic characteristics of English fricatives. *Journal of the Acoustical Society of America, 108,* 1252–1263.

Kent, R., & Moll, K. (1969). Vocal tract characteristics of the stop cognates. *Journal of the Acoustical Society of America, 46,* 1555–1559.

Klatt, D., Stevens, K., & Mead, J. (1968). Studies of articulatory activity and airflow during speech. *Annals of the New York Academy of Sciences, 155,* 42–55.

Ladefoged, P., & Maddieson, I. (1996). *The sounds of the world's languages.* Oxford, UK: Blackwell.

Narayanan, S. S., Alwan, A. A., & Haker, K. (1997). Toward articulatory-acoustic models for liquid approximants based on MRI and EPG data. Part I. The laterals. *Journal of the Acoustical Society of America, 101,* 1064–1077.

Proctor, M. I., Shadle, C. H., & Iskarous, K. (2010). Pharyngeal articulation in the production of voiced and voiceless fricatives. *Journal of the Acoustical Society of America, 127,* 1507–1518.

Pruthi, T., & Espy-Wilson, C. (2004). Acoustic parameters for automatic detection of nasal manner. *Speech Communication, 43,* 225–239.

Pruthi, T., Espy-Wilson, C. Y., & Story, B. H. (2007). Simulation and analysis of nasalized vowels based on magnetic resonance imaging data. *Journal of the Acoustical Society of America, 121,* 3858–3873.

Rong, P., & Kuehn, D. P. (2010). The effect of oral articulation on the acoustic characteristics of nasalized vowels. *Journal of the Acoustical Society of America, 127,* 2543–2553.

Serrurier, A., & Badin, P. (2008). A three-dimensional articulatory model of the velum and nasopharyngeal wall based on MRI and CT data. *Journal of the Acoustical Society of America, 123,* 2335–2355.

Shadle, C. (1985). *The acoustics of fricative consonants* (Unpublished doctoral dissertation). Massachusetts Institute of Technology, Cambridge, MA.

Shadle, C. (1990). Articulatory-acoustic relationships in fricative consonants. In W. Hardcastle & A. Marchal (Eds.), *Speech production and speech modeling* (pp. 187–209). Dordrecht, Netherlands: Kluwer Academic.

Stevens, K. (1998). *Acoustic phonetics.* Cambridge, MA: MIT Press.

Stevens, K., Fant, G., & Hawkins, S. (1987). Some acoustical and perceptual correlates of nasal vowels. In R. Channon & L. Shockey (Eds.), *In honor of Ilse Lehiste* (pp. 241–254). Dordrecht, Netherlands: Foris.

10

Speech Acoustic Measurement and Analysis

INTRODUCTION

Chapters 8 and 9 are devoted to the theoretical bases of speech acoustics, with acoustic patterns of selected speech sounds presented to illustrate the theory. A variety of techniques are available for generating the speech acoustic displays shown in Chapters 8 and 9, and for using the displays to obtain speech acoustic measurements. These displays and measurements are the subject matter of the current chapter.

The current use of the term "techniques" goes beyond consideration of the instruments used to store, analyze, and *represent* (i.e., graph) the speech acoustic signal. In this chapter, the term includes the *conceptual* tools that have been developed to make sense of vocal tract output. When a speech signal—the acoustic output of the vocal tract—is displayed in the several ways discussed below, a large amount of information is available, not all of which is relevant to each of the many reasons for studying speech acoustics. For example, some individuals study the speech signal to make inferences about the articulatory behavior that produced the signal (as discussed in Chapters 8 and 9). Others may be interested in the characteristics of the signal used by listeners to understand speech. Still others may be interested in which parts of the speech signal are the best candidates for computer recognition of speech. And, of course, many scientists have studied the speech acoustic signal to develop computer programs for high-quality speech synthesis. Sometimes, what is important about the speech signal is relevant to all four of these areas of interest, but this is not always the case. Thus, the conceptual tools that make sense of the speech signal may be specific to a particular purpose.

Computers Are Not Smarter Than Humans

Speech recognizers are computer programs that analyze a speech signal to figure out what was said. The programs use acoustic analysis and other data (such as stored information on the probability of one sound following another) to produce a set of words that represents a best "guess" about the true nature of the input signal. Many of these programs learn the patterns of a single talker's speech, and in doing so improve their recognition performance over time for that talker. Unfortunately, the improved performance does not always transfer to a new talker, whose acoustic-phonetic patterns are different enough from the original talker's to confuse the speech recognition program. Humans, it should be noted, typically have no trouble transferring their speech recognition skills from one talker to another (but—see Chapter 12 for why this statement may not be completely true).

A HISTORICAL PRELUDE

A brief history of the technology of speech acoustics research illustrates how much progress has been made in a relatively short time. A starting point is the multitalented German scientist Herman von Helmholtz (1821–1894), who in the 1850s was very much interested in explaining the acoustical basis of vowel quality. Like most phoneticians who puzzled over the relationship between "mouth positions" and different vowel qualities, Helmholtz used an ancient piece of equipment—the ear—as a spectral analyzer to determine the rules linking vocal tract shape and vocal tract output. Helmholtz's innovation in the study of vowels was to insert between the mouth of the speaker and his own ear a kind of spectral analysis tool—in some cases a series of tuning forks, in others a series of Helmholtz resonators (Figure 10–1). When he used tuning forks (see Figure 10–1, top), Helmholtz asked a laboratory assistant to configure his vocal tract in the position of a specific vowel, and then struck the tuning fork and held it close to the assistant's lips. If the tuning fork produced a very loud tone, Helmholtz assumed that the cavity inside the vocal tract was excited by the sound waves and was therefore "tuned" to the frequency of the fork. If the sound was weak, the natural frequency of the mouth cavity was assumed to be far from the frequency of the fork. Helmholtz was using the resonance principle discussed in Chapter 7, with the tuning fork serving as input, the vocal tract as resonator, and his ear as the detector of the output (see Figure 7–18 for a model of an input-resonator-output system). When a tuning fork produced a tone that resonated in the assistant's vocal tract configured for a specific vowel, Helmholtz assumed that the frequency of the fork was a "natural" frequency of that vowel. By using a whole series of tuning forks, ranging from low frequencies to high frequencies, Helmholtz constructed a diagram of the important frequencies for different vowels, or stated differently, the frequencies that distinguish the vowels from one another. In another series of experiments, Helmholtz's assistants phonated different vowels into the neck of a resonator while he listened at the other end (see Figure 10–1, bottom). By changing resonator size to sample a wide range of frequencies, Helmholtz identified which resonators, and hence which frequencies, seemed to produce the loudest sound at his ear. These frequencies were taken as the "natural" frequencies of the vowels. Both types of experiments show how the principle of resonance was applied to the problem of frequency analysis for vowels.

Helmholtz tried to circumvent a strictly *subjective* ear analysis by objective measurements, using physical instruments (i.e., tuning forks and Helmholtz resonators) with known frequency characteristics. After all, a sufficient number of tuning forks or resonators provides something like a low-tech Fourier analysis. In Helmholtz's case, however, the *perceptual* magnitude (i.e., the loudness), rather than a physical amplitude, was identified for selected frequency components in

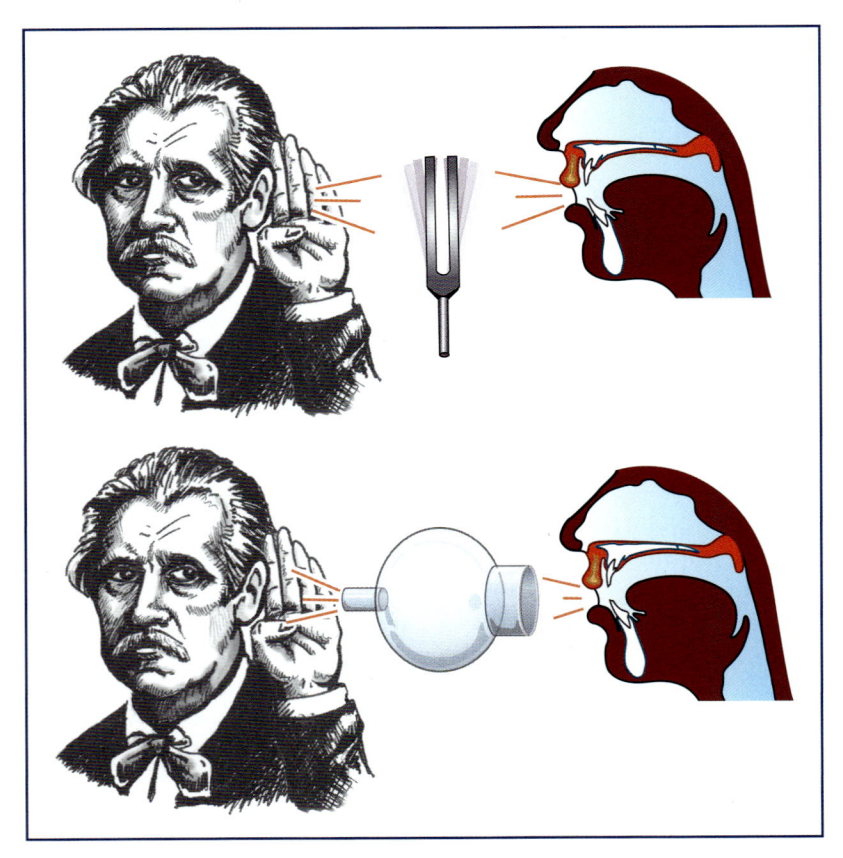

Figure 10–1. Helmholtz's experimental arrangements for determining the important frequencies of vowels. *Top panel* shows the tuning fork approach. *Bottom panel* shows the resonator approach.

the spectrum. The selected components were limited to the number of tuning forks or Helmholtz resonators available for the analysis. Even with these limitations, Helmholtz's approach was innovative and creative for the middle of the nineteenth century, long before electronic instruments were available to analyze and quantify energy at different signal frequencies.

There were other attempts, prior to the electronics age, to obtain objective data from the speech signal. For example, in the latter part of the nineteenth century, W. König knew that the acoustic output of the vocal tract was in the form of pressure waves (Chapter 7, Figure 7–2). These rapidly varying regions of high and low pressures, König reasoned, could be studied by looking at the *effect* they produced on an observable event. König found such an event in the form of a gas-fed flame like that used in chemistry labs. Figure 10–2 shows a schematic diagram of the König apparatus. Gas was fed to a chamber beneath the burner ("inflow of gas" in Figure 10–2). With a constant gas volume in the chamber the flame had a constant height. One side of the chamber consisted of a distensible (flexible) membrane, so movements of the membrane into the chamber compressed the gas and raised the height of the flame, whereas outward movements of the membrane expanded the volume of the chamber, which rarefied the gas and lowered the height of the flame. Participants in König's experiment phonated vowels into a pipe terminated by this distensible membrane, and the compressions and rarefactions of the speech wave within the pipe caused rapid pushes and pulls on the membrane. These movements made the flame dance up and down as the gas volume was alternately compressed and expanded. By filming the motions of the dancing flame during phonation of vowels, König was able to record a crude version of *speech waves*.

The conceptual basis of König's technique, of having sound waves create movement in a structure that is *transformed* into an observable event, is the basis of modern electronic recording of speech signals. For example, many microphones transform acoustic to electrical energy by means of a very thin membrane whose vibratory movement creates varying voltages in response to air pressure fluctuations of a sound wave. These varying voltages are recorded on digital tape or directly to disk, where they provide an electronic replica of the speech wave.

Devices for the transformation of aeromechanical (in this case, pressure) to electrical energy did not become readily available until the early part of the twentieth century. The great advantage of electronic devices is the ability to record and analyze a wider range of frequencies than possible using strictly mechanical devices, and the related ability to capture very accurate details of sound waves. Devices such as König's were not able to record rapidly changing details of sound waves.

Why do electronic devices extend the range of detailed frequency and amplitude analysis past that of a device like König's? As described in Chapter 7, there is an inverse relationship between frequency and period. When sound waves contain energy at higher

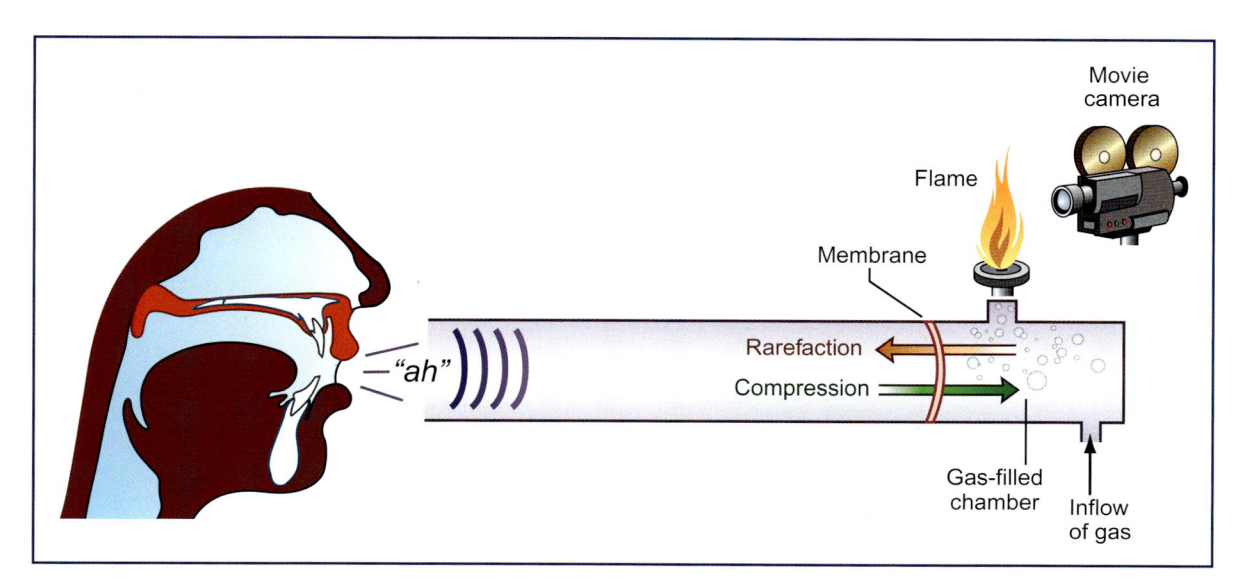

Figure 10-2. The König device for visualizing and recording pressure fluctuations in the speech wave. Compressions and expansions of the gas volume produced rises and falls in the flame height, which were filmed to obtain primitive speech waveforms.

frequencies, the motion of the air particles is very rapid (i.e., they have relatively short periods). In a device like König's, the ideal situation is for these very rapid motions of air particles to strike the membrane and set it into vibration at exactly the same high frequencies. The high-frequency motions of the membrane would be reflected in high-frequency fluctuations in flame height, and the flame would provide a precise representation of the energy in the sound wave.

Unfortunately, this is not always the case with a mechanical vibrator such as the membrane in König's device. Because the membrane has mass and therefore demonstrates inertia, it resists being accelerated by certain forces—especially those that last only a short time. The rapidly vibrating air molecules associated with high-frequency energy, and therefore short periods, result in short-lasting compressions and rarefactions. Because the membrane demonstrates inertia, it is likely to move in response to these high-frequency vibrations only a little bit, or perhaps not at all, because high-frequency forces are not applied over a long enough time interval to overcome the opposition to acceleration. Think of it this way: a short-lasting compression is applied to the membrane to compress the gas in the chamber, but the membrane does not respond immediately to the applied force because it has mass and opposes being accelerated. By the time the membrane begins to respond with inward motion, the rapidly varying pressure applied to the membrane has changed to a rarefaction phase, pulling the membrane outward, away from the gas-containing chamber and potentially enlarging the volume of gas within the chamber. In a sense, the membrane never gets a chance to respond accurately to the applied forces because of its inertial properties. The membrane acts like a filter, responding accurately with motion to lower frequency signals whose energy can be applied to it over a long enough time interval, but being insensitive to, and hence filtering out, the energy associated with higher-frequency vibration. The vibration of the membrane does not represent accurately all details of the pressure wave applied to it. The vibration of the membrane *distorts* the details of the pressure wave, and this distortion is passed on to the variation in flame height. Thus, the fluctuation in flame height over time is not an entirely accurate representation of the acoustic event.

In the case of the König device, the relatively massive membrane *transduced* the pressure waves via compression or rarefaction of the gas in the chamber. König's membrane had to be relatively massive to produce effective compressions and rarefactions of the gas molecules. When electronic recording and storage of acoustical signals became available, this problem was more or less eliminated. Electronic transducers, which form the heart of a microphone, are still membrane-like but are extremely delicate and have minimal mass. The vibrations of these transducers produce changes in the motion of *electrons* in electrical circuits. The ease of electron acceleration and deceleration (due to negligible mass) allows these thin, minimal-mass membranes to respond *faithfully* to very high frequencies in sound waves.

Early electronic recordings and analyses of vocal tract output resulted in waveforms such as those shown in Figure 10–3. A 70-ms waveform "piece" is shown for each of the four corner vowels of American English (/ɑ/, /i/, /æ/, /u/, clockwise from upper left-hand panel). These vowels were produced as sustained phonations by an adult male. The 70-ms pieces shown in the figure were extracted from the sustained sounds using computer-editing techniques. These waveforms *are* faithful representations of the pressure waves associated with the vocal tract outputs (they are "clipped" a bit at the bottom, by the picture, not the recording process) for the corner vowels, with some obvious similarities across the four waveforms. First, each waveform has a repeating period, one of which is marked in each panel. The repeating period is expected because all vowels in English are produced with nearly periodic vibration of the vocal folds. Second, each waveform shows smaller amplitude vibrations between the largest amplitude peaks. The largest amplitude peaks reflect the energy produced at the instant of vocal fold closure (see Chapter 8), and the smaller energy peaks are produced by resonances in the vocal tract. From the vowel theory presented in Chapter 8, it is known that the vocal tract resonances are different for the four corner vowels; these different resonances explain the different appearance of the four waveforms in Figure 10–3. For example, the /ɑ/ and /æ/ waveforms

---

Shouting at Early Microphones

The earliest microphone was developed in 1876 or 1877. It used a membrane that was displaced by sound waves, and the motion of the membrane was transmitted to a metal pin sitting in an acid solution. The motion of the membrane moved the pin to various depths of the acid solution, which changed the electrical characteristics of the system. Happily, this "liquid transmitter" system didn't catch on, because Alexander Graham Bell found he had to shout at the membrane to produce even a barely audible sound at the other end of the device (three miles away!).

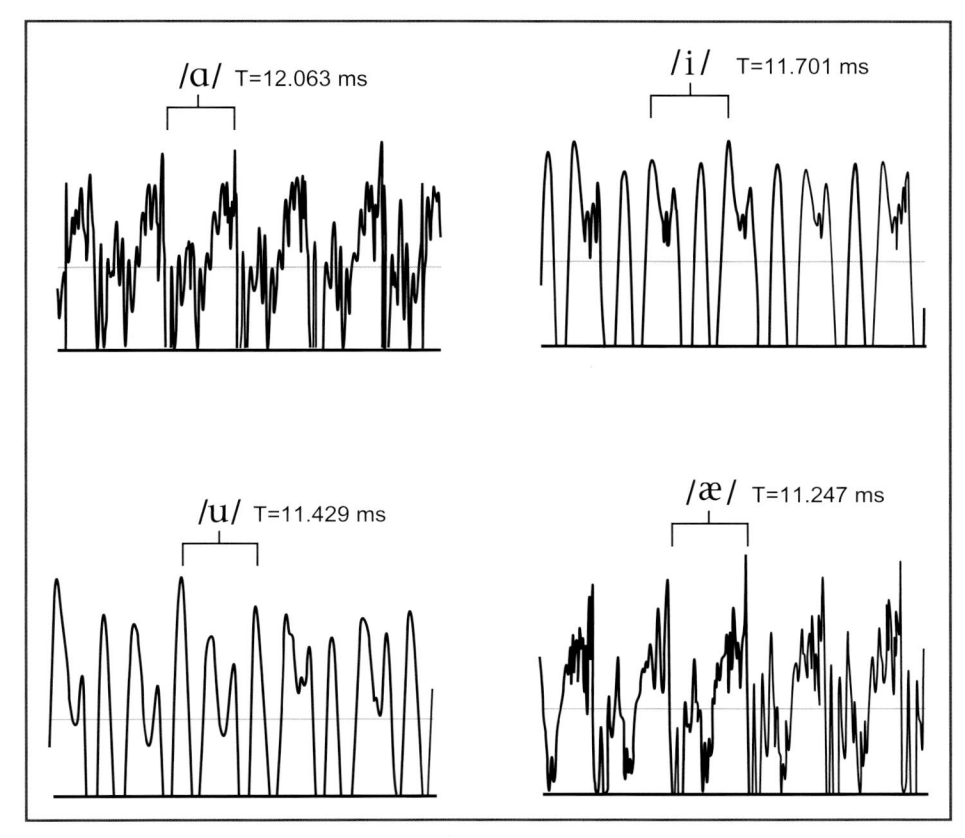

Figure 10–3. Seventy-millisecond waveform pieces from each of the four corner vowels of English. Pieces were extracted from sustained vowels. The waveforms are "clipped" a bit at the bottom, by the picture, not the recording process. Note the individual glottal pulses, and the period (T) marked on each vowel waveform. Note also the different waveform appearance depending on which vowel was produced.

seem to have more complex energy patterns within a given period compared with the /i/ and /u/ waveforms. Note the many amplitude fluctuations within the periods of the first two vowels, compared with the smaller number of amplitude peaks within the periods of /i/ and /u/.

Although the resonance patterns are reflected in the different waveform patterns displayed in Figure 10–3, the differing resonant frequencies of the vowels cannot be determined merely by looking at the waveforms. The resonant frequencies can be determined using the technique of Fourier analysis, where a complex waveform is decomposed into the frequencies and amplitudes of the component sinusoids (see Chapter 7). Originally, this may have been done with paper and pencil and the application to the measurements of the correct formulas, or with a mechanical device called a Henrici analyzer. In either case the process was tedious. As electronic devices became more sophisticated, specialized instruments were developed for automatic computation of a Fourier spectrum. These devices, called *spectrum analyzers*, took a waveform as input and stored some part of it in an electronic memory. The stored part might be a 70-ms piece such as the ones shown in Figure 10–3. The spectrum analyzer performed a Fourier analysis of that piece and showed the computed spectrum on a display screen. These analyses were quite accurate, but required a fair amount of computation time. Moreover, the spectrum results were more accurate when the stored piece was longer, rather than shorter.

The duration of the waveform undergoing analysis was of great concern for speech scientists, who even at the dawn of the electronic age had a good idea that the articulators, and hence the shape of the vocal tract, were in nearly constant motion. A discussion of the relationship between vocal tract resonances and the shape of the vocal tract is presented in Chapter 8. When the shape of the vocal tract changes, so do the resonant frequencies. During speech production, many phonetically relevant changes in vocal tract configuration are quite rapid, in some cases occurring within intervals as brief as 40 to 50 ms. For example, when a lingual stop consonant such as /d/ is released into a low vowel such as /æ/, the vocal tract changes from the consonant to vowel configuration in about 40 ms. This fast change in the shape of the vocal tract results in rapidly changing vocal tract resonances. These time-varying resonances of the vocal tract are called *formant transitions*.

Spectral analysis of rapidly changing formant transitions is often performed to determine the frequency range covered by a formant transition, or the rate of the frequency change as a function of time (that is, the slope of the frequency change). A schematic second formant (F2) transition for the syllable /bæ/, produced by an adult male speaker, is shown in Figure 10–4. The upward-pointing arrow at 0 ms indicates the beginning of the formant transition, which occurs at the first glottal pulse (vocal fold vibration) following release of the /b/. The downward-pointing arrow at 50 ms marks the end of the formant transition, or the point at which the frequency ceases changing as a function of time (note the relatively constant F2 value after the downward-pointing arrow, indicating a steady vocal tract shape for the vowel "target." This F2 transition, which covers a frequency range of 600 Hz in 50 ms, presents problems for the "static" spectrum analyzer described above. If the entire 50-ms piece of the waveform is submitted for spectral analysis, the resulting spectrum is an average of all the changing frequencies along the transition. This analysis clearly misrepresents the true vocal tract output. The "smeared" spectrum resulting from this analysis is virtually useless, especially with respect to interpretation of the articulatory behavior that produced the transition. The analysis can better match the true frequency event by picking brief temporal pieces along the transition, analyzing the spectrum of each piece, and combining the successive spectra to reconstruct the transition. This is shown by the successive, short-time pieces, along the bottom edge of the transition, each having a duration of 10 ms. As shown in Figure 10–4, a complete analysis of the transition using these 10 ms pieces requires five consecutive spectral analyses (5 pieces × 10-ms per piece = 50 ms, or the duration of the entire transition). This approach minimizes the spectral smear that occurs when the 50 ms piece is analyzed as a single interval, but even so it is not particularly attractive because: (a) the amount of work involved in separately isolating and analyzing each 10 ms piece is substantial; (b) the short-time pieces, as noted above, result in a loss of accuracy in the analysis of the frequency components; and (c) the spectral smear problem is not entirely eliminated, because each 10 ms piece covers a 120 Hz change (120 Hz for each of five 10 ms pieces = 120 × 5 = 600 Hz); a formant frequency change of 120 Hz over a 10-ms interval is a significant change in vocal tract output.

The electronically based spectrum analyzers available to early speech researchers, therefore, had notable limitations. The analyzers allowed a previously unknown precision of frequency analysis, but the requirements of the analysis (e.g., a long "piece" of the signal for precise analysis) were not well matched to many of the important features of a rapidly changing vocal tract output. Spectral analyses of long-duration speech signals can be used effectively for waveforms extracted from sustained vowels (see Figure 10–3) or some target intervals for a vowel in connected speech. In these cases, the vocal tract shape remains constant over a long time (sustained vowels) or a long enough time (targets in connected speech) to permit a reasonable, fast spectral analysis. But constancy of resonant frequencies over time is not typical of speech production. Rather, rapid frequency change over time is the rule in speech acoustics for both vowels and consonants, and almost certainly plays an important role in speech perception as well.

In summary, electronics allowed the recording and analysis of acoustic waveforms associated with vocal tract output. These electronic waveforms represented the actual fluctuations in pressure waves with a high

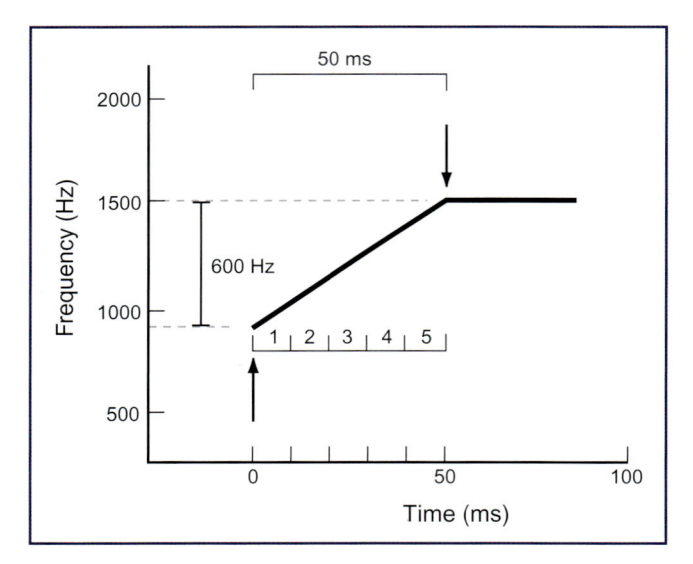

Figure 10–4. Schematic drawing showing an F2 transition for /bæ/. Upward-pointing arrow at 0 ms shows beginning of the transition. The end of the transition is shown by the downward-pointing arrow at 50 ms. The pieces spanning the duration of the transition, labeled 1 through 5, show individual 10-ms intervals that can be extracted from the transition for analysis. See text for details.

degree of accuracy but did not provide immediate (i.e., visible) access to the formants, the information critical to an understanding of vocal tract shape (see Chapter 8). Inspection of the waveform revealed the *presence* of formants, reflected in the complex vibratory features within each waveform period (see Figure 10–3), but not the actual *frequencies* of the resonances. Early spectral analyzers took pieces of waveforms and performed very accurate measures of formant (resonant) frequencies, but only for relatively long duration waveforms. Because speech production involves rapidly changing vocal tract shapes over relatively short time intervals, these were not ideal analyses. What was needed was an analyzer that was able to *display formants as a function of time*. Such an analyzer would perform a spectral analysis as a (nearly) continuous function of time and display the spectral peaks (formants) in such a way that a changing shape of the vocal tract could be inferred from a mere glance at the physical record. The development of the instrument capable of doing this kind of analysis was, in part, an ironic by-product of the human race's oldest failure of communication—war.

THE SOUND SPECTROGRAPH: HISTORY AND TECHNIQUE

Throughout the course of World War II (1939–1945), there was an increasing use of encoded messages sent between different command posts, or from central locations to troop locations on the battlefield. This encoding, or *encryption*, was necessary because the warring parties were constantly monitoring communications sent by the other side. One side employed the talents of many different people to develop codes for effective encryption of a message, and the other side employed a large staff to figure out how to break these codes. The code breakers typically worked with paper and pencil, laboring over an encoded message and working through possible decoding solutions. At some point during the war, the allies (the United States, Soviet Union, Great Britain, and France) assembled a team of linguists, puzzle and code experts, mathematicians, engineers, psychologists, and other specialists to develop an automated decoding device. The theory behind such a device was relatively simple. An encoded message, such as a radio voice transmission, would be fed into a machine that performed various types of analysis to decode the message (as in the 2014 film *The Imitation Game*). The project of the allies failed to solve the problem of automated decoding of encoded messages, but one of its products was a device called the *sound spectrograph*.

The ideal spectrum analyzer for speech, as suggested above, can display formants as a continuous function of time. This is precisely what was produced when the sound spectrograph was used to analyze speech. Scientists in the Soviet Union—*prisoner* scientists, forced to work on projects ordered by the state—developed a sound spectrograph in the late 1940s, as related by the renowned writer A. I. Solzhenitsyn (1969) in his documentary novel *The First Circle*. In the novel, Solzhenitsyn's character Major Roitman explains how the spectrograph displays the speech signal in what he calls a *voice print*:

> *In these voice prints speech is measured three ways at once: frequency, across the tape;—time, along the tape; and amplitude—by the density of the picture. Therefore, each sound is depicted so uniquely that it can be recognized easily, and everything that has been said can be read on the tape.* (p. 217)

A sample spectrogram, with a time-synchronized waveform immediately above, is shown in Figure 10–5. When Major Roitman described frequency *across the tape*, he was referring to the *y*-axis of the spectrogram, which extends in this example from 0 Hz (the baseline of the spectrogram) to just below 8.0 kHz. The *x*-axis in this spectrogram is time, corresponding to Roitman's *along the tape* dimension. In the present case, the time axis is marked off in 100-ms increments. The spectrogram shows a number of dark bands, all of which seem to vary in height (i.e., along the *y*-axis) across time. When Major Roitman described amplitude in terms of the density of the picture, he was referring to the varying darkness of different locations on the spectrogram. The darker the spectrogram at any given point in time and frequency, the greater the energy at that point. In Chapter 8, the formants of vowels were described as peaks in the spectrum, the locations in the spectrum where energy is at a maximum. Because the dark bands in the spectrogram shown in Figure 10–5 indicate locations of very high energy, they are the formants of the vowels. These dark bands vary in height (along the *y*-axis) across time, showing that the formant frequencies change substantially throughout an utterance.

Today, spectrum analyzers are digital and are programmed to the needs of speech analysis. These software packages produce spectrograms and other displays of a host of speech analyses. Figure 10–6 illustrates how the early versions of the spectrograph (the instrument) generated spectrograms (the pictures produced by the spectrograph). The operator of the spectrograph flipped a switch that caused rotation of a turntable platter as shown in Figure 10–6. Wrapped around the edge of the platter was a magnetic strip that

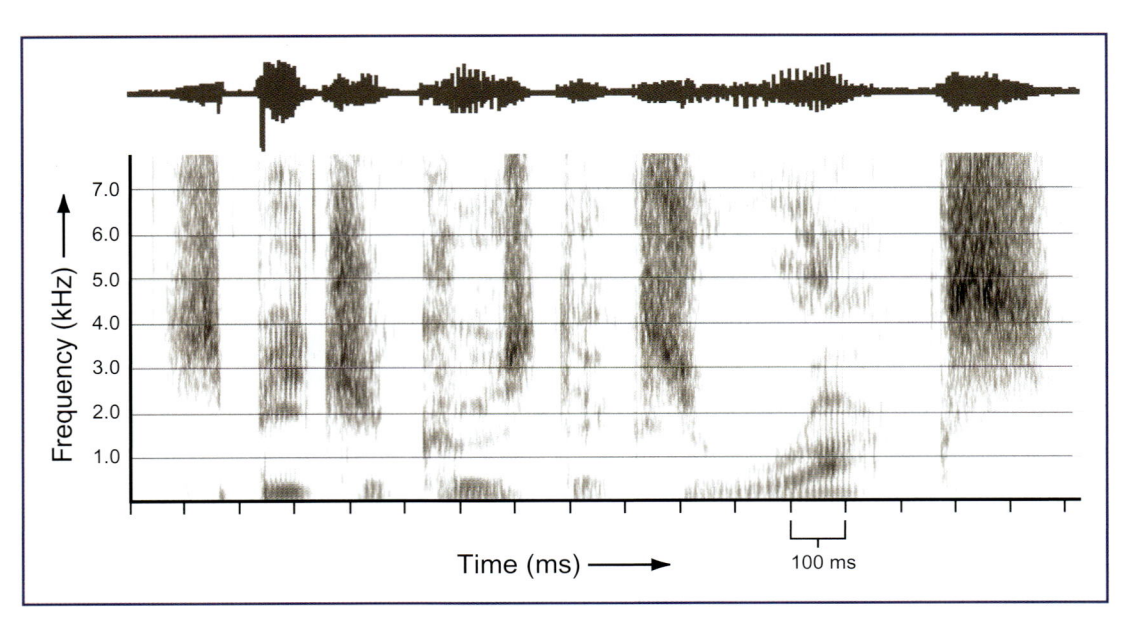

Figure 10-5. A sample spectrogram, showing time along the x-axis, frequency on the y-axis, and intensity as the darkness of the trace. The interval between each vertical tick on the time axis is equal to 100 ms, and horizontal lines running across the spectrogram from bottom to top (y-axis) mark 1000 Hz increments. The darkness of the tracing at any location indicates the relative intensity at that time-frequency coordinate. The speech waveform is above the spectrogram.

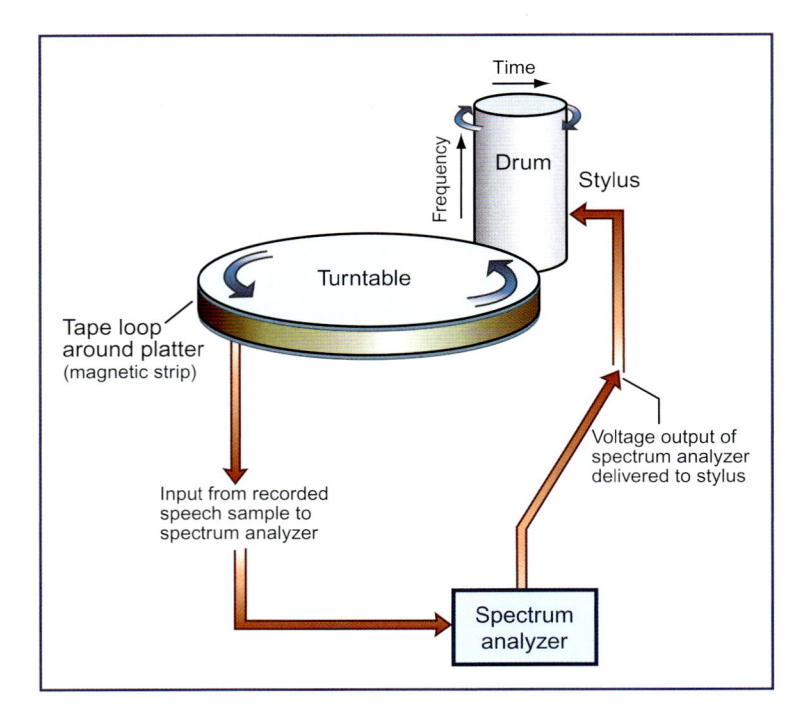

Figure 10-6. Schematic diagram of the components of the classic sound spectrograph. Speech is recorded onto the continuous magnetic tape around the turntable platter, and the magnetic fluctuations corresponding to the speech signal are passed to a spectrum analyzer. The voltage output of the spectrum analyzer is sent to a heated stylus that burns patterns onto special paper mounted on the rotating drum. See text for details.

Writing from Experience

When the world-famous writer Alexander Solzhenitsyn (1918–2008) wrote *The First Circle*, he had the firsthand experience of the *sharashka*, the Russian word for a prison camp for scientists. In the Soviet Union, many writers, artists, and politically active people were imprisoned simply for their beliefs. Most were sent to forced-labor camps, described in Solzhenitsyn's monumental work, *The Gulag Archipelago*. A very few, like Solzhenitsyn, were more fortunate and were sent to a *sharashka* to work on a scientific project. Solzhenitsyn's role in the development of the spectrograph was as a linguist. Life at a *sharashka* was infinitely better than in the regular prison camps, but Solzhenitsyn's title reveals his feelings about his time there. It is taken from the "first circle of hell" in Dante's *The Divine Comedy*.

---

served as an electronic recording medium. A speech signal[1] was recorded onto the rotating magnetic band, which functioned as a closed tape loop permitting storage of no more than about 2.5 seconds of continuous speech. The frequency and amplitude information in the speech signal, as a function of time, was stored as magnetic patterns on this loop. With the recorded signal in place on the magnetic loop, the turntable was then rotated much faster than the recording speed[2] and the magnetic patterns served as the input to a spectrum analyzer.

The spectrum analyzer performed its analysis by moving a fixed-width *analysis band*, or *filter*, across the entire frequency range. This is illustrated in Figure 10–7, which shows the hypothetical results of a Fourier analysis of the vowel /i/. Frequency is shown on the *y*-axis, increasing from bottom to top (i.e., the presentation of the spectrum is rotated 90° counterclockwise and then flipped for this example), and amplitude is shown on the *x*-axis. Each of the lines in this Fourier spectrum is a harmonic (the first three are indicated on the spectrum), and the length of each line extending to the right from the baseline indicates the relative amplitude of the harmonic (e.g., the third harmonic has greater

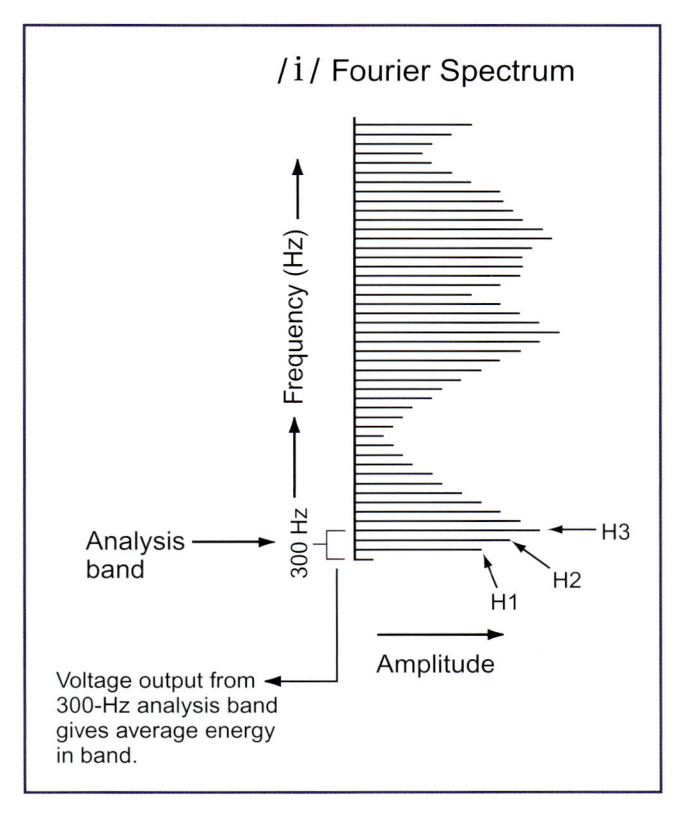

Figure 10–7. Schematic diagram showing how the spectrograph performs spectral analysis by sweeping an analysis band of fixed width (e.g., 300 Hz) across the frequency range of interest, and recording the average voltages from the analysis band as a continuous function of time and frequency. Frequency is on the *y*-axis, intensity on the *x*-axis. Each harmonic of a vowel is shown as a line extending to the right; the length of the line indicates the relative intensity of that harmonic (H1 = first harmonic [F0], H2 = second harmonic, H3 = third harmonic, and so forth).

amplitude than the second harmonic). At the bottom of the frequency scale is a small bracket that extends over a frequency range of 300 Hz. This bracket is the fixed-width (width = 300 Hz) analysis band mentioned at the beginning of this paragraph. The arrow pointing down and to the left from this analysis band is labeled *voltage output*, which is the key to the spectrum analysis performed by the spectrograph. The analysis band senses the overall energy on the magnetic tape, which

---

[1] This book is about speech, so it focuses on the use of the spectrograph to analyze speech signals. The spectrograph has been used to analyze signals produced by dolphins, birds, the act of swallowing, blood flowing through the carotid arteries, and stomachs in the process of digesting food (both efficiently and not so well!).

[2] We do not go into the details of why the turntable speed during analysis was so much faster than the turntable speed during recording; the speed difference was required for efficient analysis of the speech signal and production of the spectrogram.

it transforms into a voltage. Higher voltages are associated with greater energy, lower voltages with lesser energy. Because the analysis band covers a range of only 300 Hz, the voltage output is only for the frequencies within the band and is an average of all energy within the band. If the analysis band is swept continuously across the entire frequency range *it will provide overall voltage outputs as a continuous function of frequency*. In Figure 10–7, the arrow pointing up from the 300 Hz analysis band indicates the direction in which the band is moved continuously across the frequency range. The band starts at the lowest frequencies, where the output voltage reflects the overall energy from 0 to 300 Hz. As it moves continuously upward in frequency, the analysis band produces output voltages from the 5- to 305-Hz interval, the 10- to 310-Hz interval, and so forth. The band is always 300 Hz wide; as it moves across the frequency scale it records the average energy for successive 300 Hz bands at progressively higher frequencies, and sends these voltages as output to the stylus shown in Figure 10–6.

Recall that the magnetic patterns on the tape are fed into (i.e., serve as input to) the spectrum analyzer while the turntable is rotating. The rotation of the turntable means that the spectrum analysis is conducted as a function of time because different "pieces" of the utterance pass the analysis band at different points in time. Thus, at any instant in time, the 300 Hz analysis band provides a voltage output for the frequencies it is covering. When the analysis band is swept across the frequency range continuously, and the turntable rotates enough times to allow the analyzer to sample every instant of an utterance, the result is a set of voltages at all frequencies (i.e., within some predetermined frequency range) and at every instant in time around the tape loop. Thus, the example of Figure 10–7 is for a single instant in time—a spectral "slice in time"—and the sum of all such slice analyses results in a spectrogram of the type presented in Figure 10–5.

How does the voltage from each analysis band result in marks of varying darkness on the spectrogram? The schematic drawing of the spectrograph (see Figure 10–6) shows a drum attached to the turntable, and a stylus marking the drum. When the turntable rotates for the spectral analysis of the recorded speech signal, the attached drum rotates at the same speed. A piece of special heat-sensitive paper is wrapped around the drum, and the stylus is applied to the paper and heated in proportion to the voltage output from the analysis. As the analysis band is swept slowly across the frequency range, the stylus is synchronously transported up the vertical dimension of the spectrogram (see frequency dimension along the drum in Figure 10–6). The varying voltages from the analysis band are burned onto the special paper, with darker regions representing areas of relatively greater acoustic energy, and lighter regions representing areas of relatively lower acoustic energy. The entire process of recording a speech signal onto the tape loop, mounting the paper around the drum, and burning a complete frequency-by-time pattern onto the paper takes place over about 100 seconds. All this to obtain acoustic knowledge of no more than 2.5 seconds of speech.

The Original Sound Spectrograph: Summary

A detailed discussion has been devoted to the origins and function of the sound spectrograph for several reasons. Most importantly, the invention of this instrument initiated a scientific revolution in the study of speech production. For the first time, and with relative ease, study of the *time-varying* acoustic results of articulatory processes became possible. These time-varying characteristics were revealed most prominently by the always-changing formant frequencies. If articulator movements are changing as a function of time, and therefore changing vocal tract configuration as a function of time, the changes are reflected in formant transitions—formant frequencies that change over time. The discovery of these changes led to new ideas and insights about the behavior of the articulators in speech production.

Another reason for the detailed discussion is to (hopefully) demystify the general engineering concepts of speech acoustic analysis. An engineering degree is not necessary to understand the conceptual basis of spectrographic analysis. The amplitude and frequency characteristics of a speech signal are stored as a function of time on magnetic tape. The time-varying patterns of electromagnetic strength are submitted to a spectrum analyzer in the form of time-varying voltages (corresponding to the time-varying intensity of the magnetic fields on the tape), where voltage is proportional to sound intensity (greater voltage = greater intensity) and the speed with which the voltage changes is proportional to frequency (faster voltage changes [shorter periods] = higher frequencies). The energy in the spectrum is sampled using an analysis band, or filter, that has a bandwidth of 300 Hz that is swept continuously across the entire frequency range of interest. Because the voltage output from the analysis band is available for all frequencies and at every point in time, the spectrograph creates a total picture of the speech spectrum as a function of time. This picture is created by burning the energy patterns onto a piece of heat-sensitive paper, which results in a spectrogram. This process is summarized in Figure 10–6, by following the arrow from the turntable (the magnetic tape) all the way around to the stylus at the spectrograph drum.

Today, when scientists and clinicians make spectrograms to study speech, they do so digitally, using a desktop or laptop computer, a tablet, or smart phone. These *digital spectrograms* are displayed on screens and look like the one shown in Figure 10–5. Digital spectrograms are produced almost instantaneously after an utterance has been recorded. The computer allows a spectrogram to be generated in just a fraction of the time required to produce the burned records described. The principles discussed above for the original spectrograph are basically the same in digital spectrograms; the frequency and amplitude analysis are performed by moving a digital filter from low to high frequencies with the output being a digital magnitude that is proportional to amplitude as a function of frequency. The spectrograms shown in this textbook were produced using digital techniques, as are other forms of speech acoustic analyses. The rapid development of computer-based analysis of speech has resulted in a host of new analyses for speech acoustics, but the spectrogram remains the gold standard because it is such an immediate and rich source of information about speech production, and speech perception (see Chapter 12).

A detailed presentation of spectrograms and their interpretation is now provided. Selected information on the application of spectrographic analysis to the understanding of speech disorders is presented in Chapter 11.

Speech Acoustics as a Health Hazard?

Those of us of a certain age (your authors included), who made and analyzed spectrograms before digital spectrograms became a reality, may read the title of this sidetrack and find themselves smiling and sniffing nostalgically. As the pattern was burned onto the special paper, carbon smoke floated away from the spinning drum and filled the room with the smell of speech acoustics. That smell was something like the exhaust of a car with a corroded, burned-out muffler, seasoned with fume from an electrical fire. The wearing of light-colored clothes to the lab was discouraged—one would find fine black specks on a nice white sweater after a few hours of spectrogram-making. Some people—especially graduate students assigned to prepare spectrograms—took to wearing surgical masks in the lab.

Interpretation of Spectrograms: Specific Features

Figure 10–8 shows a spectrogram of the utterance *Peter shouldn't speak about the mugs*. A broad phonetic transcription of the sounds in the utterance is provided at the bottom of the display. Immediately above the spectrogram, on the same time scale, is the waveform of the utterance. The utterance was produced by an adult male aged 52 years, at a normal rate of speech and without special emphasis on a particular word. The utterance was chosen for its ability to showcase certain spectrographic patterns, not because it has special meaning (as far as we know, Peter does not plan on ruining a surprise birthday present of nice coffee mugs by telling the intended gift-receiver about them before the package is opened). This spectrogram was produced with the computer program *TF32*, written by Professor Paul Milenkovic of the Department of Electrical and Computer Engineering at the University of Wisconsin–Madison. *TF32* is a complete speech analysis program that includes algorithms for recording, editing, and analyzing speech waveforms, as well as displaying the speech signal as a spectrogram. Most of the speech analysis displays shown in this text were produced with *TF32* (http://userpages.chorus.net/cspeech/). Another very popular speech analysis program is Praat (http://www.fon.hum.uva.nl/praat/), which performs and displays many of the same analyses performed by TF32, as well as some unique analysis features. Praat is a free download on the Internet.

The important features of the spectrographic display in Figure 10–8 include the *x*-, *y*-, and *z*-axes; *glottal pulses*; *formant frequencies*; *silent intervals*; *stop bursts*; and *aperiodic intervals*. Each of these features is discussed below. It is important to point out that a casual glance at the spectrogram suggests a series of chunks, or *segments*, as the pattern is inspected from left to right. An individual with no training in speech acoustics, shown this spectrogram and asked to find natural "breaks" in the pattern along the time axis, probably would be able to do this easily (try it!). The chunks, or segments, are important because they often correspond roughly to speech sounds. Chapter 11 presents detailed information on the specific acoustic characteristics of the sound segments of English, and in some cases of other languages as well.

Axes

The *x*-axis is time, marked off in successive 100 ms intervals by the short vertical lines occurring at regular intervals along the baseline of the spectrogram. These 100-ms *calibration intervals* are similar in length to many

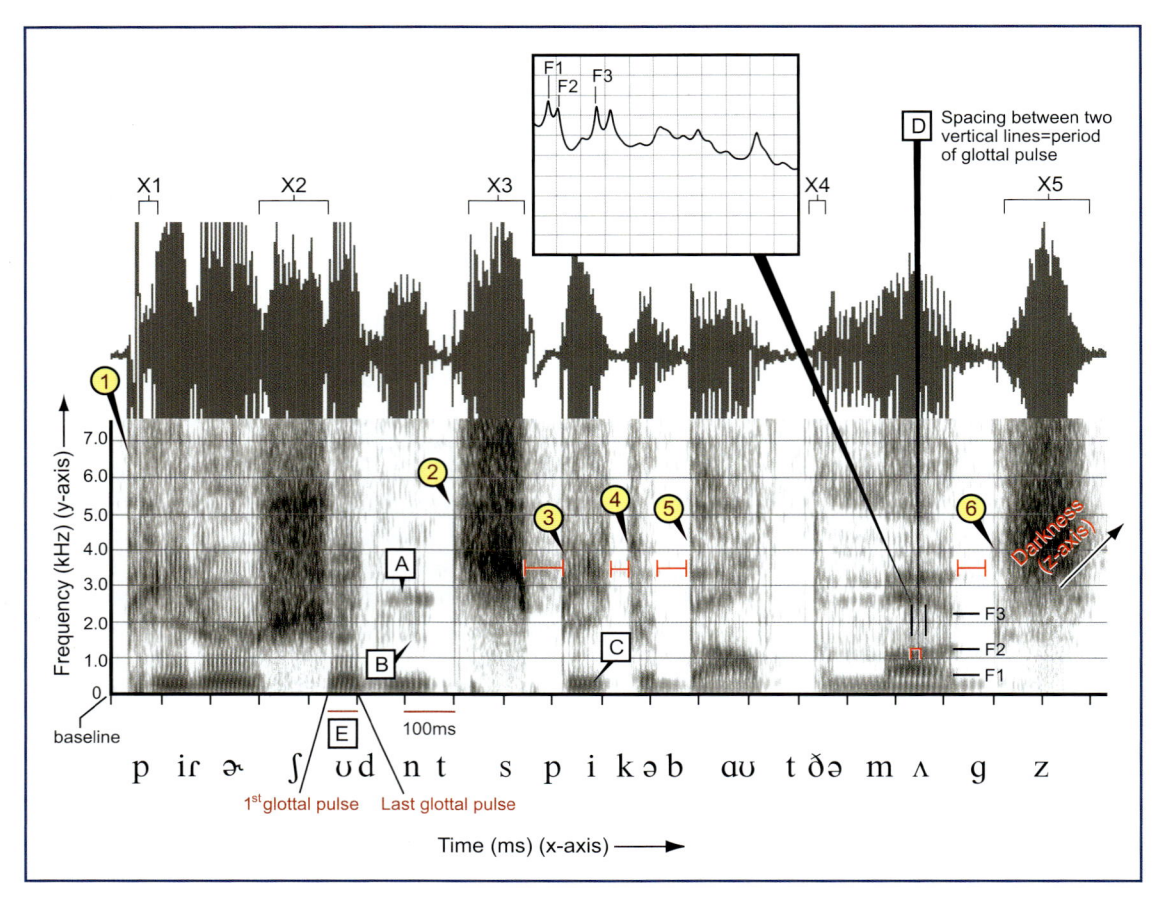

374 PRECLINICAL SPEECH SCIENCE: ANATOMY, PHYSIOLOGY, ACOUSTICS, AND PERCEPTION

Figure 10–8. Spectrogram showing important features of a spectrographic display. Follow text description for information on axes, glottal pulses, formant frequencies, silent intervals, stop bursts, and aperiodic intervals.

of the segments in this spectrogram, suggesting a relatively short time span for important events of speech production. Using these calibration intervals, it is possible to estimate the entire duration of the utterance at just under 2000 ms, or a little less than 2 s. This does not seem like a particularly long time, but it is typical for utterance durations. An utterance of 2 s duration contains many distinct segments.

The y-axis is frequency, which in the current spectrogram extends from 0 kHz to about 7.5 kHz. Calibration of the frequency axis is shown as the series of horizontal lines marked off in 1.0 kHz increments. The 0 to 8.0 kHz range is often considered a standard for spectrographic displays because most of the important acoustic energy for understanding articulatory events, as well as how the speech signal provides phonetic information in the perception of speech, is contained within this range. This is true for the most part, but spectrograms can be generated for any frequency range up to about 22 kHz. In the current text, a variety of spectrographic frequency ranges is used, depending on the purpose of the illustration.

The z-axis (indicated on the right side of the spectrogram in red print), or third dimension of the spectrogram, is intensity. Unlike time (x-axis) and frequency (y-axis), this type of spectrogram does not allow direct measurement of intensity. Rather, intensity is coded by the darkness of the pattern at any time-frequency coordinate (that is, at any point on the spectrographic display). The darkness at any time-frequency coordinate can be compared *only in relative terms* to the darkness at any other time-frequency coordinate. This kind of coding is called a *gray scale*, which allows only *ordinal* comparisons between event magnitudes. For example, the intensity of the formant indicated by arrow A, roughly at the time-frequency coordinate of 600 ms (x-axis) and 2.7 kHz (y-axis) where the segment is marked phonetically as [n], is greater (i.e., darker) than the formant above arrow B at the same segment (time-frequency coordinate of roughly 600 ms and 1.5 kHz). Similarly, the formant marked by arrow C, which occurs at a time-frequency coordinate of roughly 950 ms and 0.3 kHz where the segment is marked as [i], is slightly darker (more intense) than point A. These comparisons are not stated in terms of numbers, but only as "greater than" or "less than" relations. Time and frequency, on the other hand, can be measured directly from the spectrogram, and numerical values and differences can be determined. There are other ways to determine numerical intensity differences (e.g., difference in decibels) between different regions of a spectrogram, but not in the type of display shown in Figure 10–8.

Glottal Pulses

Certain segments in Figure 10–8 have a characteristic appearance of a series of dark, vertical lines. These segments are the ones containing the dark horizontal bands identified above as vowel formants. The lines appear to be running vertically throughout the segments containing the most obvious formants, such as the /i/ in /pi/ and the /ʊ/ in /ʃʊd/. The vertical lines are an acoustic result of vocal fold vibration, with each individual line reflecting a single glottal pulse. More precisely, in Chapter 8 the vocal tract resonances are said to be excited each time the vocal folds snap shut during a series of glottal cycles. Each of the vertical lines in the spectrogram represents these points of excitation, when the vocal folds close quickly at the end of a glottal cycle and create a pressure wave whose spectrum is shaped by the vocal tract filter. The shaping of the source spectrum by the vocal tract filter is shown on the spectrogram as darkened areas—that is, the dark bands—at the frequencies of the vocal tract resonances. Thus, the vertical lines and formants are not really different characteristics of the spectrogram. Rather, the formants are darkened areas along the vertical lines, showing where energy in the glottal source spectrum is emphasized (i.e., resonated) by the vocal tract filter.

Within any segment having a series of glottal pulses, the spacing of the lines appears to be very consistent. As described in Chapter 8, vocal fold vibration is quasi-periodic, with consecutive periods of *nearly* the same duration. The consistent spacing of the vertical lines along the time dimension (*x*-axis) of the spectrogram reflects the quasi-periodic nature of vocal fold vibration, and the spacing between any two vertical lines is equal to the period of the glottal cycle (see example D, incomplete red box in Figure 10–8 showing the distance between two glottal pulses). Although this kind of spectrogram does not provide a direct display of the F0 of vocal fold vibration, segments can be compared visually for the relative spacing of glottal pulses and, thus, their relative F0s. For example, compare the spacing of the glottal pulses in the two segments marked /i/ (in /spik/) and /ʌ/ (in /mʌgz/). The vertical lines, or glottal pulses, are closer together in /i/ compared with /ʌ/. Another way to make this comparison is to say that the number of vertical lines *per unit time* is greater for /i/ than for /ʌ/. A greater number of glottal pulses per unit time implies a shorter period and a higher F0. Thus, a quick glance at this spectrogram tells us that /i/ has a higher F0 than /ʌ/.

Formant Frequencies

The dark bands seen in the patterns with regularly spaced glottal pulses have been identified as formants. This pattern is seen for any speech sound produced with a relatively open vocal tract and voicing, including vowels, diphthongs, and semivowels (/l/, /w/, /ɹ/, /j/). Nasals are voiced and radiate sound through the open nares, producing a similar pattern. The spectrographic patterns seen above the phonetic symbols for these kinds of segments (in Figure 10–8, from left to right /i/, /ɚ/, /ʊ/, /n/, /i/, /ə/, /aʊ/, /ə/, /m/, /ʌ/) confirm this distinctive appearance.

In most cases, it is relatively easy to look at a spectrogram and determine which dark band is F1, which is F2, and so forth. The general rule is to start at the baseline (where frequency = 0 Hz) and move up the frequency scale, or *y*-axis, until the first dark band is encountered. This is the first formant, or F1. Continue up the frequency axis until the next dark band is found, which is F2. The next dark band above F2 is F3, and so forth. In Figure 10–8, the first three formants for the terminal part of the vowel /ʌ/ in the word /mʌgz/ have been identified and labeled in this way. This is the same approach used to identify formants in the spectrum plots presented in Chapter 8 (e.g., Figure 8–14), where frequency is on the *x*-axis and relative amplitude is on the *y*-axis. Starting from zero frequency on these plots, the first peak is labeled as F1, the next peak as F2, and the next as F3 (see spectrum inset, Figure 10–8, where the formant peaks are identified from a timepoint at the middle of the vowel). When formants are labeled as F1, F2, F3 ... F*n* in a spectrographic display, the peaks in the spectrogram are identified exactly as in the spectrum plots, except that the spectrogram displays frequency on the *y*-axis; in spectral displays, the spectral peaks are shown as peaks on the *x*-axis of the spectrum.

Another important difference between a spectrum plot and a spectrographic display of speech is that the spectrogram shows the formants *over time*, whereas a spectrum plot is constructed for some slice in time, or *time window*. The spectrum inset shown for the vowel /ʌ/ in /mʌgz/ was constructed for a carefully selected piece of the /ʌ/ waveform. A closer look at the formants throughout the duration of this vowel shows why the selection of a *part* of a vowel waveform is an important step in the determination of formant frequencies. All the formants, but especially F3, have changing frequency values as a function of time. At the first glottal pulse of /ʌ/, F3 is approximately 200 Hz below the 3.0 kHz calibration line, but the formant falls steadily after the temporal middle of the vowel and appears to finish, at the final glottal pulse, about 300 Hz above the 2.0 kHz line. If the question is asked, "What are the formant frequencies of the vowel /ʌ/ in the word /mʌgz/?" the answer depends on where the measurement is taken throughout the vowel. When scientists or clinicians talk about vowel formant frequencies in connected speech, they are usually referring to a set of measurements taken at or near the *temporal middle of the vowel*. In Figure 10–8, this point is indicated for the vowel /ʌ/ by the vertical line labeled "D" extending through the formant pattern. In practice, a time window of relatively brief duration (20–30 ms) is centered around a temporal midpoint and the spectral analysis is performed on the signal within this window. The interval corresponding to this window is shown by the two short vertical lines crossing the 2.0 kHz line. A line from this window extends to the inset spectrum at the top of the spectrogram. That inset spectrum shows the formant frequencies averaged across this brief window. The formants do not change much over such a brief window, so the average is not a "smear" of rapidly changing frequencies (recall the discussion of Figure 10–4).

Formant frequencies are indicated by the dark bands, but where along their *vertical extent* should the measurement be taken? At the temporal middle of the vowel /ʌ/ in /mʌgz/, the lower edge of the F2 band is slightly below 1.0 kHz, and the upper edge is above 1.0 kHz. Formant frequencies are identified by the peaks in the spectrum—that is, by single frequency values associated with energy maxima—but the formant bands cover a *range* of frequencies, so how is the single formant frequency determined? The answer is, at any given point in time such as the temporal middle of /ʌ/, *the center of the formant band, halfway between the bottom and top of the band, is taken as the formant frequency*.

The great majority of the formant frequencies shown in Figure 10–8 are changing as a function of time. When connected speech is examined, this movement is the rule rather than the exception. The constant movement of the formants during speech production reflects the constant change in the configuration of the vocal tract. One of the earliest revelations to emerge from studies of speech movements was the continuous motion of the articulators, and the absence of many "held," or static, vocal tract postures. This has made it difficult to identify *targets* for speech sounds and, indeed, has led some scientists to *deny* the existence of such targets. Nevertheless, formant frequencies measured at the temporal middle of a vowel, as in the /ʌ/ example of Figure 10–8, have often been regarded as acoustic targets for vowels.

Silent Intervals and Stop Bursts

The aeromechanical characteristics of stop consonants are presented in Chapter 9. Recall that the vocal tract is completely sealed for a brief interval, during which time a positive pressure (oral pressure, or P_o) is developed within the closed cavity. When the articulators separate, the seal is broken, pressure is released suddenly, and airflow rushes from the vocal tract (see Figure 9–16). The acoustic result of this interval of complete vocal tract closure is called a *closure interval*, *silent interval*, or *stop gap*. The sudden release of pressure is called, appropriately, a *stop burst*.

Closure intervals are usually easy to identify in spectrograms. Because the vocal tract is, in theory, completely sealed during the closure, acoustic energy should not be radiated from the vocal tract and the interval should appear as a brief blank spot, or *gap* on the spectrogram. If intensity is scaled on a spectrogram as the darkness of the trace, a white or nearly white segment on the spectrogram indicates an interval of no acoustic energy—a "silent" vocal tract. In Figure 10–8, the spectrographic appearance above the /p/ and /k/ in /spik/, the /b/ in /əbaʊt/, and the /g/ in /mʌgz/ confirms this expectation in varying degrees. The closure intervals for these stops are indicated by the red horizontal bars terminated by vertical tick marks between 3.0 and 4.0 kHz (placed in this frequency region for convenience of display only). The closure interval for the /p/ in /spik/ shows some energy between about 2.5 and 7.5 kHz, which is not uncommon when stops follow /s/ in /s/+ stop clusters. A small amount of energy is also seen in the closure interval for /k/ in /spik/. The energy in these intervals suggests an incomplete vocal tract seal during the closure interval A small amount of acoustic energy "leaks" through the mouth and sometimes, an imperfectly sealed velopharyngeal port, and is sensed by the microphone, appearing on the spectrogram as relatively weak-to-moderate aperiodic energy.

The gap for /b/ also shows a small amount of energy on the baseline, which appears to be periodic as indicated by a series of three or four small, regularly spaced pulses. Periodic energy is also seen along the baseline during the /g/ closure interval. The presence of periodic pulses during the /b/ and /g/ closure intervals makes sense because these are *voiced* stops, produced with vocal fold vibration during the vocal tract closure.

The periodic acoustic energy recorded on the baseline for these voiced stops is not radiated through either the mouth or nare openings, because these are (typically) sealed during the closure intervals. Rather, the pressure wave resulting from vibration of the vocal folds during a closure interval causes vibration of the *walls* of the vocal tract (i.e., the neck walls, the cheeks), which transmit their vibratory energy to the surrounding air. A pressure wave is propagated from the external surface of the vocal tract walls to the microphone used to record the acoustic event. This energy is seen only in the very lowest frequencies of the spectrogram because the walls of the vocal tract vibrate only at the lowest frequencies of vocal fold vibration, filtering out the higher source harmonics and preventing their energy from being sensed by the microphone (see also Chapter 4, Sidetrack on "Lubker Bumps").

As reviewed above, the termination of a closure interval is defined acoustically as a stop burst. Stop bursts are, at least in carefully articulated speech (like that elicited in many laboratory experiments), easy to identify in spectrograms. Figure 10–8 shows six of them, numbered 1 through 6. The distinctive spectrographic characteristic of a stop burst is a spike-like event—a dark, single vertical line—following a closure interval. The spectrographic feature of the dark vertical line signifying a stop burst seems to be similar to the description of glottal pulses, but there are several ways to distinguish the two acoustic events. First, as noted above, stop bursts are typically seen following a well-defined closure interval, so if one characteristic of stops is noted (i.e., the closure interval), the occurrence of a second characteristic (i.e., the burst) may be expected. Bursts 2, 5, and 6 in Figure 10–8 conform to the pattern of a burst following an obvious closure interval. Second, stop bursts often have a much broader frequency representation than nearby glottal pulses. Stop bursts typically (but not always) contain energy at frequencies where the adjacent vowel or other sounds (such as fricatives) do *not* have formant (or frication noise) energy. Note how the energy of stop bursts 1, 2, 3, and 5 extends throughout most of the vertical scale of the spectrogram. Third, bursts are not often associated with the *clear* formant structure associated with glottal pulses. This is especially exemplified by burst 2. And fourth, when a stop burst occurs in succession with a series of glottal pulses, it typically is separated from the immediately adjacent pulse by an interval that is different from the separation between consecutive glottal pulses within the vocalic event. In other words, the interval between the burst and the immediately adjacent glottal pulse is not consistent with the period of vocal fold vibration as reflected by the succeeding intervals between the regularly spaced glottal pulses. For example, the interval between burst 3 and the first glottal pulse of /i/ in /spik/ is subtly greater than the intervals between the following glottal pulses. If a vertical line on the spectrogram is a glottal pulse, and not a stop burst, it fits with the repetitive pattern of the following or preceding glottal pulses.

In practice, none of the individual criteria for identifying stop bursts should be relied on by themselves. Some or all criteria can be applied simultaneously to make the best decision about the identity of a spectrographic event. The choice of which criteria to apply may depend on the specific segment under study. The /b/ burst in /əbaʊt/ (burst 5 in the spectrogram) is a good example of how some of the criteria described above may or may not apply to a given case. First, there is a clear closure interval preceding the burst-like feature, suggesting the articulation of a stop consonant. Second, this spike has substantial energy at frequencies other than those associated with the formants of the adjacent vowel. Note, for example, the spike energy from 1.5 to 2.0 kHz, 3.5 to 4.0 kHz, and 7.0 to 7.5 kHz. The following vowel does not contain formant peaks at these frequencies. However, the next two criteria for identifying stop bursts are more ambiguous. This burst does seem to have a formant structure, with darker marks in the vicinity of F1, F2, and F3 of the adjacent vowel. And the interval between the burst and the following glottal pulse is not so different from the intervals between any of the glottal pulses in the /aʊ/ diphthong. Does the failure to meet clearly the third and fourth criteria for distinguishing a stop burst from a glottal pulse cast doubt on the identification of this acoustic event as a stop burst? Probably not, in this case, because the evidence for the closure interval is very clear, as is the evidence for voicing (glottal pulses) during the closure interval. This reasoning is convenient in this case because of the knowledge that a /b/ was intended by the speaker. Thus, a voiced closure interval is expected, and it follows that a /b/ burst is superimposed on the continuous series of glottal pulses extending through the closure interval and into the diphthong.

There are many cases, however, in which this kind of simple reasoning—which includes expectations about what has been spoken, who has spoken it, and how it has been spoken—cannot be applied. For example, acoustic analysis of disordered speech is often done with imperfect knowledge of what has been spoken. In this case, the *who has spoken the utterance* (for example, a client with a neurologically based speech disorder) and the *what has been spoken* are very much intertwined. If the client has impaired speech intelligibility and the examiner has difficulty generating a reliable gloss of the utterance, a decision about the spike-like event labeled as #5 in Figure 10–8 (is it, or is it not a burst?) becomes problematic. This may even be a problem in the speech of persons with no speech disorder, depending on *how* an utterance is produced. The utterance displayed in Figure 10–8 was spoken by one of the authors in a formal way, very unlike his speech patterns in more casual speech. In casual speaking styles, speakers often produce blurrier acoustic landmarks than those seen in Figure 10–8, and in the case of stop consonants may even omit bursts all together. This goes against textbook descriptions of stop consonant production, but Crystal and House (1988) and Byrd (1993) concluded from their acoustic analyses of connected speech that as many as 50% of stop consonants have no identifiable burst.

How is a pause distinguished from a closure interval for a voiceless stop consonant? As described above, voiceless stop closures are identifiable on a spectrogram by an interval of no energy—a silent interval—but isn't a similar or identical spectrographic display expected for a pause, during which no energy is being generated by the vocal tract?[3] Obviously, if an interval of no energy is terminated by a burst, it is likely the acoustic result of a voiceless stop closure. Not all stops, however, have bursts (see above) and in some speech disorders bursts may be present but extremely weak. The potential for confusion between pauses and voiceless stop closures, therefore, must be recognized. In the speech of individuals who are free from speech disorders, there is a general criterion for distinguishing voiceless stop closure intervals from pauses, based on the duration of the silent interval. Pauses in speech are typically no less than about 150 ms in duration, whereas voiceless stop closure intervals are typically no more than about 120 ms. To be on the conservative side, many scientists have adopted a criterion of 200 ms for the minimal duration to consider a silent spectrographic interval as a pause. Silent intervals 200 ms or greater are identified as pauses, those less than 200 ms are subject to further evaluation (using information such as the presence of a burst). This criterion is somewhat less reliable in certain speech disorders, for which very long stop closure intervals may be one result of a very slow speaking rate, quite common in many cases of motor speech disorders. In these cases, the 200-ms criterion may not be effective, and the potential for confusion between stops and pauses is increased.

Aperiodic Intervals

As described in Chapter 9, aperiodic energy is produced within the vocal tract in several different ways and is an important component of the acoustic characteristics of fricatives, stops, and affricates (affricates are covered below). Aperiodic energy is shown in a spectrogram as an interval of energy having no repeating pattern. These aperiodic intervals are most commonly associated with fricatives and the release phase of stops and affricates. Aperiodic energy may also be mixed with periodic energy for certain sound segments (such as voiced fricatives) or phonation types (such as breathy voice).

In Figure 10–8, five intervals of aperiodic energy, labeled X1, X2, X3, X4, and X5, are marked at the top of the spectrogram by horizontal bars terminated by short, downward vertical lines. These five intervals vary in duration, the range of frequencies over which energy is distributed, and intensity. The duration of each interval can be estimated by comparing the length of each horizontal bar to the length of the time calibration ticks (at 100-ms increments) at the base of the spectrogram. The short, vertical lines extending downward from the ends of each horizontal bar show the location of the operationally defined onset and offset of each interval. The range of frequencies is indicated by the locations along the *y*-axis where there are light, medium, or dark tracings, and the relative intensity of the segments is indicated by the darkness of those tracings. Based on these characteristics, intervals X2, X3, and X5 share similar characteristics, each having relatively long duration and intense energy distributed across a wide range of frequencies. In general, aperiodic intervals of relatively long duration and intense energy are the result of voiceless fricative articulations, especially those produced with a lingua-alveolar or lingua-palatal constriction (i.e., /s/ and /ʃ/, see Chapter 9). There are subtle, but important, differences in the distribution and intensity of energy for intervals X2, X3, and X5. For example, very dark tracings indicating intense energy extend from above 7.0 kHz to just above 1 kHz for segment X2, but not much lower than 2.5 kHz for segments X3 and X5. These differences are discussed in Chapter 9, where the relations of place of articulation to fricative frequency and intensity characteristics are considered.

Segments X1 and X4 differ from X2, X3, and X5, largely due to their brief durations. At its outset, seg-

---

[3]Reference is made here only to the kind of pause that is silent, typically called an *unfilled* pause. In the case of *filled* pauses, such as the many "um's" found in everyday spoken discourse, there is no confusion with a voiceless stop consonant.

ment X1 shows aperiodic energy in the form of a very brief "spike," the darkness of which is fairly constant between 0 and 7.0 kHz. This is a stop burst, and its distribution of energy across frequency is related to the place of articulation of the stop, as discussed in Chapter 9. Immediately following the burst is an interval of roughly 40 ms during which aperiodic energy is distributed broadly across frequency, but is relatively more intense in the 2.0 to 5.0 kHz range. This is the frication interval of the stop, and its distribution of energy is also related to the place of articulation. Segment X4 is very brief, showing a spike-like event that, in this case, is not associated with a stop articulation, but rather with end of the voiced fricative /ð/. Some fricatives, especially those produced at the front of the vocal tract (e.g., /θ,ð,f,v/), may show little, if any, energy on a spectrogram, and in some cases the energy that is visible is very brief, as in segment X4. Possibly, part of the "blank space" interval immediately preceding the spike-like /ð/ noise is also associated with the fricative, which typically has very low energy. Because of the preceding /t/ closure, it is impossible to determine how much of the blank interval is stop closure, and how much is a /ð/ constriction whose acoustic output is very weak and not displayed in the spectrogram.

Segmentation of Spectrograms

The process of segmenting a spectrogram involves the identification of pieces of the display that correspond roughly to phonemic or phonetic units. The distinction between "phonemic" and "phonetic" is important, because often there are more phonetic than phonemic units per spectrographic interval (see example below).

Glottal pulses play an important role in the measurement of various attributes of the spectrogram. The term *segment* has been introduced as a temporal chunk or piece of the spectrogram that is distinguishable from an adjacent chunk. These chunks also have rough correspondence with sound categories, as indicated by the phonetic symbols at the bottom of the spectrogram. When scientists and clinicians want to know something about these chunks they go past the very coarse observation of matching a given chunk with a sound type. Specifically, they are interested in making measurements to provide *quantitative information* about a segment. For example, a clinician might be interested in measuring the duration of the vowel /ʊ/ in the word /ʃʊd/, but cannot do so unless there are some rules for defining the onset and offset of the vowel. The rules for the boundaries, or onsets and offsets of many segments, often depend on the first and last glottal pulses of voiced segments. The glottal pulses shown as vertical lines in the spectrogram,

therefore, play an important role in segmentation of spectrograms. Segmentation of the vowel /ʊ/ in /ʃʊd/ is shown in Figure 10–8 as example E, where the upward-pointing lines indicate the first and last glottal pulses of the vocalic segment. The first glottal pulse is defined as the onset, or beginning of the vowel, and the last glottal pulse is defined as the offset or end of the vowel. The distance between the first and last glottal pulses along the *x*-, or time axis—the interval "E"—can be converted to time to determine the duration of /ʊ/.

The use of glottal pulses to identify onsets and offsets of segments in a spectrogram is a well-accepted practice. These rules are *operational definition*, and not the *truth*. Investigators, whether in the laboratory or clinic, use such definitions for precise and reproducible definitions of measurements and to allow other investigators to make the same measurements using the same criteria. When an investigator identifies the first glottal pulse of a vowel as the onset of the vocalic event, it does not necessarily imply a belief that this point in time is where the brain initiates a vowel, or even that the brain represents onsets and offsets of speech segments.

Segmentation of vowels is relatively straightforward when vowels are located between two obstruents. The beginning of the vowel is taken as the first "full" glottal pulse, and the end of the vowel is the last full glottal pulse. A full glottal pulse is one that extends from the baseline at least through F2 of the display. The requirement that the glottal pulse is at least as high in frequency as F2 distinguishes it from the glottal pulses seen in voiced stops, affricates, and fricatives, as well as some low-intensity pulses that extend only through F1. According to this reasoning, a glottal pulse that extends through at least F2 is visible because the vocal tract is open and therefore unambiguously vocalic. The sound energy generated by a closed vocal tract is not visible at such high frequencies because they are filtered out by the vocal tract walls. Clearly, when trying to find the acoustic boundaries of a vowel, a clinician or scientist wants to identify the first and last instants in time when the vocal tract is open.

When vowels are located before or after nasals, the "full glottal pulse" criterion cannot be used to segment the vowel from the nasal, but the change from an oral to nasal filter function (a murmur), discussed in Chapter 9, can be used to find a vowel-nasal or nasal-vowel boundary. A sudden change in intensity at the boundary between a nasal and a vowel and the sudden appearance of the low-frequency F1 characteristic of nasal cavity resonance are good criteria for this segmentation problem.

When vowels are located before or after semivowels (/ɹ,l,w,j/) or diphthongs (/aɪ, ɔɪ, aʊ, eɪ, oʊ/) the segmentation problem is very difficult because there are no natural boundaries. In general, the conservative approach in sequences such as "yellow" (/jɛloʊ/ or "I honor" (/aɪjanɚ/) is not to attempt a phonetic or phonemic segmentation. The duration of semivowels is often combined with the duration of surrounding vowels or based on segmentation boundaries that do not allow good reliability either within or across measurers.

Segmentation of obstruents is, in many cases, fairly simple. When an obstruent follows a vocalic segment (vowels, diphthongs, semivowels), the last full glottal pulse of the preceding vocalic is taken as the instant before closure of the vocal tract, and as the beginning of the closure or constriction interval. The same criterion can often be applied to nasal + obstruent sequences because nasals are voiced and have an obvious formant pattern. In the case of stops, the offset (or end) of the closure interval is taken as the burst (same for the closure offset of affricates). In the case of fricatives, the offset is taken as the end of the frication noise, or the first full glottal pulse of the following vowel. Even though this latter measurement point (the glottal pulse following the frication noise) results in a fricative interval that may be slightly longer than the actual frication, it is more reliable than locating the precise ending of the frication noise. When fricatives and stops are abutted, as in an /s/ + stop sequence, separation of the frication from the closure interval must rely on the termination of frication noise and the onset of silence (i.e., no energy in the closure interval). When two fricatives follow each other, the changing spectrum must be used to identify the end of one and beginning of the other; this is often a challenging task. When two stops follow each other, the only way to distinguish the closure intervals is if the first stop is released, producing a burst.

The case of voiceless stops provides a good example of the correspondence of measured intervals to phonemes versus phonetic segments. Take the case of voiceless stops which include a closure interval, a burst, a frication interval, and an aspiration interval. Each of these intervals can be identified as segments on the spectrogram, but they are all associated with a single stop. If these intervals can be segmented, the segmentation is labeled "phonetic" because the different segments all relate to the same phoneme (i.e., the stop). If the closure, burst, frication, and aspiration are combined and regarded as one interval, this is a "phonemic" segment. This is not a problem with segments such as vowels, where "subsegments" are not likely to be identified. However, when dealing with spectrograms produced by speakers with speech disorders, the distinction between phonetic and phonemic segments can be a problem, and it is wise to keep in mind that segmentation may result in two or more pieces that relate to the same phoneme. The opposite case is also true, that two or more consecutive phonemes may not be segmentable as two separate "pieces," as described above for vowel-vowel, vowel-semivowel, and other sequences for which clear boundaries cannot be identified.[4]

Segmentation of the utterance "The blue spot is a normal dot," spoken by a 53-year-old male, is shown

---

Can Unlabeled Spectrograms Be Segmented and Labeled?

The answer to this question is yes, and no. Speech acousticians have always been interested in their ability to examine an unlabeled spectrogram to determine the phonetic segments and ultimately the words displayed as acoustic patterns. This is an extraordinarily difficult task. Even highly experienced speech scientists are reduced to babbling confusion when asked to "read" an unlabeled spectrogram. Many years ago, a speech scientist named Dr. Victor Zue, of the Massachusetts Institute of Technology, became so good at this that a colleague made a film of him reading an unlabeled spectrogram with what seemed to be unworldly quickness. Zue trained himself for this task, spending many hours learning the subtle phonetic variants of speech sounds that trip up seasoned speech scientists. Zue and a colleague also showed that students could be trained to read unlabeled spectrograms (Zue & Cole, 1979), although not with his remarkable speed and accuracy. Interested students can visit YouTube and enter "Reading Spectrograms" in the search window (e.g., https://www.youtube.com/watch?v=TEOiAnXNFFQ) to access a series of instructional clips on spectrogram-reading skills).

---

[4]Segmentation of a spectrogram does not have to be guided by sound classes (the approach described here), although that is certainly the most typical strategy. Segmentation can be guided by the underlying vocal tract gestures, an example of which is the vocalic articulatory gesture for the /uɪ/ sequence in the utterance "The stew is good" (/ðəstuɪzgʊd/). Here the interest is in the relatively rapid and smoothly executed transition from a high-back (/u/) to a high-front (/ɪ/) configuration. These sorts of articulatory sequences, for which the "units" (segments) are defined on the basis of gestures rather than sound classes, have not been explored much in the clinical literature but are potentially of great diagnostic and theoretical value in understanding speech disorders.

in Figure 10–9. The frequency scale is "zoomed" from 0 to 4.0 kHz for better identification of segment boundaries; the waveform is shown above the spectrogram. A broad phonetic transcription is provided below the spectrogram, with phonetic symbols located along the time axis roughly in the middle of the acoustically identified segments. The vertical lines immediately below the baseline mark the segmentation boundaries, determined according to the rules outlined above. The pieces of the acoustic signal identified with these rules—the segments—are numbered in sequence from left to right. Seventeen segments are identified.

Some of the segments shown in Figure 10–9 result from straightforward application of rules. For example, segments 1, 6, 8, 10, and 16 are vowels or diphthongs, for which the identification of first and last glottal pulses is clear. Segments 3 and 12, however, have obvious glottal-pulse boundaries but include two phonemes because there is no reliable way to separate the /l/ from the /u/ in segment 3 or the /ɔ/ from the /r/ in segment 12. It appears to be relatively easy to segment the nasals (segments 11 and 13), the stops[5] (segments 2, 5, 7, 15 and 17), and the fricatives (segments 4 and 9), although the intervocalic /z/ in /ɪzeɪ/ and the /t/ in segment 7 present certain segmentation challenges.[6] The ease of segmenting any single spectrogram depends on several factors, including the speaker, the speaking style (e.g., casual vs. formal), the context in which a given sound is spoken, and so forth.

Why segment a spectrogram? This question can be answered in several different ways, but the general response is: to mark off a piece of the signal to discover its typical acoustic characteristics and similar pieces. Similar pieces would be, for example, the same phoneme produced by different speakers, or by the same speaker under different speaking conditions (e.g., stressed or unstressed, fast or slow rate, etc.). If the acoustic characteristics of well-defined pieces of the speech signal are known, computer code can be written for high-quality speech synthesizers and speech recognizers. Another reason is to provide a quantitative

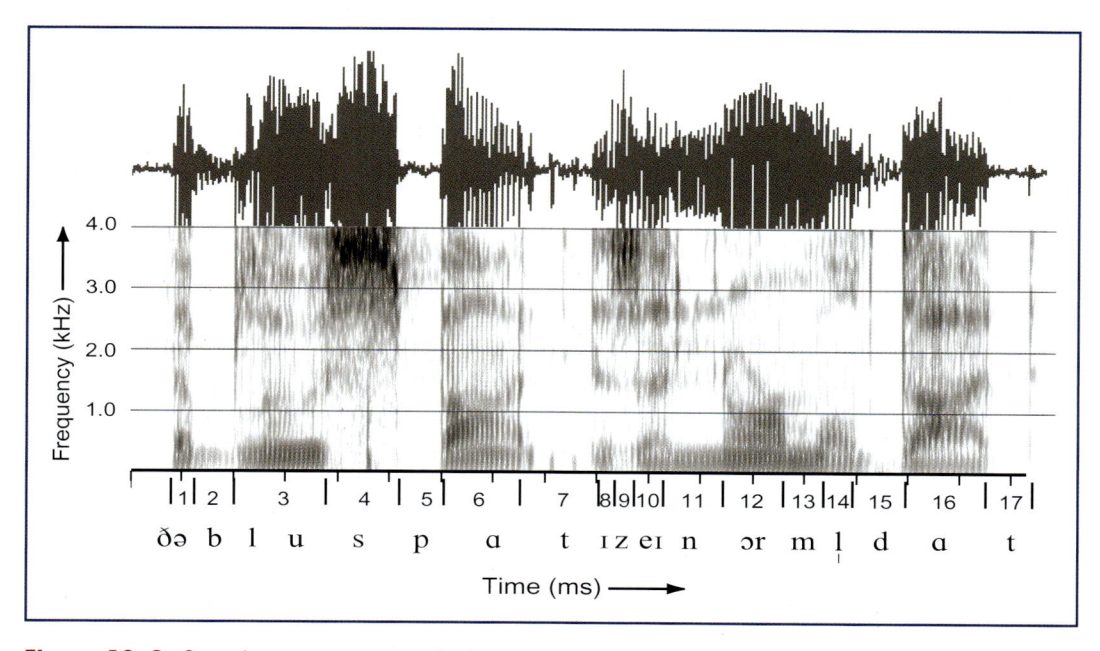

Figure 10–9. Spectrogram segmented according to the rules described in the text. The vertical lines immediately below the baseline of the spectrogram show the operationally defined onsets and offsets of the segments, and the phoneme corresponding to a segment is shown between the segment boundaries.

---

[5]In this text, when the term "stop duration" or "stop segment," is used, it refers to the closure interval. This is the conventional usage in the acoustic phonetics literature (Klatt, 1976; Umeda, 1977). The burst and voice-onset time (VOT) are sometimes allied with the stop, sometimes with the vowel, as in the discussion above of the difference between phonetic and phonemic segmentation.

[6]In English, word-final /t/ is often produced as a glottal stop (/ʔ/); the /t/ in /spɑt/ may have been produced in this way. The weak "spike" seen a little more than halfway through interval 7 of Figure 10–9 may be an example of a momentary "leak" in glottal closure (not unusual for glottal stops), and the release at the end of the stop interval has energy concentrated at the formant frequencies of the following vowel /i/, also common for glottal stop releases.

description of the articulatory problem in a speech disorder. Yet another reason is to identify the acoustic properties that should be processed optimally by a hearing instrument, be it a hearing aid, cochlear implant, or classroom-based assistive hearing device. Finally, knowledge of the acoustic characteristics of pieces of the speech signal can be incorporated into theories that attempt to explain the origin of, for example, disorders such as stuttering, apraxia of speech, and specific language impairment. When conversing with an individual who, because of a condition or disease process, cannot produce oral speech and instead uses a speech synthesizer to produce intelligible responses and engage in what we humans love to do—talk, talk, talk—it is the study of the acoustic characteristics of speech sounds—acoustic phonetics—that creates the possibility of the enjoyable experience of communicating with other people.

SPEECH ACOUSTICS IS NOT ALL ABOUT SEGMENTS: SUPRASEGMENTALS

A discussion of the techniques of speech acoustic analysis is not complete without mention of phonetic events whose characteristics extend beyond the duration of segments. These events are often called "suprasegmentals" because the pieces over which acoustic analysis is performed are longer than the duration of segment-sized events. Some authors refer to suprasegmental variables as *prosodic* variables.

A well-known example of a suprasegmental is the *fundamental frequency (F0) contour*, the variation in F0 over several segments and even across sentence-level utterances. To obtain an F0 contour, the periods of many cycles of vocal fold vibration are measured. In Figure 10–10, the segmented utterance of Figure 10–9 provides an example of an F0 contour analysis. One way to obtain the F0 contour is to measure each of the periods, convert each to F0 by $F0 = 1/T$, and graph the resulting values as a function of time. With a proper display of a speech waveform, this is an easy measurement task, but incredibly tedious. One of the authors, who performed this kind of hand analysis before the availability of speech analysis software, did a period-by-period measurement of the utterance in Figure 10–10 and completed it in about 40 minutes.

It is preferable to have an automated procedure to measure F0. Most computer programs designed for speech acoustic analysis, like *TF32* or *Praat*, include algorithms for measurement and display of F0 contours. Scientists typically refer to these algorithms as *pitch trackers*, even though the name is a technical

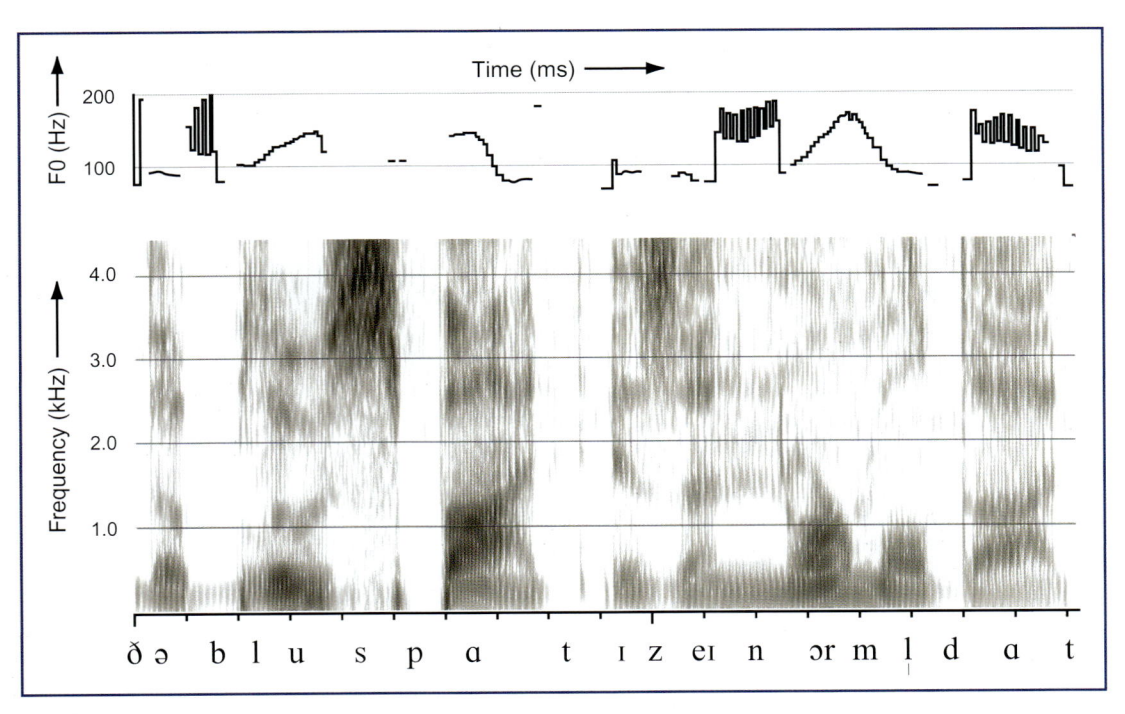

Figure 10–10. F0 contour (*top of display*) for "The blue spot is a normal dot," spoken by a 53-year-old male. The F0 data are displayed on a scale from 75 to 200 Hz. The spectrogram is shown below the F0 contour. See text for additional details.

misnomer because pitch is a perceptual phenomenon and F0 is a physical event (see Chapter 14 for information on the relationship between F0 and pitch). There are many different algorithms for the measurement of F0, each using somewhat different strategies and computations, but ultimately all perform the analysis by measuring the period of each glottal cycle. Above the spectrogram in Figure 10–10 is the F0 contour for "The blue spot is a normal dot," spoken with a small degree of emphasis on the word "normal." The F0 contour was computed automatically by *TF32* ("automatically" means selecting a command such as "perform pitch analysis") and is shown exactly as it was computed on a frequency scale of 75 to 200 Hz. Values are computed for each glottal pulse, and typically are *not* computed where there are no glottal pulses, although there are exceptions to both statements. For example, there are no values computed for the voiceless /s/ in *spot* (except for two at the end of the frication energy), which makes sense because of the absence of a periodic waveform for the voiceless fricative. However, a couple of values were computed during the /t/ closure interval of the utterance-final word *dot*. More surprising, perhaps, is: (a) the uncertain performance of this analysis throughout the /ɪzeɪ/ sequence, for which the F0 contour appears to be discontinuous, as if there are missing values; and (b) the strange behavior of the analysis for the /n/, where the F0 values seem to jump between roughly 175 and 135 Hz, giving the contour an "up and down" staircase appearance that reflects errors in computation rather than rapidly changing rates of vocal fold vibration. Surpisingly, the sequence of F0 values starting with /ɪ/ in *is* and continuing through the word-initial /n/ of *normal* (segments 8 through 11 in Figure 10–9) is continuously voiced, and in theory should yield good F0 values for each of the glottal pulses.

Errors in the computation of F0 contours illustrate certain weaknesses of most pitch tracker analysis programs. The programs tend to make errors when a glottal period estimated from the waveform is not "clear." What makes a glottal cycle unclear? The answer is, a lot of things, many of which are found in normal speech production and certainly are present in many speech disorders. For example, glottal cycles associated with breathy voice quality have both periodic and aperiodic energy and therefore present problems for F0 analysis programs. The aperiodic energy makes it difficult for the measurement algorithm to detect the beginnings and endings of individual glottal cycles. In general, F0 measurement algorithms have increasing difficulty with accurate identification of glottal periods as the level of aperiodic energy increases. In the case of the /z/ in /ɪzeɪ/, periodic energy can be seen mixed with the frication energy above 3.0 kHz, but the program "lost" the periodicity and failed to compute F0 values during the middle of the fricative. The errors during the nasal /n/ may be attributed to one or both of two factors. First, the segment has relatively low energy (compare the darkness of the formants with that of the /ɑ/s in *spot* or *dot*). Low acoustic energy often confuses F0 analysis programs because consecutive glottal cycles may not be distinct from one another. Second, some F0 analyses, like the one in Figure 10–10, generate values by first computing the formant frequencies and then subtracting them from the overall spectral analysis, leaving the part of the signal associated with vocal fold vibration. This residual part of the signal is then used to generate the F0 value (see the discussion of inverse filtering in Chapter 8, and Figure 8–3). Nasals have antiresonances, as well as resonances, and antiresonances can make the separation of resonances from glottal vibrations problematic, resulting in poor F0 estimates like the ones shown for /n/ in Figure 10–10.

The purpose of the foregoing discussion is not to dwell on the intricacies and delicate nature of F0 analysis programs. There is a larger point to be made, that automated analyses of speech acoustics are very, very fast—the F0 contour in Figure 10–10 was gen-erated with a single point-and-click maneuver and appeared on the screen in less than a second—but areprone to error, even when the speaker is "normal." The F0 analysis in Figure 10–10 is not unique in this re-spect. All "pitch trackers" suffer from the kinds of errors shown in Figure 10–10. A good F0 analysis program performs the computations rapidly, provides a display such as the one in Figure 10–10, and allows the user to examine the display for errors and *correct them* interactively. There are, therefore, two lessons to take away from this discussion: (a) programs make errors and (b) programs should allow the user to make corrections rapidly and easily. Corrections for the F0 contour shown in Figure 10–10 (not shown here) required about 5 min of time from one of your authors, well under the 40-some min required for the complete hand-analysis described above.

Despite errors in the F0 contour of Figure 10–10, the general shape is consistent with theories of prosody and previous laboratory observations. Generally, declarative utterances show an increasing F0 at the start of the utterance which quickly reaches a maximum value. For the remainder of the utterance, F0 falls gradually, reaching a lowest value at the end of the utterance. In the utterance shown in Figure 10–10, there is an F0 peak soon after the utterance begins, toward the end of the word "blue," with a value of roughly 145 Hz. Later in the utterance, another peak F0 (~170 Hz) occurs on the emphasized word "normal." This peak F0 is associated with the stressed vocalic /ɔr/ in "normal," and is often assumed to be superimposed on the gradual F0 fall following the early peak referred to above. The gradual fall of F0 from the high to low point in a declarative utterance is referred to as "declination." F0 details along the contour in Figure 10–10 are not discussed here, but a general shape description of F0 contours is amenable to a kind of contrast analysis similar to that used for segments. The general declination pattern for declarative utterances can be contrasted with the fall-rise pattern of F0 common for question utterances (e.g., "Are you going to help out?"). The shape of an F0 contour carries contrastive information concerning the grammatical and affective function of the utterance.

In *tone languages* such as Thai, Igala (a language spoken in Nigeria), and the Mandarin and Cantonese dialects of Chinese, shape of the F0 contour across a vocalic segment has the same contrastive function as, say, the difference in formant frequencies between two vowels. In these languages, different F0 contours across the vowel of a CV syllable function as phonemes. For example, in Mandarin the sequence /bɑ/ produced with a flat F0 contour means "eight," but /bɑ/ spoken with a rapid fall-rise contour means "to hold" (Catford, 2000). The specific shape of the segment-sized F0 contour changes the meaning of the sequence, even as the articulatory characteristics of the segments (that is, the /b/ and the /ɑ/) stay the same. This is analogous to the case of English where the change of a vowel from "bat" to "bit" changes the meaning of the sequence. Both the Mandarin and English cases are examples of minimal pairs, implemented using different phonetic strategies.

F0 analysis is an important area of study because (among other issues) tone languages are widespread on the planet (more people speak Mandarin than any other language in the world). At the utterance level, the contour shape has important grammatical functions. In addition, F0 variation during conversation plays an important role in conveying a speaker's emotional state, by providing signals concerning the rules of turn-taking and by marking important aspects of an individual's personality. Some of these issues, as well as a broader consideration of the acoustics of prosody, are discussed in Chapter 11.

DIGITAL TECHNIQUES FOR SPEECH ANALYSIS

This chapter is not a technical manual of hardware and algorithmic details for speech analysis, but some discussion is appropriate concerning the basics of computer analysis of speech. Digital analysis of speech has the same general goal as spectrographic analysis of speech: to produce an accurate spectral analysis as a function of time. As in the case of the F0 analysis outlined above, there are many different algorithms and hardware solutions to obtaining a quality analysis of speech waveforms. Here, the focus is on the main components and procedures for speech acoustic analysis by computer.

Spectrographic analysis using the original spectrograph from the 1950s (see Figure 10–7) or any of its several modernized models through the late 1980s required a recording of speech on some permanent medium and, of course, the instrument itself. Typically, a speech sample was recorded on a tape recorder (the tape being the permanent medium) and at some later time input to the spectrograph for production of a spectrogram. All processing of the signal—the frequency analysis, the type of display, and so forth—was done by the fixed electronic circuitry of the instrument. That circuitry processed and displayed the *continuous* fluctuations of the magnetic field's strength recorded on the tape and stored temporarily on the tape loop of the spectrograph. The word *continuous* is important to this discussion: everything in this process was based on original recordings and transformations of the signal (i.e., from voltage to magnetic field, and then back to voltage, and ultimately to the darkness of the burned pattern). The process did not change the continuous nature of the speech signal. A process such as this, in which the transforms and representations (magnetic, voltage, darkness of the trace, and so forth) are in the same form as the input signal—in this case the speech signal—is called an *analog process*. In contrast, computer analysis of speech requires a conversion of analog speech waveforms to digital representation.

Speech Analysis by Computer: From Recording to Analysis to Output

Computers—whether desktops, laptops, tablets, or smartphones—take an analog signal (the pressure waveforms and the microphone transduction of that signal, which provides an electrical replica of the pressure wave) as input to a computer disk. The computer *digitizes* the analog input signal, converting the signal to a series of discrete numbers, each of which has the form of sequences of zeros (0s) and ones (1s). The analog signal is digitized with filtering, at a specific sampling rate and bit level.

Digital Speech Samples and the Aural Flip Book

When speech is synthesized by computer, or when a natural speech signal is digitized, the computerized form of the signal is a series of discrete time points—samples—each of which can be analyzed for its spectrum characteristics. When these time points are output from a computer—when they undergo digital-to-analog conversion—the human ear will connect the discrete samples and hear them as a smoothly flowing speech signal. It is just like the flip books you enjoyed, and perhaps created, as a child (and maybe even as an adult). Each individual picture in the flip book is like a digital sample. When the stack of individual pictures is flipped, the human visual system connects the sequence of images and voilà! We have animation! Think of the process of digital-to-analog conversion as aural animation.

Energy Present, Phonetic Utility Not

The frequency range of human hearing, when the auditory system is healthy, is said to be 20 to 20,000 Hz. Do all of those frequencies above 11.0 kHz get wasted when we speak to each other? Probably not. One study (Tabain, 1998) asked the question, Does energy above 10.0 kHz help distinguish /f/ from /θ/, two sounds known to have high-frequency energy? For real words containing these two sounds the answer was no. Stated in phonetic terms, energy above 10.0 kHz did not contribute to the /f/–/θ/ contrast. Some evidence exists that infants produce some fricatives with energy reaching 14 kHz (Bauer & Kent, 1987), but these infants were not using the sounds in a contrastive way and an analysis of the reliability of the acoustic contrasts for the listener was not presented. Vowels and consonants can almost always be classified and used by listeners for phonetic decisions with frequencies no higher than 11.0 kHz.

Sampling Rate

The transformation of an analog waveform to a digital representation requires a systematic and recurring sampling of the analog signal. The samples are extracted from the time-varying speech signal by "picking off" successive pieces of the waveform and storing each of these as a series of ones and zeros. The number of times per second the computer picks off a part of the waveform and stores it in digital form is called the sampling rate. Sampling rate is expressed as samples per second, which is the same as expressing the sampling rate as a frequency. A standard sampling rate in the audio industry and in contemporary speech research is 44,100 Hz (44.1 kHz). At this sampling rate, an analog signal is digitized (represented in the computer as discrete samples) every 0.0000026 sec (2.6 μs).

For reasons that are not described in detail in this chapter, there is a relationship between the sampling rate and the highest signal frequency that can be analyzed reliably. This highest frequency is one-half the sampling rate. For example, the standard sampling rate in audio applications of 44.1 kHz allows a reliable frequency analysis up to 22.05 kHz. For the majority of phonetic analyses, including sounds with significant high-frequency energy such as fricatives and stops, and even for speech produced by children with short vocal tracts, a highest frequency for analysis of 11.05 kHz and therefore a sampling rate of 22.1 kHz is sufficient.

Filters

Digitization of speech signals requires a filter to eliminate all frequencies above one-half of the sampling rate, to eliminate errors in the process of representing analog waveforms in digital form. These filters are called *anti-aliasing* filters, to denote the problem of frequencies above the ½ boundary "masquerading" (i.e., aliasing) as frequencies below the ½ boundary (that is, frequencies that are meant to be analyzed). If frequencies above the ½ boundary were digitized, the sampling rate would mistake them as lower frequencies. The reasons for this go beyond the scope of this text. Interested readers can consult https://www.geek.com/news/geek-answers-why-do-wheels-seem-to-spin-backwards-at-high-speeds-1565327/ or any other of the many websites where explanations of the phenomenon are offered. A brief account of aliasing (and the need to filter frequencies higher than the ½ sampling rate border) is also offered in the previous edition of this textbook).

Bits

Speech waveforms need to be digitized not only along the time scale, but on the amplitude scale as well. The process of coding amplitude information as the analog signal is transformed to a digital representation is called quantization. Digital conversion of the amplitude of an analog signal depends on the number of fixed amplitude levels built in to the digitization process. For example, if a digital process has ten "levels" to represent amplitude—discrete levels for digital representation of amplitude—an amplitude of the analog waveform that doesn't match one of these ten levels is stored at the closest level. The amplitude is stored, but not at the "real" amplitude in the analog signal. This distorts the waveform in digital form, relative to its analog form, which is an undesirable outcome. If the number of digitization levels for amplitude is increased to 100, more amplitude levels are available to match, as closely as possible, the actual amplitudes in the analog signal. The number of amplitude levels available for storing amplitude variations in an analog signal is called the bit rate, and the higher the bit rate, the more accurate and better the amplitude match between the analog and digital forms of a signal. Twelve or 16 bits are typical bit rates for digitization of speech signals. Twelve bits provides 4096 amplitude levels for storage of amplitude variation in a waveform, which is sufficient to provide an accurate representation of amplitude variation in a speech signal. Even better representations of analog amplitude variation can be achieved with a bit rate of 16, which gives 65,526 amplitude levels (bit rate is calculated as 2^n, where n = number of bits, hence $2^{12} = 4096$, $2^{16} = 65,526$).

Analysis and Display

Most speech analysis programs have algorithms for display, editing, and analysis of speech waveforms. The basic display of a speech analysis program is the speech waveform, shown above the spectrograms in Figures 10–8 and 10–9. A waveform of the utterance "To feed the cat one must shoo the dog" is shown in Figure 10–11. This utterance was produced by one of the authors as a direct-to-disk recording, with a sampling rate of 22.05 kHz and 16 bits of amplitude resolution. The utterance waveform was displayed in near-real time as it was spoken, and immediately stored as a

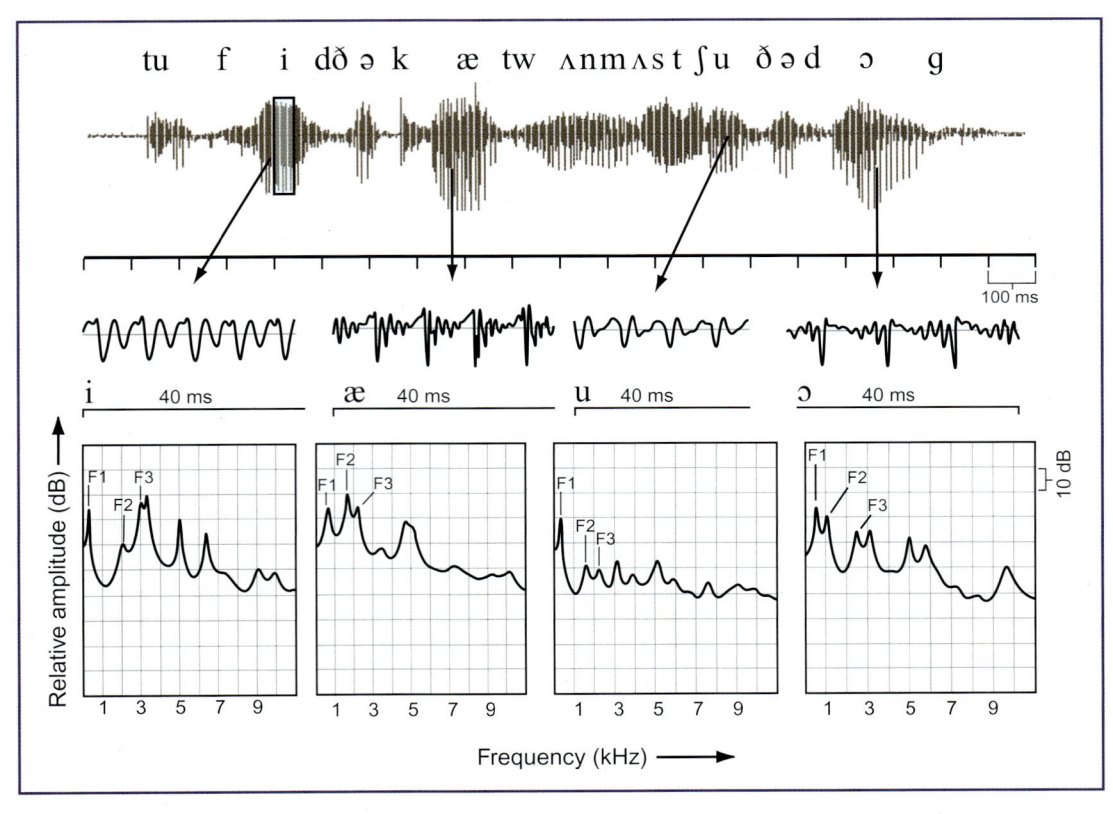

Figure 10–11. *Top*: Waveform of the utterance, "To feed the cat one must shoo the dog." Forty-millisecond pieces are extracted from each of the four corner vowels, by centering an analysis window at the temporal middle of the vowel. One such window is shown by the shaded box over the /i/ waveform. Each 40 ms waveform piece is shown in the middle row of the display, and the bottom row of panels shows the LPC spectra for each of these pieces.

file. The waveform display at the top of Figure 10–11 is essentially identical to the one that appeared on the screen as it was being recorded.

Speech analysis programs allow the user to manipulate and process waveforms in many ways, and to display the results of those processes. The typical speech analysis program allows linear predictive code analysis of formant frequencies (see below), different types of F0 and intensity measurement, computation of spectral moments (see Chapters 9 and 11), as well as other analyses beyond the scope of this book. Programs can generate a digital spectrogram, F0 contours, intensity contours, spectra for different "chunks" of a waveform, measures of voice production (jitter, shimmer, signal-to-noise ratio), and so forth. As a case study of computer analysis of speech and as a teaser for information on vowels presented in Chapter 11, consider Figure 10–11 from top to bottom as a demonstration of computer analysis of vowel formant frequencies.

The utterance whose speech waveform is shown in Figure 10–11 contains an example of each of the corner vowels of English (the phonetic symbol for the vowel in *dog* is given as /ɔ/, but the low-back corner vowel is usually thought to be /ɔ/'s near neighbor /ɑ/. In the dialect of the individual who produced the display shown in Figure 10–11, a weird farrago of Philadelphia origin and Cheesehead spirit, the vowel in *dog* sounds to most listeners as something between /ɔ/ and /ɑ/). Formant frequencies are often measured for the corner vowels to map out, in acoustic terms, the limits of vowel articulation for a given speaker. The conventional way to make formant frequency measures is to locate and segment the vowel of interest, select for analysis a relatively brief piece ("window") from the overall vowel waveform, and calculate for this piece the values of F1, F2, and F3.

The waveform editing function of *TF32* was used to isolate brief pieces of the /i/ in *feed*, the /æ/ in *cat*, the /u/ in the *shoo*, and /ɔ/ in *dog*. A shaded rectangle indicates the relatively brief, 40-ms time window of the waveform selected for analysis from the vowel /i/. In practice, these windows are not taken from a random part of the vowel waveform, but are 20 to 50 ms in duration and centered around the temporal middle of the vowel. Traditionally, "targets" for vowels have been located at their temporal midpoint and the use of a time window of 20 to 50 ms around this midpoint ensures a more stable spectral analysis than a shorter window (say, 5 ms). The 40-ms piece of the full /i/ waveform in Figure 10–11 is shown in detail immediately below the arrow pointing away from the /i/ in the full utterance. The 40-ms piece shows individual cycles of vocal fold vibration—about four cycles—expanded from their more compressed appearance in the full waveform.

[kɔrnɚ] or [kɑrnɚ] Vowels?

"Corner" vowels play a major role in speech acoustics research and in clinical applications of speech acoustics analysis. These sounds define the limits—high-front, high-back, low-front, low-back—of vowel articulation. /ɑ/ is almost always identified as the low-back corner vowel, but in some dialects /ɑ/ may be realized as [ɔ], or /ɔ/ may be realized as [ɑ] or either vowel as something between [ɔ] and [ɑ]. /ɔ/ may even involve a more extreme articulatory position compared with /ɑ/. If so, *it* should be the low-back corner vowel, not /ɑ/. English /u/, the high-back corner vowel, is even more slippery than /ɑ/ and /ɔ/, as over the last two decades it seems to be losing its lip-rounding characteristic. And not only that: /u/, the high-*back* vowel of phonetic-textbook lore, seems to have a tongue position advancing toward /i/—it is being *fronted* in many dialects. Perhaps /i/ will be like that perfect older brother, always doing the right thing, always stable, never changing. /æ/? Let's not even talk about that vowel, so pervasive and dialectally variable in American English, so rare in other languages of the world . . .

Most waveform editing functions of speech analysis programs allow a user to zoom in and zoom out on specific parts of the waveform, using cursor control and simple point-and-click maneuvers. Similar 40-ms windows around the vowel midpoints were extracted and "zoomed in" for the three other vowels. Their 40-ms pieces are shown below the arrows issuing from each of the vowels.

For these time windows, a type of analysis specific to speech analysis by computer was used to generate a spectrum from which formant frequencies were estimated. The analysis is called *linear predictive coding*, or LPC analysis. LPC analysis of speech spectra was first described in 1971 by two scientists from Bell Telephone Laboratories (Atal & Hanauer, 1971) and has become, with various refinements over the years, the standard approach to measuring formant frequencies. In Chapter 8, Figure 8–13 shows spectra for three vowels with two superimposed analyses, one a Fourier spectrum containing all the details of the harmonics and their amplitudes, the other a smooth curve showing the location of the peaks and a smooth resonance curve, minus the distracting details of the Fourier spectrum. The simplified, smoothed spectra in Figure 8–13 are LPC spectra. LPC spectra for the 40 ms windows extracted from the four corner vowels in "To feed the cat one must shoo the dog" are shown in the bottom four panels of Figure 10–11. The x-axis of each spectrum has a frequency range of 0 to 11.0 kHz, marked off by the grid lines in 1.0 kHz steps. The y-axis is marked off by grid lines in 10 dB steps. The spectra show peaks labeled F1, F2, and F3, the locations of which, for the different vowels, are consistent with expectations from the acoustic theory of vowel production and with empirical data collected from adult males (Hillenbrand, Getty, Clark, & Wheeler, 1995; and Chapter 11). The mathematical mysteries of the software that makes the analysis happen are beyond the scope of the present discussion. Rather, our emphasis is on the happy outcome of LPC analysis, which is to show the locations of the prominent frequency components (i.e., the formants) without the individual harmonic content of a Fourier spectrum. The LPC spectra along the bottom of Figure 10–11 illustrate just how obvious the peaks are in these displays, and how easy it is (in most cases) to "pick" them as F1, F2, and F3.

It is a welcome outcome to have well-defined and easily pickable peaks provided by LPC analysis, but automatic analyses—like the F0 analysis described above—run the risk of errors. Some of these errors are predictable. For example, the likelihood of erroneous formant estimates from LPC analysis increases as the speech signal becomes noisier (that is, contains more aperiodic energy), or when there is acoustic transmission through the nasal cavities. In more direct clinical terms, speakers with breathy voices or with a moderate or substantial degree of hypernasality are not the best candidates for LPC analysis. Of course, these kinds of speech characteristics are common in many different speech disorders, so the use of LPC analysis to estimate formant frequencies in clinical populations must be undertaken with a great deal of care. As in the case of F0 errors made by automatic pitch trackers, speech analysis programs that allow correction of miscalculated formant frequencies are best suited to research and clinical applications.

REVIEW

A brief history of speech analysis shows how the transduction of pressure waves produced during speech moved from mechanical to electronic transduction; the electronics age allowed recording and measurement devices to be more faithful to the details of the speech waveform.

Speech waveforms provide information on amplitude fluctuations as a function of time and allow computation of fundamental frequency (F0) for voiced sounds, but do not provide direct access to formant frequencies.

The spectrogram, a display that shows formant frequencies as a function of time, allows a user to infer changes in vocal tract configuration resulting from movement of the articulators.

Strategies are presented for how to identify from spectrograms different segment types, how to perform segmentation, and how certain conventional measurements are performed.

Much of what is known about speech acoustics has been derived from spectrographic-type analyses, including temporal (e.g., segment durations) and spectral (e.g., vowel formant frequencies and energy distribution for obstruents) characteristics.

Computer software such as *TF32* and *Praat* allows a user to generate a spectrogram, measure segmental durations, vowel formant frequencies, obstruent spectral characteristics, as well as suprasegmental characteristics such as F0 and intensity contours.

The fundamentals of computer-based analysis of speech are presented, including discussions of sampling rate, anti-aliasing filters, and quantization.

Computer-based techniques for analysis of formant frequencies are fast, reliable, automatic, and for the most part accurate except in cases where a speaker has a breathy voice quality and/or excessive nasality.

An important caution about the use of digital speech analysis techniques is the possibility of computational errors, due to a noisy source or excessive nasality; a computer program must be employed that allows expert analysis of the automatic results and correction of errors when needed.

REFERENCES

Atal, B., & Hanauer, S. (1971). Speech analysis and synthesis by linear prediction. *Journal of the Acoustical Society of America, 50,* 637–655.

Bauer, H., & Kent, R. (1987). Acoustic analyses of infant fricative and trill vocalizations. *Journal of the Acoustical Society of America, 81,* 505–511.

Byrd, D. (1993). 54,000 American stops. *UCLA Working Papers in Phonetics, 83,* 97–116.

Catford, J. C. (2000). *A practical introduction to phonetics* (2nd ed.). Oxford, UK: Oxford University Press.

Crystal, T., & House, A. (1988). The duration of American English stop consonants: An overview. *Journal of Phonetics, 16,* 285–294.

Hillenbrand, J., Getty, L. A., Clark, M. J., & Wheeler, K. (1995). Acoustic characteristics of American English vowels. *Journal of the Acoustical Society of America*, 97, 3099–3111.

Klatt, D. (1976). Linguistic uses of segmental duration in English: Acoustic and perceptual evidence. *Journal of the Acoustical Society of America*, 59, 1208–1221.

Solzhenitsyn, A. (1969). *The first circle*. New York, NY: Bantam Books.

Tabain, M. (1998). Non-sibilant fricatives in English: Spectral information above 10 kHz. *Phonetica*, 55, 107–130.

Umeda, N. (1977). Consonant duration in American English. *Journal of the Acoustical Society of America*, 61, 846–858.

Zue, V., & Cole, R. (1979). Experiments on spectrogram reading. *Acoustics, Speech, and Signal Processing, IEEE International Conference on ICASSP '79*, 4, 116–119.

Acoustic Phonetics Data

INTRODUCTION

This chapter provides a selective summary of acoustic phonetics data. The presentation is selective because the research literature is voluminous. The large quantity of data available reflects the many uses of acoustic phonetics research—the discipline of acoustic phonetics serves many masters. Acoustic phonetics data are used by linguists who wish to enhance their phonetic description of a language; by speech communication specialists who are interested in developing high-quality speech synthesis and recognition systems; by scientists who wish to test theories of speech production and prefer to use the speech acoustic approach to the interpretation of articulatory patterns rather than data obtained using one of the more invasive and time-consuming physiological approaches (such as x-ray or electromagnetic tracking of articulatory motions); by speech perception scientists who want to understand the acoustic cues used in the identification of vowels and consonants by normal hearers and persons with hearing loss and prosthetic hearing devices; and by speech-language pathologists who want information concerning a client's speech production behaviors—information that can be documented quantitatively and in some cases may be too subtle or transient to be captured by auditory analysis.

The chapter is concerned primarily with the acoustic characteristics of *speech sound segments*—the vowel and consonant segments of a language. A brief discussion of the acoustic characteristics of suprasegmentals (prosody) is also presented. The chapter does not provide coverage of the rich literature on the acoustic characteristics of voice production (phonation). Good sources for this information are Baken and Orlikoff (1999) and Titze (2000).

VOWELS

The upper part of Figure 11–1 shows a spectrogram of two vowels, /æ/ and /i/, spoken by a 57-year-old healthy male in the disyllable frames /əˈhæd/ and /əˈhid/. The /əˈhVd/ frame (where V = vowel) is famous in speech science, originally used by Peterson and Barney (1952) in their landmark study of vowel formant frequencies produced by men, women, and children. Peterson and Barney wanted to measure formant frequencies of vowels under minimal influence from the surrounding phonetic context—that is, with little or no coarticulatory effects. The most apparent way to get this kind of "pure" information on vowel articulation, and the resulting formant frequencies, is to have speakers produce isolated, sustained vowels. However, when speakers phonate sustained vowels they tend to sing, rather than speak, the vowels. Peterson and Barney designed a more natural speech task in which the unstressed schwa preceded a stressed syllable initiated by the glottal fricative /h/. The reasoning was that a segment whose initial articulation required primarily laryngeal gestures had minimal influence on the vocal tract gestures required for a following vowel. The /d/ at the end of the syllable was necessary to provide a "natural" ending to the syllable (in English, at least), as well as accommodating the production of lax vowels such as /ɪ/, /ɛ/, and /ʊ/, which in English do not occur in open syllables (with very few exceptions, such as "yeah").

The /d/ at the end of the syllable may have some influence on the vowel articulation. But Peterson and Barney (1952) made their formant frequency measurements at a location where the formants were assumed to be sufficiently distant from the /d/ to minimize its influence on the formant frequency estimates. Conveniently, this measurement location also seemed

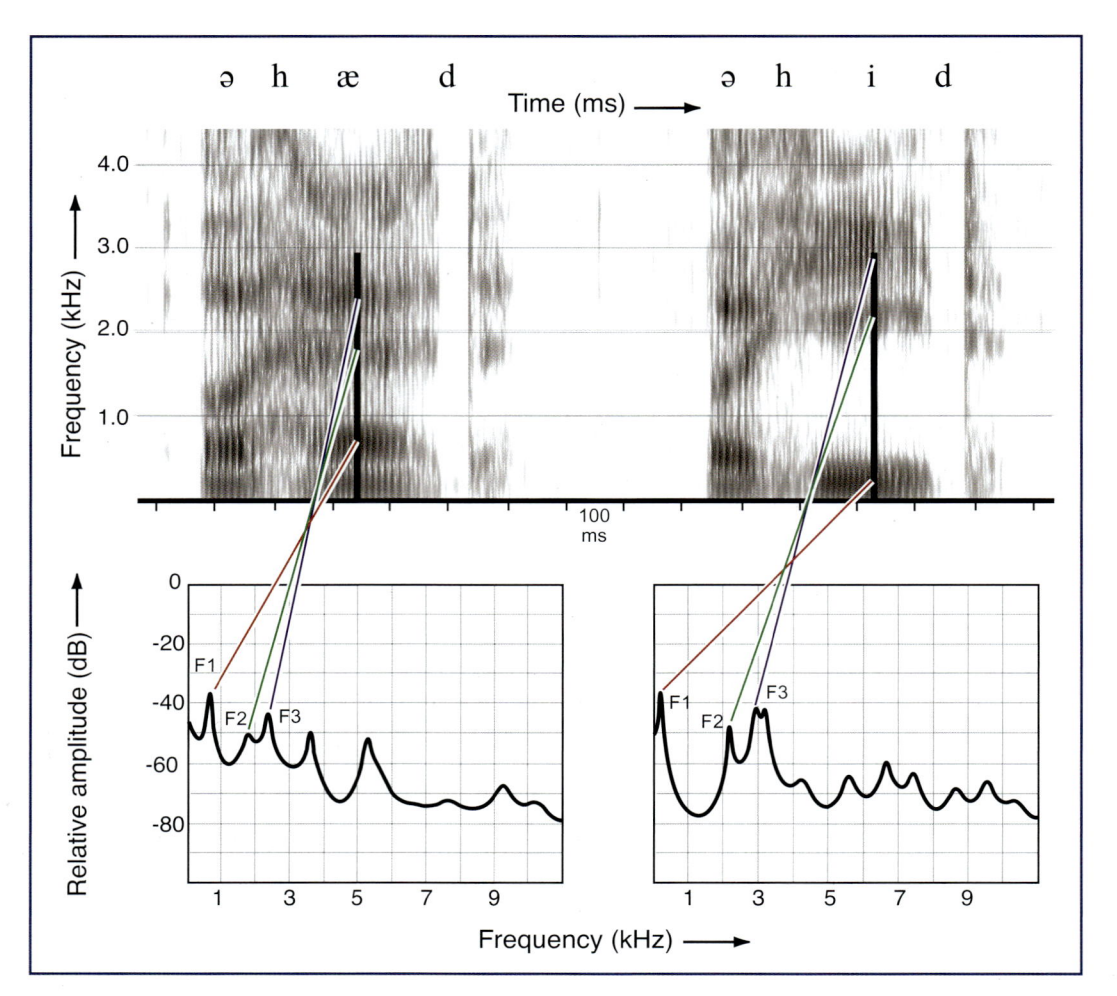

Figure 11-1. Spectrograms of two vowels (*top part of figure*), /æ/ and /i/, spoken by a 57-year-old healthy male in the disyllable frames /ə'hæd/ and /ə'hid/. Bottom part of the figure shows LPC spectra for the two vowels, measured at the temporal middle of the vowels. The colored lines (red = F1; green = F2; blue = F3) connect the middle of the formant bands on the spectrograms to the peaks in the LPC spectra.

to capture the "target" location of the vowel: the point in time at which formant frequencies were thought to coincide with the articulatory configuration aimed at by the speaker when trying to produce the best possible version of the vowel. The inclusion of the schwa as the first syllable provided some control over the prosodic pattern of the disyllable, placing stress on the /hVd/ syllable.

Forty-three years following the publication of Peterson and Barney's (1952) classic work, Hillenbrand, Getty, Clark, and Wheeler (1995) published a replication of the study using updated analysis methods. Like Peterson and Barney, Hillenbrand et al. studied men (n = 45), women (n = 48), and children aged 10 to 12 years (n = 46, both girls and boys) producing the 12 monophthong vowels of English (/i,ɪ,e,ɛ,æ,ɑ,ɔ,o,ʊ,u,ʌ,ɝ/) in an /hVd/ frame.[1] Hillenbrand et al. measured the first four formants (F1–F4) at their most stable point, in much the same way as shown in Figure 11–1 (except that F4 is not shown). The heavy vertical line through the spectrogram in Figure 11–1 shows the point in time at which the formant frequencies were measured (in

---

[1] The vowel inventory of English is not always described as having 12 monophthongs. In particular, /e/ and /o/ are diphthongized in many dialects, but less often in the upper Midwest dialects included (primarily) in the Hillenbrand et al. (1995) study. /ɝ/ is sometimes also not included as an English monophthong, but may be considered a rhotacized (/ɪ/-colored) vowel. Also note that Hillenbrand et al. did not use the schwa preceding the /hVd/ syllable, as in Peterson and Barney (1952).

these cases, roughly in the middle of the vowel duration). Formant frequencies were estimated using linear predictive code (LPC) analysis, discussed in Chapter 10. The LPC spectra for the measurement point shown on the spectrograms are provided in the lower half of Figure 11–1. Lines point from the middle of the formant bands to the corresponding peaks in the LPC spectra. For these vowels, values of the first three formant frequencies for /æ/ are approximately 700, 1750, and 2450 Hz, and for /i/ are roughly 290, 2200, and 2950 Hz.

Figure 11–2 shows Hillenbrand et al.'s (1995, p. 3104) formant frequency data in the form of an F1-F2 plot (see Peterson & Barney, 1952, Figure 8, p. 182). Each phonetic symbol represents an F1-F2 coordinate for a given speaker's production of that vowel. Two of the vowels (/e/ and /o/) are not plotted to reduce crowding of the data points. The ellipses drawn around each vowel category enclose roughly 95% of all the observable points for that vowel.

These data show how a single vowel can be associated with a wide range of F1-F2 values. For example, the vowel /i/ shows points ranging between (approximately) 300 and 500 Hz on the F1 axis and 2100 and 3400 Hz on the F2 axis. The ellipse enclosing the /i/ points is oriented upward and leaning slightly to the right. Points in the lower part of the ellipse are almost certainly from men, points in the middle from women, and points at the upper part and to the right from children. This follows from material presented in Chapters 7 and 8 on resonance patterns of tubes of different lengths, and age- and sex-related differences in vocal tract length: shorter vocal tracts have higher resonant frequencies than longer ones. The same general summary can be given for almost any vowel in this plot, even though the degree of variation and orientation of the ellipses vary from vowel to vowel.

Despite the wide variation across speakers in formant frequencies for a given vowel, Hillenbrand et al.

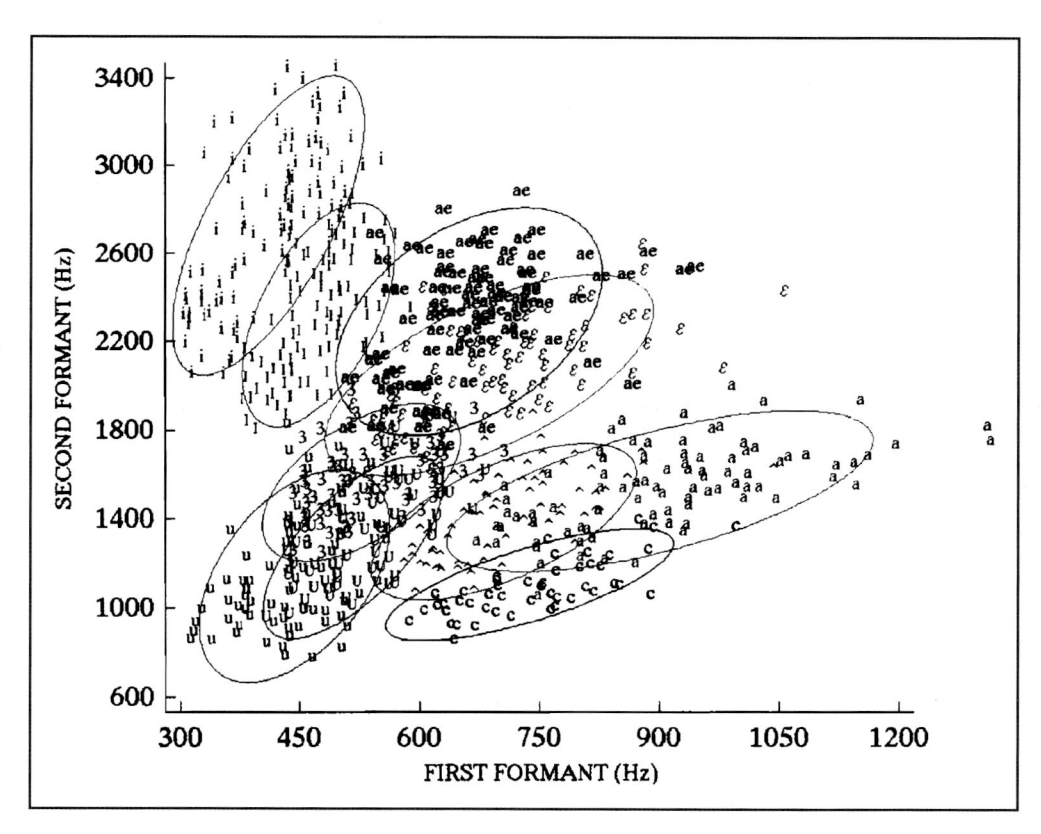

Figure 11–2. F1-F2 plot of American English vowels from Hillenbrand et al. (1995, p. 3104). Each phonetic symbol represents an F1-F2 coordinate for a given speaker's production of that vowel. Two vowels (/e/ and /o/) are not plotted to reduce crowding of the data points. The ellipses drawn around each vowel category enclose roughly 95% of all the observable points for that vowel. Reproduced with permission from Hillenbrand, J., Getty, L., Clark, M., and Wheeler, K. (1995). Acoustic characteristics of American English vowels. *Journal of the Acoustical Society of America, 97,* 3099–3111.

(1995) replicated Peterson and Barney's (1952) finding that the vowel intended by a speaker was almost always perceived correctly—consistent with the speaker's intention—by listeners. Somehow listeners heard the same vowel category even when confronted with a wide variety of formant patterns.

Figure 11–2 also shows that the formant frequency patterns of one vowel often overlap with those of another vowel. There is a small region of overlap between the ellipses of /i/ and /ɪ/, and a larger region of overlap between /æ/ and /ɛ/. In the lower left-hand part of the plot, roughly around F1 = 525 Hz and F2 = 1400 Hz, there is a three-way overlap of the vowels /u/, /ʊ/, and /ɝ/. In many cases, these areas of overlap are for vowels produced by speakers with vocal tracts of different lengths. For example, a good portion of the overlap between /æ/ and /ɛ/ seems to come from adult male /æ/ values with adult female, or child /ɛ/ values. But there are many cases where the overlap is not so clearly explained by differing vocal tract lengths. Overlapping formant frequencies for the same vowel produced by different speakers raises the question of how we hear the *same* formant frequencies produced by different speakers as *different* vowels. Hillenbrand et al.'s (1995) data, like those of Peterson and Barney (1952), demonstrate that knowing a pattern of formant frequencies does not necessarily provide sufficient information to identify the intended (spoken) vowel category. At the least, the identity of the speaker, including age, sex, and almost certainly dialect (Clopper, Pisoni, & de Jong, 2006), must be known to link a specific formant pattern to a vowel category.

Figure 11–3 plots a summary of a subset of the data reported by Hillenbrand et al. (1995). The subset includes averaged F1-F2 data from men, women, and children, for American English corner vowels that were "well identified" by a panel of listeners. Corner vowels define the limits of vowel articulation, with /i/ the highest and most front vowel, /æ/ the lowest and most front, /ɑ/ the lowest and most back, and /u/ the highest and most back. If these are the most extreme articulatory configurations for vowels in English, the formant frequencies should be at the most extreme coordinates in F1-F2 space. By including only data

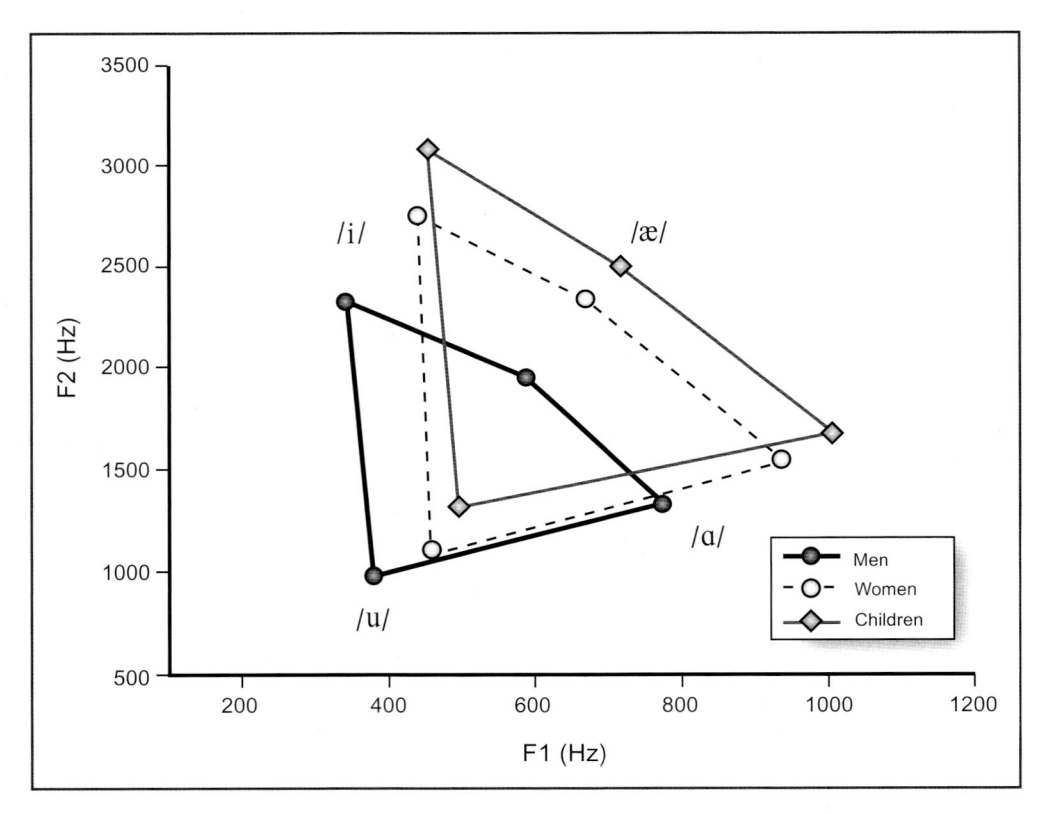

Figure 11–3. Vowel spaces constructed from corner vowels (/i/, /æ/, /ɑ/, /u/) of American English for men (*filled circles connected by solid lines*), women (*unfilled circles connected by dashed lines*), and children aged 10 to 12 years (*lightly shaded diamonds connected by solid lines*). These data are replotted from Hillenbrand et al. (1995, Table V., p. 3103) and are averages of vowels that were well identified by a crew of listeners.

It's Never That Simple, Even When It's Complex to Begin With

Students sometimes have difficulty embracing the gray areas in science; black and white answers are more comfortable. The overlap of vowel formant frequencies shown in Figure 11–2, coupled with listeners' apparent ease in identifying vowels in the overlapped areas, seems to be one of those hard-to-embrace gray areas: how do listeners do it? One possible answer is that the relationship of vowel acoustics to vowel identification is both more complex and more simple than suggested by the scatterplot in Figure 11–2. Both Peterson and Barney (1952) and Hillenbrand et al. (1995) constructed scatterplots based on F1 and F2 measured at a single point in time during vowel production. In identification experiments, however, listeners heard the *whole* vowel. What if changes in formant frequency throughout the vowel duration are important for vowel identification? If this is the case, plots such as Figure 11–2 underrepresent the mapping between vowel acoustics and vowel identification (see Hillenbrand & Nearey, 1999; Jacewicz & Fox, 2012, 2017; Nearey & Assman, 1986 for just this argument). The scientific problem is more complex because there is more to the acoustics of vowels than formant frequencies measured at a single point in time, and less complex because plots such as those in Figure 11–2 may miss the point. Think gray: it's so much more fun than thinking black and white.

---

from "well-identified" vowels, the plotted data can be regarded as excellent exemplars of these vowel categories. When average F1-F2 coordinates for each of the four corner vowels are connected by a line for each of the three speaker groups, three vowel quadrilaterals are formed. In an F1-F2 plot, the area enclosed by such a quadrilateral is called the acoustic vowel space.

Three general characteristics of these F1-F2 plots are noteworthy. First, the vowel quadrilaterals for men, women, and children move from the lower left to upper right part of the graph, respectively. This is because the vocal tract becomes progressively shorter across these three speaker groups. Second, the area of the vowel quadrilaterals—the acoustic vowel space—appears to be larger for children, compared with women, and larger for women compared with men. This probably has little to do with articulatory differences between the groups (although there may be some sex-specific articulatory effects, see Simpson, 2001), but rather is another consequence of the different-sized vocal tracts. Exactly the same articulatory configurations for the corner vowels in a shorter compared with longer vocal tract generate not only higher formant frequencies but also greater distances between F1-F2 points for the different vowels. The larger vowel space for children compared with men does not mean the children use more extreme articulatory configurations for vowels. Third, the acoustic vowel quadrilateral for one group of speakers cannot be perfectly fit to the quadrilateral for a different group by moving it to the new location (up and to the right) and uniformly expanding or shrinking it to achieve an exact match. Imagine the quadrilateral for men in Figure 11–3 moved into the position of the quadrilateral for women, followed by a uniform expansion of the male space to "fit" the female space. This attempt to scale the male quadrilateral to the female quadrilateral fails because the magnitudes of the sex-related vowel differences are not the same for each vowel. For example, note the relative closeness in F1-F2 space of the male and female /u/ compared with the other three vowels. A similar inability to scale the vowels of one group to another is seen in Figure 11–4, which is an F1-F2 plot for the lax vowels (/i/, /ʊ/, /ɛ/), based on data reported by Hillenbrand et al. (1995). The group differences in these vowel triangles are very much like the ones shown for the corner vowel quadrilaterals (Figure 11–3), including vowel-specific differences across groups. Note especially the small difference between males and females for /ʊ/ compared with the much larger male-female differences for /ɪ/ and /ɛ/. The lax-vowel triangle for men cannot be scaled in a simple way to obtain the triangle for women.

Professor Emeritus James Hillenbrand has made the vowel formant frequencies reported in Hillenbrand et al. (1995) available for public use. Interested readers are directed to https://homepages.wmich.edu/~hillenbr/voweldata.html

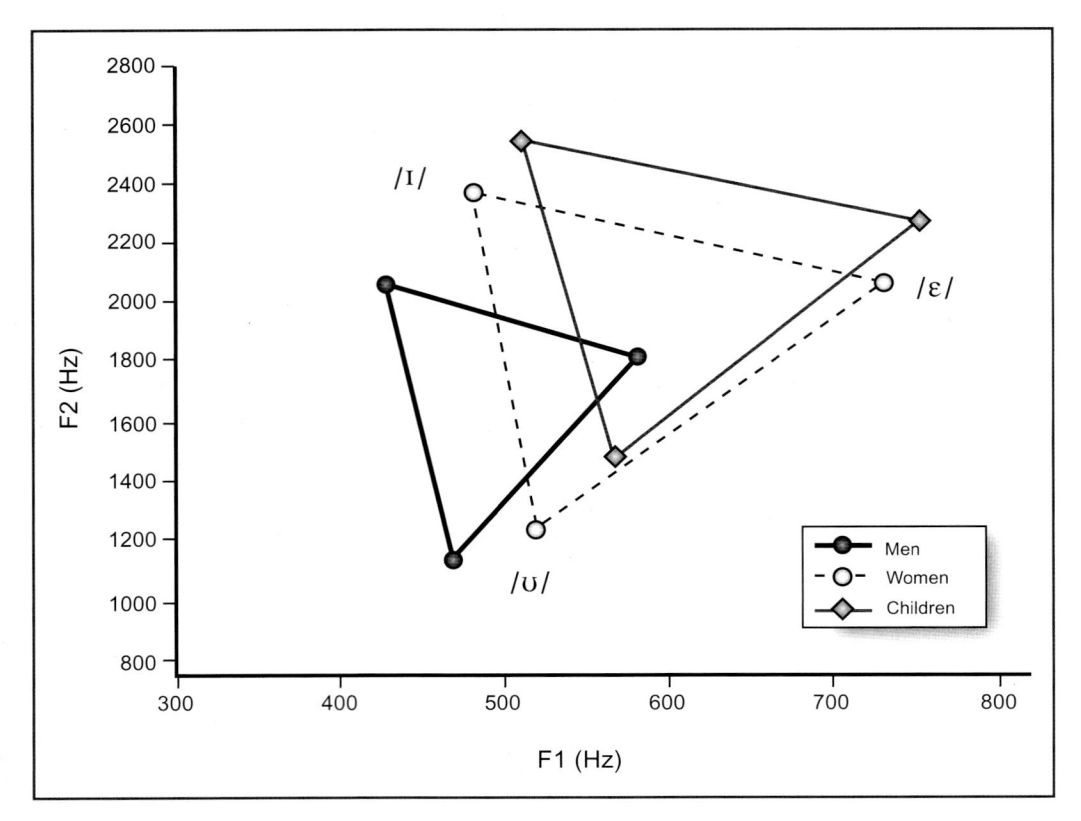

Figure 11–4. Vowel spaces constructed from three American English lax vowels (/ɪ/, /ʊ/, /ɛ/) for men (*filled circles connected by solid lines*), women (*unfilled circles connected by dashed lines*), and children aged 10 to 12 (*lightly shaded diamonds connected by solid lines*). These data are replotted from Hillenbrand et al. (1995, Table V., p. 3103) and are averages of vowels that were well identified by a crew of listeners.

The acoustic vowel space for corner vowels has potential clinical application as an index of speech motor integrity, the effects of speech therapy, and comparison of vowel articulation in different languages. Evidence from studies of speakers with dysarthria (speech disorders resulting from neurological disease; see Liu, Tsao, & Kuhl, 2005; Turner, Tjaden, & Weismer, 1995; Weismer, Jeng, Laures, Kent, & Kent, 2001), glossectomy (removal of tongue tissue, usually because of a cancerous tumor; see Whitehill, Ciocca, Chan, & Samman, 2006), cochlear implants (Chuang, Yang, Chi, Weismer, & Wang, 2012), and even neurologically normal speakers (Bradlow, Torretta, & Pisoni, 1996) suggests that the size of the acoustic vowel space is modestly correlated with independent measurements of speech intelligibility or perceptual measures of articulatory precision (Fletcher, McAuliffe, Lansford, & Liss, 2017). The size of the vowel space is smaller in persons with dysarthria (Lee, Littlejohn, & Simmons, 2017) and can be made to expand and contract with different speaking styles such as "clear speech" versus "casual speech" (Lam & Tjaden, 2013). Computation of the acoustic vowel space is often based on the assumption that the area enclosed by the formant frequencies of corner vowels in an F1 versus F2 (or F2 vs. F3) plot serves as a "proxy" for articulatory behavior (Berisha, Sandoval, Utianski, Liss, & Spanias, 2014). The idea is that larger vowel space areas reflect greater articulatory distinctions between the corner vowels, and perhaps between vowels on the "interior" of the corner vowels as well (e.g., lax vowels of English such as /ɪ/ in "bit," /ɛ/ in "bet," and /ʊ/ in "book"). Over the past fifteen years there have been many publications on the acoustic vowel space, applied to many different problems, some of which are listed above.

The correlation between the area of the acoustic vowel space and speech intelligibility (or perceptual measures of speech precision) can be interpreted in at least two ways. First, because the acoustic vowel space for corner vowels is constructed from the most extreme articulatory positions for vowels (i.e., most high and front vowel /i/, most high and back vowel /u/, and so

> **The Many Dimensions of Speech Perception**
>
> A popular research goal has been to find a reliable connection between the speech acoustic output of the vocal tract and the intelligibility of utterances. This makes sense because the treatment of many speech disorders has a central goal of making a speaker more intelligible. To meet this overall goal, treatment efforts are often aimed at improving phonetic accuracy, under the assumption that speech intelligibility is better or worse as phonetic accuracy for sound classes (vowels, fricatives, and so forth) improves or declines. This very reasonable assumption is, unfortunately, not completely true, and in fact a good deal less true than you might think (Weismer, 2008). In an effort to identify other perceptual consequences of speech disorders, researchers have developed scales for *articulatory precision*, *naturalness*, *acceptability*, *bizarreness* (we kid you not), *normalcy*, and *severity*. There are other terms, too, but let's not go on. Whether or not the terms are variants of one phenomenon—speech intelligibility—is a topic for future research.

forth), the size (area) of the space may be an index of articulatory mobility—the acoustic "proxy" mentioned above. Larger vowel space areas are thought to reflect greater differences between vocal tract configurations for the corner vowels. In speakers with motor speech disorders, as one example, larger vowel spaces are thought to reflect greater articulatory flexibility compared with smaller vowel spaces. The size of the vowel space area may indeed serve as a global index of speech motor control. In this view, one cannot claim that specific vowels in the acoustic vowel space contribute directly to speech intelligibility; the vowel space measure is a general measure of the overall severity of a speech motor control deficit. A corollary to this is that the inference from the vowel space to the degree of articulatory flexibility is connected to speech intelligibility in a general way: intelligibility increases with increases in vowel space area.

A second interpretation is that larger vowel space areas increase the acoustic difference between closely related vowels, such as /i/ versus /ɪ/ or /u/ versus /ʊ/. In other words, acoustic contrasts for vowels other than the corner vowels are more sharply defined within larger vowel spaces.[2] In this interpretation, a smaller vowel space is not simply a sign of overall speech motor control problems (as in the first interpretation) but is an important, independent component of a speech intelligibility deficit. More sharply defined contrasts among vowels allow better vowel identification, and therefore contribute to increased speech intelligibility (Liu, Tsao, & Kuhl, 2005). This may also explain why children with cochlear implants, whose auditory input is not as rich as that of children with normal hearing, produce smaller vowel spaces than normal-hearing children (Chuang et al., 2012).

There is a critical distinction between the first and second interpretations of the size of the vowel space. The second interpretation predicts an improvement in speech intelligibility for a client who, as part of a management program, learns to produce corner vowels with more extreme positions and, therefore, expands the acoustic vowel space. If the vowels are an independent component that contributes to speech intelligibility, larger vowel spaces resulting from management will be associated with more sharply defined vowel contrasts, for all vowels of a language. The better vowel contrasts result in improved speech intelligibility (Kim, Hasegawa-Johnson, & Perlman, 2011; Lansford & Liss, 2014; Liu et al., 2005). The first interpretation, that a smaller vowel space merely reflects some limitation on articulatory flexibility, does not necessarily require that the smaller vowel space be associated with reduced intelligibility. In fact, a given speaker produces vowel spaces of very different size depending on the speaking style (formal versus casual) and even the kind of speech material produced (e.g., vowels in isolated words versus vowels in an extended reading passage) without any significant loss of speech intelligibility (Kuo & Weismer, 2016; Picheny, Durlach, & Braida, 1986).

---

[2]This hypothesis is based on single-point measurements at the temporal middle of the vowel, as discussed in the text. The contrast between nearby vowels such as /i-ɪ/ and /u-ʊ/ (tense vs. lax vowels, where the tense member contributes to the corner-vowel space), rather than between lax vowels, (such as /ɪ-ɛ/) may depend on a complex set of characteristics, including duration and formant change as a function of time, rather than single point-in-time measurements (Leung, Jongman, Wang, & Sereno, 2016).

Speech Acoustics and Your Smile

In a 1980 paper delivered to the 100th meeting of the Acoustical Society of America in Los Angeles, the famous phonetician/phonologist John Ohala (now Professor Emeritus of Linguistics at UC Berkeley) proposed an acoustic explanation for smiling. By pulling the corners of the mouth back and against the teeth, Ohala argued, the vocal tract is effectively shortened. Shorter vocal tracts mean higher formant frequencies, and higher formant frequencies are associated with smaller people. Smaller people, such as children, are generally not viewed as a physical threat. Speaking while smiling—think game-show host—sends a signal that says, "I'm small, I'm not a threat, I'm friendly, like me, don't hurt me." In evolutionary terms, vocalizations while smiling eventually were dispensed with, and the soundless smile was enough to send a signal of friendliness.

It is not clear which of these interpretations is correct, or even if they should be considered opposing viewpoints. Both views may be correct to some degree. A set of data relevant to interpretation of vowel space area shows that among normal, young adult males, the area may vary dramatically with change in speaking material (Kuo & Weismer, 2016). Figure 11–5 shows vowel space areas adapted from Kuo and Weismer for a single speaker in two conditions: (1) speaking clearly in an /hVd/ frame (where V = vowel; unfilled boxes), and (2) vowels extracted from a reading passage (filled circles). This plot shows F1 on the *y*-axis and F2 on the *x*-axis, corresponding to tongue height on the ordinate (higher tongue height as values move down the ordinate, hence the higher F1 values with lower tongue height) and tongue advancement on the abscissa (greater advancement as values move to the right on the abscissa). Eight monophthongs are plotted for each of both conditions (1) and (2) with the corner vowels identified by phonetic symbols. The other vowels can be inferred from their position along the tongue height and advancement dimensions. The vowel space area in the citation speech condition (/əˈhVd/) is substantially greater than the area in the reading condition. Does the normal speaker's reduction of vowel space area in the reading condition reflect a loss of speech motor control relative to the clear speech condition? The answer is obviously no. Seven of the 10 speakers studied by Kuo and Weismer (2016) had an extensive reduction pattern like the speaker shown in Figure 11–5, to varying degrees; the remaining 3 speakers had smaller reductions in the same direction as the 7 speakers. The vowel spaces from the reading condition are comparable to those reported for speakers with amyotropic lateral sclerosis (Turner & Tjaden, 2000), and for speakers with Parkinson's disease (among others) (Whitfield & Goberman, 2014). These comparable "normal" data and data reported for speakers with speech motor control deficits resulting from neurological disease are not meant to deny the potential of vowel space area as a noninvasive, clinical index of the integrity of speech motor control and its effect on speech intelligibility. Rather, it points to caution in the interpretation of vowel space area as an index of speech motor control.

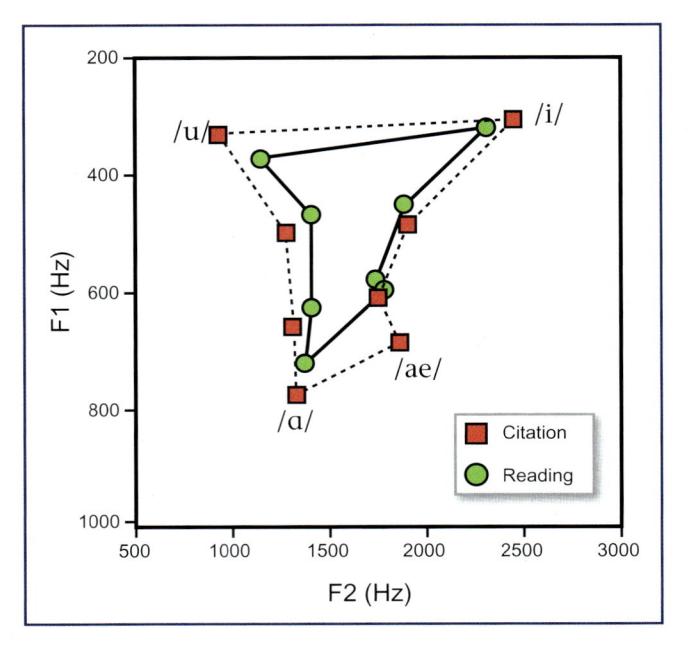

Figure 11–5. F1-F2 plot of one speaker's corner vowel productions in two speaking conditions. The conditions are citation speech in an /əˈhVd/ context (*unfilled boxes*), and passage reading (*filled circles*). F1 is on the ordinate, F2 on the abscissa, to display the formants as "within" the vocal tract. Tongue height increases upward on the ordinate and tongue advancement increases to the right on the abscissa.

Vowel Acoustics: Dialect and Cross-Language Phonetics

In recent years there has been enormous interest in *comparative acoustic phonetics*. Comparative acoustic phonetics has two main, interrelated branches. One concerns the acoustic characteristics of similar speech sounds in two or more languages or in two or more dialects of the same language. The other branch concerns the effect of native language (or dialect) phonetics (usually abbreviated as L1) on the acoustic characteristics of speech sounds in a second language (or dialect) (L2).[3] The relationship between these two branches is simple in concept, but complex in practice. Both branches are relevant to preclinical speech science. The population of the United States includes many people who speak English as an L2. Dialect variation within the United States is not subtle, and a person's dialect may be a core component of identity and culture. A significant proportion of individuals who seek the services of a speech-language pathologist and whose language or dialect does not match the clinician's presents an interesting diagnostic and treatment problem. These concerns may include the diagnosis and treatment of a developmental speech sound disorder, the influence of disease on speech production, or a desire among healthy speakers for accent modification or reduction.

Acoustic characteristics of vowels have been a major focus for both branches of inquiry. Figure 11–6 shows F1-F2 patterns for "shared" vowels, measured roughly at the temporal midpoint of the vowels, produced by adult male speakers in four languages—Madrid Spanish; American English as spoken in Ithaca, New York (presumably corresponding to the "Inland North" dialect; see Labov, 1991); modern Greek (primarily from Athens); and modern Hebrew as spoken in Israel. These four languages share the vowels /i/, /e/, /o/, and /u/. A fifth vowel, /a/ slightly advanced from American English /ɑ/, is shared by Spanish, Greek, and Hebrew. A "shared" vowel is one that phoneticians

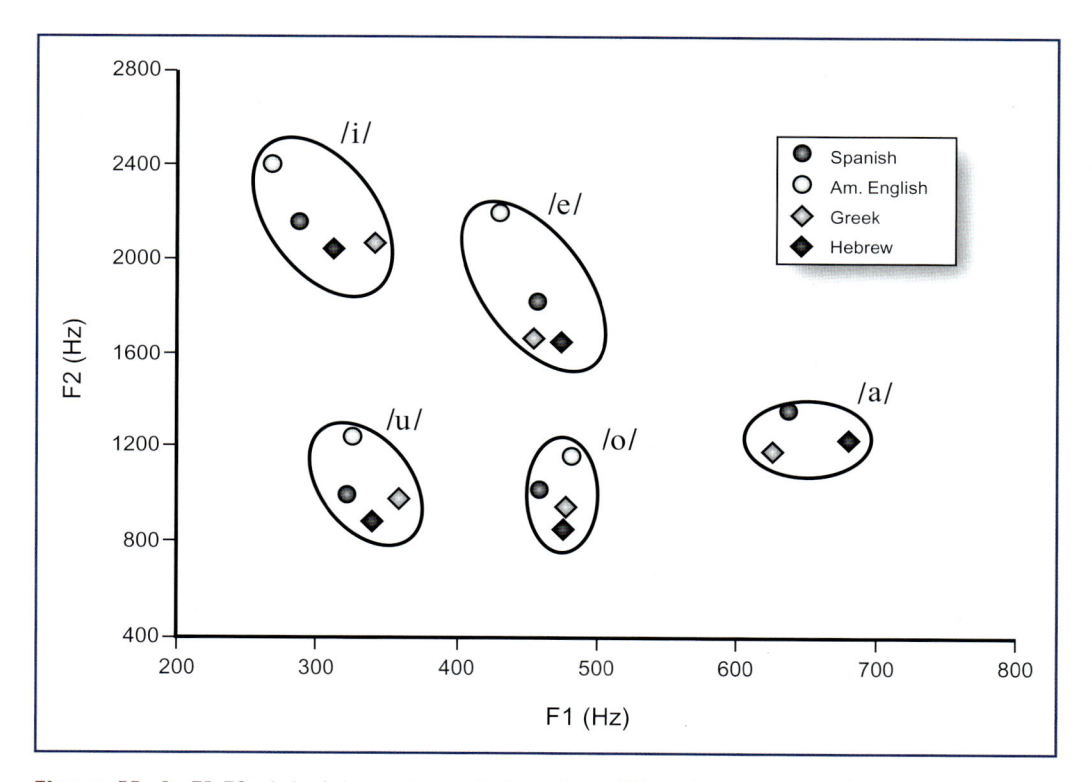

Figure 11–6. F1-F2 plot of shared vowels from four different languages. Spanish, American English, modern Greek, and Hebrew all have the vowels /i/, /e/, /o/, and /u/ in their phonetic inventories. In addition, Spanish, modern Greek, and Hebrew share the vowel /a/. Spanish data are shown by filled circles, American English data by unfilled circles, Greek data by lightly shaded diamonds, and Hebrew data by filled diamonds. The sources for the data are Bradlow (1995; Spanish and English), Jongman, Fourakis, and Sereno (1989; Greek), and Most, Amir, and Tobin (2000; Hebrew). All data are from adult male speakers.

---

[3]The "L1-L2" terminology is typically used to designate speakers of two different languages, but the usage could be generalized to two different dialects of the same language (perhaps the designation should be "D1-D2"). At least one linguist (McWhorter, 2001) argues that the differences between languages and dialects are not so clear cut, with dialects and languages (including their phonetics) blending into each other as if they were on a continuum rather than being categorically different.

transcribe with the same symbol across languages. In Figure 11–6, the F1-F2 values for shared vowels are enclosed by ellipses drawn by eye. Shared vowels in Hebrew and English (for example) have different F1-F2 values; the magnitude of these differences varies across vowels. The Hebrew-English differences for the high front vowels /i/ and /e/ are more dramatic compared with /u/ and /o/. Similar comparisons for different language pairs suggest the same conclusion: the use of the same phonetic symbol does not mean the sound has the same acoustic characteristics in different languages. Data such as these may explain why an L2 speaker's production of a vowel shared by L1 and L2 (e.g., an Israeli speaker's production of the vowel /i/ when speaking American English) can still be detected as accented by a native speaker of the L2 (Bradlow, 1995).

The cross-language comparison presented in Figure 11–6 is a simplistic one, even though it makes a valid point. The comparison is simplistic because "shared" vowels across different languages may vary in more ways than the F1-F2 values measured at a single point in time. The vowels may also differ (or be similar) by the higher (F3, F4) formant frequencies, the formant transitions going into and out of the so-called vowel steady-states, the overall vowel duration, the relation of the vowel duration to the duration of adjacent syllables, and other factors. The acoustic comparison of shared vowel sounds in different languages is potentially very complex.

Despite this complexity, a simple F1-F2 comparison of L2 vowels and their corresponding native vowels (the L1, e.g., Americans producing English) reveals a good deal about the influence of L1 on an L2 vowel system (i.e., the vowel productions of speakers learning an L2). Chen, Robb, Gilbert, and Lerman (2001) studied the formant frequencies of American English vowels produced by native speakers of Mandarin, the primary language of Taiwan and many parts of mainland China. The Mandarin vowel system includes six vowels, /i/, /e/, /u/, /o/, /a/, and /y/ (similar to a lip rounded /i/), the first four of which are also found in American English. The American English lax vowels /ɪ/, /ɛ/, and /ʊ/ are "new" for the Mandarin speaker learning English (just as /y/ would be a new vowel for the American speaker learning to produce Mandarin). Figure 11–7 shows F1-F2 data from the

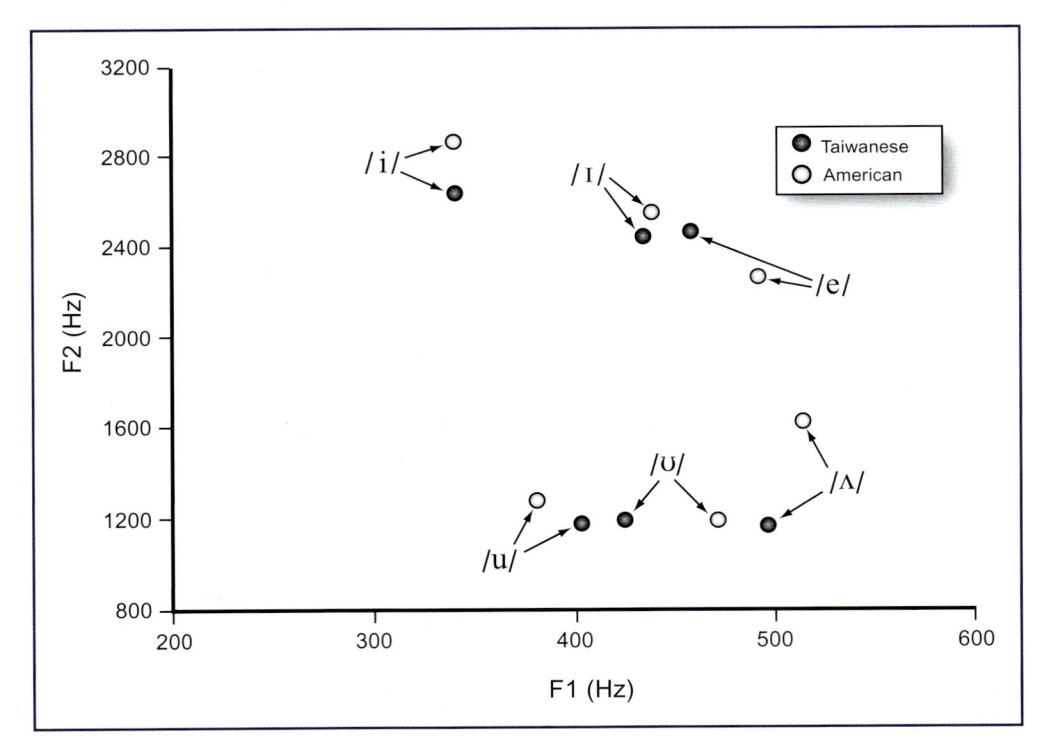

Figure 11–7. F1-F2 data for American English vowels /i/, /ɪ/, /e/, /u/, /ʊ/, and /ʌ/, spoken by adult female speakers from Taiwan whose native language is Mandarin (*filled circles*) and adult female speakers whose native language is American English (*unfilled circles*). Arrows project from each phonetic symbol to the points representing a specific, average F1-F2 coordinate for vowels produced by both groups of speakers. Data replotted from Chen et al. (2001).

Chen et al. study, specifically for the American English vowels /i/, /e/, /ɪ/, /u/, /ʊ/, and /ʌ/ produced by Taiwanese adult females whose native language is Mandarin (filled circles) and by native female speakers of American English (unfilled circles). Each plotted point is labeled with the phonetic symbol matching the American English vowel intended by the Mandarin speakers.

These data suggest several important conclusions concerning the way in which the vowel pairs [i]-[ɪ] and [u]-[ʊ] were produced by the two groups of speakers. Native speakers of English produced these vowel pairs with a fair degree of separation in F1-F2 space, as expected for vowels with categorical (that is, phonemic) status. English [i] and [ɪ] differ both in the F1 and F2 dimensions, the differences implying a somewhat more open (higher F1) and slightly more posterior tongue position (lower F2) for [ɪ]. English [u] and [ʊ] are separated only minimally along the F2 dimension, but differ by nearly 100 Hz on the F1 dimension, suggesting a more open vocal tract for the latter vowel. In contrast, the F1-F2 points for the [i]-[ɪ] and [u]-[ʊ] English vowel pairs produced by Taiwanese speakers were closer together, differing by small amounts along the F2 dimension. In the case of [u]-[ʊ], the Taiwanese points in F1-F2 space are so close to each other it appears the speakers treated the vowels as members of a single vowel category. Note also the large separation in F1-F2 category between [ɪ] and [e] for the native speakers, but the small separation between the same two vowels for the Mandarin speakers.

There are competing theories for the L1-L2 data in Figure 11–7. The Mandarin speakers produced a "new" vowel ([ɪ] in one case, [ʊ] in the other) as if it were a member of one of the "shared" vowels ([e] and [u]). Because the formant frequencies for the "shared" vowels are not identical across the two languages (see above), it may be more accurate to say the Mandarin speakers took "shared"-"new" vowel pairs and treated them as one category. The F1-F2 values for both the "shared" and "new" vowels had intermediate locations between the American's well-separated F1-F2 points for the two vowels. Think of it as a phonetic compromise when the skill of producing two nearby, but separate, vowels is not yet available to a speaker. The influence of the L1 vowel system on the L2 is to draw "new" vowels toward one of the shared vowels.

Within-Speaker Variability in Formant Frequencies

The formant frequencies plotted in Figures 11–3 to 11–8 are averages across speakers. Figure 11–2, from Hillenbrand et al. (1995), presents a more realistic picture of variability in formant frequencies for a given vowel, but this presentation shows only *across*-speaker variability. Within a speaker, vowel formant frequencies vary with a number of factors. These factors include—but may not be limited to—speaking rate, syllable stress, speaking style, and phonetic context.

Traditionally, the effects of different factors on vowel formant frequencies have been referenced to a speaking condition in which the vowel is produced in a hypothetically "pure" form, as described above. As already mentioned, in their original study of vowel formant frequencies, Peterson and Barney (1952) designed the /əˈhVd/ frame as a speech production event similar to real speech but largely free of many of the influencing factors noted above. Stevens and House (1963), in their classic paper on phonetic context effects on vowel formant frequencies, demonstrated for three phonetically sophisticated speakers (i.e., speech scientists) the lack of any difference in F1 and F2 for isolated vowels and vowels spoken in the /hVd/ frame. This result, as well as other data reviewed by Stevens and House, suggested that formant frequencies measured at the midpoint of a vowel in the /hVd/ frame are representative of vowels articulated under minimal influence from factors such as context, rate, and so forth. Because of this, vowels measured in the /hVd/ frame are often referred to as *null context vowels*.

When null context vowels are plotted in F1-F2 space together with the same vowels produced in varied phonetic contexts, at different rates, and in different speaking styles, an interesting pattern emerges. Figure 11–8 shows an F1-F2 plot for the corner vowels of American English (/i/, /æ/, /ɑ/, /u/). The formant frequencies in this plot were derived for male speakers from several different sources in the literature. Two sets of "null context" data are plotted, one from Peterson and Barney (1952; filled circles connected by solid lines), the other from Hillenbrand et al. (1995; open circles connected by dashed lines). The decision to include F1-F2 data for null context vowels from two different data sets underscores the potential variability in these kinds of measurements. The two sets of null context data are most different for the low vowels /æ/ and especially /ɑ/. The speakers in the two studies were from the same geographical region (Michigan, with a few speakers from other areas), but the recordings are separated in time by approximately 45 years. A likely explanation for the difference in the low vowel formant frequencies is changing patterns of vowel pronunciation over the second half of the twentieth century.

How do formant frequencies deviate from null context values when they are produced under different speaking conditions? The data shown in Figure 11–8

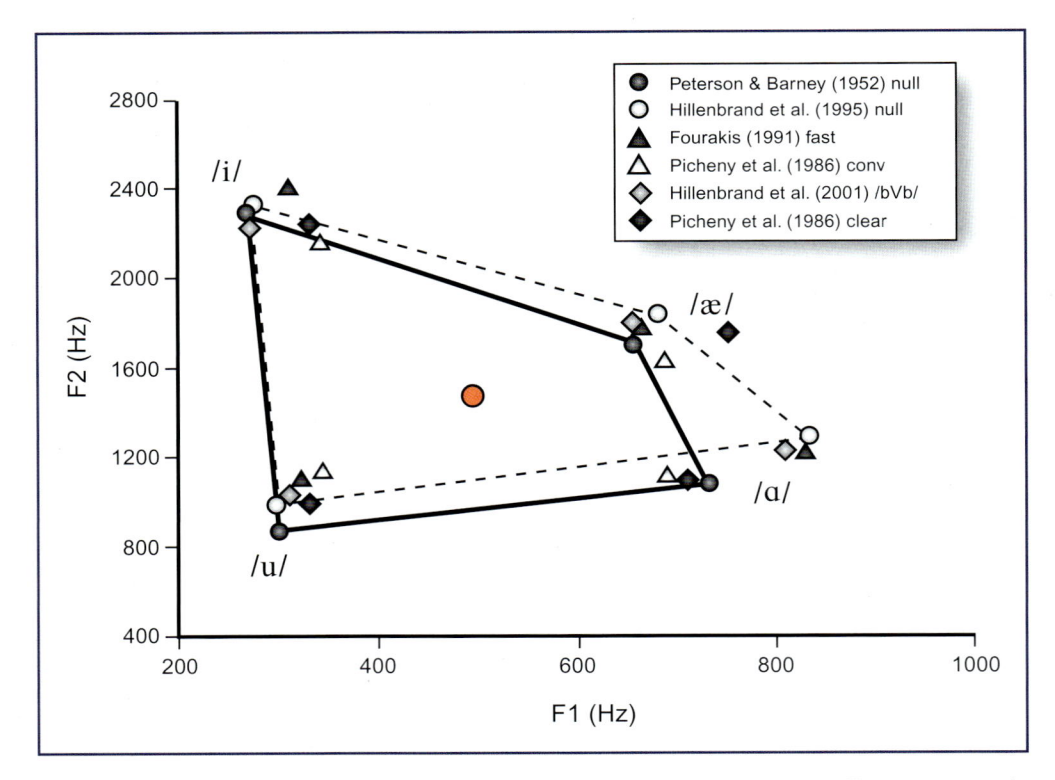

Figure 11–8. F1-F2 plot showing two vowel spaces for the "null context" corner vowels, plus corner-vowel data from studies in which the vowels were produced in other speaking conditions. Null context data are from tabled means published by Peterson and Barney (1952) and from careful pencil-and-ruler estimates of figures shown in Hillenbrand et al. (1995). Data from Fourakis (1991) are from tabled formant frequencies for fast-speech, stressed vowels averaged across various phonetic contexts. Values plotted from Picheny, Durlach, and Braida (1986) are for vowels extracted from sentence productions in conversational (*unfilled triangles*) and clear-style speech (*filled diamonds*) and were estimated from their published figures by the pencil-and-ruler technique. The same estimation technique was used to obtain the /bVb/ data from Hillenbrand et al. (2001). The red circle in the middle of the plot is the F1-F2 pattern expected from a male vocal tract with uniform cross-sectional area from glottis to lips (the expected vocal tract shape for schwa). All plotted data points are from male speakers.

include F1-F2 data for the corner vowels spoken at a fast rate, but with syllable stress (Fourakis, 1991; filled triangles), in conversational-style production of sentences (Picheny et al., 1986; unfilled triangles), in a "clear-speech" production style of sentences (Picheny et al., 1986; filled diamonds), and in a /bVb/ context (Hillenbrand, Clark, & Nearey, 2001; lightly shaded diamonds).

With certain exceptions (the Fourakis [1991] points for /ɑ/ and /i/), especially when the Hillenbrand et al. (1995) null context vowel space is used as a reference, vowels spoken in any of the other conditions tend to have F1-F2 points that are "inside" the null context vowel space. More specifically, the F1-F2 points for the different conditions move away from the null context coordinates in the direction of a point roughly in the center of the quadrilaterals, indicated by the red circle. This point plots F1 = 500 Hz, F2 = 1500 Hz, the first two formant frequencies associated with the "neutral vowel" configuration, or a vocal tract with uniform cross-sectional area from the glottis to the lips. As discussed in Chapter 8, this is the vocal tract configuration most closely associated with schwa (/ə/). The F1 = 500 Hz, F2 = 1500 Hz pattern is consistent with an adult male vocal tract with uniform cross-sectional area from glottis to lips.

One way to interpret the patterns seen in Figure 11–8 is to regard the null context formant frequencies (and underlying vocal tract configuration) for a given vowel as idealized targets. In this view, described explicitly by Bjorn Lindblom (1963, 1990), the speaker always aims for the idealized target, but misses it in connected speech because the articulators do not have sufficient time to produce the target before transitioning to production of the following sound. For example, the target vocal tract shape (the area function) for the vowel /i/ has a relatively tight constriction in the front of the vocal tract, and a wide opening in the pharyngeal region. This vocal tract shape is a significant deviation from the straight-tube configuration of schwa and fits the description of /i/ as a high-front vowel. In Lindblom's view, when a vowel such as /i/ is produced in a condition other than the null context, the idealized target is missed in a specific way, namely, by producing a vocal tract configuration (and resulting formant frequencies) that reflects a lesser deviation from the schwa configuration. It is as if all vowels are viewed as deviated vocal tract shapes (and formant frequencies) from the straight-tube configuration of schwa. Under optimal conditions, when the target is achieved, these deviations in vocal tract shape are maximal. In connected speech, however, the deviations from the schwa configuration are not as dramatic. By not producing the most extreme configuration associated with the sound, the speech mechanism has more time to produce a sequence of sounds in an efficient and intelligible way. An /i/ in connected speech is still a high-front vowel, but not quite as high and front as in the null context.

Lindblom (1963) called this phenomenon "articulatory undershoot." Undershoot, in his opinion, is a result of phonetic context (relative to the null context), increased speaking rate, reduced stress, and casual speaking style, but all these different causes are likely to be explained by a single mechanism. Simply put, the shorter the vowel duration, the greater the undershoot. Relative to the duration of a null context vowel, phonetic context (e.g., a vowel surrounded by two obstruents), increased speaking rate, reduced stress, and a casual speaking style are all associated with shorter vowel durations. In the language of phonetics, vowels experience greater reduction as vowel duration decreases, regardless of the condition, resulting in a shorter vowel duration. Although this is not a universally accepted interpretation of undershoot, it explains a good deal of variation in formant frequencies for a given vowel produced by a specific speaker. Most likely, factors other than vowel duration may, in some cases, have an independent effect on formant frequencies. For example, in Figure 11–8, the vowels /ɑ/ and /i/ from Fourakis (1991) do not fit the duration explanation of undershoot because they fall outside the null context quadrilaterals, even though the "fast condition" vowel durations were relatively short (as reported by Fourakis, 1991, Table III, p. 1821). Because these vowels were stressed, an independent effect of stress on vowel formant frequencies must be considered a possibility.

Kuo and Weismer (2016) varied speech materials so that American English vowels occurred in simple, single-syllable utterances, words in sentences, and words in long reading passages. The Lindblom-inspired logic of this manipulation was that as speech material changed from formal, simple syllables (close to the "null" vowel) to more "connected" and conversational utterances (more casual), vowel durations would shorten, resulting in an increased amount of undershoot of formant frequencies. Data were obtained from 10 adult males producing American English vowels embedded in the varied speech materials. As predicted from Lindblom's theory, the undershoot of "target" vowel formant frequencies increased as the speech material became more "casual." The degree and patterns of undershoot, however, depended on speaker and vowel. Some speakers were dramatic undershooters, some less so. In addition, the extent of undershoot across the speech materials was not the same for all vowels, and the vowel-specific patterns varied across speakers. An important lesson from the Kuo and Weismer experiment, as well as other experiments (e.g., Johnson, Ladefoged, & Lindau, 1993), is that almost any "pattern" in acoustic or articulatory phonetics, for any sound segment, is likely to have a broad range of variability when a sufficient number of speakers is studied. The across-speaker variability may be so dramatic as to challenge the identification of a well-defined acoustic and/or articulatory pattern for a given sound segment. The reader is encouraged to keep this in mind as the acoustic characteristics of speech sounds are reviewed in this chapter.

Summary of Vowel Formant Frequencies

The take-home messages from this discussion of vowel formant frequencies and their variability across and within speakers are as follows. First, sex and age have a dramatic effect on the formant frequencies for a given vowel because these variables are closely associated with differences in vocal tract size and length. In general, the longer and larger the human vocal tract, the lower the formant frequencies for all vowels. This explains why, for a given vowel, there is such a large range of formant frequencies across the population (see Figure 11–2). Second, even when vocal tract length/size factors are held constant, "target" formant frequencies for a given vowel may vary for several reasons. One reason may reflect the inherent constraints on a phonetic symbol system. Even though a vowel is transcribed as

/u/ in several different languages, the F-pattern associated with productions of this vowel category may be substantially different (see Figure 11–6). The same conclusion can be made about the same vowel produced by speakers of different dialects of the same language (Clopper, Pisoni, & de Jong, 2005). Additional reasons for variation with constant vocal tract length include the effects of phonetic context, syllable stress, speaking rate, and speaking style.

The implication of the variation in "target" formant frequencies for a particular vowel is that if one is asked the question, "What are the formant frequencies for the vowel /u/ (or any other vowel)?" an answer cannot be supplied without additional information on the speaker, the nature of the speech material, the language being spoken, the style of the speech (formal versus casual), and so forth. Even with answers to all these questions, a definitive, precise answer is probably not feasible. It is more likely that a definitive, precise answer is not necessary because vowels may be perceived by focusing on relations among the formant frequencies, rather than absolute values of individual formants. In addition, it is likely that the formant frequencies measured near the temporal middle of vowels—the so-called target values—are only part of the information critical in distinguishing among the vowels of a language (see next section).

A Note on Vowel Formant Frequencies Versus Formant Trajectories

The discussion above presented a "slice-in-time" view of vowel formant frequencies but mentioned the possible importance of formant frequency change across the duration of a vowel. When single-slice formant frequencies are supplemented with information on formant frequency change throughout the vowel nucleus, identification/classification accuracy increases, sometimes substantially (Assman, Nearey, & Hogan, 1982; Hillenbrand & Nearey, 1999; Jacewicz & Fox, 2012). Both single-slice formant frequencies *and* formant movement throughout a vowel nucleus make important contributions to vowel identity.

The complexity of the mapping from articulatory to acoustic phonetics comes as no surprise to anyone who has studied tongue, lip, and jaw motions during speech production for even the simplest consonant-vowel-consonant (CVC) syllable. Figure 11–9 shows these motions for the vowel [ɪ] in the word [sɪp] produced by a young adult female. These data were collected with the x-ray microbeam instrument, which tracked the motions of very small gold pellets attached to the tongue, jaw, and lips (see Chapter 6). In Figure 11–9 the lips are to the right and the outline of the hard palate is seen in the upper part of the *x-y* coordinate system. The motions of two lip pellets (UL = upper lip; LL = lower lip), two mandible (jaw) pellets (MM = mandible at molars; MI = mandible at incisors), and four tongue pellets (T1–T4 arranged front to back roughly from tip [T1] to dorsum [T4]) are shown for the entire duration of the vowel [ɪ]. The shaded portion on the waveform in the lower part of the figure corresponds to the duration of the motions shown in the upper part of the figure. Arrows pointing up to the waveform indicate the onset and offset of the vowel, hence the beginning and end of the displayed pellet motions. The vowel duration is 115 ms. The direction of the tongue pellet motions throughout the vowel is shown by arrows with dashed lines. The final position of each pellet, at the last glottal pulse of the vowel (the operationally defined end of the vowel) before lip closure for [p], is marked by a small circle at the end of the motion track. All tongue pellets move down throughout the vowel, with the exception of the small upward motions in T2 and T3 at the beginning of the vowel. Throughout the syllable, the mandible moves up very slightly and the lips come together, as would be expected when a vowel is followed by a labial consonant. Although this display does not show the motions as a function of time (they are spatial displays of events that unfold over time but there is no time scale, other than the knowledge that the tracks cover a time interval of 115 ms), they are more or less continuous throughout the vowel nucleus and do not have obvious steady-state portions where the motion "freezes." This is especially so for the tongue pellets, for which the downward motion is smooth and continuous from the beginning to the end of the vowel.

The continuous motions of the articulators for the short-duration vowel [ɪ] are consistent with changing formant frequencies throughout the vowel nucleus. The change in tongue position over time is associated with a change in the vocal tract area function over time, and it is the area function that determines formant frequencies. Based on these motions and the resulting formant transitions, it is not surprising that portions of the vowel in addition to the "slice-in-time" target measurement contribute to vowel identification. One future area of research is to generate better descriptions of these simple vowel motions, and to understand the role of such motions in vowel identification. This is an important area of research because of the significant contribution of vowel articulation to speech intelligibility deficits in the speech of individuals who are hearing impaired (Metz, Samar, Schiavetti, Sitler, & Whitehead, 1985) and who have dysarthria (Weismer & Martin, 1992), among other disorders.

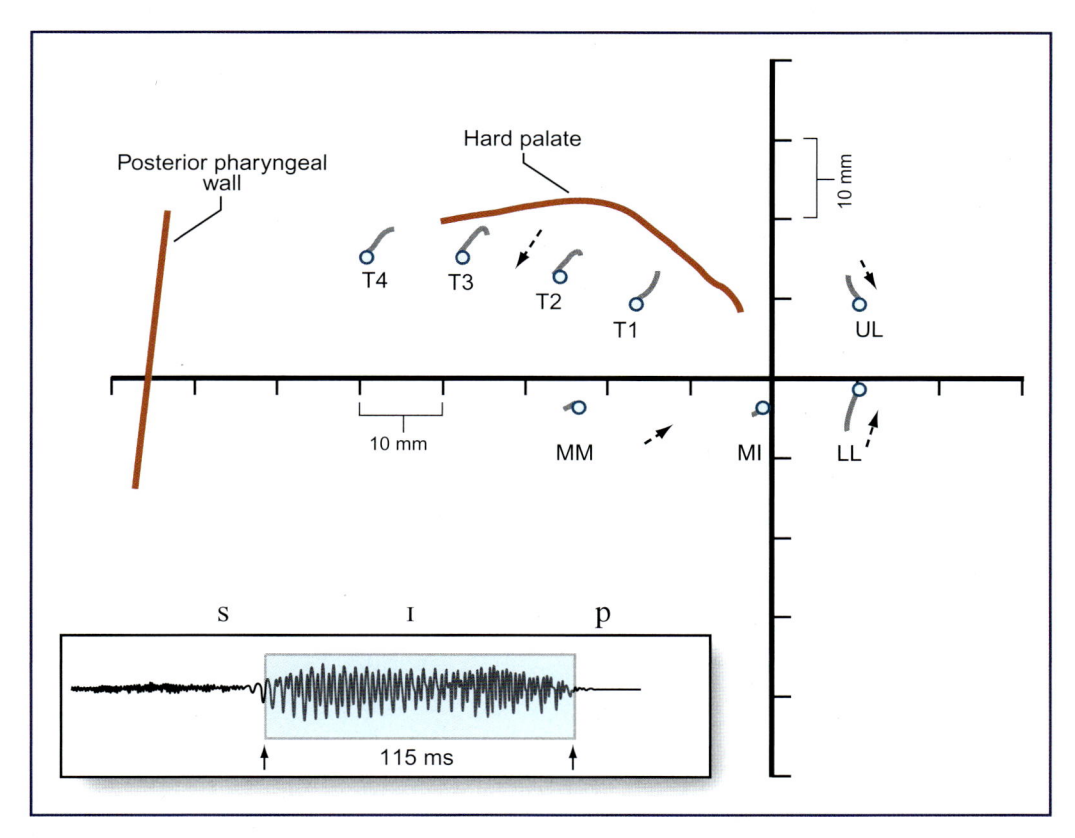

Figure 11-9. Tongue (T, in four locations), mandible (M, at the level of the molars, M, and incisors, I), and upper and lower lips (UL, LL) pellet motions throughout the vowel are shown by dashed arrows, and the final pellet positions at the end of the vowel are marked by circles at the end of the motion tracks. Data are shown in the x-ray microbeam coordinate system (Westbury, 1994), with the x-axis defined by a plate held between the teeth and the y-axis by a line perpendicular to the x-axis and running through the maxillary incisors. The interval of the speech waveform for which the motions are shown is highlighted in the lower part of the figure by the shaded box on the waveform.

Articulatory and Acoustic Phonetics

When speech scientists use the term "articulatory phonetics," they have in mind the positions and movements of the articulators, as well as the resulting configuration of the vocal tract, as they relate to speech sound production. The term "acoustic phonetics" describes the relations between the acoustic signal (resulting from those positions, movements, and configurations) and speech sounds. Many scientists have studied the relations between articulatory and acoustic phonetics, and found them to be fantastically complex. Why is this so? There are many reasons, but here are two prominent ones: first, exactly the same acoustic phonetic effect can be produced by very different articulatory maneuvers. For example, the low F2 of /u/ can be produced by rounding the lips, backing the tongue, or lowering the larynx. And second, certain parts of the vocal tract—the pharynx, for instance—are exceedingly difficult to monitor during speech production, yet play a very important role in the speech acoustic signal. Scientists who study the relations between articulatory and acoustic data often use advanced mathematical and experimental techniques to determine just how an articulatory phonetic event "maps on" to an acoustic phonetic event.

Vowel Durations

Vowel durations have been studied extensively because of the potential for application of the data to speech synthesis, machine recognition of speech, and description and possibly diagnosis of speech disorders in which timing disturbances are present. What follows is a brief discussion of the major variables known to affect vowel durations.

Intrinsic Vowel Durations

An "intrinsic" vowel duration derives from the articulation of the vowel segment itself, as opposed to an external influence (as described more fully below). The easiest way to understand this is to imagine a fixed syllable such as a CVC frame, with vowel durations measured for all vowels inserted into the "V" slot. Figure 11–10 shows three sets of vowel duration values from a CVC frame, as reported by Hillenbrand et al. (2001). In this experiment the Cs included /p,t,k,b,d,g,h,w,r,l/, in all combinations (consonants such as /h/ and /w/ were restricted to initial position). Vowel duration in milliseconds (y-axis) is presented for each vowel (x-axis), averaged across all consonant contexts (filled circles, solid lines), across vowels surrounded only by voiceless Cs (unfilled circles, dotted lines), and only by voiced Cs (lightly filled diamonds, solid lines). The pattern of durations across vowels is essentially the same for these three contexts. Because the contexts stay constant for any one of the three curves, any differences in vowel duration must be a property of the vowels themselves—precisely what is meant by an "intrinsic" property. For each of the curves, low vowels such as /æ/ and /ɑ/ have greater duration than high vowels such as /i/, /ɪ/, /ʊ/, and /u/. The differences between low and high vowel durations typically are on the order of 50 to 60 ms, a very large difference in the world of speech timing.

The explanation for the intrinsic difference in the duration of low versus high vowels has sometimes been based on the greater articulatory distance

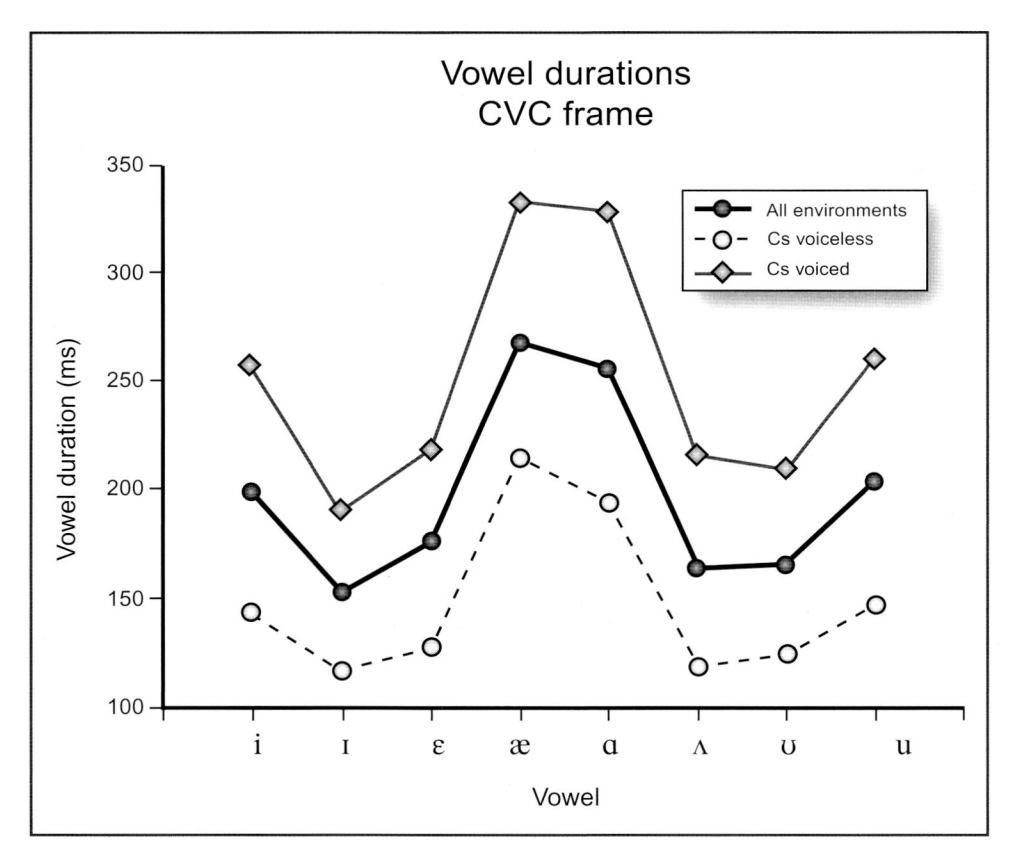

Figure 11–10. Vowel durations in fixed CVC frames for eight vowels in American English. Data are shown for environments in which C = voiceless (*unfilled circles*), C = voiced (*lightly shaded diamonds*), and for all C environments combined (*filled circles*). Data replotted from Hillenbrand et al. (2001).

required for the consonant-to-vowel-to-consonant path when the vowel is low compared with high. According to this idea, if one vowel requires articulators to travel greater distances than another vowel, it will take more time. The jaw travels a greater distance for the opening required for low versus high vowels, possibly explaining the intrinsic duration difference in low versus high vowels. This may explain part of the duration difference between low and high vowels, but doesn't account for all of the 50 to 60 ms difference.

The data in Figure 11–10 show another intrinsic vowel duration difference, between tense and lax vowels. In any one of the three consonant contexts, tense vowels are longer than their lax vowel "partners" (compare the durations of the /i/-/ɪ/ and /u/-/ʊ/ pairs for any of the three curves). The duration between tense and lax vowels has a wide range (from about 22 to 65 ms in Figure 11–10, depending on the consonant context), but always favors tense vowels when the consonant environment is held constant. This consistent difference between tense and lax vowel durations is not easy to explain, and may be related to the spectral similarity of tense-lax pairs and the resulting need to distinguish them by duration.[4]

Listeners are sensitive to the high-low and tense-lax intrinsic differences in vowel duration. When high-quality speech synthesizers are programmed, for example, the differences just described are built into the algorithms to generate natural-sounding speech.

Extrinsic Factors Affecting Vowel Durations

Many extrinsic factors influence vowel duration. What follows is a brief discussion of a few of these influences. Readers interested in comprehensive surveys of how and why vowel duration varies in speech production can consult House (1961), Klatt (1976), Umeda (1975), the series of papers by Crystal and House (1982, 1988a, 1988b, 1988c), and Van Santen (1992).

Consonant Voicing. Vowels are typically longer when surrounded by voiced compared with voiceless consonants. This effect is seen in Figure 11–10 by comparing the "C voiceless" curve (unfilled circles, dashed lines) with the "C voiced" curve (lightly shaded diamonds, solid lines). The effect varies from vowel to vowel, but a reasonable generalization from the Hillenbrand et al. (2001) data is that vowels surrounded by voiced consonants are about 100 ms longer than vowels surrounded by voiceless consonants. The voicing of both the initial and final C in the CVC frame contributes to changes in vowel duration, but the largest influence is the voicing status of the final consonant of the syllable. If the syllable frame is marked as C1VC2, a voiced C1 will lengthen a vowel by somewhere between 25 to 50 ms compared with a voiceless C1, whereas a voiced C2 will lengthen a vowel by 50 to 90 ms relative to a voiceless C2. The magnitude of these effects is lessened, perhaps greatly so, in more natural speaking conditions (Crystal & House, 1988a, 1988b).

Stress. Lexical stress is a characteristic of multisyllabic words in many languages, the best known examples in English being noun-verb contrasts such as "rebel-rebel" (/ˈrɛbl̩/-/rəˈbɛl/) and "contract-contract" (/ˈkɑntrækt/-/kənˈtræːkt/). Many other multisyllabic words have alternating patterns of stressed and unstressed syllables, as in "California" /kæləˈfɔrnjə/), where the first and third syllables have greater stress than the second and fourth syllables. When single syllables are stressed for emphasis or contrast ("Bob stopped by earlier"; "Did you say *Barb* stopped by?" "No, *Bob* stopped by"), the vowel in the emphasized syllable has greater duration than the original, lexically stressed production. All other things being equal, vowels in lexically or emphatically stressed syllables have greater duration than vowels in unstressed or normally stressed syllables (Fourakis, 1991). The magnitude of the duration difference between stressed and unstressed syllables, or between contrastively stressed and "normally stressed" syllables, is variable across speakers (Howell, 1993; Weismer & Ingrisano, 1979).

Speaking Rate. Vowel duration varies over a large range when speakers change their speaking rate. Slow rates result in longer vowel durations, fast rates in shorter vowel durations. Speaking rate also varies widely *across* speakers. Some speakers have naturally slow rates, some fast. Speakers who have habitually slow speaking rates have longer vowel durations than speakers with habitually fast rates (Tsao & Weismer, 1997).

Utterance Position. The same vowel has variable duration depending on its location within an utterance. If the duration of /i/ in the word "beets" is measured in the sentence, "The beets are in the garden" versus "The garden contains no beets," the /i/ is about 30 to 40 ms longer in the second sentence. This effect is referred to as phrase-final or utterance-final lengthening (see Klatt, 1975). The degree of lengthening depends on the

---

[4]The thinking is that /i/ and /ɪ/, and /u/ and /ʊ/ have formant frequencies that are only subtly different, so vowel duration may have evolved in phonological systems to create another cue to the tense-lax distinction. Other explanations for the tense-lax duration difference for vowels have also been proposed (Leung, Jongman, Wang, & Sereno, 2016).

"depth" of the grammatical boundary. A major syntactic boundary yields more vowel lengthening compared with a "shallower" boundary. An extreme example is the greater lengthening at a truly end-of-utterance boundary (when the speaker is finished talking)—compared with a syntactic boundary between two consecutive phrases.

Speaking Style. Over the past quarter-century, since Picheny, Durlach, and Braida (1985, 1986) introduced the notion of "clear speech" as a phenomenon worthy of experimental attention, research on the acoustics and perception of speaking style has been popular (for reviews see Calandruccio, Van Engen, Dhar, & Bradlow, 2010 and Smiljanić & Bradlow, 2011). Clear versus casual speech styles are potentially relevant to such diverse considerations as speaking to someone with a hearing impairment, to someone whose native language is different from the language being spoken, and to someone listening to a native language who is not a fully effective processor of spoken language input (such as infants or toddlers, or persons with intellectual challenges, or computers programmed to recognize speech). A clear speech style is thought to enhance acoustic contrasts that are useful to a listener or machine trying to decode and identify segmental components of the incoming signal.

When speakers produce "clear speech," they typically slow their speaking rate to produce longer vowel durations, and expand their vowel space. Whether clear speech exaggerates duration contrasts between vowels is, however, unclear. For example, in American English, vowel duration is not a critical contrastive characteristic—phoneme categories are not contrasted strictly by vowel duration—which may explain why clear speech does not clearly exaggerate the duration distinction of vowel pairs such as /ʌ/-/ɑ/ and /ɪ/-/i/, which vary in duration (the first member of each pair is typically shorter than the second member; see DeMerit, 1997) and perhaps in spectrum (formant frequencies; see footnote 4). On the other hand, there is evidence of greater lengthening of tense compared with lax vowels in clear English speech (Picheny et al., 1986), even though tense and lax vowels also have different formant frequencies. Croatian, a language in which each of five vowels may be either long or short, appears to have a tendency for clear speech to emphasize the duration difference (and thus the contrast between the long and short versions of the vowel; see Smiljanić & Bradlow, 2008). However, clear speech in Finnish, another language in which there are short and long vowels, does not seem to exaggerate the long-short vowel duration difference relative to its conversational speech difference (Granlund, Hazan, & Baker, 2012). A careful reading of the literature suggests a lot of speaker-to-speaker variability in the acoustics of speaking clearly. The question remains open of whether or not phonetic contrasts are "improved" by clear speech, if the improvements are seen for all important contrasts (e.g., between vowels, between fricatives), and if clear speech contrasts give the listener a perceptual benefit. Tuomainen, Hazan, and Romeo (2016) provide an interesting discussion of the clear speech literature.

The effects of clear speech reviewed above are becoming part of the fundamental knowledge base for speech-language clinicians, as speaking clearly is increasingly used as an approach to modifying articulatory impairment in a number of clinical populations (see, for example, Park, Theodoros, Finch, & Cardell, 2016; Lam, Tjaden, & Wilding, 2012; Whitfield & Goberman, 2017).

Are We Wired for Rate?

Imagine a large sample of talkers—say, 100 people—each of whom reads a passage from which speaking rates (in syllables per second) are measured acoustically. If the talkers were chosen randomly, you would find a huge range of "typical" speaking rates, from very slow talkers, to talkers of average rate, to very fast talkers. These experimental measurements would conform to the everyday observation that some people speak very slowly, some very rapidly. Now imagine that you chose the slowest and fastest talkers in this sample and asked them to produce the passage as fast as possible. If all talkers produced the passage at the same, maximally fast speaking rate, regardless of their "typical" rate, that would indicate that the very slow or fast "typical" rates were a kind of conscious choice on the part of individual talkers. However, if the slow talkers couldn't speak as fast as the fast talkers, that would suggest that speaking rates reflect some basic neurological "wiring" that determines the "typical" rate. This experiment was performed by Tsao and Weismer (1997), who found that the maximal speaking rates of slow talkers were, in fact, significantly less than the maximal rates of fast talkers. It seems we are not all wired the same for typical speaking rate, and probably a bunch of other stuff, as well.

DIPHTHONGS

American English has five or six diphthongs, depending on the dialect of the speaker and which authority is describing the sounds. In some dialects some or all of the six diphthongs are not always diphthongized. The six diphthongs include /aɪ/ ("guys"), /ɔɪ/ ("boys"), /aʊ/ ("doubt"), /eɪ/ ("bays"), /oʊ/ ("goes"), and /ju/ ("beauty"). /ju/ is not considered a diphthong in many phonetics textbooks, but has properties similar to the other diphthongs. Spectrograms of the first five are shown in Figures 11–11 and 11–12. Diphthongs have not been studied as extensively as vowels, possibly because the former have sometimes been considered as sequences of the latter. The symbols used to represent diphthongs, after all, are combinations of two vowels. Is the diphthong /ɔɪ/, for example, an /ɔ/ connected to /ɪ/ by a relatively rapid change in vocal tract configuration? In Figure 11–11, at least for /ɔɪ/ and /aɪ/, the spectrographic data can be studied to address this question. Figure 11–12 shows spectrograms of the diphthongs /eɪ/ and /oʊ/, discussed below.

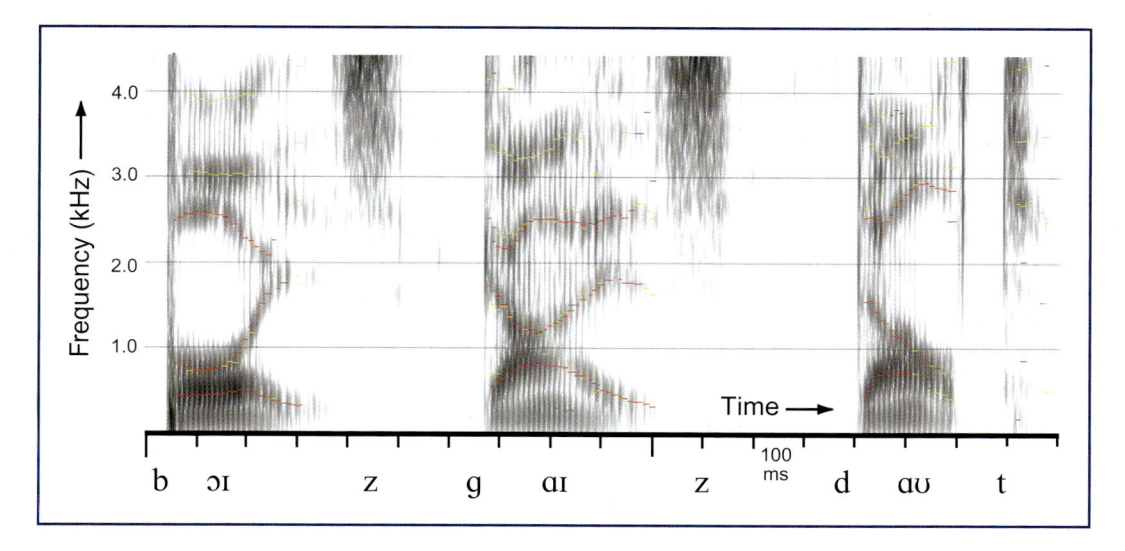

Figure 11–11. Spectrograms of the American English diphthongs /ɔɪ/, /aɪ/, and /aʊ/, spoken in the words "boys," "guys," and "doubt," respectively. LPC tracks are shown in red for F1, F2, and F3. Speaker is a 57-year-old healthy male.

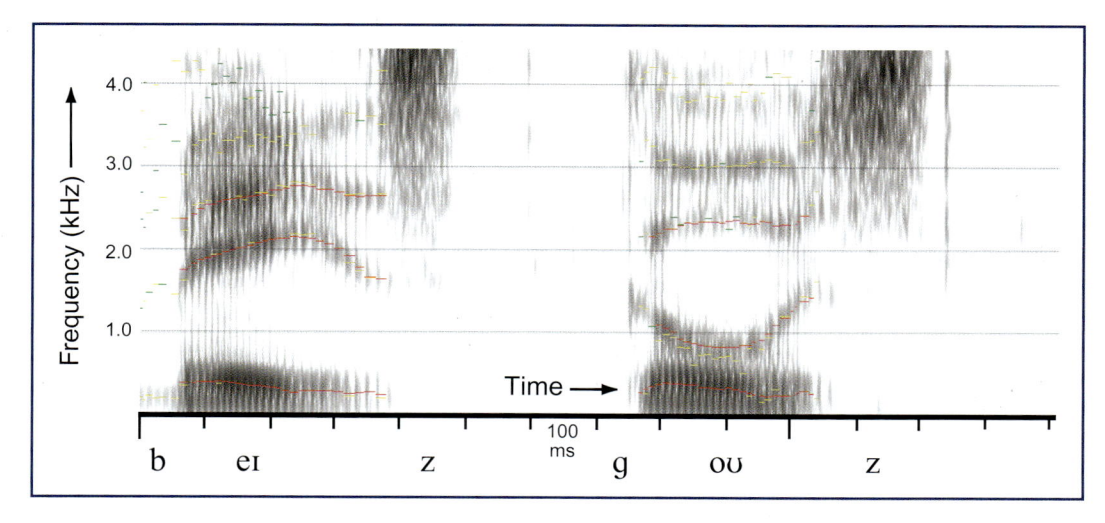

Figure 11–12. Spectrograms of the American English diphthongs /eɪ/ and /oʊ/, spoken in the words "bays" and "goes." LPC tracks are shown in red for F1, F2, and F3. Speaker is a 57-year-old healthy male.

LPC tracks for F1-F3 are shown as red dashed lines throughout the vocalic nuclei. An LPC formant track is a sequence, over time, of estimated formant frequencies based on LPC analysis. In the case of the tracks in Figure 11–11 a formant frequency is estimated at each glottal pulse throughout the diphthong. For /ɔɪ/ there is a large, rising F2 transition preceded and followed by intervals of nearly unchanging formant frequencies—these are the so-called steady states mentioned earlier. For this /ɔɪ/, the steady state preceding the large F2 transition is of greater duration than the steady state following it, the latter being very brief and perhaps only visible in F2. For the /ɑɪ/ in Figure 11–11, there is also a large F2 transition preceded and followed by steady states. The formant tracks for /ɑɪ/ are somewhat more complicated than the ones for /ɔɪ/ because of the influence of the initial /g/, which causes the initial falling (decreasing frequency) transition in F2. The steady state is the brief interval following this initial downward transition, immediately before the sharp rising transition in F2. The steady state following the transition is, as in the case of /ɔɪ/, most evident in F2.

Diphthongs: Two Connected Vowels or a Unique Phoneme?

The spectrographic data are relevant to the question of whether diphthongs are two vowels connected by a rapid change in vocal tract configuration. The research logic is simple. Measure the formant frequencies at the steady states, and the hypothesis of two connected vowels is confirmed (in part) if they are similar to the formant frequencies of the vowels indicated by the transcription. For example, are the formant frequencies for the first steady state in /ɔɪ/ like those measured for the vowel /ɔ/, and the formant frequencies for the second steady state like those for the vowel /ɪ/?

The answer seems to be no. Studies by Holbrook and Fairbanks (1962), Gay (1968), and Lee, Potamianos, and Narayanan (2014; see their Figure 7) do not support the idea of diphthongs as sequences of two vowels, for several reasons. Holbrook and Fairbanks had 20 male speakers produce each of the diphthongs in an /hVd/ frame at the end of a short sentence. They made spectrographic measurements of formant frequencies at the first and last glottal pulses of the diphthongs, as well as three additional points roughly equidistant between the initial and final points. The formant frequencies of each diphthong are represented by these five measurement points throughout the duration of the vocalic nucleus. These data are summarized in Figure 11–13, which shows averages of the five measured F1-F2 points throughout each diphthong. The direction of the arrow next to each phonetic symbol indicates the direction of the five plotted points from beginning to end of each diphthong. For example, the points for /ɔɪ/ (filled triangles) are indicated by a bent arrow pointing up. The first measurement point, at the first glottal pulse, is located at F1 ~550 Hz and F2 ~800 Hz, and the final measurement point, at the last glottal pulse, is F1 ~500 Hz and F2 ~1900 Hz. The other diphthong paths in F1-F2 space can be interpreted in the same way. Also plotted in Figure 11–12 are the F1-F2 values for the vowels /ɪ/, /ʊ/, /ɔ/, and /ɑ/ reported for adult males by Hillenbrand et al. (1995) for the same /hVd/ frame used by Holbrook and Fairbanks. The phonetic symbol for each vowel identifies its average location in F1-F2 space. The oval enclosing the symbol has no meaning other than to set off the vowel locations from the diphthong points. These vowel points were chosen because the diphthong symbols include them either as end points (/ɪ/ being the end symbol for /ɔɪ/, /ɑɪ/, and /eɪ/; /ʊ/ the end symbol for /oʊ/ and /ɑʊ/) or as starting points (/ɑ/ the start for /ɑʊ/ and /ɑɪ/; /ɔ/ the start for /ɔɪ/).

Compare the F1-F2 points for the vowel /ɪ/ with the end points for the diphthongs /ɔɪ/, /ɑɪ/, and /eɪ/. The end points for /ɔɪ/ and /ɑɪ/ are distant from the formant frequencies for monophthong /ɪ/. Although the end point for /eɪ/ is relatively closer to monophthong /ɪ/, it is substantially different in the F2 dimension. A similar analysis seems to apply to the comparison of /oʊ/ and /ɑʊ/ to the plotted point for /ʊ/. The F1-F2 starting points of /ɑɪ/ and /ɑʊ/ are a good match for monophthong /ɑ/ especially for /ɑʊ/ (filled boxes) and less so for /ɑɪ/; the plotted point for /ɔ/ is very far from the start point for /ɔɪ/.

Holbrook and Fairbanks (1962) concluded that the trajectory of diphthongs in F1-F2 space did not begin and end in well-defined vowel areas. They noted, however, that a careful examination of diphthong paths suggests little or no overlap between the five diphthongs shown in Figure 11–13. A similar conclusion was reached by Lee et al. (2014). When the starting and ending frequencies plus the direction of the F1-F2 change are considered, the five diphthongs separate nicely.

Perhaps the difficulty of representing diphthongs as two sequenced vowels should have been obvious by examining spectrograms of natural productions of the sounds. As noted earlier, initial and final steady states can be identified for /ɔɪ/ and /ɑɪ/ (see Figure 11–11), but in the case of /ɑʊ/ F1 and F2 are changing at the beginning and end of the diphthong. A similar absence of initial and final steady states is seen for /eɪ/ and /oʊ/ (see Figure 11–12). The absence of steady states in diphthongs has been noted by previous scientists (Lehiste & Peterson, 1961), and cited as

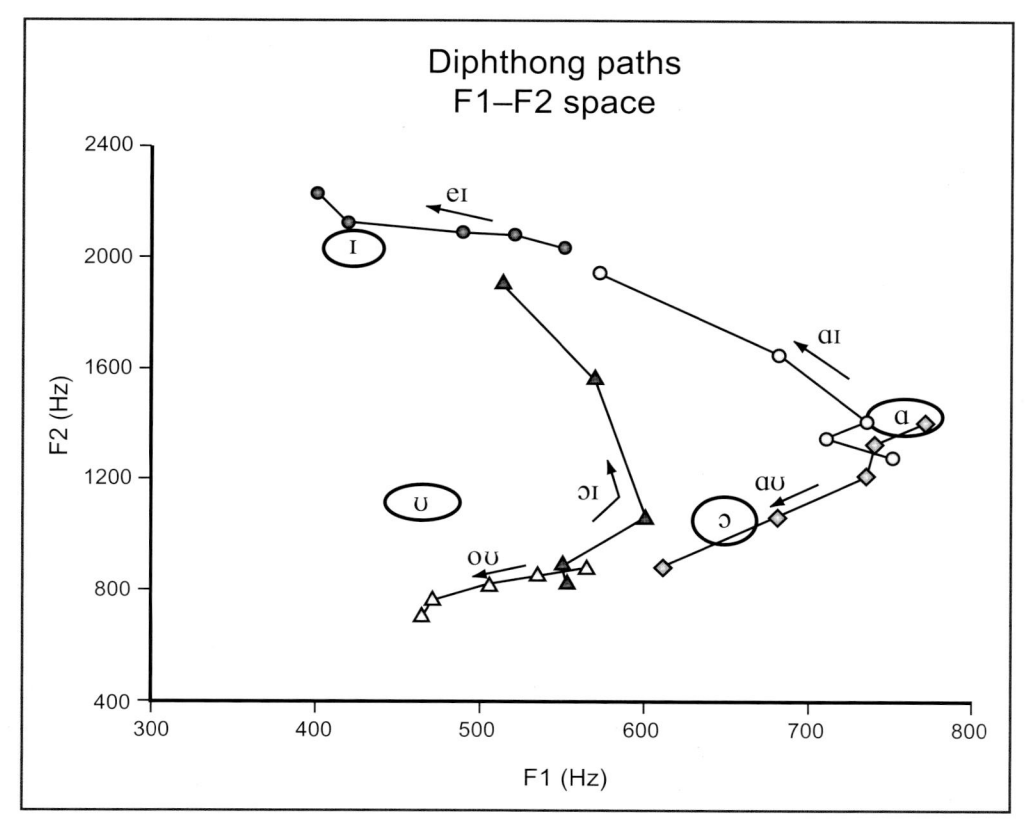

Figure 11-13. Diphthong paths in the F1-F2 plane, and F1-F2 points for four monophthongs. Each diphthong formant path is represented by five, equally spaced measurement points throughout the diphthong duration. The first point (at the beginning of the diphthong) is the one preceding the arrowhead, and the last point is the one terminating the path, in the direction indicated by the arrow (see text for a worked example). Diphthong path symbols, clockwise from /aʊ/, lightly shaded diamonds; /ɔɪ/, filled triangles; /oʊ/, unfilled triangles; /eɪ/, filled circles; and /aɪ/, unfilled circles. Diphthong data from Holbrook and Fairbanks (1962), vowel data from Hillenbrand et al. (1995).

a potential complication in classifying diphthongs as a sequence of two vowels.

If steady states are not a reliable characteristic of diphthongs, what is? A close look at Figures 11–11 and 11–12 suggests that each of the diphthongs has an identifiable, and in some cases substantial, transitional segment. The transitional segments, usually most pronounced in F2 but also seen in F1 and F3, reflect the rapid change in vocal tract shape between the initial and final parts of the diphthong.

Gay (1968) performed an experiment to determine which aspects of diphthong production varied and which remained constant across changes in speaking rate. Gay asked speakers to produce diphthongs at slow, conversational, and fast speaking rates, and measured F1 and F2 steady states at the beginning and end of the diphthongs as well as the slopes (speeds) of F2 transitions. The variation of speaking rate resulted in substantial changes in the duration of the diphthongs (see below), with stable F1 and F2 onset measurement. In contrast, the F1 and F2 offset measures (at the hypothetical "second vowel" of the diphthong) varied substantially. Of special interest was the finding that the slope of the F2 transition was essentially constant across the rate changes: "The second formant rate of change [that is, the slope] for each diphthong remains relatively constant across changes in duration and *distinct from the rates of change of the other diphthongs*" (Gay, 1968, p. 1571, emphasis added). For Gay, the slope of the F2 transition was a constant and distinguishing characteristic of diphthongs. His findings argued against the notion of diphthongs as merely sequences of two vowels connected by a transition. Rather, diphthongs appeared to be a sound class separate from vowels (see Watson & Harrington, 1999, for similar comments on the difference between vowels and diphthongs in Australian English).

> ### What's a Diphthong, What's a Vowel?
>
> Figure 11–13 makes the case that direction of movement in F1-F2 space, when included with starting and ending frequencies, separates the American English diphthongs nicely. It is as if inherent vocal tract movement characteristics must be accounted for to distinguish between diphthongs. This conceptual strategy for distinguishing between diphthongs apparently applies to some vowels as well. Like diphthongs, vowels such as /ɪ/, /ɛ/, and /ʊ/ have inherent movement characteristics (Nearey & Assman, 1986) important for their identification. These movements are expressed as formant transitions throughout the vowel. These vowels—the lax vowels, mostly—are also quite variable across dialects, and their inherent movement characteristics may be specific to particular dialects. Recently, Jacewicz and Fox (2012, see their Figures 1 and 2) plotted data for lax vowels produced by speakers from southern Wisconsin and western North Carolina, in a way similar to the diphthong data in Figure 11–12. The plot shows that, when *formant transitions* are taken into consideration for these vowels, almost always identified as monophthongs, much of the confusion among the vowels disappears. So, are /ɪ/, /ɛ/, and /ʊ/ vowels or diphthongs?

Diphthong Duration

The duration characteristics of diphthongs have not been well studied, but if asked, most speech scientists expect diphthongs to be somewhat longer than monophthong vowels in equivalent environments and speaking conditions. Data published by Umeda (1975) for a single speaker suggest that /ɑɪ/, /ɑʊ/, and possibly /eɪ/ have greater duration than monophthongs. The diphthong duration data reported for adults by Lee et al. (2014) and Tasko and Greilick (2010) are 30 to 70 ms greater than durations reported for monophthong vowels (Gopal, 1996; Klatt, 1976; Umeda, 1975) produced at conversational speaking rates. The intuition of speech scientists, at least in the case of diphthong duration in contrast to monophthong duration, appears to be correct.

NASALS

Data on the acoustic characteristics of nasals are more limited than those on vowels. There are no large-scale studies on formant and antiresonance frequencies (Chapter 9) in nasals, or their variation across speakers due to age and sex. The relatively small body of work on nasals has been concerned with the acoustic characteristics associated with nasal manner and place of production.

As discussed in Chapter 9, nasal articulations are described acoustically in two broad categories. One, the nasal murmur, concerns acoustic characteristics during the interval of complete oral cavity closure with an open velopharyngeal port. For example, the nasal murmur for /m/ occurs during the interval when the lips are sealed and sound waves travel through the open velopharyngeal port and radiate from the nostrils. During the nasal murmur, the speech spectrum includes resonances of the combined pharyngeal and nasal cavities, as well as antiresonances originating in the closed oral cavity and the sinus cavities. The second category of nasal articulation is nasalization, or the articulation of vowels (that is, with an open oral cavity) with a velopharyngeal port sufficiently open to "add" nasal resonances and antiresonances into the oral vowel resonances.

Nasal Murmurs

Figure 11–14 shows spectrographic characteristics of the nasal murmur interval for /m/ in stressed CVC syllables surrounding an /i/ (left side of upper panel) and /ɑ/ (right side of upper panel). The boundaries of the prestressed (first /m/) murmur intervals are marked below the spectrogram baseline by short, vertical bars. These murmur intervals have durations of slightly greater than 100 ms (left spectrogram) and just under 100 ms (right spectrogram). These murmur durations are likely to be typical for other speakers (see Umeda, 1977), and like other segment durations variable with speaking rate, stress, and other factors.

The nasal murmur intervals of both utterances shown in the upper panel of Figure 11–14 are clearly less intense compared with the surrounding vowels. Using the marked boundaries of the murmur intervals as reference points, note the dramatic change in intensity from vowel to murmur or murmur to vowel. The intensity difference is reflected in the relative darkness

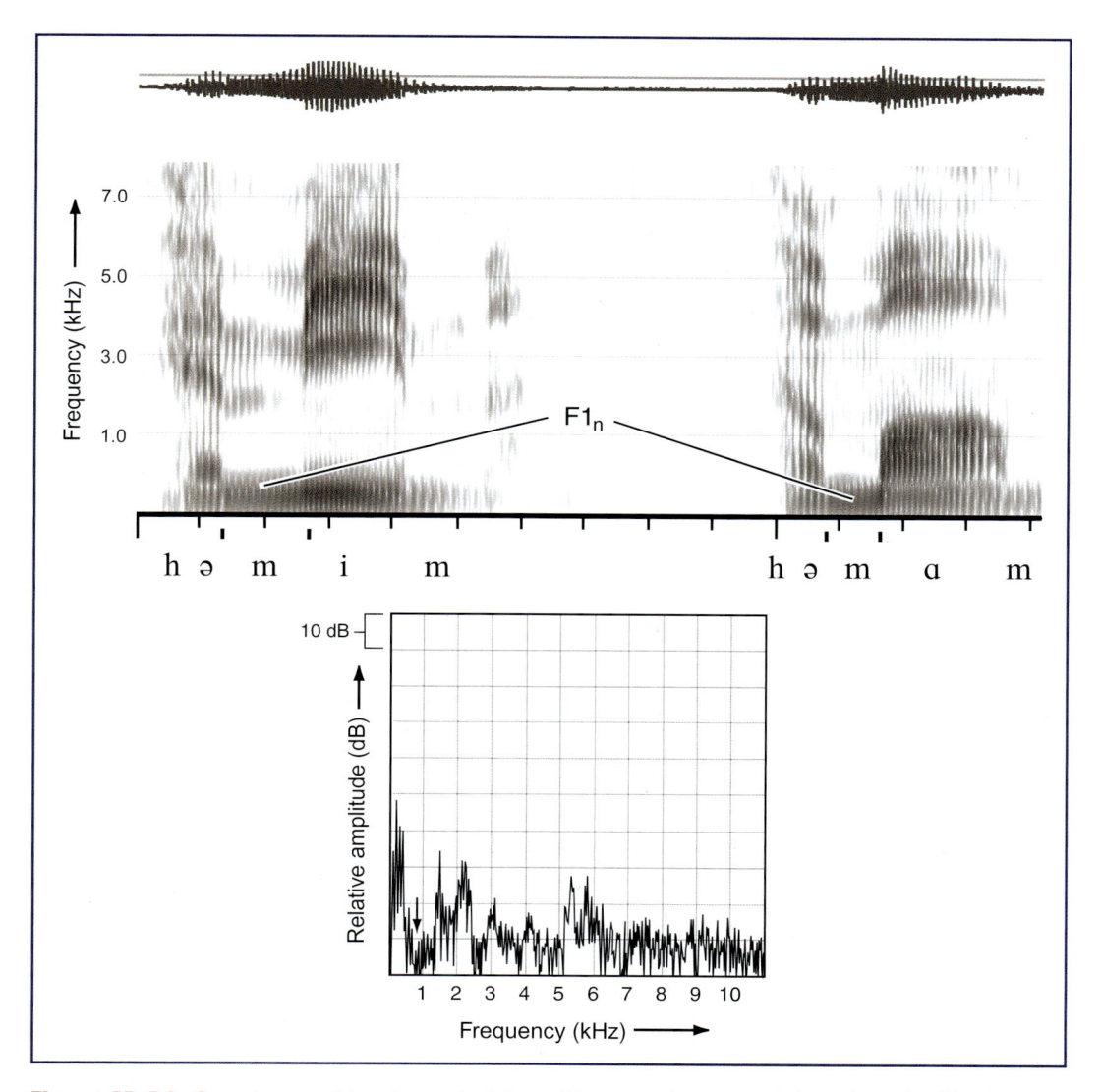

Figure 11-14. Spectrographic characteristics of the nasal murmur interval for /m/ in stressed CVC syllables surrounding an /i/ (*left side of top panel*) and /ɑ/ (*right side of top panel*). Short, vertical bars immediately below the baseline of the spectrogram mark the onsets and offsets of the nasal murmur intervals. An FFT spectrum from the middle 50 ms of the /m/ preceding the /i/ is shown in the lower part of the figure; the downward-pointing arrow indicates the approximate location of an antiresonance.

of the vowel and nasal murmur traces. As discussed in Chapter 9, nasals tend to be less intense than vowels and other sonorant sounds (such as liquids, glides, rhotics) for two reasons. One is the presence of antiresonances in the spectrum, which result in a substantial reduction of energy at the exact frequency of the antiresonance and at frequencies in the immediate vicinity of the antiresonance. An antiresonance from the middle 50 ms of the first nasal murmur of /hə'mim/ is indicated at 750 Hz by a downward-pointing arrow in the Fast Fourier Transform (FFT) spectrum shown below the spectrogram. Note the general depression of spectral energy around 1000 Hz, as well as the "white space" from 500 to 1100 Hz in the spectrogram, reflecting the broad influence of the antiresonance. Because a speech sound's total energy is the sum of all energies at all frequencies, the presence of antiresonances in nasal murmur spectra makes their overall intensity relatively low compared with vowels. The second reason for the relatively weak intensities of nasal murmurs is the greater absorption, and therefore loss, of sound energy when acoustic waves propagate through the nasal cavities (see Chapter 9). The greater absorption of sound results in wider formant bandwidths and lower peak amplitudes of resonances.

The first formant of the nasal murmur is marked in both spectrograms as $F1_n$. The subscript "n" indicates that the resonance is from the combined pharyngeal and nasal cavities (hereafter, nasal cavities). This lowest resonance of the nasal cavities is a nearly constant characteristic of nasal murmurs, with the greatest intensity among nasal formants and a frequency around 300 to 400 Hz (Fujimura, 1962). The nasal murmur spectrum contains a fair number of resonances in addition to $F1_n$, as well as antiresonances. The spectrograms in Figure 11–14 illustrate this well, with the prestressed murmur of /hə'mim/ showing an $F2_n$ around 1500 Hz (at least for the first part of the murmur), a possible pair of formants ($F3_n$, $F4_n$) around 2000 Hz, and another around 3000 Hz. In the prestressed murmur of /hə'mɑm/ (Figure 11–14, upper right panel), there is a similar pattern of resonances above $F1_n$ but of much weaker intensity compared with /hə'mim/. Fujimura described the substantial variability in patterns of nasal resonances and antiresonances, both across and within speakers. Presumably, the within-speaker variation is primarily a result of changing phonetic contexts. The differences in the nasal resonances and major antiresonance for the /i/ and /ɑ/ contexts can be seen in Figure 11–14 (antiresonance location indicated by the different white spaces in the two nasal murmurs).

It may seem odd to see spectral evidence of different vowels during a nasal murmur, for which sound transmission is fully (or almost nearly so) through the nasal cavities. Such vowel-context effects on nasal murmur spectra have been demonstrated in modeling studies based on human vocal tract and nasal tract cavity measurements. In these studies the vocal tract is represented with different vowel shapes with the velopharyngeal port set to "wide open" to see what happens to nasal spectra as the vocal tract configuration is varied. Serrurier and Badin (2008, Figure 23) present a beautiful plot showing how their model reveals subtle vowel effects on nasal murmur spectra. Such model data are consistent with the spectrographic differences shown in Figure 11–14 for /mim/ versus /mɑm/.

Perhaps one explanation for the absence of an acoustic data base for nasals comparable to vowels is the difficulty of identifying formants and antiresonances during the nasal murmur. Many nasal formants above $F1_n$ are challenging to locate because of their weak intensity, and antiresonances are often inferred from the absence of energy, rather than by something definitive in the spectrogram or spectrum.[5] An alternative approach to identifying important acoustic characteristics of nasal murmurs (or any speech sound) is to make several measures of the murmur spectrum and use those measures in an automatic classification analysis. This work is usually done by scientists interested in computer recognition of speech. They want to know which acoustic features allow the most rapid and accurate identification of individual speech sounds.

A good example of this work is found in Pruthi and Espy-Wilson (2004). These investigators were interested in machine recognition of segments having a nasal *manner* of articulation. Pruthi and Espy-Wilson (2004) noted that nasals are often confused with liquids (/l/, /r/) and glides (/w/, /j/) when computers classify speech sounds using extracted acoustic measures (that is, a computer algorithm that identifies segments through temporal and spectral measures). They designed four acoustic measures, based on consideration of the acoustic characteristics of nasal murmurs relative to those associated with the constriction interval of liquids and glides (the relatively constant formant frequencies of liquids and glides—see below), as classification parameters for nasal manner of articulation. In a sense, the selection of the four measures was a hypothesis concerning the acoustic characteristics required to identify the nasal manner of production. These measures, with a brief explanation of why they were chosen, are listed in Table 11–1.

The point of this discussion is not to consider in detail the four measures selected by Pruthi and Espy-Wilson (2004) but to demonstrate the value of their experiment for understanding critical acoustic features of speech sounds. Pruthi and Espy-Wilson, using a combination of these measures, correctly classified nasal manner of production for 94% of the more than 1000 nasal murmurs in a large database of sentences spoken by many different speakers. These measures were chosen carefully, to reflect aspects of nasal murmur acoustics previously described in the research literature. The measures also made sense in terms of the theory of vocal and nasal tract acoustics. The very successful classification performance suggests that these measures are strong candidates for further acoustic studies of nasal production and perception.[6]

---

[5]Sharp dips in an FFT spectrum (downward-pointing arrow around 750 Hz in the spectrum shown in the lower panel of Figure 11–14) or white spaces in a spectrogram can occur in the absence of an antiresonance. A definitive identification of an antiresonance depends, in part, on knowing that an antiresonance *should* be found in a spectrum—that the spectrum is derived from a speech sound whose underlying articulation involves a parallel resonator (see Chapter 9).
[6]Simply because an acoustic measure can be used in a statistical or machine recognition procedure to obtain correct classifications of the manner (or any other feature) of articulation of a speech sound does not mean that humans use the same kind of information to make

Table 11–1. Four Acoustic Measures Used by Pruthi and Espy-Wilson (2004) for Automatic Classification of Nasal Manner of Articulation

MEASURE	EXPLANATION
Energy onset/offset at vowel-nasal (liquid/glide) boundaries	Energy change from vowel to nasal or nasal to vowel is greater than from vowel to liquid or liquid/glide to vowel.
First spectral peak	Nasal murmurs have lower F1 compared with F1s of liquids and glides.
$dB_{0-320Hz}/dB_{320-5360Hz}$	Nasal murmurs have most energy concentrated below 320 Hz (at the $F1_n$), little energy above, so energy ratio would be high; liquids and glides have more energy in the 320 to 5360 Hz band, so ratio would be lower.
Energy fluctuation	Level (in dB) of energy throughout a nasal murmur is more stable than throughout the constriction interval of a liquid or glide.

Note. The measures were chosen as most likely to separate nasal manner from liquid and glide manner, because nasals are often mistaken as liquids or glides by speech recognition devices. Descriptions and explanations of the measures have been modified slightly from the original presentation.

Nasal Place of Articulation

There is a long history of documenting the acoustic correlates of place of articulation for consonants, including nasals. Much of this history is concerned with the acoustic cues used by *listeners*, not computers, to identify place of articulation. Although speech perception is considered in greater depth in the next chapter, the case of nasal place of articulation provides a good introduction to the interplay between studies of acoustic characteristics of speech sounds and their role as cues in speech perception.

Consider the following thought experiment. Imagine a CV syllable, where C = /m/ or /n/ and V = /i/, /ɛ/, /æ/, /ɑ/, /o/, or /u/. The nasals are chosen to represent the two (/m/ and /n/) that occur in syllable-initial position of English words. The vowels are chosen to sample different locations around the vowel quadrilateral, to maximize potential coarticulatory influences on murmur acoustics—that is, to create variability in murmur acoustics due to phonetic context. The complete set of 12 syllables (2 nasal consonants × 6 vowels) is spoken by several speakers and saved as computer wave files. Speech analysis programs are used to make certain measurements as well as to "pull out" from each syllable selected temporal pieces from the wave files for presentation to listeners. The waveform pieces are (1) an interval from the murmur, (2) an interval that straddles the murmur-vowel boundary (therefore containing formant transitions from the murmur release into the vowel) and (3) and interval that includes only the transitions after the murmur release. Figure 11–15 illustrates these waveform pieces with a spectrogram of the utterance /ə'mɛ/. The boundaries of the nasal murmur are indicated by the short, upward-pointing arrows at the baseline. The three waveform pieces are shown by narrow rectangles ("windows") superimposed on the spectrogram. Each window is approximately 25 ms in duration. The leftmost window is the murmur piece, the middle window the piece straddling the boundary between murmur offset and vowel onset (murmur + transition piece), and the right-hand window the transition piece—the piece of the vowel containing transitions to the vowel, immediately after the release of the murmur.

These waveform pieces can be used to address the question "Which piece(s) of the waveform, or which acoustic characteristics within each piece, allow computer and human classification of nasal place of articulation?" Stated in a different way: "Do the three pieces allow equivalent accuracy in classifying place of articulation for nasals, or is one piece 'better' than

the same decisions. But the statistical/machine data do suggest testable hypotheses for human perception experiments. One hypothesis is that listeners classify sound segments based on multiple sources of acoustic information, not just a single piece of information such as formant frequencies. This is discussed further in Chapter 12.

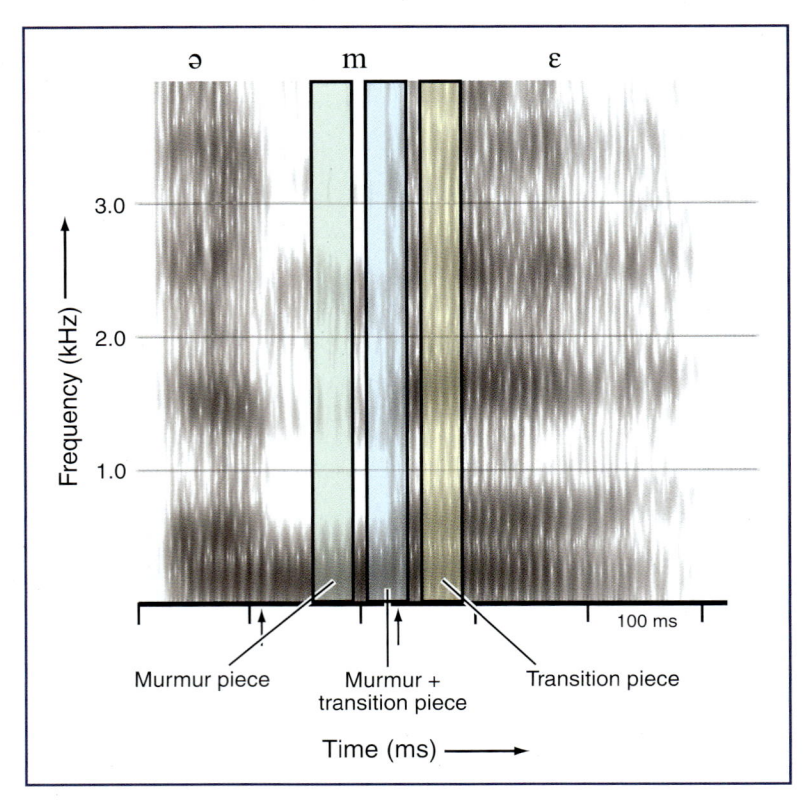

Figure 11–15. Spectrogram of the utterance /əˈmɛ/, shown with three 25-ms "windows" centered at different times. The leftmost window (*light green shading*, "murmur piece") is within the nasal murmur, the center window (*light blue shading*, "murmur + transition piece") straddles the murmur-vowel boundary, and the rightmost window (*light yellow shading*, "transition piece") is completely within the vowel, during the formant transitions from the murmur to the vowel.

another?" For example, if only the nasal murmur piece (the leftmost box) is presented to listeners, can they use this acoustic information to make accurate identification of place of articulation? Alternatively, if certain acoustic characteristics are extracted from the murmur windows for /m/ and /n/, can these be used by an automatic classification algorithm to separate the two places of articulation? These types of experiments appear several times in the speech acoustics literature (e.g., Harrington, 1994; Kurowski & Blumstein, 1984, 1987; Repp, 1986). The results of the experiments, although not always precisely consistent, suggest that *any* of these three pieces, when presented to human listeners or classified statistically, allow fairly accurate identification of place of articulation for syllable-initial nasals. Moreover, when two or more of the pieces are presented (or classified) together, the accuracy of place identification improves.

First consider the results for isolated murmurs. If nasal place of articulation can be identified (classified) accurately from just the murmur, something about its acoustic characteristics must be systematically different for labials versus lingua-alveolars. The duration of the murmur can be ruled out as a measure that separates /m/ from /n/, but there are almost certainly spectral differences between the two nasal murmurs. The spectral differences are a result of different resonances and antiresonances of the coupled pharyngeal and oral tracts. In Chapter 9, the frequency locations of the antiresonances for /m/ versus /n/ were discussed, the former having a lower region (according to Fujimura [1962], roughly 750–1250 Hz), the latter a higher region (1450–2200 Hz). The unique resonances for /m/ in Fujimura's study included a two-formant cluster in the vicinity of 1000 Hz, and for /n/ a similar cluster above 2000 Hz. Qi and Fox (1992), in an analysis of the first two resonances of nasal murmurs for /m/ and /n/ produced by six speakers, reported average second resonances for /m/ and /n/ of 1742 and 2062 Hz, respectively. Careful examination of the /m/ and

/n/ murmurs in Figure 11–16 shows formant patterns, and inferred antiresonance locations, generally consistent with the observations of Fujimura and of Qi and Fox. Both /m/ and /n/ have the expected first formant around 300 Hz, but in the frequency range above this formant, the spectra are different. Between the F1 and the next evidence of a higher resonance, both murmurs have an obvious "white space." For /m/, the white space extends roughly from 500 to 1150 Hz, and for /n/ it is located between 500 and 1600 Hz. The different antiresonance locations for the /m/ and /n/ are expected from the different cavity volumes behind the respective places of articulation (Fant, 1960). Under the assumption that the exact antiresonance frequencies are approximately in the middle of these white space ranges, their center frequencies are 850 Hz for /m/ and 1050 Hz for /n/. Immediately above the antiresonance, the /m/ murmur has a second and perhaps third resonance around 1500 Hz, and above that a resonance around 2300 Hz. In comparison, the /n/ murmur has a second resonance around 1800 Hz, and what appears to be a cluster of two resonances around 2500 Hz. Clearly, the two murmurs have different spectral characteristics. It is reasonable to expect that listeners can use these differences to identify place of articulation.[7] In Repp (1986), listeners made accurate place judgments for /m/ and /n/ when given only the murmur piece of CV syllables, and Harrington (1994) obtained excellent statistical classification for these two nasals when using acoustic information from single spectrum "slices" taken from the murmur.

The spectrograms in Figure 11–16 also show different patterns of formant transitions as the murmur is released into the following /ɛ/. There is a long history of considering formant transitions at CV boundaries as strong cues to consonant place of articulation. This history originated in the late 1940s and early 1950s, at the Haskins Laboratories, where experiments showed that synthesized formant transitions cued place of articulation in the absence of consonant spectra (Liberman, Delattre, Cooper, & Gerstman, 1954). Figure 11–16 shows spectrograms of /ə 'mɛ/ and /ə 'nɛ/, where the differences between the F2 and F3 transitions following release of the murmur are shown. Figure 11–17 shows a spectrogram of the utterance /ə 'ŋɛ/ to contrast its transitions with those in Figure 11–16. The patterns of F2 and F3 transitions over the first 40 or 50 ms following release of the murmur are unique to the different places of nasal articulation. Transitions coming out of the /m/ murmur have rising F2 and F3, from /n/ are more or less flat, and from /ŋ/ F2 falls and F3 rises. This latter pattern (see Figure 11–17) shows F2 and F3

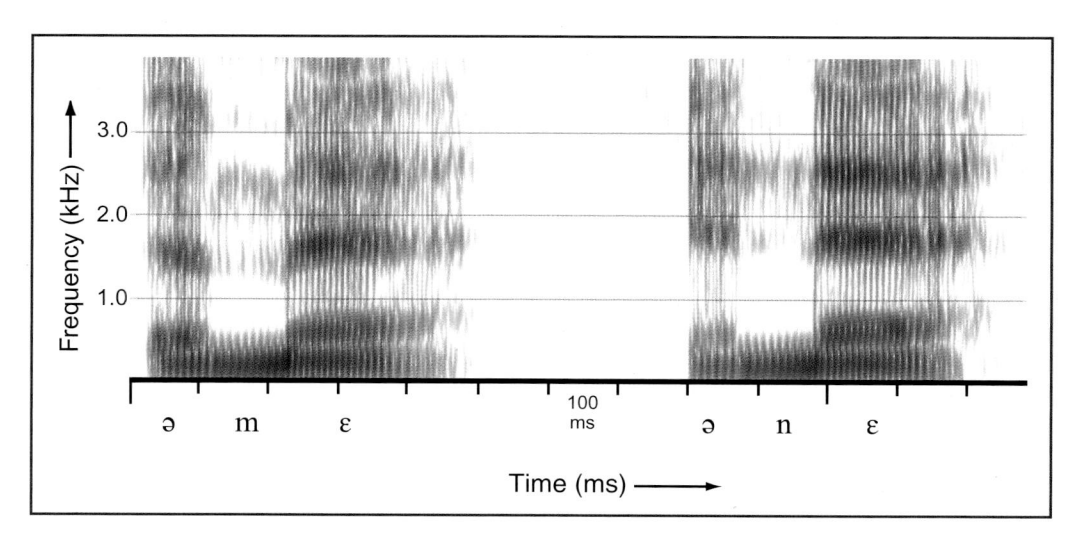

Figure 11-16. Spectrograms of the utterances /ə'mɛ/ and /ə'nɛ/, produced by a 57-year-old healthy male. Note between-place differences in the murmur spectra and the pattern of formant transitions as the nasal is released into the vowel.

---

[7]The antiresonance and upper resonance locations for the murmurs in Figure 11–16 are different from those reported by Fujimura (1962), which were based on his theoretical calculations and data from two subjects, but the spectral relations (e.g., higher antiresonance for /n/ compared with /m/, different patterns of resonance above the constant F1 at 300 Hz) are consistent with Fujimura's general description. The resonances and antiresonances for /m/ and /n/ shown in Figure 11–16 are also somewhat different from the modeling results reported by Rong and Kuehn (2010). Fujimura, and many other authors, have pointed to the wide range of variability expected across speakers for nasal murmur spectra due to variations in nasal tract and sinus cavity morphology (Dang & Honda, 1995).

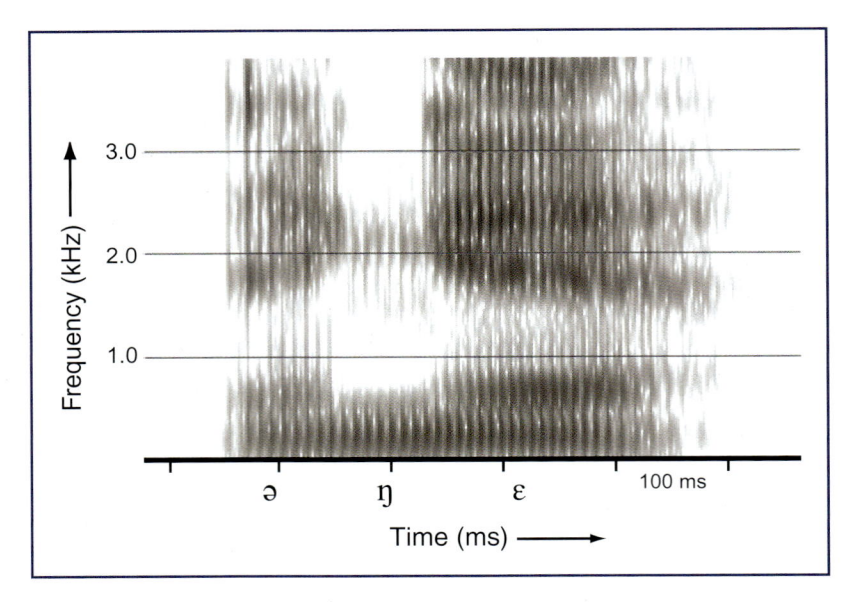

Figure 11–17. Spectrogram of the VCV utterance /ə'ŋɛ/, produced by a 57-year-old male. Note the F2-F3 transition pattern immediately following release of the nasal murmur.

starting at the murmur-vowel boundary nearly at the same frequency and separating throughout the transition. Details of these F2-F3 transition patterns depend on the identity of the vowel following the murmur, but in most cases the patterns are different for the three places of articulation. In English the velar nasal /ŋ/ does not appear in the prestressed position shown in Figure 11–17, and this is why the examples discussed above have been restricted (until now) to /m/ and /n/. The absence of /ŋ/ in word-initial position is not a physiological limitation—there are languages in which the sound can appear in this position—so the point concerning place-specific transition patterns is relevant and as shown below applies to transition characteristics of stop place of articulation.

Place of articulation information is present in these unique transition patterns, as demonstrated for listeners (Repp, 1986) and statistical classification (Harrington, 1994). The accuracy of place identification from the transitions (i.e., the "transition piece" of the spectrogram shown in Figure 11–14) is similar to the accuracy from the "murmur piece." Place information for nasals, therefore, seems to have acoustic correlates in at least two different locations throughout a CV syllable, and these correlates are sufficiently stable to be reliable for listeners and statistical classification of nasals.

Finally, in Figure 11–15 the middle "piece" straddles the boundary where the murmur ends and the transition begins. This interval has a very rapid change from the low-energy, unique resonance patterns associated with murmurs to the high-energy formant patterns for vowels. Several scientists (Kurowski & Blumstein, 1984, 1987; Seitz, McCormick, Watson, & Bladon, 1990) have argued that each place of articulation is associated with a unique frequency pattern for this rapid change. Whether or not this particular "piece" is more important in the classification of nasal place of articulation compared with the murmur or transitions alone is a matter of considerable debate.

Nasalization

Nasalization, as reviewed in Chapter 9, is a concept with broad application in general and in clinical phonetics. Nasalization of vowels, which is of concern here, involves complex acoustics resulting from the mix of oral and nasal tract formants with antiresonances originating in the sinus cavities.[8] Only a few studies have

---

[8]Recall that nasalization occurs when the velopharyngeal port is open at the same time the oral tract opens for vowel production. This combination of events is characteristic of "normal" speech production in at least two ways. First, vowels are typically not produced with perfect velopharyngeal port closure, but have variable amounts of small opening that depend on tongue height (higher the vowel, tighter the velopharyngeal closure: see Chapter 4). Second, the coarticulatory patterns of nasal-vowel and vowel-nasal sequences almost always involve some velopharyngeal port opening during the vowel that reflects the previous (in nasal-vowel sequences) or upcoming (in vowel-nasal sequences) open port requirement of the nasal consonant.

reported data on the spectra of nasalization. Theoretical treatments of vowel nasalization can be found in Feng and Castelli (1996), Pruthi, Espy-Wilson, and Story (2007), Rong and Kuehn (2010), Stevens, Fant, and Hawkins (1987), and Serrurier and Badin (2008).

Chen (1995, 1997) developed two acoustic measures of nasalization, one of which is described here. Recall that a Fourier spectrum of a vowel shows the amplitude of the consecutive harmonics (where the first harmonic = F0) produced by the vibrating vocal folds. Furthermore, the varying amplitude of the harmonics reflects, in part, the resonance characteristics of the vocal tract. When a vowel is produced with an open velopharyngeal port and is nasalized, some glottal harmonics in the region of the nasal resonances have increased amplitude (relative to the amplitudes when the vowel is not nasalized), and some harmonics in the region of oral formants have reduced amplitude, due to nearby antiresonances and damping from increased absorption of sound energy in the nasal cavities (see Chapter 9). Chen (1995) took advantage of these facts and constructed a spectral measure of nasalization in which the amplitude of the harmonic closest to the first formant was compared with the amplitude of a harmonic close to the location of the second nasal resonance. The technique is illustrated in Figure 11–18.

Figure 11–18 shows two FFT spectra, both for the middle 30 ms of the vowel /i/ in the CVC [bib] (left spectrum) and [min] (right spectrum). In both spectra, two harmonics are of interest. One, labeled "A1," is the harmonic in the immediate vicinity of the low-frequency F1 of /i/. As expected, the A1 harmonic in the two spectra has relatively high amplitude compared with the other harmonics. This makes sense because the amplitude of this harmonic is "boosted" by the typical first resonant frequency (F1) of /i/, which is approximately 300 Hz in adult males. The other harmonic of interest is the one labeled "P1." Chen (1995) identified this harmonic as "boosted" when the oral and nasal cavities are coupled via opening of the velopharyngeal port. The P1 harmonic is close to the second resonance of the nasal cavity. In theory, the amplitude of the P1 harmonic is quite low when the velopharyngeal port is closed and relatively greater when the port is open. Based on theoretical and experimental work, Chen recommended identifying the P1 harmonic by locating the FFT peak closest to 950 Hz.

Chen's (1995) index of nasalization requires measurement of the A1-P1 amplitude difference within a vowel spectrum. In Figure 11–18, the A1 and P1 *relative* Lamplitudes for [i] surrounded by [b] are roughly 0 and −45 dB, respectively, yielding an A1-P1 index of 45 dB.

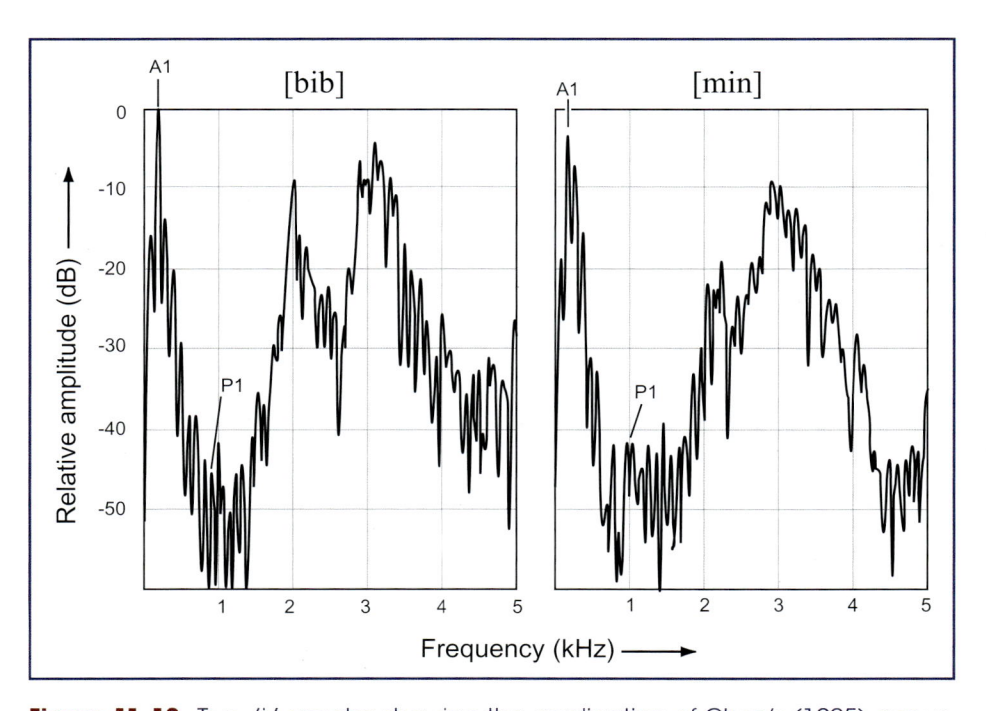

Figure 11–18. Two /i/ spectra showing the application of Chen's (1995) acoustic technique to the quantification of the degree of vowel nasalization. The left spectrum is for /i/ in a non-nasal context, the right spectrum for /i/ is in a nasal context. "A1" is the highest-amplitude harmonic in the vicinity of the F1 for /i/, "P1" a harmonic around 950 Hz, close to the second resonance of the nasal tract. The acoustic measure is the amplitude difference, in dB, between A1 and P1.

Spectrographic Challenges

Experienced acoustic phoneticians know that some spectrograms are easy to analyze, others are more difficult. The "goodness" of a spectrographic display is often predictable based on characteristics of the speaker. Talkers with very high F0s and/or breathy voices are notoriously difficult to analyze, as are persons with a lot of nasalization. The low-amplitude, broad bandwidth formants in hypernasal speech complicate the precise identification of formant frequencies (as in speakers with cleft palate and some degree of velopharyngeal insufficiency). Moreover, the most popular computer technique for formant frequency identification—linear predictive code (LPC) analysis—is based on a mathematical model that neglects the antiresonance "dips" described in Chapter 9. LPC formant estimates for a nasalized vowel are, therefore, often incorrect, and must be checked carefully on a spectrogram-by-spectrogram basis. This complicates the use of LPC analysis in many speech disorders associated with velopharyngeal insufficiency.

When [i] is surrounded by nasal consonants (right spectrum), and likely to be partially nasalized due to coarticulatory influences, A1 = −4 dB and P1 = −38 dB, giving an A1-P1 index of 38 dB. As expected, the A1-P1 index for the vowel in a nasal environment is smaller than the index when the vowel is between non-nasal consonants. In Figure 11–18 this is due to both a decrease in the amplitude of A1 and an increase in the amplitude of P1, as expected from Chen's analysis strategy.

An alternative acoustic measure of nasalization is called *nasalance*. Nasalance is a measure of the acoustic energy radiating from the nares (usually expressed as A_n, where A = amplitude and the subscript n indicates "nares") divided by the total energy emitted by the speech apparatus (i.e., $A_n + A_m$, where m = "mouth"). The nasalance value $A_n/A_n + A_m$ is obtained from an instrument called a nasometer. The nasometer uses a mask pressed firmly to the face; a dividing partition separates the nose and mouth. The upper partition (nose) and lower partition (mouth) each have separate microphones to record the energy radiated separately from the two openings (the two nares considered here as one opening). A computer measures these two values of energy and reports the value of nasalance. The idea is that higher ratios of $A_n/A_n + A_m$ indicate greater degrees of nasalization.

Nasometry values, expressed as percentages ($A_n/A_n + A_m \times 100$), are often computed for extended passages. One passage may include no nasal consonants, another may be loaded with nasals. The reason for collecting nasalance values for two passages that vary in phonetic content is to control for variation in nasalance values related to anatomical variation across speakers, rather than true variations in the degree of nasalization. The nasal-loaded passage is designed to elicit high values of nasalance, while the no-nasal passage provides an estimate of the performance of the velopharyngeal port when velopharyngeal closure is required to close the valve between the oral and nasal cavities, and especially for the many stops and fricatives in the passage. In some cases, a passage with a mix of obstruents and nasals is used to obtain a nasalance measure for speech materials that are a better match for the phonetics of typical utterances.

Nasometry is a very popular measure in research and clinical practice. The advantages of the measure include the speed of obtaining a value (especially important in clinical practice), the automatic nature of the measurement, the tendency for perceptual estimates of nasality to increase as nasalance increases, and a large number of published articles on nasalance values in various populations, including persons with normal speech structures and those with velopharyngeal insufficiency or incompetence. The popularity of nasometry can be gauged by a literature search on the term "nasalance" conducted for the previous five years from the time of this writing (August 2017). That search indicated more than 100 published articles, many of which report norms for various groups and languages.

The disadvantages of nasometry include the global nature of the measure, which is usually averaged across entire passages and yields a single number per passage, the tendency for perceptual estimates of nasality to vary imperfectly with nasalance values, and the difficulty of knowing how variation in nasalance values relates to the specific nature of velopharyngeal dysfunction (see Bunton, 2015 for initial work on this problem). A few citations for nasometry and nasalance values are Awan, Bressman, Poburka, Roy, Sharp, and Watts (2015), Bettens, De Bodt, Maryn, Luytn, Wuytz, and Van Lierde (2016), and Sweeney and Sell (2008), as well as one of the original papers on this topic, by Fletcher (1976).

SEMIVOWELS

In this chapter, /w/, /ɹ/, /l/, and /j/ are considered semivowels. /w/ and /j/ are also referred to as glides, /ɹ/ and /l/ as liquids. The latter two sounds are also called rhotic and lateral, respectively. The term "semivowel" is a convenient way to group all four sounds because it captures a shared aspect of their production. All four sounds require movement to and away from a vocal tract constriction tighter than that for vowels, but not nearly so tight as required for obstruents (fricatives, stops, and affricates). All are produced with a vocal tract open to the atmosphere, and are considered vocalics.

Constriction Interval

Figure 11–19 shows spectrograms of the four semivowels in VCV frames, where V = /ɛ/. These spectrograms suggest a few prominent acoustic features of all semivowels. All have an interval during which F1, F2, and F3 are more or less constant; all have relatively large transitions in at least one of the first three formants going into and out of these steady formant frequencies. The interval of relatively "flat" formants is called the *constriction interval*, and is assumed to correspond to the part of semivowel articulation when the vocal tract is *most* constricted. The duration of the constriction interval for each semivowel is marked in Figure 11–19 by a horizontal bar between the 1.0 and 2.0 kHz calibration lines (the precise location of the horizontal bar along the frequency scale is not important; the position is different from semivowel to semivowel to avoid obscuring formants within the constriction interval). The duration of each of the constriction intervals in Figure 11–19 is less than 100 ms, and in less carefully articulated speech is probably about 40 to 50 ms, on average (Dalston, 1975).

The constriction interval has a formant pattern like those of vowels. The relative stability of these formant

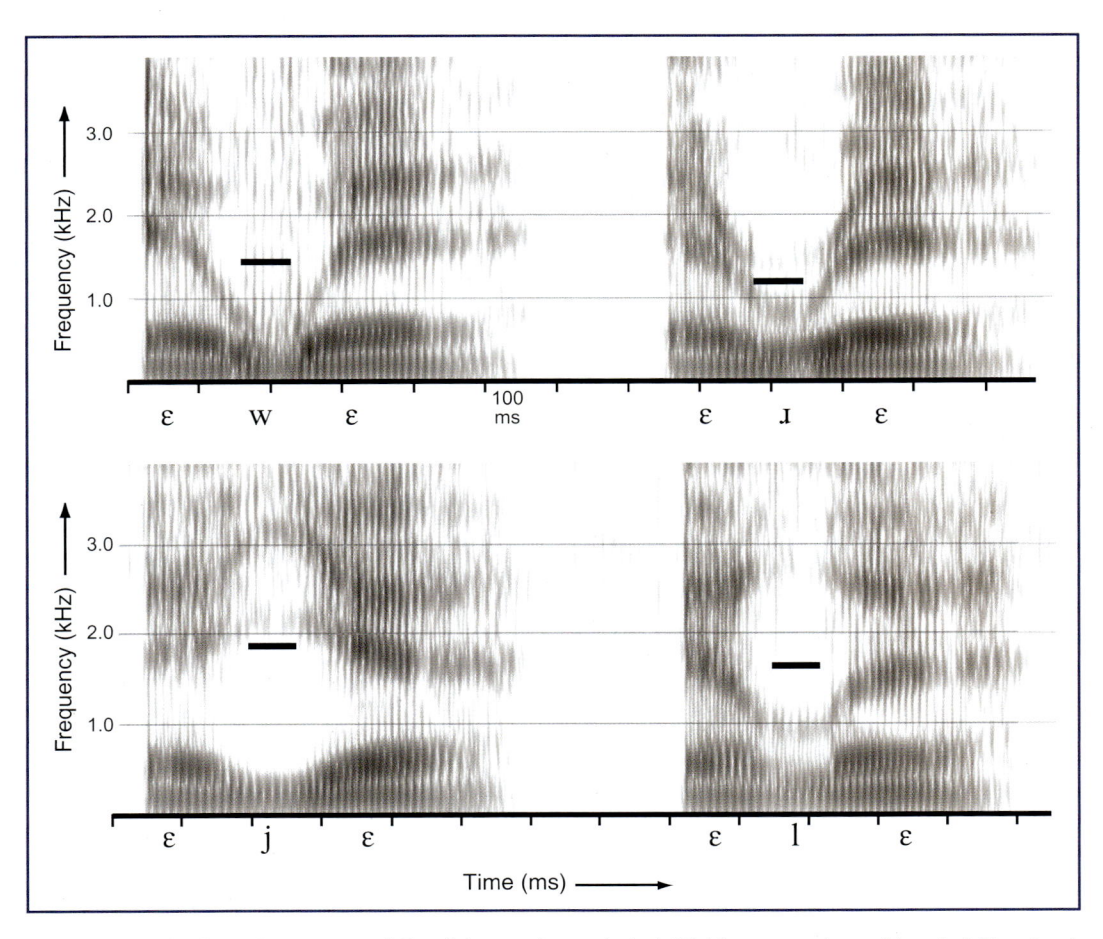

Figure 11–19. Spectrograms of English semivowels in VCV frames where V = /ɛ/. The horizontal bar located between 1.0 and 2.0 kHz in each spectrogram shows the time interval corresponding to the constriction interval of each semivowel. See text for further explanation.

frequencies allows target values to be measured for the different semivowels. Do these formant frequencies distinguish the semivowels from each other? F1 is quite similar across the semivowels, but the F2 and F3 are different for these sounds. Figure 11–20 shows how the formant frequencies of the semivowel constriction intervals in Figure 11–19 are separated in F2-F3 space. These formant frequencies, estimated by eye at the temporal midpoint of the horizontal bars in Figure 11–19, are plotted in Figure 11–20 (filled circles) together with values reported for young adult speakers by Dalston (1975; unfilled triangles = males, filled triangles = females) and Espy-Wilson (1992; unfilled squares). The values for each semivowel are consistent across the three different data sources, even though there are differences in speaker sex, age, and phonetic context (see Figure 11–20 caption). The ellipses are included to show the separation of the points for the four semivowels. Most obvious in this plot is the low F3 associated with /ɹ/, clearly different from the F3s of the other semivowels. The low F3 for /ɹ/ is usually below 2000 Hz and very close to F2. Figure 11–20 shows just such a pattern: a horizontal line at roughly 2100 Hz can be drawn across the graph to separate /ɹ/ data from the other three semivowels. Both /w/ and /l/ have a wide frequency separation between F2 and F3, as indicated by their general location in the upper left quadrant of the plot. /w/ and /l/ are distinguished from each other by the generally lower F2 and F3 of /w/ compared with /l/. This results in a greater F2-F3 separation between /l/ compared with /w/. Finally, /j/ has a much higher F2 than the other semivowels. F3 of /j/ is also higher than the F3 of /w/, /ɹ/, and /l/. /j/ appears to occupy its own corner of the F2-F3 plot, clearly separated from the other semivowels.

Formant Transitions

The pattern of formant transitions into and out of the constriction intervals also distinguishes among the semivowels. The important characteristics of these

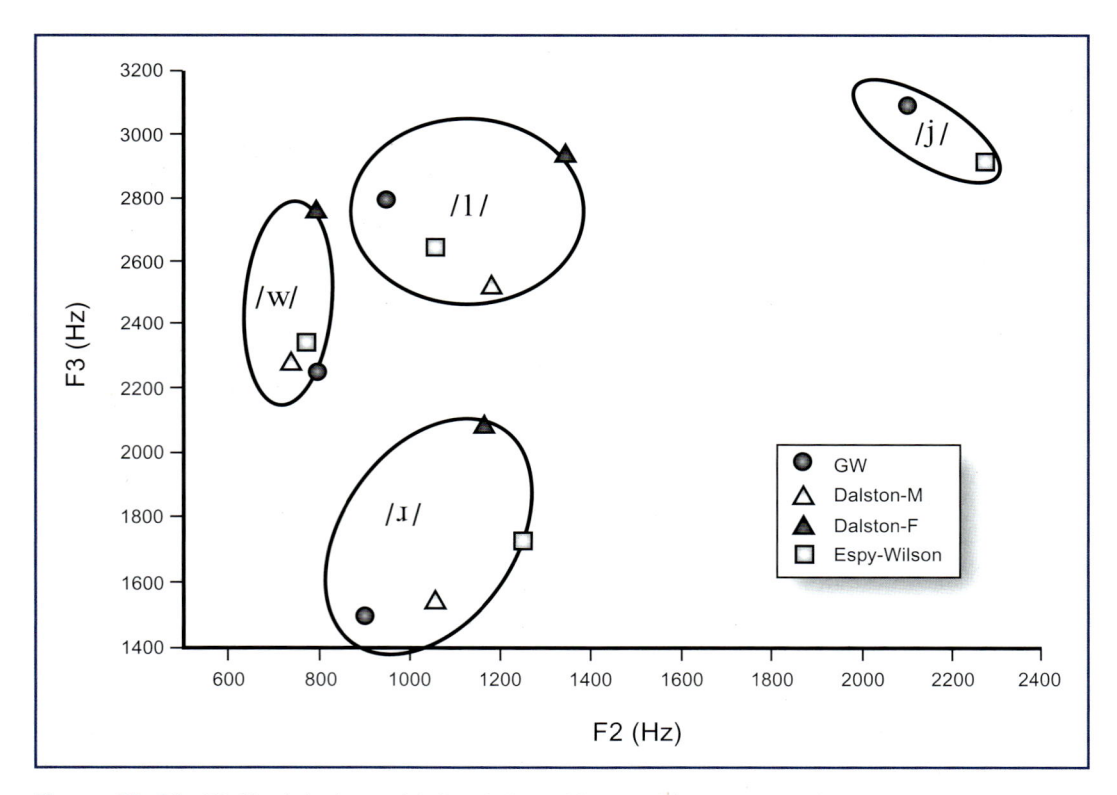

Figure 11–20. F2-F3 plot of constriction interval formant frequencies from three data sources. GW points (*filled circles*) are estimated formant frequencies (by eye) from the semivowels shown in Figure 11–19. Dalston-M and Dalston-F points (*unfilled and filled triangles, respectively*) are averages from Dalston (1975) for semivowels spoken as word-initial consonants in isolated words by three adult males and two adult females. Espy-Wilson (1992) points (*unfilled boxes*) are averages for intervocalic semivowels produced by two adult males and two adult females.

patterns are: (a) the specific formants that have large transitions into and out of the constriction interval, and (b) the direction (rising versus falling) of the transitions. For the purposes of this discussion, the direction of transitions is always referenced to the constriction interval. For example, in Figure 11–19, the VC (V = /ɛ/, C = semivowel) F1 transitions for all semivowels are falling into the constriction interval and rising for the CV part. With a special-case exception described below, the F1 transitions do not seem to distinguish among the four semivowels.

The direction of the F2 transitions into and out of the constriction interval easily separates /j/ from the other three semivowels. For /j/ the transition is rising into the constriction, and falling out of it. For /w/, /ɹ/, and /l/, there are large, falling transitions into the constriction interval, and rising transitions out of it. The magnitude of these transitions—the frequency range covered from the onset of the transition to its end—and the transition rate (transition magnitude/transition duration) are affected by the vowel context in which the semivowel is articulated. These context effects are very detailed and numerous. Interested readers should consult Espy-Wilson (1992, 1994) for relevant information.

F3 transitions allow further distinction of /w/, /ɹ/, and /l/. /ɹ/ has a large falling (VC) and rising (CV) transition. This F3 transition is often immediately above (of greater frequency than) the F2 transition. The F3 transition follows the F2 transition closely, especially just prior to and after the constriction interval. An F3 transition is often absent for /w/, or possibly has only very slight movement. The large F3 transition for /ɹ/ effectively separates its acoustic characteristics from those of /w/. The F3 transition for /l/, as shown in Figure 11–19, is rising slightly into the constriction interval and falling slightly out of it.

CV transition characteristics for semivowels are summarized in Table 11–2. When semivowels are in a symmetric VCV frame as in Figure 11–19, the VC and CV transitions are mirror images of each other. Table 11–2 uses a simple classification approach to transition type, much like that published by Espy-Wilson (1994). In this classification scheme, no two semivowels have exactly the same pattern of transitions to or from the following or preceding vowel. To be sure, the F1 and F2 transitions in this classification system are identical for /w/, /ɹ/, and /l/, but the F3 transition distin-

Table 11–2. Classification of CV Transition Type for the CV Sequence of a VCV Frame Where C = Semivowel and V = /ɛ/

SEMIVOWEL	F1	F2	F3
/w/	rising	rising	flat[a]
/ɹ/	rising	rising	rising
/l/	rising[b]	rising	falling[c]
/j/	rising	falling	falling

[a]Some may rise, some may fall depending on context.
[b]Rise may look like a "jump"; see text.
[c]Very context sensitive; some may be flat, some may rise.

guishes among them. Note, however, the qualifications in Table 11–2 concerning the F3 transition of /w/ and the F1 and F3 transitions of /l/. These transitions may be especially sensitive to the identity of the following or preceding vowels. The F1 transition for /l/ + vowel sequences often appears to "jump" from the constriction interval to the following vowel, which may be the result of a sudden change in area function from a lateral articulatory configuration to the configuration for a following vowel (Narayanan, Alwan, & Haker, 1997). Figure 11–19 shows this F1 "jump" in the CV part of /ɛlɛ/.

When the constriction interval and transition acoustics of semivowels are taken together, there is ample reason to believe the acoustic information is rich enough to distinguish among these sounds. Much like the case of nasals, if the acoustic information is sufficient to distinguish among the semivowels, an automatic classification based on these acoustic characteristics should be successful in getting the sounds "right." As reported by Espy-Wilson (1994), however, there are frequent classification confusions between /w/ and /l/. These confusions occur because /w/ and /l/ are so similar acoustically (Figure 11–20) and different phonetic contexts blur the subtle acoustic distinctions between them.[9]

Semivowel Acoustics and Speech Development

Knowledge of semivowel acoustics is important to speech-language pathologists because semivowel errors

---

[9]Speech-language pathologists are familiar with the distinction between light and dark /l/ ([l] vs.[ɫ]). Dark /l/ usually involves an articulatory configuration with a tighter constriction in the velar region or more posterior tongue position, compared with light /l/. The dark /l/ constriction interval, therefore, has a higher F1 and lower F2 compared with light /l/ (Narayanan, Alwan, & Haker, 1997). The higher F1 and lower F2 of dark /l/ may make it more confusing than the light /l/ with /w/, especially because of the lowered F2 in dark /l/ (see Figure 11–19, and notice how a lowering of F2 for /l/ would move it toward the /w/ region).

are frequent during phonological development and in speech delay. In both typical and delayed phonological development, /w/ for /ɹ/, /w/ for /l/, and /j/ for /l/ errors are not unusual. Perhaps the unique and shared gesture characteristics of semivowels, of complex vocal tract configurations and rapid articulatory movement to and away from a narrow, vocalic constriction, make the sounds more difficult to articulate than vowels and therefore more confusable as a speech motor control requirement (Boyce, 2015 offers this perspective). A different perspective is that the difficulty of mastering these sounds is not due to the similarity of their articulatory gestures, but rather to the similarity of the acoustic models of semivowels heard by the child as she is trying to connect perceptual representations of speech sounds with their production requirements. In this latter view, the child could produce the semivowels correctly if she were able to distinguish between them on a consistent basis (Person, Irwin, & Turcio, 2015 offer this perspective).

This issue has been given attention in the literature, by asking a simple question: When, for example, a child produces what appears to be a [w] for /ɹ/ error (as when a child is heard to say [wɑɪt] for the word "right"), is the error [w] acoustically similar or identical to a correctly produced [w] (when a child says [wɑɪt] for the word "white")? The question has been asked in two ways, when both the error and correct versions of the sound are obtained from the same child, or when the error sound is obtained from a single child and is compared with acoustic characteristics of the correctly produced sound collected from a group of children with normal articulation. Either approach yields the same result: the acoustics of a [w] in a [w] for /ɹ/ error (or any other substitution error) are often *not* like the acoustics of normally articulated [w] (Chaney, 1988; Dalston, 1972; Hoffman, Stager, & Daniloff, 1983). In these analyses, the error [w] is different from correct [w] by having acoustic characteristics more or less between the error sound and the correct sound. A distinction is made by the child but may be too subtle for human listeners to perceive. Even if listeners do hear a subtle distinction they may place it in a "comfortable" phoneme category—that is, to consider the distinction as a phonetic variant of a single phoneme category.

This finding is consistent with the child's ability to hear the differences between semivowels but to have a limited ability to reproduce those distinctions. Acoustic characteristics that distinguish error [w] from correct [w], even if those characteristics are not the "right" ones, provide evidence for the child's knowledge of a phonemic distinction between [w] and other semivowels. This knowledge is presumably obtained from the distinctions heard by the child, as produced by normally articulating adults and children. A more provocative finding (McAllister Byun & Tiede, 2017) demonstrates for normally articulating children age 9 to 14 years a possible linkage between a child's perceptual ability to distinguish /r/ from /w/ and his or her separation of /r/ from /w/ in production. In other words, when a child hears a clear perceptual distinction between /r/ and /w/, using carefully constructed signals organized as a continuum between the two sounds (Chapter 12), he or she is more likely to produce the distinction clearly. Perceptual contrast training, therefore, may lead to success in production of /r/-/w/ contrasts. McAllister Byun and Tiede's findings need to be replicated in younger children, and especially children who are producing an inconsistent separation between /r/ and /w/.

The acoustic analyses described above provide a level of understanding of a child's articulation behavior that may be unavailable when perceptual analyses alone are used to understand speech sound errors.[10] The /r/-/w/ distinction is not the only contrast that may benefit from the match between perceptual ability and acoustic analysis of production. Contrasts such as /l/-/w/ and /s/-/ʃ/ are also good candidates for this work, which may have substantial influence in clinical diagnostics and documentation of progress throughout therapy for children with speech sound disorders.

Semivowel Durations

Specific data on semivowel durations are difficult to provide because it is challenging to segment semivowels from adjacent vowels (see Chapter 10). When constriction intervals can be segmented from the surrounding transitions—essentially a *phonetic* segmentation, as described in Chapter 10—they have durations of 30 to 70 ms, with the majority of values toward the lower end of this range (Dalston, 1975). The duration of transitions into and out of the constriction interval are also in the 30 to 70 ms range. The combined duration of the transition and constriction intervals of semivowels may, therefore, be very brief (as short as 100 ms). This suggests very rapid, complex articulatory gestures occurring in a short amount of time, perhaps explaining, in part, why children master the contrasts of these sounds relatively late in the overall scheme of phonological development.

---

[10] The [w] for /ɹ/ examples presented here were chosen because of their clarity and frequency as errors in normal and delayed phonology. Many other examples can be described. Interested readers should consult Forrest, Weismer, Hodge, Dinnsen, and Elbert (1990), Schellinger, Munson, and Edwards (2017), Weismer (1984), and Weismer, Dinnsen, and Elbert (1981) for additional examples.

FRICATIVES

Fricatives are characterized by an interval of aperiodic energy whose spectrum and overall amplitude depend on place of articulation and, in some cases, voicing status. In English, fricatives are categorized as sibilants (/s,z,ʃ,ʒ/) and nonsibilants (/f,v,θ,ð/); the glottal fricative /h/ is discussed toward the end of this section. The sibilant-nonsibilant distinction is acoustically and perceptually meaningful because sibilants are more intense and have better-defined spectra than nonsibilants. "Better defined spectra" implies the presence of more easily identified spectral peaks and concentrations of spectral energy.

Sibilants Versus Nonsibilants: Spectral Characteristics

An illustration of the acoustic bases of the sibilant-nonsibilant distinction is shown in Figure 11–21. Spectrograms are shown of the fricatives /s/ and /f/ in a

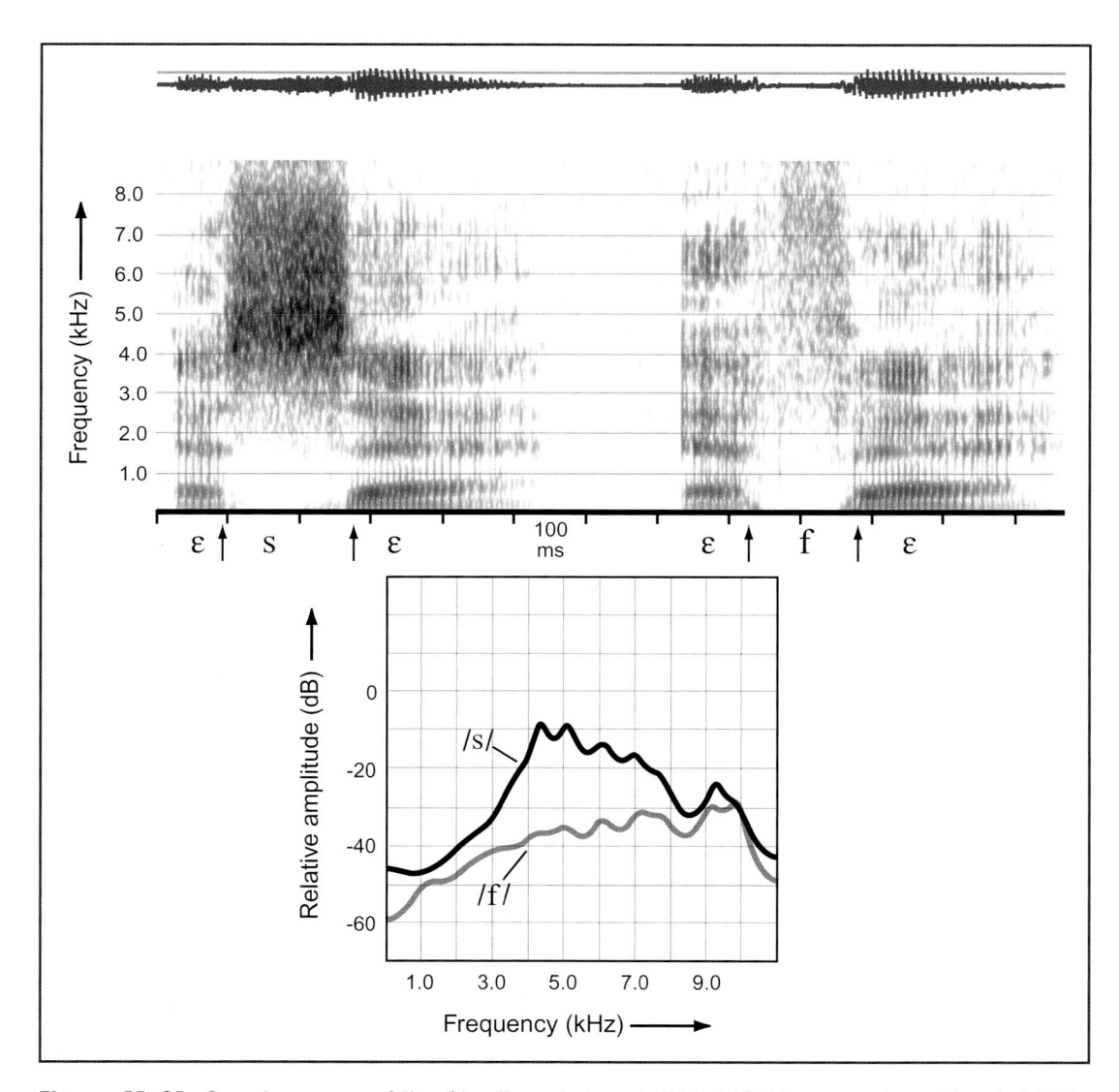

Figure 11-21. Spectrograms of the fricatives /s/ and /f/ in VCV frames where V = /ɛ/. Note the 0 to 8.4 kHz frequency range in these displays to demonstrate the characteristic higher-frequency energy of frication noise. The upward-pointing arrows indicate the onsets and offsets of the fricatives, indicated by the last glottal pulse preceding the frication noise (onset) and the first glottal pulse following the frication noise (offset), respectively. Below the spectrograms LPC spectra ranging from 0 to 11.0 kHz are shown for the middle 50 ms of the frication noise; lighter line = /f/ spectrum, darker line = /s/ spectrum.

VCV frame where V = /ɛ/. Superimposed LPC spectra for /s/ and /f/, computed over a 50-ms time interval centered at the midpoint of the frication noise, are immediately below the spectrogram. Along the baseline of the spectrogram, upward-pointing arrows show the frication onsets and offsets, based on the last glottal pulse preceding and the first glottal pulse following the frication noise, respectively (Chapter 10). The /s/ and /f/ durations are 174 ms and 154 ms, respectively.

The intensity difference between the sibilant /s/ and nonsibilant /f/ is represented in the spectrogram by the much darker frication noise for /s/. Note in the superimposed spectra the overall higher level of /s/ compared with /f/. This kind of intensity difference is consistent for any sibilant-nonsibilant comparison, such as the /ʃ/ versus /θ/ comparison.

Behrens and Blumstein (1988) reported a typical intensity difference of 14 dB between voiceless sibilant and nonsibilant frication noises. Data reported by Jongman, Wayland, and Wong (2000) suggest a slightly smaller difference of about 9 to 10 dB. The sibilant-nonsibilant intensity difference applies to voiced fricatives (e.g., /z/ vs. /v/, or /ʒ/ vs. /ð/) as well, but the difference is probably not as great as in the case of voiceless fricatives (see Jongman et al., 2000, Table V, p. 1259). The higher intensity for sibilants compared with nonsibilants is largely due to the presence of an obstacle, the teeth, in the path of the airstream emerging from the fricative constriction. As discussed in Chapter 9, the airstream striking the teeth creates a second acoustic source and boosts the overall energy of the source spectrum for sibilants. The nonsibilants /f,θ,v,ð/ are produced with little or no obstacle in front of the constriction, and, therefore, have a weaker source spectrum than sibilants.

The difference in sibilant versus nonsibilant spectra is also appreciated by studying superimposed spectra of fricatives from the two categories. The /f/ and /s/ spectra in Figure 11–21 differ by the prominence of their peaks. The /s/ spectrum has two distinct, intense peaks, one around 4.3 kHz and the other just above 5.0 kHz. Both peaks are roughly 35 dB more intense than the lowest amplitude in the /s/ spectrum. In contrast, the /f/ spectrum has its greatest peaks just above 9.0 kHz and just below 10.0 kHz, roughly 30 dB more intense than the lowest energy in its spectrum (close to 0 kHz). The /f/ spectrum is flatter than the /s/ spectrum (or the /s/ spectrum can be described as "peakier" than the /f/ spectrum). Sibilants typically have peakier spectra than nonsibilants, as shown in Figure 11–22 for the /ʃ/-/θ/ (left) and /z/-/v/ (right) contrasts.

Quantification of Fricative Spectra

As discussed in Chapter 9, quantification of the frequency characteristics of fricative spectra is not straightforward. Fricative spectra have sometimes been characterized with a single number, the peak fre-

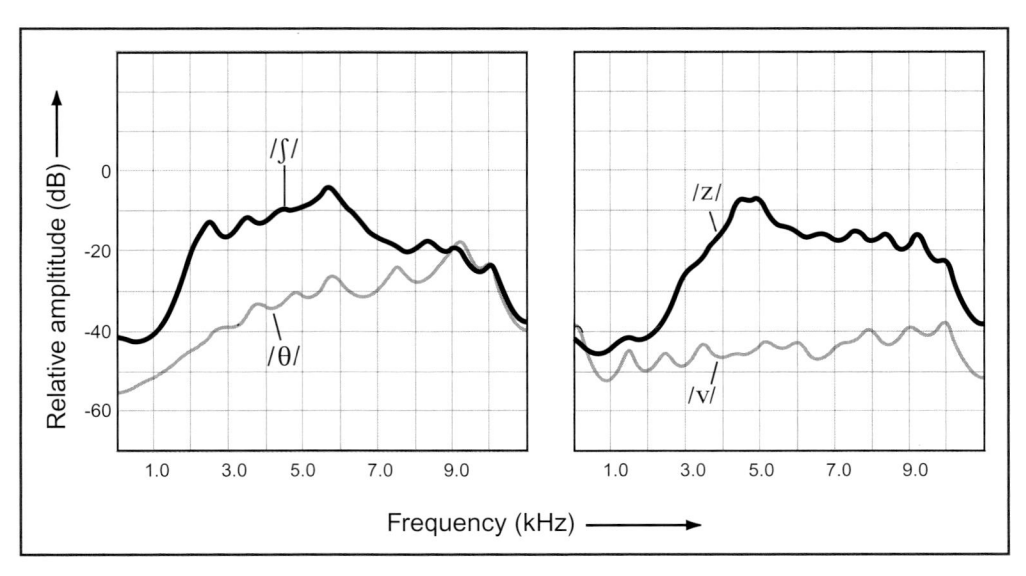

Figure 11-22. *Left panel:* LPC spectra for /θ/ (*light trace*) and /ʃ/ (*dark trace*). *Right panel:* LPC spectra for /v/ (*light trace*) and /z/ (*dark trace*). All fricatives were produced in a VCV frame where V = /ɛ/. Spectra were computed from the middle 50 ms of the frication noise.

quency, defined as the frequency in the spectrum with maximum amplitude. For example, in Figure 11–22 the peak frequency for /ʃ/ is roughly 5.8 kHz, for /θ/ 9.2 kHz, for /z/ 4.5 to 5.0 kHz (there is a broad peak spanning this frequency range), and for /v/ 10.0 kHz. Jongman et al. (2000) reported that the simple measurement of peak frequency *statistically* distinguished fricative place of articulation when data were averaged across 20 speakers. The average, peak frequencies obtained by Jongman et al. for the four places of English fricative articulation are shown in Table 11–3. These peaks decrease in frequency as place of articulation moves back in the vocal tract. As discussed in Chapter 9, this is consistent with consonant theory because the primary resonance of the vocal tract in fricative production derives from the cavity in front of the constriction. The size of this cavity increases as the place of articulation becomes more posterior. Larger resonators mean lower resonant frequencies.

The match between Jongman et al.'s (2000) peak frequency data and speech acoustic theory should be approached with a certain degree of caution. The data, averaged across male and female speakers and vowel contexts, do not capture the substantial variation in spectral details from repetition to repetition for a given speaker, and across different speakers. One of these details is the location of the peak frequency. In Figure 11–22, for example, the peak frequency of one of the author's /ʃ/ spectra (left panel) is approximately 1000 Hz higher than that of his /z/ spectrum (right panel).

Table 11–3. Average Peak Frequencies for Four Fricative Places of Articulation Reported by Jongman et al. (2000) for 20 Speakers Producing CVC Words in a Carrier Phrase

PLACE		PEAK FREQUENCY (Hz)
Labiodental	/f,v/	7733
Dental	/θ,ð/	7470
Alveolar	/s,z/	6839
Palatoalveolar	/ʃ,ʒ/	3820

Note. Data are for the first C in the CVC word. Peak frequencies were derived from spectra computed from the center 40 ms of the frication noise. Measurements were made from inspection of both FFT and LPC spectra.

Not only are these numbers inconsistent with the *direction* of the effect reported by Jongman et al., in which alveolar fricatives have higher peak frequencies compared with palate-alveolar fricatives,[11] but the actual values of the peak frequencies shown in Figure 11–22 are quite different from those listed in Table 11–3. For example, the peak frequency in Figure 11–22 for /ʃ/ is 5800 Hz, compared with the average for /ʃ/ and /ʒ/ of 3820 Hz reported by Jongman et al. (2000). Substantial intra- and interspeaker variation in fricative spectrum details has been described by Narayanan (1995). Peak frequency as a descriptor of fricative spectra may separate fricative place of articulation with statistical reliability across groups of speakers, but there is a great deal of error variation (unexplained data noise) in the statistical findings.

The measure "peak frequency" does not take advantage of a good deal of additional information in fricative spectra. For example, the fricative spectra in Figures 11–21 and 11–22 have varying shapes. Some seem to have energy "bunched up" in the middle (e.g., /ʃ/ and /z/), some have energy "tilted" to the right half of the spectrum (e.g., /f/ and /θ/), and some are nearly "flat" (e.g., /v/). These descriptions are based on the pattern of energy across all frequencies of the spectrum and go substantially past the limited information of a single frequency at which maximum energy occurs. As discussed in Chapter 9, the shape of a spectrum can be quantified using characteristics of statistical distributions. The amplitude-by-frequency information in the *entire* spectrum is used to generate four numbers that represent the spectral shape. These numbers are called *spectral moments*.

Spectral moments are the basic statistical properties of a distribution of numbers, applied to speech-sound spectra. A distribution has a mean, variance, skewness, and kurtosis. The mean is the average of all numbers in the distribution, the variance is the degree to which the numbers are dispersed about the mean, the skewness the degree of tilt of the distribution to the right or left of center, and kurtosis the extent to which the distribution is peaked or flat. When applied to speech spectra, mean = the first spectral moment (M1), variance = the second spectral moment (M2), skewness = the third spectral moment (M3), and kurtosis = the fourth spectral moment (M4).

The relationship of different distribution shapes—in the current case, spectral shapes—to number values is illustrated in Figure 11–23. At the top of the figure is

---

[11] The reversal of the direction expected from Jongman et al.'s (2000) data, and from speech acoustic theory, still holds even when the Figure 11–21 comparison is adjusted for mixing of place and voicing. Jongman et al. reported that voiced fricatives had somewhat lower peak frequencies than voiceless fricatives—about 300 Hz on average—but even when this is applied to the Figure 11–21 spectra, the peak frequency difference is still around 700 Hz, and in the wrong direction.

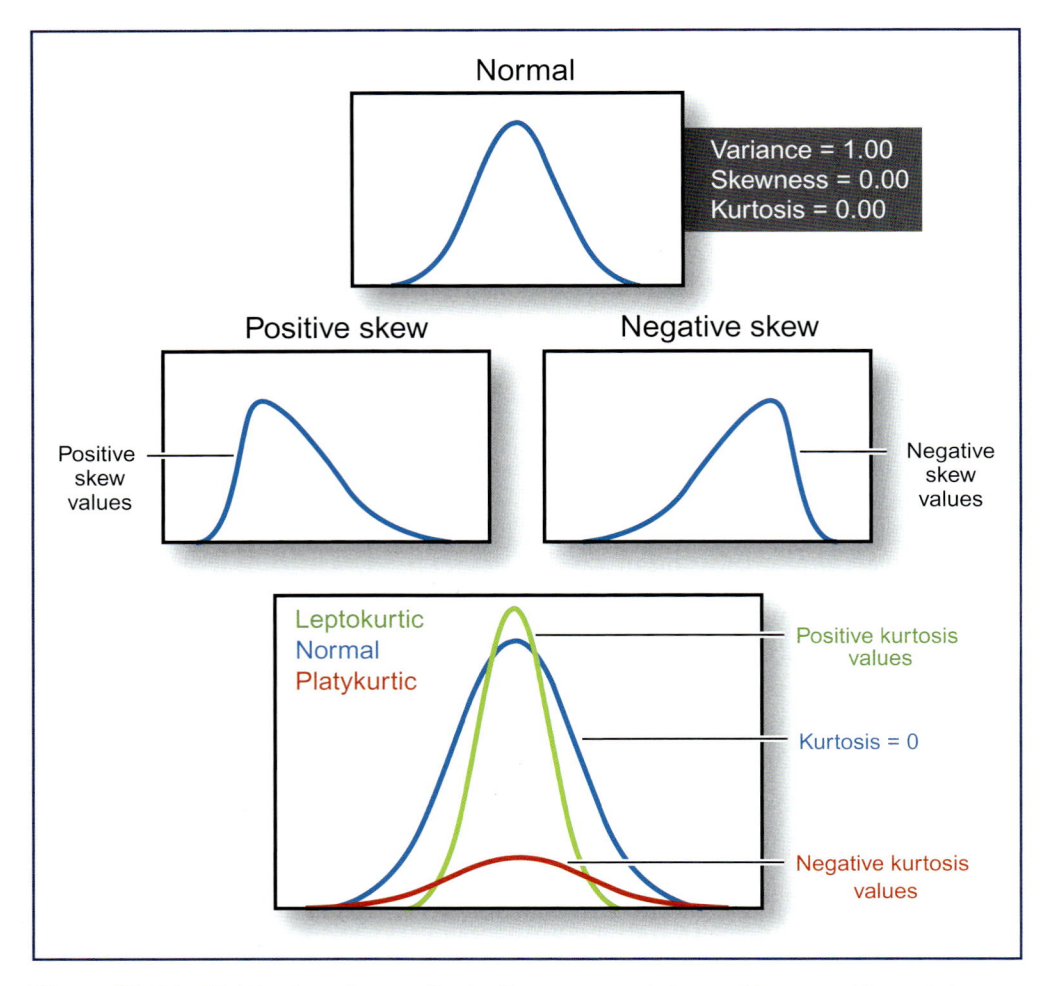

Figure 11–23. Distribution shapes illustrating a normal shape (*top graph*), and shapes showing skewness (*middle two graphs*), and kurtosis (*bottom graph*). Distributions with different variances are also illustrated in the bottom graph; see text for additional detail.

the symmetrical, normal distribution, typically described as having a mean of zero, a variance of one, and skewness and kurtosis values of zero. For present purposes, the normal distribution serves as a reference shape for other distribution shapes. The two distribution shapes immediately below the normal shape show positive (left shape) and negative (right shape) skewness. When the majority of numbers in a distribution are bunched to the left-hand side and the right-hand tail is relatively long, the value of skewness is positive. The opposite case, when numbers are bunched to the right-hand side and the left-hand tail is long, is associated with a negative value of skewness. From an acoustic phonetics perspective, the concentration of *vowel* energy in the low frequencies should produce positive skewness values. In contrast, a sound such as /s/ has the majority of energy in the higher frequencies (see the /s/ spectrum in Figure 11–21, and the discussion below of the pitfalls of spectral moments analysis) and, therefore, has a negative value of skewness.

Variations in the "peakiness" of a distribution are illustrated in the bottom panel of Figure 11–23, with the normal distribution reproduced in blue. A distribution with a more pronounced peak than normal, shown by the green curve, has a positive value of kurtosis. A shallower peak than normal, shown in red in Figure 11–23, has a negative value of kurtosis. A comparison of the /v/ and /z/ spectra in the right-hand side of Figure 11–22 provides a good contrast in kurtosis values. The /v/ spectrum is flat and has a negative kurtosis, whereas the /z/ spectrum has distinct peaks and a substantially more positive kurtosis.

The second spectral moment, variance, can be explained by considering the kurtosis shapes in the bottom panel of Figure 11–23. The very peaky distribution shown in green has its values "bunched up" near the center. This distribution has a low value of variance. In contrast, the relatively flat distribution in red has values spread across a wider range, which is associated with a higher value of variance. The /z/-/v/ spectrum comparison in Figure 11–22 shows the difference between a distribution having many values "bunched" toward the center (/z/) versus values spread across a wider range (/v/). The /v/ spectrum is expected to have a larger variance than the /z/ spectrum.

Scientists have been interested in spectral moments for fricatives as a way to supplement the peak frequency approach to quantifying fricative spectra. Early publications presenting qualitative analyses of fricative spectra (Hughes & Halle, 1956) suggested spectral shape as one possible distinguishing characteristic of fricative place of articulation. Forrest, Weismer, Milenkovic, and Dougall (1988) performed a spectral moments analysis of the four English voiceless fricatives (/f,θ,s,ʃ/) to classify place of articulation. This experiment was performed not only to determine if the moments were effective in separating the four fricatives from each other (therefore demonstrating that spectral shape was an important characteristic of fricative acoustics), but to identify which moment(s) played the primary role in successful classification. Forrest et al. found that sibilants were classified by the moments more accurately than nonsibilants, but overall the four voiceless fricatives were classified correctly only about 50% of the time. The poor classification results were attributed primarily to the frequent confusions of /f/ and /θ/ spectra. When sibilant spectra were classified incorrectly, it was often as one of the nonsibilants. Because the nonsibilant fricatives are so much less intense than the sibilants, the classification results may have been improved by the inclusion of intensity as a variable in addition to the four moments.

Jongman et al. (2000) obtained spectral moments for all English fricatives produced by men and women in a variety of vowel contexts. Their moments data, averaged across speakers and vowels, are reproduced in Table 11–4. The data for the first moment (M1), given in units of Hz, are consistent with the theoretical discussion of fricative acoustics presented in Chapter 9.[12] M1 is nearly 2000 Hz higher for /s,z/ compared with /ʃ,ʒ/, reflecting the difference in size of the resonator in front of the fricative constriction. The nearly identical M1 values for /f,v/ and /θ,ð/ are consistent with the absence of a resonating cavity in front of the constrictions for nonsibilants. The M1s for /f,v,θ,ð/ are located roughly in the center of the analyzed frequency band (approximately 1–11,000 Hz). In the absence of a resonating cavity to shape the source spectrum, nonsibilant output (source × filter) spectra often resemble the aperiodic source spectra (see Chapter 9), which are relatively flat. The flatness of the spectrum explains why the M1s are so close to 5000 Hz, close to the center frequency of the analysis band.[13]

Table 11-4. Spectral Moments Data for Fricatives

	M1	M2	M3	M4
/f,v/	5108	6.37	0.007	2.11
/θ,ð/	5137	6.19	−0.083	1.27
/s,z/	6133	2.92	−0.229	2.36
/ʃ,ʒ/	4229	3.38	0.693	0.42

Note. M1 = mean, M2 = variance, M3 = skewness, M4 = kurtosis. M1 values are in Hz, M2 values in MHz, and M3 and M4 values have no units (they are dimensionless, having been normalized). See Forrest et al. (1988) for computational details.

Source: Data from Jongman et al. (2000, Table I, p. 1257).

The M2 values listed in Table 11–4 also contrast the nonsibilants with sibilants. Sibilant spectra have much smaller variances than nonsibilant spectra, which follows from the tendency of sibilant spectra to be peaky and nonsibilant spectra to be flat.

The M3 data show a dramatic contrast between /s,z/ and /ʃ,ʒ/, the former having negative skewness, the latter positive skewness. This skewness contrast can be seen by comparing the /z/-/ʃ/ spectra displayed in Figure 11–22. The peaks for the palato-alveolar /ʃ/ are pushed to the lower-frequency, left-hand side of the spectrum, compared with the higher-frequency peaks of the alveolar /z/. The /z/ spectrum is tilted more to the right than the /ʃ/ spectrum, hence the negative skew value for /z/ relative to the positive skew value for /ʃ/. The M3 values for /f,v,θ,ð/ are very close to zero, consistent with the flatness of their spectra.

---

[12] Although the mean of a normal distribution is zero, computation of the first spectral moment is based on frequency (Hz) and is not normalized like the zero mean of the normal distribution. M1 is computed by taking each frequency in the analysis band and weighting it by its amplitude. Thus, frequencies with greater amplitude are given more weight than frequencies with lesser amplitude in determining the M1 value of the spectrum. M1 can be interpreted as the primary energy concentration within the spectrum.

[13] Spectral moments are calculated within fixed frequency bands; the end frequencies of the moments reported in Table 11–4 are 1 Hz on the low end, and 11,000 Hz on the high end. The width of the band can be varied in whatever way an investigator desires, but is typically dictated by the sampling rate and the low-pass filter cutoff frequency used when digitizing speech waveforms (Chapter 10). For example, the moments reported in Table 11–4 (Jongman et al., 2000) were derived from waveforms sampled at 22,000 Hz and filtered with a cutoff frequency of 11,000 Hz.

In contrast to the values of the first three moments, values for M4 (kurtosis) reported by Jongman et al. (2000) are less easy to connect with known or expected characteristics of fricative spectra. The M4 values in Table 11–4 suggest that /f,v/ spectra are peakier than /ʃ,ʒ/ spectra, which is at odds with the large resonance peaks observed around 2000 to 4000 Hz for /ʃ,ʒ/ compared with the flattened spectra of /f,v/.

Some time has been spent explaining spectral moments and reviewing the relationship of values reported by Jongman et al. (2000) to spectral characteristics of exemplar fricatives presented in Figures 11–21 and 11–22, as well as characteristics expected from theoretical considerations. Spectral moments are a popular way to quantify fricative and stop-burst spectra. Most speech analysis programs, such as the one used to generate the spectrograms and spectra shown in this chapter, include algorithms to compute moments or similar measures. There are, however, three problems with spectral moments to keep in mind when the measures are used as acoustic indices of fricative (or stop) production. First, the values of the moments are quite variable across different studies, and highly variable within and across speakers within a study. The intraspeaker variation is underscored in a study by Haley, Seelinger, Mandulak, and Zajac (2010), who reported ranges of the first moment (the mean) across multiple repetitions of /s/. Six of their 10 speakers had mean ranges across repetitions of 2.0 kHz or more. Intraspeaker ranges were not quite as great for /ʃ/ but were still large—at least 1.0 kHz. This is a remarkable (and somewhat disheartening) finding, that an automated analysis produces such variation in a single measurement even when the same speaker repeats the same fricative over multiple repetitions. Alternatively, the fluctuation in M1 may reflect small differences in the articulation of /s/ from repetition to repetition, or across speakers. As suggested by Haley et al., spectral moments may be of greatest value when used to contrast closely related sounds such as /s/ and /ʃ/, rather than to describe single sounds. These are important considerations because spectral moments have been applied to the speech acoustic characteristics of consonants produced by persons with speech disorders (for developmental sound errors, see McAllister Byun, Buchwald, & Mizoguchi, 2016; for motor speech disorders, see Tjaden & Martel-Sauvageau, 2017; for speech of children with cochlear implants, see Yang, Vadlamudi, Zin, Lee, & Xu, 2017). For moments data from speaker without speech disorders, see Fox and Nissan (2005), Jongman et al. (2000), Newman, Clouse, and Burnham (2001), Tabain (2001), Tabain, Butcher, Breen, and Breare (2016), and Tjaden and Turner (1997), to gain a sense of the cross-study variation in these measures.

Second, although moments quantify a lot of information in fricative spectra, they have not been successful in classifying fricative place of articulation. Forrest et al. (1988), Fox and Nissan (2005), and Jongman et al. (2000) all obtained the same results when classifying fricatives with moments (and some other variables). Typically, correct classification rates are about 90% for sibilants but only 60 to 70% for nonsibilants.[14] If spectral moments were the most inclusive and best way to represent fricative spectra, better classification rates would be obtained.

The third problem with spectral moments involves two interrelated problems. One problem is the tendency for high intercorrelations among the moments, suggesting a lack of independence of the different measures. For example, because spectral moments are computed from a fixed analysis band, an M1 (spectral mean) of higher frequency is likely to have a more negative M3 (skewness). Stated otherwise, as the concentration of energy is "pushed" to the right of the analysis band (higher M1, as in /s/) the spectrum is tilted more to the right (more negative M3). Similarly, a more positive M4 (kurtosis), reflecting a spectrum in which there are very prominent peaks, likely has a smaller M2 (variance) because the energy is concentrated in a small frequency range (see bottom graph of Figure 11–23). The extent to which the moments are intercorrelated has not been reported in the literature in a formal, large-scale analysis, but speech scientists who have used the analysis are aware of this issue.

The related problem is a lack of uniqueness between the numbers obtained in a moments analysis and the actual shape of the observed spectrum. To understand this issue, consider the following thought experiment. A speech scientist is shown a list of formant frequencies in which each row consists of F1, F2, and F3 values. Based on these three formant frequencies, the speech scientist is asked to identify a vowel category. For example, the values F1 = 310, F2 = 2000, and F3 = 2800 would most likely be assigned the vowel category /i/.

---

[14] The frequent confusions in classification experiments between /f/ and /θ/ and /v/ and /ð/ are due to the similarity of their spectra and their weak intensity. Sounds that are not easily distinguished, or in the language of phoneticians, that do not meet a reasonable criterion of acoustic contrast, are often merged over time and lose their contrastive value. In English, for example, there are many dialects where the /ɪ/-/ɛ/ distinction is not made, or perhaps made not in a way easily perceptible. In southern Indiana, for example, one both writes with a [pɪn] "pen" and wears a [pɪn] "pin"). A similar merger seems to be occurring between the labiodental and dental fricatives in African-American English, where forms such as [bof] "both" and [bɝfdeɪ] "birthday" are commonly heard (Craig, Thompson, Washington, & Potter, 2003). It is reasonable to assume the merger is being "provoked," in part, by the lack of discriminability between these sounds.

This is a fairly easy task for a person with experience in acoustic phonetics. Now, assume a similar experiment with the four spectral moments, the speech scientist's task being to select the most likely fricative category, or to draw the approximate spectral shape based on the numbers. This is a daunting task for even the most seasoned expert. The difficulty of the task derives from the lack of independence of the moment values, as described above, and because a specific moment value can be associated with very different spectral shapes.

These cautionary comments are not meant to negate the use of moments in the quantification of fricative (or affricate or stop) spectra. Spectral moments probably capture more information about a fricative spectrum than a peak frequency measure, and for certain distinctions, such as /s/-/ʃ/, seem to function well. M1, in particular, is an excellent estimate of the peak frequency of *some* fricative spectra, especially those of the lingual fricatives /s,z,ʃ,ʒ/ that tend to be relatively peaky. A claim has been made for /s/ spectra that M1 and the measurement of a single peak frequency produce essentially the same result (Iskarous, Shadle, & Proctor, 2011), but the underlying data are not shown, and even if true, the claim may not be applicable to analysis of other fricatives. Spectral moments are potentially valuable measures, but care should be taken in their use and interpretation, and their relations to other measures of fricative spectra.

Formant Transitions and Fricative Distinctions

In the earlier section on nasal acoustics, the role of formant transitions at the release (CV) or onset (VC) of the nasal murmur was discussed as an acoustic correlate of place of articulation. Interest in formant transitions as a reliable marker of place of articulation for fricatives has been driven by concerns with the lack of a consistent distinction in fricative *spectra* between /f,v/ and /θ,ð/. The fricative spectra of /s,z/ are sufficiently different from the spectra for /ʃ,ʒ/, /f,v/ and /θð/ to serve as reliable cues to place of articulation, but some other part (or parts) of the acoustic signal must contain the information to distinguish labiodentals from dental nonsibilants.[15] In an early experiment on fricative perception, Harris (1958) showed that the primary cue for the labiodental-dental distinction (/f/ vs. /θ/, or /v/ vs. /ð/) was the pattern of formant transitions at the release of the fricative. This idea has been accepted in the speech science community for many years, even in the absence of supporting data from acoustic measurements of speaker productions. As reviewed by Jongman et al. (2000), the evidence for the importance of formant transitions in distinguishing place of articulation for nonsibilant fricatives is mixed. Jongman et al. failed to identify formant transition patterns that consistently separated the four places of fricative articulation, including the critical labiodental-dental distinction.

The Ultimate Social Consequence

The literature on speech sound development makes frequent reference to the negative social consequences faced by children who have speech sound errors. These are important, but none results in such extreme punishment as was meted out for an /s/-/ʃ/ confusion to the Ephramites of biblical fame. As told in the Book of Judges in the Old Testament, a battle between the Gileadites and Ephramites resulted in the passages of Jordan being held by the Gileadites. Ephramites who desired safe passage were required to pass a verbal screening test that revealed whether or not they were friend or foe. Chapter 12, verse 6 says, "Then said they unto him, Say now Shibboleth: and he said Sibboleth: for he could not frame to pronounce it right. Then they took him, and slew him at the passages of Jordan." Verse 6 goes on to say that 42,000 fell at the time. There is no record of how many went because their speech revealed them to be foe. The concept of a specific utterance that marks a person's geographical home was borrowed from this biblical story for the TIMIT (Texas Instruments/MIT) speech database, a huge collection of utterances from many different speakers, carefully transcribed and recorded for research use by speech scientists. The dialect group of the speakers in this database is revealed by two "shibboleth sentences," designed to be phonetically sensitive to dialect variation around the United States.

---

[15]Most spectral analyses of frication noises have been confined to a highest frequency of 10.0 to 11.0 kHz, so there is always the possibility that /f,v/ can be distinguished from /θ,ð/ on the basis of spectral features above 10 kHz. Tabain (1998) examined just this hypothesis for speakers of Australian English and found no evidence for consistent spectral distinctions between the labiodental and dental fricatives in the frequency region above 10.0 kHz.

Fricative Duration

The literature on fricative duration has produced a fair amount of agreement on some basic facts. First, voiceless fricatives are longer than voiced fricatives, all other things being equal. This qualifier is important, because such factors as position-in-word (e.g., /ʃæk/ "shack" versus /kæʃ/ "cash"), stress level of the syllable in which the fricative occurs, speaking rate, immediate phonetic context (e.g., /sæk/ "sack" versus /stæk/ "stack"), among other variables, modify the duration of a fricative segment. Second, among the voiceless fricatives and possibly also voiced fricatives, sibilants have slightly greater duration than nonsibilants.

Figure 11–24 is a spectrogram of the syntactically well-formed but semantically curious utterance "Two scenes at the zoo failed to verify the shame." This utterance was constructed to illustrate fricative duration measures. Precise measures of fricative duration were made using TF32 (Milenkovic, 2001), guided by the segmentation rules presented in Chapter 10. The durations for the eight fricatives marked in Figure 11–24 are provided in the caption. Fricative onsets and offsets are marked by arrows at the spectrogram baseline, and a horizontal bar connecting the base of the arrows shows the duration (solid lines = voiceless fricatives; dotted lines = voiced fricatives). The two voiceless sibilant durations (/s/ = 165 ms, /ʃ/ = 162 ms) are clearly a good deal longer than the voiceless nonsibilants (/f/ = 114 ms; /f/ = 130 ms). And although one /z/ (in "zoo") has a duration of 127 ms, each of the other three voiced fricatives have durations less than 100 ms. Even these single examples of fricatives, in a connected-speech utterance (compared with citation forms; see below) with variation in phonetic context and stress level, show patterns of duration largely consistent with the generalizations noted above. Voiceless fricatives are longer than voiced fricatives, sibilants are longer than nonsibilants.

A summary of published fricative duration data is provided in Table 11–5. Consideration of these data does not contradict the two generalizations about fricative duration, but it does show that the magnitude of the voiceless/voiced and sibilant/nonsibilant difference varies a good deal across studies. For example, among the three studies in which both /s/ and /ʃ/

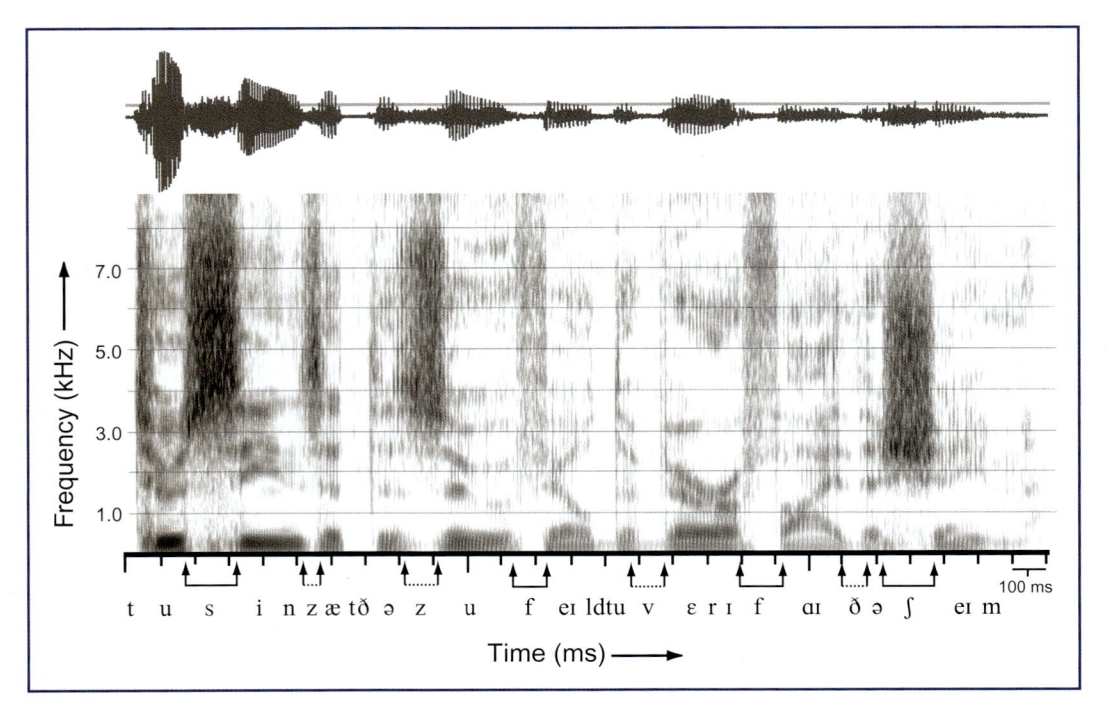

Figure 11–24. Spectrogram of the utterance "Two scenes at the zoo failed to verify the shame," constructed to show aspects of fricative duration. Eight fricatives in the utterance have been marked for duration; from left to right the fricative durations (all in milliseconds) are /s/ = 165; /z/ = 59; /z/ = 127; /f/ = 114; /v/ = 88; /f/ = 130; /ð/ = 71; and /ʃ/ = 162 (the /ð/ in /t ð ə/ ("at the") was not measured because the preceding stop makes it impossible to locate the /ð/ onset). Solid horizontal bars connecting the onset and offset arrows are for voiceless fricatives, dotted bars for voiced fricatives.

Table 11–5. Selected Fricative Durations from Sources in the Literature

	/f/	/v/	/θ/	/ð/	/s/	/z/	/ʃ/	/ʒ/
Umeda[a]	122	78	119		129	85	118	85
Baum & Blumstein[b]	149	116	134	107	174	152		
Behrens & Blumstein[c]	149		134		174		175	
Crystal & House[d]			72	41				
Jongman et al.[e]	166	80	163	88	178	118	178	123

Note. All data are for prestressed (fricatives preceding stressed vowels) fricatives, and are reported in milliseconds.
[a]Umeda (1977); $N = 1$ speaker, connected speech (reading).
[b]Baum & Blumstein (1987); $N = 3$ speakers, citation form syllables.
[c]Behrens & Blumstein (1988); $N = 3$ speakers, citation form syllables.
[d]Crystal & House (1988d); $N = 6$ speakers, connected speech (reading).
[e]Jongman et al. (2000); $N = 20$ speakers, citation form syllables.

were compared with /f/ and /θ/ durations (Behrens & Blumstein, 1988; Jongman et al., 2000; Umeda, 1977), only one (Behrens & Blumstein, 1988) reported findings supporting a decisive difference between sibilant and nonsibilant durations. The difference is slightly more convincing for the voiced sibilant-nonsibilant difference. Similarly, the difference in fricative duration for voiceless versus voiced stops is quite large in some studies (Jongman et al., 2000) and more subtle in others (Baum & Blumstein, 1987).

Two questions arise from this review of fricative duration. First, are there good explanations for the two general effects identified above? Is there a straightforward reason why sibilants would be longer than nonsibilants, and voiceless fricatives longer than voiced fricatives? Second, why do fricative duration values, and the magnitude of the sibilant-nonsibilant and voicing effects vary so much across studies?

Explanations for the effects are tentative but may reveal something about the relationship of fricative duration measures to underlying speech physiology. More specifically, the process of making the measurements from acoustic records may explain part or all of the effects. For example, the longer duration of sibilants, compared with nonsibilants, may reflect the longer-duration, turbulent noise sources for sibilants. Sibilants have more intense frication noise than nonsibilants largely because of the obstacle (teeth) effect. Perhaps the turbulent source is not only stronger, but also active over a longer period of time for /s,z,ʃ,ʒ/ compared with /f,v,θ,ð/. This may be a reasonable explanation when scientists use the onset and offset of *frication noise* as the criterion for marking the bound-

---

The World of Fricatives and Other Fricative-Centric Matters

A textbook cannot cover everything, so here is a short list of fricative issues we are not presenting. We're dispensing with references here: the reader can confirm the list provided here by typing "fricatives" into a database search engine, allowing waves of fricative acoustic research to flow and wash and surge and crash over them. (1) Fricatives have been studied in many languages, including (at least) Bantu, Catalan, American English, French, German, Greek, Italian, Japanese, and Mandarin; (2) Fricatives have been studied across development in young children, also in many languages; (3) Fricatives have been studied for their sensitivity to phonetic context; (4) Fricatives have been studied in many speech disorders, including dysarthria, speech sound disorders, cleft palate, and in persons with cochlear implants; and (5) fricatives have been studied with mechanical and computer-modeling techniques. An intimidating list.

aries of a fricative duration (e.g., Baum & Blumstein, 1987; Behrens & Blumstein, 1988; Jongman et al., 2000). The possible impact of this approach is illustrated by the subtle case shown in Figure 11–25, which shows two VCVs spoken by one of the authors with V = /ɑ/ and C = /θ/ (left) and /ʃ/ (right). Every attempt was made to produce these VCVs at the same rate and with stress on the second syllable. The vertical lines mark off the frication interval, defined by the onset (left line) and offset (right line) of the visible frication noise. When the measurements are made with maximal time expansion of the spectrographic display (to provide the best temporal resolution), the frication intervals of /θ/ and /ʃ/ were 114 and 124 ms, respectively. This difference is consistent with the sibilant-nonsibilant duration difference reported by Umeda (1977) and Jongman et al. If the duration of the frication noise is taken to reflect directly the duration of the fricative articulatory configuration, data shown in Table 11–5 and Figure 11–25 suggest that sibilants are longer than nonsibilants.

Fricative durations measured from spectrographic or waveform displays, however, may not capture the entire duration over which a fricative configuration is maintained. Turbulent airflow, the source of aperiodic energy seen in acoustic displays of fricatives, occurs when airflow of sufficient magnitude is driven through a sufficiently narrow constriction or strikes an edge of a sharp object. It is easy to imagine a situation in which a fricative configuration is maintained but aperiodic energy either is not generated or is of such weak intensity as to be undetected in a spectrographic or waveform display. For example, the lingual nonsibilants /θ/ and /ð/ have broad, loose constrictions (Tabain, 2001), which are often not sufficiently tight to generate turbulence, even though the fricative configuration is produced. Moreover, the conditions under which such loose constrictions occur may be more likely at the onset and offset of the fricative, when the constriction is being formed and released, respectively.

One way to address the possible mismatch of onset and offset of frication noise versus onset and offset of fricative *configuration* is to measure fricative durations from the last glottal pulse preceding the frication noise to the first glottal pulse following the noise. From an articulatory point of view, this makes sense because the last glottal pulse preceding frication is often timed to coincide with the onset of the supraglottal constriction (see review in Weismer, 2006 and below). In Figure 11–25, /θ/ and /ʃ/ durations measured with the glottal pulse criterion (boundaries marked by upward-pointing arrows) are 130 and 133 ms, respectively. Weismer (1980), using the glottal pulse criterion to measure fricative durations for nine speakers, reported average, citation-form durations for /f/, /s/, and /ʃ/ of 180, 189, and 182 ms, respectively. These means were statistically indistinguishable from each other.

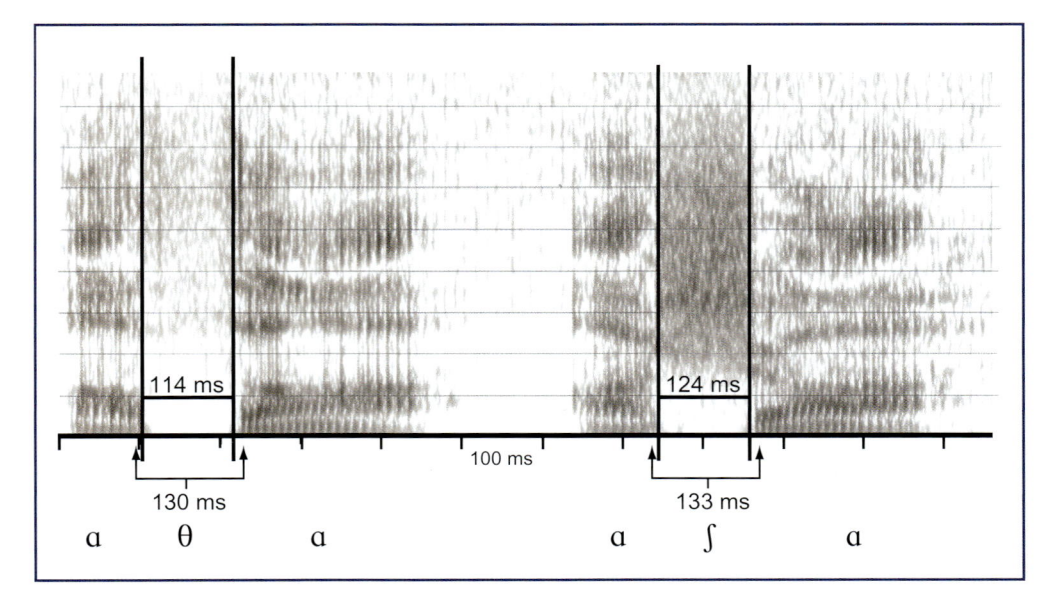

Figure 11–25. Spectrograms of the utterances /ɑθɑ/ (*left*) and /ɑʃɑ/ (*right*), illustrating the measurement of fricative duration under two criteria, one where the onsets and offsets of frication noise define the segment boundaries (*vertical lines running the length of the spectrogram*), the other where the preceding and following glottal pulses define the segment boundaries (*upward-pointing arrows*).

These considerations are offered to the reader in the spirit of an interesting scientific problem, rather than an endorsement of one measurement approach relative to another. The scientific problem shows how a measurement decision may affect conclusions about underlying articulatory processes. This issue also shows how interpretation of acoustic data requires a good working knowledge of speech physiology. In the current case, the relevant physiology concerns the aeromechanics associated with fricative production.[16]

Laryngeal Devoicing Gesture and Fricative Duration

The second effect for fricative durations, of consistently longer voiceless compared with voiced fricatives, also requires a working knowledge of speech physiology. Data in Table 11–5 from Umeda (1977) and Jongman et al. (2000) suggest that voiceless fricatives in the prestressed position (in a CV or VCV frame where the vowel following the fricative is stressed) are nearly twice the duration of voiced fricatives. Why should there be such a large difference between the durations of cognate fricatives? The answer is likely found in the different laryngeal behavior for voiceless versus voiced fricatives.

Voiceless fricatives require the laryngeal devoicing gesture (LDG), an opening-closing movement of the vocal folds observed in many languages for virtually all voiceless obstruents (e.g., Hirose, 1977; Löfqvist, 1980). The LDG differs from the opening-closing motions of the vocal folds during phonation in two important ways. First, the opening and closing movements of the LDG are produced under muscular control—the *posterior cricoarytenoid* muscle producing the opening, the *interarytenoid* (perhaps assisted by the *lateral cricoarytenoid*) the closing; the *cricothyroid* muscle may also be activated for the opening, to stiffen the folds and contribute to the cessation of phonation (Hirose, 1976; Löfqvist, Baer, McGarr, & Story, 1989). In contrast, the opening and closing movements during phonation are the result of aerodynamic and mechanical forces acting against the background forces exerted by laryngeal muscles (see Chapter 3). Second, the opening plus closing motions of the LDG produce a very long event compared with the short-duration opening and closing motions of a single cycle of vocal fold vibration. The LDG typically has a duration of roughly 120 to 150 ms, whereas an example of a "long" period for one phonatory cycle would be roughly 10 ms (for an F0 = 100 Hz, a rather low average speaking fundamental frequency). The long duration of the LDG is critical to understanding the relatively long duration of voiceless compared with voiced fricatives.

The laryngeal and supralaryngeal events shown schematically in Figure 11–26 for a VCV, where C = /f/, /θ/, /s/, or /ʃ/, explain the relatively long duration of voiceless fricatives. Laryngeal events are shown as a function of time on the line labeled Ag, or area of the glottis (see Chapter 8). These kinds of data are collected through an endoscope positioned directly above the vocal folds and connected to a recording device. The opening and closing motions of the vocal folds produce closely related variations in the area of the glottis (i.e., the area of the opening between the vocal folds). Upward deflections of the trace reflect opening of the vocal folds, downward deflections reflect closing of the vocal folds. The baseline represents full vocal fold approximation, such as occurs at the end of every phonatory cycle. The short duration cycles of opening-closing movements are the phonatory cycles associated with the vowels and the long-duration, larger opening-closing movement is the LDG. The time course of the LDG can be compared to events on the line labeled "Timing of fricative configuration." This is a schematic representation of the onset, duration, and offset of the grooved fricative configuration made by the tongue in contact with parts of the palate, or between the lower lip and upper teeth. This contact is shown as a raised box meant to represent the timing of the fricative configuration relative to the laryngeal events depicted on the top line. When the joint timing of laryngeal and supralaryngeal events is considered, the following conclusions can be drawn. First, the onset of the fricative configuration is synchronous with the onset of the LDG. Second, the offset of the fricative configuration, presumably when the fricative is released into the following vowel, occurs approximately at the same time as the return of the vocal folds to the phonation-ready position, the closed position that permits aerodynamic and mechanical forces to create repeated oscillations of the vocal folds for phonation. Third, the LDG exceeds 100 ms, as indicated by comparison of its duration to the time scale indicated above the trace. In Figure 11–26, the duration of the LDG is labeled as the "voiceless interval."

---

[16]There is, at least in theory, a simple answer to the problem posed here. When fricative configurations are evaluated *directly* (by electropalatography techniques, or perhaps x-ray or electromagnetic techniques), are sibilant configurations longer than nonsibilant configurations, all other things being equal? This seems to be a straightforward question that might have been answered over the last 60 years of speech research, but, in fact, an answer requires very precise technical tools and measurement decisions. This is a fancy way to say that the relevant experiment has not been done.

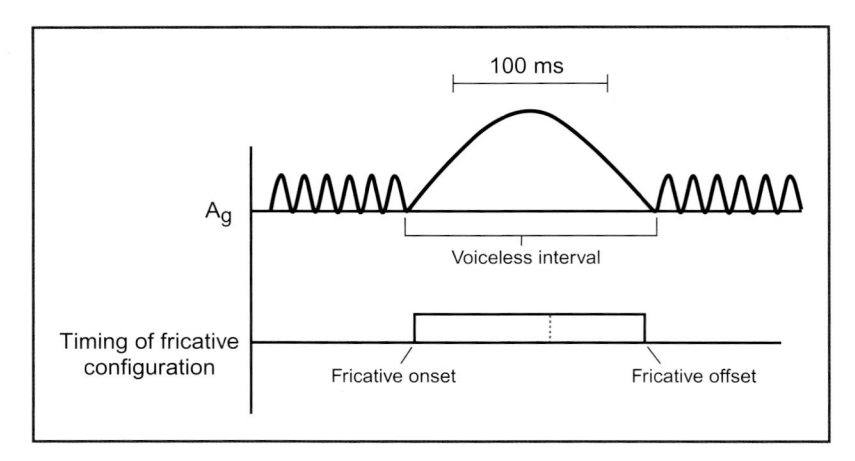

Figure 11–26. Schematic representation of laryngeal and supralaryngeal events for a VCV utterance in which C = a voiceless fricative. A_g = area of the glottis. Upward movement on this trace indicates opening motions of the vocal folds, downward movement closing motions of the folds. The short-duration cycles are phonatory motions of the folds, the long-duration motion is the LDG. Voiceless interval = the duration of the laryngeal devoicing gesture. "Timing of fricative configuration" indicates the onset, duration, and offset of the supralaryngeal configuration required for fricative production. See text for additional details.

The LDG appears to be executed as a programmed gesture for production of voiceless obstruents. "Programmed," as used in this context, means that once the gesture is initiated it follows a more or less fixed amplitude and time course. The gesture does not seem to be subject to precise voluntary control (Löfqvist, Baer, & Yoshioka, 1981), supporting the idea that its amplitude and duration are relatively fixed, at least for a given stress condition and speaking rate. If the LDG is implemented for production of a voiceless fricative and if its "programmed" duration is substantially in excess of 100 ms as shown in Figure 11–26, the duration over which the fricative configuration is maintained also must be in excess of 100 ms and, in fact, must nearly match the duration of the LDG. This is because an earlier release of the fricative, such as the point in time shown in Figure 11–26 by the dotted, vertical line, slightly past the most open point in time of the LDG, results in a substantial period of aspiration noise. The aspiration noise extends from the time of fricative release until the LDG brings the vocal folds back to midline in preparation for phonation. This is not desirable because aspiration noise following release of an English obstruent is a hallmark of voiceless stops, as well as the single voiceless affricate. An extended interval of aspiration noise following a fricative may result in misidentifications of fricatives as stops or affricates.

The duration of the supralaryngeal fricative configuration must be matched to the duration of the LDG—that is, to the voiceless interval duration. Because voiced fricatives are not produced with an LDG, their duration is not required to be so long. The duration of most voiced fricatives is in the neighborhood of 100 ms, and often 15 to 20 ms less.

/h/ ACOUSTICS

/h/ is often described as a glottal fricative because an aperiodic, continuant-type source is generated in and around the glottis. The glottis is partially or largely open during the production of /h/, and the aperiodic source is produced when the air jet emerging from the constriction between the vocal folds strikes the edges of the ventricular folds and epiglottis, generating turbulent airflow (Stevens, 1998, pp. 428–436). This is like the teeth-obstacle model presented above for fricatives /s/, /z/, /ʃ/, and /ʒ/, except in the case of /h/ the obstacles are structures immediately above the vocal folds.

The source-filter acoustics for /h/ are complex (Stevens, 1998). Here, /h/ acoustics are summarized in a few major points with reference to spectrograms of the utterances "Ohio" (/ohaɪjo/) and /əˈhɛ/ (Figure 11–27). In both utterances, /h/ is in the intervocalic position, and the approximate onsets and offsets of the /h/-intervals are indicated by upward-pointing arrows at the spectrographic baseline. The /h/-interval contains aperiodic energy, as expected when the

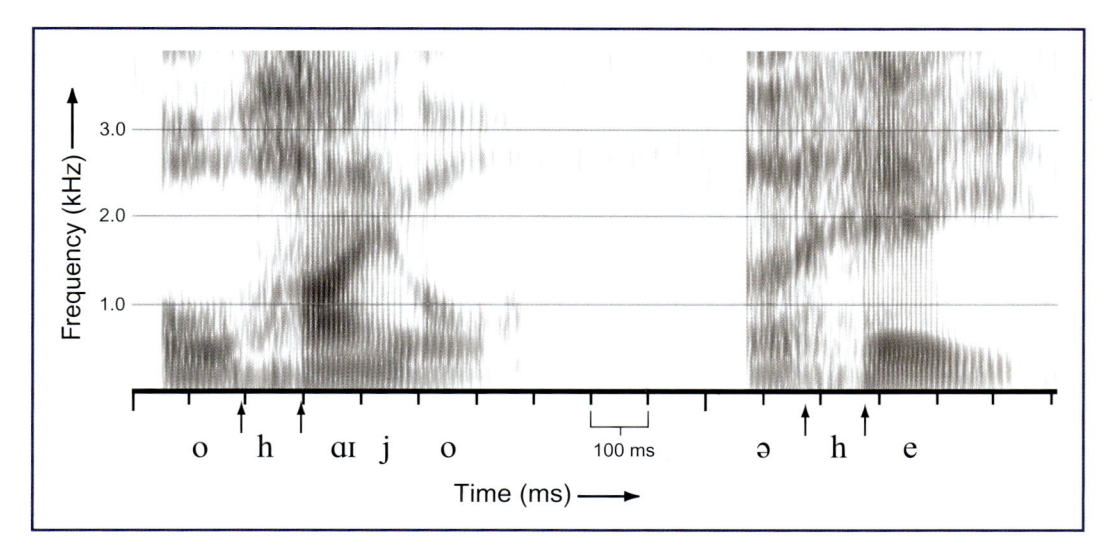

Figure 11-27. Spectrograms of the utterances /ohaɪjo/ (*left*) and /əˈhɛ/ (*right*), illustrating the acoustics of /h/. The onsets and offsets of the /h/ interval are indicated by upward-pointing arrows.

sound source is the result of turbulent airflow. Careful examination of the /h/-intervals indicates evidence of relatively weak glottal pulses—compared with the pulses in the surrounding vowels—mixed in with the noise. Intervocalic /h/ often has a combination of aperiodic and weak, periodic energy, suggesting that the abducted vocal folds are vibrating loosely, with minimal or absent closed phases (Ladefoged, 2005).

Formants can be detected during the /h/-intervals. These regions of dark, aperiodic-plus-voicing energy line up with the formants of the following (and to some extent, preceding) vowel (Robb & Chen, 2009). This makes sense under the assumption that /h/ is produced with the vocal tract shape of the surrounding vowel(s), except with a largely aperiodic source.

Perhaps this is why Ladefoged (2005, p. 58) described /h/ as a "noisy vowel." The most complete treatment of the formant structure of /h/-intervals is found in Lehiste (1964, pp. 141–180).

A dramatic feature of this noisy, formant-bearing interval is the relative weakness of energy around F1 compared with the much more intense energy of the upper formants. This intensity difference is shown for both /h/s in Figure 11–27. The weak energy in the F1 region of the /h/ noise is the result of sound absorption in the trachea. Interestingly, this fact explains why a person with a breathy voice may also suffer intelligibility problems as a result of indistinct vowels. The loss of F1 energy resulting from vocal fold vibration in which there is poor closure, a physiological correlate

Survival of the Phonetic Fittest

Speech and language are constantly changing, always evolving. This is the case in phonetics, where "strong" phonetic segments maintain their contrastive identity, weak phonetic segments do not. In Chapter 9 and footnote 14 of the current chapter the ongoing merger of the /f/-/θ/ contrast in African American English was cited as one such case. /h/ qualifies as phonetically "weak" for the same reason as /f/ and /θ/—it has very low amplitude. The sound is, therefore, subject to possible disappearance from sound inventories or deletion in connected speech. The weak energy of /h/ gives it poor survival potential due to low audibility and especially in noisy or difficult communication settings. Mielke (2003) reported an experiment in which Turkish speakers deleted /h/ at fast speaking rates, but only in phonetic environments where the /h/ energy was most likely to be extremely weak and hard to perceive. It is almost as if speakers recognized the phonetic conditions in which /h/ was likely not to be heard, and took advantage of this knowledge by deleting the sound production from their utterances. /h/ deletion is common in other languages as well, the best known example being Cockney English (Norman, 1973).

of breathy voice, may contribute in a significant way to loss of vowel distinctiveness. The effect of a breathy voice on communication may, therefore, be more than just a voice problem. The effect may extend to segmental (acoustic) integrity and, as noted above, speech intelligibility.

STOPS

Stop consonants enjoy a special status in speech acoustics. Their acoustic characteristics have been the subject of much study and debate, and their role in the perception of speech has a very long and contentious history. Stops are also attractive for acoustic-phonetic study because they are the only consonant type to occur in virtually *all* languages of the world (Ladefoged & Maddieson, 1996). Within languages, stops are among the most frequently occurring consonant segments (Maddieson, 1997).

Spectrograms illustrating the basic properties of stop consonants are shown in Figure 11–28. The stops /t/ and /d/ are shown in V'CV frames, where V = /ɑ/. The upper spectrograms show the stops produced with stress on the second syllable (/ɑ'tɑ/, /ɑ'dɑ/), whereas the lower spectrograms show stops with stress on the first syllable (/'ɑtɑ/, /'ɑdɑ/). The frequency range for these spectrograms is roughly 0 to 8.5 kHz.

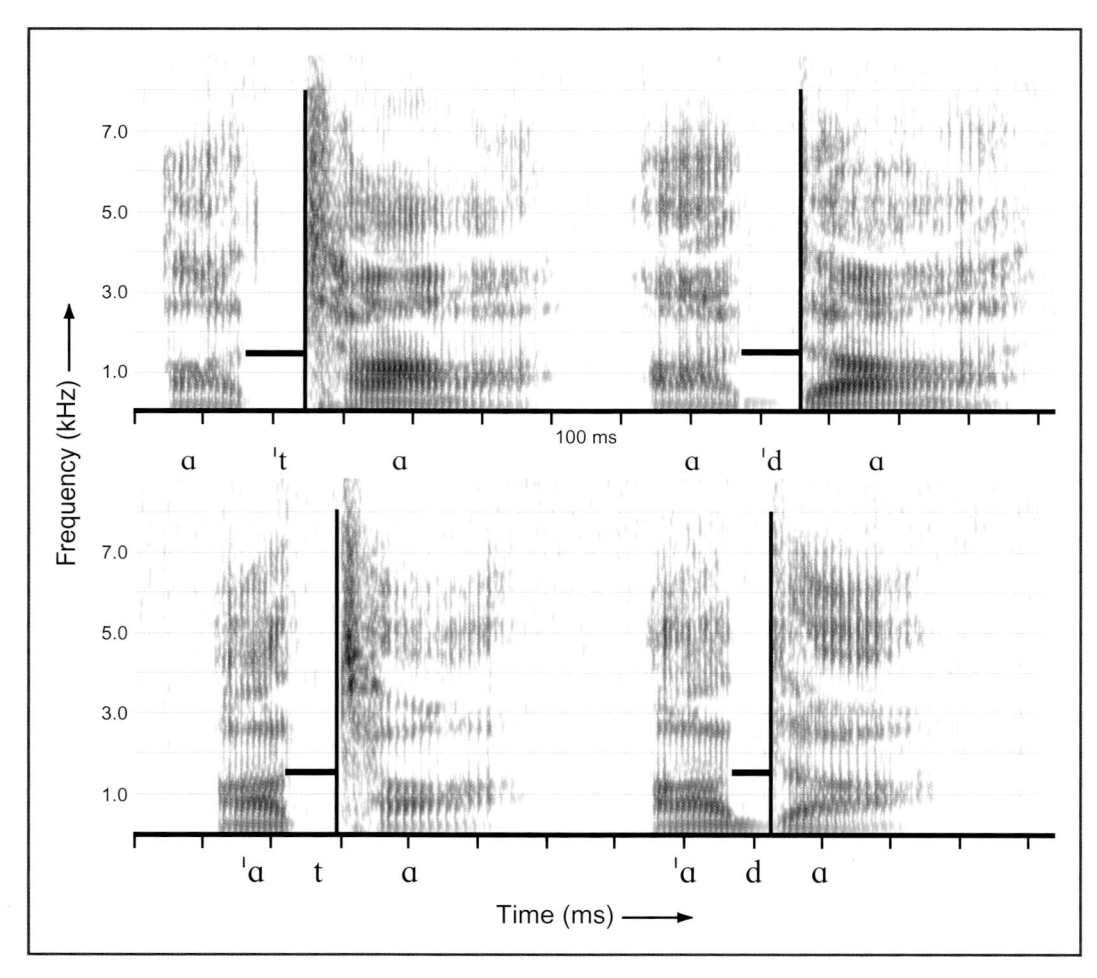

Figure 11–28. Spectrograms of the utterances /ɑ'tɑ/ and /ɑ'dɑ/ (*top*) and /'ɑtɑ/ and /'ɑdɑ/ (*bottom*). Each stop has a closure interval consisting of no energy (voiceless stops) or a small amount of periodic energy on the baseline (voiced stops). The duration of each closure interval is shown by the length of the heavy, horizontal bar between 1.0 and 2.0 kHz. The vertical line at the end of each closure interval shows the location of the burst. The ticks on the baseline are each separated by 100 ms (see top spectrogram).

Closure Interval and Burst

As discussed in Chapters 9 and 10, the familiar acoustic markers—the manner cues—of a stop consonant are a closure interval followed by a burst. The closure interval corresponds to the interval during which the vocal tract is completely sealed by the closed velopharyngeal port and the contact between the lips (for /p/ and /b/) or between the tongue and points along the palate (for /t/, /d/, /k/, and /g/). Closure intervals are indicated in Figure 11–28 by the heavy horizontal bars placed midway between the first and second frequency calibration lines. Spectrographically, closure intervals for voiceless stops appear as the white (no energy) intervals seen in Figure 11–28. For voiced stops, the closure interval is white with periodic energy along the baseline indicating vibration of the vocal folds (see /d/ closures in Figure 11–28).

Closure Interval Duration

In connected speech, including sentences and extended reading passages, closure intervals for any of the stop consonants are rarely greater than 70 ms, the majority having durations of around 60 ms (Byrd, 1993; Crystal & House, 1988b). When closure duration measures are made for more formal utterances, such as CVCs or other simple syllabic frames, sometimes called "citation forms" (and sometimes produced in carrier phrases such as "Say _ again"), the values are often longer than 70 ms but rarely exceed 100 ms (Luce & Charles-Luce, 1985; Stathopoulos & Weismer, 1983). The spectrograms in Figure 11–28 were produced in citation form.

A fair amount has been written about variation in closure durations due to stop voicing and place of articulation. Various sources in the literature claim that stop closure durations are longer for voiceless compared with voiced stops, and become increasingly shorter as place of articulation moves back in the vocal tract (that is, /p/ closures are longer than /t/, which, in turn, are longer than /k/). The claims for the voicing effect are most interesting, because they have their origin in a famous perceptual experiment reported by Lisker (1957). Lisker measured for a single speaker the closure durations of a small number of /p/s and /b/s in words such as "rapid-rabid," "staple-stable," and "rupee-ruby." For this intervocalic, post-stressed environment, Lisker measured average /p/ and /b/ closure durations of 120 and 75 ms, respectively. He then showed, using tape-splicing techniques, that an original "ruby" utterance (with glottal pulses eliminated in the closure interval) having a stop closure duration of 65 ms could be made to sound like "rupee" by lengthening the closure interval, leaving all other aspects of the signal unchanged. Lisker showed the reverse effect by systematically shortening an original 130 ms closure interval for /p/ in "rupee," which produced "ruby" responses at relatively short durations even though the closure interval contained no glottal pulses. Lisker concluded from these and other experiments that "closure durational differences play a major role in the voiced-voiceless stop distinction *in the type of context studied*" (1957, p. 48, emphasis added).

Lisker's (1957) carefully conducted and interpreted experiment was overgeneralized by subsequent scientists who studied the link between stop voicing and closure duration. First and foremost, Lisker was careful to restrict his conclusion to the specific context of intervocalic, post-stressed stop consonants (as in /'rupi/ versus /'rubi/, with stress on the first syllable). Selected closure duration data from the literature are summarized in Table 11–6, where values are included both for individual places of articulation (first six columns of data) as well as averaged across place but within voicing category (last two columns). The phonetic context and conditions under which stop closure durations were measured are described in the notes at the bottom of the table. These data support only a very subtle version of Lisker's proposed voicing effect on stop closure durations, especially when data are taken from connected speech. For example, Umeda (1977) reported only a 6 ms difference between the closure durations of voiceless and voiced stops for the 'VCV environment (see the two right-hand columns in Table 11–6 for Umeda, note b). Luce and Charles-Luce (1985) reported larger differences in the 'VCV environment (27 ms when the stop was followed by a vowel, 18 ms when the stop was followed by an /s/; see Table 11–6, notes e and f). The four speakers studied by Luce and Charles-Luce produced CVC citation forms in carrier phrases. Similar findings were reported by Stathopoulos and Weismer (1985; Table 11–6, note d). Even so, the effects reported by Luce and Charles-Luce and Stathopoulos and Weismer are of substantially lesser magnitude than the closure duration difference (~60 ms) used by Lisker as a starting point for typical voiceless and voiced stops. What is clear, however, is that the voiceless-voiced difference for closure durations does not extend to stops generally, across different contexts. Crystal and House (1988b), and Byrd (1993) reported voiceless stop closure durations to be between 2 and 6 ms longer than voiced stops in connected speech (Table 11–6, notes g and h), a difference of insufficient magnitude to serve as a useful perceptual cue to the voicing status of a stop.

The preceding discussion of closure duration as a potential marker of the voicing status of a stop consonant does not include the likely effect of periodic

Table 11-6. Selected Stop Closure Durations from Sources in the Literature

	p	b	t	d	k	g	Voiceless	Voiced
Umeda[a]	89	90	77	83	69	69	78	81
Umeda[b]	67	57	25	26	61	53	51	45
Stathopoulous & Weismer[c]	96	92	82	76	72	68	83	79
Stathopoulous & Weismer[d]	87	66	44	41	71	56	67	54
Luce & Charles-Luce[e]	93	61	68	51	84	52	82	55
Luce & Charles-Luce[f]	89	77	89	62	75	60	84	66
Crystal & House[g]	66	55	—	—	61	60	54	52
Byrd[h]	69	64	53	52	60	54	59	56

Note. All data are reported in milliseconds.
[a]Umeda (1977); N = 1 speaker, connected speech (long reading passage), V'CV environment.
[b]Umeda (1977); N = 1 speaker, connected speech (long reading passage), 'VCV environment.
[c]Stathopoulos & Weismer (1983); N = 6 speakers, CVCVC citation forms in carrier phrase, V'CV environment.
[d]Stathopoulos & Weismer (1983); N = 6 speakers, CVCVC citation forms in carrier phrase, 'VCV environment.
[e]Luce & Charles-Luce (1985); N = 4 speakers, CVC citation forms in long carrier phrases, closure for second C measured preceding vowel /ɪ/, stops, therefore, in 'VCV environment, with C = word final.
[f]Luce & Charles-Luce (1985); N = 4 speakers, CVC citation forms in long carrier phrases, closure for second C measured preceding fricative /s/, position , therefore, in 'VC/s/ environment, with C = word final.
[g]Crystal & House (1988b); N = 6 speakers, connected speech (two reading passages), data for /p,b,k,g/ are for stops in prevocalic, word-initial position; voiced/voiceless data are for stops in all positions.
[h]Byrd (1993); N = 630 speakers, connected speech (sentences), all phonetic contexts pooled.

energy during the closure interval on perception of the voicing status of a stop. Lisker (1957) was careful to qualify his perceptual findings with the same concern, as he had eliminated glottal pulsing during the closure interval as a potential cue to the voicing status of the labial stop in the "rupee-ruby" pair. Voiceless stops as produced by speakers who are free from speech disorders typically have no glottal pulsing during the closure interval. Occasionally, one or two glottal pulses extend from a preceding vowel into the beginning of a voiceless closure interval, as can be seen along the baseline of /ˈɑtɑ/ in Figure 11–28. In the case of voiced stops, voicing of the closure interval is often incomplete. The typical pattern, illustrated nicely by /ɑˈdɑ/ in Figure 11–28, is for voicing to be present at the start of the closure interval and terminate some milliseconds prior to the burst; in the /ɑˈdɑ/ example of Figure 11-28, voicing terminates roughly 30 ms prior to the burst. As discussed in Chapter 9, this may occur when the oral air pressure developed in the vocal tract approximates the magnitude of the tracheal pressure. An insufficient pressure difference across the vocal folds prevents phonation; it makes sense for the pressure difference to become insufficient later rather than earlier in the closure interval.

Flap Closures

The case of /t/ and /d/ in the intervocalic, post-stressed position of words is particularly interesting, and serves to illustrate how the style of speech—formal versus less formal—can influence speech segment durations. The single speaker studied by Umeda (1977) produced /t/ and /d/ closure durations of 25 and 26 ms in the 'VCV context, respectively (Table 11–6, note b). For the same context, Luce and Charles-Luce (1985) reported /t/ and /d/ closure durations of 68 and 51 ms (see Table 11–6, note e). At first glance, Umeda's (1977) values seem too short compared with closure durations in Table 11–6. In fact, they are almost identical to intervocalic, post-stressed flap durations (/t/ = 26 ms; /d/ = 27 ms) reported by Zue and LaFerriere

(1979) for six speakers producing words such as "rater" (/reɪɾɚ/) and "matter" (/mæɾɚ/). Luce and Charles-Luce's much longer intervocalic, post-stressed closure durations for /t/ and /d/ almost certainly reflect, in part, the more formal speech style associated with citation form. Luce and Charles-Luce's lingua-alveolar closure durations also reflect the word-final position from which their stop closure durations were measured (see Table 11–6, notes e and f). As Byrd (1993) reported, flaps occur in this word-final position when they are intervocalic and post-stressed, but are more likely to occur when the lingua-alveolar stop is located *within* a word (e.g., flaps are expected in the words "rooter" and "ruder," but perhaps not so frequently in "root a lot," where the lingua-alveolar stop occurs in word-final position).

Closure Duration and Place of Articulation

Data in Table 11–6 can be used to evaluate the effect of place of articulation on stop closure duration. When closure duration values in the two columns for labial stops are compared with the lingua-alveolars and dorsals, there is a tendency for labials to have the longest durations. Differences between lingua-alveolar and dorsal closure durations are less convincing.

Stop Voicing: Some Further Considerations

The acoustics of stop consonant voicing are complex. A famous article by Lisker (1986) listed *16* potential acoustic measures that may differentiate /p/ and /b/ in minimal pairs such as "rapid" versus "rabid." It seems there are multiple "candidate" acoustic cues to the voicing distinction for stop consonants. According to Lisker, the notion of "candidate" cues for stop voicing means that they *may* signal the difference between voiced and voiceless stops, but are not *all* necessary to make the distinction a good one. In fact, the cues that may signal the voicing status of a stop are context dependent. This context dependency includes not only the location of the stop relative to other sounds (e.g., word-initial or word-medial) and the prevailing stress pattern (e.g., pre- or post-stressed), but also the relational status of the candidate cues to the voicing distinction. Lisker provides an excellent example of the latter dependency, noting that even though the duration of the closure interval can signal the difference between "rabid" and "rapid," it does not do so even at long durations if the [b] closure interval is fully voiced. In this case, the word is heard as "rabid" no matter how long or short the closure interval.

It seems as if the presence or absence of glottal pulses during the closure interval is the logical cue for distinguishing voiced from voiceless stops. The absence of glottal pulses during a voiceless closure interval is almost always the case, but the presence of glottal pulses during the closure interval of a voiced stop is a more complicated phenomenon. First, as discussed earlier, glottal pulses do not always occur throughout the entire closure interval of a voiced stop. The pulses may begin at the onset of the closure interval but terminate well before the stop is released. Depending on how much of the closure interval is voiced (i.e., contains periodic energy generated by the vibrating vocal folds) as well as the intensity of the pulses that are present, the closure may have a voiced or voiceless quality when judged by a listener. In the absence of consideration of other potential cues to the stop voicing distinction, voiced stops may be considered more vulnerable to perceptual errors (i.e., voiceless-for-voiced stop errors) compared with voiceless stops (voiced-for-voiceless errors). Interestingly, literature on stop voicing errors in dysarthria and apraxia of speech is consistent with this asymmetry. Speakers with speech motor control problems are more often heard to produce voiceless-for-voiced than voiced-for-voiceless errors (Marquardt, Reinhart, & Peterson, 1979; Platt, Andrews, & Howie, 1980).

The potential ambiguity of a partially voiced closure interval may be reduced or eliminated as a result of the value(s) of one or more of the other cues to stop voicing. The best-studied cue to stop voicing is voice onset time (VOT), defined as the time interval between the burst and the first glottal pulse of a following vowel. Because the value of VOT is grossly correlated with the presence or absence of glottal pulses within the closure interval, VOT may remove any ambiguity concerning the voicing status of a stop. This is true in English for stops preceding stressed vowels. Why should the value of VOT be associated with the presence versus absence of glottal pulses within the closure interval?

Laryngeal Devoicing Gesture, Stop Closures, and Voice Onset Time

The laryngeal devoicing gesture, discussed above with reference to the voicing distinction for fricatives (see Figure 11–26), explains the absence of glottal pulses within the stop closure interval. Figure 11–29 repeats the schematic presentation of Figure 11–26, but with the vocal tract timing (labeled as "Timing of stop closure") appropriate for a voiceless stop closure . The LDG is identical to the one shown in Figure 11–26 for a voiceless fricative. Note the synchronized onsets of the LDG and supralaryngeal closure, as well as the LDG

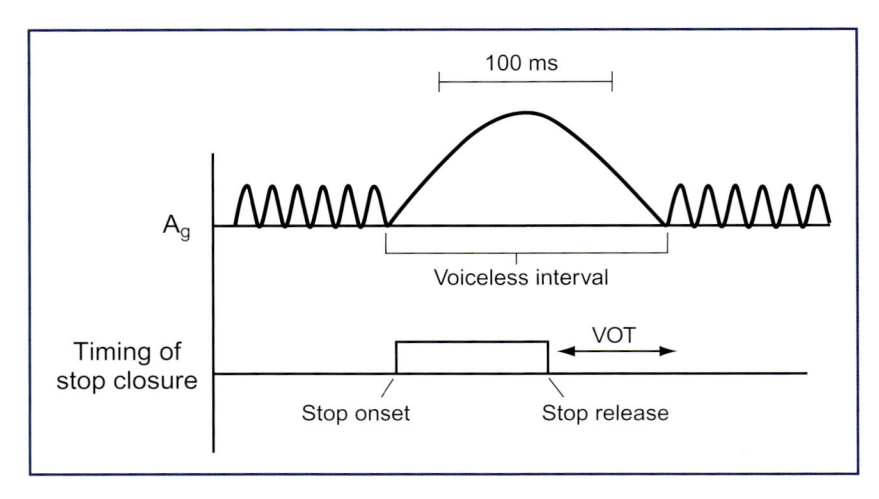

Figure 11–29. Schematic representation of laryngeal and supralaryngeal events for a VCV utterance in which C = a voiceless stop. A_g = area of the glottis. See Figure 11–26 legend for other details. "Timing of stop closure" indicates the onset, duration, and offset of the supralaryngeal closure for stop consonant production.

duration of well over 100 ms. All this is the same as in Figure 11–26. The striking difference in Figure 11–29, compared with Figure 11–26, is the release of the stop consonant closure interval roughly 60 to 70 ms after its onset (compared with the fricative constriction over the entire duration of the LDG in Figure 11–26). The earlier release for stops, which occurs shortly after the widest separation of the vocal folds during the LDG, means that a significant interval of time elapses between the stop release and the point in time when the vocal folds are brought together to resume vibratory activity. This interval is the VOT, and its relatively long duration results because the stop is released well before the LDG has completed its opening-closing movement. The release of the stop before the vocal folds are in the phonation-ready position results in frication and aspiration noise, as described in Chapter 9. This is why voiceless stops with long VOTs are also called aspirated stops.

Voiced stops do not have an LDG. During the closure interval, the vocal folds remain in the midline, in the phonation-ready position. The vocal folds vibrate and generate glottal pulses within the closure interval provided there is a sufficient pressure differential (tracheal pressure minus pharyngeal pressure) across the glottis. Even if vocal fold vibration ceases halfway through the closure interval, when the supralaryngeal stop closure is released, the vocal folds are near or in the midline position and ready to resume vibration almost immediately. This is why the value of VOT is grossly correlated with the presence versus absence of glottal pulses within a stop closure interval. The complete absence of glottal pulses throughout the closure interval implies the presence of the LDG, which in turn results in a relatively long VOT. Glottal pulses within the closure interval, even if ceasing well before the stop release, imply the absence of the LDG and the readiness of the vocal folds to resume vibrating soon after the stop release.

VOT values have been reported many times since the classic study of Lisker and Abramson (1964). These authors defined the measure and showed how it varied in different languages and speaking conditions. Reviews of VOT data are available in Auzou et al. (2000), Cho and Ladefoged (1999), and Weismer (2006). Figure 11–30 summarizes VOT data for English by showing typical values along with selected factors known to modify the measured values. The VOT continuum shown in Figure 11–30 ranges between −30 and 50 ms and is marked off in 10-ms steps. Immediately above the horizontal time continuum phonetic symbols are placed to indicate typical VOT values for stops in sentences, as reported by Lisker and Abramson for four speakers. For example, Lisker and Abramson (their Table 17) reported average VOTs for /p/, /t/, and /k/ of 28, 39, and 43 ms, respectively. Each of the voiced stops has two entries along the VOT time line. One set is in the positive part of the continuum (7, 9, and 17 ms for /b/, /d/, and /g/, respectively), the other shows the three sounds grouped together with an arrow pointing to values more negative than −30 ms. Lisker and Abramson (1964) noted that some utterance-initial voiced stops are produced with glottal pulses *before* their release, and designated these as *prevoiced* with negative VOT values. Just as positive VOT values represent the delay between the burst and first

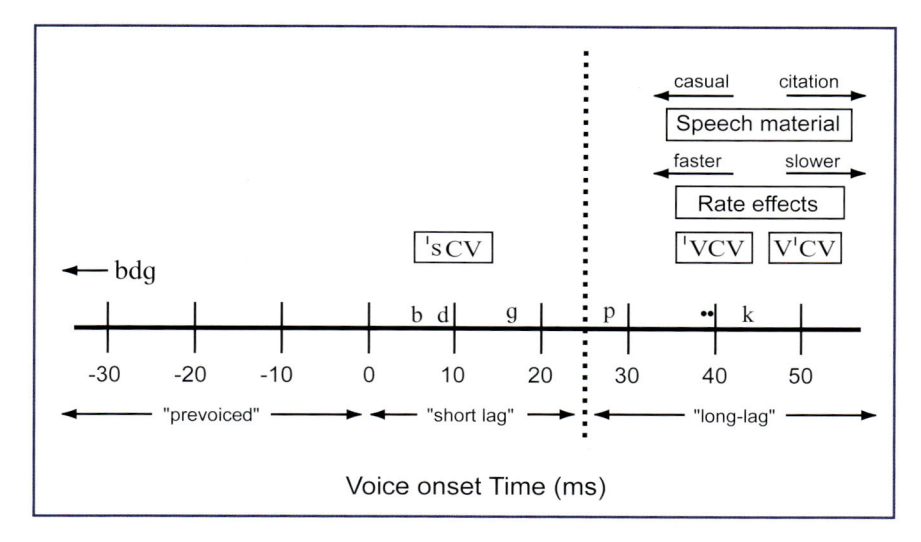

Figure 11–30. Graphic summary of VOT data from English speakers. A VOT continuum ranging from −30 to +50 ms is shown, and effects are indicated by the phonetic symbols and boxes above the continuum line. See text for additional detail.

glottal pulse of the following vowel, negative VOT values represent the time by which glottal pulses within the closure interval *precede* the burst.

Both positive and negative VOT values are common in voiced stop production. As noted above, negative VOTs are associated with stops produced in the utterance-initial position (no speech sounds preceding the stop); intervocalic voiced stops often have glottal pulses during the closure interval, but these are not considered prevoiced. When voiced stops have glottal pulses that are not continuous throughout the closure interval, the VOT is often positive, but very short, as shown in Figure 11–30. The prevoiced, voiced stops reported by Lisker and Abramson all had VOTs more negative than −30 ms, the last negative value on the continuum shown in Figure 11–30.

Figure 11–30 shows a vertical dotted line at 25 ms along the VOT continuum. This line designates a boundary between typical positive VOTs for voiced and voiceless stops. Voiceless stops can be expected to have VOTs exceeding 25 ms (*long-lag* VOTs), whereas voiced stops have VOTs less than 25 ms (*short-lag* VOTs) (Weismer, 2006).

The boxes above the VOT continuum and to the right of the 25 ms boundary identify factors that cause VOT to vary in systematic ways. These boxes are in the long-lag range of the VOT continuum because the effects are most prominent for voiceless stops, with much smaller effects on the short-lag VOTs of voiced stops. VOT is affected by the position of a voiceless stop relative to a stressed vowel. Longer VOTs are measured when the stop precedes, compared with follows, a stressed vowel. The box containing the V'CV frame has been placed to the right (longer VOTs) of the 'VCV box to indicate this effect. In fact, VOTs for voiceless stops in 'VCV frames may be so short as to place them in the short-lag range (Umeda, 1977). The effect of speaking rate on VOT, indicated in Figure 11–30 by the box and arrows immediately above the stress effects, are predictable from the direction of rate change. Slower rates produce longer VOTs for voiceless stops (shown by the arrow pointing to the right), and faster rates produce shorter VOTs (left-pointing arrow) (Kessinger & Blumstein, 1997). The reduction (shortening) of long-lag VOTs at very fast speaking rates is rarely so dramatic as to encroach on the short-lag range (Kessinger & Blumstein, 1997; Summerfield, 1975). Finally, the topmost box indicates that speaking style affects the value of long-lag VOTs. Longer VOTs for voiceless stops are produced in more formal speaking styles, sometimes referred to as citation form or "clear" speech (Krause & Braida, 2004; Smiljanić & Bradlow, 2005). Casual speech styles yield shorter VOTs. The difference between formal and casual speaking styles is likely to involve a difference in speaking rate. Formal speaking styles typically have slower rates than casual styles (Picheny et al., 1986).

A special case of VOT modification for voiceless stops is indicated by the "sCV" box above the short-lag range. "sCV" stands for prestressed s + stop clusters, in words such as "<u>s</u>top," "<u>s</u>kate," "<u>s</u>peech," "a<u>s</u>tounding." Voiceless stops in s + stop clusters have short-lag

> ### Seeking Phonetic Clarity
>
> One of your authors conducted a PubMed search for the number of publications on "acoustics of clear speech" over the period spanning from August 2012 to August 2017. The search, using a conservative criterion for papers on clear speech, resulted in 30 peer-reviewed publications. Another conservative estimate, going back to one of the original papers on clear speech (Picheny, Durlach, & Braida, 1985), turns up about 80 publications on this topic. Why so much interest in a speaking style well known to (as one example) actors? The original intent was to identify the acoustics of a speaking style that may be directed to persons with hearing loss. The idea was that clear speech may enhance the acoustic characteristics that define and separate phonetic categories and prosodic events. And it does. Clear speech enhances the separation between vowel formant frequencies and the range and speed of formant transitions, reduces (slows) speaking rate, increases the peakiness of fricative spectra and the burst prominence of stops, increases VOT for voiceless stops, increases the overall energy (SPL) of utterances and the "swings" in F0 contours (the latter making the utterances more "melodic"). No wonder that clear speech has been explored as a possible solution to producing intelligible speech in noise and as a therapy technique for persons with articulatory disorders.

VOTs (Umeda, 1977), as illustrated by the spectrograms in Figure 11–31. The first two words in this spectrogram are "peach" and "speech," with the VOT measurement for the two /p/s shown along the baseline. The left-hand boundary of these intervals is the /p/ burst, the right-hand boundary the first glottal pulse of the following vowel. The 55-ms VOT for the /p/ in /pɪtʃ/ fits the long-lag expectation for voiceless stops, whereas the 10 ms VOT for /p/ in /spɪtʃ/ illustrates the short-lag outcome of producing a voiceless stop in an s + stop cluster. This shortening effect on VOT seems to require that the s + stop cluster is part of one syllable (Davidsen-Nielsen, 1974). In Figure 11–31, the rightmost spectrographic pattern is for the sequence /lɛs#pɪtʃ/, where the s + stop cluster crosses a word boundary (symbolized by "#"). In this case, the VOT for /p/ is in the long-lag range, essentially the same as the /p/ VOT in "peach."

In summary, in many cases the value of VOT can be used as a correlate of the voicing status of a stop

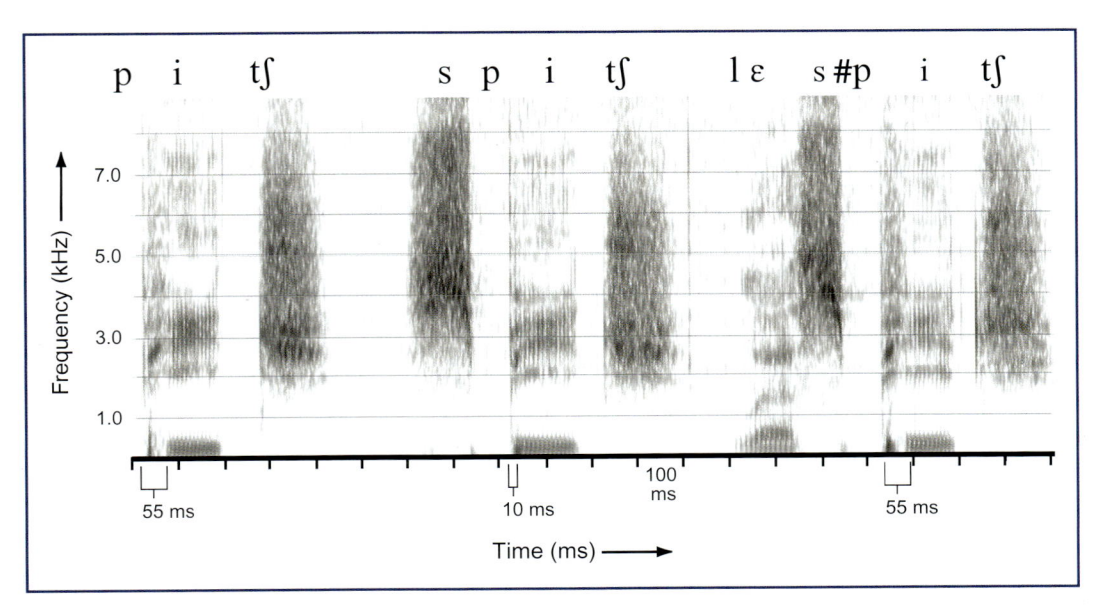

Figure 11–31. Spectrograms of the utterances /pɪtʃ/, /spɪtʃ/, and /lɛs#pɪtʃ/, showing how VOT varies when preceded by an /s/ in the same syllable (/spɪtʃ/) and across a word boundary (/lɛs#pɪtʃ/). VOT intervals are shown on the baseline.

consonant. Long-lag stops are typically voiceless, and short-lag stops are typically voiced. The "mismatches" between VOT values and the voicing status for stops usually occur only when voiceless stops have a VOT in the short-lag range. This can occur when voiceless stops are in the post-stressed position of a word, and occurs with near certainty when a voiceless stop is part of an s + stop cluster within a single syllable.

VOT is critical in the phonetic characteristics of languages other than English. Many languages have stop voicing distinctions, but "cut up" the VOT range in different ways compared with English. For example, Korean has a three-way voicing distinction for each place of articulation, with a VOT range of roughly +20 to 120 ms "cut up" in three ways for the contrast (Cho, Jun, & Ladefoged, 2002). Like English, French has a two-way voicing contrast but divides the VOT continuum differently than English. The voiced stops of French all have negative VOTs (i.e., they are prevoiced), and *short-lag*, positive VOTs for voiceless stops (Kessinger & Blumstein, 1997). The voiceless stops of French are therefore described as voiceless but unaspirated. Cho and Ladefoged (1999) provide an excellent analysis and interpretation of how different languages exploit the VOT continuum to "implement" their unique voicing contrasts.[17]

Bursts

Material presented in Chapter 9 describes the burst as the acoustic result of the sudden and rapid loss of oral air pressure at the release of a stop constriction. In practice, the isolation of a burst from the following frication interval (see Chapter 9) is difficult. Theoretical analysis (Stevens, 1998; and see Johnson, 2003) suggests a duration of less than 5 ms for the true burst interval of a stop. In the acoustic phonetics literature, the term "burst" is often used in a broader sense to include the burst plus the following 10 to 20 ms into the frication interval. This broader use is justified by the following summary of material from Chapter 9.

Although the aeromechanical bases of the burst source and frication source are different, their spectra are similar. Because both source spectra are shaped significantly by the resonator in front of the source, the output spectra for the "true" burst and the following frication interval tend to be similar. The use of the term "burst" to include the burst plus a brief part of the frication interval is, therefore, not a case of mixing apples and oranges. In this chapter, the term "burst" is used in this broader sense of the 20 to 30-ms interval following the burst "spike" seen on waveforms and spectrograms.

Bursts are considered one of the hallmarks of the stop manner of production. In laboratory experiments involving citation-form speech, stops are almost always produced with a clear burst. In connected speech such as reading and spontaneous speech, a significant number of stop consonants have no identifiable burst even when perception suggests a "good" stop has been produced (Byrd, 1993; Crystal & House, 1988c). This is another example of how speech style can modify acoustic phonetic phenomena.

Stop bursts have been the focus of a great deal of research. The spectrum of stop bursts has been studied to determine if each of the three places of stop articulation in English is associated with a unique spectral shape. This problem was framed early in the history of speech acoustics research by Halle, Hughes, and Radley (1957), who measured spectra for stop bursts in simple CV syllables, where C = each of the English stops and V = /i/, /ɪ/, /æ/, /ɑ/, and /u/. Their analysis was similar to those shown in Figure 11–32, where speech waveforms produced by one of the authors are shown for /pʌ/, /tʌ/, and /kʌ/. In each waveform a 20 ms increment beginning at the burst is marked off for spectral analysis. Halle et al. isolated these 20 ms intervals and for each one computed a Fourier spectrum over a frequency range of 250 to 10,000 Hz (the Fourier spectra shown in Figure 11–32 have a slightly wider frequency range, namely 0 to 11,000 Hz).

Halle et al.'s (1957) observations concerning the spectral shape of these burst intervals have been replicated (with some minor differences) in several studies. They described labial bursts as having a primary concentration of energy in the lower frequencies; lingua-alveolar bursts with flat spectra or an emphasis of energy in the high frequencies (by which they meant above 4.0 kHz); and dorsal stops as having prominent energy peaks in the midfrequency regions, roughly between 1.5 and 4.0 kHz. In Figure 11–32, the /p/ burst has a relatively flat spectrum between 0 and 5.0 kHz and decreasing energy between 5.0 and 11.0 kHz. The /t/ burst has clearly increasing energy from 0 to

---

[17]Voicing contrasts may be implemented in several different ways, including manipulation of the VOT continuum. This is not to say that VOT is the only way to contribute to a voicing contrast, just one of the more popular, at least among speech scientists who enjoy measuring it and perhaps among speakers of different languages, too (Kingston & Diehl, 1994). The popularity of VOT as a measurement in languages of the world can be gauged by the results of a citation search performed by one of your authors on August 16, 2017. He used "Voice onset time" as the key words in the *Linguistics and Language Behavior Abstracts* (LLBA) database and received over 800 "hits" extending back to the 1970s. That's a lot of research on VOT.

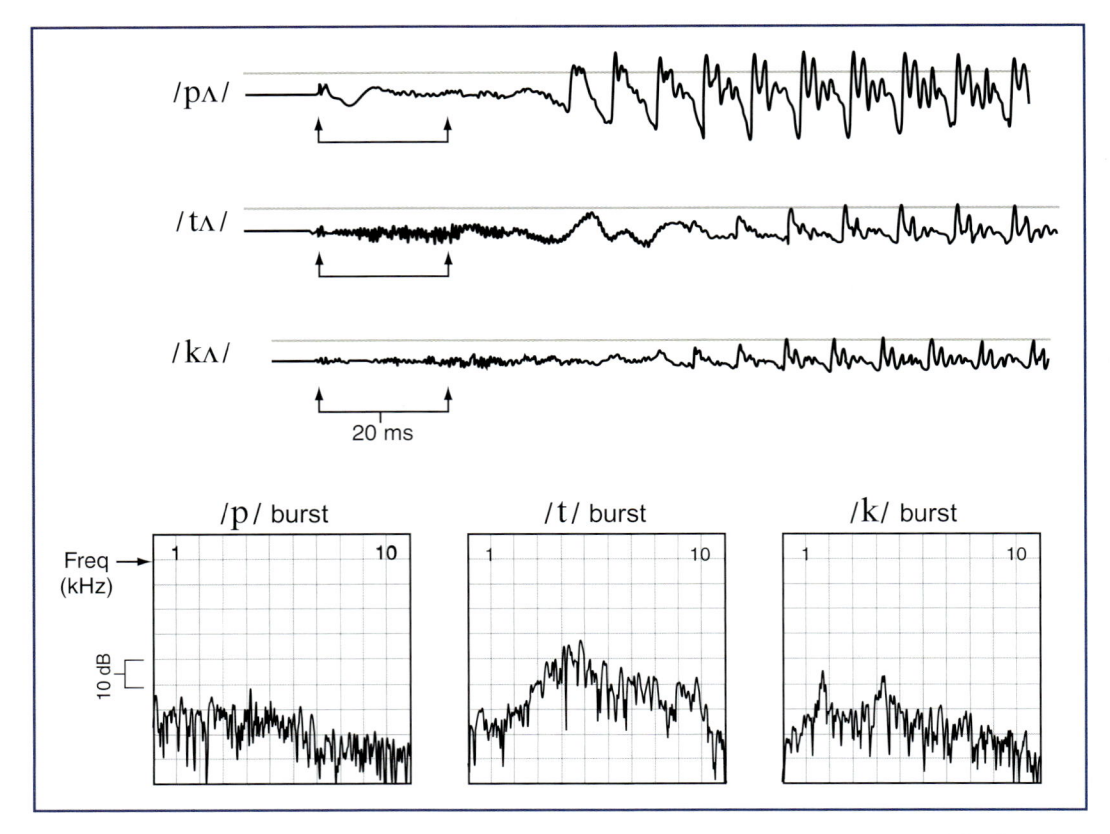

Figure 11–32. Waveforms (*three upper traces*) and spectra (*lower three panels*) for the stop consonants and initial part of vowels in /pʌ/, /tʌ/, and /kʌ/. A 20-ms interval, beginning at the stop burst, is indicated in the upper three traces by the horizontal line whose endpoints are marked by upward pointing arrows. This is the interval over which Halle et al. (1957) computed spectra for the stop burst. The Fourier spectra shown at the bottom of the figure are computed for the 0 to 11 kHz range. Each division along the frequency axis is a 1.0 kHz increment, each division along the intensity axis a 10 dB increment.

5.0 kHz and decreasing energy at the higher frequencies, and the dorsal burst has two large, midfrequency peaks of energy, one around 1.8 kHz and the other at 4.2 kHz. Despite the difference in speakers and the slightly different range of analyzed frequencies, the spectral shapes in Figure 11–32 are consistent with the major summaries of stop burst spectral shape offered by Halle et al. Based on these observations, stop place of articulation seems to be differentiated by the spectrum of the stop burst. If this is true, listeners presumably can use this information to identify place of articulation for stop consonants.

Perhaps it seems obvious that the burst has unique spectral characteristics for the three different places of articulation. After all, the acoustic theory of speech production predicts different resonant frequencies depending on the location of a constriction in the vocal tract. The different constriction locations for the three places of articulation are accompanied by differences in vocal tract shape over the first few milliseconds following the release of a stop. Reliable differences in stop burst spectra as a function of place of articulation are therefore expected from the acoustic theory of consonant production (Chapter 9).

Acoustic Invariance for Stop Place of Articulation

Speech scientists use the term *acoustic invariance* to refer to the stable, place-specific acoustic characteristics discussed in this chapter. An acoustically invariant characteristic of a speech sound is one that is always found in the spectrum, or the manner in which the spectrum changes as a function of time, regardless of who is producing the utterance or under what conditions the utterance is spoken.

This view, although attractive and apparently logical, may be partially or largely complicated by the well-known phenomenon of coarticulation. There are different ways to define coarticulation, but a conventional definition makes the point: coarticulation is the influence of one segment on another. Stated otherwise, the articulatory (and hence acoustic) characteristics of a speech sound segment depend on the articulatory (acoustic) characteristics of adjacent, and in some cases nonadjacent, segments. In the case of stop burst spectra, the important question is: how stable is the spectrum for a specific stop place of articulation when the following vowel (or any preceding or following segment) varies? If stop burst spectra vary in a significant way depending on the following vowel, the claim of unique spectral characteristics for the three different places of stop articulation may be difficult to defend. Vowel-induced variation could result in highly variable stop burst spectra for a given place of articulation, with too little acoustic stability to serve as a reliable cue to place identification.

Figure 11–33 shows an example of a vowel effect on a burst spectrum. Two spectra are shown, both calculated for a 26 ms interval starting at the burst of the /t/ in /ɑti/ (light trace) and /ɑtu/ (dark trace). The analysis band is limited to 0 to 5 kHz and the spectra have been smoothed using LPC analysis (see Chapter 10). These two spectra have obvious differences but are also very similar in an important way. The main difference between the spectra is the emphasis of lower frequencies for /tu/ compared with /ti/. The /tu/ spectrum has large peaks at 2.8 and 3.7 kHz, whereas the /ti/ spectrum lacks well-defined peaks below 4.0 kHz but has steadily increasing energy up to 5.0 kHz, where a peak is present. Stated more generally, the /t/ burst followed by /u/ has more low-frequency energy compared with the /t/ burst followed by /i/, at least for this 0 to 5.0 kHz analysis band. In coarticulatory terms, this makes sense because the formants of /u/ have concentrated energy in the low frequencies, with low F1 and F2), whereas the formants of /i/ have more high-frequency concentration with high F2 and F3 (see previous section on vowel formant frequencies). These different concentrations of vowel energy influence the concentration of energy in the burst spectra.

The commonality in these two spectra is the steadily increasing energy from 0 to nearly 4.0 kHz, despite the difference in the location of prominent peaks. In this analysis band, both spectra are tilted to the higher frequencies. Perhaps the gross, upward tilt for /t/ bursts is the critical acoustic correlate to this place of articulation, always present even when the following vowel influences details of peak frequency location and amplitude. The auditory system may strip away "local" spectral detail and use the gross spectral shape to identify stop place of articulation.

In a classic acoustic phonetics study, Blumstein and Stevens (1979) attempted to demonstrate the uniqueness of such spectral shapes for the three different places of stop articulation. After examining LPC burst spectra (0–5.0 kHz analysis band) for a 26-ms interval starting at the burst, Blumstein and Stevens designed "spectral templates" for each of the three stop places of articulation (see Chapter 10). The templates were constructed to allow spectral variation in the burst spectrum due to speaker differences and coarticulation while preserving the more global spectral shape that presumably was the constant, or invariant acoustic characteristic. The templates were named *diffuse-falling* for bilabials, *diffuse-rising* for lingua-alveolars, and *compact* for dorsals. Examples of LPC spectra consistent with these templates are shown in Figure 11–34.

According to Blumstein and Stevens (1979), the diffuse-falling template fit most of the bilabial bursts, the diffuse-rising template the lingua-alveolar bursts, and the compact template the dorsal bursts. The diffuse-falling template had peaks between 0 and 5.0 kHz of roughly equivalent magnitude or with somewhat decreasing energy as frequency increased. In contrast, the diffuse-rising template showed peaks increasing in amplitude with increasing frequency. Both the diffuse-falling and diffuse-rising templates were likely to

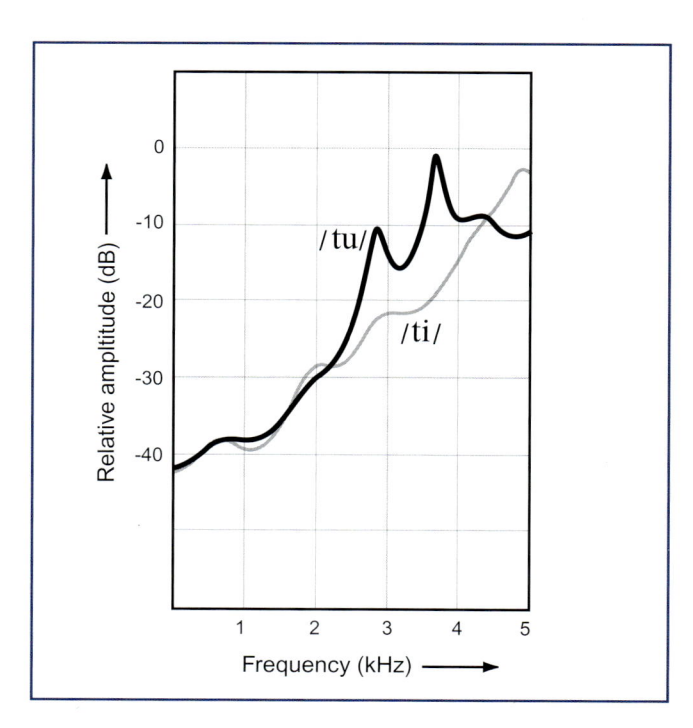

Figure 11–33. Two LPC spectra (0–5.0 kHz) for /t/ bursts produced before an /u/ (*dark line*) and an /i/ (*light line*). A comparison between these spectra shows the effects of vowel coarticulation on /t/ burst acoustics.

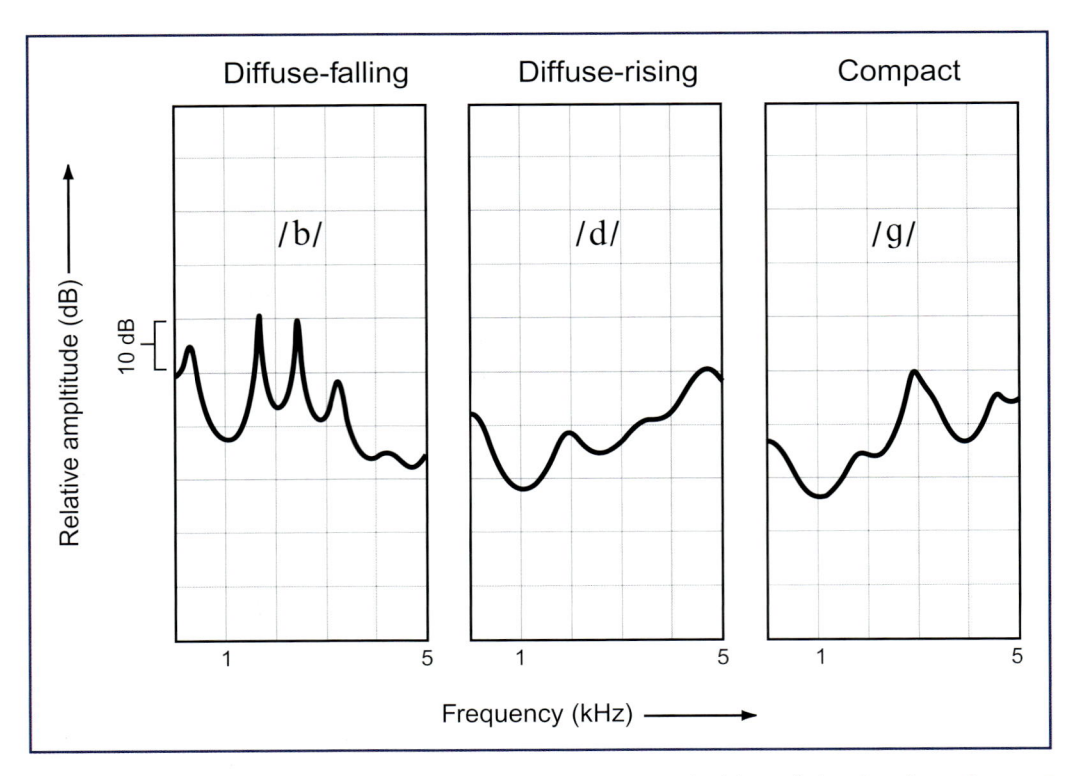

Figure 11–34. Examples of burst spectra fitting the spectral templates for stop place of articulation, based on 26-ms burst spectra (LPC). The three templates—diffuse falling, diffuse rising, compact—were developed by Blumstein and Stevens (1979).

have multiple peaks of energy (energy diffusely spread across the spectrum), but with essentially opposite tilts. In contrast, the compact template had energy focused in a single, prominent midfrequency peak somewhere between 1200 and 3500 Hz. Burst spectra shown in Figure 11–34 for the voiced stops /b/, /d/, and /g/, followed by the vowel /ɛ/, are generally consistent with these descriptions. It is not difficult to see the /b/ burst spectrum as flat or falling at higher frequencies, the /d/ burst as rising, and the /g/ burst as having a central peak of energy around 3.0 kHz. The stops from which these bursts were extracted were produced by one of the authors in V'CV frames, and the spectral analysis was derived from a 26-ms interval starting at the burst, as in the Blumstein and Stevens study.

Blumstein and Stevens' (1979) description of place-specific spectral templates for stop consonant bursts is very much consistent with the more qualitative observations of Halle et al. (1957). Blumstein and Stevens, however, were the first scientists to quantify the *consistency* of these spectral templates in the classification of stop place of articulation. After the templates were finalized, six speakers produced 900 CV stops where C = /b,d,g,p,t,k/ and V = /i,e,a,o,u/, in all combinations and with each combination repeated five times (6 stops × 5 vowels × 5 repetitions × 6 speakers = 900 stops). Every stop was produced with a variety of vowels to create burst spectrum variation due to coarticulation. Stevens and Blumstein asked the following two questions: (1) even with vowel-induced variation (see example in Figure 11–33), do the templates capture a consistent spectral characteristic related to place? and (2) are these consistencies found for different speakers? LPC spectra were prepared for each of the 900 stops and then *visually* classified by fitting each spectrum to each template and judging it as a match or not a match.

The results of this analysis procedure can be stated in simple terms, even if the interpretation is not so simple. Roughly 85% of the burst spectra were both correctly matched to the "correct" place template and correctly rejected by the "incorrect" templates. The last point needs clarification. Each burst spectrum was compared with *each* template and a decision of "match" or "no match" was made. A match was recorded when a burst spectrum from a specific place of articulation fit that place's template, and no match was recorded when the same burst did not fit the two other place templates. The no match decision meant that a template "rejected" a real spectrum from a different place of articulation.

Is an 85% "correct match" and "correct rejection" performance sufficient to support the presence of invariant spectral characteristics for stop place of articulation? Blumstein and Stevens (1979) thought so, concluding that their visual spectrum-matching experiment demonstrated the existence of acoustic invariants for stop place of articulation, at least in CV syllables and for a limited number of speakers using a carefully articulated speech style. Later experiments measuring different types of smoothed (LPC) burst spectra also demonstrated successful classification of place of articulation (85–95% correct rates), either by visual matching or using automatic (statistical) classification procedures (Forrest et al., 1988; Kewley-Port, 1983; Kobatake & Ohtani, 1987; Nossair & Zahorian, 1991). There is a good deal of research support for Blumstein and Stevens' conclusion. The question, therefore, is not whether classification of stop place from burst spectra can be done with reasonable success, but *is the success good enough* and *why does the answer to this question matter?*

Acoustic Invariance and Theories of Speech Perception

The answer to the question of acoustic invariance for stop place of articulation is important because of the profound role it has played in the development of theories of speech perception. Here, a summary of the issues is provided. More detail is provided in Chapter 12.

Early in the history of speech research, many speech scientists did not believe there were consistent acoustic characteristics for a given stop place of articulation. The influence of different vowels on stop consonant acoustics was thought to be too great to allow a constant to remain in the acoustic signal for a given place of articulation. Interestingly, this conclusion of "no acoustic invariance" (note the curious, double negative; despite the literary inelegance, this is a famous phrase in the speech science literature) was mostly derived from a series of well-known *perceptual* experiments conducted at the Haskins Laboratories (located originally in New York City, now for many years in New Haven, Connecticut). These experiments used a device called a *pattern-playback machine* (see Chapter 12) to convert painted replicas of spectrographic patterns into sound. This device allowed an experimenter to create spectrographic patterns of any type to determine how the patterns affected a listener's perception of sound identity.

When the Haskins scientists painted a pattern based on a real spectrogram, they typically did not reproduce every spectrographic detail. The painted patterns were like stick figures or schematic representations of real spectrographic patterns. In the course of preparing these patterns and presenting them to listeners, the scientists discovered something interesting. They could elicit perception of a stop-vowel syllable with a pattern having only F1-F2 transitions and the steady states of the following vowel. Surprisingly, the burst was not necessary to create the auditory impression of a stop consonant (see Liberman, Cooper, Shankweiler, & Studdert-Kennedy, 1967 for a review of this work and relevant citations; and Story & Bunton, 2010 for a modern version and interpretation of this experiment).

Examples of two burstless, painted patterns are shown in Figure 11–35. The schematic F1 and F2 in both patterns show transitions followed by a steady state, the latter defined as the interval during which the formant frequencies of the vowel remain at constant frequencies (that is, when they are not changing over time). When the pattern on the left was converted to sound and played to listeners, they heard /di/. The pattern on the right was heard as /du/. If the transition portions were eliminated and only the steady states played to listeners, they clearly heard the vowels /i/ (left) and /u/ (right).

Note in Figure 11–35 the very different F2 transition for the perception of the /d/ in /di/ versus /du/. After examination of these two patterns, the reader may ask the following question relevant to the discussion of acoustic invariance: Why did two such different patterns of formant transitions result in the perception of the *same* stop consonant? The Haskins scientists determined, in fact, that for any place of articulation

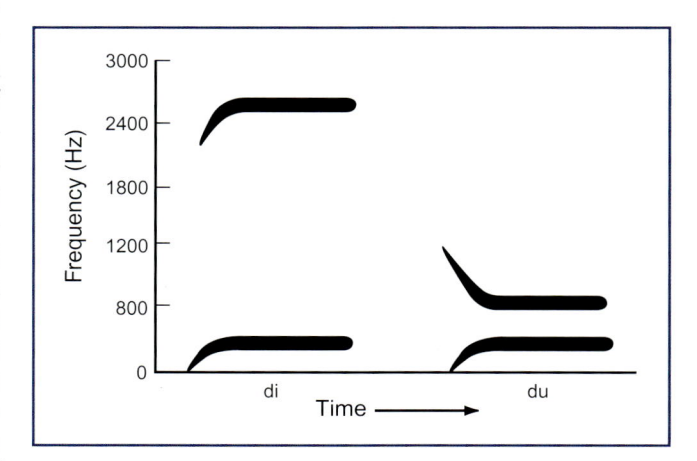

Figure 11–35. Burstless, painted patterns of formant transitions and steady states used in early Haskins Laboratories experiments to elicit perception of the consonant /d/ in two vowel environments. Adapted from Liberman et al. (1967).

a wide variety of F2 transition patterns was associated with the perception of the same stop. The different F2 transitions depended on which vowel was paired with a specific stop consonant. If the vowel context had such a profound influence on the acoustic characteristics related to place of articulation of a stop, the Haskins scientists argued that there was no acoustic invariance for the place feature of stop consonants. This conclusion led to a theory of speech perception, discussed more fully in Chapter 12, that downplays (if not eliminates) a primary role for auditory acoustic analysis in the perception of speech.

Blumstein and Stevens (1979), as well as other investigators who have had success in classifying stop place of articulation using the burst spectrum, argued against this position. The demonstrated ability, in different studies, to assign 85% to 95% of burst spectra to the "correct" place of articulation pointed to sufficient acoustic invariance for important perceptual decisions, at least in the case of stop place of articulation. Researchers interested in the issue of acoustic invariance, or the lack of it, could reasonably argue that the Haskins studies were bound to find what appeared to be unmanageable variability in the acoustic properties of a given stop consonant. This is because the Haskins scientists focused almost all attention on the transition patterns, not the spectrum of the burst interval. In defense of the Haskins scientists, however, they did recognize the importance of the burst spectrum for *some* vowel contexts (Liberman et al., 1967), but never investigated the actual stability of those burst spectra in spoken utterances. The Haskins conclusions concerning the lack of acoustic invariance for stop acoustics were based almost exclusively on perceptual, not production, experiments.

Story and Bunton (2010) showed that a model of vocal tract acoustics has certain "hot spots" for stop consonant articulation, and the resulting pattern of formant transitions into and out of the closure interval. Story and Bunton identified regions in and around the bilabial (/p, b/), lingua-alveolar (/t, d/), and dorsal (/k, g/) places of articulation that affect the pattern of F1, F2, and F3 transitions in unique and consistent ways, regardless of which vowel is adjacent to a particular stop. In this view, there is a nearly invariant, place-specific pattern in the *transitions* that is almost completely due to laws relating vocal tract configuration changes, from stops to vowels, to a pattern of formant frequency transitions. In effect, Story and Bunton's results suggest that not only did the Haskins scientists ignore an acoustic event (the stop burst) that has place-specific, invariant characteristics, but even the events deemed to be too variable across vowels: the transitions into and out of the closure interval. These transitions were also not investigated thoroughly, and when examined carefully have their own invariant characteristics.

Locus Equations

Another approach to acoustic invariance for stop consonant place of articulation combines measures that reflect both consonant and vowel production. This work, reported over the years by Sussman, Lindblom, and their colleagues (e.g., Lindblom, Agwulele, Sussman, & Cortes, 2007; Lindblom & Sussman, 2012; Modarresi, Sussman, & Lindblom, 2005; Sussman, McCaffrey, & Matthews, 1991), is based on two measures, as shown in Figure 11–36A. Spectrograms of 10 vowels, all preceded by /b/, are shown. For each syllable, a red horizontal bar crosses the first glottal pulse following the /b/ release; this is the F2 onset, or the initial F2 value of the vowel. F2 onset reflects the vocal tract configuration at the instant of vocal tract opening. This measure is regarded as an acoustic estimate of the preceding consonant target in the same way that the F2 value at the temporal middle of a vowel is considered a measure of the vowel target. The F2 target is indicated by an interval marked by the yellow horizontal line. This measure is taken within this interval, as close as possible to a "steady" F2 (not changing as a function of time).

Examination of the F2 onsets shows that they are not at a fixed frequency across the different vowels. The F2 onsets vary because they are "pulled" in the direction of the varying F2 targets. For example, the top row of spectrograms shows five front vowels from highest (/i/) to lowest /æ/. Based on the tongue height rule (Chapter 8), the F2 target decreases as the vowel becomes more open. The highest F2 target is observed for /i/, the lowest F2 target for /æ/, with the F2 target declining systematically for the intervening vowels (/ɪ/, /eɪ/, /ɛ/). The F2 onset is higher when the vowel target has a higher F2 (as in /i/) and decreases as the F2 target decreases. This pattern is seen (with one exception, /eɪ/) from left to right in the top row of Figure 11–36A. The F2 onset is therefore sensitive to the F2 target of the following vowel. The back vowels in the lower part of Figure 11–36A show a similar pattern, although not as "clean" as the front vowels.

Figure 11–36B shows a plot of F2 onset by F2 target for the 10 vowels preceded by /b/. Each vowel is shown as a plotted point. Across the 10 vowels, the points cluster closely around a linear function, showing the variation of F2 onset with F2 target. The higher the F2 target, the higher the F2 onset. The linear function, computed by a simple "best fit" mathematical equation,

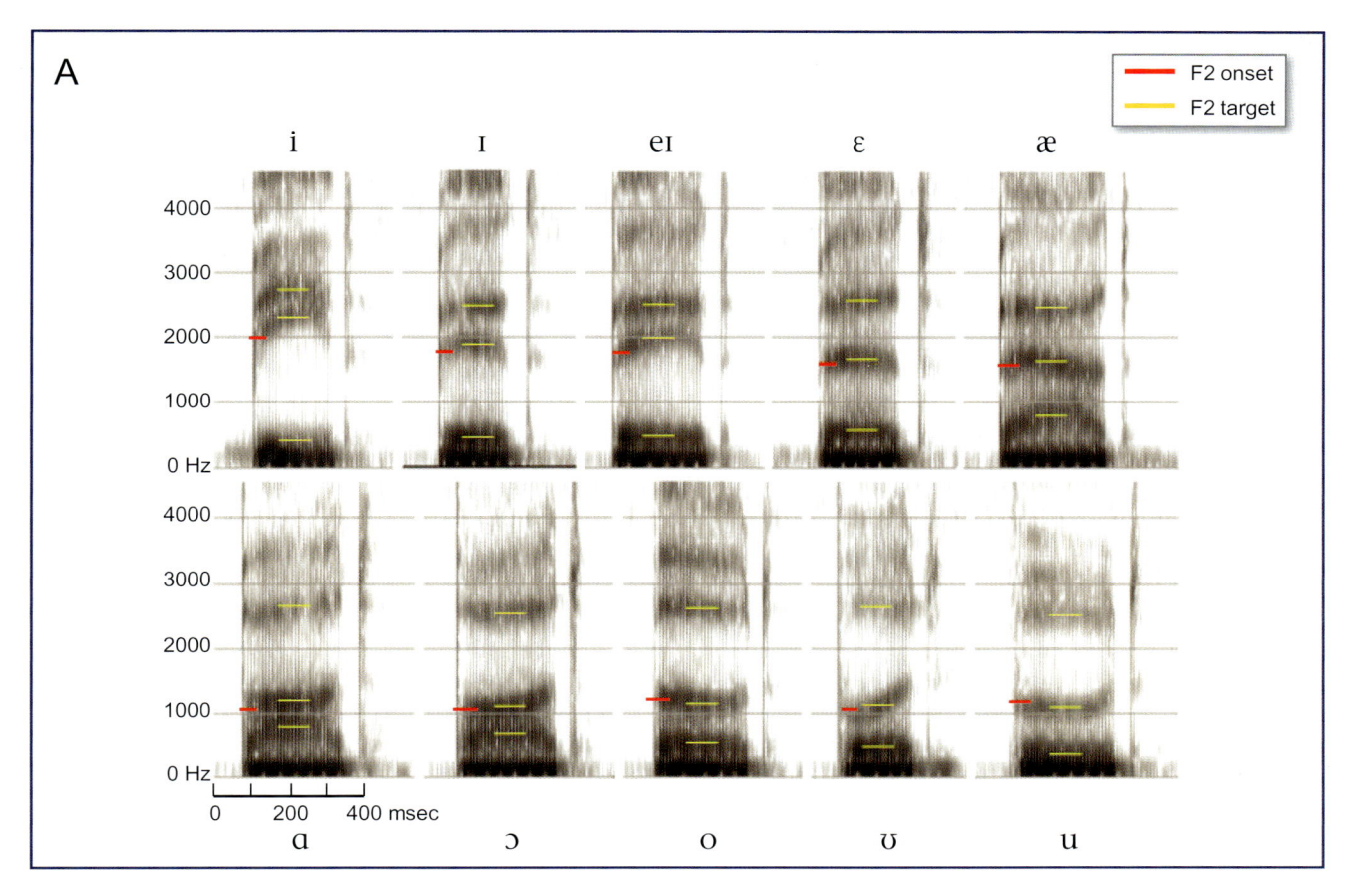

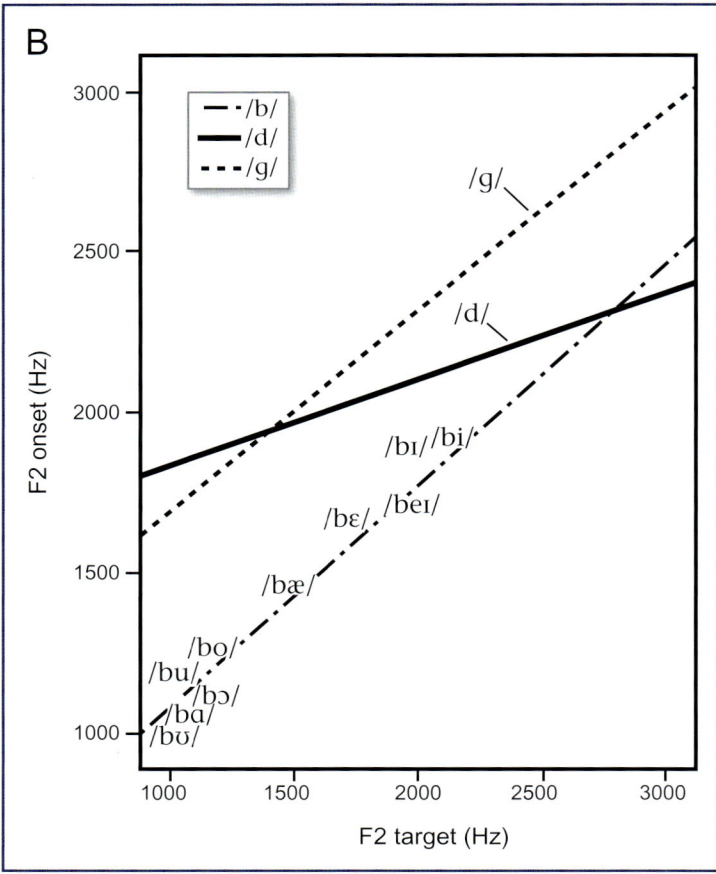

Figure 11–36. A. Spectrograms of /bV/ syllables in which V = one of 10 vowels. For each syllable, the horizontal red bar crosses the first glottal pulse following release of the /b/, where the F2 onset measure is made. The yellow horizontal bar is a brief interval within which the F2 target measure is made. **B.** Linear fits of F2 onset versus F2 target. Individual points plus the linear fit are shown for the /b/ function, with measures taken from the spectrograms in part **A**. Only the linear fits are shown for /d/ and /g/. See text for details. Spectrogram and permission courtesy of Dr. Robert Hagiwara, University of Manitoba.

> ### Locus Pocus
>
> Locus equations and their interpretation as an acoustic invariant have been generalized to place of articulation of fricatives and affricates, to stops in other languages (that may have more than the three places of stop articulation of American English), and most importantly, to speech disorders. The slopes of the three linear functions shown in Figure 11–36B are regarded by some scientists as an index of the degree of coarticulation (alternatively, gesture overlap; see Chapter 5) between the consonant and vowel. The greater the slope, the greater the coarticulation between the two segments. In Figure 11–36B the steeper slope for /b/ compared with /d/ and /g/ makes sense, because during the closure interval for /b/ the tongue is free to go through motions and reach positions appropriate for the following vowel. In lingual /d/ and /g/, the motions and positions required for the stop closures limit (but do not completely eliminate) anticipation of the vowel gestures. A disruption of coarticulation has been hypothesized in several speech disorders (dysarthria, apraxia of speech, stuttering), and locus equations have been used to address these hypotheses. Yet another example of the potential of basic speech science to have relevance to clinical issues.

represents the relationship between F2 onset and F2 target as a strong one. The plotted points are located close to the best fit line, which justifies the description of a strong relationship. F2 target "pulls" on F2 onset in a predictable way. The strength of the relationship can be gauged by the correlation between the two variables, which is often at least 0.90, as reported in many studies (see summary in Sussman, Fruchteer, Hilbert, & Sirosh, 1998).

Figure 11–36B also shows best fit lines for /d/ and /g/; the individual plotted points for these two stops are omitted from the graph to reduce clutter. The relationship between F2 onset and F2 target, across vowels, is also linear and very strong for these stops (Lindblom & Sussman, 2012).

The functions for these best fit lines are called *locus equations* (Lindblom & Sussman, 2012; Sussman, McCaffrey & Matthews, 1991). The *locus* is the F2 onset, the index described earlier of the consonant configuration at the immediate release of the stop. How do locus equations for the three voiced stop consonants address the issue of acoustic invariance?

Sussman et al. (1998) argue that acoustic invariance for stop place of articulation is found in the slope and y-intercepts of the linear functions. Because the locus lines (the linear functions) connect F2 onsets with F2 targets, they are like transitions from the consonant to the vowel, albeit simplified by the connection of only two frequency points. The /b/ and /g/ functions are different from the /d/ function by virtue of their steeper slopes, and even though the /b/ and /g/ slopes are similar, their functions have very different y-intercepts (about 1000 Hz for /b/, 1650 Hz for /g/). According to Sussman et al., the differences in the locus functions reflect invariant acoustic characteristics for stop place of articulation. It is as if listeners base their decisions about place of articulation on the unique parameters (slope and y-intercept) of the functions. Moreover, the locus equation concept has been extended to the area of speech perception (Sussman et al., 1998). This is discussed in Chapter 12.

Acoustic Invariance at the Interface of Speech Production and Perception

The issue of acoustic invariance has focused on stop consonants, but a more general question is the stability of the acoustic characteristics for *any* speech sound. A given sound may have very different acoustic characteristics, in both the temporal and spectral domains, depending on who produces the speech sample and the conditions under which it is produced. A speech sound has acoustic variability depending on the age, dialect, sex, size, and possibly race of the speaker. In addition, phonetic context, speaking rate, and speaking style have major effects on a speech sound's acoustic characteristics. If the acoustic characteristics of a speech sound are so variable, exactly what is meant by the term "acoustic invariance"?

The Haskins scientists apparently defined acoustic invariance in a very strict way. For them, almost any degree of acoustic variability of a speech sound (such as the cues for place of articulation of stops) was an undesirable aspect of the speech signal as a reliable cue for listeners. Blumstein and Stevens (1979), and several others who followed them, had a slightly looser approach to this problem. These scientists allowed that a sufficient degree of acoustic invariance was demonstrated when a relatively small percentage of stops (5–15%) was misclassified according to their analysis criteria. This work has sometimes been criticized for two reasons, one having to do with the arbitrary nature of the analysis criteria, the second with the failure to explain the classification errors and how they are treated in the perception of speech.

Arbitrary analysis criteria can be illustrated with the following questions: Does the 26-ms burst interval used by Blumstein and Stevens (1979) bear any relationship to the way the auditory system processes speech spectra? Is there good evidence for spectral shape analysis by the auditory system? Does the auditory system use a straightforward frequency analysis as suggested by Blumstein and Stevens, and others, or does it change the way frequency is represented as the signal travels the auditory pathways from the ear canal to the auditory cortex? These questions are not pursued in detail in this chapter; the answers to the questions are not simple and in many cases are controversial.

The second issue, of classification errors and how they are handled, has not been addressed. Five to 15% does not seem like a lot of errors, but how often do listeners experience such perceptual errors when listening to speech? The answer is, not very often at all, unless speech is being produced and perceived in a very noisy environment or is heard by a listener with a hearing loss. So, how are classification errors explained within a perspective on "normal" speech perception?

An alternative view to this problem has been formulated by Lindblom (1990). For Lindblom, the issue is not the strict acoustic invariance of a specific speech sound, but rather how much its acoustic characteristics can vary and still remain distinctive relative to neighboring sounds. Lindblom (see also Moon & Lindblom, 1994) pointed to the known variability in acoustic characteristics of speech sounds as an asset, not a liability. Speakers often vary the precision with which they produce sound segments. Under more formal circumstances, they produce speech very carefully, but in casual situations are likely to be rather imprecise. As described above, a clear speech style is characterized by acoustic characteristics of speech sounds that are maximally distinct from each other (Ferguson & Kewley-Port, 2007). Casual speech styles decrease the distance between these acoustic characteristics but leave them sufficiently distinct to retain their contrastive function. A good example of this effect would be the relative expansion and collapse of the F1-F2 vowel space under different speaking conditions (see Figure 11–7 and associated discussion). Variability in the acoustic characteristics of a class of speech sounds is allowable provided it does not compromise the speaker's need to be understood and the listener's requirement for speech signals that meet the criterion of phonemic contrast. The speaker, according to Lindblom, calibrates just how much phonetic contrastivity a listener requires in a specific listening environment. Articulatory behavior is then adjusted to meet those requirements. This view seems more consistent with natural communication situations than one in which a very narrow definition of acoustic invariance is required for the acoustic characteristics of speech sounds.

Stops (Still) Win the Prize

On January 8, 2008, one of the authors searched the *Linguistics and Language Behavior Abstracts*, a database devoted to published papers in all aspects of linguistics, including phonetics. The goal was to identify the numbers of publications on different types of consonants, to compare the scientific interest in the various speech sounds (excluding vowels, always a speech scientist's favorite). This search, conducted in 2008 for the first edition of this textbook, was for peer-reviewed articles published from 1950 to January 8, 2008. Updated searches were conducted on October 4, 2012, and August 17, 2017, for the second and current editions of this text. The results, given by keyword and number of hits in parentheses with the first number representing the 2008 search, the second number the 2012 search, and the third number the current text, were stops (1658, 3965, 9663), fricatives (879, 1785, 3792), nasals (507, 2143, 4286), affricates (329, 566, 1250), and liquids (271, 648, 1710). We can add rhotics to these numbers (109, 205, 323). Among consonants, scientists still love stops the most, which may be partially explained by their domineering frequency of occurrence in languages of the world. The rankings of the other speech sounds is pretty much the same as it was in 2012. Will speech scientists ever say "Stop that!" and focus relatively more attention on other sounds? Those poor affricates. Stay tuned.

AFFRICATES

As noted in Chapter 9, affricates have aspects of both stop and fricative articulation. Affricates have not been studied extensively in English, and only a limited amount of work on affricate acoustics has been completed (see Stevens, 1993). What is known is that the frication interval of the English affricates /tʃ/ and /dʒ/ is longer than the frication interval of the stop component and shorter than the typical duration of the fricative component. Moreover, the stop closure duration of affricates tends to be slightly shorter than the closure duration of singleton stops. Also, place of articulation of the English affricates is slightly posterior to the place of articulation for lingua-alveolar stops and fricatives (Fletcher, 1989). This means that the frication spectrum and pattern of formant transitions into and out of an English affricate are likely to be different than the pattern for either lingua-alveolars or dorsals, as discussed above (see Stevens, 1998 for further information).

ACOUSTIC CHARACTERISTICS OF PROSODY

Prosody encompasses intonation, rhythm, stress, pause, and even grammatical function. The relevant acoustic measures include phrase-level F0 and intensity contours, relative timing measures of multisyllabic utterances, pause occurrence and duration, and local (segmental) changes in F0, intensity, duration, and vowel quality that are used to signal syllable stress.

Phrase-Level F0 Contours

Figure 11–37 shows a spectrogram of close to 9 s of speech produced by an adult female reading a standard passage ("The Hunter Passage"; see Crystal & House, 1982). Immediately above the spectrogram is an F0 trace, generated automatically by TF32 and edited for obvious F0-estimation errors (see Chapter 10). The speaker read the following: "In late fall and early spring the short rays of the sun call a true son of the out of doors back to the places of his childhood." The phrases in this utterance, separated according to very coarse grammatical phrase rules, are shown in Figure 11–37 above the F0 trace. The orthographic transcription of each phrase extends roughly over the time span corresponding to the acoustic signal for the phrase. The organization of the F0 trace within each of these phrases is consistent with the description of phrase-level, F0 contours provided years ago by Lehiste (1970) in her famous book, *Suprasegmentals*. Lehiste noted that, for declarative phrases, an F0 peak typically occurs near the beginning of the phrase, followed by a gradually declining F0 to the lowest value at the end of the phrase. In Figure 11–37 the peak (highest) F0 values within a phrase are indicated by black arrows, the low F0 values by red arrows. Each "phrase" is a grammatical unit, and the peak F0 occurs near the beginning of the unit, often during the first content word. The lowest F0 within each phrase typically occurs during the phrase-final word. The tendency of F0 to start high and then decline steadily throughout

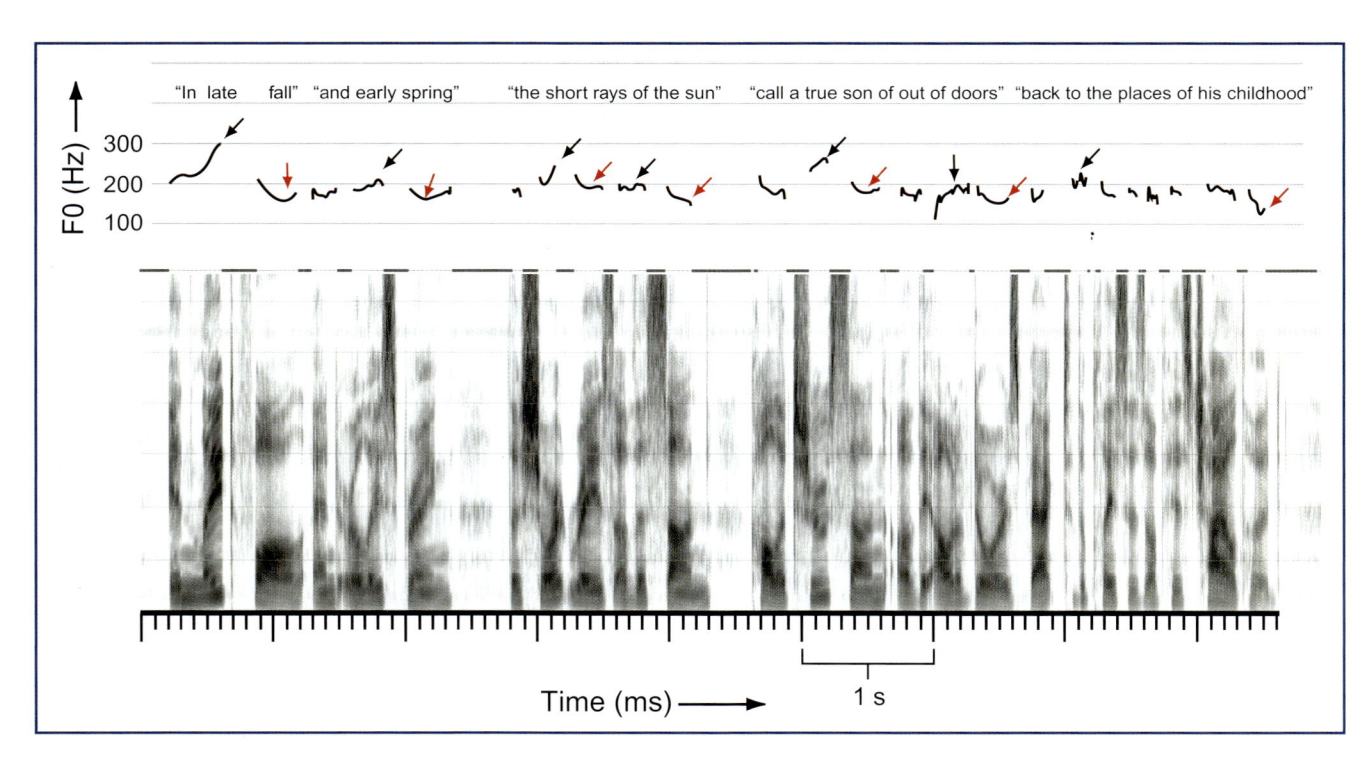

Figure 11–37. Spectrogram (*lower part of figure*) and time-synchronized F0 contour (*upper part of figure*) showing F0 variation across five phrases from a connected reading by an adult female. Within each phrase, the dark arrows point to the approximate location of the highest F0, the red arrow to the lowest F0. See text for additional information.

an utterance is called F0 *declination*. Each of the phrases in Figure 11–37 shows F0 declination; the details vary with each phrase, but the general pattern is present. Similar observations of F0 patterns across grammatical phrases were made by Lea (1973) in his extensive study of read and spontaneous utterances.

In Figure 11–37, the highest F0 value (~300 Hz) throughout the *entire* utterance occurs at the beginning, during the first content word ("late"). The lowest F0 value (~120 Hz) of the utterance occurs on the final syllable of the final word ("childhood"). It seems the structure of this sequence of phrases may be organized at a "supraphrase" level, as if a larger-scale declination was planned by the speaker across the sequence of several phrases. A half-decade following the publication of *Suprasegmentals*, Lehiste (1975) described this "supraphrase" declination of F0 as if a paragraph containing several phrases was organized as a prosodic unit with individual phrases as subunits.

The F0 contours shown in Figure 11–37 are for declarative phrases. Interrogative phrases have different F0 contours. An interrogative F0 contour typically has a *rising* F0 at the end of an utterance, not the falling F0 shown within and across the phrases in Figure 11–37. The utterance-final rise of F0 is a cue to the listener, along with other cues (lexical, syntactic, situational), that a question is being asked. F0 contours may also rise at the end of a declarative utterance when the speaker intends to continue talking. These F0 rises are less dramatic than the rise for questions, but they are effective in signaling the listener that the talker is not finished (Lea, 1973). When a talker is finished and wants to signal the listener to respond, he or she is likely to produce a phrase-final F0 contour with a very steep and rapid fall.

F0 contours may also be modified by the level of stress produced on a specific syllable or syllables throughout a phrase or series of phrases. In English, multisyllabic words have lexical stress patterns (such as "frequency" /ˈfrikwənsi/ and "approach" /əˈproʊtʃ/) in which one or more syllables has greater stress than the other syllables. In words such as "frequency" and "approach," the stressed syllable typically has a higher F0 than the unstressed syllable or syllables. The magnitude of the F0 difference between stressed and unstressed syllables is variable across speakers (Howell, 1993; Sereno & Jongman, 1995). Syllables can also be stressed to focus attention on a specific word within an utterance. For example, in the utterance "Put these two back" (Wang, Kent, Duffy, & Thomas, 2005), speakers can add stress to any of the words (e.g., "Put THESE two back" versus "Put these TWO back") to signal their importance in conveying a message. This is called sentence stress (sometimes emphatic stress, or contrastive stress), and the syllable receiving extra emphasis typically has a higher F0 compared with the syllables spoken without extra stress.

As in the case of lexical stress, the magnitude of the F0 difference between the emphatic and normally stressed syllable is variable across speakers (McRoberts, Studdert-Kennedy, & Shankweiler, 1995; Wang et al., 2005). More is said in the section titled "Stress" about the role of F0 in both lexical and sentence stress.

A phrase-level F0 contour is also affected, albeit at a subtle (but systematic) level, by the identity of the specific segments in a phrase. For example, all other things being equal, the F0 of high vowels is 7 to 15 Hz higher than the F0 of low vowels (Lea, 1973; and see Whalen & Levitt, 1995). Also, the F0 following a voiceless consonant is up to 20 Hz higher than the F0 following a voiced consonant (Ohde, 1984; Silverman, 1987). These influences of segmental identity on F0 contours may appear to be small, but listeners can detect them as deviations from the "base" contour (gradually declining or rising) (Silverman, 1987).

Finally, F0 contours are subject to a variety of paralinguistic influences. The term *paralinguistics* is used to describe nonverbal aspects of speech, usually related to prosodic variation, that convey emotion and physiological status. Paralinguistic aspects of vocal communication can be thought of as a backdrop against which a message is transmitted. This vocal backdrop conveys a meaning in parallel to the meaning conveyed by the spoken words. For example, the same words can be spoken in a happy and sad way; happy versus sad is conveyed partially by F0 contours. Studies of variation in F0 contours with natural emotional variation are challenging because they require an experimenter to be there when there is an emotional change, and to identify reliably which emotional state is the correct description for a speaker. Scientists have developed paralinguistic models of F0 contours using actors to simulate different emotions and measuring the resulting variation in phrase-level F0. This work has revealed subtle changes between the F0 contours of simulated emotions such as anger, joy, and sadness (Bänziger & Scherer, 2005). "Sad" F0 contours tend to be flatter than angry or joyful F0 contours, but there is no clear evidence of sharp (categorical) distinctions between them (see review in Pell, 2001).

In summary, phrase-level F0 contours are subject to a number of influences. The basic form of declarative and interrogative contours is clear, as are segmental influences on local F0 changes throughout an utterance. A general understanding of F0 contours and the influences on them is important because prosody plays a role in clinical issues. For example, F0 variation across words or phrases has been identified as a potentially important aspect of diagnosing developmental verbal apraxia (Shriberg et al., 2003) and characterizing neurogenic speech disorders in adults (Kent & Rosenbek, 1982). Treatment of persons with various speech disorders may have to account for paralinguistic influences on F0 contours, as in Parkinson disease, where depression seems to be a component of the disease.

Phrase-Level Intensity Contours

Phrase-level intensity contours have not been studied as extensively as F0 contours, but clinical considerations suggest the need for more data on this aspect of prosody. In a connected speech sample, an intensity contour varies over time primarily because consonants are less intense than vowels. An estimate of typical intensity differences between consonants and vowels is 7 to 14 dB. The degree to which consonants are less intense than vowels depends on many factors, including type of consonant and type of vowel, position of the consonant in a word, syllable stress level, overall vocal effort level, and sex of the speaker (Fairbanks & Miron, 1957). In more recent data from conversational speech, the standard deviation of intensity across utterances (pauses, and therefore "minimum" or theoretically zero intensity intervals, were excluded in this analysis) was found to be about 6.5 dB (Rosen, Kent, Delaney, & Duffy, 2006). This number is consistent with the low end of the 7 to 14 dB range reported by Fairbanks and Miron because the standard deviation reflects intensity variation across an utterance between relatively high-intensity vowels and lower-intensity consonants.

Figure 11–38 shows a relative intensity trace, scaled in decibels, for the same utterance shown in Figure 11–37. Selected relative intensities have been marked to show the typical differences between consonants (red arrows) and vowels (black arrows). For example, in the phrase "the short rays of the sun," the relative intensity of /ʃ/ is about 6 dB less than the intensity of the following vocalic segment /ɔr/, and the relative intensity of /s/ is about 12 dB less than the following /ʌ/. Note also the very low, relative intensities of two stop closure intervals (upward-pointing, red arrows), consistent with a closed vocal tract that radiates little or no energy.

The clinical potential of phrase-level intensity contours is that a measure such as the standard deviation

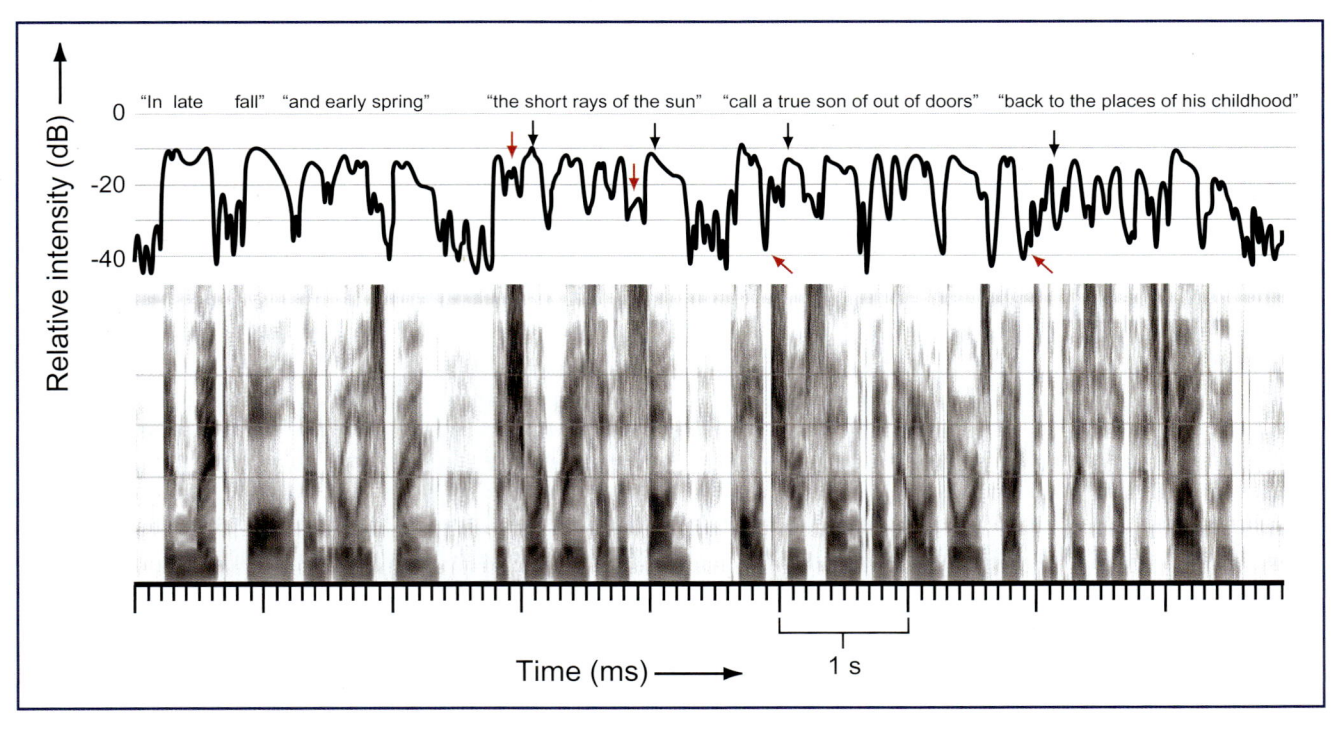

Figure 11–38. Spectrogram (*lower part of figure*) and time-synchronized intensity contour (*upper part of figure*) showing intensity variation across five phrases from connected reading by an adult female. Selected vowel intensities are shown by downward-pointing dark arrows; selected consonant intensities are shown by downward-pointing red arrows. The two slanted upward-pointing red arrows indicate intensities during stop closure intervals.

> **Paralinguistics Trivia, Literally**
>
> Paralinguistics is the branch of linguistics concerned with how utterances are spoken—their loudness, melody, rate, even voice quality. These utterance characteristics can convey mood, intent, and personality characteristics. Kimble and Seidel (1991) used a game of trivia to study the confidence with which people answered questions. They approached this as a paralinguistic question, hypothesizing that more confident answers (as rated by the responders) would have greater speech intensity (i.e., the answers would be louder) and be delivered faster than less confident answers. The data, as reported by Kimble and Seidel, supported the hypothesis. Casual observation suggests that politicians, bullies, and certain radio-show hosts and their guests already understand this effect.

may serve as an index of the degree to which *segmental contrast* is maintained in a client's speech. In typical speech, acoustic boundaries between consonants and vowels are often "sharp," resulting in sudden changes in energy (i.e., intensity). The sharpness of these boundaries, or the sudden contrasts in energy between consonants and vowels, help listeners identify the presence of a succession of segments. When these sharp boundaries are dulled, perhaps because a speaker does not make tight consonant constrictions or produces low-energy vowels, the listener's task becomes more difficult. In a sense, the listener loses the segmental landmarks that allow rapid and efficient sound identification and ultimately the ability to access the words that have been spoken (Mattys & Liss, 2008; Stevens, 2002). The reduction or loss of segmental landmarks is a problem in many speech disorders.

Stress

English has multisyllabic words in which one syllable (sometimes two) is (are) stressed relative to the others. "Dictionary pronunciation," or more technically "lexical stress," is a description of which syllables in a word are stressed and which are not stressed. Lexically stressed syllables often have higher F0, greater intensity, longer duration, and perhaps a less reduced vowel formant pattern compared with unstressed syllables (Fry, 1955; Lea, 1973; Sereno & Jongman, 1995). This generalization applies not only to noun-verb pairs in which the segments are the same (such as noun "rebel" /ˈrɛbl̩/ versus verb "rebel" /rəˈbɛl/, or noun "survey" /ˈsɜrveɪ/ versus verb "survey" /sɚˈveɪ/), but also to the F0 pattern for a multisyllabic word such as "Escanaba" /ɛskəˈnɑbə/. The same combination of acoustic variables may also be used for sentence stress, as defined above.

Kochanski, Grabe, Coleman, and Rosner (2005) reviewed the long history of research efforts to determine how the several acoustic variables associated with stress combine to produce a listener's perception of syllable prominence. The term *prominence* is used to refer to syllables that "stand out" for a listener—it is a perceptual term. Prominence and stress are often used interchangeably, but technically they are different.[18] As Kochanski et al. noted, many scientists regard the relative value of F0 or movement of the F0 contour (e.g., a rapid increase in F0) to be a primary correlate of stress. The evidence on which this claim is based, however, is slim and typically derived from unnatural speaking situations (single words, or highly formal sentence readings). Howell (1993) showed that different speakers use very different combinations of F0, intensity, duration, and vowel formant frequencies to produce stressed syllables in two-syllable words. Speakers did not follow a rule in choosing one phonetic "solution," such as raising F0, to make a syllable prominent. Similar variation across speakers in the use of F0, duration, and intensity for lexical stress patterns can be found in data published by Sereno and Jongman (1995). Kochanski et al. examined various kinds of speech in British and Irish English, including spontaneous speech samples, in which prominent syllables were marked by two experienced phoneticians. They used statistical classifiers, as discussed above for classification of nasals, rhotics, stops, and fricatives, to determine which acoustic measures were most successful in identifying the prominent syllables. F0 measures had only a weak role in successful classification of prominent syllables. Syllable intensity and duration measures were far more successful in classifying the syllables marked as prominent.

The findings of Kochanski et al. (2005) are instructive for clinical strategies seeking to use stress to treat and understand speech disorders. Apparently, a patient who has difficulty stressing syllables for lexical stress or for sentence stress has multiple ways to make

---

[18] A technical difference between stress and prominence is that stress is phonological and prominence is achieved by phonetic solutions. Presumably, there are several *phonetic* solutions to making a syllable prominent (F0, intensity, duration, vowel quality), and any one or a combination of these ways may satisfy the *phonological* requirement of prominence for a stressed syllable.

a syllable prominent. Some studies have attempted to average acoustic measures related to stress to achieve a "composite" index of stress as a classifier of speech disorders. For example, Shriberg et al. (2003) averaged measures of F0, intensity, and duration to construct an acoustic index of lexical stress for bisyllabic word forms as a possible unique marker for children with apraxia of speech. The composite acoustic measure treated all acoustic measures related to stress as equal in the contribution to making a syllable prominent, an assumption not consistent with the information reviewed above. The inconsistency is not only in the potentially greater contribution of intensity and duration, compared with F0, to the perception of stress (Kochanski et al., 2005), but also in the varied use of the measures across speakers to make a syllable prominent (Howell, 1993; Sereno & Jongman, 1995). Similarly, some studies (Penner, Miller, Hertrich, Ackermann, & Schumm, 2001) have evaluated the ability of speakers with Parkinson's disease to use F0 as an indicator of sentence stress, but have not included other potential acoustic correlates of prominence (intensity, duration, vowel quality) in their analyses. This may result in an incomplete representation of the prominence-producing capabilities of a group of speakers.

The point of this discussion is not to be overly critical of the cited studies. Rather, it highlights the complexity of stress/prominence, both as production and perception phenomena. A growing awareness of the importance of prosodic control in communication disorders requires a careful and complete understanding of the relevant phenomena (Blake, 2007; Caspar, Raphael, Harris, & Geibel, 2007; Lenden & Flipsen, 2007).

Rhythm

Rhythm is the patterning of segment or syllable durations across an utterance. If the unit of speech timing is taken to be a syllable, English is said to have a rhythm in which long and short-duration syllables alternate with each other. The long syllables are the stressed ones, the short syllables are unstressed. The alternation between long and short syllables is not usually a pattern of one long/one short/one long/one short (and so on), but rather a sequence of one long followed by several short syllables. This repeating pattern of one stressed syllable followed by several unstressed syllables is why English is referred to as a *stress-timed language*. A strict view of a stress-timed language requires the duration *between* stressed syllables in an utterance to be nearly constant. Stated otherwise, in a connected discourse, the time required to produce a stressed syllable and all the unstressed syllables that follow is nearly identical to the time required to produce another

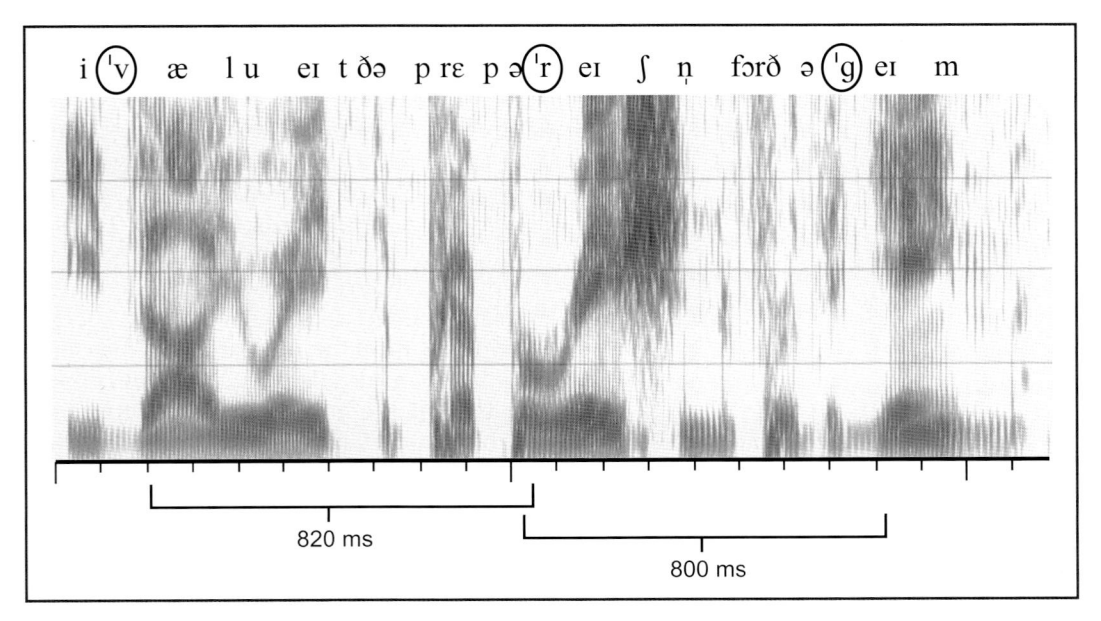

Figure 11-39. Spectrogram of the utterance "Evaluate the preparation for the game" as an illustration of stress timing in English. The stress marks in the phonetic transcription show the stressed syllables of the succeeding phrases, and two stressed-syllable-plus-unstressed-syllable intervals are measured at the bottom of the spectrogram, one for the first "stress group," the next one for the second "stress group." See text for additional details.

stressed syllable and its following unstressed syllables. A simple example of this idea is shown in Figure 11–39, where a spectrogram of the utterance "Evaluate the preparation for the game" is shown together with a time-aligned phonetic transcription. The stressed syllables in this utterance (/væ/ in "evaluate," /reɪ/ in "preparation," /geɪ/ in "game") are indicated in the phonetic transcription; the consonants preceding the stressed syllables are enclosed in ovals. At the bottom of the spectrogram there are two time intervals, the first of 820 ms between the onset of the first glottal pulse of the stressed /æ/ and the first stressed /eɪ/, the second of 800 ms between the initial glottal pulses of the first and second stressed /eɪ/s. The nearly identical time intervals between the consecutive stressed intervals of this brief utterance seem consistent with the idea, stated above, of a stress-timed language. Note also the several short-duration, unstressed syllables following the first two stressed syllables. As Lehiste (1973) demonstrated, absolute *isochrony*—the phenomenon of equal time intervals between stressed syllables—does not exist, but speakers may approximate isochrony in production and listeners may hear these approximations as more isochronous than they really are (Lehiste, 1977).[19]

This summary of speech rhythm as an aspect of prosody is important because certain speech disorders exhibit rhythmic abnormalities. For example, speakers of English with diseases of the cerebellum may produce speech with a rhythm that distorts the normal approximation to stress timing by making *all* syllables roughly equal in duration. This eliminates the normal duration difference between stressed and unstressed syllables and results in perception of "metered" or "scanned" speech (Darley, Aronson, & Brown, 1975). In "scanned" speech, listeners report that each syllable sounds metered out in a fixed (relatively constant) time interval, as if a metronome were timing the speaker's output. Scientists interested in speech rhythm disorders have adopted an acoustic measure (or a variation of it) originally developed by Low, Grabe, and Nolan (2000) for use in second language acquisition (rhythmic differences between languages can cause substantial difficulty for the second language learner). This acoustic measure is called the *Pairwise Variability Index* (PVI). The formula for the PVI is available in Low et al.; here it is sufficient to describe the logic of the measure. If the vowels of consecutive syllables have very different durations, as would be expected in a stress-timed language such as English, the measure reflects this with a "high-difference" value computed over many syllables. If, on the other hand, the vowels of consecutive syllables have very similar durations, as in ataxic dysarthria or syllable-timed languages (e.g., Spanish, for which the duration between consecutive syllables, rather than stressed syllables, is nearly constant), the measure yields a "low-difference" value. The PVI is, therefore, an acoustic measure of the relative duration difference between consecutive syllables in connected speech. Measures such as the PVI show great potential as a diagnostic marker for different types of speech disorder (see Henrich, Lowit, Schalling, & Mennen, 2006; Liss, LeGendre, & Lotto, 2010; Liss, White, Mattys, Lansford, Lotto, Spitzer, & Caviness, 2009).

REVIEW

For the speech-language pathologist, there is much that can be learned and documented about an individual's speech production problem, using the techniques of acoustic phonetic analysis.

Acoustic phonetic analysis is noninvasive, and a tremendous amount of scientific literature on typical speakers and speakers with disorders is available for comparison to a client's data.

Speech analysis can be implemented rather easily and relatively inexpensively on a desktop or laptop computer.

The audiologist who diagnoses and treats hearing loss with hearing aids or implantable devices should have a working knowledge of acoustic phonetics and its link to speech intelligibility.

Acoustic characteristics of vowels, diphthongs, nasals, semivowels, fricatives, stops, and affricates are described with respect to formant frequencies, antiresonances, formant transitions, spectral shapes, segment durations, and segment intensities.

Several approaches to measurement of segment characteristics are described and evaluated.

Suprasegmental (prosodic) characteristics including F0 and intensity contours, and speech rhythm are presented.

Acoustic characteristics of lexical and sentence stress are presented and shown to be variable across speakers.

Acoustic phonetics is an increasing presence in both the speech-language pathology and audiology literature, and a working knowledge of theory and data will serve the clinician well as she or he strives for excellence in service delivery.

---

[19]For advanced reading on the phenomenon of isochrony and rhythmic variation across language, see Port (2003) and White and Mattys (2007).

REFERENCES

Assman, P., Nearey, T., & Hogan, J. (1982). Vowel identification: Orthographic, perceptual, and acoustical factors. *Journal of the Acoustical Society of America, 71,* 975–989.

Auzou, P., Özsancak, C., Morris, R., Jan, M., Eustache, F., & Hannequin, D. (2000). Voice onset time in aphasia, apraxia of speech and dysarthria: A review. *Clinical Linguistics & Phonetics, 14,* 131–150.

Awan, S. N., Bressman, T., Poburka, B., Roy, N., Sharp, H., & Watts, C. (2015). Dialectical effects on nasalance: A multicenter, cross continental study. *Journal of Speech, Language, and Hearing Research, 58,* 69-77.

Baken, R.J., & Orlikoff, R.F. (1999). *Clinical measures of speech and voice (speech science),* (2nd ed). Boston, MA: Cengage Learning.

Bänziger, T., & Scherer, K. (2005). The role of intonation in emotional expression. *Speech Communication, 46,* 252–267.

Baum, S., & Blumstein, S. (1987). Preliminary observations on the use of duration as a cue to the syllable-initial fricative consonant voicing in English. *Journal of the Acoustical Society of America, 82,* 1073–1077.

Behrens, S., & Blumstein, S. (1988). Acoustic characteristics of English voiceless fricatives: A descriptive analysis. *Journal of Phonetics, 16,* 295–298.

Berisha, V., Sandoval, S., Utianski, R., Liss, J., & Spanias, A. (2014). Characterizing the distribution of the quadrilateral vowel space area. *Journal of the Acoustical Society of America, 135,* 421–427.

Bettens, K., De Bodt, M., Maryn, Y., Luytn, A., Wuytz, F. L., & Van Lierde, K. M. (2016). The relationship between Nasality Severity Index 2.0 and perceptual judgments of hypernasality. *Journal of Communication Disorders, 62,* 67–81.

Blake, M. (2007). Perspectives on treatment for communication deficits associated with right hemisphere brain damage. *American Journal of Speech-Language Pathology, 16,* 331–342.

Blumstein, S., & Stevens, K. (1979). Acoustic invariance in speech production: Evidence from measurements of the spectral characteristics of stop consonants. *Journal of the Acoustical Society of America, 66,* 1001–1017.

Boyce, S. E. (2015). Articulatory phonetics for residual speech sound disorders: A focus on /r/. *Seminars in Speech and Language, 36,* 257–270.

Bradlow, A. (1995). A comparative acoustic study of English and Spanish vowels. *Journal of the Acoustical Society of America, 97,* 1916–1924.

Bradlow, A., Torretta, G., & Pisoni, D. (1996). Intelligibility of normal speech I: Global and fine-grained acoustic-phonetic talker characteristics. *Speech Communication, 20,* 255–272.

Bunton, K. (2015). Effects of nasal port area on perception of nasality and measures of nasalance based on computational modeling. *Cleft Palate-Craniofacial Journal, 110,* 110–114.

Byrd, D. (1993). 54,000 American stops. *UCLA Working Papers in Phonetics, 83,* 97–116.

Calandruccio, L., Van Engen, K., Dhar, S., & Bradlow, A. R. (2010). The effectiveness of clear speech as a masker. *Journal of Speech, Language, and Hearing Research, 53,* 1458–1471.

Caspar, M., Raphael, L., Harris, K., & Geibel, J. (2007). Speech prosody in cerebellar ataxia. *International Journal of Language and Communication Disorders, 42,* 407–426.

Chaney, C. (1988). Acoustic analysis of correct and misarticulated semivowels. *Journal of Speech and Hearing Research, 31,* 275–287.

Chen, M. (1995). Acoustic parameters of nasalized vowels in hearing-impaired and normal-hearing speakers. *Journal of the Acoustical Society of America, 98,* 2443–2453.

Chen, M. (1997). Acoustic correlates of English and French nasalized vowels. *Journal of the Acoustical Society of America, 102,* 2360–2370.

Chen, Y., Robb, M., Gilbert, H., & Lerman, J. (2001). Vowel production by Mandarin speakers of English. *Clinical Linguistics & Phonetics, 15,* 427–440.

Cho, T., Jun, S-A., & Ladefoged, P. (2002). Acoustic and aerodynamic correlates of Korean stops and fricatives. *Journal of Phonetics, 30,* 193–228.

Cho, T., & Ladefoged, P. (1999). Variation and universals in VOT: Evidence from 18 languages. *Journal of Phonetics, 27,* 207–229.

Chuang, H-F., Yang, C-C., Chi, L-Y., Weismer, G., & Wang, Y-T. (2012). Speech intelligibility, speaking rate, and vowel formant characteristics in Mandarin-speaking children with cochlear implant. *International Journal of Speech Language Pathology, 14,* 119–129.

Clopper, C., Pisoni, D., & de Jong, K. (2005). Acoustic characteristics of the vowel systems of six regional varieties of American English. *Journal of the Acoustical Society of America, 118,* 1661–1676.

Craig, H., Thompson, C., Washington, J., & Potter, S. (2003). Phonological features of child African American English. *Journal of Speech, Language, and Hearing Research, 46,* 623–635.

Crystal, T., & House, A. (1982). Segmental durations in connected-speech signals: Preliminary results. *Journal of the Acoustical Society of America, 72,* 705–716.

Crystal, T., & House, A. (1988a). The duration of American-English vowels: An overview. *Journal of Phonetics, 16,* 263–284.

Crystal, T., & House, A. (1988b). The duration of American-English stop consonants: An overview. *Journal of Phonetics, 16,* 285–294.

Crystal, T., & House, A. (1988c). Segmental durations in connected-speech signals: Current results. *Journal of the Acoustical Society of America, 83,* 1553–1573.

Crystal, T., & House, A. (1988d). A note on the durations of fricatives in American English. *Journal of the Acoustical Society of America, 84,* 1932–1935.

Dalston, R. (1972). *A spectrographic analysis of the spectral and temporal acoustic characteristics of English semivowels spoken by three-year-old children and adults* (Doctoral dissertation). Northwestern University, Evanston, IL.

Dalston, R. (1975). Acoustic characteristics of English /w,r,l/ spoken correctly by young children and adults. *Journal of the Acoustical Society of America, 57,* 462–469.

Dang, J., & Honda, K. (1995). Acoustic characteristics of the paranasal sinuses derived from transmission characteristic measurement and morphological observation. *Journal of the Acoustical Society of America, 100,* 3374–3383.

Darley, F., Aronson, A., & Brown, J. (1975). *Motor speech disorders.* Philadelphia, PA: W. B. Saunders.

Davidsen-Nielsen, N. (1974). Syllabification in English words with medial sp, st, sk. *Journal of Phonetics, 2,* 15–45.

DeMerit, J. L. (1997). *Acoustic and perceptual effects of clear speech on duration-dependent vowel contrasts* (Unpublished doctoral dissertation). University of Wisconsin–Madison, Madison, WI.

Espy-Wilson, C. (1992). Acoustic measures for linguistic features distinguishing the semivowels /wjrl/ in American English. *Journal of the Acoustical Society of America, 92,* 736–757.

Espy-Wilson, C. (1994). A feature-based semivowel recognition system. *Journal of the Acoustical Society of America, 96,* 65–72.

Fairbanks, G., & Miron, M. (1957). Effects of vocal effort upon the consonant-vowel ratio within the syllable. *Journal of the Acoustical Society of America, 29,* 621–626.

Feng, G., & Castelli, E. (1996). Some acoustic features of nasal and nasalized vowels: A target for vowel nasalization. *Journal of the Acoustical Society of America, 99,* 3694–3706.

Ferguson, S., & Kewley-Port, D. (2007). Talker differences in clear and conversational speech: Acoustic characteristics of vowels. *Journal of Speech, Language, and Hearing Research, 50,* 1241–1255.

Fletcher, S. (1989). Palatometric specification of stop, affricate, and sibilant sounds. *Journal of Speech and Hearing Research, 32,* 736–748.

Fletcher, S. G. (1976). "Nasalance" vs. listener judgments of nasality. *Cleft Palate Journal, 13,* 31–44.

Fletcher, A. R., McAuliffe, M. J., Lansford, K. L., & Liss, J. M. (2017). Assessing vowel centralization in dysarthria: A comparison of methods. *Journal of Speech, Language, and Hearing Research, 60,* 341–354.

Forrest, K., Weismer, G., Hodge, M., Dinnsen, D., & Elbert, M. (1990). Statistical analysis of word-initial /k/ and /t/ produced by normal and phonologically disordered children. *Clinical Linguistics & Phonetics, 4,* 327–340.

Forrest, K., Weismer, G., Milenkovic, P., & Dougall, R. (1988). Statistical analysis of word-initial voiceless obstruents: Preliminary data. *Journal of the Acoustical Society of America, 84,* 115–124.

Fourakis, M. (1991). Tempo, stress, and vowel reduction in American English. *Journal of the Acoustical Society of America, 90,* 1816–1827.

Fox, R. A., & Jacewicz, E. (2017). Reconceptualizing the vowel space in analyzing regional dialect variation and sound change in American English. *Journal of the Acoustical Society of America, 142,* 444–459. doi:10.1121/1.4991021

Fox, R., & Nissan S. (2005). Sex-related acoustic changes in voiceless English fricatives. *Journal of Speech, Language, and Hearing Research, 48,* 753–765.

Fry, D. (1955). Duration and intensity as physical correlates of linguistic stress. *Journal of the Acoustical Society of America, 27,* 765–768.

Fujimura, O. (1962). Analysis of nasal consonants. *Journal of the Acoustical Society of America, 34,* 1865–1875.

Gay, T. (1968). Effect of speaking rate on diphthong formant movements. *Journal of the Acoustical Society of America, 44,* 1570–1573.

Gopal, H. S. (1996). Generalizability of current models of vowel duration. *Phonetica, 53,* 1–32.

Granlund, S., Hazan, V., & Baker, B. (2012). An acoustic phonetic comparison of the clear speaking styles of Finnish-English late bilinguals. *Journal of Phonetics, 40,* 509–520.

Haley, K. L., Seelinger, E., Mandulak, K. C., & Zajac, D.J. (2010). Evaluating the spectral distinction between sibilant fricatives through a speaker-centered approach. *Journal of Phonetics, 38,* 548–554.

Halle, M., Hughes, G., & Radley, J-P. (1957). Acoustic properties of stop consonants. *Journal of the Acoustical Society of America, 29,* 107–116.

Harrington, J. (1994). The contribution of the murmur and vowel to the place of articulation distinction in nasal consonants. *Journal of the Acoustical Society of America, 96,* 19–32.

Harris, K. (1958). Cues for the discrimination of American English fricatives in spoken syllables. *Language and Speech, 1,* 1–7.

Henrich, J., Lowit, A., Schalling, E., & Mennen, I. (2006). Rhythmic disturbance in ataxic dysarthria: A comparison of different measures and speech tasks. *Journal of Medical Speech-Language Pathology, 14,* 291–296.

Hillenbrand, J., Clark, M., & Nearey, T. (2001). Effects of consonant environment on vowel formant patterns. *Journal of the Acoustical Society of America, 109,* 748–763.

Hillenbrand, J., Getty, L., Clark, M., & Wheeler, K. (1995). Acoustic characteristics of American English vowels. *Journal of the Acoustical Society of America, 97,* 3099–3111.

Hillenbrand, J., & Nearey, T. (1999). Identification of resynthesized /hVd/ utterances: Effects of formant contour. *Journal of the Acoustical Society of America, 105,* 3509–3523.

Hirose, H. (1976). Posterior cricoarytenoid as a speech muscle. *Annals of Otology, Rhinology, and Laryngology, 85,* 334–343.

Hirose, H. (1977). Laryngeal adjustments in consonant production. *Phonetica, 34,* 289–294.

Hoffman, P., Stager, S., & Daniloff, R. (1983). Perception and production of misarticulated /r/. *Journal of Speech and Hearing Disorders, 48,* 210–215.

Holbrook, A., & Fairbanks, G. (1962). Diphthong formants and their movements. *Journal of Speech and Hearing Research, 5,* 38–58.

House, A. (1961). On vowel duration in English. *Journal of the Acoustical Society of America, 33,* 1174–1178.

Howell, P. (1993). Cue trading in the production and perception of vowel stress. *Journal of the Acoustical Society of America, 94,* 2063–2073.

Hughes, G., & Halle, M. (1956). Spectral properties of fricative consonants. *Journal of the Acoustical Society of America, 28,* 303–310.

Iskarous, K., Shadle, C. H., & Proctor, M. I. (2011). Articulatory-acoustic kinematics: The production of American English /s/. *Journal of the Acoustical Society of America, 129,* 944–954.

Jacewicz, W., & Fox, R. A. (2012). The effects of cross-generational and cross-dialectal variation on vowel identification and classification. *Journal of the Acoustical Society of America, 131,* 1413–1433.

Johnson, K. (2003). *Acoustic and auditory phonetics.* Oxford, UK: Blackwell.

Johnson, K., Ladefoged, P., & Lindau, M. (1993). Individual differences in vowel production. *Journal of the Acoustical Society of America, 94,* 701–714.

Jongman, A., Fourakis, M., & Sereno, J. (1989). The acoustic vowel space of modern Greek and German. *Language and Speech, 32,* 221–248.

Jongman, A., Wayland, R., & Wong, S. (2000). Acoustic characteristics of English fricatives. *Journal of the Acoustical Society of America, 108,* 1252–1263.

Kent, R., & Rosenbek, J. (1982). Prosodic disturbance and neurologic lesion. *Brain and Language, 15,* 259–291.

Kessinger, R., & Blumstein, S. (1997). Effects of speaking rate on voice-onset time in Thai, French, and English. *Journal of Phonetics, 25,* 143–168.

Kewley-Port, D. (1983). Time-varying features as correlates of place of articulation in stop consonants. *Journal of the Acoustical Society of America, 73,* 322–335.

Kim, H-H., Hasegawa-Johnson, M., & Perlman, A. (2011). Vowel contrast and speech intelligibility in dysarthria. *Folia Phoniatrica et Logopaedica, 63,* 187-194.

Kimble, C., & Seidel, S. (1991). Vocal signs of confidence. *Journal of Nonverbal Behavior, 15,* 99–105.

Kingston, J., & Diehl, R. (1994). Phonetic knowledge. *Language, 70,* 419–454.

Klatt, D. (1975). Vowel lengthening is syntactically determined in a connected discourse. *Journal of Phonetics, 3,* 129–140.

Klatt, D. (1976). Linguistic uses of segmental duration in English: Acoustic and perceptual evidence. *Journal of the Acoustical Society of America, 59,* 1208–1221.

Kobatake, H., & Ohtani, S. (1987). Spectral transition dynamics of voiceless stop consonants. *Journal of the Acoustical Society of America, 81,* 1146–1151.

Kochanski, G., Grabe, E., Coleman, J., & Rosner, B. (2005). Loudness predicts prominence: Fundamental frequency lends little. *Journal of the Acoustical Society of America, 118,* 1038–1054.

Krause, J., & Braida, L. (2004). Acoustic properties of naturally produced clear speech at normal speaking rates. *Journal of the Acoustical Society of America, 115,* 362–378.

Kuo, C., & Weismer, G. (2016). Vowel reduction across tasks for male speakers of American English speakers. *Journal of the Acoustical Society of America, 140,* 369–383.

Kurowski, K., & Blumstein, S. (1984). Perceptual integration of the murmur and formant transitions for place of articulation in nasal consonants. *Journal of the Acoustical Society of America, 76,* 383–390.

Kurowski, K., & Blumstein, S. (1987). Acoustic properties for place of articulation in nasal consonants. *Journal of the Acoustical Society of America, 81,* 1917–1927.

Labov, W. (1991). The three dialects of English. In P. Eckert (Ed.), *New ways of analyzing sound change* (pp. 1–44). New York, NY: Academic Press.

Ladefoged, P. (2005). *Vowels and consonants* (2nd ed.). Oxford, UK: Blackwell.

Ladefoged, P., & Maddieson, I. (1996). *The sounds of the world's languages.* Oxford, UK: Blackwell.

Lam, J., & Tjaden, K. (2013). Acoustic-perceptual relationships in variants of clear speech. *Folia Phoniatrica et Logopaedica, 65,* 148–153.

Lam, J., Tjaden, K., & Wilding, G. (2012). Acoustics of clear speech: Effect of instruction. *Journal of Speech, Language, and Hearing Research, 55,* 1807–1821.

Lansford, K. L., & Liss, J.M. (2014). Vowel acoustics in dysarthria: Speech disorder diagnosis and classification. *Journal of Speech, Language, and Hearing Research, 57,* 57–67.

Lea, W. (1973). Segmental and suprasegmental influences on fundamental frequency contours. In L. M. Hyman (Ed.), *Consonant types and tone* (pp. 15–70). Los Angeles, CA: University of Southern California.

Lee, J., Littlejohn, M. A., & Simmons, Z. (2017). Acoustic and tongue kinematic vowel space in speakers with and without dysarthria. *International Journal of Speech-Language Pathology, 19,* 195–204.

Lee, S., Potamianos, A. and Narayanan, S. (2014). Developmental acoustic study of American English diphthongs. *Journal of the Acoustical Society of America, 136,* 1880–1894.

Lehiste, I. (1964). Acoustical characteristics of selected English consonants. *International Journal of American Linguistics, 30,* 1–197.

Lehiste, I. (1970). *Suprasegmentals.* Cambridge, MA: MIT Press.

Lehiste, I. (1973). Rhythmic units and syntactic units in production and perception. *Journal of the Acoustical Society of America, 54,* 1228–1234.

Lehiste, I. (1975). The phonetic structure of paragraphs. In A. Cohen & S. Nooteboom (Eds.), *Structure and process in speech perception* (pp. 195–206). New York, NY: Springer-Verlag.

Lehiste, I. (1977). Isochrony reconsidered. *Journal of Phonetics, 5,* 153–163.

Lehiste, I., & Peterson, G. (1961). Transitions, glides, and diphthongs. *Journal of the Acoustical Society of America, 33,* 268–277.

Lenden, J., & Flipsen, P. Jr. (2007). Prosody and voice characteristics of children with cochlear implants. *Journal of Communication Disorders, 40,* 66–81.

Leung, K. K. W., Jongman, A., Wang, Y., & Sereno, J. A. (2016). Acoustic characteristics of clearly spoken English tense and lax vowels. *Journal of the Acoustical Society of America, 140,* 45–58.

Liberman, A., Cooper, F., Shankweiler, D., & Studdert-Kennedy, M. (1967). Perception of the speech code. *Psychological Review, 74,* 431–761.

Liberman, A., Delattre, P., Cooper, F., & Gerstman, L. (1954). The role of consonant-vowel transitions in the perception of stop and nasal consonants. *Psychological Monographs, 68,* 1–13.

Lindblom, B. (1963). Spectrographic study of vowel reduction. *Journal of the Acoustical Society of America, 35,* 1773–1781.

Lindblom, B. (1990). Explaining phonetic variation: A sketch of the H&H theory. In W. Hardcastle & A. Marchal (Eds.),

Speech production and speech modeling (pp. 403–440). Dordrecht, Netherlands: Kluwer Academic.

Lindblom, B., Agwuele, A., Sussman, H. M., & Cortes, E. (2007). The effect of emphatic stress on consonant vowel coarticulation. *Journal of the Acoustical Society of America, 121*, 3802–3813.

Lindblom, B., & Sussman, H. M. (2012). Dissecting coarticulation: How locus equations happen. *Journal of Phonetics, 40*, 1-19.

Lisker, L. (1957). Closure duration and the intervocalic voiced-voiceless distinction in English. *Language, 33*, 42–49.

Lisker, L. (1986). "Voicing" in English: A catalogue of acoustic features signaling /b/ versus /p/ in trochees. *Language and Speech, 29*, 3–11.

Lisker, L., & Abramson, A. (1964). A cross-language study of voicing in initial stops. *Word, 20*, 384–442.

Liss, J. M., LeGendre, S., & Lotto, A. J. (2010). Discriminating dysarthria type from envelope modulation spectra. *Journal of Speech, Language, and Hearing Research, 53*, 1246–1255.

Liss, J. M., White, L., Mattys, S. L., Lansford, K., Lotto, A. J., Spitzer, S. M., & Caviness, J. N. (2009). Quantifying speech rhythm abnormalities in the dysarthrias. *Journal of Speech, Language, and Hearing Research, 52*, 1334–1352.

Liu, H-M., Tsao, F-M., & Kuhl, P. (2005). The effect of reduced vowel working space on speech intelligibility in Mandarin-speaking young adults with cerebral palsy. *Journal of the Acoustical Society of America, 117*, 3879–3889.

Löfqvist, A. (1980). Interarticulator programming in stop production. *Journal of Phonetics, 8*, 475–490.

Löfqvist, A., Baer, T., McGarr, N., & Story, R. (1989). The cricothyroid muscle in voicing control. *Journal of the Acoustical Society of America, 85*, 1314–1321.

Löfqvist, A., Baer, T., & Yoshioka, Y. (1981). Scaling of glottal opening. *Phonetica, 38*, 236–251.

Low, L., Grabe, E., & Nolan, F. (2000). Quantitative characterizations of speech rhythm: Syllable-timing in Singapore English. *Language and Speech, 43*, 377–401.

Luce, P., & Charles-Luce, J. (1985). Contextual effects on vowel duration, closure duration, and the consonant/vowel ratio in speech production. *Journal of the Acoustical Society of America, 78*, 1949–1957.

Maddieson, I. (1997). Phonetic universals. In W. Hardcastle & J. Laver (Eds.), *The handbook of phonetic sciences* (pp. 619–639). Oxford, UK: Blackwell.

Marquardt, T., Reinhart, J., & Peterson, H. (1979). Markedness analysis of phonemic substitution errors in apraxia of speech. *Journal of Communication Disorders, 12*, 481–494.

Mattys, S. L., & Liss, J. M. (2008). On building models of spoken word recognition: When there is as much to learn from natural "oddities" as artificial normality. *Perception and Psychophysics, 70*, 1235–1242.

McAllister Byun, T., Buchwald, A., & Mizoguchi, A. (2016). Covert contrast in velar fronting: an acoustic and ultrasound study. *Clinical Linguistics & Phonetics, 30*, 249–276.

McAllister Byun, T., & Tiede, M. (2017). Perception-production relations in later development of American English rhotics. *PLoS One, 12*, e0172022. doi:10.1371/journal.pone.0172022

McRoberts, G., Studdert-Kennedy, M., & Shankweiler, D. (1995). The role of fundamental frequency in signaling linguistic stress and affect: Evidence for a dissociation. *Perception and Psychophysics, 52*, 159–174.

McWhorter, J. (2001). *The power of Babel: A natural history of language*. New York, NY: Henry Holt.

Metz, D., Samar, V., Schiavetti, N., Sitler, R., & Whitehead, R. (1985). Acoustic dimensions of hearing-impaired speakers' intelligibility. *Journal of Speech and Hearing Research, 28*, 345–355.

Mielke, J. (2003). The interplay of speech perception and phonology: Experimental evidence from Turkish. *Phonetica, 60*, 208–229.

Milenkovic, P. (2001). *TF32* [Computer program]. Retrieved from http://user pages.chorus.net/cspeech/

Modarresi, G., Sussman, H. M., Lindblom, B., & Burkingame, E. (2005). Locus equation encoding of stop place: Revisiting the voicing/VOT issue. *Journal of Phonetics, 33*, 101–113.

Moon, S-J., & Lindblom, B. (1994). Interaction between duration, context, and speaking style in English stressed vowels. *Journal of the Acoustical Society of America, 96*, 40–55.

Most, T., Amir, O., & Tobin, Y. (2000) The Hebrew vowels: Raw and normalized acoustic data. *Language and Speech, 43*, 295–308.

Narayanan, S. (1995). *Fricative consonants: An articulatory, acoustic, and systems study* (Doctoral dissertation). University of California, Los Angeles.

Narayanan, S., Alwan, A., & Haker, K. (1997). Toward articulatory-acoustic models for liquid approximants based on MRI and EPG data. Part I. The laterals. *Journal of the Acoustical Society of America, 101*, 1064–1077.

Nearey, T. M., & Assman, P. F. (1986). Modelling the role of inherent spectral change in vowel identification. *Journal of the Acoustical Society of America, 80*, 1297–1308.

Newman, R., Clouse, S., & Burnham, J. (2001). The perceptual consequences of within-talker variability in fricative production. *Journal of the Acoustical Society of America, 109*, 1181–1196.

Norman, L. (1973). Rule addition and intrinsic order. *Minnesota Working Papers in Linguistics and Philosophy of Language, 1*, 135–159.

Nossair, Z., & Zahorian, S. (1991). Dynamic spectral shape features as acoustic correlates for initial stop consonants. *Journal of the Acoustical Society of America, 89*, 2978–2991.

Ohala, J. (1980). *The acoustic origin of the smile*. Paper presented at the 100th meeting of the Acoustical Society of America, Los Angeles.

Ohde, R. (1984). Fundamental frequency as an acoustic correlate of stop consonant voicing. *Journal of the Acoustical Society of America, 75*, 224–230.

Park, S., Theodoros, D., Finch, E., & Cardell, E. (2016). Be clear: A new intensive speech treatment for adults with nonprogressive dysarthria. *American Journal of Speech-Language Pathology, 25*, 97–110.

Pell, M. (2001). Influence of emotion and focus location on prosody in matched statements and questions. *Journal of the Acoustical Society of America, 109*, 1668–1680.

Penner, H., Miller, N., Hertrich, I., Ackermann, H., & Schumm, F. (2001). Dysprosody in Parkinson's disease: An investigation of intonation patterns. *Clinical Linguistics & Phonetics, 15*, 551–566.

Person, J. L., Irwin, J. R., & Turcio, J. (2015). Perception of speech sounds in school-aged children with speech sound disorders. *Seminars in Speech and Language, 36,* 224–233.

Peterson, G., & Barney, H. (1952). Control methods used in a study of the vowels. *Journal of the Acoustical Society of America, 24,* 175–184.

Picheny, M., Durlach, N., & Braida, L. (1985). Speaking clearly for the hard of hearing I: Intelligibility differences between clear and conversational speech. *Journal of Speech and Hearing Research, 28,* 96–103.

Picheny, M., Durlach, N., & Braida, L. (1986). Speaking clearly for the hard of hearing II: Acoustic characteristics of clear and conversational speech. *Journal of Speech and Hearing Research, 29,* 434–446.

Platt, L., Andrews, G., & Howie, P. (1980). Dysarthria of adult cerebral palsy. II. Phonemic analysis of articulation errors. *Journal of Speech and Hearing Research, 23,* 41–55.

Port, R. (2003). Meter and speech. *Journal of Phonetics, 31,* 599–611.

Pruthi, T., & Espy-Wilson, C. (2004). Acoustic parameters for automatic extraction of nasal manner. *Speech Communication, 43,* 225–239.

Qi, Y., & Fox, R. (1992). Analysis of nasal consonants using perceptual linear prediction. *Journal of the Acoustical Society of America, 91,* 1718–1726.

Repp, B. (1986). Perception of the [m]-[n] distinction in CV syllables. *Journal of the Acoustical Society of America, 79,* 1987–1999.

Robb, M. P., & Chen, Y. (2009). Is /h/ phonetically neutral? *Clinical Linguistics & Phonetics, 23,* 842–855.

Rong, P., & Kuehn, D. P. (2010). The effect of oral articulation on the acoustic characteristics of nasalized vowels. *Journal of the Acoustical Society of America, 127,* 2543–2553.

Rosen, K., Kent, R., Delaney, A., & Duffy, J. (2006). Parametric quantitative acoustic analysis of conversation produced by speakers with dysarthria and healthy speakers. *Journal of Speech, Language, and Hearing Research, 49,* 395–411.

Schellinger, S. K., Munson, B., & Edwards, J. (2017). Gradient perception of children's production of /s/ and /θ/: A comparative analysis of rating methods. *Clinical Linguistics & Phonetics, 31,* 80-103.

Seitz, P., McCormick, M., Watson, I., & Bladon, A. (1990). Relational spectral features for place of articulation in nasal consonants. *Journal of the Acoustical Society of America, 87,* 351–358.

Sereno, J., & Jongman, A. (1995). Acoustic correlates of grammatical class. *Language and Speech, 38,* 57–76.

Serrurier, A., & Badin, P. (2008). A three-dimensional articulatory model of the velum and nasopharyngeal wall based on MRI and CT data. *Journal of the Acoustical Society of America, 123,* 2335–2355.

Shriberg, L., Campbell, T., Karlsson, H., Brown, R., McSweeny, J., & Nadler, C. (2003). A diagnostic marker for childhood apraxia of speech: The lexical stress ratio. *Clinical Linguistics & Phonetics, 17,* 549–574.

Silverman, K. (1987). *The structure and processing of fundamental frequency contours* (Doctoral dissertation). Cambridge University, Cambridge, UK.

Simpson, A. P. (2001). Dynamic consequences of differences in male and female vocal tract dimensions. *Journal of the Acoustical Society of America, 109,* 2153–2164.

Smiljanić, R., & Bradlow, A. (2005). Does clear speech enhance the voice onset time contrast in Croatian and English? *Journal of the Acoustical Society of America, 118,* 1900.

Smiljanić, R., & Bradlow, A. R. (2008). Stability of temporal contrasts in conversational and clear speech. *Journal of Phonetics, 36,* 91–113.

Smiljanić, R., & Bradlow, A. (2011). Bidirectional clear speech perception benefit for native and high-proficiency nonnative talkers and listeners: Intelligibility and accentedness. *Journal of the Acoustical Society of America, 130,* 4020–4031.

Stathopoulos, E., & Weismer, G. (1983). Closure duration of stop consonants. *Journal of Phonetics, 11,* 395–400.

Stevens, K. (1993). Modelling affricate consonants. *Speech Communication, 13,* 33–43.

Stevens, K. (1998). *Acoustic phonetics.* Cambridge, MA: MIT Press.

Stevens, K. (2002). Toward a model for lexical access based on acoustic landmarks and distinctive features. *Journal of the Acoustical Society of America, 111,* 1872–1891.

Stevens, K., Fant, G., & Hawkins, S. (1987). Some acoustical and perceptual correlates of nasal vowels. In R. Channon & L. Shockey (Eds.), *In honor of Ilse Lehiste* (pp. 241–254). Dordrecht, Netherlands: Foris.

Stevens, K., & House, A. (1963). Perturbation of vowel articulations by consonantal context: An acoustical study. *Journal of Speech and Hearing Research, 6,* 111–128.

Story, B. H., & Bunton, K. (2010). Relation of vocal tract shape, formant transitions, and stop consonant identification. *Journal of Speech, Language, and Hearing Research, 53,* 1514–1528.

Summerfield, Q. (1975). How a full account of segmental perception depends on prosody and vice versa. In A. Cohen & S. Nooteboom (Eds.), *Structure and process in speech perception* (pp. 51–66). New York, NY: Springer Verlag.

Sussman, H. M., Fruchtman, D., Hilbert, J., & Sirosh, J. (1998). Linear correlates in the speech signal: The orderly output constraint. *Behavioral and Brain Sciences, 21,* 241–299.

Sussman, H. M., McCaffrey, H., & Matthews, S. (1991). An investigation of locus equations as a source of relational invariance for stop place categorization. *Journal of the Acoustical Society of America, 90,* 1309–1325.

Sweeney, T., & Sell, D. (2008). Relationship between perceptual ratings of nasality and nasometry in children/adolescents with cleft palate and/or velopharyngeal dysfunction. *International Journal of Language and Communication Disorders, 43,* 265–282.

Tabain, M. (1998). Non-sibilant fricatives in English: Spectral information above 10 kHz. *Phonetica, 55,* 107–130.

Tabain, M. (2001). Variability in fricative production and spectra: Implications for the hyper- and hypo- and quantal theories of speech production. *Language and Speech, 44,* 57–94.

Tabain, M., Butcher, A., Breen, G., & Breare, R. (2016). An acoustic study of multiple lateral consonants in three Central Australian languages. *Journal of the Acoustical Society of America, 139,* 361–372.

Tasko, S. M., & Greilick, K. (2010). Acoustic and articulatory features of diphthong production: A speech clarity study. *Journal of Speech, Language, and Hearing Research, 53,* 84–99.

Titze, I. (2000). *Principles of voice production.* Denver, CO: National Center for Voice nd Speech.

Tjaden, K., & Martel-Sauvageau, V. (2017). Consonant acoustics in Parkinson's disease and multiple sclerosis: Comparison of clear and loud speaking conditions. *American Journal of Speech-Language Pathology, 26,* 569–582.

Tjaden, K., & Turner, G. (1997). Spectral properties of fricatives in amyotrophic lateral sclerosis. *Journal of Speech, Language, and Hearing Research, 40,* 1358–1372.

Tsao, Y-C., & Weismer, G. (1997). Interspeaker variation of habitual speaking rate: Evidence for a neuromuscular component. *Journal of Speech, Language and Hearing Research, 40,* 858–866.

Tuomainen, O., Hazan, V., & Romeo, R. (2016). Do talkers produce less dispersed phoneme categories in a clear speaking style? *Journal of the Acoustical Society of America, 140,* EL320–EL326.

Turner, G. S., & Tjaden, K. (2000). Acoustic differences between content and function words in amyotrophic lateral sclerosis. *Journal of Speech, Language, and Hearing Research, 43,* 769–783.

Turner, G., Tjaden, K., & Weismer, G. (1995). The influence of speaking rate on vowel space and speech intelligibility for individuals with amyotrophic lateral sclerosis. *Journal of Speech, Language, and Hearing Research, 38,* 1001–1013.

Umeda, N. (1975). Vowel duration in American English. *Journal of the Acoustical Society of America, 58,* 434–445.

Umeda, N. (1977). Consonant duration in American English. *Journal of the Acoustical Society of America, 61,* 846–858.

Van Santen, J. (1992). Contextual effects on vowel duration. *Speech Communication, 11,* 513–546.

Wang, Y., Kent, R., Duffy, J., & Thomas, J. (2005). Dysarthria associated with traumatic brain injury: Speaking rate and emphatic stress. *Journal of Communication Disorders, 38,* 231–260.

Watson, C., & Harrington, J. (1999). Acoustic evidence for dynamic formant trajectories in Australian English vowels. *Journal of the Acoustical Society of America, 106,* 458–468.

Weismer, G. (1980). Control of the voicing distinction for intervocalic stops and fricatives: Some data and theoretical considerations. *Journal of Phonetics, 8,* 427–438.

Weismer, G. (1984). Acoustic analysis strategies for the refinement of phonological analyses. In M. Elbert, D. Dinnsen, & G. Weismer (Eds.), *Phonological Theory and the Misarticulating Child, ASHA Monographs, 22,* 30–52.

Weismer, G. (2006). Speech disorders. In M. Traxler & M. Gernsbacher (Eds.), *Handbook of psycholinguistics* (pp. 93–124). Oxford, UK: Blackwell.

Weismer, G., Dinnsen, D., & Elbert, M. (1981). A study of the voicing distinction associated with omitted, word-final stops. *Journal of Speech and Hearing Research, 46,* 320–327.

Weismer, G., & Ingrisano, D. (1979). Phrase-level timing patterns in English: Effects of emphatic stress location and speaking rate. *Journal of Speech and Hearing Research, 22,* 516–533.

Weismer, G., Jeng, J-Y., Laures, J., Kent, R., & Kent, J. (2001). Acoustic and intelligibility characteristics of sentence production in neurogenic speech disorders. *Folia Phoniatrica et Logopaedica, 53,* 1–18.

Weismer, G., & Martin, R. (1992). Acoustic and perceptual approaches to the study of intelligibility. In R. Kent (Ed.), *Intelligibility in speech disorders* (pp. 67–118). Amsterdam, Netherlands: John Benjamin.

Westbury, J. (1994). *X-ray microbeam speech production database user's handbook.* Madison, WI: University of Wisconsin.

Whalen, D., & Levitt, A. (1995). The universality of intrinsic F0 of vowels. *Journal of Phonetics, 23,* 349–366.

White, L., & Mattys, S. (2007). Rhythmic typology and variation in first and second languages. In P. Prieto, J. Mascaró, & M-J. Solé (Eds.), *Segmental and prosodic issues in romance phonology. Current issues in linguistic theory series* (pp. 237–257). Amsterdam, Netherlands: John Benjamin.

Whitehill, T., Ciocca, V., Chan, J., & Samman, N. (2006). Acoustic analysis of vowels following glossectomy. *Clinical Linguistics & Phonetics, 20,* 135–140.

Whitfield, J. A., & Goberman, A. M. (2014). Articulatory-acoustic vowel space: Application to clear speech in individuals with Parkinson's disease. *Journal of Communication Disorders, 51,* 19–28.

Whitfield, J. A., & Goberman, A. M. (2017). Articulatory-acoustic vowel space: Associations between acoustic and perceptual measures of clear speech. *International Journal of Speech-Language Pathology, 19,* 184–194.

Yang, J., Vadlamudi, J., Yin, Z., Lee, C. Y., & Xu, L. (2017). Production of word-initial fricatives of Mandarin Chinese in prelingually deafened children with cochlear implants. *International Journal of Speech Language Pathology, 19,* 153–164.

Zue, V., & LaFerriere, M. (1979). Acoustic study of medial /t,d/ in American English. *Journal of the Acoustical Society of America, 66,* 1039–1050.

12

Speech Perception

INTRODUCTION

Speech perception is a multifaceted and complicated topic that depends in important ways on information presented in Chapters 7 to 11. The study of speech perception, however, has its own jargon and theoretical content. The complications occur partly because there are several competing theories of speech perception, and partly because it is not always clear how experimental data bear on a choice between those theories. The same data, or at least the same general form of data, can be used to support two theories that provide opposing accounts of speech perception. This is somewhat different from speech acoustics, where a single theory seems to explain the major phenomena, and the relation of data to theory is fairly straightforward.

The goal of this chapter is to present a review of speech perception that has potential relevance to clinical applications. Because history is very important to a proper understanding of the scientific study of speech perception, the early days of speech perception research are reviewed to show how these beginnings dictated the course of thinking in the area for the past half-century, indeed to the present day. The major theories of speech perception are reviewed, together with selected experiments whose results are consistent (or inconsistent) with these theories. We discuss the differences in traditional approaches to speech perception, which focus on segment identity (or identity of several segments in sequence), and the recognition of spoken words. The idea of spoken word recognition as a key part of speech perception is introduced. The chapter concludes with a review of speech intelligibility and its direct relevance to clinical practice in speech and hearing diagnosis and management.

EARLY SPEECH PERCEPTION RESEARCH AND CATEGORICAL PERCEPTION

As reviewed by Cole and Rudnicky (1983), scientists in the late nineteenth and early twentieth centuries were interested in speech perception. Systematic work in this area, and the creation of speech perception research as a flourishing scientific discipline, began in the late 1940s and early 1950s. Scientists at Haskins Laboratories—initially in New York City, later and currently in New Haven, Connecticut—employed an early kind of speech synthesizer to perform experiments on the perception of speech. The scientists who developed the synthesizer—Franklin Cooper, Alvin Liberman, and John Borst—were already familiar with the spectrogram, at that time a relatively new way to display speech acoustic events (Chapter 10). Cooper, Liberman, and Borst (1951) described a machine that allowed them to use spectrographic features of natural speech, such as vowel formant frequencies, formant transition characteristics, and stop burst spectra, and manipulate them in small steps for presentation to listeners. Such a device, they reasoned, would allow them to identify the important acoustic cues for the identification of specific speech sounds.

A diagram of this speech synthesizer, called a *pattern-playback* machine, is shown in Figure 12–1. The machine used the principle that fluctuations in light can be transformed into sound waves, under the proper conditions. Figure 12–1 shows how a light source was directed at a rotating wheel that was a circular film negative. On this negative a series of rings were arranged to produce frequencies from 120 Hz to 6000 Hz, in a consecutive-integer harmonic series. The rotating circle was aptly called a "tone wheel."

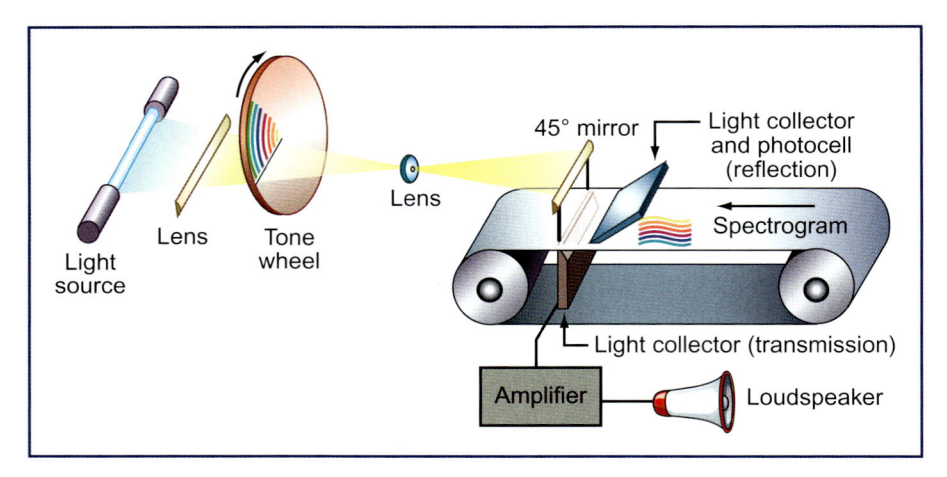

Figure 12–1. Schematic drawing of the pattern-playback machine, an early speech synthesizer used by scientists at Haskins Laboratories to perform speech perception research. See text for details.

A spectrographic pattern was painted on a transparent sheet (such as the overhead transparencies used in classroom presentations before the advent of computer-based presentations) and mounted on a movable surface exposed to light coming through the tone wheel. As light passed through the harmonic rings on the film negative, the painted spectrogram was transported by a moving belt through the machine. The dark parts of the spectrogram reflected certain of the "light frequencies" generated by the wheel, whereas the clear parts of the spectrogram generated no reflection. The movement of the belt simulated the time dimension of speech. The reflected light frequencies, changing over time as the belt moved, were transmitted to a device that converted the reflections to sound (the light collector in Figure 12–1). These sound waves were amplified and output by a loudspeaker, producing the speech-like sounds resulting from the time-varying patterns of light reflection.

The key to understanding how the device was used to create small changes in spectrographic patterns is this: the clear sheet on which the spectrographic representation was painted reflected whatever pattern the investigator desired; any type of "speech signal" could be painted. The Haskins scientists asked the question, how are these different patterns heard? Cooper and colleagues (1951) performed a set of experiments with the pattern-playback machine in which they discovered that a two-formant pattern with proper F1 and F2 transitions elicited perception of stop-vowel syllables, even though stop bursts were *not* included in the painted pattern. Such patterns—like stick figure representations of real speech signals—are shown in Figure 12–2 for the voiced (top) and voiceless (bottom) set of English stop consonants. The portion of the signals between the dotted, vertical lines shows the transitions, or changing formant frequencies as a function of time. The steady states of F1 and F2 were painted to elicit perception of the vowel /ɑ/. For the voiceless stops, the F1 transition was "cut back" in time relative to the F2 transition. More is said about this later.

When the top patterns in Figure 12–2 were transported by the moving belt and their reflected light converted over time to sound, most listeners heard the leftmost pattern as /bɑ/, the middle pattern as /dɑ/, and the rightmost pattern as /gɑ/. Cooper and colleagues (1951) selected these patterns to mimic the ones they had seen in spectrograms of natural speech. They already knew the F2 transition was different for the three places of stop consonant articulation in English, at least when the stops were followed by /ɑ/. The finding that a *burstless* pattern elicited the perception of stop consonants, with the correct place of articulation dependent on the pattern of transitions shown in Figure 12–2, was somewhat of a surprise.

The /bɑ/-/dɑ/-/gɑ/ Experiment

Cooper and his colleagues (1951) asked the question: What happens to listeners' perception when the *starting frequency* of F2 is changed in small and systematic steps over a large range of frequencies? Using the pattern-playback machine, the scientists painted a series of two-formant patterns varying only in the F2 start-

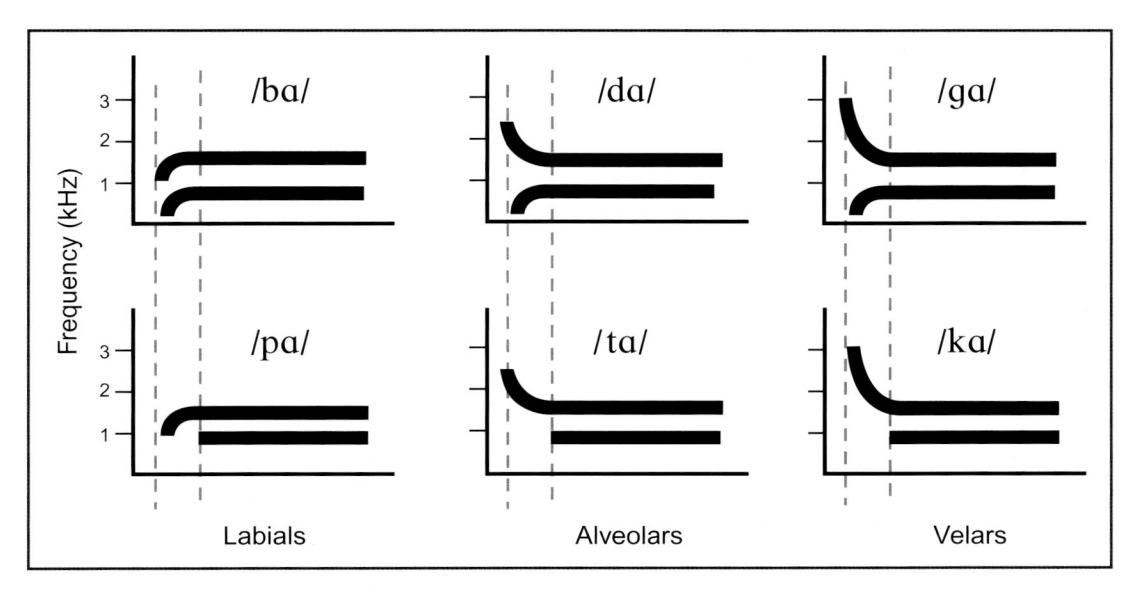

Figure 12–2. Two-formant, painted patterns used in pattern-playback experiments. These patterns, like stick figure representations of real spectrograms, were heard as stop-vowel syllables (*top,* /ba/, /da/, /ga/; *bottom,* /pa/, /ta/, and /ka/ from left to right), even though there were no stop bursts painted as part of the pattern.

ing frequency.[1] The result was a series, or *continuum*, of stimuli, like those shown in Figure 12–3.

Each of these two-formant stimuli is labeled with a number, ranging from −6 to +6. The stimulus labeled 0 had no F2 transition, and the two *endpoint* stimuli had the most extreme F2 transitions—that is, transitions covering the widest range of frequencies but moving in opposite directions. Stimulus −6 had the lowest starting frequency and, therefore, an extensive, rising F2 transition (where the transition starts at a lower frequency and moves to a higher one). As an example, the measurement point for the F2 starting frequency is shown for stimulus −6; F2 starting frequency is located at the beginning of the painted F2 for all stimuli. Stimulus +6 had the highest starting frequency and, therefore, a very extensive, falling F2 transition. The other features of these stimuli were constant across the entire continuum, including the rising F1 transition and the voice bar preceding it. The voice bar was a low frequency part of the painted patterns, seen as the flat bar before the F1 transitions; this ensured that all phonologically voiced stops were heard as voiced. The previous discussion of the three patterns in Figure 12–2 suggests that endpoint stimulus −6 was heard as /ba/ and endpoint stimulus +6 as /ga/. This series of stimuli tested the listeners' response to systematic variations in F2 starting frequency between these two extremes. How did listeners respond to the other stimuli along the continuum?

Cooper and colleagues (1951) first obtained *identification data* from listeners. In this experiment, listeners were asked to label the presented stimuli. Listeners had three labels from which to choose: /b/, /d/, or /g/. Each stimulus was presented several times to each member of a crew of listeners, and the results were plotted as the percentage of /b/, /d/, or /g/ responses across the series of stimuli. A typical plot of the results is shown in Figure 12–4.

In this plot, stimulus number (see Figure 12–3) is on the *x*-axis, which is also labeled "F2 starting frequency" because the different stimulus numbers indicate different starting frequencies. The percentage of /b/ (pink boxes), /d/ (white boxes), and /g/ (blue boxes) labels for each stimulus number is on the *y*-axis. A quick glance at these identification results shows that stimuli from −6 to −3 were heard almost exclusively as /b/, stimuli from −1 to +2 as /d/, and stimuli from +4 to +6 as /g/. A few stimuli, such as −2 and +3, were ambiguous, but −2 was only ambiguous for /b/ and /d/ responses (no /g/ responses) and +3 was

---

[1] This is not strictly true: when the starting frequency of the F2 transition is changed in small steps, the slope of the second formant transition is also changed when the vowel target formants are held constant, as they were in these experiments. This detail of the early Haskins experiments is not pursued further in this chapter.

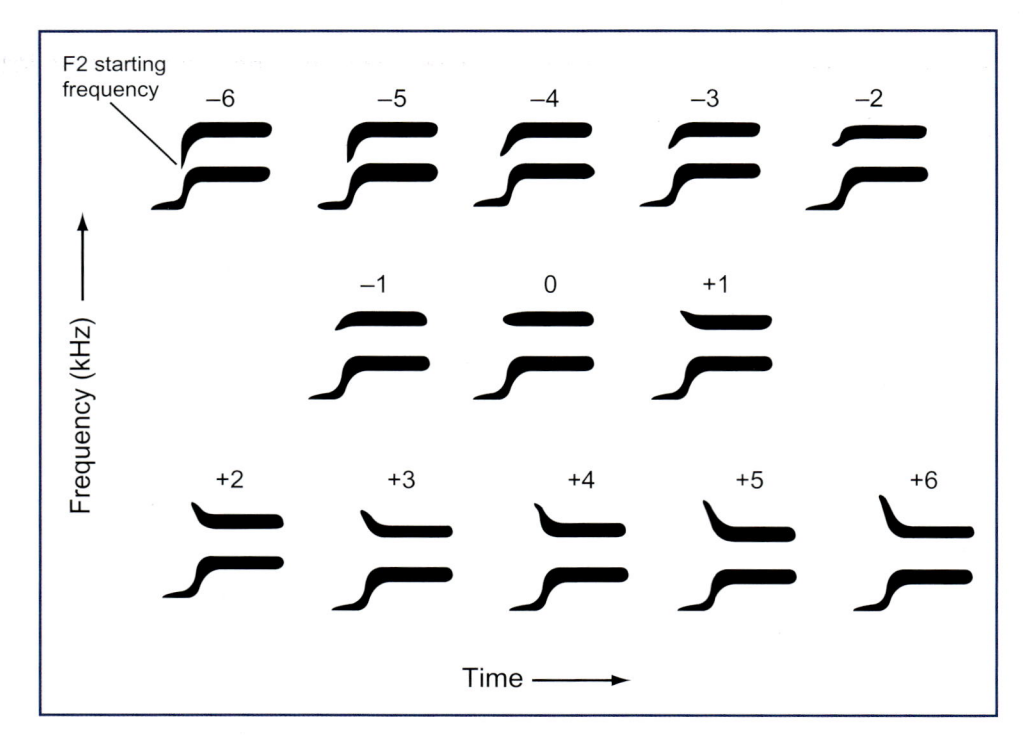

Figure 12-3. Series of stimuli painted for pattern-playback experiments on the effect of F2 transition starting frequency on perception of stop consonant place of articulation. Stimulus "–6" had the lowest F2 starting frequency, and stimulus "+6" had the highest F2 starting frequency. Each stimulus from "–6" to "+6" increased the F2 starting frequency by a small increment. The flat portion in each stimulus preceding the F1 transition ensured that the stop was heard as voiced. After Liberman, Harris, Hoffman, and Griffith (1957).

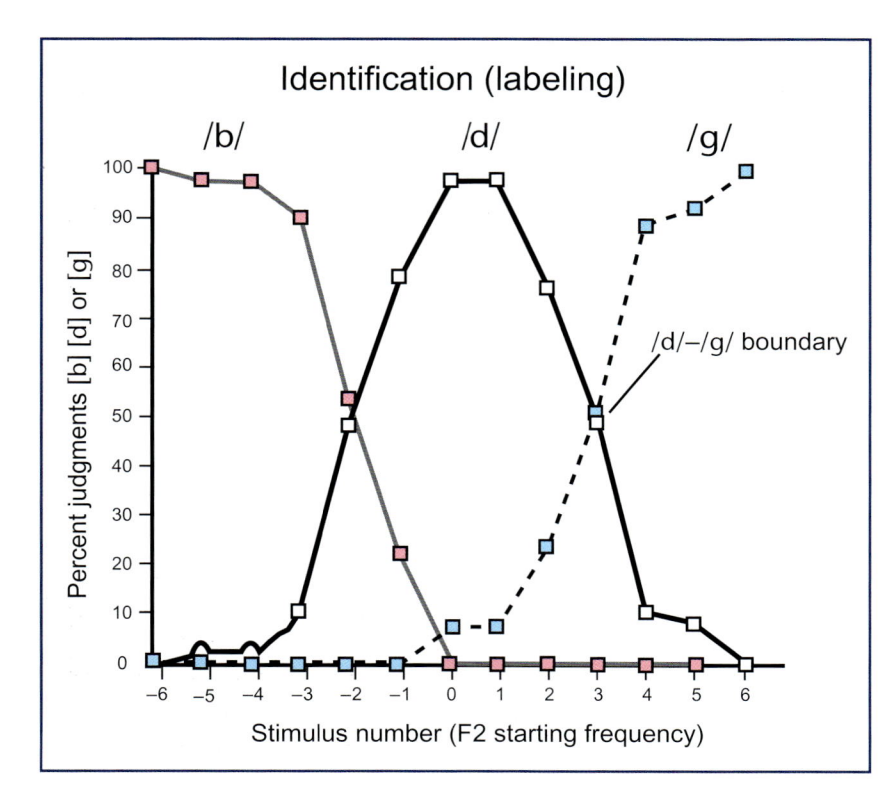

Figure 12-4. Identification (labeling) data for the two-formant stimuli shown in Figure 12-3 and described in text. The x-axis is labeled "F2 starting frequency" but the values along the axis are the stimulus numbers shown in Figure 12-3. The y-axis is the percent judgments of /b/, /d/, or /g/ labels as a function of F2 starting frequency (stimulus number). /b/ responses are shown by pink boxes, /d/ labels by white boxes, /g/ labels by blue boxes. The boundary between the /d/ and /g/ categories is labeled. The boundary for the /b/-/d/ categories follows the same rule as the stimulus where half the responses are for one category, half for the adjacent category. See text for interpretation. Figure adapted from Liberman et al. (1957).

only ambiguous for /d/ and /g/ responses (no /b/ responses). The boundary of the /d/ and /g/ categories is labeled in the figure; the boundary for the /b/-/g/ categories follows the same principle (50% /b/ responses, 50% /d/ responses).

The take-home message from this experiment was that relatively continuous variation of the physical stimulus—the starting frequency of the F2 transition—did not result in a continuous change in the perceptual response. Rather, place of articulation seemed to be perceived *categorically*, with a series of adjacent stimuli yielding one response, as in the case of stimuli −6 through −3 producing a percept of /b/, followed by a sudden change in response pattern to /d/ at the next step along the continuum (e.g., at stimulus −2). The same pattern was observed between /d/ and /g/. When the labeling functions for two adjacent phonemes (like /b/ and /d/, or /d/ and /g/) changed suddenly, they crossed at a point where 50% of the responses were for one label, and 50% for the adjacent label (see Figure 12–3). For this stimulus, the labeling appeared to be at chance levels—the listeners responded to the stimulus as if making a guess between the two adjacent labels such as /b/ or /d/, or /d/ and /g/. This 50% point was called the phoneme boundary and was taken to indicate the stimulus defining the categorical distinction between two sounds.

Categorical Perception: General Considerations

The finding that stop place of articulation was perceived categorically, not continuously, has had a profound effect on speech perception research and theory. Categorical perception is discussed here more thoroughly before returning to the interpretation of the /bɑ/-/dɑ/-/gɑ/ experiment described above.

Categorical perception is demonstrated when continuous variation in a physical stimulus is perceived in a discontinuous (i.e., categorical) way. The study of psychological reactions to variations in physical stimuli is called *psychophysics* (see Chapter 14). Categorical perception is an example of a psychophysical phenomenon. A schematic illustration of categorical perception, and how it contrasts with the psychophysical phenomenon of *continuous perception*, is shown in Figure 12–5.

Both graphs in Figure 12–5 show hypothetical relationships between a continuously varying physical variable (*x*-axis) and a perceptual (psychological) response (*y*-axis). The perceptual response in this case is a number assigned by the perceiver to the magnitude or quality of each stimulus along the physically varying continuum. In the left-hand graph, each change of the physical variable from a lower to higher value elicits a corresponding change in the perceiver's mind and, therefore, on the number scale. This results in the straight-line, 45-degree function relating the changes in the physical stimulus to changes on the psychological scale. The function in the left-hand graph is labeled "continuous perception" because a given increment along the physical scale always results in the same increment along the perceptual scale.

The right-hand graph shows a different relationship. Here the continuous variation of the physical stimulus is the same as in the left-hand graph, but the perceptual response is much different. The initial

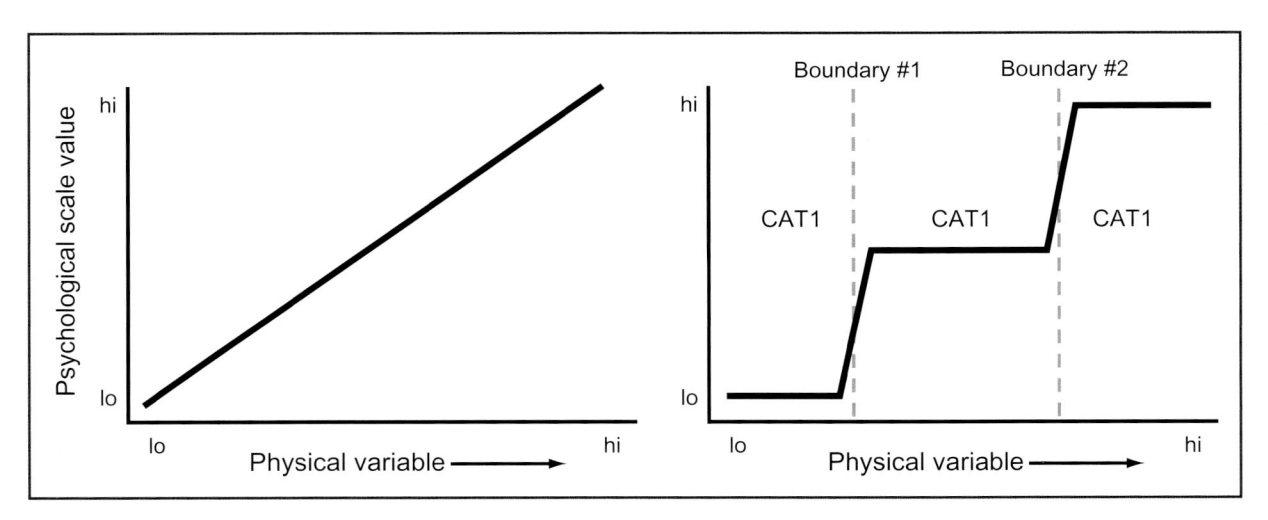

Figure 12–5. Two schematic graphs showing the difference between continuous (*left*) and categorical (*right*) psychophysical functions. Variation in the physical stimulus is shown on the *x*-axes, variation in the psychological reaction on the *y*-axes. See text for discussion.

changes in the physical stimulus, beginning at the lowest values, produce *no change* in the psychological scale value. The listener treats the different stimuli as belonging to a single psychological event. When the stimulus reaches the value indicated by the first vertical dotted line, the perceptual scale "jumps" to a higher number. The new psychological number remains the same even as the physical stimulus continues to increase. The same thing happens at the second dotted line, where the perceptual scale value jumps to yet another higher value and remains at that value as the physical stimulus increases in magnitude.

The vertical dotted lines in the right-hand graph are labeled "Boundary 1" and "Boundary 2." The lines indicate locations along the physical stimulus continuum where a small change in the value of the stimulus results in a sudden, large change in the perceptual response. Alternatively, as noted above, it is a stimulus at which 50% of the responses are for one category, and 50% for the other, as if the responses were based on chance (guessing). The function in the right-hand graph shows categorical perception because the two boundaries separate the psychological reaction to a continuously varying stimulus into three categories, labeled CAT1, CAT2, and CAT3. In categorical perception, the *same* increment along the physical stimulus produces very different psychological responses, depending on whether the increment is within a category versus straddling a category boundary. Within a category, a small change along the physical continuum leads to little or no difference in the psychological response. The same change in a physical stimulus *across* a category boundary results in a major change in the psychological response.

This simple description of the difference between continuous and categorical perception applies directly to the pattern-playback results for stop consonant place of production, shown in Figure 12–4. The F2 starting frequency was changed continuously from low to high values, but listeners heard only categories, not smoothly changing phonetic events. The categorical labeling functions shown in Figure 12–4 are consistent with the schematic illustration of categorical perception shown in Figure 12–5. Small changes in the F2 starting frequency, beginning from the lowest value, all yielded /b/ responses. At a certain point along the physical continuum of F2 starting frequencies the *same* change resulted in a sudden shift to /d/ responses. The perception of place of articulation for stop consonants appeared to be categorical even though the starting frequency of F2 was changed continuously.

Labeling Versus Discrimination

One more experiment was required to verify the categorical perception of stop consonant place of articulation. The categorical perception functions shown in Figure 12–4 were obtained in an experiment in which listeners heard a stimulus and labeled it as either /b/, /d/, or /g/. The resulting categorical perception functions may have reflected nothing more than the listeners' restriction to just three response categories. For example, listeners were not permitted to respond, "This stimulus sounds as if it is midway between a /b/ and /d/ (or between a /d/ and /g/)," even though it was possible some stimuli sounded this way. If such responses were available to the listeners, the functions may not have looked as categorical as those shown in Figure 12–4.

To address this potential problem, the labeling experiment was followed by a *discrimination experiment*. As indicated above in the discussion of Figure 12–5, in a true categorical perception function, an increment of fixed magnitude in the physical stimulus may result in either no psychological change or a large psychological change, depending on where the increment is located along the entire physical continuum. A fixed physical increment between two stimuli, located *within* a category determined by a labeling experiment, should produce little or no psychological change. The same increment located *across* a category boundary should produce a large psychological change. In a discrimination experiment, a true categorical perception function is determined when listeners cannot discriminate two different stimuli chosen from within a category, but easily discriminate two stimuli chosen *across* a category boundary (one chosen from one category, the other from the adjacent category). *The physical difference between the two stimuli is the same in both cases, but the psychological reaction to the difference between the stimuli is radically different.*

Following the labeling experiments, Cooper and colleagues (1951) performed these discrimination experiments. The discrimination experiments produced the expected results. When listeners were asked if two stimuli (presented one after the other) were the same or different, they said "same" for stimuli chosen within a category, and "different" when stimuli were chosen from adjacent categories (i.e., when one stimulus was immediately to the left of a category boundary determined in the labeling experiments, and the other to the right). This result was obtained even when the actual physical difference between the two judged stimuli was the same. The categorical labeling functions (see Figure 12–4) were confirmed by the discrimination experiment.

Categorical Perception: So What?

What was important about the demonstration of categorical perception for place of articulation? Liberman, Cooper, Shankweiler, and Studdert-Kennedy

(1967), in their famous paper "Perception of the Speech Code," pointed to categorical perception as a cornerstone of the *motor theory of speech perception*. Listeners do not hear the continuous changes in F2 starting frequency, at least until a category boundary is reached, because they cannot *produce* continuous changes in place of articulation. Consideration of the different places of articulation for English stops shows why Liberman and his colleagues reasoned this way. How do you produce a stop between a bilabial /b/ and a lingua-alveolar /d/? Or between a /d/ and dorsal /g/? The places of articulation for stops are essentially categorical, allowing no "in-between" articulatory placements.[2]

The motor theory was built on the idea that speech perception was constrained by speech production. In this view, categorical production of a speech feature, such as place of articulation for stops, limits speech perception to the same categories. Detection of acoustic differences within categories is therefore not possible. Liberman et al.'s (1967) focus on the role of speech production in speech perception, however, extended beyond the demonstration of categorical perception. Recall from Chapter 11 the discussion of pattern-playback experiments in which very different F2 transition patterns cued the perception of a single stop consonant (/d/, in the case covered in Chapter 11; see Figure 11–34). Liberman et al. reviewed several experiments in which a great deal of acoustic variability, primarily due to varying phonetic context, was associated with perception of a single stop consonant. In Chapter 11, this was described as the "no acoustic invariance" problem. Liberman et al. regarded the lack of acoustic invariance for a given stop consonant as a problem for a theory of speech perception in which listeners based their phonetic decisions on information in the acoustic signal. Instead, the constant factor in speech perception, at least for stop consonants, was thought to be the *articulatory* characteristics of a stop consonant. A stop such as /d/ may have varying acoustic characteristics—especially as seen in the F2 transition, and possibly also in the burst—depending on the identity of a preceding or following vowel, but the lingua-alveolar place of articulation remains constant across all phonetic contexts. For Liberman et al., it made more sense for listeners to base their phonetic decisions on these constant articulatory characteristics, rather than the highly variable speech acoustic signal.

It is one thing to claim that speech is perceived by reference to articulation; it is another to say exactly how this is done. Liberman et al. (1967) argued for a

> **Mirror, Mirror, in the Brain**
>
> When the motor theory was first proposed, the brain mechanisms for the (hypothesized) special module were unknown. Experiments were done to show that the likely location of the module was in the left hemisphere (Studdert-Kennedy & Shankweiler, 1970), but these were perception experiments and the inference to actual brain mechanisms involved a long interpretative leap. Fast forward to the twenty-first century and the use of imaging and stimulation techniques to uncover brain function for complex behavior (like speech), and we have the concept of "mirror neurons." These are neurons that appear to be active during both the production and perception of action. When someone produces a gesture (such as a speech gesture), the *perceiver* of that gesture has greater activity in the neurons that are involved in *producing* the gesture. The motor neurons are said to "mirror" the perception of the gesture. Perhaps this is the brain basis of the species-specific speech module proposed in motor theory (see Watkins & Paus, 2004).

species-specific mechanism in the brain of humans— a specialized and dedicated module for the perception of speech. An important component of this claim was the link between speech production and perception, specifically the "match" between the capabilities of the speech production and speech perception mechanisms. The match was proposed as an evolutionary, *encoded* form of communication. The encoding is on the speech production side of communication; the decoding is provided by the special perceptual mechanism in the brain of humans. For Liberman et al. the tight link between speech perception and production was part of the evolutionary history of *Homo sapiens*.

There is more to the motor theory. Specifics are provided by Liberman et al. (1967) on how speech production is encoded in the acoustic signal emerging from a speaker's mouth, and how this signal is decoded by the human brain to recover articulatory behaviors. The original motor theory was later revised in an important way as described by Liberman and Mattingly (1985). In the original motor theory, the focus was on the encoding and decoding of place of articulation for stops

---

[2]This may not be completely true. It seems as if stops can be made between the English locations for /d/ and /g/, by retroflexing the tongue and making the point of articulation posterior to the typical lingua-alveolar location (or anterior to the typical dorsal location for /g/; in fact, some languages have stops that are made in this way). Other "in-between" possibilities can also be imagined.

(and by extension, to other obstruents and possibly nasals as well). The revised motor theory changed the articulatory invariant to gestures, rather than positions. In the revised motor theory articulatory gestures, such as the tongue gesture from a stop to a following vowel, are encoded by production and then decoded by the species-specific perceptual module.

For the purposes of this chapter, details of the differences between the original and revised motor theories are not critical. The phenomenon of trading relations in phonetic identification, and how it fits into the revised motor theory, is taken up later in the chapter. Both the original and revised motor theories share the idea of a special speech module, and both have faced strong scientific challenges. What is critical for both versions of the theory are two general claims: (a) speech perception is a species-specific human endowment; and (b) the speech acoustic signal associated with a given sound is far too variable to be useful for speech perception, but the underlying articulatory behavior is not, hence the claim that speech is perceived by reference to articulation.

Speech Perception Is Species Specific

The ability to speak and form millions of novel sentences is exclusive to humans. It makes sense that a theory of speech *perception* as a capability "matched" to speech production is regarded by many scientists as an exclusively human capability. The notion of co-evolved mechanisms for production and perception of vocalizations, and especially of dedicated perceptual mechanisms "tuned" to species-specific vocalizations, is not limited to humans, however. There is evidence in monkeys, bats, and birds (and other animals) of perceptual mechanisms matched to the specific vocalizations produced by each of these animals (Andoni, Li, & Pollak, 2007; Davies, Madden, & Butchart, 2004; Miller & Jucszyk, 1989). The possible existence of such a match in humans is consistent, in principle, with evolutionary principles derived from the study of vocal communication in other animals.

"In principle" evaluations of a theory are fine, but they do not go far enough. A theory should be testable, either by natural observation or experimentation. Karl Popper (2002a, 2002b), a famous philosopher of science, argued that a theory can only be considered "scientific" if it can be disproved by a proper experiment. According to Popper, these experiment-based "falsifications" of a theory are the basis of scientific progress. Popper first published these ideas in the 1935 German edition of *The Logic of Scientific Discovery*. The book was published in English translation in 1959. Popper's ideas have had a profound influence on modern science in general, and specifically on the motor theory of speech perception.

The Motor Theory of Speech Perception: Proofs and Falsifications

Can the motor theory be falsified? The scope of the present chapter does not allow a detailed answer to this question, but there have been attempts to falsify the claims of the motor theory. Some of these experiments are described below. For a detailed and challenging article on the issue of falsifying the motor theory of speech perception, see Galantucci, Fowler, and Turvey (2006).

Categorical Perception of Stop Place of Articulation Shows the "Match" to Speech Production

The motor theory was criticized for failing to explain why certain individuals who could not speak (as in some cases of cerebral palsy, or other neurological diseases) were able to perceive speech in a normal way. This complaint was misguided, however, because the motor theorists never argued for the ability to *produce* speech as a requirement for normal speech perception abilities. To the contrary, the species-specific module for speech perception was thought to be innate (Liberman & Mattingly, 1985)—a property of the human brain at birth. The demonstration of categorical perception in infants as young as 1 month of age was taken as evidence for this innate mechanism, and hence as strong support for the motor theory of speech perception. The infant categorical perception functions were very much like those obtained from adult listeners, even though infants do not produce speech. The categorical perception functions were obtained in infants by taking advantage of something infants do quite well, which is to suck for long periods of time. Over time, as babies suck, the strength of the suck varies with the degree of novelty in their environment. If the environment remains the same, sucking becomes less intense. The introduction of a novel stimulus (e.g., something seen, heard, smelled) results in a sudden increase in suck strength, frequency, or both. Early studies of infant speech perception used sucking behavior to assess babies' reactions to speech stimuli within and across speech sound categories. Categorical perception functions, closely resembling those obtained from adults, were obtained in infants with the sucking paradigm. An excellent review of early infant speech perception research and methods is found in Eimas, Miller, and Jusczyk (1990).

> **What About Talking Birds?**
>
> The motor theory is species specific to humans. The link between articulatory and speech perception capabilities is special because humans are the only species who produce speech sounds for communication. But wait. What about talking birds?—mynahs, crows, budgerigars (small parrots, often called parakeets), and African Greys, for example. Talking birds produce speech using a very different apparatus from humans—they have no lips, and do not produce a sound source at the larynx but rather have a sound-producing mechanism deep in their chests called a syrinx. Yet the major question is not, "Can these birds articulate?" (because they obviously produce intelligible speech, even if mimicked), but "When they articulate, can they make *voluntary* adjustments to produce different speech sounds?" If the answer is "Yes, they make such adjustments," then the species-specific claim of motor theory runs into some difficulty. Patterson and Pepperberg (1998) made just this claim for an African Grey parrot named Alex (1977-2007, https://en.wikipedia.org/wiki/Alex_(parrot)). An opposing view, that the speech produced by talking birds is nothing more than non-inventive mimicry, was expressed by Lieberman (1996).

An apparent falsification of the motor theory was, ironically, a logical outgrowth of the findings in infants. If nonspeaking infants had categorical perception of sound contrasts, perhaps the same would be true of animals. Perhaps the reason infants showed the effect had little to do with a species-specific speech perception mechanism, but instead reflected some general property of mammalian auditory systems. In fact, work by Kuhl and her colleagues (Kuhl, 1986; Kuhl & Miller, 1975; Kuhl & Padden, 1983) and others demonstrated categorical perception for voice onset time (VOT) and stop place of articulation in chinchillas and monkeys, respectively. If categorical perception is the result of a special linkage between human speech production and perception, as claimed by Liberman et al. (1967), the finding of categorical speech perception in animals is a falsification of the linkage specifically, and the motor theory in general. A kinder interpretation of the animal data is that they raise questions about the motor theory but do not falsify the theory in an absolute way. Miller and Jusczyk (1989) summarized this position in this way: "*In principle, there are many ways to arrive at the same classification of a set of objects. Hence, the fact that the animals can achieve the same classification does not prove that they use the same means to do so as humans*" (pp. 124–125, emphasis added). The data may be the same in adult humans, human infants, and animals, but not necessarily because of a common mechanism. This is an example of the same findings (categorical perception of speech signals) supporting opposing theoretical views.

Duplex Perception

The possibility of a special speech-perception module in the brains of humans does not, of course, eliminate the need for general auditory function. A host of everyday auditory perceptions requires analysis by mechanisms external to the speech module. Presumably, a speech signal "automatically" engages the speech module; the option is not available to "turn it off" for short periods of time, even if this would occasionally be a nice idea. Other auditory signals engage "general" (non-modular) auditory mechanisms for analysis and perception. The idea of a separation[3] between mechanisms for speech perception versus general auditory perception was explored experimentally to prove the existence of the speech module.

The schematic spectrograms in Figure 12–6 (adapted from Whalen & Liberman, 1987) illustrate the physical basis of *duplex perception*, the phenomenon in which the speech module *and* general auditory mechanisms seem to be activated simultaneously by one signal (Mann & Liberman, 1983; Whalen & Liberman, 1987). The upper graph shows a schematic spectrogram, with fixed patterns for F1 and F2, and two different transitions for F3. The steady-state formant frequencies are appropriate for the vowel /ɑ/, and the F1 and F2 transitions convey the impression of a stop consonant preceding the vowel. Synthesis of this F1-F2-F3 pattern with a rising F3 transition causes listeners to hear /gɑ/. A falling F3 transition cues the perception of /dɑ/. The different perceptual effects of the rising versus falling F3 transition are consistent with naturally produced /gɑ/ and /dɑ/ syllables.

---

[3]"Separation" may be too weak to describe what the motor theorists meant by a speech perception module. The motor theorists, and other cognitive scientists who investigated the role of modules in various aspects of cognition, viewed these mechanisms as dedicated to a single process, and isolated from other processes. The speech module envisioned by motor theorists was not only separable from other auditory processes, but insulated from other auditory processing because there was no neural traffic between the two. The speech module was impermeable to general auditory processes, and vice versa.

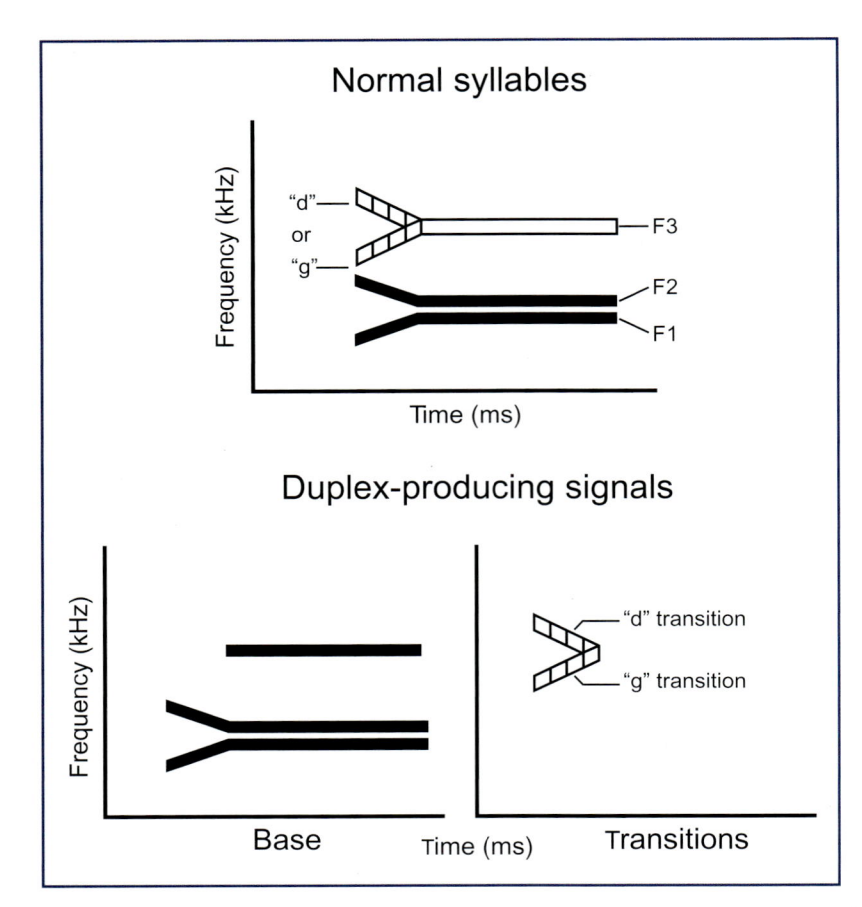

Figure 12-6. Signals used in duplex (speech) perception experiments. Top graph shows three-formant patterns, with fixed patterns for F1 and F2. The third formant has either a rising transition (producing a percept of /ga/) or falling transition (producing a percept of /da/). When the F3 transitions are presented alone, as shown in the lower right-hand panel of the figure, they sound like rising or falling bird "chirps" or whistles. When the three-formant pattern is presented without the F3 transition (the base, lower left-hand panel of the figure), listeners hear an ambiguous /da/ (compared with the clear /da/ heard when the falling F3 transition is in place). Playing the base into one ear and an F3 transition into the other ear results in simultaneous perception of the "good" syllable (either /da/ or /ga/, depending on which F3 transition is played) plus the nonspeech "chirp." The same effect can be produced with both signals in one ear and the isolated F3 transition played at a fairly high level. The "duplex" in "duplex perception" is the simultaneous perception of a speech and nonspeech event from the same signal.

If the F3 transition portion (either the rising or falling one) is edited out from the schematic signal in the upper part of the figure and played to listeners, the brief signal (~50 ms in duration) sounds something like a bird chirp or whistle glide. In the case of the transition for /g/, the pitch of this "chirp" rises quickly, and for /d/ it falls quickly. The isolated transitions are shown in the lower right-hand graph in Figure 12–6. Regardless of exactly how people hear these isolated transitions—as "chirps," quick frequency glides (*glissandi*, in musical terms), or outer space noises—they are *not* heard as phonetic events.

This situation suggests something of a perceptual mystery. Listeners hear the three-formant pattern at the top of Figure 12–6 as either /g/ or /d/, depending on whether the F3 transition is rising (/g/) or falling (/d/). But when that brief, apparently critical F3 transition is isolated from the spectrographic pattern and played to listeners, they hear something with absolutely no phonetic quality.

What do people hear when presented with the spectrographic pattern *minus* an F3 transition? In Figure 12–6, this pattern is referred to as the "base," which listeners hear as a not-very-clear /d/, different from the unambiguous /d/ heard when the falling F3 transition is in place.

The phenomenon of duplex perception, and its relationship to the concept of a special speech perception module in the brains of humans, can now be explained. Consider the base and either one of the isolated transitions shown in Figure 12–6 as two separate signals and imagine one of these signals (the base) delivered to one ear, and the other (an isolated transition) delivered to the other ear. This experimental arrangement is shown in the cartoon of Figure 12–7, where the "base" is sent to a listener's right ear and one of the "isolated transitions"—the one appropriate to either /g/ or /d/—is sent to the left ear. The isolated F3 transition is delivered to the left ear with proper timing relative to the F1 and F2 transitions in the base, meaning the transition is sequenced properly in time relative to the base (as in the top graph of Figure 12–6, showing the "complete" patterns for either /d/ or /g/).

What did listeners hear when the experiment depicted in Figure 12–7 was performed? Mann and Liberman (1983), among others, showed that listeners heard a "good" /da/ or /ga/ (depending on which F3

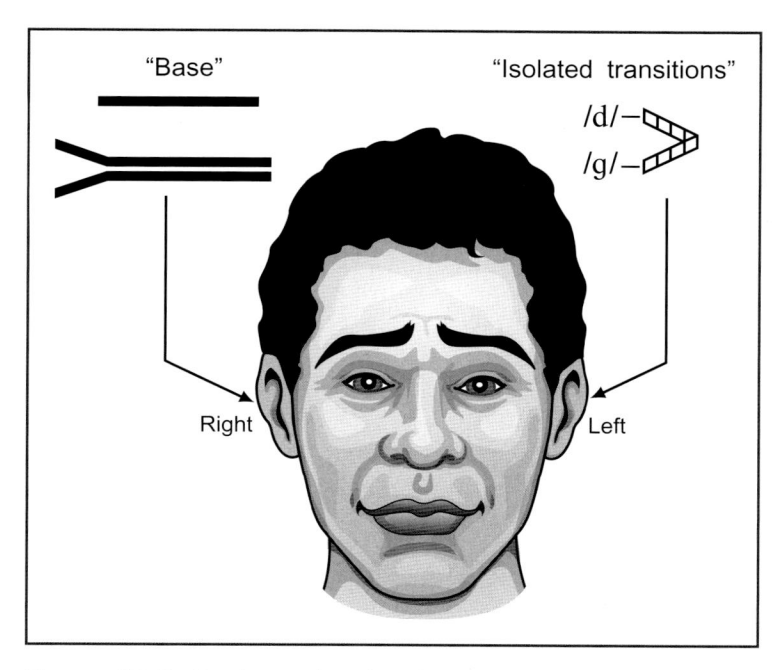

Figure 12-7. Cartoon showing how the duplex perception experiment was performed. The base was delivered to one ear, the isolated F3 transition to the other ear. Alternatively, both signals were delivered to the same ear and the presentation level of the isolated transition was increased until listeners heard both the "good" syllable and the chirp.

transition was played) *plus* a chirp. The simultaneous perception from the same signal of two events—speech and nonspeech—suggested the term "duplex perception." Duplex perception seemed to show the human listener operating simultaneously in the special speech mode and in the general auditory mode. The perception of the "good" /dɑ/ or /gɑ/ was the result of the "base" and the "isolated transition" combining somewhere in the nervous system, automatically engaging the speech mode of perception. At the same time, the isolated F3 transition was processed as a chirp by general auditory mechanisms. The F3 transition did double duty, engaging two different kinds of hearing mechanism at the same time. One of those mechanisms, according to Mann and Liberman and Whalen and Liberman (1987), must be the specialized speech perception module proposed as the centerpiece of the motor theory. As Whalen (1997) pointed out, the perception was not "triplex," which would have included three ambiguous signals with the missing F3 transition (the percept when only the base was presented to listeners), the clear /dɑ/ or /gɑ/ (depending on which F3 transition was used), and the chirp. Listeners heard only two events, the clear syllable and the chirp. The ambiguous phonetic percept elicited by the base was gone.

This experimental finding seemed to be a strong endorsement of a species-specific module for perceiving speech. What other explanation could account for the same signal (the F3 transition) evoking two simultaneous perceptions, one clearly phonetic and consistent with previous studies on the role of the transition in cuing /g/ or /d/, the other clearly non-phonetic and consistent with the direction of the frequency glide (rising versus falling)? Duplex perception seemed like ironclad evidence for a special mode for perceiving speech, distinct from general auditory processes. However, an experiment reported by Fowler and Rosenblum (1991) cast doubt on this interpretation.

Fowler and Rosenblum (1991) recorded the acoustic signal produced by the closing of a metal door. They computed a spectrum of this acoustic event, like the one shown in the upper graph of Figure 12–8. Then they separated the spectrum into two parts, a lower frequency part (from 0–3.0 kHz) and a higher frequency part (from 3.0–11.0 kHz; see lower left and lower right graphs in Figure 12–8). This separation was accomplished by filtering the original signal (0–11.0 kHz) to obtain the 0 to 3.0 kHz and 3.0 to 11.0 kHz parts. Fowler and Rosenblum presented these three signals (the original, "full" signal; the 0–3.0 kHz part; and the

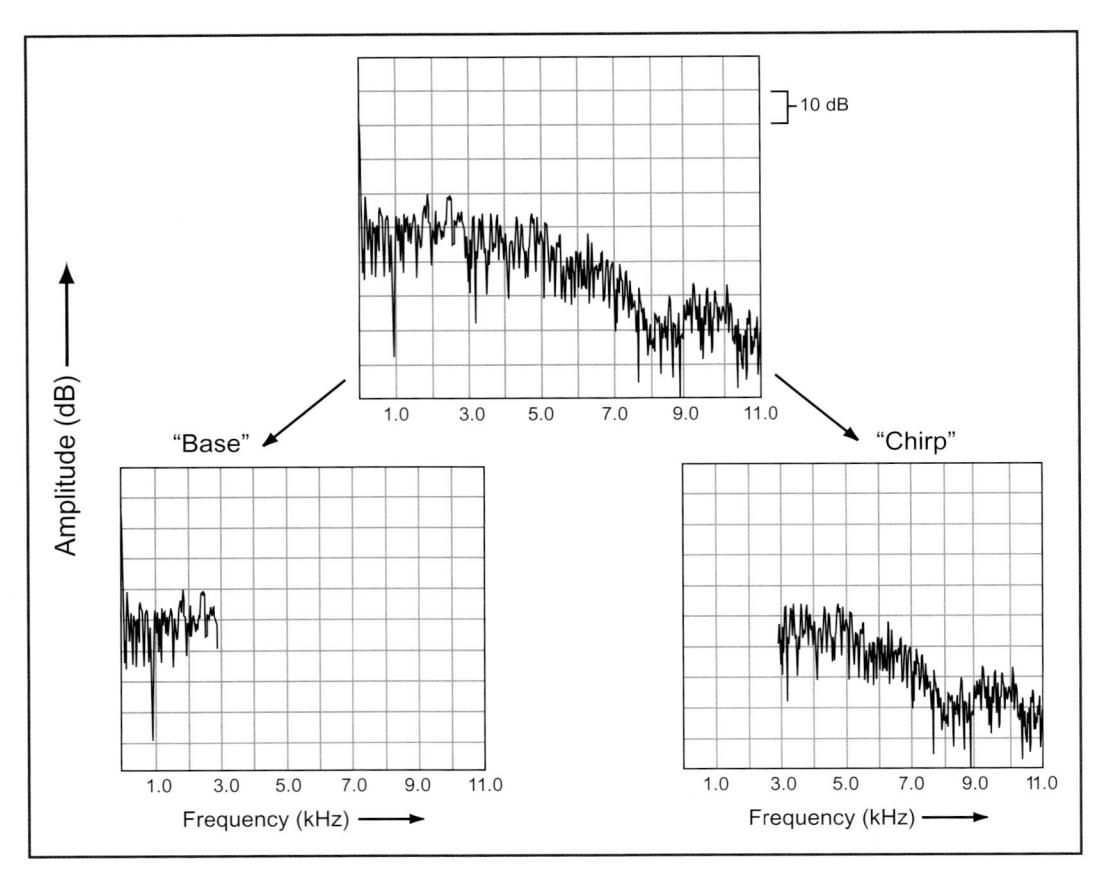

Figure 12-8. Spectra like those used by Fowler and Rosenblum (1991) to demonstrate duplex perception for a nonspeech event. Top spectrum is for the acoustic event associated with a slamming metal door. The bottom two spectra are the result of filtering the top spectrum in two ways: a low-pass filter, allowing only frequencies from 0 to 3.0 kHz to be heard (*bottom, left*), and a high-pass filter, allowing only the frequencies from 3.0 to 11.0 kHz to be heard (*bottom, right*). The 0 to 3.0 kHz spectrum is analogous to the base, the 3.0 to 11.0 kHz spectrum is analogous to the chirp. When the two bottom signals are played at the same time and the 3.0 to 11.0 kHz signal has sufficient intensity, listeners hear a slamming metal door and a shaking can of rice (or jangling keys) at the same time, demonstrating duplex perception for a nonspeech signal.

3.0–11.0 kHz part) to listeners for separate identification. Listeners reported hearing a metal door closing or some "hard collision" for the full signal (upper graph of Figure 12–8), a duller, wooden door-closing sound for the 0 to 3.0 kHz signal (lower left graph, Figure 12–8), and a shaking can of rice, a tambourine, or jangling keys for the 3.0 to 11.0 kHz signal (lower right graph, Figure 12–8).

Fowler and Rosenblum (1991) took advantage of a variation of the duplex perception finding. Whalen and Liberman (1987) discovered that a duplex perception was obtainable when the base and isolated F3 transition were delivered to the same ear, provided the isolated F3 transition was increased in intensity relative to the base. When the "chirp" intensity was relatively low in comparison with the "base," listeners heard a good /da/ or /ga/ depending on which F3 transition was used. As the F3 "chirp" was increased in intensity, a threshold was reached at which listeners heard both a good /da/ or /ga/ *plus* a "chirp." Listeners perceived the signal as duplex, as in the earlier experiments in which the "base" and "chirp" were in opposite ears. Fowler and Rosenblum repeated this same-ear experiment, but using signals lacking phonetic content, in this case the slamming metal door signal split into a base and chirp, as described above. Relatively low "chirp" intensities (the 3.0–11.0 kHz part of the signal) in combination with the "base" (the 0–3.0 kHz signal) produced a percept of a slamming metal door, consistent with the percept elicited by the original, intact signal (top spectrum in Figure 12–8). As the "chirp" intensity was raised, a threshold was reached at which listeners heard the slamming metal door *plus* the shaking can of rice/tambourine/jangling keys. Fowler and Rosenblum thus evoked a duplex percept exactly parallel to the one described above for /dɑ/ and /gɑ/, except in this case for nonspeech sounds.

If the original duplex perception findings (Liberman & Mattingly, 1985; Mann & Liberman, 1983; Rand, 1974; Whalen & Liberman, 1987) provided compelling evidence for a special speech perception module in humans, the demonstration of duplex perception for a slamming metal door is strong evidence *against* the idea of the speech module. As Fowler and Rosenblum (1991) pointed out, if the phonetic part of duplex perception (i.e., the "good," unambiguous signal) was regarded as the output of a special speech module, the perception of a slamming metal door plus the shaking can of rice when the 3.0 to 11.0 kHz signal was raised to a sufficient intensity was evidence of a special human module for, the perception of door-slamming, and metal door slamming at that. It is hardly absurd to imagine a human biological endowment for perceiving speech signals as an evolutionary adaptation, but the existence of a brain module dedicated to the perception of a slamming metal door is a non-starter. Perhaps there is a special biological endowment for perceiving speech, but duplex perception is not the critical test for its existence.

Acoustic Invariance

The lack of acoustic invariance for speech sounds was an important catalyst for the development of the motor theory of speech perception. As discussed in Chapter 11, Blumstein and Stevens (1979) performed an acoustic analysis of stop burst acoustics that led them to reject this central claim of the motor theorists. Blumstein and Stevens used the stop burst spectrum to classify correctly 85% of word-initial stop consonants in a variety of vowel contexts. They regarded this finding as a falsification of the motor theorists' claim that there was too much context-conditioned acoustic variability to allow listeners to establish a consistent and reliable link between speech acoustic characteristics and phonetic categories. For the motor theorist, consistency associated with speech sound categories was found in the underlying articulatory behavior for specific sounds, even when the context of a sound was changed. The "underlying articulatory gesture" was the neural code for generating the gesture. This code was assumed to be "fixed" regardless of its phonetic context. Whatever changes occurred to the *actual* articulatory gestures—the observed, collective movements of the lips, tongue, mandible, and so forth—were not relevant to the motor theory. In the motor theory, perception of speech depended on these more abstract neural commands, higher up in the process, that were not coded for phonetic context. The phonetic context effects (see Chapter 11, Figure 11-33) were stripped away by the special speech module, leaving the abstract commands for just the phoneme (original motor theory) and/or gesture (revised motor theory). These invariant commands were assumed to be part of the special speech module.

Blumstein and Stevens' (1979) apparent falsification of the lack of acoustic invariance for sound categories is a bit more involved than a simple demonstration of consistency between a selected acoustic measure (such as the shape of a burst spectrum) and a particular sound. Liberman and Mattingly (1985), in a very fine review of why they believed the acoustic signal was not sufficiently consistent to establish and maintain speech sound categories in perception (where "categories" = "phonemes"), identified complications with so-called auditory theories of speech perception. Auditory theories claim that information in the speech acoustic signal is sufficient, and sufficiently consistent, to support speech perception. These theories regard the auditory mechanisms for speech perception to be the same as mechanisms for the perception of environmental sounds, music, or any acoustic signal. One specific auditory perspective on speech perception (Diehl, Lotto, & Holt, 2004; Kingston & Diehl, 1994) claims that speakers control their speech acoustic output to produce speech signals well matched to auditory processing capabilities. Another auditory perspective, described in Chapter 11, is based on locus equations which represent formant transitions that provide reliable information on place of articulation for stops and fricatives.

Why were Liberman and Mattingly (1985) so adamant in rejecting auditory theories of speech perception? First, Liberman and Mattingly pointed to what they termed "extraphonetic" factors that cause variation in the acoustic characteristics of speech sounds. These factors include (among others) speaking rate and speaker sex and age. The speaker sex/age issue is particularly interesting because the same vowel has widely varying formant frequencies depending on the size of a speaker's vocal tract (Chapter 11). An auditory theory of speech perception either requires listeners to learn and store all these different formant patterns or must employ some sort of cognitive process to place all formant patterns on a single, "master" scale. This issue, of how one hears the same vowel (or consonant) when so many different-sized vocal tracts produce it with different formant frequencies, is called the "speaker (or talker) normalization" problem (interesting papers on speaker normalization are found in Johnson & Mullenix, 1997; see also Adank, Smits, & van Hout, 2004; and see discussion below). The motor theory finesses this problem by arguing that the perception of different formant transition patterns is mediated by a special mechanism that extracts intended articulatory gestures and "outputs" these gestures as the percepts. For example, the motor theory assumes that the intended gestures (the neural code for the gestures) for the vowel in the word "bad" are roughly equivalent for men, women, and children, even if the outputs of their different-sized vocal tracts are different. The special speech perception module registers the same intended gesture for all three speakers, and hence the same vowel perception (or the same consonant perception). The motor theory makes the speaker normalization problem go away.

A second reason to reject auditory theories, according to Liberman and Mattingly (1985), is the interesting case of trading relations in the acoustic cues for a given sound category. For any given sound, there are at least several different acoustic cues that can contribute to the proper identification of the sound. As Liberman and Mattingly pointed out, none of these individual values are necessarily critical to the proper identification of a sound segment, but the *collection* of the several values may be. Among these several cues, the acoustic value of one can be "offset" by the acoustic value of another to yield the same phonetic percept. For example, Figure 12–9 shows spectrograms of a single speaker's production of the words "say" and "stay." These two words can be described as a minimal-pair opposition defined by the presence or absence of the stop consonant /t/. In "stay" (but not "say") there is the obvious silent closure interval of approximately 60 to 90 ms, but the "say"-"stay" opposition also involves a subtle difference in the starting frequency of the F1 transition for /eɪ/. Figure 12–9 shows the F1 starting frequency in "stay" to be somewhat lower than the starting frequency in "say" (compare frequencies labeled "F1 onset"). The lower starting frequency in "stay" is consistent with theoretical and laboratory findings of F1 transitions pointing toward the spectrographic baseline—that is, 0 Hz—at the boundary of a stop consonant and vowel (Fant, 1960). The difference is subtle but measurable.

In a frequently cited experiment, Best, Morrongiello, and Robson (1981) performed a clever manipulation of these two cues to the difference between "say" and "stay." The two cues—the closure interval and the lower F1 starting frequency following the stop closure—were used to demonstrate the "trading relations" phenomenon. Figure 12–10 shows one version of the stimuli used by Best and her colleagues. The gray, stippled interval represents the voiceless fricative /s/, the narrow rectangles the closure intervals for /t/, and the two solid lines the F1-F2 trajectories for /eɪ/. Best et al. synthesized these sequences in two ways, one with an F1 starting frequency of 230 Hz (Figure 12–10, left side), the other with an F1 starting frequency of 430 Hz (Figure 12–10, right side). Best et al. changed the duration of the stop closure interval between 0 (no closure interval) and 136 ms, sometimes with the lower F1

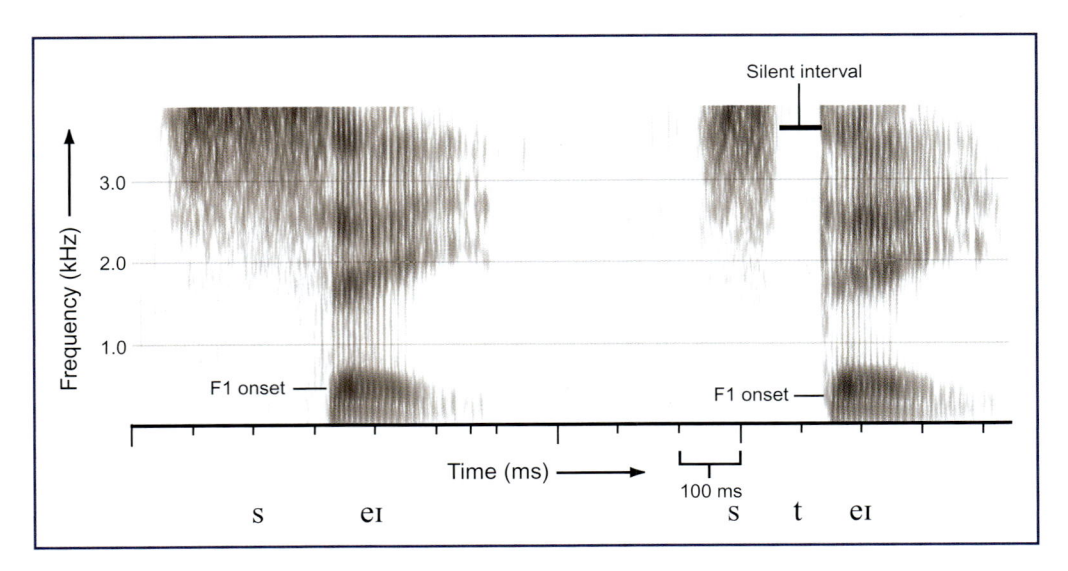

Figure 12-9. Spectrograms of the utterances "say" and "stay" showing two acoustic differences that distinguish the syllables with and without the /t/. One difference is the presence of the silent interval (closure interval) for /t/ (*right*), the other is the slightly lower F1 starting frequency in "stay" compared with "say." See text for details.

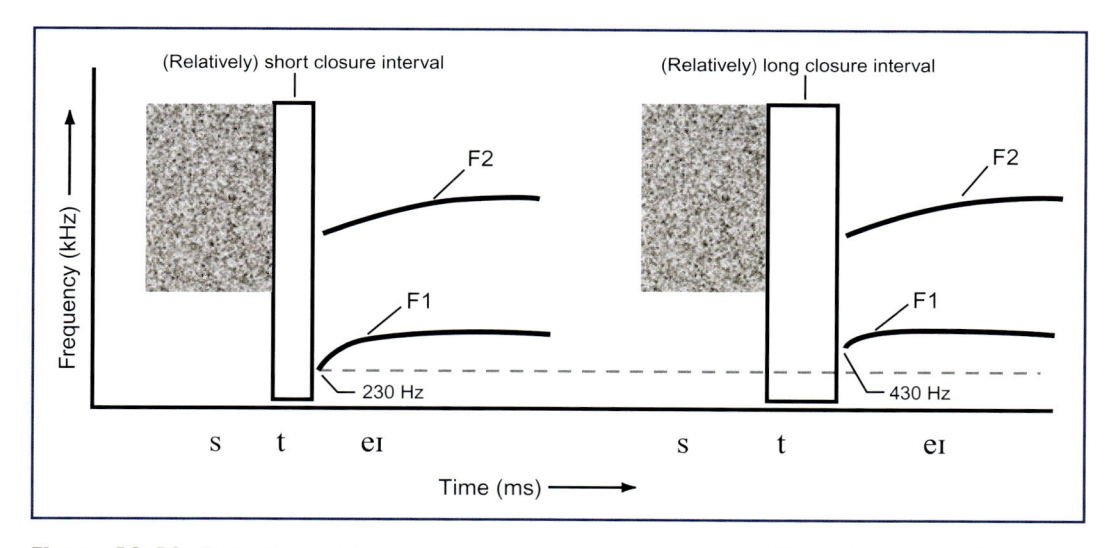

Figure 12–10. Two schematic spectrograms, showing how two different cues can "trade off" against each other to maintain a single phonetic percept. The phonetic percept is the presence of the stop consonant /t/ between /s/ and /eɪ/. The two cues manipulated in these schematic spectrograms are: (a) the duration of the closure interval (the width of the narrow rectangles), and (b) the starting frequency of the F1 transition. Longer closure intervals and lower F1 starting frequencies tend to produce more /t/ responses. The tendency for more /t/ responses with longer closure intervals can be offset by a higher starting frequency for F1. In the left spectrogram, a shorter closure requires a lower F1 starting frequency for the /t/ percept. In the right spectrogram, which shows a longer closure interval, the F1 starting frequency can be higher.

starting frequency, and sometimes with the higher F1 starting frequency. When the pattern was synthesized with one of the longer closure intervals, close to 136 ms, listeners clearly heard the sequence as "stay." When the pattern was synthesized with a very short or nonexistent closure interval, "say" was heard. None of this is surprising and is consistent with the spectrographic patterns shown in Figure 12–9.

The interesting findings occurred when the length of the closure interval between the /s/ and /eɪ/ was rather short (~30–50 ms) and resulted in roughly equal "say" and "stay" responses. For these stimuli, the presence or absence of a /t/ closure was ambiguous. Best et al. (1981) determined that when the F1 starting frequency was the higher one (430 Hz in Figure 12–10), a longer closure interval was required for listeners to hear "stay." When the F1 starting frequency was the lower one (230 Hz in Figure 12–10), a shorter closure interval allowed the listeners to hear "stay." In other words, the two cues to the presence of a /t/ between the /s/ and /eɪ/ seemed to "trade off" against each other to produce the same percept—a clear /t/ between the fricative and the following vowel. "Trading relations" is the term used for any set of speech cues that can be manipulated in opposite directions to yield a constant phonetic percept.

Speech Synthesis and Speech Perception

The pattern-playback machine allowed speech scientists to synthesize speech signals, but the quality of these signals was—let's be gracious—not particularly good. Developments in computer technology, knowledge of acoustic phonetics, and the sophistication of software codes have greatly improved speech synthesis. Current synthetic speech signals are so good they sometimes cannot be distinguished from natural speech. These developments have allowed speech perception researchers to make very fine adjustments in signals to learn about speech perception while avoiding the problem of the fuzzy speech signals produced by the pattern-playback machine. In 1987, Dennis Klatt from the Massachusetts Institute of Technology published a wonderful history of speech synthesis and provided audio examples of synthetic speech signals from 1939 to 1987 (Klatt, 1987). You can hear these examples at http://www.cs.indiana.edu/rhythmsp/ASA/Contents.html

For Liberman and Mattingly (1985), the trading relations phenomenon proved the point about the inability to connect a specific acoustic characteristic with a specific sound category. The potential, multiple acoustic cues to a given phonetic category were simply too numerous to be used by a listener to develop and maintain the category identification. In the case of "say"-"stay," the lower versus higher F1 starting frequency, or the precise duration of the closure interval, was not by itself sufficient to serve as an acoustic constant of a phonetic category. The *collection* of these several cues, however, reflected the underlying gesture for the sound category. Small variations in one cue could be compensated for by variations in a different cue, but in the end the sum of these various cues yielded a single percept. In support of Liberman and Mattingly's theoretical cause, trading relations have been demonstrated for many different phonetic distinctions. It is not just a "say"-"stay" phenomenon (see Repp [1982] and Repp and Liberman [1987] for reviews of trading relations in phonetic perception).

The trading relations experiment takes advantage of the categorical perception method by varying a stimulus continuum (in the case above, between "say" and "stay") and finding a specific stimulus along the continuum where 50% of the responses are "say" and 50% "stay." This is the category boundary for the "say"-"stay" contrast, and modifications of parts of the signal cause changes in the boundary as described above. Stimulus continua for many phonetic contrasts have been used in speech perception research, including /s/-/ʃ/, /s/-/z/, and /r/-/w/, among others. The stimuli are synthesized to construct a signal continuum with endpoints that are excellent exemplars of the two sounds (e.g., clear /s/, clear /ʃ/ for an /s/-/ʃ/ continuum). As the stimuli are adjusted to be less like an endpoint (less /s/-like, less /ʃ/-like), the respective signals are ultimately adjusted to produce a middle stimulus that is ambiguous, as if halfway between the endpoints. For this stimulus, 50% of the responses are one of the endpoint percepts, and 50% the other endpoint percept. The 50-50 percept defines the phoneme boundary.

Categorical perception as a method to study speech perception is sometimes thought of as outdated. Some people think of it as a method associated with the motor theory of speech perception. As reviewed below in the section "Speech Perception and Word Recognition," the method is used in contemporary research to identify the influence of the lexicon on phonetic perception.

The Competition: General Auditory Explanations of Speech Perception

An obvious approach to understanding speech perception is to regard the speech acoustic signal as a sufficiently rich source of information for a listener's needs. In this view, the speech acoustic signal contains reliable, learnable information for the identification of sounds, words, and phrases intended by a speaker. A *general auditory explanation* of speech perception seems simple, and perhaps the logical starting point—like a default perspective—for scientists who study speech perception. Contrary to this apparent logic, general auditory explanations have fought an uphill scientific battle since the motor theory was formulated in the 1950s.

The information presented above describes the reasons for the development of the original and revised motor theories of speech perception. Those reasons led to one overarching assumption concerning speech perception. A special perceptual processor is required because general auditory mechanisms were not up to the task of perceiving speech. In contrast, a central theme of general auditory explanations of speech perception is that special perceptual mechanisms are not required.

As in the published work on the motor theory, a set of reasons in support of a general auditory account of speech perception has been carefully articulated in the scientific literature. These are summarized below.

Sufficient Acoustic Invariance

As noted earlier, Blumstein and Stevens (1979) demonstrated a fair degree of acoustic consistency for stop consonant place of articulation, and many of the successful automatic classification experiments described in Chapter 11 imply consistency in the acoustic signal for vowels, diphthongs, nasals, fricatives, and semivowels. Recall from Chapter 11 that Lindblom (1990) argued for a more flexible view of speech acoustic variability. In this view, listeners do not need *absolute* acoustic invariance for a speech sound, but only enough to maintain discriminability from neighboring sound classes.

General auditory accounts of speech perception rely on this more flexible view of acoustic distinctiveness for the perception of speech sounds. Presumably, an initial front-end acoustic analysis of the speech signal by general auditory mechanisms is supplemented by higher-level processing which resolves any ambiguities in sound identity. The front-end analysis is like a hypothesis concerning the identity of the sequence of incoming sounds, based on initial processing of the incoming acoustic signal. The higher-level processes include knowledge of the context in which each sound is produced, plus syntactic, semantic, and pragmatic constraints on the message. Listeners bring more to the speech perception process than a capability for acoustic analysis. These additional sources of knowledge considerably loosen the demand for strict acoustic invariance for each sound segment.

Scientists often refer to the front-end part of this process as "bottom-up" processing, and the higher-level knowledge affecting perception as "top-down" processing. The top-down processes influence the bottom-up analyses, taking advantage of the rich source of information in the auditory signal. Stevens (2005) has proposed a speech perception model in which bottom-up auditory mechanisms analyze the incoming speech signal for segment identity and top-down processes resolve ambiguities emerging from this front-end analysis. When an account of speech perception is framed within the general cognitive abilities of humans, including top-down processes, a role for general auditory analysis in the perception of speech becomes much more plausible (Lotto & Holt, 2006). In this view, the lack of strict acoustic invariance for speech sounds cannot be used as an argument against a primary role of general auditory mechanisms in speech perception.

Recall from Chapter 11 the discussion of locus equations. Chapter 11 presents the equations as acoustic measurements of F2 onset and F2 target that have unique slopes and y-intercepts for the three places of stop consonants. These two parameters yielded unique linear functions for each of the three stop places of articulation in English. Fruchter and Sussman (1997) explored the perceptual value of locus equations by varying the parameters in small steps and presenting the resulting linear functions to listeners for identification of /b/, /d/, and /g/. This approach is similar to the early experiments performed by the Haskins Lab scientists when they varied F2 onset in small steps and determined that listeners responded to these variations with categorical labels.

Fruchter and Sussman (1997) found that the varying combinations of F2 onset and F2 target were not heard as continuous variations, but were clustered in the categories /b/, /d/, and /g/, consistent with the acoustic measurements that separated the three stops. This is an auditory explanation of the perception of place of articulation, but with a twist. The twist, described by Sussman, Fruchter, Hilbert, and Sirosh (1998), is that many animals have special neural mechanisms for connecting two acoustic events and using those connections to establish categories (see Andoni & Pollak, 2007). In the case of locus equations, the two events are the F2 onset and F2 target and the connection between them forms the linear functions shown in Chapter 11. Sussman et al. argued that these connections may be species-specific and matched to vocalization characteristics of the different species. The perceptual basis of locus equations is like a combination of auditory and special speech module theories: processing of auditory information (the combinations of F2 onset and F2 target) and special, specific mechanisms to use the information to establish categories such as stop place of articulation.

Replication of Speech Perception Effects Using Nonspeech Signals

Many categorical perception effects have been demonstrated using synthetic speech stimuli. Several of these experiments are reviewed above. There are also demonstrations of similar effects using nonspeech signals. Categorical perception of speech signals has been a centerpiece of the original and revised motor theory. The demonstration of the same effects with nonspeech signals, however, seems to damage the proposed link between speech production and speech perception implied by findings of categorical perception for speech signals.

The approach employed by scientists interested in a general auditory theory of speech perception is to reproduce a categorical perception effect for speech signals using nonspeech signals. If the results of a nonspeech experiment are the same as a speech experiment, the categorical perception effect can be attributed to general auditory, not perceptual, mechanisms specialized for speech. A well-known example of such an experiment was published by Pisoni (1977), who showed that categorical perception functions for the voiced-voiceless contrast were probably due to auditory, not speech-special mechanisms.

Pisoni (1977) reviewed speech perception experiments in which labeling and discrimination data suggested categorical perception of voiced and voiceless stops. A typical set of data for this experiment is shown in Figure 12–11, where VOT is plotted on the x-axis and labeling (red points, left axis) and discrimination (blue points, right axis) are plotted as two y-axes. In this experiment, the stimuli are synthesized to sound like stop-vowel syllables, with all features held constant except for VOT. Assume the transitions are synthesized to evoke perception of a bilabial stop and that VOT is varied in 5-ms steps from lead values (negative VOT values) to long-lag (positive) values. Figure 12–11 shows a VOT continuum ranging from −10 ms to +50 ms. For each VOT value, listeners are asked to label the stimulus as either /b/ or /p/. In the discrimination experiments, two stimuli from the VOT continuum are presented, always separated by 20 ms along the continuum (e.g., one stimulus with a VOT of 0 ms, the other with a VOT of 20 ms). In the discrimination experiment, listeners are asked if the stimulus pairs are the same or different. The results in Figure 12–11 show only /b/ labels for stimuli with VOTs from −10 ms to +15 ms, half /b/ and half /p/ labels for the stimulus with VOT = 20 ms, and all /p/ labels for stimuli with VOT = 30 ms

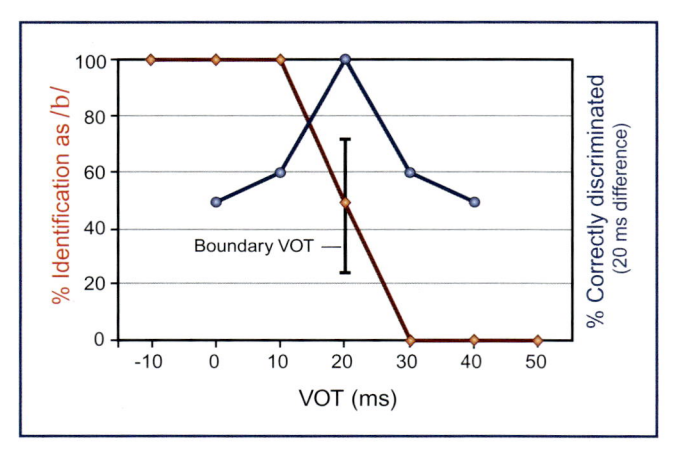

Figure 12–11. Labeling (identification) and discrimination functions for a VOT continuum, showing the expected pattern for an interpretation of categorical perception of the voicing distinction for stops. The x-axis is VOT. Two y-axes are shown, one for identification (left y-axis, red points), one for discrimination (right y-axis, blue points). The categorical boundary, where the labeling function shifts rapidly between /b/ and /p/, is shown as 20 ms. Discrimination across this 20 ms boundary is 100%. Within the categories it is close to chance (50%).

or more. The change from /b/ to /p/ labels occurs quickly in the 20 to 30 ms range of VOTs, as required for an interpretation of categorical perception. The discrimination data (blue points) show perfect discrimination when the two VOT stimuli cross the labeling "boundary," but much poorer discrimination when the two stimuli are within a category. These labeling and discrimination VOT data meet the requirements for categorical perception as reviewed above. The interpretation of categorical perception of VOT was consistent with the motor theory of speech perception. Speakers cannot produce *continuous* changes in VOT, so they cannot perceive them.

Pisoni (1977) knew that the synthesis of VOT differences for the same place of stop articulation involved variable asynchronies between two acoustic events (in natural speech, the burst and the onset of voicing). Examination of Figure 12–2 shows that the two-formant patterns for the three cognate pairs /ba-pa/, /da-ta/, and /ga-ka/ differ in the onset time of the first formant relative to the second formant. Listeners were made to hear the voiceless member of each pair by delaying the onset of the first formant by approximately 50 ms relative to the onset of the second formant. A synthetic VOT continuum was generated in early studies by varying the starting time of the first formant relative to the starting time of the second formant, without a stop burst. Pisoni mimicked these asynchronies with nonspeech stimuli like those shown in Figure 12–12. Each stimulus consisted of a pair of sinusoids, one at a lower frequency (500 Hz), the other at a higher frequency (1500 Hz). Stimulus 1 shows the two tones with simultaneous onsets, which mimic simultaneous onset of the first two formant frequencies, or VOT = 0 ms. Stimuli 2 through 6 have increasing asynchronies between the two tones, with the onset of the lower-frequency tone lagging that of the higher-frequency tone by increasing amounts. The stimulus progression from 2 through 6 mimics increasing positive VOTs.[4]

Each two-tone stimulus using the sinusoids was played to listeners who participated in both labeling and discrimination experiments. Pisoni (1977) found that unless the starting times of the two tones differed by more than 20 ms, listeners categorized (labeled) the two-tone pair as the same event. A sudden change in the listeners' perception of the stimulus pairs occurred when the onset of the lower tone began at least 20 ms later than the onset of the higher tone. In Figure 12–12, stimuli 1 through 5 were heard as the "same" event, and stimulus 6 was heard as two different events. This 20 ms "boundary" for classifying the tone pairs (see dashed line = 20-ms for stimulus 6) as one event, versus two events, was very close to the VOT boundary obtained for synthesized speech signals, where the first formant was delayed relative to the second formant. As in the speech experiments, discrimination experiments showed that pairs of stimuli chosen within a category were not discriminated as different; pairs of stimuli across the categorical boundary were discriminated. Based on the findings with nonspeech signals, Pisoni concluded that the VOT boundary for the experiments with *speech* signals did not reflect a special speech mechanism such as that proposed by motor theorists. The same boundary was demonstrated with nonspeech signals, suggesting analysis of VOT differences by a general property of auditory mechanisms (see Hirsh, 1959).

Many other experiments in which phonetic effects are mimicked with nonspeech signals have been reported in the literature (see Diehl et al., 2004 for a summary). In general, categorical perception effects or

---

[4]Readers will note that the manipulation of VOT in the synthetic speech signals of Figure 12–2, and the mimic signals illustrated in Figure 12–12, depend on modification of an acoustic variable that is somewhat different from the typical definition of VOT. VOT for natural speech signals is defined as the time difference between a stop burst and the onset of vocal fold vibration for the following vowel. The synthetic signals used to construct VOT continua for the speech signals used by motor theorists typically did not have a burst. Rather, the percept of the voiced-voiceless contrast was elicited with the "F1 cutback" technique described in the text and illustrated in Figure 12–2.

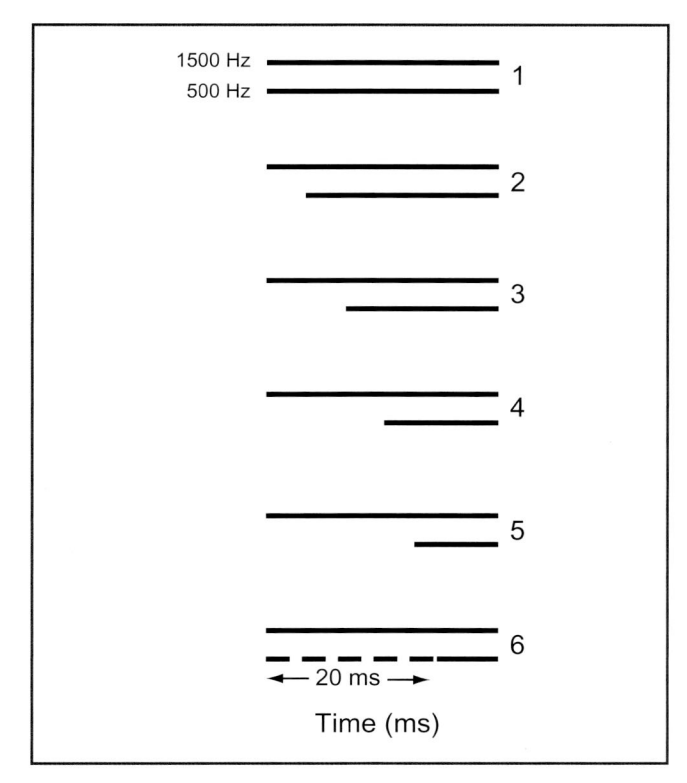

Figure 12–12. Illustration of stimuli used by Pisoni (1977) to demonstrate categorical perception of sinusoid tone pairs whose relative onsets simulated the VOT continuum shown in Figure 12–11. The onset of the lower-frequency sinusoid was either simultaneous with that of the higher-frequency sinusoid (stimulus 1) or was delayed in small steps (stimuli 2–6). Listeners labeled stimuli 1 through 5 as the same event and could not discriminate between any of these tone pairs. Stimulus 6 was labeled as a different event from the other five and was discriminated from them as well.

context effects demonstrated with speech signals can be demonstrated equally well when nonspeech signals (tones, noise intervals, etc.) mimic the speech conditions. Auditory theorists regard these findings as evidence for the ability of general auditory mechanisms to do the important, "front-end" work in speech perception. These theorists reject the idea of a special module for speech perception.

An interesting variation on this style of experiment has been reported by Laing, Liu, Lotto, and Holt (2012). These researchers showed that the categorization of a speech segment such as /g/ or /d/ was affected by the frequency range of a sequence of tones (that is, *nonspeech* signals) preceding the stop. The listeners' choice of /d/ vs. /g/ was affected *systematically* by whether the preceding tone sequence occupied a higher, versus lower, frequency range. A theory of speech perception that separates the mechanism for perceiving speech signals from the perceptual mechanism for other auditory signals is inconsistent with this finding. A motor theory of speech perception cannot explain why the frequency range of a sequence of tones has a systematic effect on the choice of a sound as /d/ or /g/. This is another possible example of falsification of the motor theory.

Animal and Infant Perception of Speech Signals

Auditory theorists point to the demonstration in animals of categorical perception for many speech sound contrasts, as well as the ability of animals to learn phonetic contrasts when properly trained, as evidence for the use of general auditory mechanisms in the perception of speech (Diehl, Lotto, & Holt, 2004; Kluender, 1994; Kluender & Kiefte, 2006). An argument for a special speech-perception mechanism in animals does not make sense because animals do not speak. The ability of animals to learn phonetic contrasts, when trained to do so, points to the ability of human infants to use their substantially more powerful cognitive resources to do the same thing. If infants can use phonetic input from their environment to develop sound categories, the logical appeal of a species-specific module for speech perception decreases dramatically.

Saffran and Thiessen (2007) have summarized evidence for the human infant's use of phonetic data from the environment (e.g., speech produced by parents and others) in the development of sound categories. Saffran and Thiessen's viewpoint about such learning is consistent with the philosophy of auditory theorists, who believe general auditory mechanisms are used in speech perception. Saffran and Thiessen argue for general (not special) cognitive mechanisms in a child's learning of speech and language. These cognitive mechanisms allow the child to build an enormous phonetic data base which is used to organize regularities within the data. Those regularities can be imagined to include phoneme categories, word forms, word boundaries, and so forth. This idea of *statistical learning* is a theoretical approach to child speech and language learning that is very popular among language development scientists (Newport, 2016).

An interesting extension of this line of thought concerning speech perception abilities is the possibility that such learning influences speech production as well (Lehet & Holt, 2017). Lehet and Holt's work was performed with adult participants; relevant data on 4- and 5-year-old children have been reported by Richstmeier and Goffman (2017). A clear link between statistical learning in speech perception and production among children who are developing speech and language would be very interesting.

> **That Cute Cuddly Infant Is Really a Statistical Model-Builder**
>
> Professor Jenny Saffran of the University of Wisconsin–Madison asks the question, "How do infants, when listening to connected speech, learn where one word ends and the next begins?" This interesting question is even more compelling because speakers do not "mark" the ends and beginnings of words with special acoustic effects. The sounds all run together. So how do infants figure this out?—how do they learn to identify where words begin and end? Saffran (2003) proposed that, over time, infants compile the phonetic input in their environment as a statistical model of which sound sequences are likely to begin words, to straddle words, and to end words. The model is basically a set of probabilities of which sound sequences are heard as word beginnings versus endings. Saffran points out that this kind of "statistical learning" is seen with all kinds of input—not just speech—and even among animals. This learning perspective on speech sound perception is at odds with the innate, species-specific mechanisms proposed by motor theorists. Like cookies and clicks on the Internet, watch what you say in the presence of a 6-month-old.

The Competition: Direct Realism

A theory of speech perception called direct realism (Fowler, Galantucci, & Saltzman, 2003) is an alternative to both the motor theory and a general auditory approach. The direct realism perspective on speech perception is not easy to explain in the absence of substantial background information (which is not pursued here). Some scientists (Cleary & Pisoni, 2001) question the utility of direct realism as a theory because it is hard to understand how reasonable experimental tests can be made to support or falsify it.

The direct realism perspective on speech perception takes its inspiration from the pioneering work of the psychologist J. J. Gibson (1904–1979). Gibson's theoretical and experimental focus was on visual perception. Gibson (1968, 1979) rejected the idea of cognitively driven, "constructed" percepts. He did not like the idea of perception in which percepts—often referred to as the "objects" of perception—were mediated by cognitive operations to produce a representation of the external world. Rather, he proposed the idea that animals, including humans, perceive the visual layouts of environments directly, by linking the stimulation of their senses (by light waves, in the case of vision) with the sources of the stimulation. For example, when perceivers are exposed to the patterning of light reflected from a chair, they perceive the chair directly, rather than interpreting through neural mechanisms the light patterns reaching their eyes. Gibson's view was that objects in the environment structure the medium through which they are conveyed to the senses. A chair structures the medium (light waves) by the patterns of light reflected from it, and humans presumably learn that structure and perceive the chair directly, without cognitive mediation. Direct realists argue that the objects of perception are not the proximal stimulation, which in the example above is the light reflections at the eye, from the chair, but rather the distal source of the light reflection. In this example, the distal source is the chair.

More specifically, in Gibson's view, perceivers do not "process" and "encode" the light waves via cognitive operations whose output is a symbolic representation. Gibson coined the term "ecological psychology" for this view of perception. The term is consistent with a "realist" (i.e., ecologically valid) view of how organisms perceive objects. For Gibson, much of the experimental psychologist's vocabulary, including terms found in information processing models such as "encoding" and "representation," were not much more than a convenient set of descriptive terms. For Gibson, the terms did not have ecological validity—that is, they did not represent "real" things, "real" mechanisms that were the stuff of perception.

The motor theory of speech perception requires operations of a special module to convert (decode) an unstable acoustic signal into a stable articulatory representation. In the motor theory, the objects of speech perception are the articulatory characteristics (either places of articulation or articulatory gestures over time) of phonemes or phoneme sequences as transformed by the special processor. On the other hand, a general auditory approach to speech perception requires some processing stages to match the incoming acoustics to stored templates or features or a statistical model of acoustic speech signals (Klatt, 1989; Massaro & Chen, 2008; Stevens, 2005). The object of speech perception in the auditory theory is the speech acoustic signal, plus other sources of sensory information (such as visual information from a speaker's face during speech). In both cases, cognitive operations of varying degrees of automaticity are required for perception of incoming sounds. Fowler (1986, 1996; Fowler, Shankweiler, & Studdert-Kennedy, 2016, especially pp. 138–143), the leading proponent of direct realism in speech perception, rejects cognitive "constructions" in the perception of speech sounds. Fowler agrees with the Gibsonian idea that scientists should reject the idea of perception driven by cognitive processes that produce an "output symbol." In the case of speech perception, the simplest example of such a symbol is a phoneme. Rather, Fowler argues for direct perception of articulatory gestures. In this case, the objects of speech perception are articulatory gestures, such as movements of the tongue or jaw. The gestures are the distal source and the pressure wave produced by articulatory movement and that reaches the ears is the proximal stimulation. Movements of the articulators, in Fowler's view, structure the medium (air) through which the information is transmitted to the ears. Listeners track this structure as phonetic gestures unfold over time. The perception of these gestures is direct, not mediated by other processes. Listeners literally hear articulatory gestures (or, on another interpretation, the sounds they hear *are* the articulatory gestures). The parallel with Gibson's (1969, 1970) view of visual perception is easy to see.

How is direct realism different from the motor theory? Both theories focus on perception of articulatory gestures, but motor theory requires a special, completely automatic mechanism (a module) to transform acoustic signals into articulatory behavior. Direct realism proposes no special mechanisms, and, in fact, claims that direct perception applies to visual, auditory, haptic (sense of touch), and presumably olfactory and gustatory (taste) perception. In all cases, the source of the stimulation is what is perceived, because that source structures the medium through which it is conveyed.

How is direct realism different from an auditory approach to speech perception? This is a more interesting question, and one with a more complicated (and hotly debated) answer (see Diehl & Kluender, 1989; the exchange between Lotto and Holt [2006] and Fowler [2006], and between Fowler et al. [2006] and Massaro and Chen [2008]). The simplest answer is that in direct realism, listeners hear the articulatory gestures, whereas in a general auditory approach, listeners hear the acoustic signal, not the gestures that produced the signal.

Does a comparison between the auditory and direct realism theories of speech perception reveal an advantage of the direct realist perspective?[5] As reviewed in Chapter 11, the speech acoustic signal for a given sound varies depending on its phonetic context (and other factors as well). For example, /s/ spectra in the utterances [su] and [si] are quite different, because speakers typically produce some lip rounding during the /s/ in [su], but not [si]. The acoustic effect of lip rounding during the /s/ in [su] is to emphasize much lower frequencies in the aperiodic fricative spectrum, compared with the /s/ spectrum in [si]. Direct realists argue that a general auditory approach to speech

---

Growing Up in the 1950s and Speech Perception

Many of us who grew up in the 1950s went to the picture show every Saturday and sat through double features of perfectly awful science fiction movies. The music meant to convey the weirdness of on-screen aliens was equally awful, usually a kind of multitonal whistling you might associate with attempts to tune in a distant radio station. Professor Robert Remez of Barnard University and his colleagues used similar sounds to prove a point about speech perception. They looked at the first three formants of a natural utterance and mimicked their time-dependent frequency changes using sinusoids (you can hear these signals, plus the sentences they were based on, at http://www.haskins.yale.edu/featured/sws/swssentences/sentences.html). When listeners heard these sounds, some described them as suggested above—weird outer space signals. But when people were told to listen to the signals as if they were speech, many heard the sentence as originally spoken, even though the signal was composed of only three time-varying sinusoids. Remez and his associates concluded that this finding disproved the idea of a speech-specific module that was automatically engaged by speech signals. They reached this conclusion because the three-sinusoid replica of speech formants could not have been produced by a human vocal tract. It was as if listeners could hear the signals as speech, if instructed to do so. A dedicated speech perception module would not allow that kind of choice (see Pardo & Remez, 2006, pp. 207–208).

---

[5]Many direct realists, including Fowler (Fowler et al., 2003), believe that their theory is preferable on *philosophical* grounds, in addition to any scientific advantages that may be demonstrated. Direct realism unifies perceptual behavior across the senses, discards the (in their view) awkward theoretical constructs of cognitive psychology (such as the notion of mental representations, or specialized modules), and may be easier to integrate with general evolutionary theory than the "constructed perceptions" of so many psychological theories.

perception is cumbersome and overly complicated because a listener must learn and store all these different variants of spectra for a given sound. They are correct in arguing that the effects of coarticulation result in acoustic variation for each speech sound. In direct realism, listeners are not burdened with the learning and storage problem of these many spectral and temporal variations because they "hear" the lingual fricative gesture combined, or coproduced (the two gestures produced at the same time), with the lip rounding gesture. Moreover, in direct realism the degree to which two articulatory gestures, such as lingual and labial gestures, are coproduced, or overlapped, is perceived directly. In a general auditory approach, the large number of variations (for example, of how much of the /s/ in [su] is lip-rounded) introduces acoustic variability for a given sound that may complicate the learning of speech sound categories and the mature form of speech perception. Direct realists see their theory of speech perception as much simpler than general auditory approaches. Scientists usually prefer theories that are simple, compared with more complex theories involving lots of add-ons (such as cognitive processes and massive storage needs).

VOWEL PERCEPTION

To this point the discussion has been almost exclusively about consonants. The early speech perception work was driven by research on consonants, especially stops. The motor theory was based on consonant perception, but made reference to vowel perception to support the theory. Categorical perception was reported for stop place of articulation, and later for fricative place of articulation, and for VOT. The theoretical support for the link between categorical perception and place of articulation, and VOT, was the inability to produce articulations between categories of place and voicing. This prompted the need for a special mechanism to match production to perception. The encoded categorical sounds of production required a decoder for perception of the categories.

But what about vowels? Early attempts to demonstrate categorical perception for vowels (e.g. a categorical function between vowel pairs like /i/-/ɪ/) were not successful, and later efforts demonstrated only a weak categorical effect for vowels compared with the strong effects for consonants (Kronrod, Coppess, & Feldman, 2016). For motor theorists, weak (or no) categorical effects for vowel distinctions made sense. The logic of the continuous perception of vowels followed directly from the logic of categorical perception of stop place of articulation and other consonant contrasts. Humans are limited to categorical production of stop or fricative place, and to the voiced-voiceless distinction for stops and fricatives and affricates; perception must be limited to those production categories. Humans can produce *continuous* variations in vowels, as in the continuous lowering of the tongue (or of the jaw, or of both) from /i/ to /ɪ/, or between any closely related vowel pair. The ability to produce continuous variation in vowels does not require a categorical mechanism to perceive them. The argument sounds reasonable, at least within the context of the motor theory. However, it is not strictly true that vowels can be produced continuously (Kent, 1974; Repp & Williams, 1985).

Vowel perception has been studied extensively. The structure of the discussion to follow is to consider vowel perception within the framework of the three theories of speech perception presented earlier.

Motor Theory (Original and Revised)

The original motor theory of speech perception focused on the need for a special perceptual mechanism for consonants, and payed little attention to vowels. Vowels did not require the special mechanism because it was assumed they could be produced continuously across a series of vowels. This awkward aspect of the original motor theory was cleared up by the revised motor theory, in which the objects of speech perception are articulatory gestures. These gestures involved vocalic parts of speech signals. For example, a gesture from a stop to a vowel is realized acoustically as a set of formant transitions in the direction of vowel targets. The gestures contributing to contrasts between words such as "say" and "stay," described earlier, also produce an important acoustic effect on the F1 onset frequency of the vowel following the "s" or "st." These acoustic effects of consonant-vowel formant transitions and/or formant onset frequencies, however, have long been considered as products of consonant production rather than essential features of vowels (e.g., Sussman et al., 1998; van Son & Pols, 1996). A reasonable conclusion is that the perceptual identification of vowel identity does not play an important role in, or is explained by, the original or revised motor theories.

Auditory Theories

Special perceptual mechanisms are not required in auditory theories of speech perception. Vowels and consonants are not treated differently in auditory theories, although there may be differences in the way the auditory mechanism processes and categorizes the two sound classes.

A vowel system, and the acoustic characteristics of the segments within the system, can be established over the course of phonetic learning by auditory exposure to thousands of vowels. Phonetic learning of vowels is a part of language development in children, and in adults is a component of new language acquisition in which the second language has a different vowel system compared with the native language. Auditory theories of speech perception have a learning component (sometimes implicit) by which the massive statistical database accumulated over so much exposure to speech sounds results in a template, or prototype of a vowel category. Along the learning trajectory in language development an acoustic template is organized for a vowel category. As the template is refined and stabilized, incoming speech signals are compared to these templates. If there is a good match between an incoming signal and a template a decision for vowel identity is confirmed.

The templates do not have to be rigid, and the match between them and the incoming signals do not have to be perfect; variability is permitted. In fact, there is evidence that a vowel category may have good and not-so-good acoustic representatives yet still be classified within that category (Kuhl, Conboy, Coffey-Corina, Padden, Rivera-Gaxiola, & Nelson, 2008; for an opposing view, see Lively & Pisoni, 1997).

The vowel templates are often conceptualized in terms of formant frequencies at the temporal middle of a vowel (Chapter 11). These frequencies are thought to represent the "target" formants for a vowel. It is easy to imagine such brain representations of vowel acoustics, developed and refined over time. And there are multiple studies showing that vowels are well identified from synthesized signals with steady (non-changing frequencies) F1 and F2 (see review in Johnson, 2005).

In connected speech, of course, formant frequencies are rarely steady (Chapter 10). A simplified auditory theory of speech perception, however, may envision a process in which the auditory system "picks" formants from the temporal middle of the vowel, analyzes their frequencies and compares them to stored data for all vowels of the language. The assumption in such a process is that the formant frequencies halfway between the onset and offset of the vowel represent the vowel target.

There are problems with this view. Why would vowel acoustic templates be developed only for the target formant frequencies? Auditory measurement of target formant frequencies at the temporal middle of the vowel would require an analysis window centered around the midpoint (Chapter 10). The width of the window (in duration) is short to avoid spectral smearing of the type described in Chapter 10. Short measurement windows may be no more than 20% of the overall vowel duration. Such "slice-in-time" sampling of vowel acoustics ignores frequency change throughout the vowel.

Formant frequency changes throughout a vowel are likely important to vowel identification. The degree of this importance was evaluated by Hillenbrand and Nearey (1999), who showed that the identification of vowels whose formant frequencies changed naturally (or after speech synthesis) over time were identified better than synthesized, "flat formant" versions of the vowels. The flat-formant, synthesized vowels were identified fairly well (about 70%–75% correct, on average), but the same vowels with natural variation in formant frequencies were identified with 90% to 95% accuracy. The natural variation of formant frequencies across a vowel's duration clearly adds to the accurate identification of a vowel category, even if the flat-formant versions provide a good amount of information to listener (see Johnson (2005); and Nearey & Assman, 1986).

Normalization

Speech scientists have been concerned for decades with acoustic variability and the difficulties it presents for a theory of speech perception. They have sought ways to normalize the speech acoustic signal produced by *any* speaker. The ideal result of normalization is an auditory process that represents the acoustic characteristics of speech sounds on a common scale, reducing or eliminating the variability due to the factors described above. This is called *speaker* normalization. A full treatment of normalization of vowel acoustics for speech perception is available in Johnson (2005), which serves as the basis for the current discussion.

An example of normalization is the use of formant frequency ratios, rather than individual formant frequencies, as the acoustic representation of vowels. Perhaps the auditory system analyzes vowels by their overall spectral shape (like the tube resonance curves described in Chapters 7 and 8), rather than just the peaks (formants) in the spectrum. Formant frequencies for a given vowel are different depending on the length of the vocal tract, but formant ratios may be more constant for different vocal tract lengths. The ratios may reflect more about a common vowel spectrum shape across speakers; they certainly are less variable across speakers compared with individual formant frequencies. The auditory system may process the acoustic signal for vowels using ratios such as F2/F1 and F3/F2, rather than the single formant frequencies F1, F2, and F3.

The formant ratio approach has support in the research literature. The ratio approach is consistent with the idea that formant frequencies for a given vowel produce a pattern of stimulation on the basilar membrane, the part of the cochlea containing cells responsible for hearing sensation (Chapter 13), This is in contrast to individual points of stimulation as would be the case for individual formant-frequency analysis. This pattern can be moved up and down the basilar membrane, which is to say up and down the frequency range important for speech perception (roughly 50–12,000 Hz). The exact frequencies stimulated on the basilar membrane are not critical for vowel perception; the pattern of stimulation is critical, and it is similar regardless of vocal tract length. Formant ratios normalize the effect of vocal tract length on vowel acoustics and place the formant frequency patterns on a common scale for most, if not all speakers.

A different aspect of the normalization issue is referred to as *talker* normalization. Talker normalization is a calibration, by a listener, of an individual talker's vowel space. The concept of talker normalization is related to two interesting findings. First, frequencies of a speech or nonspeech signal preceding a vowel affects the identification of a vowel. A low frequency signal preceding a vowel produces a different effect on vowel identification compared with a preceding high-frequency signal. It is as if the frequency of the signal preceding the vowel establishes frequency expectations for the listener that are carried over to the vowel identification (recall the effect of preceding frequency signals on the identification of consonant-vowel transitions, reported by Laing, Liu, Lotto and Holt, 2012).

The second finding is that the intelligibility of a list of words is better when the words are spoken by a single talker, as compared with two or more talkers. A list of words produced by the same male talker has higher intelligibility than the same list produced by a male and female talker, either alternating every other word, or more dramatically, varying unpredictably across the list. The interpretation of this finding is that listeners "tune" their expectations for vowel acoustics to a specific talker. When the talker is switched the listener's tuning is not quite right for the new vocal tract length, and listening errors are made. The tuning adjustment is made quickly, but the effect of the mistuning—more identification errors—is real.

Auditory theories gain credibility when normalization of acoustic characteristics, either by transforming the raw acoustic information to a common scale, or by listener calibration of a talker's vowel space, or both, are included in the theory. Normalization reduces or eliminates some of the difficulties associated with large variability in formant frequencies resulting from factors such as vocal tract length.

Direct Realism

In the direct realism theory of speech perception, articulatory gestures are perceived directly. No special mechanisms are required to make perceptual decisions concerning phonetic events. An apparent advantage of this perspective is that the acoustic variability for a given vowel, which seems to make auditory theories cumbersome with the need to "know" all the possible variations of the vowel's formant frequencies both within and across speakers (e.g., Figure 11–2), becomes a non-issue. The directly-perceived gestures for the vowel may have variable formant frequencies, especially across speakers whose vocal tract lengths are very different (e.g., men versus children), but the gestures are nearly the same. Adult men have much longer vocal tracts than five-year-old children and therefore different formant frequencies for any vowel, but the articulatory gestures for both groups are nearly the same for any vowel. According to this view, children use articulatory gestures for /i/ similar to those used for the same vowel produced by adult men. The gestures can be perceived directly across age and sex and are not affected by the acoustic variability for the vowel from speaker to speaker and other sources of acoustic variation as discussed earlier.

Unfortunately, it is not true that different speakers use the same articulatory gestures for a specific sound. Using direct measures of speech movement, Johnson, Ladefoged, and Lindau (1993) showed substantial articulatory variation for the same vowel across different speakers. Similarly, significant speaker-to-speaker variability of tongue movements for American English "r" before vowels was reported by Westbury, Hashi, and Lindstrom (1998). There does not appear to be across-speaker stability of articulatory gestures for vowels or the sonorant "r" (sonorant = vowel-like). Direct realism does not have a ready answer at the level of articulatory gestures to get around the variable acoustic characteristics of a given vowel or other vowel-like sounds.

A SUMMARY OF SPEECH PERCEPTION THEORIES

Table 12–1 is a summary of the three theories of speech perception presented above. Other theories exist, but these three are the major ones debated in the literature. At least one of the theories—the motor theory of speech perception—requires a special human endowment in the brain to perceive speech. The other two—the auditory theory and the theory called direct realism—do not require special mechanisms to perceive speech, at least not in the strict sense of dedicated areas of brain

Table 12–1. Summary of Three Theories of Speech Perception

THEORY	OBJECTS OF SPEECH PERCEPTION	MECHANISMS	COGNITIVE PROCESSES?
Motor theory	Articulatory positions/gestures[a]	Species-specific module, co-evolved with speech production	Yes[b]
Auditory theory	Speech acoustic signal	General auditory mechanisms (not special to speech)	Yes[c]
Direct realism	Articulatory gestures[d]	Direct perception of sources (changes in vocal tract configuration over time) that structure the medium (air)	No

[a] Objects of perception in original motor theory (Liberman et al., 1967) are articulatory positions for obstruents; in the revised motor theory (Liberman & Mattingly, 1985) objects are articulatory gestures. Both assume there is a species-specific special mechanism for speech perception.
[b] Assuming the speech module is considered a "dedicated" cognitive processor.
[c] Top-down influences on bottom-up data analysis; top-down influences involve many cognitive processes.
[d] Does not require special, speech-specific mechanisms.

tissue being "wired" exclusively, and innately, for the perceptual processing of speech sounds, words, and even sentence forms.

What is the current state of this debate? The three theories have often been presented as mutually exclusive—if you believe one, you don't believe the others, even any parts of the others—but there have been recent attempts to merge some of the ideas of two of the theories. Scientists have taken advantage of developments in brain imaging techniques to study infants, who turn out to be good test cases for the unqualified idea of a completely innate mechanism for processing speech and language. If the mechanism for speech perception is a dedicated, human-specific module, lateralization to the left hemisphere (in the great majority of people) of the brain for speech perception (see Chapter 15) is present at birth and remains more or less constant throughout the first year of life as the child passes from a prelingual to language-using individual. On the other hand, if speech perception skills have an extensive basis in learning, with exposure to speech acoustic signals shaping the way the brain processes speech and language input, the degree of brain lateralization should shift across the first year of life. This shift might be from a symmetrical pattern of brain activation around birth to an increasingly left-lateralized pattern as the child develops within a language environment. Minagawa-Kawai, Cristià, and Dupoux (2011) reviewed the available evidence from brain imaging studies in infants listening to linguistic (and nonlinguistic) input, and concluded that there is a shift, over the first year of life, to the left-lateralized pattern observed in most adults. Minagawa-Kawai et al. argue for a hybrid theory of brain activity for speech perception. Babies, in this view, use the special computational skills of the left hemisphere to process speech signals and categorize them in a linguistically meaningful way. Notice the way the preceding sentence is written: the use of acoustic signals for speech perception is key to learning speech, as suggested by auditory theories, but "special computational skills" of the left hemisphere are used to organize speech categories at all levels of language (phonetic, phonemic, morphemic, lexical, and so forth). The specialized computational skills mentioned by Minagawa-Kawai et al. may or may not be *speech* specific, but they certainly are specific to constructing categories for all things needing categorization (music, for example). These computational and categorizing skills are well matched to the category needs of developing speech and language skills. If this sounds like a game with words to avoid the "special speech module" idea, perhaps it is, but the point is the attempt to move from extreme and opposing theoretical positions to a middle view that recognizes the strengths of both extreme positions.

Speech Perception and Word Recognition

The three major theories (or approaches) discussed above are concerned with phonetic perception. They attempt to account for speech sound identification. Speech sound identification is clearly an important part of speech perception, but just as clearly the goal of speech perception is to recognize words, their combinations, and ultimately the message they convey.

Speech sound identification, however it is accomplished, is seen by many scientists as the "trigger" that initiates the process of word identification. One way to think about the link between sound and word identification is to imagine the lexicon as consisting of word "units" represented by strings of abstract phonological symbols (phonemes). Spoken word recognition occurs when the incoming sounds are identified and well matched to one of these stored word units.

This view glosses over some important considerations in speech perception. First, the analysis of speech acoustic information, prior to phonetic identification and phonemic representation, is not independent of lexical effects. In a famous study, Ganong (1980) constructed a VOT continuum for the first stop in a consonant-vowel-consonant (CVC) sequence. In theory, a VOT continuum for the nonword CVs /dɑ/-/tɑ/, with the best exemplar of /dɑ/ at one end and of /tɑ/ at the other end, has classic categorical perception functions (see Figure 12–11) like those described above for stop place of articulation. As VOT is increased from short values (voiced) to longer values, the responses are all (or nearly all) /d/ until the VOT has a value at which there is a sharp decrease in /d/ identifications and sharp increase in /t/ identifications. The /d/ and /t/ functions cross at this VOT value, usually around 20 to 30 ms, where 50% of the responses are /d/ and 50% are /t/. These are chance identification responses; the VOT value at this crossover point produces a maximally ambiguous perceptual response.

Ganong (1980) modified the continuum used in many categorical perception experiments by changing the endpoints. At one end he placed a real CVC word ("dash"), at the other end a CVC nonword ("tash"). Stimuli along the continuum differed only by the VOT of the /d/-/t/ contrast. The vowel and final consonant were the same for all stimuli along the continuum. The listeners' task in responding to stimuli along the continuum was to write down the initial stop they heard—/d/ or /t/. When the real word "dash" was at one end of the continuum and the nonword "tash" at the other, a significant increase was observed for /d/ responses to the maximally ambiguous VOT. In other words, the VOT that resulted in 50% "t" and 50% "d" responses for a "da-ta" continuum was associated with a greater percentage of "d" responses along the VOT continuum when one endpoint was the real word "dash."

Ganong's (1980) experiment showed an effect of lexical status on phonetic decisions. A view of speech perception as a strictly phonetic analysis preceding higher levels of analysis (such as phoneme and word decisions) is not consistent with these findings. In a strictly phonetic analysis with no influence from higher levels of processing, the presence of a word at one end of the continuum and a nonword at the other should not change the chance responses at the maximally ambiguous VOT for a "da-ta" continuum. The effect of lexical status on phonetic analysis is an example of top-down processing.

Another implication of Ganong's work is that speech perception is more than: (1) acoustic analysis of speech signals, (2) matching that analysis with a string of phonemes, (3) putting the phoneme string together and (4) identifying the word that matches the sound sequence suggested by acoustic analysis. Top-down processes (such as the Ganong effect; see sidetrack on Having an Effect) interact with processing of the incoming acoustic signal. For example, spoken word recognition does not require a complete acoustic analysis of all sounds in a word. Listeners make decisions concerning word identity before all incoming sounds are analyzed. This is especially the case for longer, multisyllabic words (Dahan & Magnuson, 2006; Nooteboom & van

---

Having an Effect

Scientists achieve historical fame when a significant finding known as an "effect" is named after them. From the world of mysticism and paranormal phenomena we have the "Carpenter effect," so named because a nineteenth-century physician (named Carpenter, of course) argued that thoughts may result in small movements of the body even though the movements are not voluntary. Hmm. The famous "Hawthorne effect" (you will find it in almost any text on experimental design) is the tendency for people to have their behavior change simply by being in an experiment. The experiment may not affect them, but they affect the experiment. The Hawthorne effect is critically relevant to the design of drug trials, in which the possible effect of a drug is controlled by informing members of both the control and experimental group (control group gets a sugar pill, experimental group gets the drug) that they may or may not be in the experimental group. When study members are told they might be receiving a drug, they may feel better even if they receive the control group sugar pill. Ganong's 1980 findings are almost always referred to as the "Ganong effect"—lexical items affect the processing of speech acoustic signals even before phoneme decisions are made.

der Vlugt, 1988). Spoken word recognition unfolds over time, by a *continuous* process of lexical activation as sound analysis and top-down information become increasingly available as the acoustic signal enters the auditory system (Dahan & Gareth Gaskell, 2007; Grosjean, 1980; see review in Samuel, 2011).

"Lexical activation" is the process by which a candidate set of words is activated by the incoming acoustic signal. The activation is typically by the acoustic signal associated with word-onset sounds. The candidate set of words initially includes all words in a listener's lexicon that begin with the initially identified phonetic segment. As the acoustic input continues and more sounds are available to the listener, the number of word candidates decreases—the word-recognition process including both bottom-up and top-down processes brings a listener closer to the complete word. The acoustic analysis is the bottom-up part of spoken word recognition. As the acoustic analysis is under way, top-down processes eliminate lexical candidates. As more acoustic analysis is performed, fewer lexical items are potential matches to the spoken word. The recognition of a word is complete when both bottom-up and top-down processes converge on a decision that can be made (and probably is made) before all acoustic information corresponding to the word has been analyzed. The influence of bottom-up and top-down processing is in both directions; bottom-up processing influences higher-level decisions (such as lexical candidates), and top-down processing influences the interpretation of the acoustic analysis. Top-down processes may include, but are not limited to, a listener's knowledge of possible word candidates with a similar phonetic structure (see below) or similar frequencies of occurrence, the meaning of previously recognized words in an extended utterance, the topic under discussion, and even the identity of the person who is speaking.

There is a disagreement concerning the specific processes involved in transforming an initial sound analysis to an abstract word representation. For example, when a man and woman speak the same word, the acoustic analysis may require transformation to a common "acoustic space" before it can be mapped onto abstract phonological and word symbols. This follows from the different vocal tract lengths of men, women, and children, which result in different resonances for the same sound (Chapter 11, and discussion above of the revised motor theory).

A final issue is that the acoustic signal for each sound is variable depending on such factors as dialect, speaking rate, speech style (formal vs. casual), and immediate phonetic context (Chapter 11). How are these factors handled in moving from sound analysis to an abstract, phonological representation of words? A popular concept in the contemporary speech perception literature is "phonetic recalibration," where the acoustic boundary for two contrasting phonemes (such as the /r/-/w/, /s/-/ʃ/, or /b/-/d/ contrasts) is reset depending on factors such as dialect, speaking rate (Kraljic & Samuel, 2005), or even listening to or learning a new language (Reinisch, Weber, & Mitterer, 2013). Boundaries between phonetic categories are flexible, depending on many factors associated with acoustic variability for a single sound (or pair of sounds in the case of a contrast). Phonetic recalibration, which is an elaboration of the Ganong effect, is an example of a top-down process in speech perception. The Ganong effect and the demonstration of phonetic recalibration are dependent on the categorical perception method, in which the label for an ambiguous speech signal along a continuum is evaluated for response shifts based on the continuum endpoints or other factors mentioned above.

SPEECH INTELLIGIBILITY

The concept of speech intelligibility is well known to speech-language pathologists and audiologists. Tests of speech intelligibility have been developed for audiometric evaluation (Martin & Greer, 2015) and to estimate the impact of a speech disorder on a speaker's effectiveness in communicating an oral message to listeners. Speech intelligibility tests for speech disorders are also used to estimate the severity of a speech motor control deficit (Kent, 1992; Weismer, 2008; Yorkston, Beukelman, Strand, & Bell, 1999). Speech intelligibility scores are measures of speech perception, but in most cases the design of speech intelligibility tests has not been guided by contemporary principles derived from speech perception theory.

Speech intelligibility tests were originally designed to measure the effectiveness of speech transmission over communication systems, such as telephone land lines. Tests most often consisted of lists of single words, although sentence tests were also developed. These tests were intended to assess *only* the relationship between the acoustic characteristics of the speech signal and the percentage of words (or sentences) correctly heard by listeners. The design of the tests assumed that under controlled conditions, the primary variable contributing to the percentage intelligibility score was the integrity of the medium through which the acoustic signal was transmitted (e.g., a telephone line, or in contemporary terms, a cell signal and the reception of the device). In addition, the type of speech sounds used in the test words had an important role in the speech intelligibility score. Typically, the integrity of the speech signal was defined at the sound segment level. When acoustic characteristics of individual speech sounds were in good shape, speech intelligibility scores were expected to be high. Disruption of speech sound acoustics, by a low presentation level, filtering (restriction of frequencies transmitted by the communication system), or competing noise, lowered the speech intelligibility score in proportion to the extent of the disruption (Weismer, 2008). Moreover, speech presented in noise caused a reduction of speech intelligibility scores roughly in proportion to the relative levels of the speech signal and the noise (the signal-to-noise [S/N] ratio).

When early investigators considered the effect of sound segments on speech intelligibility scores, they made an important assumption. If each segment in a word, or the same word in a sentence, had excellent acoustic characteristics, the intelligibility score was expected to be nearly perfect, at least in a quiet listening enviroment. Easy identification of the sounds led to easy identification of the words composed of these sounds, and a near-perfect intelligibility score. As reviewed by Weismer (2008), this assumption is not correct, especially when intelligibility tests are used as an index of severity of a communication impairment in speech disorders. Apparently, word recognition does not depend fully on the integrity of the component sound segments, consistent with lexical identification as the primary goal of speech perception (see previous section "Speech Perception and Word Recognition").

The original concept of speech intelligibility was extended past the evaluation of a communication system, to the case of a person with a *hearing* disorder. Speech reception tests (SRTs) measure the audiometric threshold for two-syllable words called spondees, such as *baseball, greenhouse,* and *crowdsource* (the term "spondee" is used to describe meter in poetry, where a word has two equally stressed syllables). The SRT is therefore the presentation level at which spondees become just intelligible. A speech discrimination (SD) score is the percentage of correctly identified words presented 25 to 40 dB above the speech reception threshold. This is a low presentation level relative to a person's SRT,[6] but listeners with normal hearing understand between 90% and 100% of the words in the test. People with hearing loss often have SD scores much lower than 90% to 100%. In SD tests, the listener is the focus of the test results.

Another use of speech intelligibility tests is to evaluate the *speaker* (sender). When speech is impaired and the communication system (medium) and receiver are in good shape, a speech intelligibility score serves as an index of the speaker's communication impairment. Speech intelligibility tests developed specifically for the evaluation of speech impairment were initially designed for speakers with hearing impairment and dysarthria (Monsen, 1983; Weismer & Martin, 1992). Kent, Weismer, Kent, and Rosenbek (1989) reviewed these tests and concluded that most were indices of severity of speech impairment. Listener characteristics were potentially part of the evaluation of speech severity, as Monsen demonstrated for speech intelligibility among persons with severe to profound hearing impairment. In these experiments, intelligibility scores depended on factors extrinsic to the speaker. These factors included the identity of the listener (the degree of experience with the specific speech characteristics of persons with hearing impairment or dysarthria) and the phonological and (in the case of sentence tests) syntactic complexity of the test utterances. Additional extrinsic factors also contribute to variation of speech intelligibility scores for individuals with normal hearing or with a speech impairment, or for those individuals with hearing loss and/or a cochlear implant. An older but still-relevant review of these factors was published by Pickett (1983).

The statement, "Mr. Jones has a speech intelligibility score of 75%" is nearly impossible to interpret unless additional information is available about the test, the listening conditions (including the specific speech materials), and the listeners. This potential ambiguity may limit the utility of the measure even for simple estimates of speaker severity.[7] However, even with problems of interpretation, speech intelligibility measured as percentage words or sentences heard correctly continues to be a gold standard in research and clinics. A popular semi-standardized, widely used test of intelligibility was developed and published by Yorkston and Beukelman (1980), and refined over the years. Several tests are available with their instrument, including word and sentence intelligibility materials.

The relationship of word and sentence intelligibility scores is interesting. In a classic study, Miller, Heise, and Lichten (1951) assessed the intelligibility of single words and those same words in sentences, at various signal-to-noise ratios (S/N ratios). The single words and sentences containing those words were "mixed" with noise before presentation to listeners; the S/N ratios are the speech signal levels relative to noise levels. When

---

[6]Speech discrimination tests may be administered to an individual at several presentation levels, which is thought to yield a better estimate than a single level of the individual's hearing ability for speech.

[7]These limitations can be eliminated by national or international standards for speech intelligibility testing of persons with speech disorders, but these do not exist at the current time.

the single words and words in sentences are compared at the same S/N ratio, the words in sentences are more intelligible. Figure 12–13 is an adaptation of Miller et al.'s Figure 3 (p. 335), showing word and word-in-sentence intelligibility as a function of S/N ratio. At an S/N ratio of +6 dB, intelligibility for words and sentences is roughly 60% and 85%, respectively. When the S/N ratio is +12 dB, the corresponding intelligibilities were 65% and 90%. Words in sentences had better intelligibility than the same words in isolation apparently because the sentences provided a context for the words, making them more predictable than they were in isolation. The same pattern of better sentence intelligibility than word intelligibility was reported by Yorkston and Beukelman (1981, Figure 1, p. 299) for 10 of 13 speakers with dysarthria, and recently by Snell and Grainger (2017). The context in which words are presented adds another variable to those that affect intelligibility scores.

"Explanatory" Speech Intelligibility Tests

Kent et al. (1989) extended the interpretation of speech intelligibility testing by isolating the specific phonetic problems that contributed to intelligibility deficits (see also Miller, 2013). This idea emerged from a common clinical observation that two individuals with the same overall speech intelligibility score (e.g., 60%) may have very different reasons for the intelligibility deficits. For example, one individual's intelligibility deficit may primarily be a result of velopharyngeal inadequacy, whereas another's may largely derive from problems with consonant place of articulation. The Kent et al. test is a single-word, multiple choice instrument in which the response alternatives are related to the target by carefully manipulated phonetic contrasts. An individual with a speech disorder produces the word list, which is then presented to a panel of listeners for word identification. The analysis of the data includes not only the total number of incorrect words, but the phonetic contrast errors underlying the incorrect choices. This latter analysis generates a profile of "vulnerable" contrasts—those frequently involved in mismatches between the speaker's intended word and the listener's choice among the response alternatives (usually four per word) that are phonetically similar to the intended word. These "vulnerable" contrasts can, in theory, be targeted in therapy because they presumably have the largest effect on speech intelligibility. Identification of "vulnerable" contrasts then becomes a prescription for primary attention in speech-language management. The concept of "vulnerable" contrasts also provided an explanation for why the same overall intelligibility score might be obtained for two individuals whose speech disorders sound so different. Even though the total number of words heard correctly by listeners is the same for these two persons, the speakers differ in their "vulnerable" contrasts, which suggest different therapy priorities.

The original speech intelligibility tests were described earlier as a way to test the contribution of segmental (sound segments) speech signal integrity to the goodness of a communication system. There is a direct link between this idea and the phonetic contrast approach to speech intelligibility testing. In the original approach, speech intelligibility scores reflected the sum of the acoustic characteristics of speech sounds in the test words. Any degradation of the acoustic characteristics of a specific sound contributed to a decrease in an overall speech intelligibility score. The greater the number of sounds affected (degraded) by the communication system, the lower the intelligibility score. Similarly, the phonetic contrast approach of Kent et al. (1989) considered speech intelligibility as a sum of "good" phonetic contrasts produced by the speaker. The smaller the number of these "good" contrasts (the greater the number of "vulnerable" contrasts), the lower the speech intelligibility score. In addition, the ability

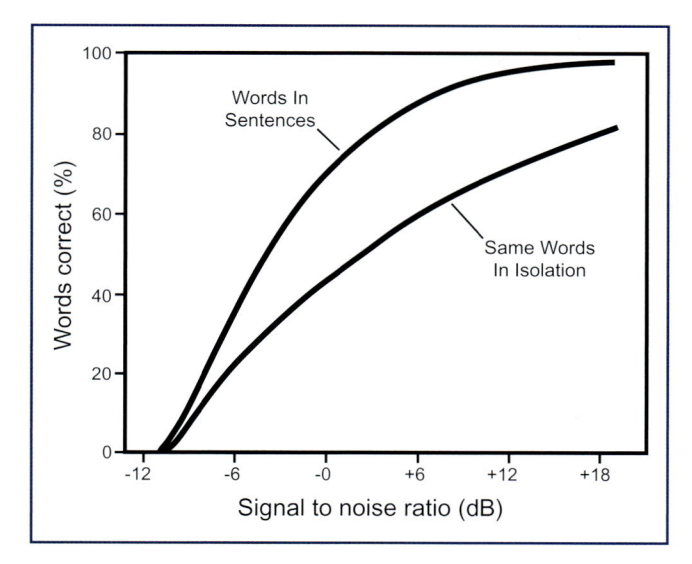

Figure 12–13. Increase ("growth") of word and sentence intelligibility (y-axis, in percentage correct) with increases in signal-to-noise ratio (x-axis, in S/N ratio). The intelligibility score is for the same words, presented either as single words or in sentences. The words and sentences are mixed with noise for presentation to listeners. Equal intensity for speech signals and noise is represented by a signal-to-noise of 0 dB. At a given S/N ratio the words in sentences are more intelligible than words in isolation. Figure adapted from Miller, Heise, and Lichten (1951).

to identify specific "vulnerable" contrasts provided an explanation of the intelligibility deficit. This explanation took the form of the phonetic contrasts that contributed heavily to an intelligibility deficit.

Different individuals with motor speech disorders had different "vulnerable" contrasts, as revealed by the Kent et al. (1989) test (Weismer & Martin, 1992). Although the concept of the Kent et al. test seems sound, there are problems in the interpretation of "vulnerable" contrasts. Specifically, the idea that the "good" phonetic contrasts sum to produce the intelligibility score is overly simple. This is because the different phonetic contrasts, such as the high-low and front-back contrasts for vowels, the voiced-voiceless and palatal-alveolar contrasts for consonants, and the glottal-null (e.g., "hate" vs. "ate") contrast for syllable shape, are apparently *not* independent. A simple way to say this is, if one of these contrasts is revealed to be vulnerable, the others are likely to be vulnerable as well (Weismer & Martin, 1992). Even though the contrasts appear to have different "vulnerabilities" in different speakers or clinical populations, they are all highly correlated with each other and may not furnish the kind of prescription for management imagined when the test was developed. This prescription would be to teach a small number of contrasts to achieve intelligibility gains, but if most the impaired contrasts are correlated in the degree to which they are impaired, it seems as if any of these vulnerable contrasts could be targeted for therapy.

The speech intelligibility tests described above are probably of greatest use when a single speaker's progress (or decline) is tracked across therapy or progression of a disease. In these cases, all measures involve the same individual, who serves as his or her own control in evaluating the effects of management or disease progression. What is needed are measures of speech intelligibility motivated by more sophisticated knowledge of speech perception, and especially by factors that truly tap into language comprehension (see sidetrack on "Intelligibility in the Ear"). For example, the ability of listeners to identify word onsets in connected speech produced by persons with speech disorders, and to access the lexicon to extract the meaning of a client's message, is a next step in enhancing the clinical relevance of measures of speech intelligibility.

Scaled Speech Intelligibility

Aspects of speech perception, including speech intelligibility, can be scaled. There is a long history of assigning numbers to reflect perceived magnitudes of speech perception characteristics (see review in Weismer, 2008). Scaling of speech perception shares similarities with the scaling of sound attributes discussed in Chapter 14. In addition to scaled speech intelligibility, perceptual scaling of speech dimensions includes speech normalcy, speech acceptability, naturalness, hypernasality, articulatory imprecision, and voice qualities such as breathiness, hoarseness, roughness, and strain. The present discussion is confined to the scaling of intelligibility, but the principles are applicable to scaling of any of these speech dimensions.

Speech intelligibility is scaled often in the research literature, and in clinical practice. Equal-appearing

---

Intelligibility in the Ear

Speech intelligibility tests that evaluate the severity of a speaker's speech problem (as in Parkinson's disease or following a stroke) or the effect of a structural problem on intelligibility (as in cleft palate) are often viewed as tests of the integrity of the speech apparatus. In fact, listeners bring their own skills to the speech perception process. For example, English speakers produce a pattern of alternating stressed and unstressed syllables (Chapter 10). Liss and her colleagues (Liss et al., 2000) showed how speech motor control problems can disrupt lexical access strategies employed by listeners. These speech production problems include departures from the rhythmic characteristics of English. Listeners whose native language is English use stressed syllables produced by the speaker to initiate a search of the lexicon. What about languages such as Spanish, Korean, and Mandarin Chinese, in which spoken utterances do not have an alternating pattern of stressed and unstressed syllables? How do English-speaking listeners who hear a pattern of equally stressed syllables identify the syllables that best initiate a lexical search? Mismatches of listening skills between two languages (as when a native speaker of English listens to a native speaker of Korean who is learning English as a second language) suggest that speech perception is as much in the ear of the listener as it is in the mouth of the speaker. Rhythmic mismatches between speaker output and listener skills are only one example of listener factors that affect speech intelligibility. (See Monsen, 1983; and Rosemann, Gießing, Özyurt, Carroll, Puschmann, & Thiel, 2017.)

interval scales are those in which a range of numbers is spaced equally along a line, with the endpoints defined from normal to most severe. Darley, Aronson, and Brown (1969a, 1969b), in their famous study of the perceptual characteristics of motor speech disorders, used a seven-point, equal-appearing interval scale to collect data on several speech dimensions, including intelligibility. Listeners heard a speech sample (a word, a sentence, or even a paragraph reading) and assigned a number along the seven-point range to correspond with their impression of the magnitude (the severity) of a specific speech dimension (imprecise articulation, distorted vowels, and so forth).

Equal-appearing interval scales are simple, can be administered quickly, and probably reflect the potential effects of all aspects of speech production (articulation, voice quality, prosody) on speech intelligibility. Single word tests and even sentence intelligibility tests in which listeners write down the words they hear, and intelligibility is expressed as a percentage of correctly heard words, are primarily dependent on the articulatory characteristics of segments making up the words and sentences. To the extent that factors such as voice quality and prosody (and perhaps other unknown factors) affect speech intelligibility, equal-appearing interval scales seem to have an advantage over percentage-correct measures. Presumably, nonsegmental factors such as voice quality can contribute to scaled speech intelligibility and may not be captured well by word and/or sentence intelligibility tests that use percentage correct measures.

The use of equal-appearing interval scales in the scaling of speech intelligibility, or any speech percept, is not without problems. First, the equal steps between numbers along the scale may imply that a difference between, for example, a scale value of 4 and 5 is psychologically equivalent to the difference between 5 and 6. In other words, the "mapping" from the speech signal to the numbers on the scale is assumed to be approximately linear. The functions that relate variation in a speech signal to a psychological impression of intelligibility are rarely linear, however. Some scientists distrust equal-appearing interval scales because they seem to force this assumption on the listener. A similar problem with equal-appearing interval scales in studies of nonspeech auditory percepts such as loudness and pitch is discussed in Chapter 14.

A second, related problem is the issue of floor and ceiling effects and how the endpoints of the scale are anchored. Scientists and clinicians often use terms such as "normal" and "most severe" to define the ends of an equal-appearing interval scale. Recorded examples of an utterance with "normal" intelligibility (1 on the scale) and most unintelligible (7 on the scale) are provided to listeners. These endpoint examples are called anchors. Unfortunately, there are no standards for anchors, and scientists and clinicians do not agree on how to anchor scale endpoints or even if the endpoints should be anchored. A typical problem with anchors is the case of an utterance deemed by a listener to be more unintelligible than the "most unintelligible" anchor used to define the end of the scale. This is called a floor effect—you can't go lower than the floor. The same problem may apply to the "most intelligible" side of the scale—the listener has no place to go when an utterance seems to be more intelligible than the "most intelligible" anchor. This is called a ceiling effect. Ceiling and floor effects, and the use of equal-appearing intervals along the scale, may (and often do) distort the true underlying process of perceiving intelligibility variation, or variation of any speech or voice dimension.

Equal-appearing interval scales are not particularly reliable, either within judges or across judges. When the same judge scales the same utterances for speech intelligibility, at different times, an error of one scale value is often taken as an acceptable criterion for scaling reliability. Exact number matches using equal-appearing interval scales are not common, and some measurement error must be tolerated. However, because a difference of one number in the middle of a 7-point scale means three numbers can represent, in terms of reliability, the same percept—that is, a 3, 4, and 5 are taken as the same measurement of intelligibility, when the original scale value is 4—it is reasonable to question the intrinsic value of these scales. After all, on a seven-point scale an error across three numbers is a nearly 50% error relative to the entire scale.

A well-studied scaling technique that avoids the linearity and endpoint problems of equal-appearing interval scales is called direct magnitude estimation (DME). In DME, listeners hear a sequence of speech stimuli varying in intelligibility and they assign numbers to each stimulus to reflect the magnitude of the speech intelligibility deficit (or any speech dimension). One version of DME uses an anchor stimulus, usually selected by the experimenter to represent a speech intelligibility deficit midway between perfectly intelligible and absolutely unintelligible. An alternate version of DME does not provide an anchor for the scaling exercise; listeners are asked to attach a number—any whole number—to the first stimulus, with all subsequent numbers using the previously assigned number as a reference. In either case of DME scaling, listeners are told to assign the numbers as *ratios* relative to a defined anchor, or to the immediately preceding stimulus. For example, in the case of anchored DME, a speech sample midway between perfectly intelligible and perfectly unintelligible may be pre-assigned the number 10. The listener hears this anchor several times throughout the sequence of speech samples as a reminder of an utterance whose intelligibility has a value of 10. Each utterance is then scaled to reflect the intelligibility of that sample relative to the anchor. When listeners perceive a stimulus as twice as intelligible as the midpoint anchor, they are told to assign it a number of 20. An utterance perceived as half as intelligible as the anchor receives a scale value of 5. Any subjective ratio is allowable, so any number can be assigned to a speech sample. Listeners are also instructed to do ratio scaling when an anchor is not used. Readers may be surprised to learn that listeners perform this task relatively easily and reliably and that anchored and unanchored versions of DME often produce very similar results for the same set of stimuli (see Schiavetti, 1992; and Weismer, 2008).

DME is viewed as a partial solution to the scaling problems associated with equal-appearing interval scales. In DME, there are no endpoints on the scale. Listeners are free to use any range of numbers which eliminates the floor and ceiling effects imposed by an equal-appearing interval scale. Moreover, there is no linearity assumption, and in fact the ratio nature of DME is thought to be more consistent with the nonlinear relationships of many perceptual magnitudes to variations in a physical signal (see Chapter 14). Extensive studies of DME reliability are not available, but in one study original and repeat estimates of the same set of stimuli resulted in an average error of about 5% of the full scale of numbers (Turner & Weismer, 1993).

Like equal-appearing interval scales, DME provides a global estimate of speech intelligibility. Like equal-appearing interval scales, DME scale values are presumably affected by factors in addition to the articulatory component of intelligibility. DME correlates well with estimates of intelligibility derived from single word tests but spreads out intelligibility estimates for speakers with very similar levels of single-word (percentage-correct) intelligibility (Weismer, Yunusova, & Bunton, 2012). The greater range of intelligibilities estimated by DME compared with single word tests is probably due to DME values reflecting aspects of voice quality, prosody, and so forth.

Speech intelligibility is a complicated topic. Interested readers are referred to Weismer and Martin (1992), Liss (2007), and Weismer (2008) for reviews of some main issues in understanding how speech intelligibility is linked to specific speech production problems.

Phonetic Transcription

Speech-language pathologists are expected to have skill in phonetic transcription. Phonetic transcription is a speech perception task in which a listener generates a symbol or sequence of symbols to represent spoken sounds.

In the speech-language pathology clinic, phonetic transcription is used to document sound pattern errors in clients who have developmental speech delay or other types of sound acquisition disorders. Researchers use phonetic transcription to answer questions concerning the nature of speech sound development in typically developing children and children with childhood conditions that may affect speech. These conditions include hearing impairment, cleft palate, speech delay, and childhood apraxia of speech, as well as many others. Phonetic transcription may also be used for adults with acquired speech sound disorders

Phonetic transcription as a speech perception skill is not just a matter of learning the symbol system (https://en.wikipedia.org/wiki/International_Phonetic_Alphabet). To develop the skill, an expert transcriber is trained by listening and transcribing utterances produced by different speakers, including those with no speech problem and those with different kinds of speech disorders. During skill acquisition, the trainee checks his symbols against transcription of the training utterances performed by an expert transcriber.

Phonetic transcription can be "broad," in which the phonetic symbols are made to match the spoken word as a sequence of major phonetic categories (e.g., "prosecute" → /prasəkjut/) or "narrow" to refine the broad transcription (e.g., "prosecute" → /pʰrasəkjutʰ/). We may assume "prosecute" was spoken carefully by the evidence of aspiration (ʰ) following the two stops, and especially the word-final stop. In more casual speech, word-final stops are typically not released and therefore not aspirated. The forward-pointing symbol beneath the vowel /u/ indicates fronting of the tongue root, as if the tongue position for the /u/ were more forward than the typical textbook description of /u/ as a high *back* vowel.

Phonetic transcription is notoriously unreliable—two skilled transcribers often use different symbols for identical sounds in the same spoken word. The lack of reliability is found in broad transcription, and more prominently in narrow transcription. A review of reliability problems in phonetic transcription is provided by Mayo, Gibbon, and Clark (2013).

Because phonetic transcription is based on perceptual processes in listening to speech, it is an interesting exercise to ask how transcription fits in with the theories discussed above. The motor theory claims that a special processor transforms the acoustic input to an articulatory representation. This representation is presumably in categorical forms, at least for stops, fricatives, and affricates. Many transcription errors or disagreements occur for sounds that seem to be between two places of articulation. These sounds may truly be produced with places of articulation that are not exactly "on target." For example, a stop produced between an alveolar and dorsal (e.g., between /d/ and /g/) presents a transcriber with a problem. Narrow transcription may help in this case, indicating either a backed alveolar or a fronted dorsal. But it is not clear how the specialized processor handles this sort of problem. Is the processor endowed with all possible articulations, even when they are not consistent with the phonemic categories of a language?

Direct realism has a similar problem, although a recent adjustment of the theory (Fowler, Shankweiler, & Studdert-Kennedy, 2016) makes it more amenable to transcription of sound segments, although not necessarily of distorted sound segments. In direct realism, listeners hear articulatory gestures directly, without mediation of cognitive processes. There are no linguistic symbols in direct realism, at least not as the output of direct perception of gestures. In the case of a stop made between the places of articulation for /d/ and /g/, the underlying gestures are presumably unknown to the listener—they have not been heard before or at least on only a few occasions. What does a transcriber do when the articulatory gesture or set of gestures (Chapter 5, p. 201) deviate from what is known? Perhaps the novelty of the gestures explains why transcribers often disagree for both normal and disordered speech: hearing a new set of articulatory gestures, transcribers are confused and record a symbol for a phonetic segment that is close to the unfamiliar gesture. The gestures are still heard directly, but the transcription processes are confused. Guesses are made, but they are not systematic. This results in transcription disagreements. The refinement of gesture theory referred to above (Fowler et al., 2016) allows acoustic stability for segments, directly related to the set of articulatory gestures that are responsible for generating the acoustic signal. The theory revision claims that the acoustic stability reflects the time history of gestures as they unfold over time, rather than being identified with a single slice in time. This is the link between the underlying gestures and the acoustic stability now promoted by Fowler et al. The "objects of perception" are the time changes in the speech acoustic signal, sometimes referred to as spectro-temporal change—spectra that change as a function of time. This is hardly a new idea (Kewley-Port, 1983; Soli, 1981; Van Tassell, Soli, Kirby, & Widen, 1987), except for the explicit link between gestures and their "structuring" of the acoustic signal, which leads to direct perception of articulatory gestures. The direct realist view has not confronted the issue of how direct perception of articulatory gestures is learned by children, or by adults learning phonetic transcription or even a new language.

The auditory theory seems to be the best match for transcription of normal and disordered speech. The auditory theory is based on analysis that is not different from the auditory analysis of other signals in the environment. There is no special processor, and the objects of perception are not articulatory gestures. Auditory analysis may be based on stored "templates" for sound segments, these templates being learned in childhood and developed and refined as children mature. This process may be similar to developing perceptual templates in second-language learning, where new templates are learned for the perception of speech. The templates can be represented as time histories (spectro-temporal templates), as in direct realism. In auditory theory, however, the objects of speech perception are the acoustic signals associated with sound production, not the gestures that "structured" the acoustic signal.

The auditory theory seems consistent with the uncertainties of phonetic transcription. There is evidence of a range of acoustic patterns consistent with a specific sound category, with some acoustic patterns judged as "excellent" versions of the sound and others judged as poor representatives (Miller, 1994). In Miller's own words, "These findings [of different acoustic patterns representing the same sound segment] indicate that the listener's representation of the phonetic categories of language includes fine-grained detail about phonetic form" (1994, p. 282). The fine-grained details reflect the varying "goodness" of the acoustic patterns. These patterns produce "less good" examples of a sound class as the acoustics move away from an excellent acoustic representation of the sound. Perhaps transcription is unreliable, especially when the acoustic representations are in-between two sound categories, such as the /d/-/g/ example, or are sufficiently far from an excellent exemplar as a result of a speech disorder. Under these circumstances, listener judgments of a sound category seem likely to be more variable because of uncertainty, at least when compared with the judgment of excellent versions of the sound.

WHY SHOULD SPEECH-LANGUAGE PATHOLOGISTS AND AUDIOLOGISTS CARE ABOUT SPEECH PERCEPTION?

Some of the information presented in this chapter may seem far removed from the daily concerns of speech-language pathologists. A good deal of research on speech perception, whether at the phonetic or word-recognition level, may appear both narrowly academic and exceedingly theoretical. In practice, however, speech-language pathologists and audiologists are frequently concerned with speech perception issues. After all, clients engage the services of speech-language pathologists to be understood better—to be more intelligible—and audiologists have as a top priority improving clients' ability to understand speech. When a speech-language pathologist plans a program of remediation for a person with a speech disorder, the plan should include a goal of making the client's sounds and words more accessible to the listener. Similarly, audiologists diagnose the type and degree of hearing loss so that decisions on amplification or cochlear implants match the processing characteristics of these devices to the details of a client's perceptual capabilities. Communication disorders are as much in the ear of the listener as they are in the mouth of the speaker. An understanding of speech perception processes in the typical listener can assist speech-language pathologists and audiologists in developing a remediation plan.

Three examples make this clear. First, persons with damage to the cerebellum, a part of the brain that plays an important role in regulating sequential motor behavior (among other things), often have a speech disorder called ataxic dysarthria. *Dysarthria* is the term used for speech production disorders associated with neurological damage, and *ataxia* signifies a set of motor symptoms and signs typically associated with damage to the cerebellum or fiber tracts connecting the cerebellum to other parts of the central nervous system (Chapter 15). Among speakers of English, a speech production sign in ataxic dysarthria is an inability to regulate the long-short-long-short patterning of syllable durations in a multisyllabic utterance (see Chapter 11). Listeners use this patterning of syllable durations to make decisions concerning word onset locations (Cutler, Dahan, & van Donselaar, 1997), a critical aspect of lexical access in speech perception, as discussed above. When listeners hear speech with an unusual pattern of syllable durations, their ability to identify word onsets and, therefore, to access the words intended by the speaker is compromised. In ataxic dysarthria, reduced word onset identification by normal listeners has been demonstrated and linked to this disruption in syllable timing patterns (Liss, Spitzer, Caviness, Adler, & Edwards, 2000). Unless a speech-language pathologist understands something about the link between neural disease, speech timing problems, and lexical access as an important part of speech perceptual processing, therapy efforts may be directed primarily to a more traditional aspect of clinical management (such as speech sound therapy or perhaps voice therapy). A focus on the speech timing issue may have a much greater benefit in improving the client's ability to make herself understood. The knowledge of spoken word recognition, which depends on an understanding of speech perception, may direct a clinician to plan therapy that is likely to benefit both the speaker and the listener.

Second, an understanding of basic principles of speech perception and word recognition allows a clinician to exploit knowledge concerning typical listening strategies and therefore maximize the effect of speech therapy. Standardized articulation tests evaluate the goodness of consonant production in the initial, medial, and final positions of a word. For example, articulation of the /s/ sound can be tested in word-initial position (e.g., "sock"), word-medial position ("messy"), and word-final position ("bus"). One outcome of standardized articulation testing may be the identification of articulatory problems for a sound in all word positions, but with more errors in word-final position compared with word-initial position. These results may suggest a therapy plan initially aimed at practice on word-final consonants, but this plan is poorly matched to the needs of listeners: speech perception research has shown that listeners typically use word onsets to recognize words in continuous speech (see review in Astheimer & Sanders, 2011). Extensive therapeutic effort devoted to the articulation of word-final consonants may result in well-produced consonants in that word position but with little improvement in the effective transmission of a message.

Third, one goal of audiometric testing is the identification of the frequencies of hearing loss in clients. Many clients have a significant hearing loss at some

---

Speech Perception: A Lost Soul in Clinical Training Programs

It is an odd fact that material on speech perception is not a highlight of preclinical or masters-level training in speech-language pathology. At the least, training in speech perception should be emphasized as much as training in the anatomy and physiology of normal and disordered speech. Communication disorders are ultimately disorders in the listener's ear. A quick look at the clinical literature on voice disorders, craniofacial anomalies, motor speech disorders, developmental phonological disorders, and fluency disorders shows the degree to which perceptual judgments by clinicians and even family members of a client play a major role in understanding diagnosis and management of the disorder. Long live knowledge of speech perception theory in the speech-language pathologist's clinical toolbox!

frequencies, but not at others. Significant hearing loss in the higher frequencies (e.g., 4000–8000 Hz) compared with lower frequencies (e.g., 250–2000 Hz) is likely to affect the processing of high-frequency speech sounds such as /s/, /ʃ/, and /t/. When a hearing aid is programmed for optimal speech understanding, knowledge of speech perception is important in matching the amplification characteristics of the aid to hearing loss patterns across frequency. A high-frequency hearing loss may be best matched by a hearing aid that provides good amplification at high frequencies and minimal amplification at low frequencies.

REVIEW

The modern era of speech perception research was initiated by experiments using the pattern-playback machine, a device that synthesized speech signals and was used to create small changes in the signals to evaluate the effect on listeners' phonetic decisions.

The concept of acoustic invariance for speech sounds—or the lack of it—plays a central role in the various theories of speech perception.

The motor theory of speech perception was based on the finding of categorical perception for stop consonant place of articulation.

Additional findings, including duplex perception and trading relations, were used to support the original and revised motor theory.

Motor theory was based on the idea that speech production and perception in humans were part of a special "code," and required a special mechanism in the brain for the perception of speech.

Categorical perception can be demonstrated in infants and animals, findings that may be interpreted as support for, or against, the motor theory.

The general auditory approach competes with motor theory as an explanation for speech perception and takes the perspective that the speech acoustic signal is sufficiently consistent to support speech sound perception, and that general auditory mechanisms (not special mechanisms) are used in the perception of speech signals.

Direct realism, a competing theory inspired by J. J. Gibson's ecological approach to perception, claims that articulatory gestures are perceived directly (not by special mechanisms), and that listeners hear articulatory gestures, not acoustic representations of speech sounds that must be processed by cognitive mechanisms for proper recognition.

Recent results from the research literature suggest that both general auditory mechanisms and brain mechanisms with properties well suited to rapid processing and formation of categories are used to establish linguistic categories for the perception of speech.

Studies showing that the responses to ambiguous stimuli along a synthesized or real contrast continuum are affected by the presence or absence of real words at one end of the continuum suggest top-down processes in speech perception that interact with the bottom-up processes of acoustic analysis.

Speech perception involves not only the perception of speech sounds, but the access of words from the lexicon by a combination of bottom-up and top-down processes.

Speech intelligibility testing, a subtype of the general category of speech perception phenomena, has a clear role in speech-language pathology and audiology, even though specific tests have rarely been constructed according to principles derived from the speech perception literature.

The most common estimates of speech intelligibility use word or sentence tests, in which the scores are expressed as percentages of correctly heard words, or scaling techniques in which listeners attach numbers to the magnitudes of a speech intelligibility deficit.

Phonetic transcription is another test of speech perception and partly of speech intelligibility and may be related to one or more of the theories of speech perception.

Familiarity with theoretical perspectives and empirical findings in the area of speech perception is important to the clinical practice of speech-language pathologists and audiologists.

REFERENCES

Adank, P., Smits, P., & van Hout, P. (2004). A comparison of vowel normalization procedures for language variation research. *Journal of the Acoustical Society of America, 116,* 3099–3107.

Andoni, S., Li, N., & Pollak, G. (2007). Spectrotemporal fields in the inferior colliculus revealing specificity for spectral motion in conspecific vocalizations. *Journal of Neuroscience, 27,* 4882–4893.

Astheimer, L. B., & Sanders, L. D. (2011). Predictability affects early perceptual processing of word onsets in continuous speech. *Neuropsychologia, 49,* 3512–3516.

Best, C., Morrongiello, B., & Robson, R. (1981). Perceptual equivalence of acoustic cues in speech and nonspeech perception. *Perception and Psychophysics, 29,* 191–211.

Blumstein, S., & Stevens, K. (1979). Acoustic invariance in speech production: Evidence from measurements of the spectral characteristics of stop consonants. *Journal of the Acoustical Society of America, 66,* 1001–1017.

Cleary, M., & Pisoni, D. (2001). Speech perception and spoken word recognition: Research and theory. In E. Goldstein (Ed.), *Blackwell handbook of perception* (pp. 499–534). Oxford, UK: Blackwell.

Cole, R., & Rudnicky, A. (1983). What's new in speech perception? The research and idea of William Chandler Bagley, 1874–1946. *Psychological Review, 90*, 94–101.

Cooper, F., Liberman, A., & Borst, J. (1951). The interconversion of audible and visible patterns as a basis for research in the perception of speech. *Proceedings of the National Academy of Sciences, 37*, 318–325.

Cutler, A., Dahan, D., & van Donselaar, W. (1997). Prosody in the comprehension of spoken language: A literature review. *Language and Speech, 40*, 141–201.

Dahan, D., & Gareth Gaskell, M. (2007). The temporal dynamics of ambiguity resolution: Evidence from spoken word recognition. *Journal of Memory and Language, 57*, 483–501.

Dahan, D., & Magnuson, J. (2006). Spoken word recognition. In M. Traxler & M. Gernsbacher (Eds.), *Handbook of psycholinguistics* (2nd ed., pp. 249–283). New York, NY: Academic Press.

Darley, F., Aronson, A. E., & Brown, J. (1969a). Differential diagnostic patterns of dysarthria. *Journal of Speech and Hearing Research, 12*, 246–269.

Darley, F., Aronson, A. E., & Brown, J. (1969b). Clusters of deviant speech dimensions in the dysarthrias. *Journal of Speech and Hearing Research, 12*, 462–496.

Davies, N., Madden, J., & Butchart, S. (2004). Learning fine-tunes a specific response of nestlings to the parental alarm calls of their own species. *Proceedings of the Royal Society of London B, 271*, 2297–2304.

Diehl, R. L., & Kluender, K. R. (1989). On the objects of speech perception. *Ecological Psychology, 1*, 121–144.

Diehl, R., Lotto, A., & Holt, L. (2004). Speech perception. *Annual Review of Psychology, 55*, 149–179.

Eimas, P., Miller, J., & Jusczyk, P. (1990). On infant speech perception and the acquisition of language. In S. Harnad (Ed.), *Categorical perception: The groundwork of cognition* (pp. 161–195). Cambridge, UK: Cambridge University Press.

Fant, G. (1960). *Acoustic theory of speech production*. The Hague, Netherlands: Mouton.

Fowler, C. (1986). An event approach to the study of speech perception from a direct-realist perspective. *Journal of Phonetics, 14*, 3–28.

Fowler, C. (1996). Listeners do hear sounds, not tongues. *Journal of the Acoustical Society of America, 99*, 1730–1741.

Fowler, C. (2006). Compensation for coarticulation reflects gesture perception, not spectral contrast. *Perception and Psychophysics, 68*, 161–177.

Fowler, C., Galantucci, B., & Saltzman, E. (2003). Motor theories of perception. In M. Arbib (Ed.), *The handbook of brain theory and neural networks* (pp. 705–707). Cambridge, MA: MIT Press.

Fowler, C., & Rosenblum, L. (1991). The perception of phonetic gestures. In I. Mattingly & M. Studdert-Kennedy (Eds.), *Modularity and the motor theory of speech perception* (pp. 33–59). Hillsdale, NJ: Lawrence Erlbaum.

Fowler, C. A., Shankweiler, D., & Studdert-Kennedy, M. (2016). Perception of the speech code revisited: speech is alphabetic after all. *Psychological Review, 123*, 225–250.

Fruchter, D., & Sussman, H.M. (1997). The perceptual relevance of locus equations. *Journal of the Acoustical Society of America, 102*, 2997–3008.

Ganong, W. F., III. (1980). Phonetic categorization in auditory word perception. *Journal of Experimental Psychology: Human Perception and Performance, 6*, 110–125.

Gibson, J. (1968). *The senses considered as perceptual systems*. Boston, MA: Houghton Mifflin.

Gibson, J. (1979). *The ecological approach to visual perception*. Boston, MA: Houghton Mifflin.

Grosjean, F. (1980). Spoken word recognition processes and the gating paradigm. *Perception and Psychophysics, 28*, 267–283.

Hillenbrand, J. M., & Nearey, T. M. (1999). Identification of resynthesized /hVd/ utterances: Effects of formant contour. *Journal of the Acoustical Society of America, 105*, 3509–3523.

Hirsh, I. (1959). Auditory perception of temporal order. *Journal of the Acoustical Society of America, 31*, 759–767.

Johnson, K. (2005). Speaker normalization in speech perception. In D. B Pisoni & R. E. Remez (Eds.), *Handbook of speech perception* (pp.363–389). Malden, MA: Blackwell.

Johnson, K., Ladefoged, P., & Lindau, M. (1993). Individual differences in vowel production. *Journal of the Acoustical Society of America, 94*, 701–714.

Johnson, K., & Mullenix, J. (1997). *Talker variability in speech processing*. New York, NY: Academic Press.

Katz, J. (Ed.). (2002). *Handbook of clinical audiology* (5th ed.). Baltimore, MD: Lippincott Williams & Wilkins.

Kent, J., Kent, R., Rosenbek, J., Weismer, G., Martin, R., Sufit, R., & Brooks, B. (1992). Quantitative description of the dysarthria in women with amyotrophic lateral sclerosis. *Journal of Speech and Hearing Research, 35*, 723–733.

Kent, R. D. (1974). Auditory-motor formant tracking: A study of speech imitation. *Journal of Speech, Language, and Hearing Research, 17*, 203–222.

Kent, R. (Ed.) (1992). *Intelligibility in speech disorders: Theory, measurement, and management*. Amsterdam, Netherlands: John Benjamin.

Kent, R., Weismer, G., Kent, J., & Rosenbek, J. (1989). Toward phonetic intelligibility testing in dysarthria. *Journal of Speech and Hearing Disorders, 54*, 482–499.

Kewley-Port, D. (1983). Time-varying features as correlates of place of articulation in stop consonants. *Journal of the Acoustical Society of America, 73*, 322–335.

Kingston, J., & Diehl, R. (1994). Phonetic knowledge. *Language, 70*, 419–454.

Klatt, D. (1987). Review of text-to-speech conversion for English. *Journal of the Acoustical Society of America, 82*, 737–793.

Klatt, D. (1989). Review of selected models of speech perception. In W. Marslen-Wilson (Ed.), *Lexical representation and process* (pp. 169–226). Cambridge, MA: MIT Press.

Kluender, K. (1994). Speech perception as a tractable problem in cognitive science. In M. Gernsbacher (Ed.), *Handbook of psycholinguistics* (pp. 173–217). San Diego, CA: Academic Press.

Kluender, K., & Kiefte, M. (2006). Speech perception within a biologically realistic information-theoretic framework. In M. Traxler & M. Gernsbacher (Eds.), *Handbook of psycholinguistics* (2nd ed., pp. 153–199). London, UK: Elsevier.

Kraljic, T., & Samuel, A. G. (2005). Perceptual learning for speech: is there a return to normal? *Cognitive Psychology, 51*, 141–178.

Kronrod, Y., Coppess, E., & Feldman, N.H. (2016). A unified account of categorical effects in phonetic perception. *Psychonomic Bulletin and Review, 23*, 1681–1712.

Kuhl, P. (1986). Theoretical contribution of tests on animals to the special mechanisms debate in speech. *Experimental Biology, 45*, 233–265.

Kuhl, P. K., Conboy, B. T., Coffey-Corina, S., Padden, D., Rivera-Gaxiola, M., & Nelson, T. (2008). Phonetic learning as a pathway to language: New data and native language magnet theory expanded (NLM-e). *Philosophical Transactions of the Royal Society B, 363*, 979–1000.

Kuhl, P., & Miller, J. (1975). Speech perception by the chinchilla: Voiced-voiceless distinction in alveolar plosive consonants. *Science, 190*, 69–72.

Kuhl, P., & Padden, D. (1983). Enhanced discriminability at the phoneme boundaries for place of articulation in macaques. *Journal of the Acoustical Society of America, 73*, 1003–1010.

Laing, E. J. C., Liu, R., Lotto, A. J., & Holt, L. L. (2012). Tuned with a tune: Talker normalization via general auditory processes. *Frontiers in Psychology, 3*, 1–9.

Lehet, M., & Holt, L. L. (2017). Dimension-based statistical learning affects both speech perception and production. *Cognitive Science, 41*, 885–912.

Liberman, A., Cooper, F., Shankweiler, D., & Studdert-Kennedy, M. (1967). Perception of the speech code. *Psychological Review, 74*, 431–461.

Liberman, A., Harris, K., Hoffman, H., & Griffith, B. (1957). The discrimination of speech sounds within and across phoneme boundaries. *Journal of Experimental Psychology, 54*, 358–368.

Liberman, A., & Mattingly, I. (1985). The motor theory of speech perception revised. *Cognition, 21*, 1–36.

Lieberman, P. (1996). Some biological constraints on the analysis of prosody. In J. Morgan & K. Demuth (Eds.), *Signal to syntax: Bootstrapping from speech to grammar in early acquisition* (pp. 55–66). Hillsdale, NJ: Lawrence Erlbaum.

Lindblom, B. (1990). Explaining phonetic variation: A sketch of the H&H theory. In W. Hardcastle & A. Marchal (Eds.), *Speech production and speech modeling* (pp. 403–440). Dordrecht, Netherlands: Kluwer Academic.

Liss, J. (2007). The role of speech perception in motor speech disorders. In G. Weismer (Ed.), *Motor speech disorders* (pp. 187–219). San Diego, CA: Plural.

Liss, J., Spitzer, S., Caviness, J., Adler, C., & Edwards, B. (2000). Lexical boundary error analysis in hypokinetic and ataxic dysarthria. *Journal of the Acoustical Society of America, 107*, 3415–3424.

Lively, S. E., & Pisoni, D. B. (1997). On prototypes and phonetic categories: A critical assessment of the perceptual magnet effect in speech perception. *Journal of Experimental Psychology: Human Perception and Performance, 23*, 1665–1679.

Lotto, A., & Holt, L. (2006). Putting phonetic context effects into context: A commentary on Fowler (2006). *Perception and Psychophysics, 68*, 178–183.

Mann, V., & Liberman, A. (1983). Some differences between phonetic and auditory modes of perception. *Cognition, 14*, 211–235.

Martin, F. N., & Clark, J. G. (2015). *Introduction to audiology* (12th ed.). London, UK: Pearson.

Massaro, D. W., & Chen, T. H. (2008). The motor theory of speech perception revisited. *Psychonomic Bulletin & Review, 15*, 453–457.

Mayo, C., Gibbon, F., & Clark, R. A. J. (2013). Phonetically trained and untrained adults' transcription of place of articulation for intervocalic lingual stops with intermediate acoustic cues. *Journal of Speech, Language, and Hearing Research, 56*, 779–791.

Miller, G. A., Heise, G. A., & Lichten, W. (1951). The intelligibility of speech as a function of the context of the test materials. *Journal of Experimental Psychology, 421*, 339–345.

Miller, J., & Jusczyk, P. (1989). Seeking the neurobiological basis of speech perception. *Cognition, 33*, 111–137.

Miller, J. L. (1994). On the internal structure of phonetic categories: A progress report. *Cognition, 50*, 271–185.

Miller, N. (2013). Measuring up to speech intelligibility. *International Journal of Language and Communication Disorders, 48*, 601–612.

Minagawa-Kawai, Y., Cristià, A., & Dupoux, E. (2011). Cerebral lateralization and early speech acquisition: A developmental scenario. *Developmental Cognitive Neuroscience, 1*, 217–232.

Monsen, R. (1983). The oral speech intelligibility of hearing impaired talkers. *Journal of Speech and Hearing Disorders, 48*, 286–296.

Nearey, T. M., & Assman, P. (1986). Modeling the role of vowel inherent spectral change in vowel identification. *Journal of the Acoustical Society of America, 80*, 1297–1308.

Newport, E. L. (2016). Statistical language learning: Computational, maturational, and linguistic constraints. *Language and Cognition, 8*, 447–461.

Nooteboom, S., & van der Vlugt, M. (1988). A search for a word-beginning superiority effect. *Journal of the Acoustical Society of America, 84*, 2018–2032.

Pardo, J., & Remez, R. (2006). The perception of speech. In M. Traxler & M. Gernsbacher (Eds.), *Handbook of psycholinguistics* (2nd ed., pp. 201–248). Amsterdam, Netherlands: Elsevier.

Patterson, D., & Pepperberg, I. (1998). Acoustic and articulatory correlates of stop consonants in a parrot and a human subject. *Journal of the Acoustical Society of America, 103*, 2197–2215.

Pickett, J. M. (1983). Theoretical considerations in testing speech perception through electro auditory stimulation. *Annals of the New York Academy of Sciences, 425*, 424–434.

Pisoni, D. (1977). Identification and discrimination of the relative onset time of two complex tones: Implications for voicing perception in stops. *Journal of the Acoustical Society of America, 61*, 1352–1361.

Popper, K. (2002a). *Conjectures and refutations: The growth of scientific knowledge*. London, UK: Routledge Classics.

Popper, K. (2002b). *The logic of scientific discovery*. London, UK: Routledge Classics.

Rand, T. (1974). Dichotic release from masking for speech. *Journal of the Acoustical Society of America, 55*, 678–680.

Reinisch, E., Weber, A., & Mitterer, H. (2013). Listeners retune phoneme categories across languages. *Journal of Experimental Psychology: Human Perception and Performance, 39*, 75–86.

Richstmeier, P. T., & Goffman, L. (2017). Perceptual statistical learning over one week in child speech production. *Journal of Communication Disorders, 68*, 70–80.

Repp, B. (1982). Phonetic trading relations and context effects: New experimental evidence for a speech mode of perception. *Psychological Bulletin, 92*, 81–110.

Repp, B., & Liberman, A. (1987). Phonetic category boundaries are flexible. In S. Harnad (Ed.), *Categorical perception: The groundwork of cognition* (pp. 89–112). Cambridge, UK: Cambridge University Press.

Repp, B. H., & Williams, D. R. (1985). Categorical trends in vowel imitation: Preliminary observations from a replication experiment. *Speech Communication, 4*, 105–120.

Rosemann, S., Gießing, S., Özyurt, J., Carroll, R., Puschmann, S., & Thiel, C. M. (2017). The contribution of cognitive factors to individual differences in understanding noise-vocoded speech in young and older adults. *Frontiers in Human Neuroscience, 11*, 294. doi:10.3389/fnhum.2017.00294

Saffran, J. (2003). Statistical language learning: Mechanisms and constraints. *Current Directions in Psychological Science, 12*, 110–114.

Saffran, J., & Thiessen, E. (2007). Domain-general learning capacities. In E. Hoff & M. Shatz (Eds.), *Handbook of language development* (pp. 68–86). Cambridge, UK: Blackwell.

Samuel, A. G. (2011). Speech perception. *Annual Review of Psychology, 62*, 49–72.

Schiavetti, N. (1992). Scaling procedures for the measurement of speech intelligibility. In R. D. Kent (Ed.), *Intelligibility in speech disorders: Theory, measurement, management* (pp. 11–34). Amsterdam, Netherlands: John Benjamin.

Snell, J., & Grainger, J. (2017). The sentence superiority effect revisited. *Cognition, 168*, 217–221.

Soli, S. D. (1981). Second formant transitions in fricatives: Acoustic consequences of fricative-vowel coarticulation. *Journal of the Acoustical Society of America, 70*, 976–984.

Stevens, K. (2005). Features in speech perception and lexical access. In D. Pisoni & R. Remez (Eds.), *The handbook of speech perception* (pp. 125–155). Malden, MA: Blackwell.

Studdert-Kennedy, M., & Shankweiler, D. (1970). Hemispheric specialization for speech perception. *Journal of the Acoustical Society of America, 48*, 579–594.

Sussman, H. M., Fruchter, D., Hilbert, J., & Sirosh, J. (1998). Linear correlates in the speech signal: The orderly output constraint. *Behavioral and Brain Sciences, 21*, 241–259.

Turner, G. S., & Weismer, G. (1993). Characteristics of speaking rate in the dysarthria associated with amyotrophic lateral sclerosis. *Journal of Speech and Hearing Research, 36*, 1134–1144.

van Son, R. J. J. H., & Pols, L. C. W. (1996). A comparison between the acoustics of vowel and consonant reduction. *Institute of Phonetic Sciences Proceedings, 20*, 13–25.

Van Tassell, D. J., Soli, S. D., Kirby, V. M., & Widen, G. P. (1987). Speech waveform envelope cues for consonant recognition. *Journal of the Acoustical Society of America, 82*, 579–594.

Watkins, K., & Paus, T. (2004). Modulation of motor excitability during speech perception: The role of Broca's area. *Journal of Cognitive Neuroscience, 16*, 978–987.

Weismer, G. (2008). Speech intelligibility. In M. Ball, M. Perkins, N. Müller, & S. Howard (Eds.), *Handbook of clinical linguistics*. Oxford, UK: Blackwell.

Weismer, G., & Martin, R. (1992). Acoustic and perceptual approaches to the study of intelligibility. In R. Kent (Ed.), *Intelligibility in speech disorders: Theory, measurement, and management* (pp. 67–118). Amsterdam, Netherlands: John Benjamin.

Weismer, G., Yunusova, Y., & Bunton, K. (2012). Measures to evaluate the effects of DBS on speech production. *Journal of Neurolinguistics, 25*, 74–94.

Westbury, J. R., Hashi, M., & Lindstrom, M. J. (1998). Differences among speakers in lingual articulation for American English /ɹ/. *Speech Communication, 26*, 203–226.

Whalen, D. H. (1997). What duplex perception tells us about speech perception. In K. Singer, R. Eggert, & G. Anderson (Eds.), *CLD33: The panels* (pp. 435–446). Chicago, IL: Chicago Linguistic Society.

Whalen, D., & Liberman, A. (1987). Speech perception takes precedence over nonspeech perception. *Science, 237*, 169–171.

Yorkston, K. M., & Beukelman, D. R. (1981). Assessment of intelligibility of dysarthric speech. *Journal of Communication Disorders, 13*, 15–31.

Yorkston, K., Beukelman, D., Strand, E., & Bell, K. (1999). *Management of motor speech disorders in children and adults* (2nd ed.). Austin, TX: Pro-Ed.

13

Anatomy and Physiology of the Auditory System

INTRODUCTION

This chapter presents an integrated description of the anatomy and physiology of the auditory mechanism. The information presented here can be found in greater detail in textbooks and hundreds of journal publications; here information from Abele and Wiggins (2015), Barin (2009), Dallos (1973), Goldberg et al. (2012), Goutman, Elgoyhen, and Gomez-Casati (2015), Hudpseth (2014), Lemmerling, Stambuk, Mancuso, Antonelli and Kubilis (1997), Luers and Hüttenbrink (2016), Olson, Duifhuis and Steele (2012), Pickles (2013), and Volandri, Di Puccio, Forte, and Manetti (2012) has been used to organize a contemporary description of the relevant structures and functions of the auditory and vestibular systems.

A comprehensive understanding of the auditory mechanism is critical to anyone interested in pursuing a career in audiology, speech-language pathology, hearing or speech science, or any other career related to communication. There are several reasons for this. First and foremost, children learn speech and spoken language through their auditory mechanism. Second, an understanding of the normal auditory mechanism allows appreciation for the way in which various diseases and conditions affect hearing. Third, knowledge of the auditory mechanism is essential to understanding the design and purpose of formal tests of hearing—the types of tests an audiologist performs to identify and diagnose a hearing problem. Even the simplest evaluation of hearing, such as a pure-tone audiometric test (when a single-frequency tone is presented through headphones and the person being tested is asked to raise a hand each time it is heard) is designed with knowledge of the anatomy and physiology of the cochlea, the end organ of hearing, and central auditory pathways. Other, more advanced evaluations of the hearing mechanism also use sound energy to estimate the status of different parts of the auditory system. Some of these diagnostic tests require no behavioral response from the listener; that is, they depend on physiological reactions to sound energy that can be measured automatically. Others, like the pure-tone audiometric test, are designed to elicit a behavioral reaction to sound energy characteristics controlled by a tester. This latter class of tests depends on a knowledge of the discipline called auditory psychophysics, the topic of Chapter 14. Fourth and finally, assistive hearing devices, ranging from a behind-the-ear hearing aid to a cochlear implant, are based on principles of normal auditory structure and function. It is the understanding of such principles that makes possible the design of devices that can help override the limitations of an impaired auditory mechanism.

Discussions of peripheral auditory anatomy typically classify structures as belonging to one of three major divisions: the outer ear, the middle ear, and the inner ear. Much of the peripheral auditory mechanism is encased in the temporal bone, one of the several bones forming the skull. The discussion of the inner ear also includes material on the vestibular system, which is technically not part of the peripheral auditory mechanism but is closely related to the cochlea. The chapter concludes with discussion of the neural component—the auditory nerve and auditory pathways—of the system.

TEMPORAL BONE

Figure 13–1 shows the complex shape and notable landmarks of the temporal bone. Figure 13–1A provides a view of the lateral (side) surface of the temporal bone

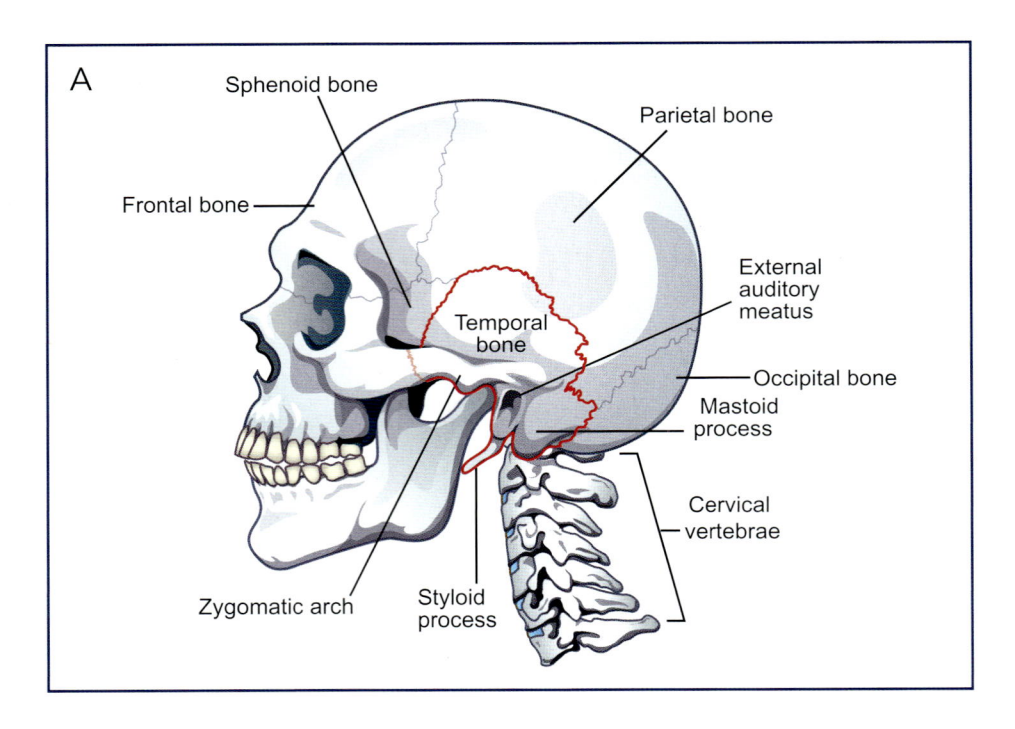

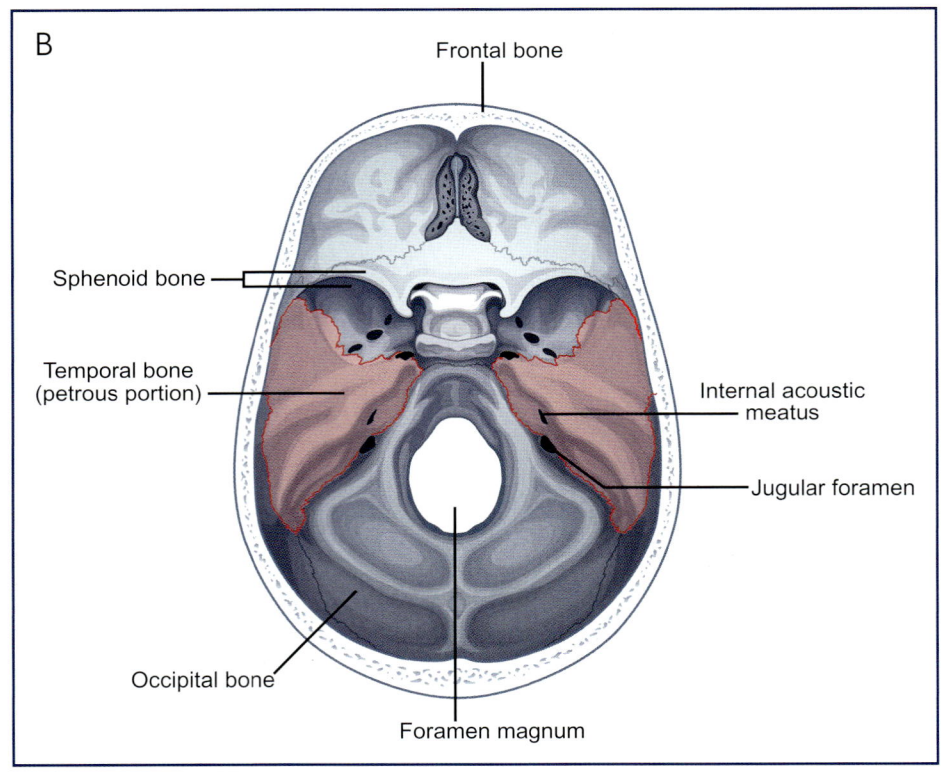

Figure 13-1. A. Sagittal view of skull showing the boundaries of the temporal bone, in red. **B.** Interior of the base of the skull, viewed from above with top half of skull removed. *continues*

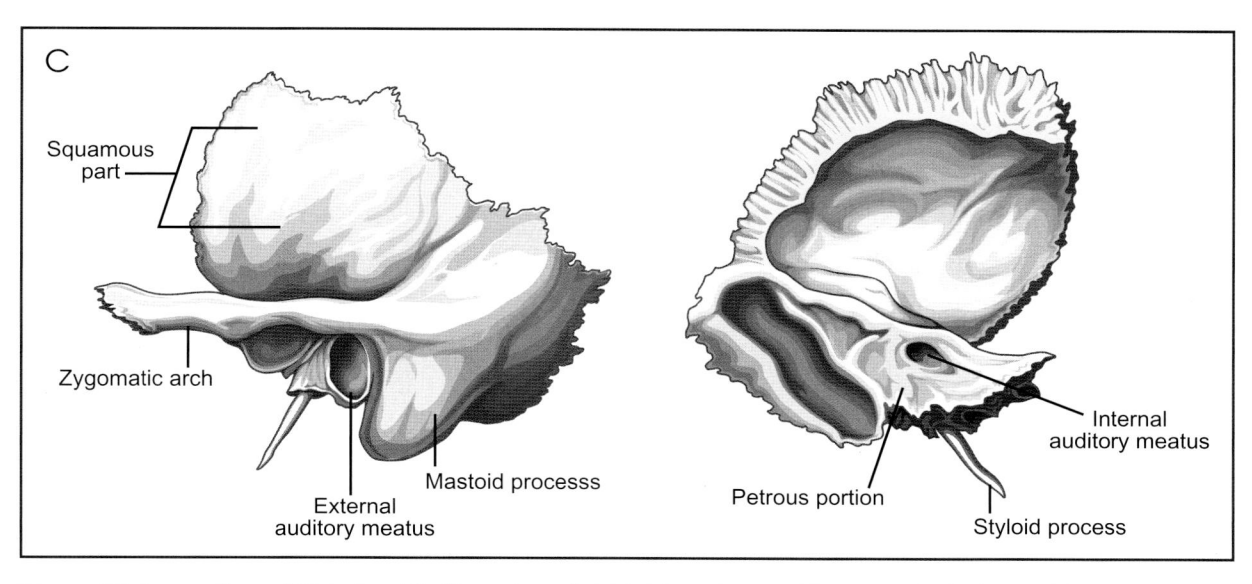

Figure 13–1. *continued* **C.** Lateral (*left*) and medial (*right*) surfaces of the complexly shaped temporal bone.

(boundary sutures shown by the red trace). The temporal bone shares boundaries with the occipital bone in back, the parietal bone above, and the sphenoid bone in front. The mastoid process of the temporal bone is behind and slightly below the bony external auditory meatus, the small tube leading from the outside of the skull to the tympanic membrane (eardrum); the entrance of this tube is seen when looking at the side of the head into the ear. The outer part of the tube is enclosed in cartilage, and the remaining two-thirds of the external auditory meatus is enclosed in the temporal bone. Deep to the mastoid process, within the mastoid bone, are air-filled cells that communicate with the air-filled middle ear cavity.

Figure 13–1B shows the interior base of the skull from above as if the top half has been removed. Note the position of the temporal bone relative to the sphenoid bone (in front) and occipital bone (behind). The temporal bone projects toward the midline, forming part of the base of the skull. The temporal bone has a broad lateral base and narrows to a blunt tip at its medial termination point. The more medial part is called the petrous part of the temporal bone. (The petrous part is not visible on the lateral surface of the temporal bone as shown in Figure 13–1A.) The petrous part of the temporal bone encases the structures of the inner ear and forms several walls of the middle ear cavity. Note the opening of the internal auditory meatus, a narrow canal roughly 10 mm in length through which nerve fibers run from the cochlea (inner ear structure of hearing) and vestibular apparatus (inner ear structure of eye-head coordination and balance) on their way to the brainstem. The opening of the internal auditory meatus into the base of the skull is in the posterior part of the petrous portion of the temporal bone. Auditory nerve fibers running in the opposite direction, from the brainstem to the cochlea, also travel through the internal auditory meatus as part of the auditory nerve, as well as nerve fibers associated with the facial nerve (cranial nerve VII). The primary blood supply to the inner ear, the labyrinthine artery which is a branch of the basilar artery which ascends the ventral surface of the brainstem (see Chapter 15), also travels to the cochlea and vestibular apparatus through the internal auditory meatus. The nerve fibers plus the labyrinthine artery emerge at the inner opening of the internal meatus.

The complexity of the temporal bone is best appreciated in Figure 13–1C, which shows it disarticulated from the other bones of the skull. The lateral surface of the bone is shown on the left, the middle surface on the right. The right-hand image shows the petrous part of the temporal bone with its wedge-like projection into the middle part of the skull base.

PERIPHERAL ANATOMY OF THE AUDITORY SYSTEM

Figure 13–2 shows an artist's rendition of the peripheral anatomy of the auditory system. The phrase "peripheral anatomy of the auditory system" refers to all structures involved in audition that extend from the pinna to the entry point of the auditory nerve into the brainstem. The structures are shown as if the head has been cut into front and back halves, with the front half

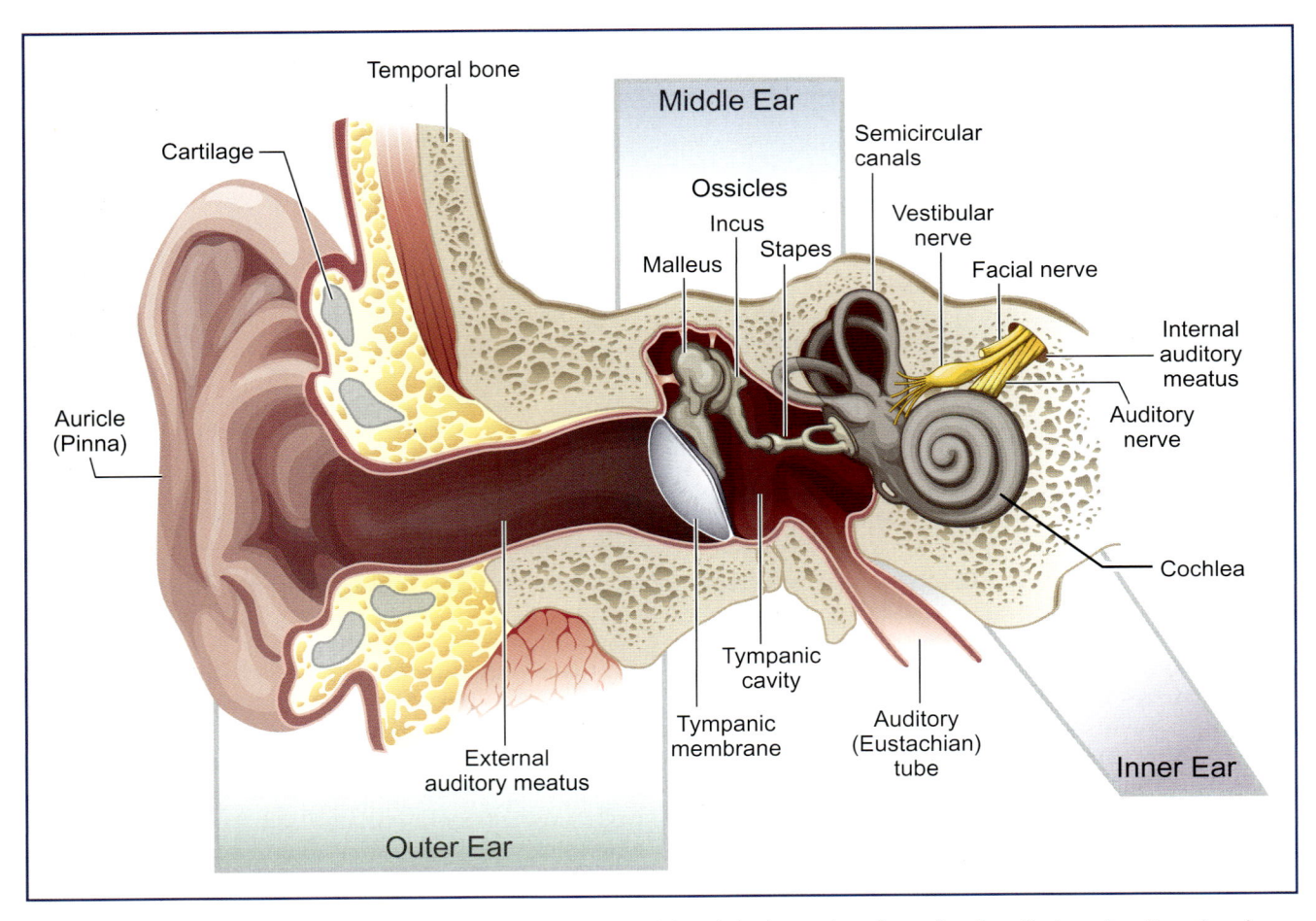

Figure 13-2. Coronal-plane view (head cut in front and back halves, view from the front) showing the structures of the peripheral auditory system and their divisions into the outer, middle, and inner ear.

removed. The image shows the peripheral auditory mechanism separated into three major parts: the outer ear, the middle ear, and the inner ear. The outer ear plus middle ear are components of the conductive part of the auditory mechanism; the inner ear and auditory nerve are the sensorineural parts of the mechanism. The tympanic membrane is included as a component of both the outer and middle ears, because one side of the membrane faces the external auditory meatus and the other side faces the middle ear cavity. Figure 13–3 is a schematic chart of these divisions. Both Figures 6–2 and 6–3 should be referred to frequently throughout the following sections.

OUTER EAR (CONDUCTIVE MECHANISM)

The outer ear includes the pinna (or auricle) and the opening into the external auditory meatus (abbreviated EAM in Figure 13–3; also called the external auditory canal). Part of the tympanic membrane (eardrum)—the sheet of tissue that terminates the external auditory meatus—is also considered a structure of the outer ear. The tympanic membrane is the boundary between the outer and middle ear.

Pinna (Auricle)

The pinna (also called the auricle) is composed of cartilage and fat tissue. In humans, the pinna collects and directs sound energy into the external auditory meatus, toward the tympanic membrane (eardrum). In most humans, the pinna is not a movable body part, at least not to the extent as in animals (like your cat) that use muscles to aim their pinnae, with great flexibility, at interesting sounds.

Careful examination of a human pinna shows many creases, folds, and cavities. Anatomists have names for all these features, perhaps as many as 15 (or more) anatomical landmarks on and within the pinna.

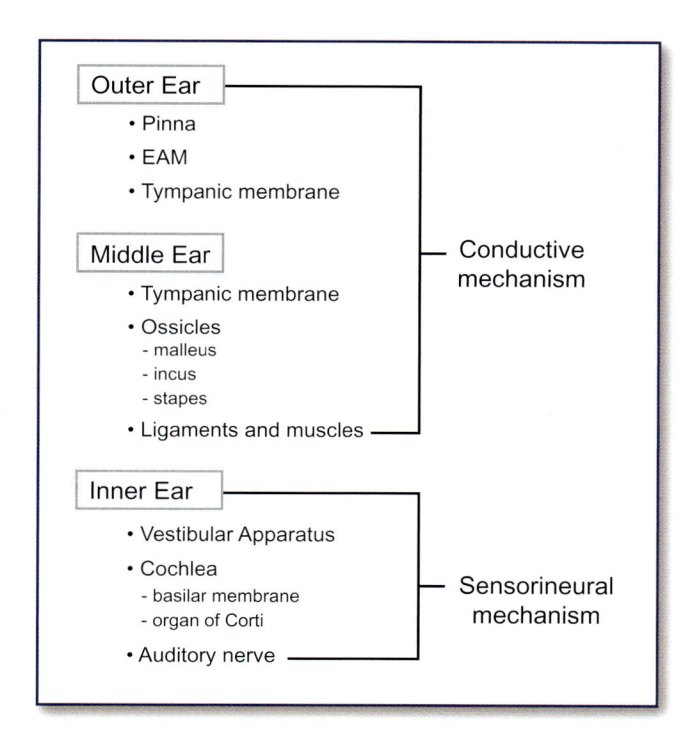

Figure 13-3. Schematic diagram summarizing anatomical components of the outer, middle, and inner ear and their relationship to the functional distinction between conductive versus sensorineural auditory components.

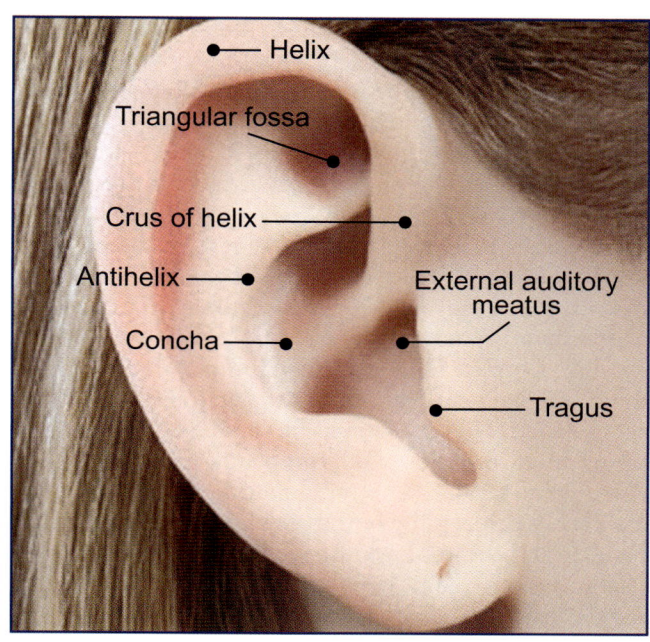

Figure 13-4. Photograph of human pinna (right ear) with labeled landmarks.

Figure 13–4 shows a human pinna with seven labeled landmarks. Pinna morphology varies a great deal across individuals; the seven chosen landmarks in this figure are observed in most individuals.

In humans, the shape and structures of the pinna play a role in the ability to localize sound sources that are higher or lower relative to a horizontal plane running through the head, at the level of the tragus. What is known is that the pinna, because of its shape and morphological characteristics, modifies the amplitudes of frequency components of sound waves striking the head. These subtle modifications provide cues to the location of a sound source in the up-down dimension.

The concha is the shallow depression in the pinna, a sort of foyer to the external auditory meatus. As shown in Figure 13–4, the concha may be separated into two chambers by a raised bar of cartilage that is a continuation of the crus of helix, the helix being the folded edge of the pinna. The concha collects sound waves and directs them into the external auditory meatus.

Inside the helix and anterior to it is the antihelix, a ridge of cartilage that follows the curve of the helix from the bottom to near the top of the pinna. As the antihelix approaches the top of the pinna, it splits into two ridges, often in a "Y" pattern, leaving the triangular fossa as the small cavity between them. This fossa serves primarily as an anatomical landmark, sometimes used to identify embryological malformations of the external ear.

The tragus is a small, rounded projection from the front of the external ear, toward the rear of the head. Apart from its obvious value as a prominent anatomical landmark, the tragus plays a role in locating sound sources in the up-down and front-back dimensions relative to the head.

The role of the pinna in sound localization may be small in humans, but in some cases significant. Chapter 14 presents information on how anatomical characteristics of the pinna may affect cues to the localization of sound in the up-down dimension relative to the head. The substantial amount of variation in pinna anatomy across individuals may account partially for findings in the literature of substantial cross-person variability of sound localization skills.

External Auditory Meatus (External Auditory Canal)

The external auditory meatus is a tube extending from the interior of the pinna, seen as a small opening in the concha (see Figure 13–4), to the tympanic membrane. *Meatus* is a Latin term meaning opening or canal. The entrance of the external auditory meatus, into which you fit your earphones or earplugs, is easy to see in most people. In adults, the external auditory meatus is roughly 2.5 cm in length and 0.7 cm in diameter, although these dimensions vary quite a bit across individuals (in this chapter, all anatomical sizes, areas, and dimensions are for young adults). The external auditory meatus is not a straight, level tube; rather it runs slightly "uphill" (see Figure 13–2) and has a small bend between its opening and the tympanic membrane, where it ends. The bend is backward (and, thus, is not discernible in Figure 13–2) and occurs in many people at the location where the canal's surrounding tissue changes from cartilage to bone. You may have noticed that your medical practitioner, when inserting an otoscope (ear scope) into your ear canal, gently pulls the pinna toward the back of the head. The practitioner does this to straighten out the natural bend in the tube for a more direct view of the tympanic membrane. The bend in the external auditory meatus is also a barrier to foreign objects moving easily from the outer ear to the delicate tissues of the tympanic membrane; in this sense, the shape of the canal serves a protective function. As can be seen in Figure 13–2, the part of the external auditory meatus close to the concha is surrounded by cartilage, which is a continuation of the tissue that makes up much of the pinna. The remaining length of the ear canal is encased by part of the temporal bone. The external auditory meatus ends as a closed tube at the tympanic membrane.

The primary auditory function of the external auditory meatus is to conduct sound energy from the concha to the tympanic membrane. The sound energy is in the form of molecule-sized pressure waves, as described in Chapter 7. The external auditory meatus acts like a resonator, causing sound energy at certain frequencies to vibrate with greater amplitude compared with the amplitude at other frequencies. Specifically, the external auditory meatus of an adult amplifies vibratory amplitude (sound wave energy) at frequencies around 3300 Hz. The specific resonant frequency at which the sound energy is "boosted" is determined by the length of the tube. The greater the length of the external auditory meatus, the lower its resonant frequency (Chapter 7). The resonant frequency is consistent with resonance characteristics of a tube closed at one end. Like all resonators, the boost in energy is not only at the peak frequency, but at surrounding frequencies as well.

The external auditory meatus protects the tympanic membrane and is a conduit for the removal of dead tissue away from the tympanic membrane. The tympanic membrane is protected by cerumen (ear wax) that is secreted by sweat glands in the cartilaginous walls of the external auditory meatus. The fluid produced by these microscopic glands mixes with a substance called sebum to create cerumen. This waxy mixture drains into the walls of the ear canal by sliding down tiny hairs that emerge from the cartilage and project into the canal. Cerumen lubricates the ear canal, presents a barrier to larger foreign objects (insects, for example), and may also block the movement of bacteria or fungal agents toward the tympanic membrane.

The dead tissue that is removed through the external auditory meatus comes from the tympanic membrane. The tympanic membrane has three tissue layers. The layer on the lateral side (that is, facing the pinna) is a continuation of the skin of the external auditory meatus, which has a superficial layer composed of keratinized epithelium. These superficial cells lack a nucleus

Getting a Boost

Imagine an experiment in which a pressure wave (sound wave) made up of frequencies of equal energy between 1 and 10,000 Hz is introduced at the entrance to the ear canal (external auditory meatus). Now imagine placing a very small, sensitive microphone deep in the ear canal, precisely at the location where the ear canal ends at the tympanic membrane. You might think that the microphone would pick up the same sound that entered the ear canal. But think again. We know that the ear canal is a tube open at one end (at the concha) and closed at the other end (at the tympanic membrane) and that such tubes have specific resonant frequencies, depending on their length. The ear canal is a tube roughly 2.5 cm long and closed at one end; by the quarter-wavelength rule the primary (lowest) resonant frequency is 3300 Hz. This means that the pressure wave arrives at the microphone at the tympanic membrane with an energy boost at 3300 Hz, and to a lesser degree at frequencies immediately surrounding the computed resonant frequency. The change in the spectrum of a sound from one location to another is called a *transfer function*. The flat spectrum (equal energy at all frequencies) introduced at the pinna opening of the ear canal is transformed by the acoustic characteristics of the external auditory meatus to a spectrum at the tympanic membrane favoring frequencies at and around 3300 Hz.

or other small organs (often called organelles) that are typical of other tissue cells in the body. They are called "keratinized" because they are essentially dead cells (hence the lack of a nucleus and organelles typically involved with metabolic functions). The keratinized cells serve a protective function, with the outermost layer continuously "shedding." The shed cells do not pile up in front of the tympanic membrane, but rather are carried down the incline of the external auditory meatus and dispersed as they approach the concha.

Tympanic Membrane (Eardrum)

The tympanic membrane, or eardrum, is shown in Figure 13–5. The tympanic membrane is the boundary between the outer and middle ear. The foundation of that boundary is bone. The circular perimeter of the tympanic membrane is linked to the bony foundation via a cartilage-ligamentous ring called the annulus (which is whitish in appearance compared with the slightly darker skin-tone of the ear canal). The annulus fits into a small circular, bony depression at the boundary of the outer and middle ear, anchoring the tympanic membrane in place.

Figure 13–5 depicts the right tympanic membrane as seen through an otoscope. The otoscope has a viewing lens and a light source to illuminate the ear canal and the tympanic membrane. As a result of the shallow conical shape of the tympanic membrane and its tilt with the lower half farther from the scope than the upper half, light reflects off the normal tympanic membrane as a "cone of light" that is directed forward, downward, and to the right. The cone of light directed to the right of the observer, as in Figure 13–5, is typical when viewing the right ear; the cone is directed to the left when viewing the left tympanic membrane. Parts of the middle ear bones (ossicles—malleus, incus, and stapes) can be seen through the membrane.

In the otoscopic view, the tympanic membrane looks more or less flat—not conical, not tilted along its top-to-bottom axis relative to the observer. The cone shape and the tilt are seen in the cross-sectional rendition of the tympanic membrane in Figure 13–2. The tympanic membrane has the shape of a flattened bowl with a conical base that points into the middle ear cavity. The "tip" of the inverted cone is called the umbo, and serves as the point of attachment for the lower end of the malleus, one of the three middle ear bones described below.

As noted above, the tympanic membrane is composed of a three-layer sheet of tissue. The layer at the termination of the external auditory meatus is composed of epithelial tissue that is a thinned continuation of the skin lining the canal. The layer of tissue facing the middle ear cavity is also very thin epithelium, but with a different cell structure than the layer facing the external auditory meatus: the layer facing the middle ear has an epithelial structure much like the mucosal tissue that covers the upper airways. The middle layer is the primary vibratory component of the tympanic membrane and is composed of fibrous tissue interlaced with collagen fibers. The highly elastic collagen fibers are arrayed throughout the middle layer in many different directions (from center to edge, radially, horizontally), forming a dense interlacing of tissue having complex vibratory capability. This middle layer is highly sensitive to very small pressures exerted by the vibrating air molecules that create sound waves, but capable of resisting extremely high static (non-vibratory) pressures such as those encountered in a poorly pressurized airplane cabin.

The three-layer tissue structure is called the *pars tensa* and makes up nearly the entire surface area of the tympanic membrane. The exception is a small region in the upper part of the membrane called the *pars flaccida* (shown in Figure 13–5; the pars flaccida is also called *Shrapnell's membrane*), which lacks the middle, fibrous layer present in the rest of the tympanic membrane.

The overall thickness of the three layers of the tympanic membrane is little more than one-tenth of a millimeter (equal to 0.0001 meter). The membrane has a diameter of roughly 8 to 10 mm and a surface

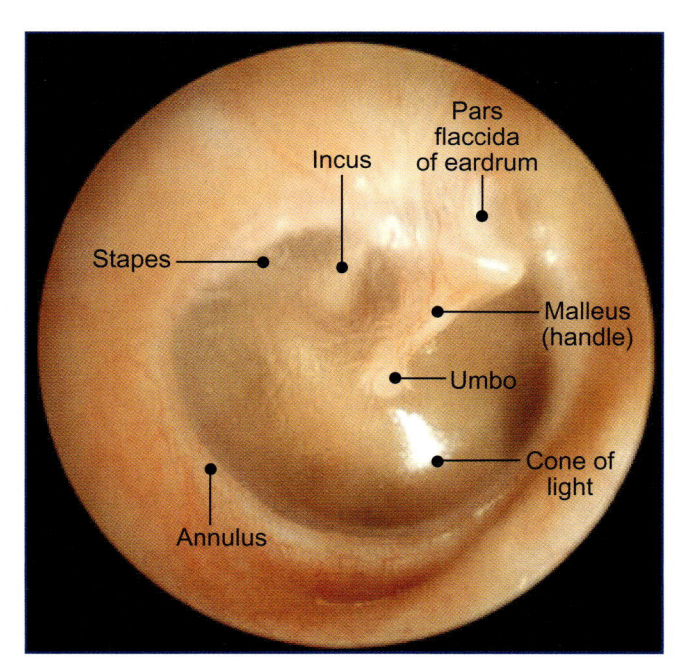

Figure 13–5. View of the right tympanic membrane as seen through an otoscope.

area of about 55 mm². The surface area of the tympanic membrane plays an important role, described below, in how the middle ear mechanism transforms sound energy from the medium of air (in the external auditory meatus) to the medium of fluid (in the cochlea).

MIDDLE EAR (CONDUCTIVE MECHANISM)

The middle ear is a tiny (1–2 cm³) air-filled cavity lined with a mucous membrane and surrounded by bone. Figure 13–6 shows the size of a cube with sides 1.15 cm in length; the volume of such a cube is 1.52 cm³, giving a fair idea of the tiny volume of the middle ear cavity (the volume is variable across humans and may even be smaller—within a range of 0.5 to 1 cm³—in many individuals; see Stepp & Voss, 2005). The middle ear cavity is complexly shaped and contains tiny, movable bones (ossicles), ligaments, two muscles, nerves, and the proximal end of a tube that leads to the nasopharynx.

The middle ear can be seen in coronal section in Figure 13–2. This two-dimensional illustration shows the lateral boundary of the cavity (the medial surface of the tympanic membrane plus the bone above it), the medial boundary (the bony covering of the inner ear, best defined by the region around and below the attachment of the footplate of the stapes into the oval-shaped "window" of the bony labyrinth—the bony encasement of the inner ear structures), and the bony floor and roof of the cavity. The section does not provide a good view of the posterior wall of the cavity or the front of the cavity, the latter cut away for the illustration.

The middle ear cavity can be conceptualized as having six surfaces—medial, lateral, superior, inferior, posterior, and anterior—much like a cube can be described with its six surfaces except that these surfaces are irregular and of unequal area. Figure 13–7 presents a schematic representation of the middle ear cavity with five of its six surfaces labeled with selected structures. The view is directed toward the medial wall of the middle ear cavity. The sixth surface is the lateral surface of the middle ear cavity, largely made up of the tympanic membrane. For this illustration the lateral surface has been cut away to allow a view of the middle ear cavity from lateral-to-medial. The different surfaces, or cavity walls, are referred to throughout the discussion of middle ear anatomy. To anticipate a fuller discussion of landmarks on the walls of the middle ear (tympanic) cavity: the medial wall shows the oval and round windows of the bony labyrinth, the prominence of the facial canal, and the promontory; the lateral wall is defined almost completely by the tympanic membrane; the superior wall, or roof of the middle ear cavity, is a thin bony plate called the tegmen tympani, separating the middle ear cavity from the cranial cavity (the space inside the skull); the posterior wall contains the aditus in its upper part and lower on the wall the pyramidal eminence, a minuscule, cone-shaped protuberance containing the stapedius muscle, which sends out a tendon to attach to the stapes (only the muscle and tendon are shown, not the bony casing); the inferior surface is a thin, plate-like bone separating the middle ear cavity from the internal jugular vein; and the anterior wall shows the location of the bony opening of the auditory (eustachian) tube and the bony canal housing the *tensor tympani* muscle, which sends out a tendon to attach to the malleus. Each of these features is discussed below.

Chambers of the Middle Ear

The middle ear cavity is often partitioned into an upper chamber, called the epitympanum (also referred to as the attic of the middle ear), a middle chamber,

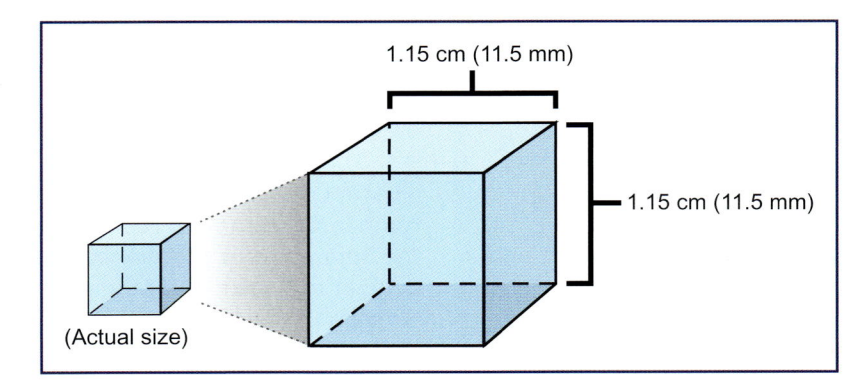

Figure 13–6. Volume of middle ear cavity in the form of a cube. Actual size is shown at the left, with an expanded cube at the right shown for illustration purposes. Approximate dimensions are for the real (*left*) cube.

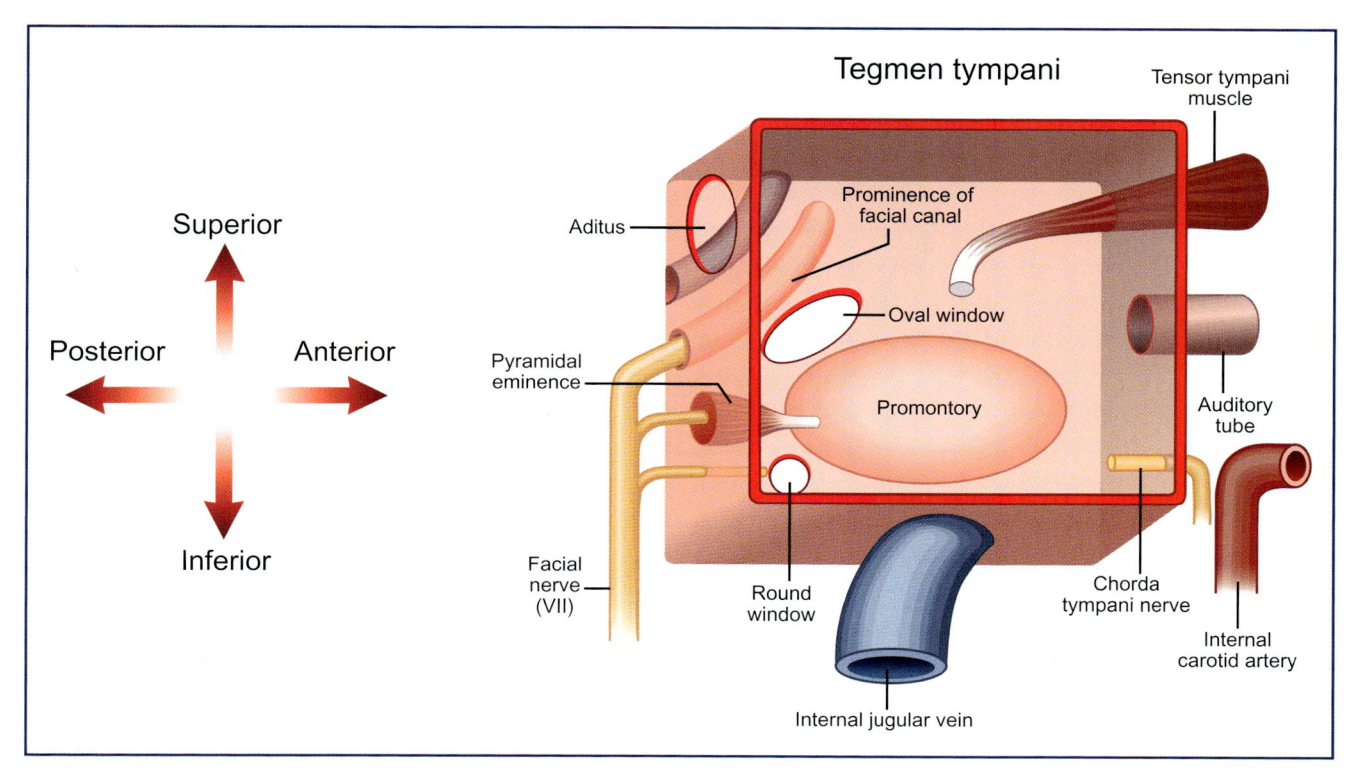

Figure 13–7. Schematic representation of the middle ear cavity, looking in from the tympanic membrane, which has been removed. Structures on the posterior, anterior, superior, inferior, and medial walls are shown.

the mesotympanum, and a lower chamber, the hypotympanum. There are no clear-cut boundaries between these chambers. Nevertheless, the epitympanum is typically regarded as the chamber above the tympanic membrane and contains the head of the malleus and the body of the incus (note in Figure 13–2 their location in the small, upper cavity of the middle ear). The epitympanum also includes an opening in its posterior wall (see Figure 13–7) called the aditus, which is directed posteriorly to the antrum, an airspace deep within the mastoid bone. The aditus and antrum allow the air in the middle ear cavity to communicate with air-filled cells of the mastoid bone. The aditus, antrum, and cells of the mastoid are shown in the coronal view of Figure 13–8. In this simplified view, the bony, ligamentous, and muscular structures have been removed from the middle ear cavity.

The mesotympanum is the space between the top and bottom edge of the tympanic membrane. The mesotympanum contains the malleus and long process of the incus, as well as the stapes and the oval and round windows (openings into inner ear, described below). The oval and round windows are features of the medial wall of the tympanic cavity (see Figure 13-7).

The hypotympanum, or lowest space of the cavity, does not contain functional components of the middle ear but is directly above the internal jugular vein (see Figure 13–7), an important part of the cardiovascular system by which blood is drained from the head. The inferior surface of the middle ear cavity—that is, the floor of the cavity—is separated from the internal jugular vein by a thin plate of bone. Just below this thin plate the internal jugular vein makes a right-angle turn along its pathway from the posterior part of the brain to larger arteries in the chest. Knowledge of the hypotympanum's relationship to this venous structure is critical to patient safety during middle ear surgery.

Ossicles and Associated Structures

The ossicles are the three smallest bones in the human body. They extend across the middle ear cavity from the tympanic membrane to the oval window of the cochlea. The individual ossicles plus their articulated configuration are shown in Figure 13–9. To appreciate the miniaturized size of these bones, consider that all three fit (at the same time) quite easily on the lower half of the surface of a penny (see actual size cube in Figure 13–6).

The *malleus* (also called the "hammer") has a handle-like part called the manubrium, which is attached

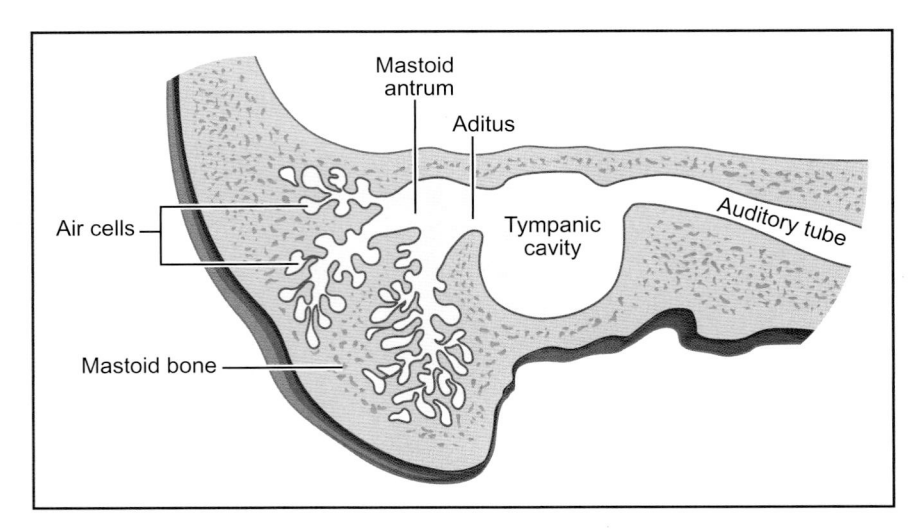

Figure 13–8. The aditus, mastoid antrum, and air-filled cells in relation to the middle ear cavity.

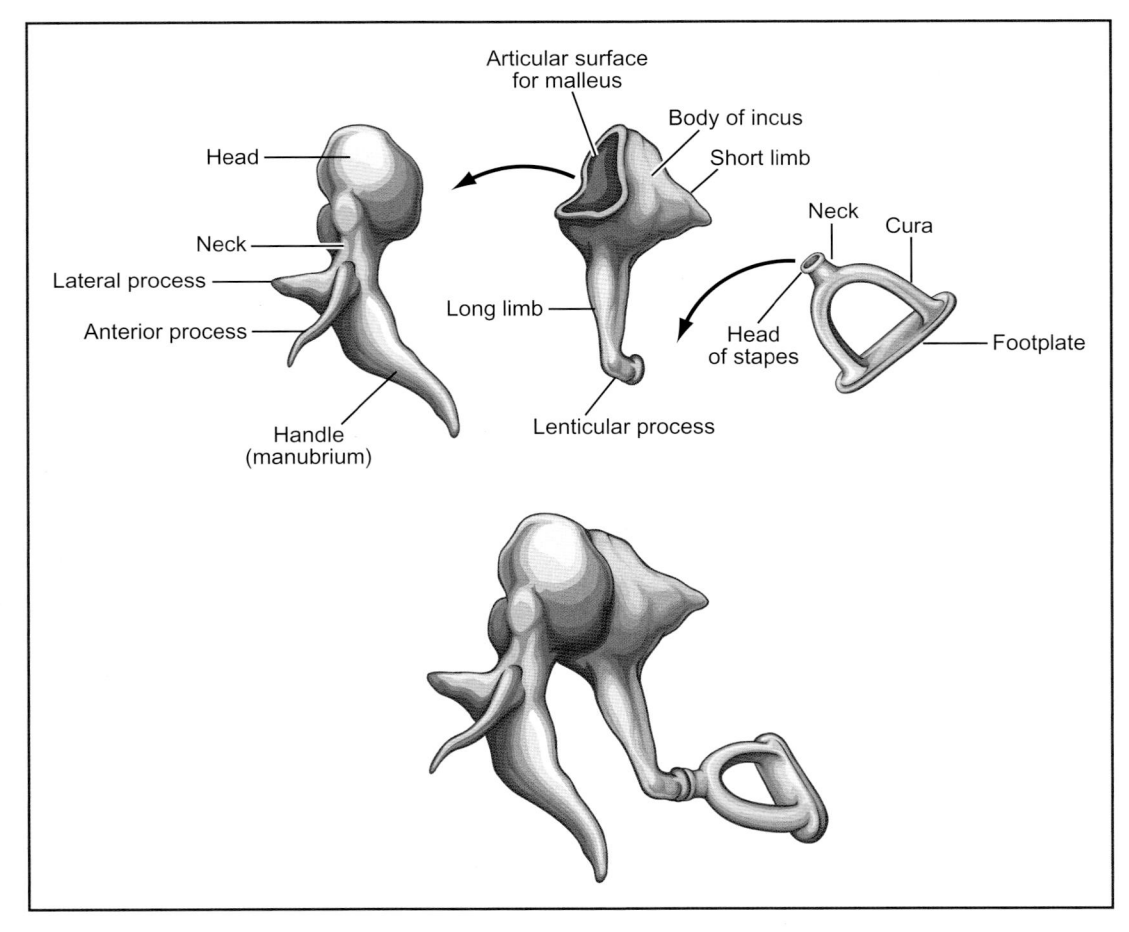

Figure 13–9. The ossicles shown as individual, disarticulated bones (*top*) from left ro right the malleus, incus, and stapes, and in their fully articulated configuration (*bottom*).

along its length to the tympanic membrane. The lowest point of attachment, at the inferior end of the handle, is called the umbo. The umbo is a prominent landmark on the tympanic membrane when it is viewed through an otoscope (see Figure 13–5). At the top of the handle is a short neck, and above that the head of the malleus. A curved edge on one side of the head of the malleus is the point of articulation with the incus.

The incus (or anvil) is the middle ossicle. The incus has a short body that issues two processes, one short and stubby, the other long and ending in the hook-like lenticular process. The body of the incus contains a curved surface for its articulation with the malleus, fitting into the curved surface of the malleolar head. The hook-like end of the long limb of the incus, the lenticular process, is a subtle modification of the bone that forms a joint with the stapes.

The stapes (or stirrup) is the most medial and smallest ossicle. The very short head of the stapes is attached to the lenticular process of the incus to form the incudo-stapedial joint. A short neck connects the head of the stapes to two arches, the anterior and posterior crura, which extend from the neck and attach to an oval-shaped base, the footplate of the stapes. The stapes fits into the oval window, an opening cut into the bony casing of the inner ear (see Figure 13–7). The footplate is held in that window by a fibrous ligament, the annular ligament (like the one securing the tympanic membrane to its circular, bony frame) that adheres to the perimeter of the footplate and attaches to the bony perimeter of the oval window.

The malleo-incudal and incudostapedial joints are synovial, meaning they are both joined together by a fibrous capsule filled with synovial fluid. Synovial fluid, a relatively viscous (thick) secretion from the capsule cells, reduces friction between the articulating surfaces of the joints as they move against each other. Movement at these joints is associated with the conduction of sound vibration from the tympanic membrane to the cochlea, as well as with displacement of the ossicular chain when static (non-vibrating) pressures are applied to the tympanic membrane. The malleo-incudal joint is more strongly linked than the incudo-stapedial joint. When there is a break in the ossicular chain, such as might occur when the skull is fractured, separation of the ossicles is much more likely to occur at the incudostapedial joint.

Surprisingly, the precise role of the ossicular joints in the conduction of sound energy from the tympanic membrane to the footplate of the stapes is unknown. Especially because birds, one of our more direct evolutionary forebearers, have a single ossicle that responds to sound energy with piston-like (rigid body) movements, it is fair to ask how the evolution of a single-ossicle transmission system to a three-ossicle system benefits human auditory capabilities. What is known is that the three ossicles do not move as a strictly rigid, uniform system (see Nakajima et al., 2005 and Volandri et al., 2012 for excellent reviews). Rather, there is some independence of ossicle motion during vibration by sound waves, with most of the non-piston-like movement, observed in experiments in which two ossicles are seen to have somewhat separate motions when they vibrate, occurring at the incudomalleolar joint. Such semi-independent motion of individual ossicles, however, has yet to be shown as providing a clear auditory advantage over the simpler, single-ossicle system.

Ligaments of the Middle Ear

The ossicles are anchored to the walls of the middle ear cavity by several ligaments (as well as muscles, described in the next section). There are six ligaments in the middle ear cavity, three associated with the malleus, two with the incus, and one with the stapes. Figure 13–10 shows a coronal view of the ligaments and muscles of the middle ear.

The malleal ligaments include the anterior, lateral, and superior ligaments. The anterior malleal ligament has one attachment on the anterior wall of the tympanic cavity and the other at the neck of the malleus. Because the view in Figure 13–10 is coronal, from the front of the head, only one point of attachment is indicated. The lateral malleolar ligament has an attachment on the lateral wall of the middle ear cavity, just above the tympanic membrane, and another on the lower part of the head of the malleus. The superior malleolar ligament is attached to the "roof" of the middle ear cavity (tegmen tympani) and the superior part of the head of the malleus.

The incus is supported by the posterior and superior ligaments. The posterior incudal ligament attaches the short limb of the incus to the posterior wall of the middle ear cavity, very close to the entrance (aditus) to the mastoid bone. The superior incudal ligament extends from the roof of the tympanic cavity to the body of the incus. Only one ligament attaches to the stapes. This is the annular ligament, which anchors the perimeter of the stapes footplate to the bony oval window.

Together these six ligaments (along with the muscles, described below) stabilize the ossicular chain and permit its piston-like motions (on an axis through the umbo to the footplate of the stapes) as well as motions of the joints that may be partially independent of the piston action. The ligaments are important to the efficient functioning of the ossicular chain in transmitting sound energy from the tympanic membrane to the fluid in the cochlea.

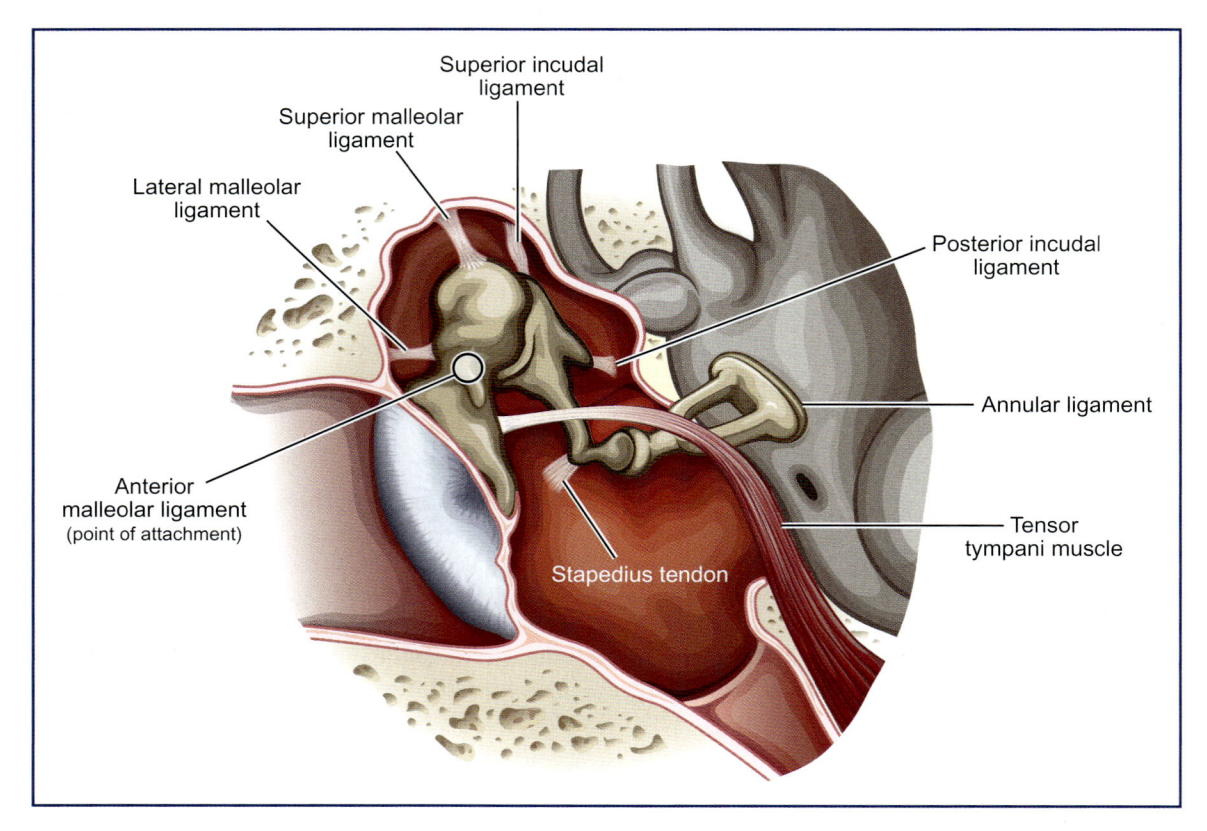

Figure 13–10. View of the right middle ear, showing points of attachment for six ligaments and two muscles.

Muscles of the Middle Ear

The two muscles of the middle ear cavity are the *tensor tympani* and the *stapedius* (see Figure 13–10). The *tensor tympani* muscle originates within a bony canal in the front wall of the middle ear cavity, just above the bony portion of the auditory tube (the tube that connects the middle ear cavity to the nasopharynx, also called the eustachian tube). The muscle fibers run backward along this bony canal, toward the middle ear cavity, and at the opening into the cavity give off a tiny tendon. This tendon makes a sharp turn toward the lateral wall of the tympanic cavity and inserts to the neck of the malleus. Contraction of the *tensor tympani* muscle pulls the handle of the malleus medially and forward, retracting the tympanic membrane into the middle ear cavity. This action may stiffen the tympanic membrane and the ossicular chain, thereby reducing the vibratory efficiency of the conductive mechanism. The muscle is thought to provide a protective function for excessive movement of the entire conductive mechanism, which may cause damage to structures of the inner ear. Contraction of the *tensor tympani* muscle can occur in response to very high intensity sounds or even during chewing. The *tensor tympani* muscle is innervated by a motor branch of the trigeminal nerve (cranial nerve V).

Fibers of the *stapedius* muscle originate in a tiny conical hole in the posterior wall of the middle ear cavity and give way to a tiny tendon that inserts to the posterior crus and neck of the stapes. In Figure 13–10 only the tendon is shown, because the muscle fibers are hidden within the pyramidal eminence (see Figure 13–7). When the muscle contracts, it pulls the stapes away from its "fit" into the oval window, the movement allowed by the flexibility of the annular ligament. The precise nature of the pull is to tilt the footplate away from the oval window, with the front part of the footplate most affected. Contraction of the *stapedius* muscle stiffens the entire ossicular chain and is thought to protect the inner ear from excessive displacement of the footplate into the fluid of the inner ear. The *stapedius* muscle plays a significant role in the acoustic reflex, which is thought to protect inner ear structures from damage due to excessively high sound levels. The *stapedius* muscle is innervated by a motor branch of the facial nerve (cranial nerve VII) and is a key component of the acoustic reflex (see below).

A Bone to Pick

Scientists don't always agree. Although the complicated arrangement of the ossicles seems to be in the service of efficient transmission of sound energy from the tympanic membrane to the cochlea, there are dissenters who have a bone to pick with this traditional view. Luers and Hüttenbrink (2016) argue that the ossicular arrangement in humans, with moving joints and strangely oriented extensions, is not specialized for sound transmission, but rather serves the combined functions of responding to molecule-size pressure variations—sound waves—*and* protection against the wide range of "ambient" static pressures that may exceed sound pressures by a million (or more) times. Why do they argue so? First, joint movement at the malleo-incudal and incudo-stapedial joints is different when responding to sound vibrations compared with large, non-sonic pressures (such as in an airplane cabin). The joint movements observed in response to large, static pressures seem to be exactly what you would expect if the ossicles were moving to limit displacement of the stapes into the oval window. These movements have a lot of joint rotation, unlike the more piston-like movement of the ossicular chain during sound vibration. Second, reconstructive otosurgeons (surgeons who "rebuild" damaged structures of the middle ear) have found that the most effective middle ear prosthesis for a person with a missing ossicle (or two) is a *straight strut*. In other words, when re-creating a pathway for sound between the tympanic membrane and the oval window, they do not mimic the contortions and complex articulations of the healthy ossicles; rather, they simply connect the two ends with a straight column of surgical material. The result is excellent sound transmission across the middle ear. Third, and finally, the ossicles of an owl's ear are basically arranged in a straight line—and the hearing of owls is known to be exquisite. This suggests that a complicated, human-like ossicle arrangement is not required for excellent sound transmission from tympanic membrane to cochlea. This bone of contention about the middle ear bones is not all bad. Such controversies keep science healthy and moving forward.

Auditory (Eustachian) Tube

The auditory tube (known also as the eustachian tube, after the sixteenth-century Italian anatomist Bartolomeo Eustachi) is shown in Figure 13–2 as a bone-encased, open tube in the lower, anterior wall of the middle ear cavity. The tube extends downward, forward, and medially from this bony part, becomes cartilaginous along its path, and terminates in a closed but flexible end in the nasopharynx at roughly the same level as the nostrils. The total length of this tube in adult humans is about 3.8 cm (1.5 inches). When the tube opens, it connects air in the middle ear cavity to air in the nasopharynx.

The nasopharynx end of the auditory tube is usually closed, but can be opened by swallowing, yawning, or chewing. The opening of the auditory tube is by muscular means, and likely includes simultaneous contraction of the *tensor veli palatini* muscle, the *superior constrictor* muscle, and the *levator veli palatini* muscle (Okada et al., 2018; and see Chapter 4). Immediately after the tube is opened, it springs back to the closed position due to the elasticity of the tissue. Intermittent opening of the auditory tube is important to expose air in the middle ear cavity to atmospheric pressure, which is typically the pressure in the nasopharynx when the mouth, velopharynx, or both are open. This intermittent opening of the auditory tube maintains atmospheric pressure in the middle ear cavity. Under normal circumstances, pressure at the surface of the tympanic membrane facing the external auditory meatus is also atmospheric. Therefore, in a healthy ear, pressure on both sides of the tympanic membrane (the external ear canal side and the middle ear side) is atmospheric. Under these pressure conditions, the tympanic membrane is at its rest position and produces the most efficient vibratory activity in response to sound energy. A pressure imbalance across the tympanic membrane pushes the membrane outward (greater pressure in middle ear cavity compared with external auditory meatus) or inward (greater pressure in external auditory meatus compared with middle ear cavity), either of which stiffens the tympanic membrane and ossicles and reduces the vibratory efficiency of the conductive mechanism. When the auditory tube does not open intermittently, as may occur in the case of a middle ear infection, pressure in the middle ear cavity may decrease relative to pressure in the external auditory meatus and push the tympanic membrane inward, away from its rest position, thereby stiffening the conductive mechanism. This results in a temporary conductive hearing loss that resolves when the infection clears. When a bulging or retracted tympanic membrane is viewed through an otoscope, the cone of light may be dimmer or completely absent.

Medial and Lateral Wall Views of the Middle Ear: A Summary

Figures 13–11 and 13–12 offer summary views of the middle ear structures. Figure 13–11 shows middle ear structures as viewed from the inner ear, looking out to the eardrum; this view looks toward the lateral wall of the middle ear cavity and associated structures. Anterior is to the left and superior to the top. The stapes has been removed to provide a direct view of the lenticular process of the incus as well as the attachment of the handle of the malleus to the tympanic membrane. Note the *tensor tympani* muscle within the bony canal just above the auditory tube, and its tendinous attachment to the handle of the malleus. The internal carotid artery, the main supply of blood to the cerebral hemispheres of the brain, is seen just in front and below the tympanic membrane (see also Figure 13–7). Cranial nerve VII (the facial nerve) is posterior to the tympanic membrane and runs in a bony canal in the back wall of the middle ear cavity. It gives off a branch called the chorda tympani that runs between the malleus and incus before exiting the skull (just below the bottom portion of the nerve as shown; the top portion of the vertical section of nerve has been cut). The chorda tympani carries taste sensation from the anterior two-thirds of the tongue into the main bundle of fibers of cranial nerve VII, which travels through the internal auditory meatus to the brainstem.

Figure 13–12 shows middle ear structures viewed from the vantage point of the tympanic membrane, looking toward the medial wall of the middle ear cavity. In this view, the incus and malleus have been removed; anterior is to the right. The crura of the stapes are shown clearly. The promontory is the bony casing of the basal turn of the cochlea. Note the attachment of the *stapedius* muscle to the posterior wall of the middle ear cavity at one end, and its distal tendon to the neck of the stapes at the other end. The proximal tendon of the stapedius muscle, arising from a tiny foramen in the posterior wall of the middle ear cavity, cannot be seen in this image. The bony casing (prominence) of one of the semicircular canals is also shown. Note the course of the facial nerve after it exits the brainstem and internal auditory meatus to enter the bony casing of

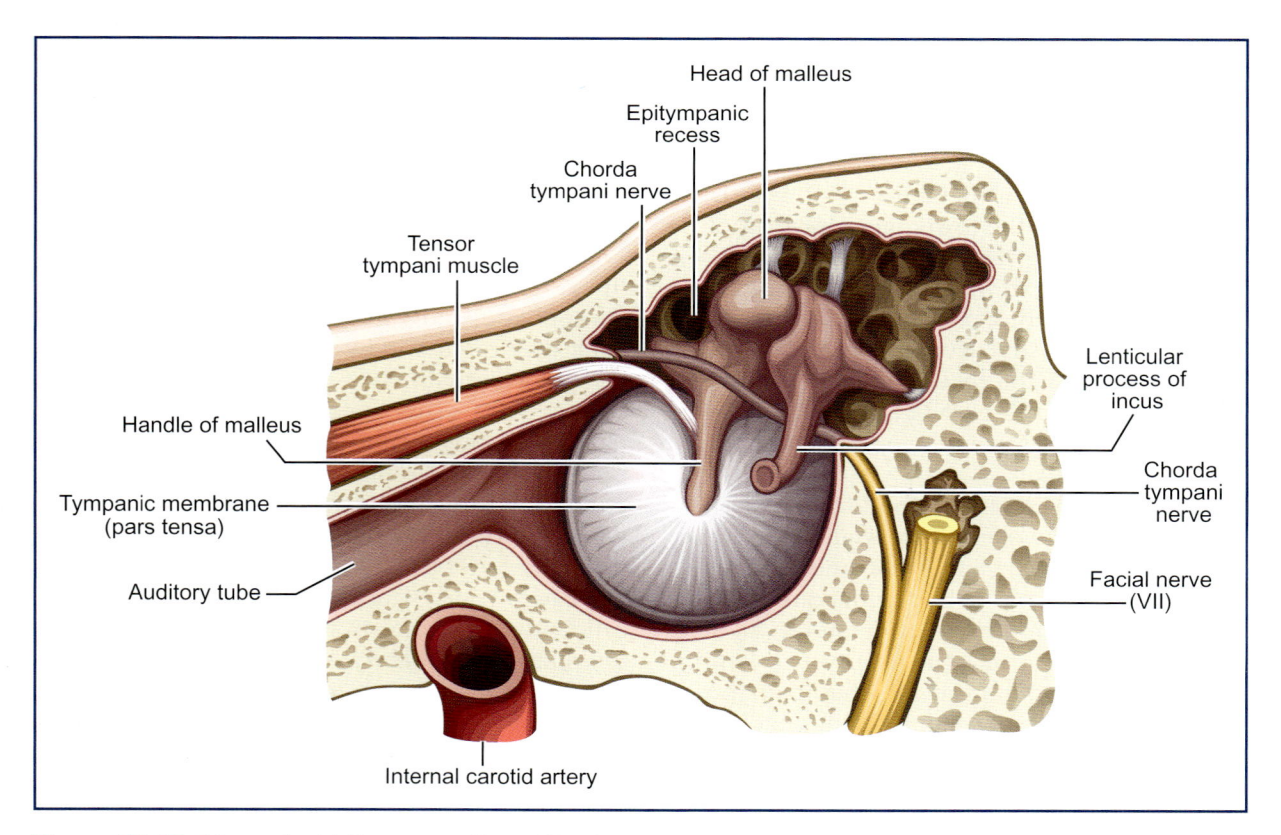

Figure 13–11. View of middle ear cavity as if looking at the structures from the inner ear, toward the tympanic membrane. The stapes has been removed for better viewing.

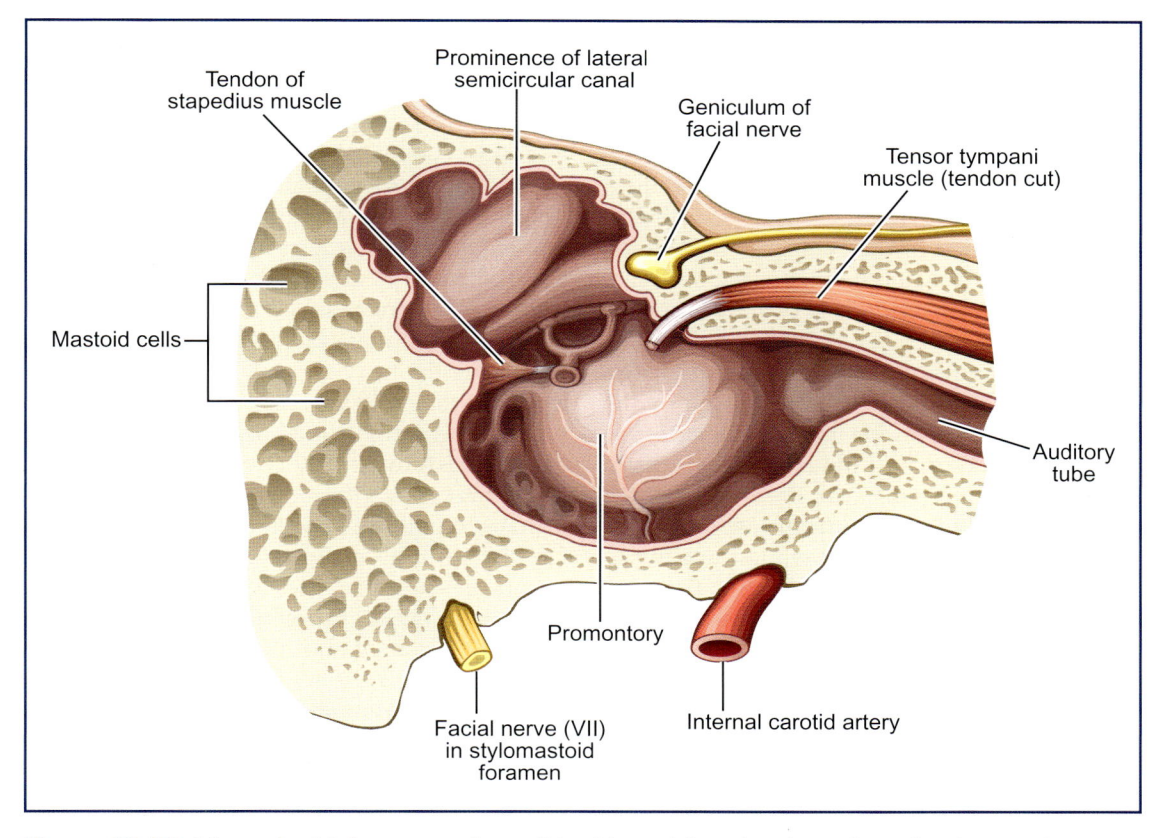

Figure 13–12. View of middle ear cavity as if looking at the structures from the tympanic membrane, toward the inner ear. In the view, the malleus and incus have been removed.

the middle ear. The nerve runs horizontally and then turns south, as it were, toward its exit from the skull. Figure 13–12 shows the beginning of the turn (with bone cut away and the nerve exposed), labeled the geniculum of the facial nerve. From the geniculum the facial nerve descends in the bony casing of the middle ear, exiting the skull through the stylomastoid foramen, one of the many openings in the base of the skull through which cranial nerves pass from inside to outside the skull (or from outside to inside).

The oval and round windows are not labeled in Figure 13–12 but are shown in this medial-wall view of middle ear. The footplate of the stapes fits into the oval window, so the window can't actually be seen, but its location can be inferred. The round window is the opening immediately below the tendon of the stapedius muscle.

Transmission of Sound Energy by the Conductive Mechanism

The ossicles transmit vibratory energy from the tympanic membrane to the cochlea, one of the three major structures of the inner ear. This transmission is possible because the ossicles are physically connected to the tympanic membrane on one end (where the malleus is attached) and the cochlea on the other end (where the footplate of the stapes fits into the oval window).

Although details of the cochlea have not yet been discussed, an understanding of the role of the ossicles in hearing requires the knowledge that the cochlea is composed of fluid (liquid)-filled chambers. Movement of this fluid is necessary to change the position of sensory receptors (hair cells) and in so doing cause auditory nerve fibers to "fire" and send impulses to the brain, where they are processed and interpreted as auditory events. The footplate of the stapes, which fits into the vestibule of the bony labyrinth that houses the cochlea, displaces the fluid when sound pressure variations in the external auditory meatus are transmitted across the tympanic membrane and ossicular chain.

The ossicular chain has special properties that solve the impedance mismatch between the air within the external auditory meatus versus the fluid (liquid) inside the cochlea. The term *impedance mismatch* refers to the difference in displacement (movement) of two media (such as air and liquid) given the same applied force. Fluid such as that contained within the inner ear has much greater impedance (opposition to movement) than air. Thus, a force applied to the fluid results in much less displacement than the same force applied to air molecules. The ossicles function to match the impedance of airborne sound energy to the fluid mechanism in the cochlea. They do this by amplifying the sound energy applied to the tympanic membrane so that it is much greater when it reaches the footplate of the stapes. This amplification is accomplished in at least three ways.

The primary amplification of sound energy from the tympanic membrane to the cochlea is based on the force of the energy exerted on the tympanic membrane and footplate of the stapes, and the large difference in the areas of these respective surfaces. Pressure, defined as force per unit area, is an important aspect of the strength of a sound wave. A sound wave traveling in the external auditory meatus applies force to the tympanic membrane, which has an area of roughly 55 mm^2. That force is transmitted across the ossicles and applied to the footplate of the stapes, which has an area of roughly 3 mm^2. The area of the footplate of the stapes is therefore nearly 20 times smaller than the area of the tympanic membrane. Because the force applied to the tympanic membrane by the sound wave travels across the ossicles to be applied to a much smaller area at the footplate of the stapes, the pressure (force/area) at the footplate of the stapes is much greater than it is at the tympanic membrane. The gain in pressure due to the area difference between the tympanic membrane and stapes footplate produces an amplification of approximately 23 to 25 decibels (dB) (which corresponds to a pressure gain of roughly 15:1–18:1). This is the primary way the impedance mismatch between air and fluid is overcome in sound transmission from the external auditory canal to the cochlea.

Sound is also amplified by the middle ear when movement of the ossicles applies a lever force between the malleus and the footplate of the stapes. During tympanic membrane vibration, a very small force applied to the malleus is "levered" to the incus, thus increasing the force exerted by the incus. The effective length of the malleus (effective with respect to its lever potential) is roughly 1.3 times the effective lever length of the incus, creating the hypothesized lever effect. The lever effect is transferred to the stapes and added to the primary effect of the area difference described above. Opinions differ on the extent of the lever effect, but a sound pressure increase of 1 to 3 dB is possible. Some authors (Luers & Hüttenbrink, 2016) have argued that the orientation of the malleus and incus makes the lever effect unlikely as a mechanism to increase energy across the ossicular chain.

A third, possible mechanism for increasing energy from the tympanic membrane to the footplate of the stapes derives from the conical shape of the tympanic membrane. Some authors have argued that small displacements of the tympanic membrane are made larger as they travel to the pointed tip (at the umbo) of the membrane. It is as if the displacements are focused down to the umbo and amplified in the process. The

No Ossicles??

What would happen if we didn't have ossicles? We wouldn't be able to hear as well. Your ossicle-less ear would have a tympanic membrane and a cochlea separated by an air-filled middle ear cavity. Vibrations of air molecules in your outer ear would be transmitted via the tympanic membrane to the air in your middle ear; these molecule vibrations would strike the membrane of the oval window, behind which is the cochlear fluid. Would the fluid in your cochlea be displaced by these sound waves? The answer is "yes," but ineffectively because of the huge impedance mismatch between air and liquid. The ossicle-less ear may transmit sound waves to the round window as well; in this case, the sound pressure strikes both the oval and round windows (discussed later in the text), pitting one sound pressure (applied to the scala vestibuli, via the footplate of the stapes) against an equal sound pressure (applied to the scala tympani, via the round window). The two pressures are equal but applied in opposed directions, so the basilar membrane is not displaced. In either case, the vibration at the tympanic membrane does not produce much (if any) displacement of the basilar membrane. If you have ducked your head under water in a swimming pool and listened to people talking outside the pool, you have experienced this effect. Their speech sounds muffled and indistinct. This is because the sound waves traveling through the air strike the surface of the water and are mostly reflected away. In the ossicle-less ear, much of the sound energy transmitted to the middle ear cavity bounces off the oval window, or off both windows. No ossicles?? Expect a conductive hearing loss of 50 to 60 dB.

possible gain in sound pressure due to this mechanism is thought to be 1 to 2 dB.

Even with the potential controversies surrounding the latter two contributions to solving the impedance mismatch between air and fluid, the tympanic membrane and ossicles clearly transform vibratory energy applied to the tympanic membrane to a pressure at the footplate of the stapes that is effective in displacing the fluid of the cochlea. The "natural" proof of this is the substantial conductive hearing loss associated with an auditory mechanism that lacks ossicles (see sidetrack called No Ossicles??).

In addition to its impedance matching function, the ossicular chain serves to emphasize certain frequencies. The ossicular chain has a resonant frequency around 1000 to 1500 Hz, which means that it vibrates best at these frequencies and selectively "boosts" their energy. Together with the energy "boost" provided by the resonance of the external auditory meatus (around 3300 Hz), the range of frequencies between 1000 and 3500 Hz is amplified relative to other frequencies that travel through the outer and middle ear. These frequency boosts lead to greater auditory sensitivity in the 1000 to 3500 Hz range, which is beneficial to the perception of speech because much of the important energy in the speech signal—energy that serves as cues to phonetic identity—occurs within this frequency range.

These facts concerning transmission of sound energy across the conductive mechanism provide examples of the interdependent nature of structure and function. Anatomical characteristics such as the relative areas of the tympanic membrane and footplate of the stapes, the relative length of "arms" of two ossicles, and the mass and stiffness of the linked ossicular chain help determine amplitude and frequency transmission as the acoustic signal is transferred from the external auditory meatus to the cochlea.

INNER EAR (SENSORINEURAL MECHANISM)

The inner ear is housed in a complex, hollowed-out structure called the bony labyrinth (also called the otic capsule), located deep within the petrous portion of the temporal bone. The bony labyrinth of the right ear is depicted in Figure 13–13. When the bony labyrinth is viewed from the perspective of the tympanic membrane (looking toward the center of the head), the semicircular canals are at the back, the vestibule in the middle, and the cochlea is at the front.

There are two openings into the vestibule of the bony labyrinth. The upper opening is called the oval window, where the footplate of the stapes is attached and held in place by the annular ligament. The lower opening is the round window, which is covered by a membrane similar in structure (although not identical) to the tympanic membrane. When the footplate of the stapes moves inward it displaces fluid, called *perilymph*, that fills much (but not all) of the cochlea. The fluid displacement wave travels through cochlea scalae (or channels) and in doing so exerts force on the round window, causing it to bulge slightly. The movable membrane covering the round window plays an important role in the cochlea's function of transforming hydraulic energy (energy associated with displacement of fluid) into neurochemical and electrical energy. The neurochemical energy produces electrical energy in the form of action potentials. The pattern

---

The Umbo and Its Tiny Ways

The tiny volume of the middle ear cavity, 1 to 2 cm³, is illustrated in Figure 13–6. Not very large, is it? Now consider that the ossicles, housed within this tiny chamber, have linear lengths of no more than 8 mm (usually the malleus) and as short as 3 mm (stapes). Moreover, this miniaturized stuff is embedded in a hard, bony casing—the petrous portion of the temporal bone—making direct experiments on ossicular motion in living, healthy humans close to impossible. An alternative approach to studying the function of middle ear structures of humans is to extract temporal bones from cadaveric material, prepare them carefully for observation, and replicate as closely as possible conditions in the living human (e.g., proper hydration and temperature). Then, sophisticated technology must be employed to make measurements of structural motion in response to applied sound energy. Such research measurements were reviewed by Volandri et al. (2012), who reported that peak-to-peak displacements at the umbo (the entire back and forth excursion) recorded during high-intensity sound input were roughly 100 *nano*meters—about 1/10,000th of a millimeter. The magnitude of these displacements varied by frequency, with the greatest displacements occurring around 1000 Hz. These very tiny motions explain why we have used the term *molecule-sized vibrations* to refer to sound waves and the resulting vibrations of the tympanic membrane and ossicles.

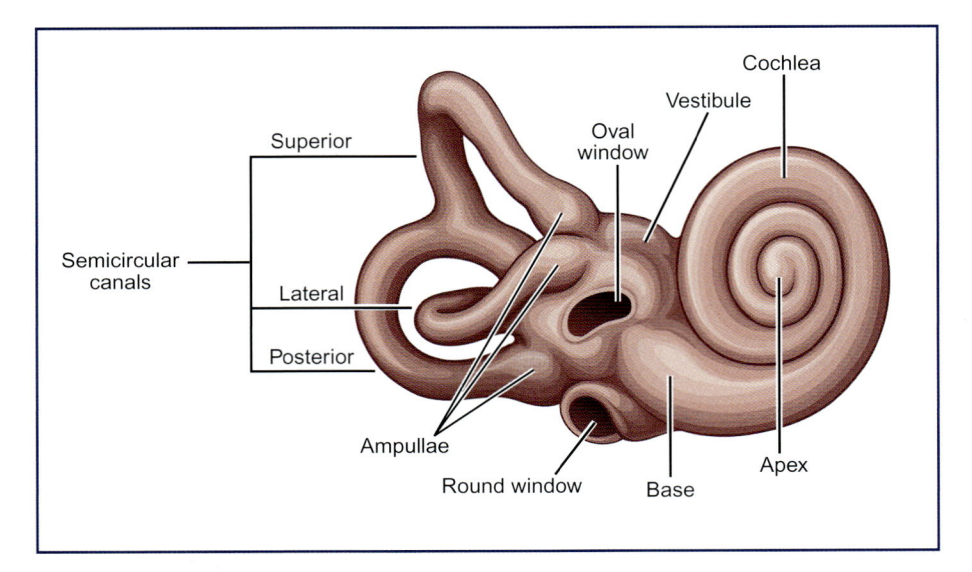

Figure 13–13. Bony labyrinth of the right ear. The semicircular canals are to the left, the cochlea to the right, and the vestibule is in the middle. The spiral of the cochlea rises from base to tip, although that is not shown in this drawing because of the perspective. Note the oval and round windows cut into the vestibule.

of action potentials in the auditory nerve is the first step in neural coding of frequency, intensity, and timing of the acoustic information entering the auditory system. Neurotransmitters and action potentials are discussed in Chapter 15.

The bony labyrinth includes three major structures. These are the semicircular canals, the vestibule, and the cochlea. Structures within the semicircular canals and vestibule are associated with the vestibular system; structures within the cochlea are associated with the auditory system. The focus in this chapter is on the cochlea, but some introductory information on the vestibular system is presented to highlight similarities of the structures within the bony labyrinth.

Vestibular System

The vestibular system is a complex array of peripheral and central structures that detect and code motion of the head in space, as well as relative to the body. The detection of motion of the head in space plays a role in the coordination of gaze and head motion, of gaze and posture, and in the highly sophisticated regulation of complex actions (such as athletic gestures) that evolve over time and through space (Cullen, 2012). The vestibular system also incorporates sophisticated detection of gravitational forces on the head into the coding of head position and motion. What follows is a basic account of the function of the vestibular system.

The peripheral structures of the vestibular system include five sensory organs, as well as the nerve fibers connecting these organs to first synapses in a ganglion. The five sensory organs of the vestibular system are contained within the three bony semicircular canals plus the utricle and saccule, the latter two located in the vestibule of the bony labyrinth (not labeled in Figure 13–13). The neural structures include the nerve fibers attached to sensory organs in these five structures, Scarpa's ganglion, and the vestibular portion of the auditory-vestibular nerve (cranial nerve VIII). Each of these is described briefly below.

The Fluidity of Language

This chapter uses the term *fluid* several times to describe the contents of the bony and membranous labyrinth. The text makes this terminology a bit more precise by indicating that, in the case of cochlear contents, the fluid is a liquid. Technically, any gas (like air) is also a fluid; thus, the claim that the cochlea is a fluid-filled structure could mean it is filled with air, which, as you know by now, is not the case. We use the term *fluid* in the lay sense, but the distinction between the fluid air and a liquid fluid is an important one, in part because air has much lower impedance compared with the liquid in the cochlea (which has an impedance close to that of water). Thus, if you want to be absolutely precise in your language, use the term *liquid* to describe the cochlear contents.

Semicircular Canals

Three semicircular canals make up the most posterior part of the bony labyrinth. One semicircular canal is oriented in the superior-inferior dimension, one extends posteriorly, and one extends laterally. Note in Figure 13–13, which shows the bony labyrinth on the right side of the head, that each canal is oriented at right angles to the other two. In addition, the superior and posterior canals are oriented at 45-degree angles to the midsagittal plane of the head, and the lateral canal is oriented at a 30-degree angle relative to the transverse plane of the head. At the base of each semicircular canal is a dilation, or widening of the bony cavity; these are called the ampullae (plural of ampulla).

Each of the bony canals contains perilymph and endolymph. The perilymph has a chemical composition like that of cerebrospinal fluid. Within the perilymph is a membrane that follows the contours of the bony canals, including the swelling at their bases. This membrane separates the perilymph from the endolymph. Endolymph is chemically different from perilymph. Endolymph contains a high concentration of potassium (K+) ions and low concentration of sodium (Na+) ions; the reverse is true of perilymph.

The ampulla of each semicircular canal contains within the fluid an epithelial tissue layer. This epithelium is continuous with the membrane wall of the duct containing endolymph (that is, the membrane wall that separates the perilymph from the endolymph). The hair cells that respond to angular acceleration (and deceleration) of the head are embedded within this epithelium. Multiple stereocilia—like small hair filaments—protrude from the tips of each hair cell and extend into the endolymph. The hair cells and their multiple stereocilia are covered by a gel called the cupola. This sensory receptor—the membrane, the hair cells and their stereocilia protruding into the endolymph, and the cupola—is called the crista ampullaris (Figure 13–14). Note in this high-magnification photograph the epithelial membrane separating the perilymph from the endolymph.

The stereocilia of each hair cell are arranged by height, from longest to shortest, and their tips are connected by structures called tip links, as depicted schematically in Figure 13–15. The figure shows six stereocilia projecting from each hair cell but typically there are many more. When the head turns in one direction, the endolymph in the semicircular canal and its ampulla on that side are displaced. The fluid displacement causes mechanical displacement of the tip-linked stereocilia relative to their "rest position" embedding in the cupola. When the shortest of the tip-linked stereocilia tilts *toward* the longest stereocilium for a given hair cell, potassium (K+) channels in the hair cell membrane are literally pulled open by the "stretch" of the stereocilia, allowing the high concentration of K+ in the endolymph (as well as other positively charged ions) to rush inside of the cell, causing it to be depolarized (see middle panel of Figure 13–15). This depolarization causes other intracellular processes to induce release of a neurotransmitter into the synaptic cleft between the hair cell base and dendrites of attached nerve fibers. The neurotransmitter binds to receptor sites on those dendrites, which open K+ channels and initiate an action potential in the nerve fiber (see Chapter 15). This neural code for the head turn is not complete without corresponding, paired information from the other side of the vestibular apparatus: the hair cells of the matched semicircular canal on the other side of the head are displaced in the opposite direction, with the tip-linked stereocilia tilted *away* from the longest stereocilium (see Figure 13–15, right panel). This causes the hair cell membrane to close most or all of its K+ channels, hyperpolarizing the cell and preventing it from evoking an action potential in the attached nerve fiber. It is as if the head turn evokes a "yes-no" code: a head turn to one side produces a nerve fiber action potential on the side of the turn ("yes"), but suppresses an action potential on the side opposite the turn ("no"). This paired pattern of impulses is the basic information code on the direction, velocity, and acceleration of a head turn.

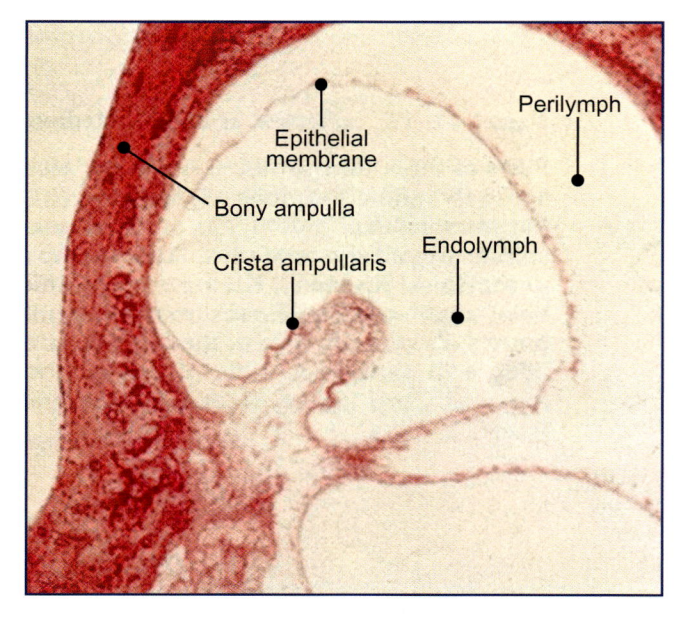

Figure 13–14. High magnification photograph of the sensory receptor, the crista ampullaris, within the ampulla of each semicircular canal. Note how the crista ampullaris protrudes into the endolymph, as well as how the epithelial membrane separates the perilymph from the endolymph.

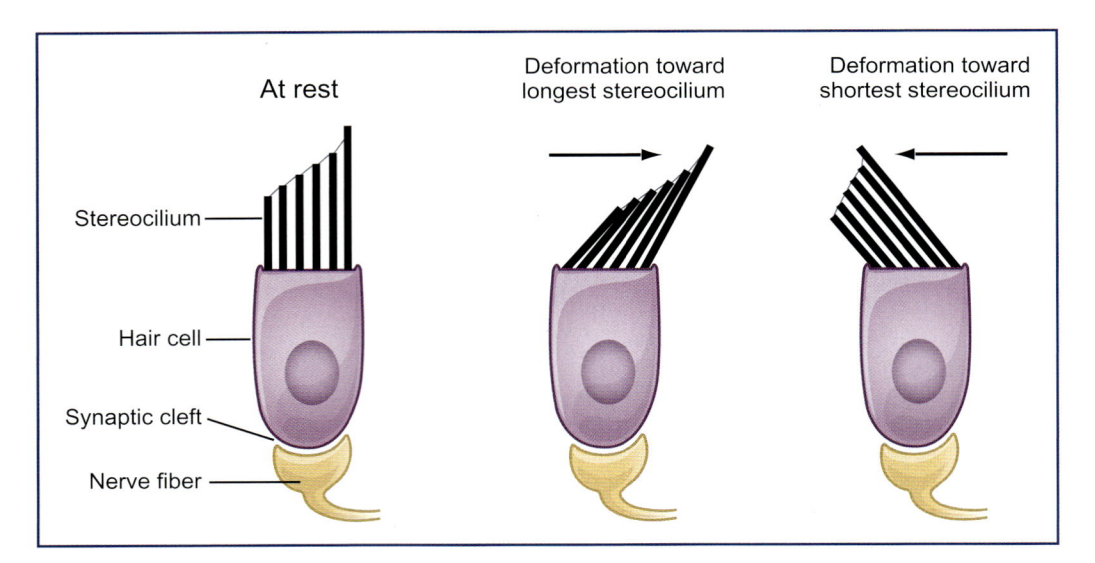

Figure 13–15. Artist rendition of three hair cells in the crista ampullaris. Stereocilia protrude from each hair cell and can be bent by displacement of the fluid within the ampulla. The stereocilia of a hair cell are connected by tip links so that the multiple stereocilia move as a unit when they are displaced. The left hair cell shows the stereocilia at rest (no displacement of the stereocilia). The middle hair cell shows the stereocilia deflected by fluid displacement in the ampulla in the direction of the longest stereocilium; this depolarizes the hair cell and causes the attached nerve to generate an action potential. The right hair cell shows the stereocilia displaced in the direction of the shortest hair stereocilium. This hyperpolarizes the hair cell, inhibiting it from causing an action potential in the hair cell.

Vestibule: Saccule and Utricle

Within the vestibule of the bony labyrinth are the saccule and utricle. These structures contain sensory organs very much like the crista ampullaris, but with some important differences. It is often said that the saccule and utricle sense "linear acceleration" of the head, the former along the horizontal plane, the latter relative to the sagittal plane. A simpler way to state this is that they encode information on the degree of head tilt front to back (saccule) and side to side (utricle).

The sensory organs in the saccule and utricle are called the maculae (singular = macula). The macula is similar to the crista ampullaris in having an epithelial membrane through which hair cells protrude, each hair cell giving off multiple stereocilia embedded in a gel-like substance. The gel-like substance in the saccule and utricle is called the otolithic membrane. The macula differs from the crista ampullaris in having crystals, or tiny stones, resting on top of the otilithic membrane. These crystals are called otoliths, and their weight and mass (and, therefore, added inertia when the stereocilia are displaced by head motion) make the sensory organ of the saccule and utricle very sensitive to small degrees of head position change, as well as to acceleration of the motion.

The transformation of mechanical energy to neurochemical/neuroelectrical energy in the saccule and utricle is like the process described above for the ampullae of the semicircular canals. Side-to-side (utricle) or forward-and-backward (saccule) movement of the head cause displacement of the endolymph in these two structures, which deforms the stereocilia relative to their embedded location in the otolithic membrane. Deformation of the stereocilia opens up K^+ and other positive ion channels in the hair cell membrane, which is a signal for the release of neurotransmitter into the synaptic cleft between the base of the hair cells and the dendrites of the nerve fibers. The nerve fibers are depolarized and send an action potential to Scarpa's ganglion. Scarpa's ganglion, located just inside the proximal (closer to the medial plane of the body) entrance to the internal acoustic meatus, is the first synapse for nerve fibers from both the ampullae of the semicircular canals and the utricle and saccule.

Summary: Vestibular Structures and Mechanisms

The vestibular system includes the three semicircular canals, plus the saccule and the utricle. Nerve fibers from the base of the hair cells in these structures are gathered together to form the vestibular portion of the auditory-vestibular nerve (cranial nerve VIII), making a first synapse in Scarpa's ganglion. The nerve continues through the internal auditory meatus, emerges from the medial opening of the bony canal, and enters the brainstem at the junction of the medulla and pons. The detection of hair cell motion in the ampullae of the semicircular canals, and in the saccule and utricle, is the basis of the nerve fiber activity that encodes the rotation, position, and acceleration of the head relative to the body.

The semicircular canals, saccule, and utricle function together to provide information on the complex positions and motions of the head; rarely are these motions one-dimensional. In addition, information arising from the peripheral vestibular system is coordinated with motion of the eyes, with the prevailing posture of the body (including gravitational forces), and even with cognitive "sets" (such as the different "sets" for walking over flat versus rocky surfaces). For a comprehensive review of all aspects of vestibular structure and function, the reader is referred to Goldberg et al. (2012).

Cochlea

The cochlea (meaning "snail") is a bony, spiral structure embedded within the petrous part of the temporal bone. In humans, the cochlea makes two and a half turns as it curls upward from its base to its apex. The widest part of the snail—at its base—is approximately 10 mm, its height from base to apex is about 5 mm, and in humans its length when uncoiled is about 35 mm (Pickles, 2013).

The bony cochlea is best appreciated in two views. The first view (Figure 13–16) is a section of the bony cochlea cut from tip to base, into back and front halves. This is technically a horizontal section because the

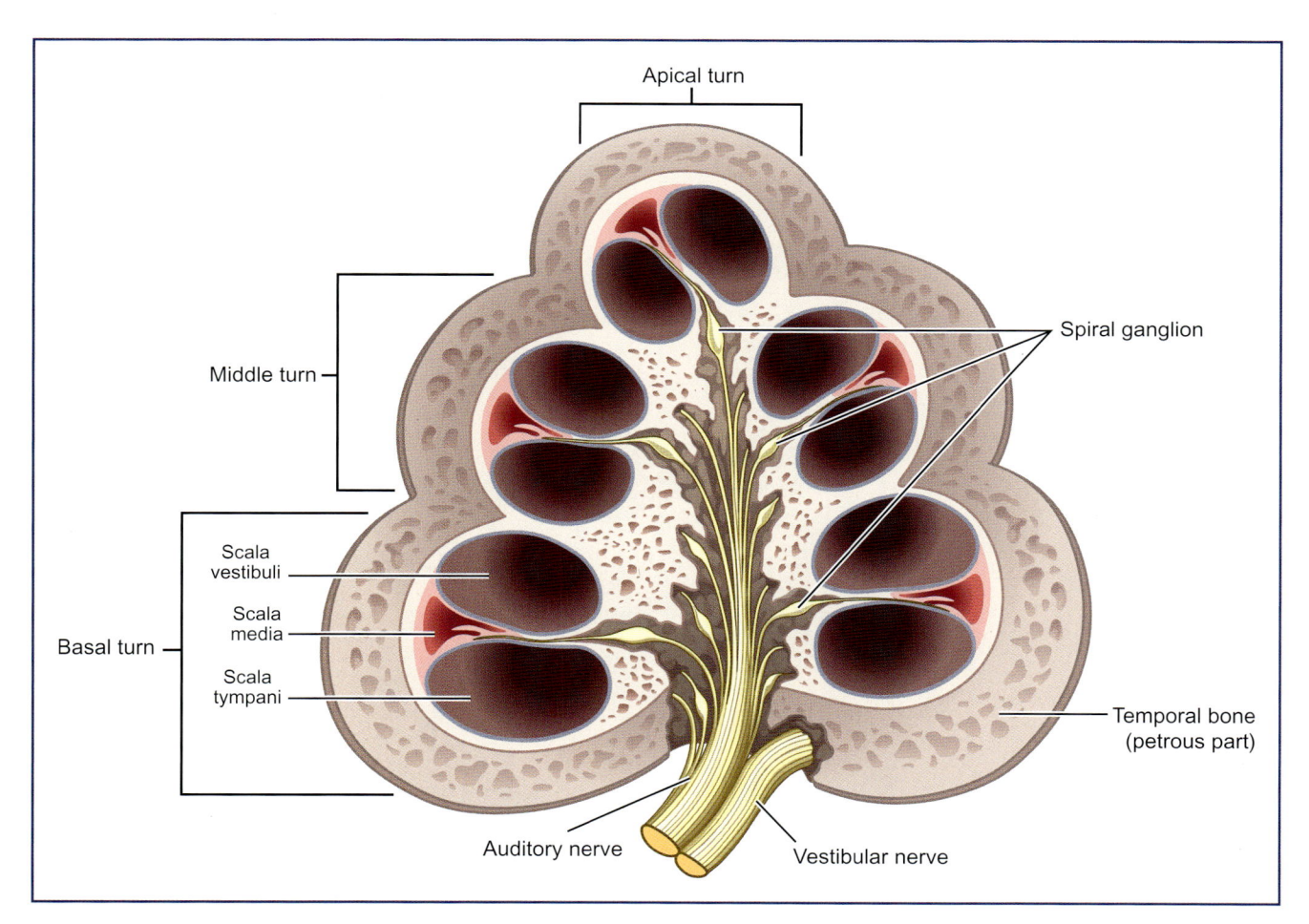

Figure 13–16. The cochlea cut into back and front halves, with a view of the back half. The drawing shows three ducts at each of three turns of the cochlea from base to tip. The spiral ganglion and nerve fibers are shown in the modiolus, the bony, hollowed-out core of the cochlea.

cochlea is oriented in the head as if the tip is pointing along the horizontal axis. The back half of the cochlea is shown in this view. On either side of the center of the slice, two "triplets" of ducts are seen, one triplet at the base (labeled "basal turn" in the figure), the other just above it (labeled "middle turn"). The top triplet of ducts is at the apical turn of the cochlea, at the very tip of which the two outside ducts—the scala vestibuli and scala tympani—are connected. The center "core" section of the cut is called the modiolus (not labeled in Figure 13–16). The turns of the bony cochlea wrap around this center core as they spiral to the apex. The modiolus contains the nerve fibers that innervate the hair cells. It also contains ganglion cells where fibers emerging from the cochlea make their first synapse before continuing to the internal auditory meatus as the auditory part of the auditory-vestibular nerve.

From base to tip, the modiolus sends out two bony shelves toward the outer edges of the spiraling cochlea. These shelves are called the spiral lamina, whose bony extensions serve as the divider between the two outer ducts—the scala vestibuli and scala tympani (labeled only for the basal turns in Figure 13–16). The spiral lamina does not extend to the lateral, bony border of the cochlea. Rather, as described below, membranes extending from the end of the bony lamina to the inside of the lateral border of the cochlea create the third duct sitting between the scala vestibuli and scala tympani. This third duct is called the scala media, or alternately the cochlear duct. All three ducts are filled with fluid.

The second way to appreciate the structure of the cochlea is by studying a zoomed view of the ducts in the cochlea. The zoomed view of the bony cochlea in Figure 13–17 is from its basal turn. From top to bottom the ducts are the scala vestibuli, scala media, and scala tympani. At the beginning of the basal turn of the scala vestibuli, near the section shown in the figure, is the oval window. The termination of the basal turn of the scala tympani is the round window. The two membranes that extend from shelves of the spiral lamina to the outer edge of the cochlea, and enclose the scala media, are called Reissner's membrane (dividing the scala vestibuli from the scala media) and the basilar membrane (dividing the scala tympani from the scala

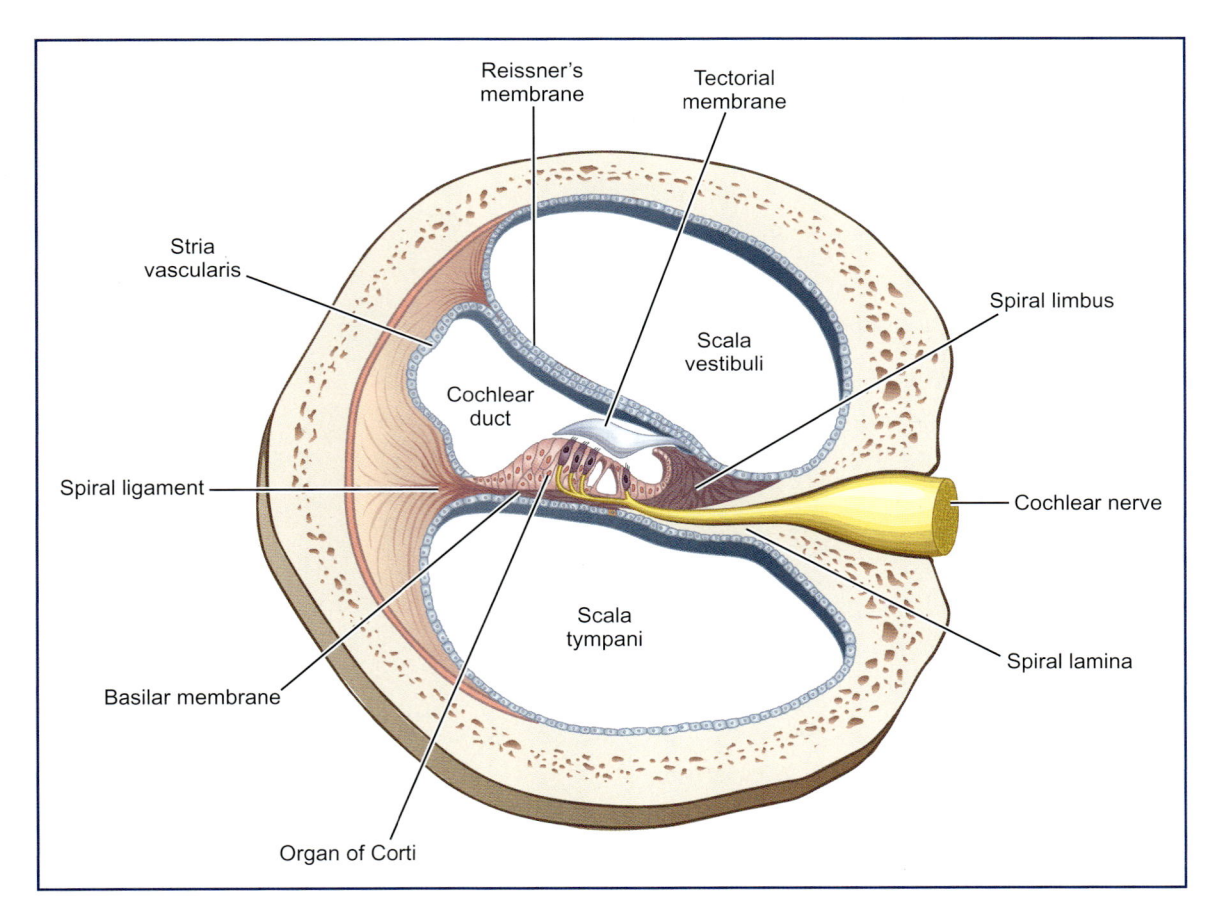

Figure 13–17. Zoom view of cochlear scalae from the basal turn of the cochlea.

media). Reissner's membrane extends from its attachment to the upper shelf of the spiral lamina to attach to the upper part of the spiral ligament covering the inside of the bony cochlea. The basilar membrane extends from the lower shelf of the spiral lamina to attach to the spiral ligament at the inner edge of the bony cochlea (see Figure 13–17). The spiral limbus is the upper, thickened part of the spiral lamina.

The scala media, the space bounded by Reissner's membrane and the basilar membrane, is called the membranous cochlea because its boundaries are defined by membranes, compared with the scala vestibuli and scala tympani, which both have outer, bony boundaries as well as a bony boundary close to the modiolus. Note at the outer edge of the scala media the stria vascularis, a vascular-cellular network that provides blood to the organ of Corti (see below) and maintains the chemical content of the endolymph.

The outer, bony turns of the cochlea enclosing the scala vestibuli and scala tympani are lined on the inside by an epithelial membrane. The fluid in the scala vestibuli and scala tympani is called perilymph, which has a chemical composition rich in sodium (Na+) and low in potassium (K+), similar to the chemical properties of cerebrospinal fluid. In contrast, the scala media is filled with endolymph, a fluid with a chemical composition rich in K+ and scarce in Na+, more or less the reverse of perilymph. The different chemical constituents of perilymph and endolymph in the cochlea are like the differences discussed above for the perilymph and endolymph of the membranous vestibular structures.

The chemical composition of endolymph is critical to the transduction of mechanical energy into chemical energy, which occurs when displacement of the basilar membrane caused by fluid waves in the cochlea results in deformation of the hair cells within the scala media. Ultimately, the chemical changes induced by bending of hair cells results in electrical changes which generate impulses in the auditory fibers of cranial nerve VIII.

The cochlear duct includes many smaller structures critical to the function of the cochlea. Among the most important of these is the organ of Corti, which sits atop the basilar membrane and includes hair cells. In addition, the scala media has a complement of other supporting structures described below. These structures play an important role in the transformation of sound energy into neural signals.

Fluid Motion within the Scalae: A Broad View

As noted above, the scala vestibuli and scala tympani are connected at the apex (tip) of the cochlea. The passageway where the two ducts communicate is called the heliocotrema. This connection allows fluid displacement caused by vibration of the footplate of the stapes into and out of the oval window to displace fluid throughout the scala vestibuli and transmit this motion to the scala tympani. The fluid displacement into the scala tympani results in a bulging of the round window (the termination of the scala tympani).

Figure 13–18 illustrates the general characteristics of fluid displacement in the cochlea by showing the structure as if it were uncoiled and the ducts of the cochlea were extended in a straight line. The basilar membrane, the dividing partition between the scala media and scala tympani, is shown as the flat structure in pink whose width varies from very narrow at the base to increasingly wide as it approaches the tip. The basilar membrane does not quite reach the end of the tip of the cochlea; the apical opening between the two outer ducts is the heliocotrema. The top channel in this view—the duct associated with the oval window—is the scala vestibuli, and the bottom channel is the scala tympani.

Fluid motion in the scala vestibuli and scala tympani takes the form of waves. Broadly speaking, there are pressure differences in these waves between the scala vestibuli and scala tympani, which cause the basilar membrane to be displaced in ways that depend on the location and pattern of the pressure differences. The organ of Corti, on the basilar membrane, responds to these waves with displacement of the hair cells. Movement of the basilar membrane and the organ of Corti in response to fluid displacement is a critical part of the sensory function of the cochlea.

Hair Cells and Associated Structures

The basilar membrane and organ of Corti with its hair cells are shown in Figure 13–19 as a cross-section at a single "slice" along the scala media. It is as if the unrolled cochlea of Figure 13–18 has been cut along its length, in the same way a loaf of bread is sliced at one point along its length. The view is directly into the contents of the scala media. The scala vestibuli and scala tympani, although not drawn in this magnified image, are at the top and bottom, respectively.

To appreciate the magnification of this image relative to the size of the actual organs, consider that the nearly vertical structures labeled "inner hair cell" and "outer hair cells" are roughly 30 micrometers (0.000030 meters, around 1/1000th of an inch) in length and 10 micrometers in diameter. Figure 13–19 shows many different cell types forming the organ of Corti. Several of these serve a support function, giving stability to the organ of Corti. These support cells include (but are not limited to) Deiters cells and pillar cells. Deiters cells, not labeled in Figure 13–19, are at the base of

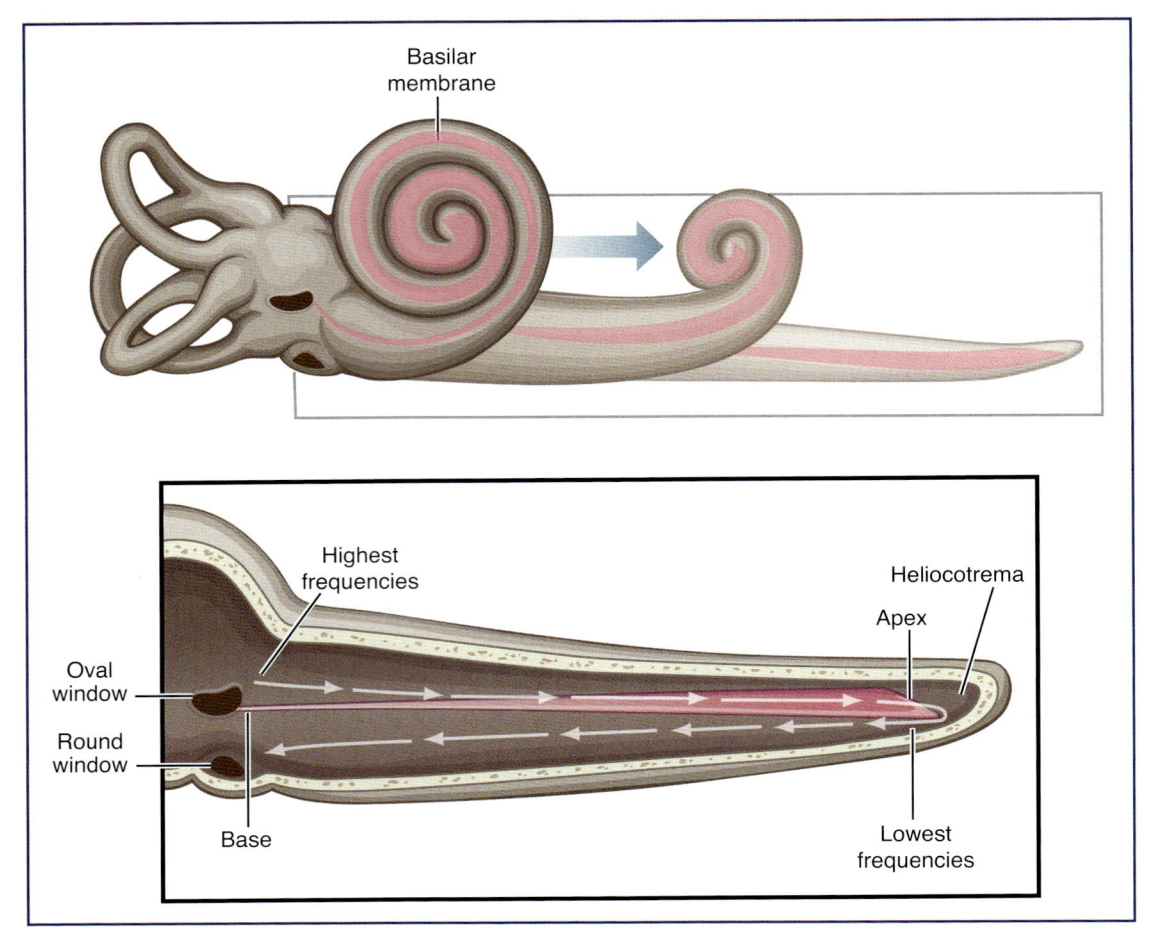

Figure 13–18. The cochlea as if unrolled (*top*) to form a straight tube (*bottom*). In the bottom image the scala vestibuli is the top duct (above the pink basilar membrane) and the scala tympani is the bottom duct. The basilar membrane is shown as the pink partition, narrow and stiff at the base and wide and floppy at the apex.

the outer hair cells and surround the inner hair cells. The pillar cells, also unlabeled in Figure 13–19, are the angled walls of the triangular space labeled "tunnel of Corti." These support cells play a role in the mechanical behavior of the hair cells, mostly by stabilizing the organ of Corti and ensuring that deformation of hair cells during fluid displacement permits them to undergo chemical changes that are converted into electrical energy and ultimately neural impulses. The support cells and tissue projections from them also reach up from the basilar membrane to form a continuous membrane connecting the apices (tops) of the inner and outer hair cells, from one side to the other of the scala media. This is the reticular membrane, which seals off the part of the organ of Corti below the hair cells from the rest of the scala media.

The outer hair cells are typically in rows of three (sometimes rows of four, or even five) and the inner hair cells form a single row. The outer hair cells are on the side of the cochlear duct facing the outer wall of the cochlea. On that wall is the stria vascularis (see Figure 13–17), the structure that provides blood to the organ of Corti and regulates the chemical (ionic) composition of the perilymph. The inner hair cells are on the side of the scala media facing the modiolus (center) of the cochlear spiral. The triangular space separating the inner and outer hair cells is called the tunnel of Corti, which contains a fluid similar to perilymph (typically referred to as corticolymph). Above the hair cells is a gel-like structure called the tectorial membrane, with one end fixed at the modiolus and the other end floating in endolymph (see also Figure 13–17).

At the top of each hair cell are tufts of hairy-looking extensions, called stereocilia. Stereocilia are tiny filaments extending from the tips of the hair cells. As in the vestibular system, the stereocilia projecting from

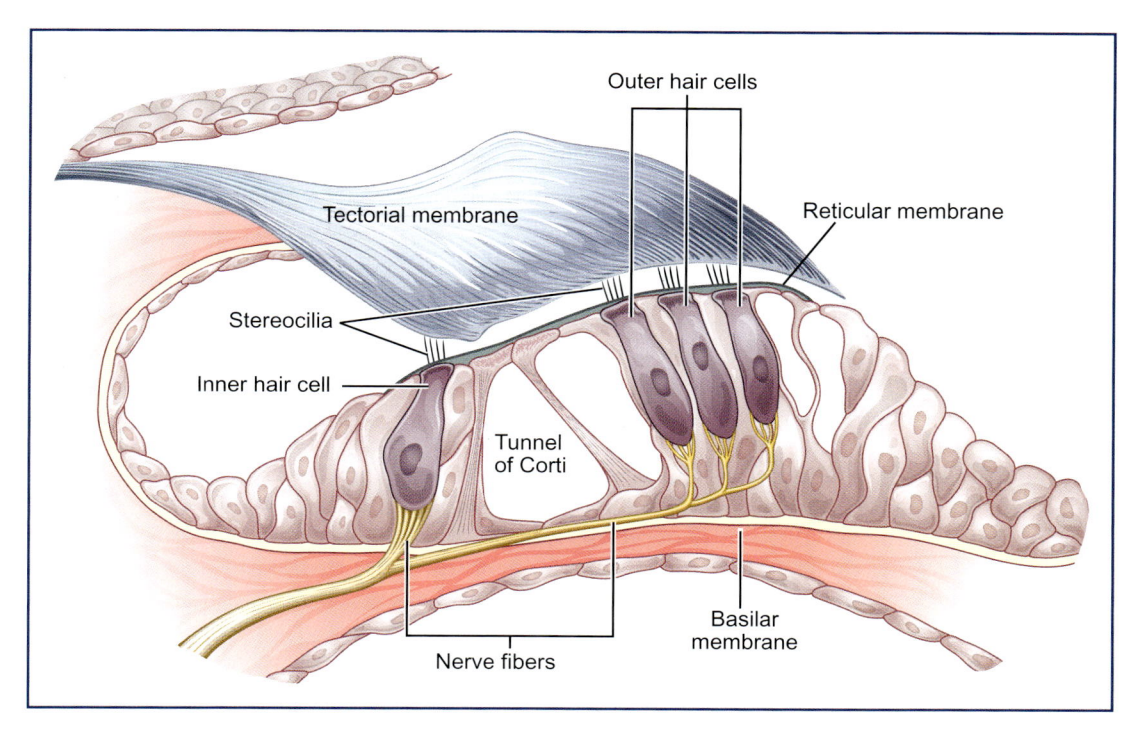

Figure 13–19. Drawing of organ of Corti, and other components of the sensory organ of hearing, as well as the nerves attached to the bottom of the hair cells.

the tip of a single hair cell are ordered from longest to shortest. Also similar to the vestibular system, the stereocilia projecting from a single hair cell are connected, or linked to one another by small filaments at the tip (see Figure 13–15). The functional result of these tip links is that when the stereocilia are deformed from their resting position, they move as a unit, either toward the longest stereocilium or toward the shortest one. The stereocilia of the outer hair cells are embedded within the tectorial membrane above them; the stereocilia of inner hair cells are not necessarily embedded in the tectorial membrane but are loosely contained within it by a shallow groove in the underside of the membrane.

The reticular membrane plays an important role in separating the fluid components of the cochlear duct. Specifically, the reticular membrane seals off the contents of the organ of Corti below the tips of the hair cells from the contents above it. The stereocilia and the tectorial membrane are suspended above the reticular membrane, in endolymph, whereas the main hair cells and supporting cells such as Deiters cells and pillar cells are in corticolymph, below the reticular membrane. The chemical makeup of the endolymph is essential to the depolarization of hair cells that results when the stereocilia are deformed in the direction of the longest one.

Inner Hair Cells. The hair cells within the organ of Corti are critical to auditory sensation, much like the rods and cones of the retina, the end organ of vision, are critical to visual sensation. Although both the inner and outer hair cells contribute to hearing sensitivity, they do so in very different ways.

Stereocilia of the inner hair cells are deformed by fluid motion within the cochlea. The hydraulic motion (movement of the fluid within the cochlea) displaces the stereocilia which causes chemical changes within the hair cell. These chemical changes modify the electrical charge within the hair cell, a release of a neurotransmitter that depolarizes the nerve cell, which sends an impulse down the axon, toward the spiral ganglion. Note in Figure 13–19 how the inner hair cells have nerve fibers (shown in yellow) extending from their base and are gathered into a larger bundle as they move to the left of the image, toward the modiolus. Nerve fibers from the base of the inner hair cells have their first synapses in the spiral ganglion. The ganglion cells send auditory nerve fibers through the internal auditory meatus to the brainstem. Because the nerve fibers from the inner hair cells send impulses from the peripheral end organ of hearing to the central nervous system, they are referred to as the afferent component of the auditory nerve.

The inner hair cells and the nerves to which they are connected perform a frequency and amplitude analysis of the acoustic pressure wave that initiated displacement of fluid in the cochlea. In humans, these analyses are exquisitely precise. The perceptual result of this frequency analysis is discussed in Chapter 14.

Outer Hair Cells. The outer hair cells are also connected to the central nervous system by nerve fibers, specifically by efferent fibers descending from the brainstem. Nerve tracts (bundles of fibers) emerge from brainstem nuclei and exit the brainstem to run in the auditory nerve and terminate at the base of the outer hair cells. The outer hair cells, stimulated by impulses from brainstem cells, vibrate and in so doing amplify and tune the response of the inner hair cells to the displacement of cochlear fluid. The outer hair cells are often referred to as the *cochlear amplifier*. This is because the efferent signals from the central nervous system appear to cause movement of the outer hair cells that affects the displacement of the basilar membrane, and therefore the deformation of the inner hair cells. The effect of the efferent system is, by its mechanical effect on basilar membrane motion, to amplify very small movements of the membrane and to sharpen the frequency analysis. The amplification is particularly effective for sounds with very little energy. A cochlea without outer hair cells would be a cochlea with poor sensitivity to the wide range of sound energies in the environment, including speech and music.

The arrangement of the inner and outer hair cells along the basilar membrane is critical to understanding how the cochlea performs its frequency analysis. The unrolled cochlea in Figure 13–18 shows the basilar membrane to be narrow at its base (the left end of the membrane in the figure) and increasingly wider as it extends to the apex of the cochlea. The narrow base of the basilar membrane is very stiff, and the wide apical end is relatively floppy. The hair cells at the base (narrow part) of the membrane are sensitive to the *highest* frequencies humans can hear (about 20,000 Hz). Moving away from the base toward the tip of the basilar membrane, the hair cells are sensitive to increasingly lower frequencies until at the tip they are sensitive to the *lowest* frequencies humans are capable of hearing (about 20 Hz). Frequency, therefore, is represented tonotopically along the basilar membrane such that the location of a hair cell along the membrane specifies its frequency sensitivity. The tonotopic organization of frequency sensitivity along the basilar membrane is linked to the concept of fluid displacement in the cochlea as a traveling wave.

Traveling Waves

The tonotopic arrangement of hair cells running from base to apex of the basilar membrane raises the question of how different locations along the membrane are stimulated when vibratory motions of the conductive mechanism are transferred to the cochlear fluid. The explanation of the cochlear response to vibration requires an understanding of how nerve fibers associated with different frequencies are made to fire and are dependent on the wave motion of fluid in the cochlea.

Georg von Békésy (1899–1972), a Hungarian physicist and engineer, observed the cochlea's response to sinusoidal sound energy in several mammals, including humans. Békésy observed that when the footplate of the stapes vibrated in response to sound energy introduced into the external auditory meatus, perilymph in the scala vestibuli was displaced and a fluid wave traveled from the base of the cochlea to its apex. Most importantly, Békésy observed that the location of maximum wave amplitude varied from base to apex depending more or less directly on the frequency of the sound energy. When frequency was low, the wave amplitude built up gradually and reached its peak near the apex of the basilar membrane, some distance from the oval window. In contrast, high frequency sound energy produced a fluid wave that built to a peak at short distances from the oval window (that is, near the base), with a quickly decreasing amplitude as the wave moved from its crest toward the apex. In his world-famous 1928 paper, Békésy described this fluid movement and its varying amplitude as a traveling wave.

Figure 13–20 shows a schematic view of two different traveling waves in an uncoiled representation of the cochlea. The top representation of the unrolled cochlea shows a straight line (no wave) from base (where the stapes fits into the oval window) to apex. This is the theoretical case when there is no sound transmitted across the conductive mechanism, and therefore no traveling wave in the cochlea (see sidetrack called Air Molecules Do Not Rest). The middle pattern shows a traveling wave for a relatively low frequency sound, a 400 Hz sinusoid, captured at a single instant in time. As expected from the tonotopic arrangement of hair cells, the greatest amplitude of this traveling wave is relatively close to the apex of the cochlea. Note the broad displacement of the wave below the peak displacement of the wave (that is, away from the peak toward the base). The bottom pattern in the figure shows a large-amplitude wave closer to the base, with a rapidly decreasing amplitude as the wave moves past this crest and toward the apex. This is like the traveling wave pattern observed for a 4000 Hz sinusoid.

Throughout his experiments, Békésy observed the tendency for the basilar membrane to be maximally deformed at a location that depended on the frequency of the incoming sinusoid. The peaks of the traveling waves vary by frequency partially due to the mechanical differences in the tissue along the membrane: the

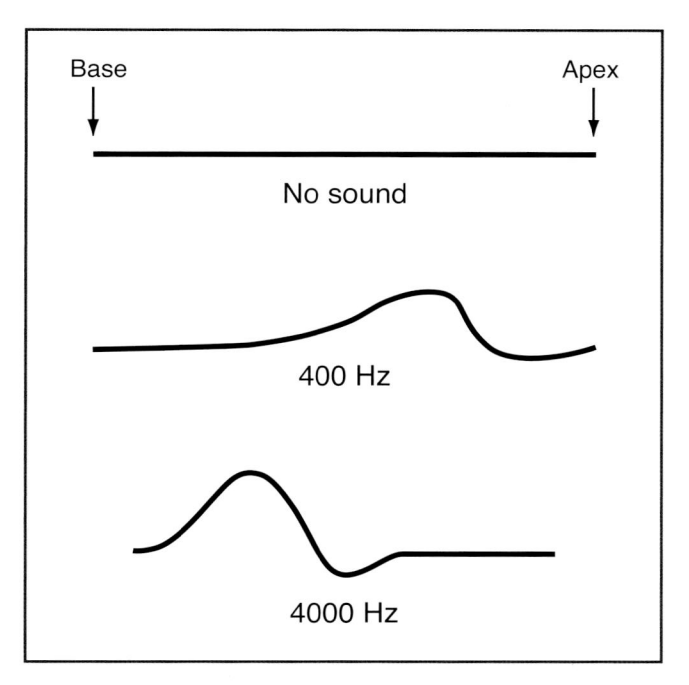

Figure 13-20. Schematic representation of the traveling wave along the basilar membrane in response to a 400 Hz tone (*middle*) and a 4000 Hz tone (*bottom*). The top line shows the reference pattern of no sound (and therefore no traveling wave).

stiff base of the membrane moves better at higher frequencies and the floppy apex moves better at lower frequencies. However, even though Békésy observed clear evidence that the peak (greatest displacement) of the traveling wave was frequency dependent, a given sinusoid seemed to produce a broad length of displacement even at frequencies distant from the peak. The notion that frequency analysis in the cochlea is based on the location of the maximum displacement of the traveling wave, and its stimulation of specific frequencies according to the tonotopic arrangement of the basilar membrane, is called the *place theory* of frequency analysis. The place theory is discussed further in Chapter 14.

Békésy called the cochlear displacement patterns traveling waves because they literally traveled through the perilymph of the cochlea; that is, it took time for the fluid to move from the base to the apex of the cochlea. Of course, the time delay between displacement of the stapes and arrival of the wave at the apex of the cochlea is extremely brief (on average, about 0.000090 second; 90 microseconds, or 90 μsec). The fact that there is any delay of fluid motion between the base and apex supports the idea of a fluid wave moving over time from the point of origin (the oval window) to the apex of the cochlea.

The nature of the traveling wave also suggests that, for a given frequency, wave patterns such as those in Figure 13–20 are snapshots in time. Even for

---

Air Molecules Do Not Rest

The absence of a traveling wave does not mean that air molecules at the tympanic membrane are at rest, waiting for a friendly force to bump them and put them into motion. These are the molecules that if set into vibration send energy across the ossicles, causing displacement of the stapes into the oval window to initiate a traveling wave. A group of air molecules that are not subjected to an applied force still move around with tiny motions, bumping into one another over and over. These small motions are not systematic; they are random in direction and displacement. This is called brownian motion, and it has been studied by famous physicists, including Albert Einstein. Brownian motion occurs in fluids (liquids and gases). Hence, there is brownian motion of liquid fluid within the cochlea. At any single "slice in time" the molecules may appear to be slightly compressed in one location, and slightly rarefied in another. Over time, however, at rest the average distance between any two molecules in the group is the same as the average distance between any two other molecules—mathematically, the molecules all appear to be at their rest positions. Molecules in fluid have a motion schedule that is 24/7, but one that averages out to "no motion" over time. This is why we refer to the rest position of the basilar membrane, and the fluid within the cochlea (see Figure 13–20), as "theoretical."

---

the same, single frequency—a sinusoid—the wave has a different appearance depending on the instant in time when the traveling wave pattern is captured. The waves "build up" over time, even if the relevant time intervals are extremely brief. For example, the 4000 Hz wave may look somewhat different if the snapshot is taken very close to the onset of the sound, or later when the sound has been continuously stimulating the peripheral auditory system.

When the basilar membrane is displaced, so are the stereocilia projecting from the tips of the hair cells. More precisely, the displacement of the basilar membrane causes the stereocilia associated with a single hair cell to be deformed in such a way as to be "pulled" in the direction of the longest stereocilium. In the case of a high-frequency sinusoid, the large amplitude displacement toward the base of the cochlea causes greater deformation of the stereocilia of hair cells in this region, which results in the firing of high-frequency nerve fibers (discussed more fully below).

This description of traveling waves, based on Békésy historical experiments and other similar experiments over the past 90 years, is simplified. It is correct only in the broad sense (which does not diminish its impact on the understanding of auditory processes). The broad sense is that sound energy delivered to the cochlea from vibration of the stapes results in a traveling wave in the cochlear fluids, which causes the basilar membrane to be displaced and the stereocilia projecting from hair cells to be deformed. The greatest (peak) displacement of the basilar membrane, and therefore greatest deformation of the stereocilia, depends on the frequency of the incoming sound energy. This fits well with the concept of tonotopic arrangement of hair cells. In Békésy's experiments, the traveling wave also had substantial displacements in locations away from the peak displacement, suggesting that a single-frequency acoustic input stimulated large portions of the basilar membrane and the hair cells within the organ of Corti.

This latter conclusion from Békésy's work, that the traveling wave for a single-frequency acoustic event affects a broad length of the basilar membrane, has been shown by more recent research to be incorrect in certain important ways. The details of why the conclusion is not correct serve as an excellent object lesson in how experimental technique and its limitations may affect scientific observation even when research is conducted in an exemplary, careful way. First, the temporal bones available to Békésy were cadaver material, and therefore different from living tissue especially in hydration and temperature characteristics. Second, because the tissue was dead the chemical composition of cochlear fluids deviated from those in the living cochlea. Although these problems were addressed in the experiments, to the degree possible at the time (early and mid-twentieth century), the traveling waves observed under these conditions differed from living traveling waves. A related problem was the decreased sensitivity of these dead tissues to sound energy. Békésy was required to use very high sound energy inputs at the stapes to elicit motion of the basilar membrane. In more contemporary work, scientists have been able to induce traveling waves in living animals at low sound-level inputs. An important outcome of these more modern experiments is that the "shape" of the traveling wave—its "peakiness" and broadness—is different at low sound-level inputs, compared with high-level inputs. Low-level inputs produce a traveling wave that does not have a broad pattern of displacement, such as the traveling waves observed by Békésy. Rather, the traveling waves induced by low-level, sinusoidal inputs have displacements more localized to the hair cells corresponding in placement along the basilar membrane to the frequency of the input signal. Figure 13–21 shows two schematic traveling waves in response to a 400 Hz sinusoid at high sound levels (solid line) versus low sound levels (dashed line). The right-hand edge of the figure represents the base of the cochlea, and the label "24 mm" above the peak of the traveling wave indicates the location along the basilar membrane where the peak occurs. Both traveling waves have maximum displacement at the same location along the basilar membrane, as expected, but at low sound levels the membrane displacements at frequencies other than 400 Hz are less than they are at higher sound levels. Also, the slope of the travel-

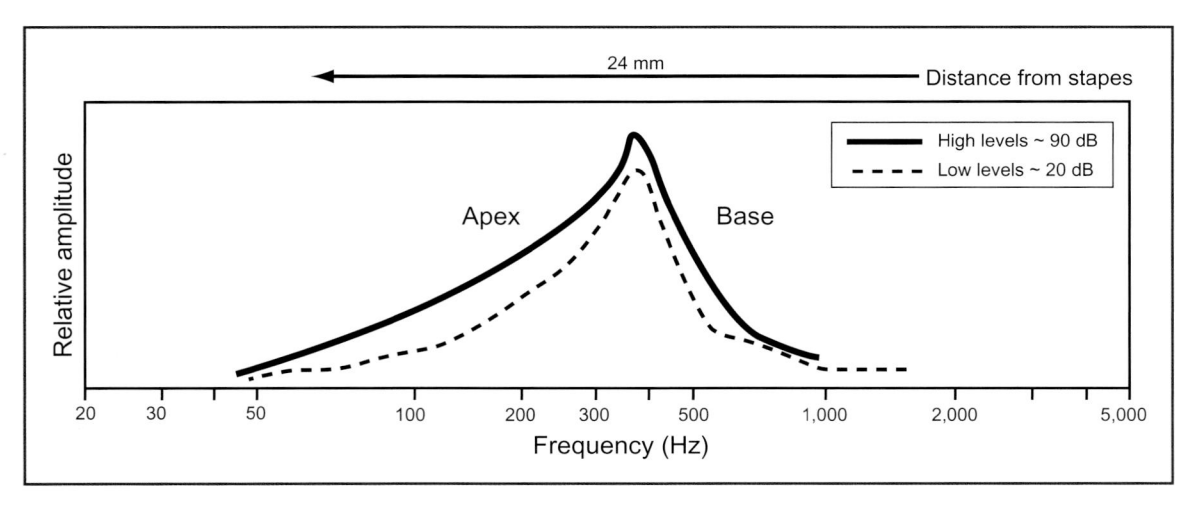

Figure 13–21. Two traveling waves with peak displacements evoked by the same frequency (400 Hz) at two different sound levels. Note the greater amplitude and broader range of displacements associated with the high—compared with low—level sound.

> **Waving It to a More Advanced Course**
>
> The reader may have noticed that there is no explanation of why the traveling wave has peak displacements at different locations along the basilar membrane, depending on the input frequency. As one alternate hypothesis, why doesn't *any* displacement of the perilymph, by stapes vibration at any frequency, always result in a traveling wave with a peak displacement at the same location along the basilar membrane? A full explanation is beyond the scope of this chapter, but physical laws explain why a high-frequency tone evokes a traveling wave with a peak toward the base of the cochlea, and a low-frequency tone evokes a traveling wave with a peak toward the apex, and so forth for other frequencies. The explanation involves the interaction between the frequency of the input vibration, the varying stiffness of the basilar membrane, and the inertial characteristics of cochlear fluid (Pickles, 2013). For more on the traveling wave, stay tuned further down the path of your education.

ing wave from the peak is steeper for the low level compared with the high level. In living mammals, therefore, and for relatively low level sounds, the traveling wave is sharply tuned around the frequency of the sound (assuming a sinusoidal input signal). Pickles (2013) has an excellent review of the historical and contemporary observations of the traveling wave.

The Traveling Wave Is Transformed to Action Potentials

The inner hair cells are mechanoelectrical transducers. When the traveling wave deforms the basilar membrane at a specific location along the cochlea, the stereocilia in that region are deformed by the fluid displacement. Recall that the stereocilia for a given hair cell are arranged by length and are connected by "tip links." For an individual hair cell, the deformation of its stereocilia is a group deformation and because of the tip links, the stereocilia move as a unit. This deformation is typically a "pull" in the direction of the longest stereocilium. This is the "mechano" part of mechanoelectrical transduction.

At rest the hair cells are polarized, with a potential inside the cells roughly 45 to 70 mV less than the potential in the endolymph. Much of this resting potential is due to the concentration of positive ions in the extracellular fluid (fluid outside the cell membrane). The ion gradient (difference in ions across the membrane) favors the movement of positively charged potassium ions (K+) and other positive ions from the extracellular fluid to the intracellular fluid (fluid inside the cell). At rest, however, the hair cell membrane blocks the passage of these positive ions into the intracellular fluid. When the stereocilia are pulled sufficiently in response to fluid motion, the pull causes specialized membrane pores or channels to open, almost like a pull on closed shutters. The opened channels are specialized to allow the K+ and other positive ions to cross the membrane. The hair cell is depolarized when the positive ions rush into it, which creates a very brief reversal of the resting potential (see Chapter 15). Depolarization of the hair cell causes the contents of neurotransmitter packets to be dumped into the synaptic cleft between the base of the hair cell and the dendrites of afferent auditory nerves. The neurotransmitter depolarizes the nerve fiber, evoking an all-or-none action potential which travels along the fiber in the direction of the central nervous system. This depolarization is the "electrical" part of the mechanoelectrical transduction.

AUDITORY NERVE AND AUDITORY PATHWAYS (NEURAL MECHANISM)

Each auditory nerve fiber exits the base of an inner hair cell (see Figure 13–19) and makes a connection (synapse) with the nerve cell bodies of the spiral ganglion, located in the modiolus (see Figure 13–16). Cell bodies in the spiral ganglion send axons to the central nervous system, where they have synapses with cell bodies that make up auditory brainstem nuclei.

The auditory nerve includes all nerve fibers that run between the cochlea and the brainstem. The central auditory pathways are those nuclei and tracts (bundles of axons) that conduct auditory information between the brainstem and the cortex, and that descend into the brainstem as part of the efferent auditory system. The central auditory pathways are *dedicated* in the sense that the nuclei and tracts are specialized for processing of auditory signals. The notion of dedicated nervous system structures does not mean the structures lack communication with other neural systems. Indeed, central auditory structures communicate extensively with cortical and subcortical structures serving speech motor control (as one example). Nevertheless, the central auditory pathways are specialized for the auditory analysis and processing of acoustic events in the environment.

Auditory Nerve and Associated Structures

The auditory nerve forms into a bundle as nerve fibers emerge from the spiral ganglion. Just like hair cells on the basilar membrane, the auditory nerve is arranged tonotopically. In the case of the inner hair cells, the outside fibers (fibers on the surface) of the nerve bundle are from the base of the cochlea, and therefore carry impulses resulting from high-frequency stimulation of the hair cells. From the surface of the nerve bundle to its core, the fibers carry information from increasingly lower frequencies. Fibers at the core of the auditory nerve carry information on very low frequencies, originating in inner hair cells from the apex of the basilar membrane.

Efferent Auditory System

The afferent portion of the peripheral auditory system makes intuitive sense—like all the senses, signals pass from the environment through peripheral structures (such as the outer and middle ear) to the inner hair cells and eventually through nerve fibers to the central nervous system. The purpose of the efferent auditory system is less intuitive, and in fact the details of its function remain controversial, although auditory scientists agree on its importance. What follows is a summary of the lower brainstem anatomy and assumed function of the efferent auditory system. The efferent auditory system also comprises central nervous system structures that include the cortex, medial geniculate nucleus of the thalamus, inferior colliculus in the midbrain, and cochlear nuclei in the pons/medulla (Terreros & Delano, 2015). This corticofugal pathway (descending from the cortex through central nervous system structures to deliver nerves to the auditory periphery) parallels the ascending structures shown in Figure 13–24 (later in this chapter), but in the opposite direction. An in-depth discussion of auditory corticofugal structures and functions is beyond the scope of this textbook. The focus in this section is on the lower brainstem part of the corticofugal pathway.

The superior olivary complex is a group of nuclei located in the pons, and a component of the ascending (from brainstem to cortex) central auditory pathways. The medial cluster of cells in the superior olivary complex, on either side of the midline of the pons, also send descending fibers to the cochlea, via the auditory nerve, to innervate the base of the outer hair cells. Cells from both sides of the medial nuclei in the superior olivary complex innervate each cochlea. Based on an image in Cooper and Guinan (2006), Figure 13–22 shows the contralateral connections from the medial nuclei to outer hair cells as blue lines, and the ipsilateral connec-

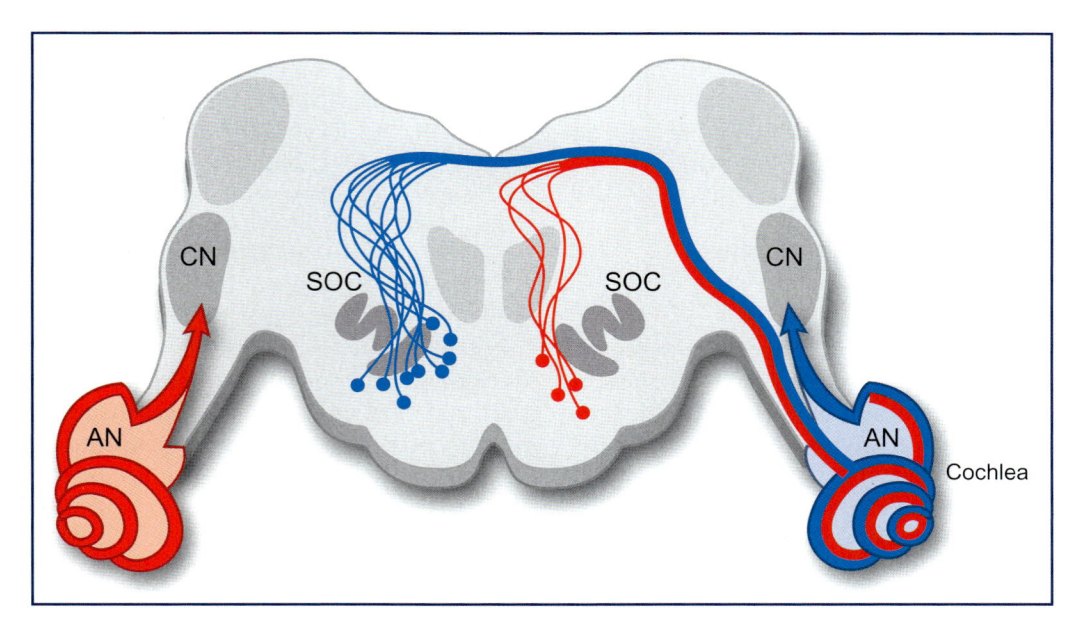

Figure 13–22. Organization of the lower brainstem part of the efferent auditory system. Neurons in the medial part of the superior olivary complex (SOC) in the brainstem send axons to synapse with both ipsilateral and contralateral outer hair cells in the cochlea. Connections are shown for only one cochlea; organization is the same for the other brainstem circuits and cochlea. AN = auditory nerve; CN = cochlear nucleus. Based on Cooper and Guinan (2006, Figure 1).

tions as red lines. The figure shows these connections only for one cochlea, but the contralateral-ipsilateral innervation pattern applies to the other cochlea as well.

What is the function of the efferent auditory system? There is general agreement that the efferent connections stimulate motion of the outer hair cells that directly affects the mechanical properties of the basilar membrane. Specifically, efferent neural stimulation of the outer hair cells affects details of the traveling wave, such as the location of peak displacement of the wave as well as the shape of the wave (Cooper & Guinan, 2006). The efferent auditory system has been shown to both amplify and attenuate (decrease) motion of the basilar membrane. The system may serve a protective function by preventing too much amplification of basilar membrane motion, and may also produce enhanced motion for very soft sounds.

A clear effect of the efferent auditory system is to sharpen the shape, and therefore frequency selectivity, of the traveling wave. The efferent auditory mechanism modifies the mechanical effects of the traveling wave to produce a more sharply tuned displacement of the basilar membrane, and therefore more precise frequency analysis by the inner hair cells and their attached nerve fibers. Experiments in animals have shown that cutting the efferent connections from the superior olivary complex to the outer hair cells greatly reduces the sharpness of the traveling wave, and therefore the precision of inner hair cell frequency analysis. The precise mechanisms that allow the efferent auditory system to modify basilar membrane displacement patterns are not well understood. The following section expands the idea of precision of frequency analysis by the auditory portion of the auditory-vestibular nerve.

"Tuning" of the Peripheral Frequency Response

The tonotopic arrangement of the hair cells and auditory nerve fibers has been described, as well as the way in which the traveling wave reflects the frequency of sound energy. The location along the basilar membrane of peak displacement of the traveling wave determines which hair cells are deformed, which in turn determines which nerve fibers are depolarized to conduct signals to the brainstem. A reasonable question is: How specific is the pattern of nerve fiber depolarization when the simplest kind of acoustic signal—a "pure tone"—is the input to the cochlea?

The answer to this question is complicated, but can be addressed with an introduction to the concept of frequency tuning curves. Imagine an experiment in which a series of pure tones ranging from very low to very high frequency are introduced to the cochlea while monitoring the firing rate (number of impulses, or action potentials, per second) of a single nerve fiber attached to an inner hair cell. This single nerve fiber is selected from a predetermined hair cell location along the basilar membrane, which means that something about the frequency characteristic of the hair cell/nerve fiber is known. For example, a nerve fiber attached to a basal-turn hair cell is known to be a high-frequency fiber, and a nerve fiber attached to a hair cell close to the apex is known to be a low-frequency fiber. The exact frequency of the selected nerve fiber may not be known—its determination is part of the experiment. Specialized, miniaturized recording devices are attached to the selected nerve fiber to record the number of depolarizations per second, called the firing rate, in response to a range of pure-tone frequencies. The experimental technique introduces each frequency at a very low sound energy (usually measured in decibels) and increases the energy until the fiber fires at a predetermined threshold rate. The goal of the experiment is to determine the threshold curve, based on this threshold firing rate, for a single fiber at a variety of input frequencies. These experiments have been performed in mammals such as cats and chinchillas (see Heil & Peterson, 2015 for a review) but, as described in Chapter 14 on auditory psychophysics, can be estimated in humans from behavioral data.

One set of data, for a fiber connected to a hair cell closer to the base of the basilar membrane than to its tip, is shown in the left plot of Figure 13–23. The x-axis shows the pure-tone input frequency from 0.1 Hz to 10.0 kHz and the y-axis shows the level of energy (in dB sound pressure level [SPL]) required to reach the firing rate threshold for action potentials in the measured nerve fiber. The input frequency axis (x-axis) is scaled logarithmically to accommodate the wide range of frequencies studied in this experiment. Points along the curve that are lower on the y-axis are associated with firing thresholds for action potentials that occur at lower input energy—they have lower SPL thresholds, or stated otherwise, are more sensitive to input energy. A plot such as this is called a tuning curve.

The tuning curve shown in Figure 13–23 shows the inverted "tip" of the curve to be located at approximately 6000 Hz; the fiber has the lowest threshold at this input frequency. These "tip" frequencies are called characteristic frequencies, and the nerve fiber associated with this tuning curve tip can be called a 6000 Hz fiber. Very importantly, the nerve fiber is clearly responsive to other frequencies as well, although with lesser sensitivity than the characteristic frequency. The fiber does respond to input energy at 4000 Hz, as one example, but requires about 40 dB greater energy to meet the firing threshold compared with the threshold at 6000 Hz. The fiber even responds to a sinusoid at 1000 Hz,

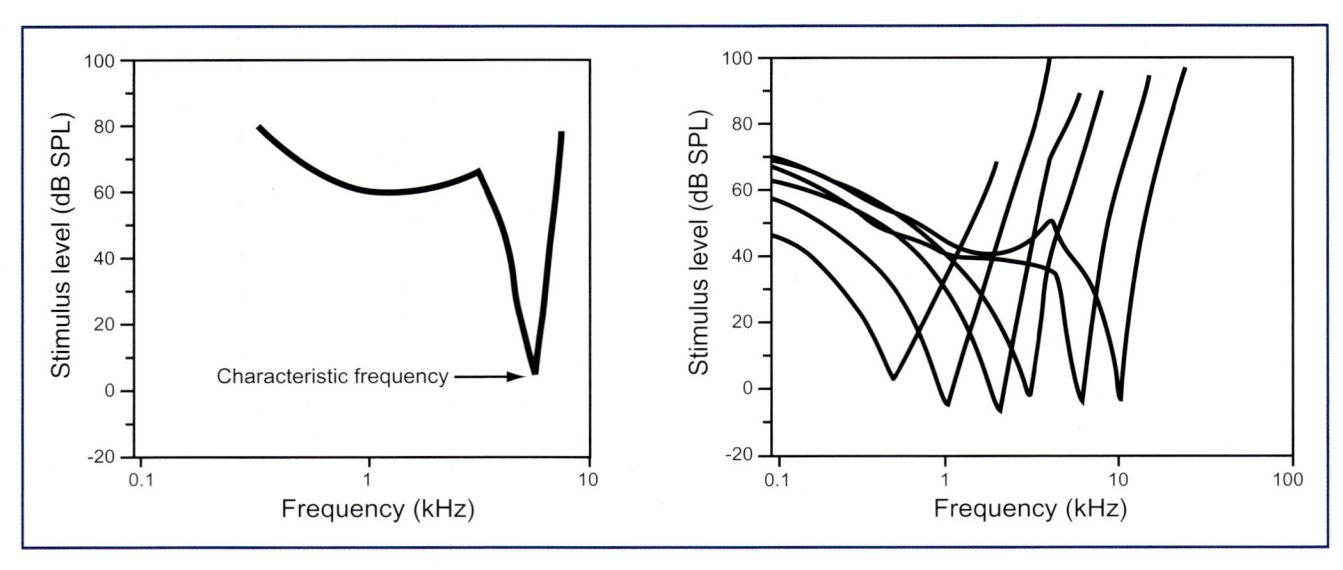

Figure 13–23. Tuning curves derived from a single auditory nerve fiber with a characteristic frequency (*left panel*) and from six individual nerve fibers with six different characteristic frequencies (*right panel*).

but requires close to 60 dB of energy to meet the threshold. The take-home message is that individual nerve fibers (and by inference, the hair cells to which they are attached) have characteristic frequencies but are sensitive to a range of frequencies. The sensitivity of the nerve fiber to frequencies surrounding the characteristic frequency decreases rapidly as the difference between the characteristic frequency and input frequency becomes greater. In support of this, note the very steep slopes along the curve on either side of the characteristic frequency.

When the experiment is repeated for many fibers selected for their varying locations along the basilar membrane, and therefore their different expected characteristic frequencies, the resulting tuning curves have both similarities and differences. The right side of Figure 13–23 shows six tuning curves for nerve fibers with characteristic frequencies of 0.5, 1.0, 2.0, 4.0, 6.0, and 10.0 kHz, moving from left to right along the frequency scale. The curves for different characteristic frequencies have similar shapes, with some differences as well. All curves have shallower slopes below the characteristic frequency compared with above it. This asymmetry suggests that above the characteristic frequency of a given nerve fiber, its sensitivity drops off much more quickly than frequencies below the characteristic frequency. Stated otherwise, a given nerve fiber is more sensitive to frequencies below its characteristic frequency than to frequencies above it.

One other aspect of tuning curves not obvious in the right panel of Figure 13–23 is that the absolute range of frequencies that causes reliable stimulus-evoked nerve fiber activity is greater for fibers with high characteristic frequencies, compared with fibers with low characteristic frequencies. Visual comparison of the six curves to verify this claim is complicated by the logarithmic scale of the *x*-axis (frequency scale), for which equal linear distances are associated with increasing absolute frequency differences as you move from the left to right end of the frequency scale. It is a fact, however, that nerve fibers with high characteristic frequencies (toward the basal end of the basilar membrane) respond to a broader range of frequencies than nerve fibers with low characteristic frequencies (toward the tip of the basilar membrane). These differences between tuning curves, depending on their characteristic frequencies, are reconsidered in the next chapter, which deals with the psychological aspects of auditory function.

Ascending Auditory Pathways

The term *ascending auditory pathways* refers to structures in the nervous system that carry auditory impulses from the auditory nerve to the auditory cortex. It also refers to efferent pathways—nerve fibers carrying information from the central nervous system to the cochlea. The efferent system is covered briefly above. The focus in this section is on the afferent auditory pathways.

Figure 13–24 illustrates the ascending auditory pathways in the human brain. The auditory nerve on one side of the head (in this case, the right ear, if the head is facing the viewer) is shown entering the

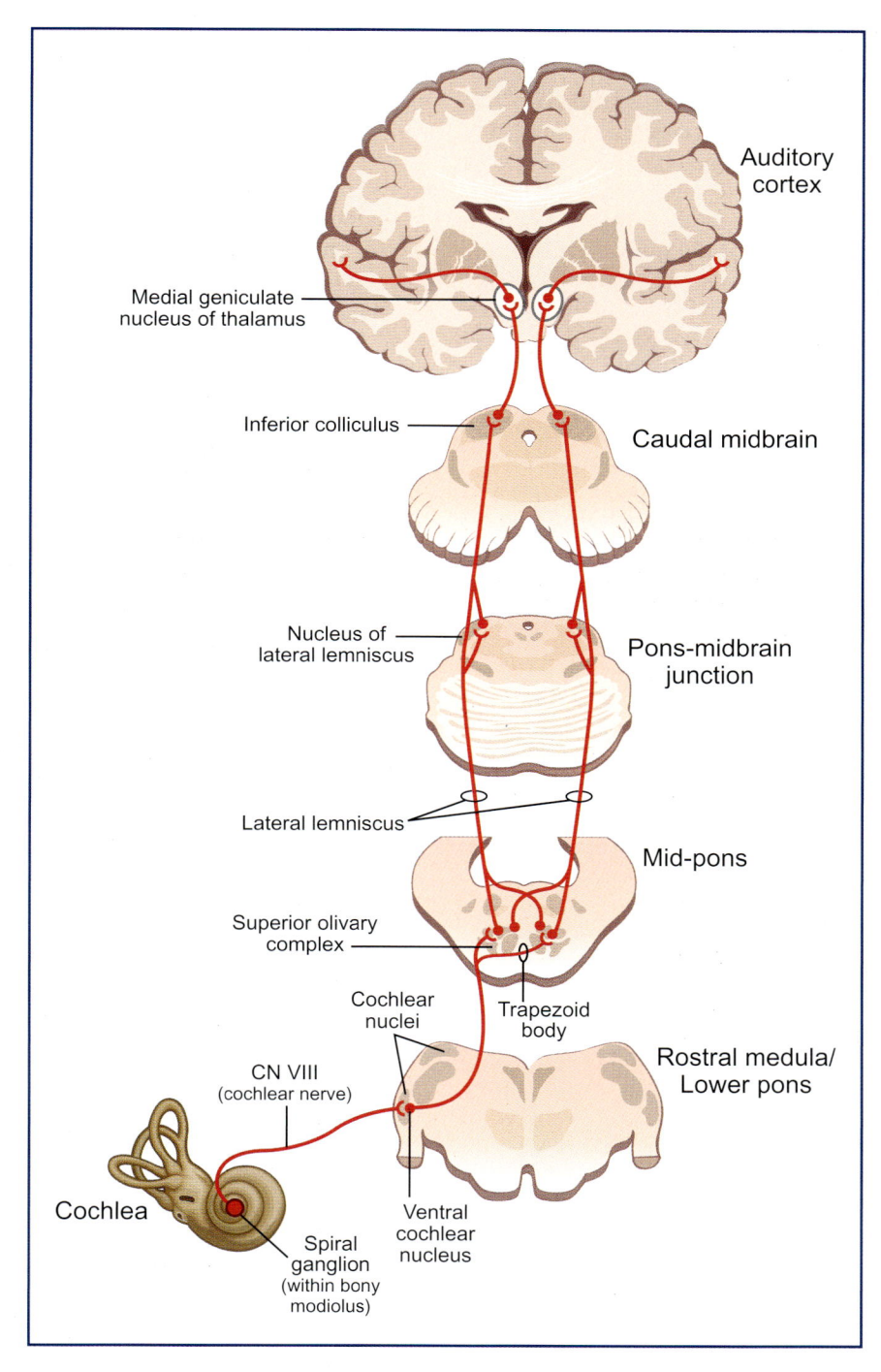

13. ANATOMY AND PHYSIOLOGY OF THE AUDITORY SYSTEM   537

Figure 13-24. The ascending central auditory pathways, from the cochlear nuclei to the primary auditory cortex.

brainstem at the level of the rostral (upper part) of the medulla. The description that follows also applies to the auditory pathway from the left ear. As the auditory nerve enters the brainstem, its fibers make synapses with clusters of cells called the cochlear nuclei. Cells in the cochlear nuclei give off axons (projections extending from the bodies of nerve cells) that enter the pons and cross the midline of the brainstem in a fiber bundle called the trapezoid body. Many of these fibers make synapses in cells of the superior olivary complex of the pons, which give off ascending fibers in an auditory tract called the lateral lemniscus. Along the course of the lateral lemniscus, near the junction of the pons and midbrain, are nuclei of the lateral lemniscus in which some ascending fibers have synapses. These fibers, as well as the ones that do not make synapses in the nuclei of the lateral lemniscus, climb to the midbrain where synapses are made with cells of the inferior colliculus, which in turn send fibers to cells of the medial geniculate body of the thalamus. Fibers from the medial geniculate body project to the cortex where they make synapses in the primary auditory cortex of the temporal lobe. The central auditory pathways, including all cell groups (nuclei) and axon bundles (fiber tracts) maintain tonotopic arrangement from the brainstem to the cortex. Primary analysis in the auditory cortex is sent to auditory association cortex in the temporal and parietal lobes for analysis of complex events such as speech, music, and environmental sounds. Additional information on the auditory cortex and auditory association cortex is provided in Chapter 15.

Most of the fibers from the cochlear nuclei cross over to the other side of the brainstem and eventually ascend in the opposite-side lateral lemniscus. Still, a large number of fibers (perhaps 25% of all auditory ascending fibers) stay on the same side as the side of entry of the auditory nerve. Although not shown in the figure, there are additional locations along the auditory pathways in the brainstem where fibers travel between cells on the two sides.

The fact that both cochleae supply nerve fibers to both sides of the brain allows for the exquisite binaural (two-eared) capabilities of the auditory system. These capabilities include, most notably, the ability to localize sources of sound in space with tremendous precision as well as the capability to isolate a single sound source among many competing sources. A good example of the latter skill is the ability to focus on the speech of a single person in a room where many people are talking at the same time (the "cocktail party effect), discussed in more detail in Chapter 14).

Acoustic Reflex

The auditory pathways include a reflex arc that implements the acoustic reflex (also called the middle ear muscle reflex: see Mukerji, Windsor, & Lee, 2010). The acoustic reflex may involve the *tensor tympani* muscle, but in a less direct way compared with the *stapedius* muscle. The following discussion focuses on the *stapedius* muscle as the primary muscular component of the acoustic reflex.

One function of the acoustic reflex appears to be protection of the cochlea from damage due to excessive displacement forces exerted by the footplate of the stapes (Borg, Counter, & Rösler, 1984). These very high displacement forces are associated with very high sound levels, such as those resulting from explosions or gunshots, loud machinery (e.g., the sound waves generated by a jet engine), or amplified sound waves (e.g., at a concert of your favorite or most disliked band). It is well known that the acoustic reflex is not elicited by low sound levels, such as those associated with many everyday sonic events. The acoustic reflex occurs in most humans with normal hearing at sound levels of roughly 80 to 95 dB sound pressure level (like the sound energy generated by heavy traffic on a highway and reaching a listener at a distance of about 30 feet; Wiley, Oviatt, & Block, 1987). The acoustic reflex threshold level varies in the human population and depends on precisely how the reflex is elicited (for example, with pure tones versus acoustic events with many frequencies). Most typically, the reflex occurs below the level at which listeners say that sound is uncomfortable or causes pain. For the purposes of this discussion, we can agree that the sound energy that elicits the acoustic reflex is perceived by listeners to be quite loud.

Figure 13–25 presents a diagram of the known anatomy of the acoustic reflex. This neuroanatomical circuitry is activated when a high-energy sound wave causes very large displacement of the stapes footplate into the perilymph of the scala vestibuli. This produces a traveling wave in the cochlea with large displacements at many locations along the basilar membrane, which presumably is encoded in auditory nerve activity as an acoustic event of excessively high energy, above some "safety threshold." The encoded, "too much energy" information reaches the cochlear nucleus, where the auditory nerve makes synapses just after it enters the brainstem. The cochlear nucleus has connections with the facial motor nucleus of the pons, on the same side, although the precise anatomy of these connections remains unclear (Mukerji et al., 2010). Fibers also appear to run from the cochlear nucleus on the side of entry of the auditory nerve to the superior olivary complex on the same side, and to the facial motor nucleus on the other side of the brainstem. Like the cochlear nucleus, the superior olivary complex has connections with the facial nerve on the same side (the ipsilateral connection), as well as a "crossed" connection with the cochlear nucleus on the other side of the brainstem (the contralateral connection). The crossed connections explain how an excessively strong acoustic input in one ear evokes the reflex in both ears. The ipsilateral loops are shown in Figure 13–25 by red highlights, the contralateral loops by green highlights.

Motor neurons in the facial motor nucleus (or just around the edge of the facial motor nucleus) send

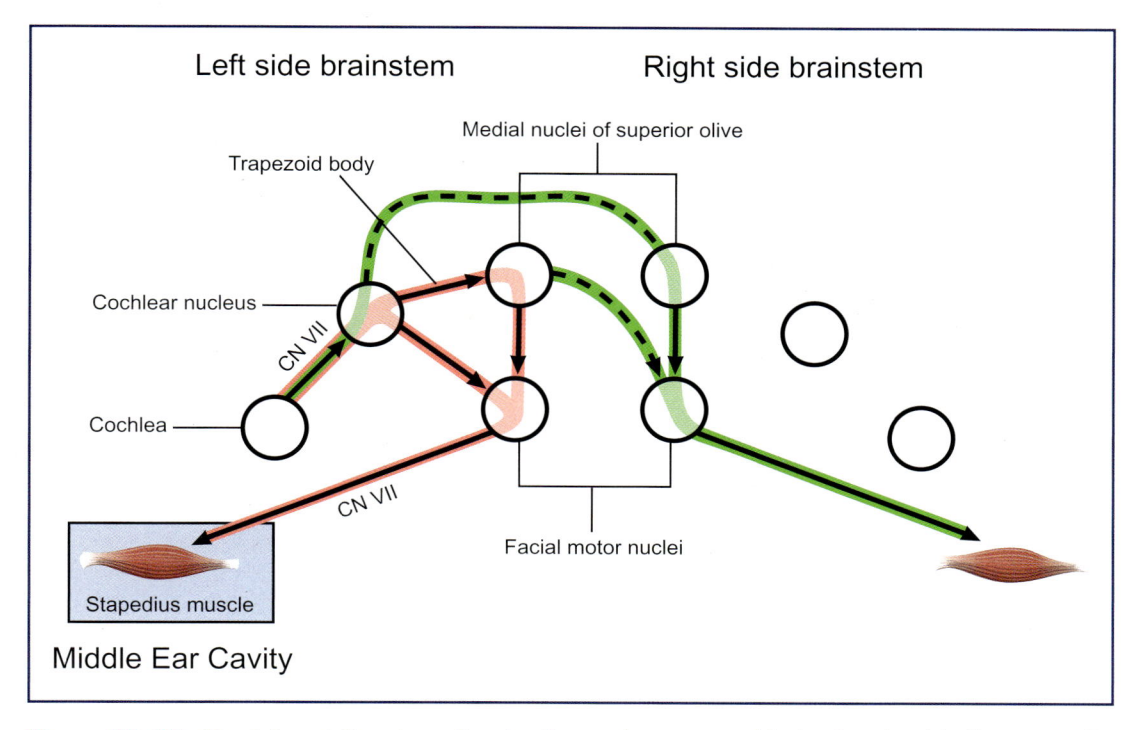

Figure 13–25. Nuclei and fiber bundles (pathways) presumed to be involved in the acoustic reflex. Ipsilateral (*red*) and contralateral (*green*) connections are shown for the left ear only; neural circuitry for the right ear is a mirror image of the structures shown in the figure.

fibers via the facial nerve (cranial nerve VII) to control contraction of the *stapedius* muscle. The *stapedius* muscle contracts, pulling the front edge of the footplate of the stapes away from the oval window, stiffening the ossicular chain and limiting transmission of excessive acoustic energy from the conductive mechanism to the cochlear fluids. The protection is required to prevent damage to the hair cells, which can result from exposure to an excessively strong traveling wave.

In healthy auditory systems, the acoustic reflex is always bilateral, as shown in Figure 13–25 by the ipsilateral and contralateral loops for the reflex pathways. Although there is agreement that the acoustic reflex can protect the cochlea by stiffening the ossicular chain in response to very strong sound energy, there are reasons to question this idea. When the time is measured between the onset of a very strong acoustic event and the reflex *mechanical* effect of stiffening the ossicular chain, the minimal interval is roughly 100 ms (1/10th of a second). This is very fast, but for a 500 Hz tone just above the threshold for elicitation of the acoustic reflex, the stiffening begins only after about 50 cycles of vibration have made it through the middle ear to the cochlea (see sidetrack on this page). Any protection against cochlear damage from high-energy sound is welcomed, of course, but this kind of delay seems

What's Up with 1/10th Second?

What do we mean by the mechanical effect of the acoustic reflex, and how do we know it requires about 100 ms to occur? A technique called impedance audiometry employs measures of sound level in the external auditory meatus to estimate stiffness of the conductive mechanism. When a loud sound is introduced into the external ear, the *stapedius* muscle contracts, pulling on the stapes and stiffening the conductive mechanism. Impedance audiometry can measure the time between the introduction of the loud sound and the beginning of increased stiffness, which is typically about 100 ms. Why does the text say that the stiffening begins only after 50 cycles of a very loud 500 Hz tone? The period of 500 Hz is 2 ms ($T = 1/f$), thus 50 cycles × 2 ms = 100 ms. Fifty cycles of a very loud sound seems to be time enough to cause damage to hair cells. It doesn't mean the acoustic reflex is not protective of cochlea from excessive sound energy; it just may not be so effective over the initial tens of milliseconds of the acoustic overload.

What Did You Say?

Tests of hearing are designed based on knowledge of the auditory system. For example, in pure-tone audiometry, tones of a single frequency (so-called pure tones) are used to estimate the response of the hair cells at different locations along the basilar membrane. Because of the tonotopic arrangement of the hair cells from base to apex of the cochlea, single-frequency tones allow an examiner to assess the health of the hair cells very precisely at different locations throughout the cochlea. There are also techniques for assessing the stiffness of the conductive mechanism (outer and middle ear). These stiffness evaluations, all performed at the entrance to the ear canal with minimal discomfort to the person being tested, are used to diagnose many auditory disorders ranging from middle ear infections, which are very common in childhood, to possible diseases of the auditory nerve, which may be reflected in poorly functioning or absent acoustic reflexes. One more example is the use of electrodes placed on the scalp to measure the amplitudes and timing of electrical activity of cell groups within the auditory pathways of the central nervous system, as nervous system analysis of an acoustic signal makes its way from the auditory nerve to the auditory cortex. Clearly, audiological tests reflect an intimate knowledge of the structure and function of the auditory system.

---

to expose the cochlea to at least some danger. This is especially true for impulse-like, high-level sonic events such as explosions and gunshots. Impulse-like sonic events occur quickly and produce very high energy over a very short period of time (for example, the sound waves of small arms fire at a distance of 10 cm may reach 120 dB over a 3 to 5-ms interval: Dezelak et al., 2016). It may be, therefore, that the acoustic reflex is especially effective in protecting the cochlea from sustained acoustic events with very high energy. Even this protection is not complete, as it is well known that chronic exposure to high-level acoustic events results in damage or death of hair cells, and hearing loss.

REVIEW

Knowledge of the structure and function of the auditory mechanism is critical to those who plan to become communication specialists to understand normal hearing, as well as the effect of auditory disease on hearing; this knowledge is also important to understanding how children learn language and how formal evaluations of hearing are designed and interpreted.

Most of the peripheral auditory mechanism and auditory nerve is housed within the temporal bone, a complex bone of the skull.

The peripheral auditory mechanism can be subdivided into the conductive mechanism, comprising the outer and middle ear, and the sensorineural mechanism, comprising the inner ear and auditory nerve.

The outer ear includes the pinna, external auditory meatus, and the part of the tympanic membrane that faces the external auditory meatus.

The pinna (or auricle) is a cartilaginous structure that is attached to the side of the head and contributes to the ability to locate a sound source.

The external auditory meatus (or external auditory canal) is approximately 2.5 cm long and 0.7 cm in diameter and extends from the pinna to the tympanic membrane, in which cerumen (ear wax) is produced and through which sound waves are directed to the tympanic membrane.

The external auditory meatus has a resonant frequency of roughly 3300 Hz, which explains in part the very acute sensitivity of the human auditory mechanism in this frequency region.

The tympanic membrane (or eardrum) is a small (area of about 55 mm^2) three-layered structure, the middle layer of which is sensitive to the very small pressure variations associated with sound waves.

The middle ear is an air-filled cavity, sometimes divided into three chambers, that lies between the outer ear and inner ear and contains three small ossicles (bones), several ligaments, and two muscles.

The ossicles are the malleus (which attaches to the tympanic membrane), incus, and stapes, the latter of which connects by means of its footplate to the oval window of the inner ear).

Connected to the ossicles are ligaments that tether the ossicles to different structures and to each other (at joints) and two muscles, the *tensor tympani* muscle, which attaches to the malleus, and the *stapedius* muscle, which attaches to the stapes, both of which serve to stiffen the ossicular chain when they contract.

The auditory tube (or eustachian tube), a 3.8-cm (1.5-inch) tube that runs from the anterior wall of the middle ear to the nasopharynx, is bony and open toward the middle ear and cartilaginous and flexible toward the nasopharynx, where it is usually closed, but can be opened to equalize the pressure in the middle ear.

The tympanic membrane and ossicles minimize the impedance mismatch between the air in the outer ear and the fluid (liquid) in the inner ear by the substantial area difference between the tympanic membrane and the oval window, and by the lever actions of the ossicular chain.

The inner ear is housed within the bony labyrinth of the temporal bone and contains the semicircular canals, vestibule, and cochlea, all structures that communicate with the central nervous system via cranial nerve VIII (auditory-vestibular nerve).

Three semicircular canals, each oriented at right angles to the other two, contain hair cells that bend when the head moves and cause the vestibular part of cranial nerve VIII to fire and send information about head orientation and head movement to the brain.

The vestibule contains the oval window as well as the utricle and saccule, which include hair cells that send signals to the brain about the relative position and acceleration of the head.

The cochlea is the spiral-shaped end organ of hearing that converts sound into neural signals and contains many important structures, including the scalae, basilar membrane, organ of Corti, and hair cells.

Within the cochlea are three membranous, fluid-filled ducts called the scala vestibuli (containing perilymph), cochlear duct (or scala media, containing endolymph), and scala tympani (containing perilymph), the first and last of which are connected at the heliocotrema, at the tip of the cochlear spiral.

The scala media duct is separated from the scala tympani by the basilar membrane and from the scala vestibuli by Reissner's membrane.

On top of the basilar membrane sits the organ of Corti, which contains a row of inner hair cells and at least three rows of outer hair cells, some of the ends of which are embedded in the tectorial membrane which sits above the hair cells.

Movement of fluid in the cochlea (caused by pressure changes transmitted through the outer and middle ear to the scala media) deforms inner hair cells and causes them to depolarize and fire.

The outer hair cells, referred to as the "cochlear amplifier," are stimulated by efferent neural signals originating in the brainstem that cause them to vibrate and amplify the movement of the basilar membrane to very soft sounds, as well as increase the response sensitivity of frequency analysis by the inner hair cells.

Hair cells are arranged tonotopically along the basilar membrane, ranging from those that respond best to the highest frequency that can be detected by humans (20,000 Hz) at its narrow base to those that respond best to the lowest detectable frequency (20 Hz) at its wide apex.

As discovered by Georg von Békésy in the early 1900s, the hair cells are stimulated by traveling waves of fluid displacement that are transmitted through the cochlear fluid, the highest amplitude of which is frequency dependent, with high-frequency sounds creating waves that peak near the base of the basilar membrane and low-frequency sounds creating waves that peak near the apex of the basilar membrane.

When inner hair cells are deformed by a traveling wave, they depolarize and send a signal through their associated nerve fibers, which carry the signal to a ganglion and then on to the brainstem via the auditory part of cranial nerve VIII.

The auditory nerve portion of cranial nerve VIII carries afferent fibers from inner hair cells and efferent fibers to outer hair cells, with the neural fibers arranged tonotopically just like the hair cells.

The auditory pathways consist of tonotopically arranged tracts and clusters of cell bodies that carry auditory signals from the brainstem to the cortex, with information from both ears included in both ascending pathways.

The acoustic reflex is a protective mechanism that reacts to very loud sounds and prevents traveling waves of excessive amplitude, with possible damage to the hair cells; contraction of the *stapedius* muscle in response to high sound energy is caused by a neural loop of auditory nerve fibers, to auditory brainstem stimuli and the facial motor nucleus, the latter of which innervates the *stapedius* muscle via cranial nerve VII (facial nerve), which pulls the stapes away from the oval window.

REFERENCES

Abele, T. A., & Wiggins, R. H. III (2015). Imaging of the temporal bone. *Radiological Clinics of North America*, 53, 15–36.

Barin, K. (2009). Clinical neurophysiology of the vestibular system. In J. Katz, L. Medwetzky, R. Burkard, & L. Hood (Eds.), *Handbook of clinical audiology* (6th ed., pp. 431–466). Baltimore, MD: Lippincott, Williams, & Wilkins.

Békésy, G. v. (1928). Zur Theorie des Hörens; die Schwingungsform der Basilarmembran. *Physik Zeits*, 29, 793–810.

Borg, E., Counter, S. A., & Rösler, G. [1984]. Theories of middle ear-muscle function. In S. Silman (Ed.), *The acoustic reflex: Basic principles and clinical applications* (pp. 63–99). Orlando, FL: Academic Press.

Cooper, N. P., & Guinan, J. J. Jr. (2006). Efferent-mediated control of basilar membrane motion. *Journal of Physiology*, 576, 49–54.

Cullen, K. E. (2012). The vestibular system: Multimodal integration and coding of self-motion for motor control. *Trends in Neuroscience*, 35, 185–196.

Dallos, P. (1973). *The auditory periphery: Biophysics and physiology*. New York, NY: Academic Press.

Gelfand, S. A. (2002). The acoustic reflex. In J. Katz (Ed.), *Handbook of clinical audiology* (5th ed., pp. 205–232). Philadelphia, PA: Lippincott, Williams, & Wilkins.

Goldberg, J. M., Wilson, V. J., Cullen, K. E., Angelaki, D. E., Broussard, D. M., Buttner-Ennerver, J., . . . Minor, L. B. (2012). *The vestibular system: A sixth sense*. New York, NY: Oxford University Press.

Goutman, J. D., Elgoyhen, A. B., & Gomez-Casati, M. E. (2015). Cochlear hair cells: The sound-sensing machines. *FEBS Letters, 589*, 3354–3361.

Heil, P., & Peterson, A. J. (2015). Basic response properties of auditory nerve fibers: A review. *Cell and Tissue Research, 361*, 129–158.

Hixon, T. J., Weismer, G., & Hoit, J. D. (2014). *Preclinical speech science: Anatomy, physiology, acoustics, perception* (2nd ed.) San Diego, CA: Plural.

Hudpseth, A. J. (2014). Integrating the active process of hair cells with cochlear function. *Nature Reviews Neuroscience, 15*, 600–614.

Lemmerling, M. J., Stambuk, H. E., Mancuso, A. A., Antonelli, P. J., & Kubilis, P. S. (1997). CT of the normal suspensory ligaments of the ossicles in the middle ear. *AJNR American Journal of Neuroradiology, 18*, 471–477.

Luers, J. C., & Hüttenbrink, K-B. (2016). Surgical anatomy and pathology of the middle ear. *Journal of Anatomy, 228*, 338–353.

Mukerji, S., Windsor, A. M., & Lee, D. J. (2010). Auditory brainstem circuits that mediate the middle ear muscle reflex. *Trends in Amplification, 14*, 170–191.

Nakajima, H. H., Ravicz, M. E., Merchant, S. N., Peake, W. T., & Rosowski, J. J. (2005). Experimental ossicular fixations and the middle ear's response to sound: Evidence for a flexible ossicular chain. *Hearing Research, 204*, 60–77.

Okada, R., Muro, S., Eguchi, K., Yagi, K., Nasu, H., Yamaguchi, K., Miwa, K., & Akita, K. (2018). The extended bundle of the tensor veli palatini: Anatomic consideration of the dilating mechanism of the Eustachian tube. *Auris Nasus Larynx, 45*(2), 265–272.

Olson, E. S., Duifhuis, H., & Steele, C. R. (2012). Von Békésy and cochlear mechanics. *Hearing Research, 293*, 31–43.

Pickles, J. O. (2013). *An introduction to physiology of hearing* (4th ed.). Leiden, Netherlands: Brill NV.

Stepp, C. E., & Voss, S. E. (2005). Acoustics of the human middle-ear space. *Journal of the Acoustical Society of America, 118*, 861–871.

Terreros, G., & Delano, P. H. (2015). Corticofugal modulation of peripheral auditory responses. *Frontiers in Systems Neuroscience, 9*, 134. doi:10.3389/fnsys.2015.00134

Volandri, G., Di Puccio, F., Forte, P., & Manetti, S. (2012). Model-oriented review and multi-body simulation of the ossicular chain of the human middle ear. *Medical Engineering & Physics, 34*, 1339–1355.

Wiley, T. L., Oviatt, D. L., & Block, M. G. (1987). Acoustic immittance measures in normal ears. *Journal of Speech and Hearing Research, 30*, 161–170.

14

Auditory Psychophysics

AUDITORY PSYCHOPHYSICS

Auditory psychophysics (also called psychoacoustics) is a branch of science that is concerned with the effects of physical stimuli (in this case, sound waves) on the psychological responses of humans. The term "psychophysics" is relevant to any biological system that transduces and processes physical attributes of events in the environment and transforms them into sensations and perceptions. Such systems include visual, olfactory, tactile, taste, and, of course, auditory systems.

The "physics" part of "psychophysics" refers to characteristics of the physical stimulus, the "psycho" part to the psychological responses to the composition and change of the physical stimulus. On the psychological side of the term, there has been a tendency to equate "sensation" with peripheral (outside the central nervous system) and perhaps brainstem responses to a physical stimulus. The term "perception" has been reserved for the more elaborated psychological processes taking place at subcortical and cortical levels.

Why is a chapter on auditory psychoacoustics necessary, separate from a chapter on characteristics of acoustic signals (Chapter 7)? If acoustic signals are simply conveyed by the peripheral and central structures of the auditory system in their physical form of frequencies, amplitudes, durations, and other features, knowledge of acoustic signal characteristics would be sufficient. However, the auditory system, like other sensory-perceptual systems, is not passive; it not only transmits, but also transduces, transforms, and codes signal characteristics to produce psychological responses to sound that are not mere reflections of the signal. The pinnacle of these complicated processes is the way in which speech acoustic signals are transformed to speech and language perception. In the current chapter, only non-speech auditory psychophysics are discussed (Chapter 12 focuses on the perception of speech).

The topics covered in this chapter include the psychophysics of thresholds and loudness, pitch, timbre, time, and sound source localization. The presentation is tailored to students with no background in auditory psychophysics, with the assumption that the previous chapter on auditory anatomy and physiology has been studied carefully. An excellent source of in-depth information on auditory psychophysics is Moore (2013).

PSYCHOPHYSICS OF LOUDNESS

Loudness is a psychological phenomenon that is *related* to the physical magnitude of sound energy but is not the same as the physical quantity. Whereas the magnitude of sound energy can be measured by an instrument, such as a sound level meter, loudness cannot. Loudness is a sensation or perception that can only be measured by listener responses. Students are encouraged to read the Appendix to Chapter 7, which explains the use of the term "decibels" (dB) to express the sound pressure level (SPL) of a sound wave. SPL is a measure of the physical magnitude of sound.

Auditory Thresholds

The determination of the lowest sound energy that humans can detect has a long history, extending at least back to 1933 when Sivian and White reported results of careful measurements on 14 participants with normal hearing (see Sivian & White's review of work prior to their publication, pp. 299–304 and pp. 308–312). Sivian and White (1933) used sinusoids of relatively long duration (at least 1 second) to obtain data on a quantity they called *minimal audible field* (MAF). By this they meant the minimal sound intensity audible to listeners with normal hearing as they sat 1 meter in front of a loudspeaker that delivered the tones. In other words,

Bringing the Bird to Auditory Threshold Testing

Determination of minimal audible field, or its non-identical twin minimal audible pressure (where the sound is delivered by a headphone covering the pinna or via a tube in the ear canal), is a highly technical business. Many variables affect the measurement of thresholds, ranging from the equipment used to generate and deliver tones to the individual characteristics of a person's head—in particular, the pinna. Another variable is the room in which a participant is tested. For the six lowest frequencies they tested, Sivian and White used sinusoids to establish minimal audible field. In the case of frequencies at 1100 Hz and higher, the signal used to establish minimal audible field was a "warble tone." These are nearly sinusoidal signals whose frequency varies subtly around a single frequency at a constant rate (e.g., five warbles per second). A warble tone is a bit like a sinusoid enhanced with a small degree of vibrato. Why use warble tones at the higher test frequencies? First, Sivian and White thought the warbles were more interesting to listeners and less likely to contribute to the substantial fatigue so common in psychoacoustic experiments; listening carefully for a long time is hard work. Second, sinusoids presented in more or less closed rooms result in standing pressure waves where multiple peaks and valleys of pressure are distributed across the listening space in a "frozen" pattern. The sound waves reflect off walls in a way that places the peaks and valleys of pressures in precisely the same location as the original wave. This results in "standing" waves of high and low pressures across the room. For higher frequencies, the precise placement of a listener's head might locate the test ear at a peak or valley of the standing pressure wave, which affects the threshold estimate. Warbling a sinusoid does not allow standing waves to be "caged" in the test room.

they wanted to determine the threshold for sound detection in a sound field, for multiple frequencies.

A sound field is a listening environment in which the ears are not covered by earphones. For this experiment, Sivian and White (1933) placed their listeners in a heavily sound-absorbent enclosure to reduce extraneous environmental noise as much as possible. The purpose of this was to establish minimal detectable sound energy as if the limits of hearing detection were being estimated. The collection of auditory threshold data under nearly optimal listening conditions is, in fact, a standard approach to one aspect of the clinical assessment of hearing capabilities.

Listeners signaled with a button when they heard a tone. The experimenter controlled the frequency, intensity, and duration of the tones. Thresholds were obtained for 21 discrete frequencies between 100 Hz and 15,000 Hz. At each frequency, the threshold was determined by first presenting the signal at a level (intensity) that was clearly audible; this established the pattern of the listener pressing the button when he or she heard the tone. The experimenter then lowered the intensity in systematic steps, in separate presentations, where each tone had a duration of roughly two seconds. The intensity was decreased until the listener stopped responding, apparently because the intensity was insufficient to elicit a response. The tone intensity was then raised slightly until a response was again obtained, lowered slightly to eliminate the response, raised again to elicit a response, and so on, until the experimenter recorded the signal intensity corresponding to the "just audible" responses. The intensity at this "just audible" level was recorded as the threshold for that frequency.

The minimal audible file curve in Figure 14–1, labeled "Threshold", is not taken directly from Sivian and White (1933), but rather is a composite of their results and those of other scientists (Killion, 1978). The x-axis is frequency, scaled logarithmically (base 10) to reflect the large range of tested frequencies on an axis of reasonable length, and the y-axis is SPL in dB with a reference pressure of 20 µPa (micropascal, or the smallest average pressure that humans can hear in their most sensitive frequency range; see Appendix to Chapter 7). The "0 dB" level on the y-axis does not indicate the absence of sound energy, but rather a measured sound pressure equivalent to the standard reference pressure (20 µPa). If SPL = $20 \log p_1/p_0$, where p_1 = the measured pressure and p_0 = the reference pressure, when $p_1 = p_0$ the pressure ratio is "1" (log of 1 = 0) which gives "0 dB." Thus, it is possible for a threshold to be negative when the sound pressure measured at threshold is less than the reference pressure. In clinical practice, negative thresholds are found frequently among young adults with normal hearing. The threshold curve shown in Figure 14–1 is the binaural, sound-

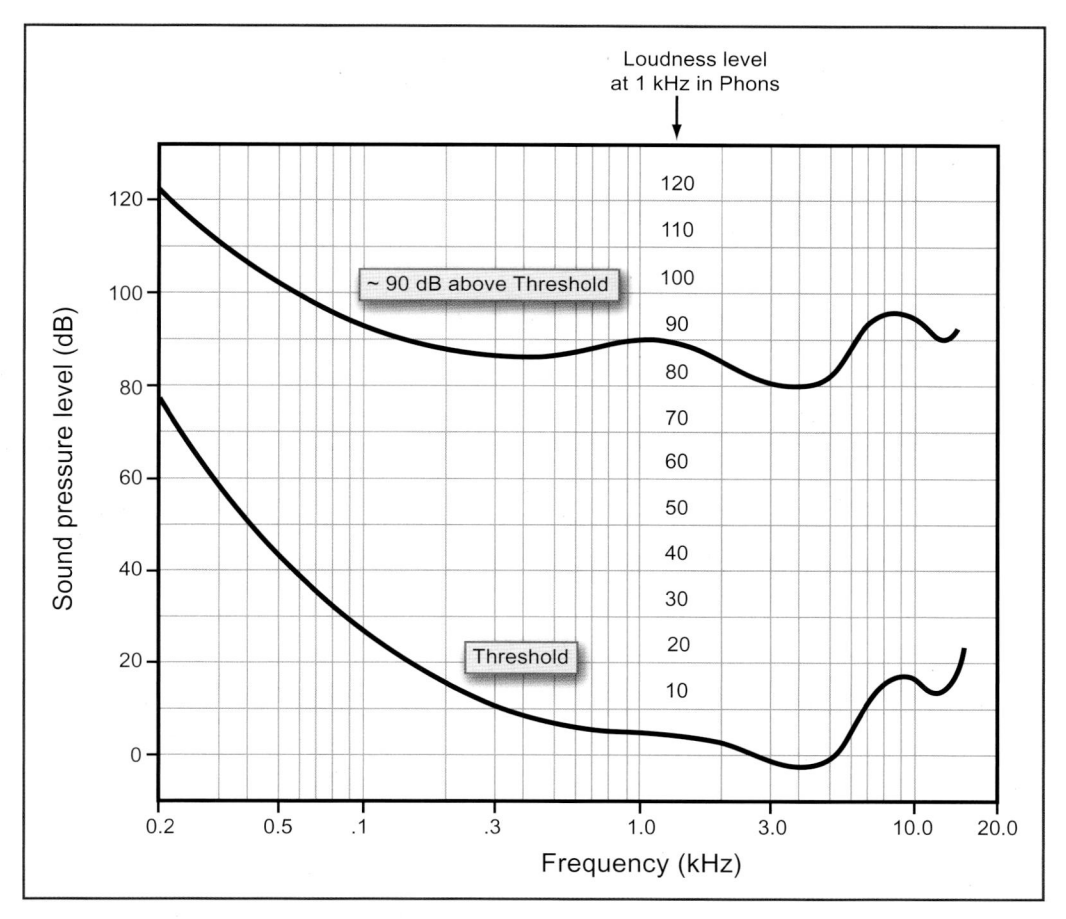

Figure 14-1. Minimal audible field (*lower curve*) as determined in Sivian and White's (1933) experiment and similar experiments performed by other scientists. The upper curve (labeled ~90 dB above threshold) is discussed in the text, as is the term "phon."

field sensitivity curve of the normal human auditory system as a function of frequency.

Two features of the minimal audible field (threshold) curve in Figure 14–1 are critical to the present chapter. First, *the SPL at auditory threshold varies across signal frequency*. Specifically, a much greater SPL is required to reach threshold at low and high frequencies compared with the SPL at thresholds for midrange frequencies (roughly 1000–5000 Hz). For example, threshold at 100 Hz requires a sound pressure of approximately 28 dB re: 20 µPa (reference pressure), whereas the sound pressure required for threshold at 3000 Hz is just a little below the reference pressure of 20 µPa (that is, the threshold at 3000 Hz is just below 0 dB).

The fact that the SPL required to reach auditory threshold varies across frequencies has direct application to clinical evaluation of hearing. An audiometer is the instrument used in audiology clinics to establish sensitivity to sinusoids. The audiometer has the same calibrated steps of SPL (usually ranging from 0 to 110 dB) for each frequency. When an examiner delivers a sinusoid (pure tone) to a listener at a dial reading of 0 dB, the SPL generated by the audiometer corresponds to the average threshold level at the selected frequency, as determined from a large population of normal-hearing young adults. This means that the 0 dB setting on an audiometer is associated with varying output SPL for different frequencies. The varying SPLs at 0 dB, across frequencies, are very similar to the minimal audible field thresholds shown in Figure 14–1. This is why the dB levels on the intensity controls of an audiometer, and the levels shown on an audiogram (a record of a patient's thresholds as a function of frequency) are referred to as dB hearing level (HL). Two frequencies with a common HL setting (same number on the audiometer dial for level; for example, 25 dB HL) deliver signals with different SPLs. These different SPLs are most prominent across frequency when sound levels are near threshold

(0 dB HL). As the sound level increases, the differences across frequency become less dramatic (see below, discussion of the 90 dB curve in Figure 14–1).

The second important aspect of the threshold curves in Figure 14–1 is that the most sensitive region for hearing is between 1000 and 5000 Hz (Moore, 2013). The resonant frequencies of the external auditory meatus (~3300 Hz) and the ossicular chain (~1400 Hz) make a significant contribution to this frequency region of maximum sensitivity (Chapter 13).

Is it possible to determine just how much the conductive resonances (of the external auditory meatus and the ossicles) contribute to auditory thresholds? The answer is "yes." In clinical testing, pure-tone thresholds are most frequently determined under headphones or with insert loudspeakers (where the sound output is delivered to the tympanic membrane by a narrow tube extending into the external auditory meatus from a firm seal at the entrance to the canal). Whether by earphone or tube, the open end of the external auditory meatus is closed and the resonant characteristics of the meatus are modified. The 1/4-wavelength rule no longer applies to the resonance because the tube is now closed at both ends. In theory, the threshold around 3500 Hz under an earphone should be higher (less sensitive) compared with the 3500 Hz threshold in a sound field. This is precisely what has been found: in the region between 3000 and 4000 Hz minimal audible field thresholds are 10 to 15 dB lower (more sensitive) than thresholds determined under earphones or with a probe tube.

Thresholds obtained under headphones or with insert tubes are higher (worse) at virtually all frequencies when compared with thresholds obtained in the sound field, but the differences are most notable in the region centered around the resonance of the external auditory meatus. Even when thresholds are obtained in the sound field (no headphones or insert loudspeakers) with the external auditory meatus of only *one* ear occluded with cotton, the minimal audible field threshold is worse than when both ear canals are open.

A general conclusion concerning auditory thresholds is that many factors influence the threshold measured at any frequency. Courses on audiometry provide additional information on how, in the clinical setting, these factors are controlled. The information on auditory thresholds provided above is necessary for discussion of the more advanced psychoacoustic phenomena presented below.

Equal Loudness Contours for Sinusoids

Another way to think about the threshold curve in Figure 14–1 is as an equal-loudness contour. The contour shows the SPLs required to just reach audibility across different frequencies, so it follows (as an example) that equal loudness of tones at 3000 Hz and 100 Hz is achieved at threshold when the intensity of the 100 Hz tone is roughly 28 dB greater than that of the 3000 Hz tone. This underscores an interesting psychophysical fact, that equal sound energy does not imply equal loudness. Note the distinction between the terms "sound energy" and "loudness." "Sound energy" is a physical quantity, measured for magnitude in dB by an instrument such as a sound level meter. "Loudness" is a psychological quantity, reported by a listener in response to a physical stimulus or inferred from a loudness match between two tones. Sound energy and loudness are not the same.

Details of equal-loudness contours differ across sound energy levels. The contour labeled "~90 dB above threshold" in Figure 14–1 shows the SPLs across frequency that result in equal loudness when the signal level is roughly 90 dB above threshold at 1000 Hz. This curve was generated by using the 90 dB SPL signal at 1000 Hz as a standard and determining the SPL required at other frequencies to match the loudness of the 1000 Hz tone. The use of 1000 Hz as a standard for loudness matches between two frequencies, at any level of presentation, is common.

The 90 dB equal loudness contour shows that there is equal loudness of the 100 Hz and 3000 Hz tones when the former is roughly 13 dB greater in intensity (or sound energy, or level) than the intensity of the 3000 Hz tone. As noted in the previous paragraph, at threshold the sound level difference for equal loudness of the two frequencies is about 28 dB, or 15 dB greater for equal loudness of the same frequencies at 90 dB. An eyeball comparison of the "~90 dB above threshold" and "Threshold" contours shows the higher-intensity contour to be relatively compressed across frequency, compared with the threshold contour. In general, SPL differences for equal loudness between frequencies become progressively diminished—the contour becomes flatter—as the overall level of presentation is increased.

The Psychophysical Function Relating SPL to Scaled Loudness of Sinusoids

How is the perceptual phenomenon of loudness related to the physical energy of a sound wave? This problem has occupied hearing scientists for a long time, and the history of research on this question points to the difficulty of answering it in a simple way. In this section a summary of loudness perception of sinusoids is provided; Marks and Florentine (2011) published a detailed, technical account of the history and contemporary status of research on loudness.

Loudness, in lay terms, is the perceived magnitude of a sound. People with normal hearing usually can agree on the difference between a soft and a loud sound—the loud sound has greater magnitude than the soft sound. These same people can also probably agree on the difference between a very soft and a soft sound, or between a loud and an extremely loud sound, using the concept of different magnitudes.

Scientists prefer to refine these lay comparisons by developing a simple formula that relates changes in perceived loudness of sinusoids to changes in the amount of energy in an acoustic signal. Measurement of the physical energy in an acoustic signal is not controversial; a proper instrument (such as a sound level meter) provides a value in decibels that, with careful calibration and the use of a standard reference pressure (20 µPa), gives reliable, reproducible results (because the standard reference pressure of 20 µPa is almost always used for sound levels in air, dB SPL values are given without the reference pressure). In contrast, the measurement of loudness, in which numbers are assigned to different SPLs or loudness matches are used to generate scales for the perception of sound magnitude, is complicated and controversial. Two well-established loudness scales, phons and sones, are described here.

Phons

A loudness scale is inherently subjective; there is no definitive way to know if the numbers generated by a listener reflect her perception of the loudness of a sound. Moreover, perceived loudness may be affected by factors other than variation in SPL. For example, loudness perception may be influenced by a sound's frequency, its spectral complexity (the pattern of amplitudes as a function of frequency in a multifrequency acoustic signal), and even the way in which a series of sounds is presented to the listener (Marks & Florentine, 2011). Efforts to investigate how loudness varies with SPL have simplified the problem to understand the relation of SPL to loudness.

An early approach to the scaling of loudness used a physical standard to serve as a reference point for perceptual judgments. The concept of "phons" was used to develop one type of loudness scale. In a sense, phons have been discussed above, but the term and its definition have not. A phon is a unit of loudness level that is tied to a specific frequency presented at a particular SPL. For example, a 1000 Hz tone presented at 40 dB SPL is said to have a loudness level of 40 phons. Similarly, a 1000 Hz tone presented at 60 dB SPL is said to have a loudness level of 60 phons. Recall the minimal audible field (threshold) and 90 dB loudness curves shown in Figure 14–1. Both are "equal loudness contours." As noted above, the substantial variation of SPL at threshold, across frequency, shows that the same loudness requires a different SPL depending on the signal frequency. For the ~90 dB equal loudness contour, it appears that a 3000 Hz sinusoid presented at 80 dB SPL sounds equally loud as a 1000 Hz sinusoid presented at 90 dB SPL. The 1000 Hz sinusoid at 90 dB SPL has a loudness level of 90 phons (following the logic above), as does the 3000 Hz sinusoid presented at 80 dB SPL.

Another way to think about equal loudness contours and phons as a loudness level is to imagine an experiment in which a 3000 Hz tone is presented at 80 dB SPL and the listener is asked to adjust the loudness of a reference tone of 1000 Hz until its loudness matches the 3000 Hz tone. The dB SPL for the 1000 Hz sinusoid selected by the listener as the loudness match for the 3000 Hz tone is the loudness level in phons for the 3000 Hz signal. In this example, a typical listener with normal hearing adjusts the 1000 Hz sinusoid to 90 dB SPL to match the loudness of the 3000 Hz sinusoid presented at 80 dB SPL. Using the 1000 Hz tone as the reference, the loudness level of the 3000 Hz sinusoid is 90 phons. Note that phons are expressed as a loudness *level* (not as loudness), in dB units. A set of equal loudness contours in 10 dB increments from threshold (0 dB) to 120 dB at 1000 Hz is shown in Figure 14–2 (adapted from Fletcher & Munson, 1933).

The phon scale is not a "direct" scale of loudness, because the loudness of a tone is dependent on a loudness *match* to another tone. Nor are phons just like dB on an intensity level (IL) or SPL scale: they are expressed as loudness levels. Phons are a perceptual phenomenon, whereas IL or SPL are physical properties. Phons played a role in the development of a more direct scaling of loudness, described in the next section.

Sones

An influential loudness scale, called the sone scale, was developed by the famous psychophysicist S. S. Stevens (1906–1973), who based his work on research from the early twentieth century. A sone is a unit of loudness. The foundation of this scale was the simple idea that listeners were likely to judge the relative loudness of two sinusoids as a ratio, as in the simple case of perceiving one sinusoid to be twice as loud as another sinusoid (or one sinusoid to be half as loud as another sinusoid). Consider an experiment in which a reference sinusoid at a known SPL is presented to a listener and assigned a number such as "1" or "10." Next, tones of the same

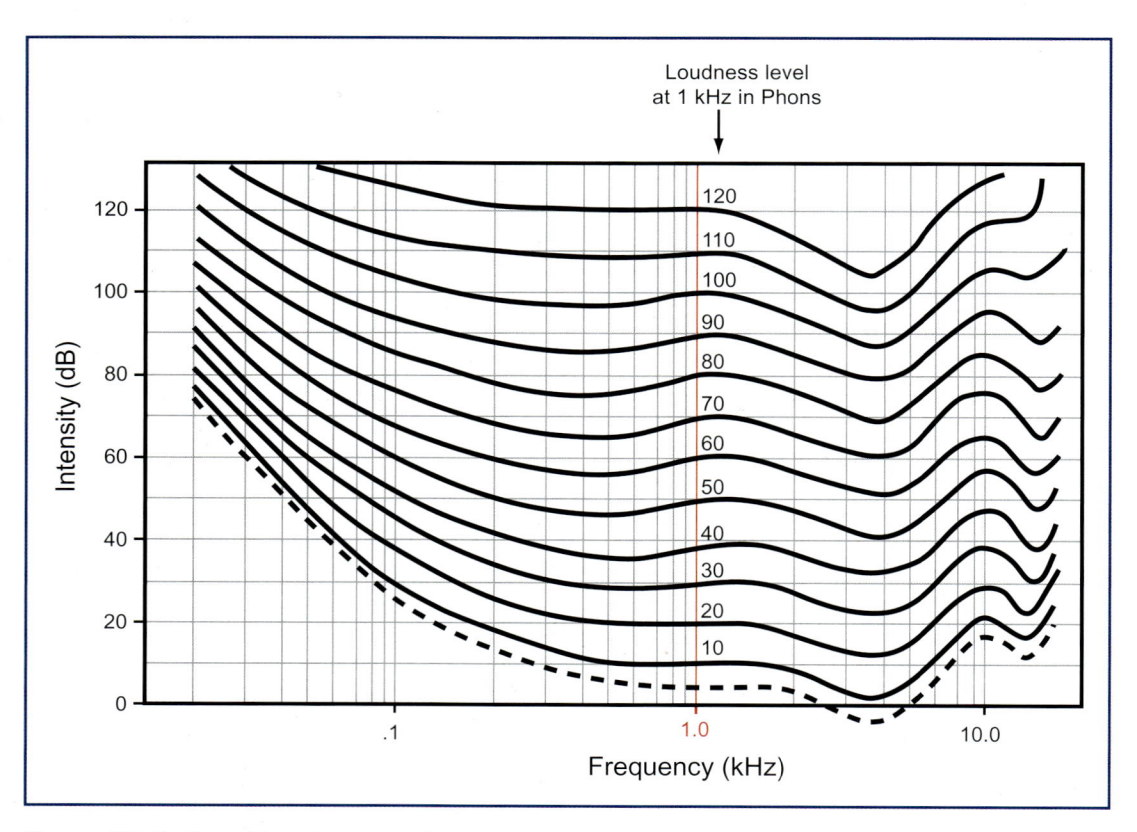

Figure 14–2. Equal loudness contours across frequency (in kHz) according to presentation level in dB. The equal loudness contours are referenced to the SPL at 1000 Hz (*vertical red line*) and are presented in 10 dB steps from threshold (*dashed line*) to 120 dB.

frequency but having different SPLs than the reference tone are presented to the listener, who is asked to assign numbers to them as ratios relative to the loudness of the reference. Under these conditions, the SPL that produces a sound perceived to be twice as loud as the reference tone should be assigned a number twice that of the reference number of "1" or "10" (whichever one is chosen for the experiment—any number can be used as the reference). An extension of this simple idea was the presumed ability of listeners to assign numbers to a tone presented at many different SPLs, and to assign the numbers as ratios to the standard stimulus, whatever the ratio may be (i.e., 1.3:1, 1.8:1, 2.0:1, and so forth). The SPLs of the presented stimuli were known, of course, so combining the known physical (SPL) variation of the tone with the numbers assigned to them allowed Stevens to construct a mathematical function relating perceived loudness (according to the ratio scaling) to SPL.

Why was Stevens interested in doing such experiments? One compelling reason was his knowledge, from previous work and laboratory experience, that ratios of the perceptual experience of loudness differed from ratios along the SPL scale. As described in an influential paper, Stevens (1955) knew that if a "standard" 1000 Hz sinusoidal tone was presented at 50 dB SPL, listeners (on average) would report a comparison tone presented at 58 to 60 dB SPL as twice as loud as the standard; a comparison tone presented at 38 to 40 dB SPL would be reported as half as loud as the standard tone. These 2:1 and 1:2 loudness ratios did not correspond to 2:1 and 1:2 ratios of sound energy (i.e., a 100 dB SPL sinusoidal tone was much more than twice the loudness of a 50 dB SPL tone). The SPL and loudness scales were not interchangeable.

In many of his experiments, Stevens arbitrarily assigned a value of 1 sone to the loudness of a 1000 Hz tone presented to a normal-hearing listener at 40 dB SPL re: 20 µPa. Additional experiments were conducted with standards at different SPLs (e.g., 20 db SPL). Stevens collected number assignments of the loudness of tones of different presentation levels relative to the loudness of the standards. He then plotted and "fit" the data, which means he applied mathematical functions to the bivariate (two-variable) data that provided the best fit. When the number estimates of loudness

—the sones—were plotted against SPL, the function was curved (Figure 14–3, left panel). When the sone scale was converted to a logarithmic (base 10) scale, the log-log plot (dB is already a log scale; see Appendix on decibels in Chapter 7) revealed a straight line relating perceived loudness to SPL. This straight line suggested that the perception of loudness was related to dB SPL by a constant proportion between any two stimuli along the SPL range. Figure 14–3 shows some sample data in a sone-SPL plot (left) and with sones transformed to logs (right panel).

Figure 14–4, adapted from Stevens (1955, Figure 4), and Buus and Florentine (2001), shows an example of data obtained with an 80 dB SPL standard. The data shown are based on magnitude estimates—the assignment of numbers corresponding to perceived loudness, relative to the 80 dB SPL standard—plotted as a function of SPL for a 1000 Hz tone. Listeners were told to

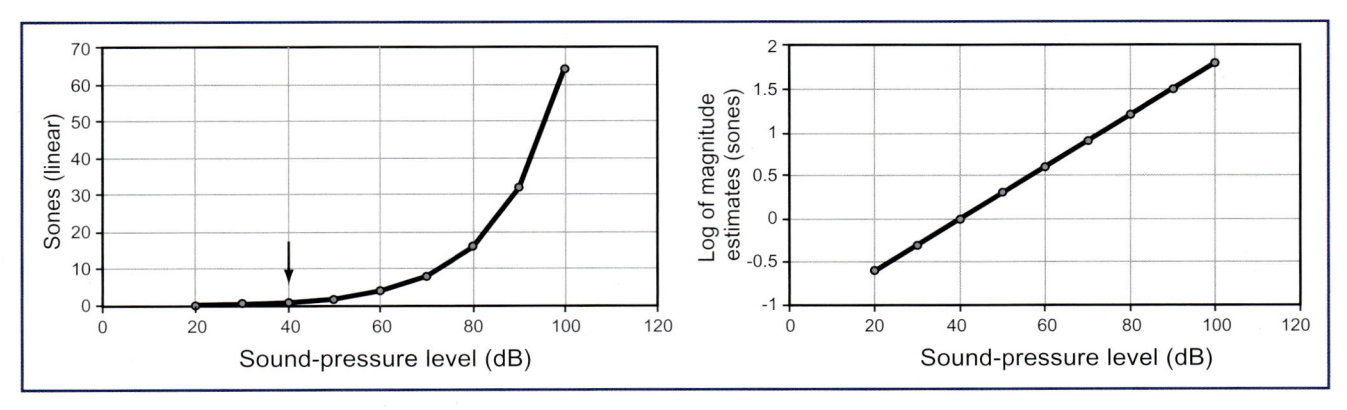

Figure 14-3. Sones plotted as a function of sound pressure level, with sones on a linear scale (*left plot*) and sones converted to logarithms (*right plot*). The reference tone is shown by the arrow in the left-hand plot.

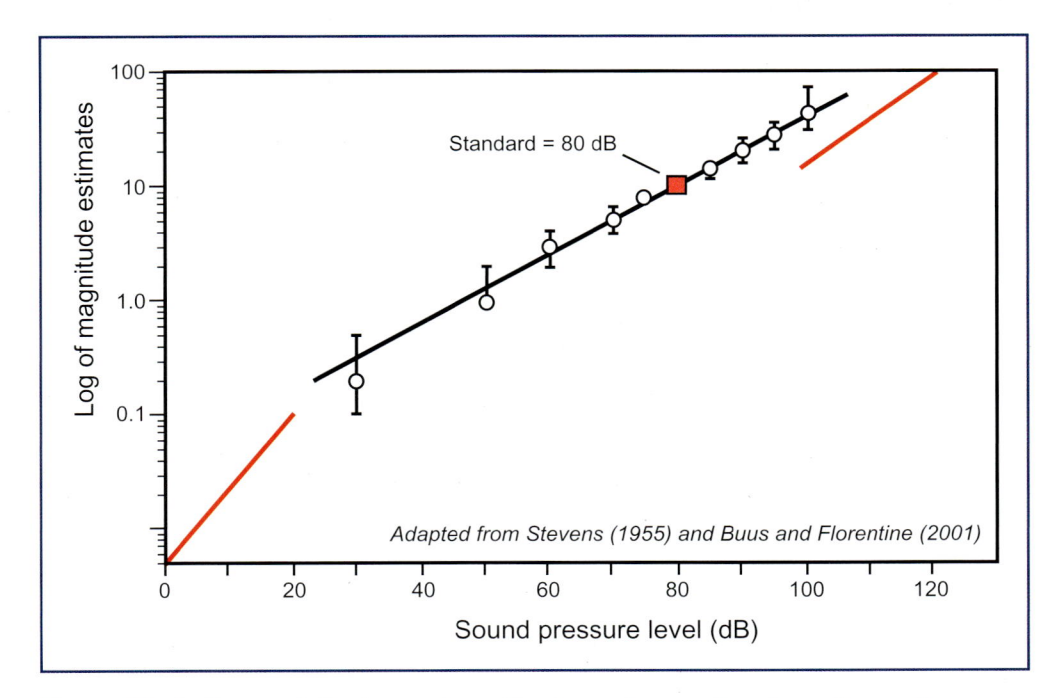

Figure 14-4. Sones plotted on a logarithmic scale as a function of sound pressure level for an 80 dB SPL, 1000 Hz tone standard. The black line in midrange SPLs is based on Stevens (1955), while the red lines near the threshold and at very high SLPs are based on Buus and Florentine (2001).

assign a value of "10" to the standard and to scale loudness of all stimuli relative to this standard value. Thus, a tone that was perceived as half the loudness of the standard was to be assigned a value of "5," a tone twice as loud as the standard a value of "20," and so forth. For this plot the magnitude estimates (sones) have been log-transformed, as in the right plot in Figure 14–3. The straight black line, the mathematical best-fit function, appears to fit the 10 plotted points quite well and is consistent with a power function relating perceived loudness to SPL. Functions such as the one in Figure 14–4 are the basis of Stevens' famous and very influential power law. Stevens presented a simple equation to summarize the law (here presented in terms of sound pressure level, not sound intensity):

$$L = k * SPL^{0.6}$$

where L = perceived loudness, SPL = sound pressure level in dB, and "k" is a constant determined by the units used for loudness estimation and other experimental variables. For the remaining discussion "k" is ignored, so for the present purpose $L = SPL^{0.6}$.

The exponent of 0.6 in this equation—the power to which SPL is raised to obtain perceived loudness— is the slope of the log-log function relating units of perceived loudness to units of sound pressure level. The slope of the black line is less than "1", as indicated by the exponent; a twofold change in SPL does not correspond to a "twice loudness" judgment. In fact, and as noted above, along the middle part of the SPL range, an increase of roughly 10 dB results in a twofold increase in loudness. A twofold increase in loudness does not nearly require a twofold increase of SPL; in fact, a twofold increase of SPL produces a huge increase in loudness, far more than "twice the loudness." Stevens' power law was based on carefully designed research and exerted a monumental influence on hearing science and audiology. An important conclusion reached from this work is that perceived loudness does not "grow" in an additive way with SPL.

There are questions and concerns with Stevens' power function, ranging from the degree to which the fitted log-log function reflects loudness judgments of individual subjects (versus the "group" data on which the functions were based), the extent to which the functions are determined by the specific methods used to elicit loudness judgments, and of course the ability to generalize from loudness judgment of sinusoids to more complex sounds such as noise, multitone acoustic events, and even speech signals. Clearly, loudness functions change depending on these factors.

Recent research shows that even for simple tones Stevens' power law is not precisely correct (Florentine & Epstein, 2006). Across the midrange of sound pressure levels (e.g., 20–70 dB) the function resembles the one described by Stevens, with perhaps a slightly shallower slope (i.e., a smaller exponent). Close to threshold, however, the log-log function has a much steeper slope compared with midrange SPLs, and at very high SPLs the function is also steeper but not to the same degree as the function at threshold (Buus & Florentine, 2001). This means that near threshold, small SPL differences yield more rapid (greater) increases in loudness than the same small differences in the 20 to 70 dB range (the same for the SPL-loudness relationship at very high SPLs). The fact that the "growth rate" of loudness near threshold and at very high SPLs is different from loudness growth across midrange SPLs suggests that for the entire range of SPL, a more complicated formula than Stevens' power law is required to relate SPL to perceived loudness of tones. The short red lines in Figure 14–4 show approximate slopes of the loudness-SPL function close to threshold (lower left of plot) and at very high SPLs (upper right of plot).

Loudness of Complex Sounds

Complex sounds, defined in Chapter 7, have energy at more than one frequency, and typically at many frequencies. Although pure-tone (single-frequency) signals are used extensively in auditory research and as an important part of the clinical evaluation of hearing, sounds in the world are complex. In this brief introduction to the loudness of complex sounds, the concept of auditory filters is introduced followed by comments on the loudness of two different types of complex sound. Readers interested in a more advanced understanding of this topic are referred to Florentine, Buus, and Bonding (1978) and Moore (2013).

The Peripheral Auditory System Is a Series of Bandpass Filters

A general discussion of filters is presented in Chapter 7; here they are summarized and related to auditory psychophysics. A filter is any device or computer program that permits some objects (which may include vibrating air molecules or time-varying voltages) to pass through it while blocking others. For example, the filter in your home furnace permits passage of air molecules but blocks passage of larger molecules, including those that form dust and plant pollens. In acoustics a filter is a physical device, software code, or anatomical/physiological process that allows certain frequencies to pass through while blocking the passage of other frequencies. Acoustic filters can be configured in many ways. Some may allow low frequencies to pass through while blocking high frequencies, whereas others do the opposite. Or, the acoustic filter can be one that allows a range, or "band," of frequencies to pass while blocking all frequencies below and above this band. Many scientists believe that the peripheral auditory system processes the human range of audible frequencies through a series of bandpass filters arranged across the basilar membrane from base to tip.

The concept of auditory bandpass filters was introduced in the preceding chapter, although the term "auditory filter" was not used. When neural tuning curves were described and illustrated (Figure 13–23), a neuron attached to a hair cell was said to have a characteristic frequency—the one with the lowest firing threshold. Frequencies above or below the characteristic frequency required more sound energy to make the neuron fire. As frequencies moved farther away from the characteristic frequency, the neuron-firing threshold became increasingly higher, until a frequency was reached which failed to elicit an action potential from the neuron. The neural tuning curve shown in Figure 13–23 is basically a bandpass filter turned upside down, with the "best" passage of energy at the characteristic frequency, and increasingly reduced passage of energy—for the neuron under study—as frequency becomes more distant from the characteristic frequency.

Neural tuning curves are derived from animal experiments. Very clever, non-invasive experiments in humans have demonstrated the same types of auditory filters by using auditory masking. Imagine an experiment in which a threshold is determined in a human for a tone of 2000 Hz. This threshold is obtained in the standard way, which is to say that the listener only hears the test tone; otherwise the listening channel is quiet. After the threshold is determined, a noise signal is played simultaneously with the 2000 Hz tone. The noise signal is composed of many frequencies which are not related harmonically and have time-varying amplitudes and phases. The noise is designed such that the average energy in a small range of frequencies is equivalent to the average energy in any other similarly sized range. For example, if a noise signal includes frequencies from 1800 to 2200 Hz, the average energy within the frequency range 1800 to 1805 Hz is equivalent to the energy within the frequency range 2100 to 2105 Hz (or 2000–2005 Hz, 1900–1905 Hz, and so forth). This description is consistent with the discussion of white noise presented in Chapter 7, of average energy within any range of frequencies, and in fact across the entire frequency band of the noise. The important difference in the current case is the band-limited nature of the 1800 to 2200 Hz noise; white noise typically has (in theory) an infinitely wide bandwidth.

Think of this 400 Hz noise band, ranging from 1800 to 2200 Hz, as derived from a white noise with energy filtered out below 1800 Hz and above 2200 Hz.

Now imagine an even narrower band of noise, one centered at 2000 Hz and having a width of 50 Hz. The 50 Hz band ranges from 1975 to 2025 Hz. This noise band is presented simultaneously with the 2000 Hz pure tone, and an experimenter determines the noise presentation level that just makes the 2000 Hz tone inaudible. In this example, the 2000 Hz tone is *masked* by the narrowband noise, requiring additional energy in the 2000 Hz tone, relative to its energy at threshold in quiet, to make it just audible again. Assume the level of the tone must be raised 1 dB relative to the quiet (unmasked) threshold to make it audible in the presence of this noise signal. The new threshold is called a masked threshold. The narrowband noise signal presented simultaneously with the 2000 Hz tone makes the previously audible tone inaudible by "hiding" it until its level is increased to make it audible again.

The interesting part of this experiment comes with the next step, when the bandwidth of the noise signal is increased (made wider). Because the average energy is the same and constant for all frequencies within the noise signal and the overall noise level is the sum of all these individual component energies, widening the bandwidth increases the overall level of the noise. If the noise signal is widened to 100 Hz, still centered at the 2000 Hz frequency (the noise extends from 1950–2050 Hz), the auditory system is stimulated by greater noise energy than it was by the 50 Hz wide noise. The tone is once again masked by the wider noise bandwidth. To make the tone audible again, its level must be increased, perhaps by another 1 dB. This new masked threshold is roughly 2 dB greater than the threshold in quiet. As the width of the noise band is progressively increased, so is the SPL required to reach threshold for tone detection. This makes sense because a greater bandwidth is associated with a greater noise level.

When the noise bandwidth reaches a certain value the threshold does not increase even though the bandwidth is increased. In fact, even further increases in noise bandwidth do not affect the masked threshold. In one such experiment, the increase in threshold for a 2000 Hz tone was roughly 4 dB for increases in noise bandwidth up to 400 Hz, centered around the 2000 Hz tone. Noise bandwidths wider than 400 Hz failed to produce further increases in the masked threshold of the 2000 Hz tone (Schooneveldt & Moore, 1989).

The interpretation of this result, and results from many other similar experiments, is that the tone threshold does not increase past a certain noise bandwidth, even though the level of noise continues to increase, because the bandwidth of the noise exceeds the frequency range of an auditory filter. The auditory filter around (in this case) 2000 Hz has a frequency range that rejects energy relatively distant from the its center frequency. The center frequency is analogous to the "characteristic frequency" of the neural tuning curves discussed in Chapter 13. Schooneveldt and Moore (1989) estimated the width of the filter centered around 2000 Hz to be about 400 Hz. When the noise bandwidth was increased beyond 400 Hz, the energy of the whole noise band affected the motions of the basilar membrane and the associated neural responses, but did not affect the output of the auditory filter with a center frequency of 2000 Hz.

The change in threshold of the 2000 Hz tone with changes in the width of a noise band centered at 2000 Hz is shown schematically in Figure 14–5, panels (a) through (e). Panel (a) shows the threshold in quiet to be roughly 2 dB SPL re: 20 μPa (see Figure 14–1 for minimal audible field at 2000 Hz). In panels (b), (c), and (d) the width of the noise band is increased symmetrically around 2000 Hz, which increases the overall energy of the noise band and causes the threshold of the 2000 Hz tone to increase. When the noise bandwidth is increased past 400 Hz, the threshold of the 2000 Hz tone remains the same, as can be seen by comparing the heights of the vertical red lines in panels (d) and (e). Energy within the 400 Hz band around 2000 Hz seems to be processed "together"—that is, the energy of both the target signal plus the masker is processed together—whereas energy outside this band has little or no effect on the output of this auditory filter.

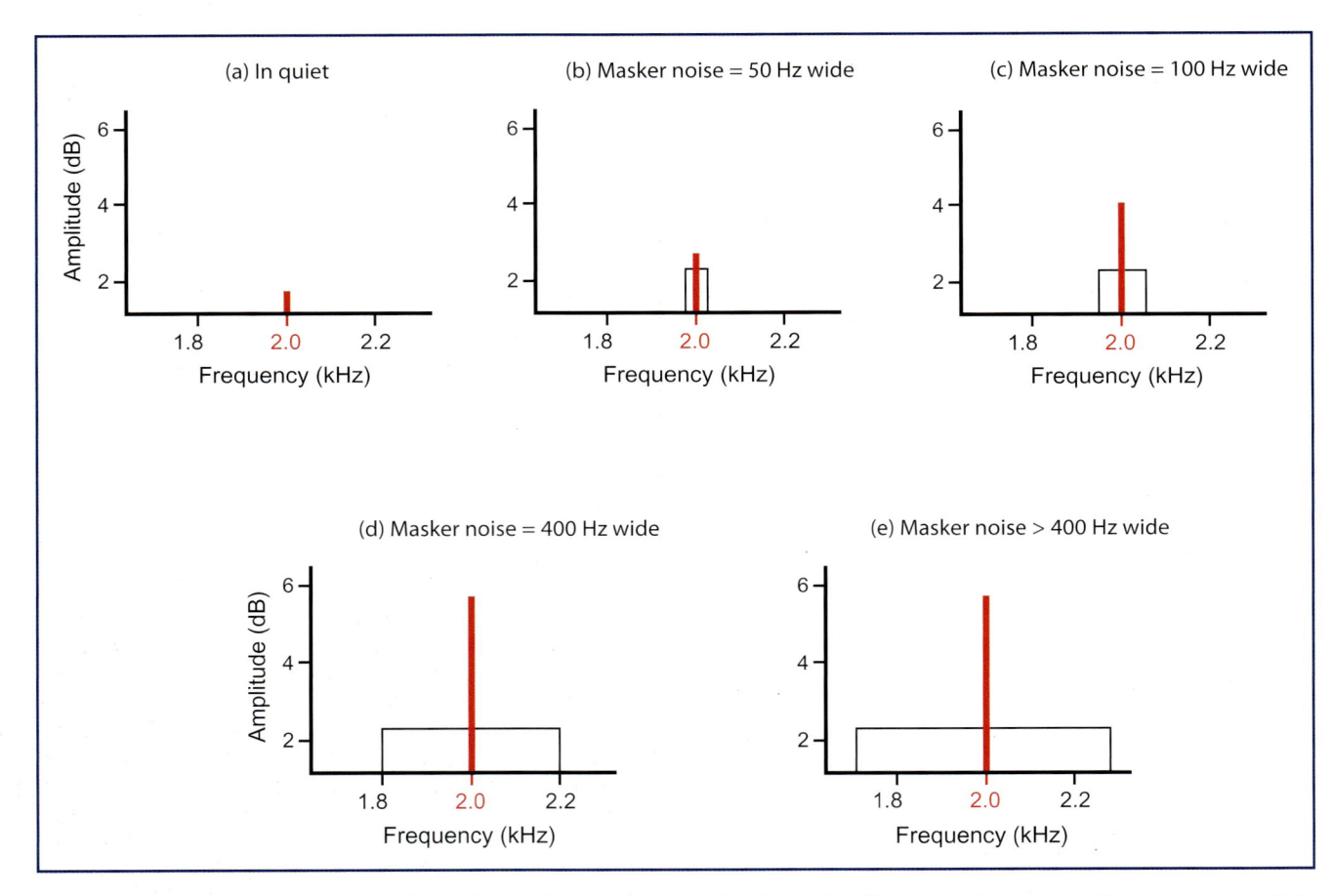

Figure 14–5. Schematic illustration of how increases in noise bandwidth around a center frequency result in increasingly higher detection thresholds for a pure tone at the center of the noise band (2000 Hz in this case), but only up to a specific bandwidth. Further increases in the width of the noise band do not cause higher pure tone (sinusoid) detection thresholds. The height of the vertical red line shows the SPL required for detection of the 2000 Hz tone; the black rectangle shows the width of the noise band centered symmetrically around 2000 Hz. **A.** Threshold of the 2000 Hz tone in quiet. **B.** Masked threshold for a noise band with a width of 50 Hz. **C.** Masked threshold for a noise band with a width of 100 Hz. **D.** Masked threshold for a noise band with a width of 400 Hz. **E.** Masked threshold for noise bandwidths greater than 400 Hz.

Another way to demonstrate auditory filters in the peripheral auditory system is to obtain psychoacoustical tuning curves (PTCs) from human listeners. PTCs are obtained using masking of one signal by another but in a way somewhat different from the method described above. In a typical experiment (see Kluk & Moore, 2004 for an example), the signal is a pure tone and the masker is a narrow band of noise. The tone is fixed at a single frequency and a low level of presentation (often 10 dB above the quiet threshold for the tone). The level of a fixed-width, symmetrical narrow band of noise, centered at the frequency of the test tone, is adjusted to determine the threshold of the test tone in noise. Under this condition, the level of the noise band required to make the signal inaudible should be fairly low—the center frequency of the noise is the same as the test tone, so the levels of both signals are very close to the quiet threshold.

The threshold of the test tone is then determined, repeatedly, in the presence of the noise band centered at each of many frequencies, below and above the frequency of the test signal. For example, assume the frequency of the test tone is 1000 Hz and the noise band has a width of 160 Hz. When the noise band is centered at the test frequency, the noise covers the frequency range 920 to 1080 Hz (a range of 80 Hz on either side of the 1000 Hz test signal). The noise band is then moved to align its center at 950 Hz (a noise band range of 870–1030 Hz). The question is, what level of the noise masker centered at 950 Hz is required to just make the 1000 Hz test tone inaudible, and then barely audible (that is, to determine the detection of the test tone with the noise band in its new frequency location)? The noise band is moved again, this time to a center frequency of 750 Hz (a noise band range of 670–830 Hz). Now, what is the level of the noise masker required to make the test tone just barely audible? When this experiment is done for many center frequencies of the constant-bandwidth noise band, a threshold curve for the 1000 Hz test tone is determined. As might be expected, the SPL of the noise band required to mask the 1000 Hz test tone increases as the center frequency of the fixed-width noise band moves away from the test tone frequency.

Figure 14–6 shows psychophysical tuning curves (PTCs) from Kluk and Moore (2004) for a 1000 Hz tone obtained from three listeners using the methods described immediately above. The x-axis is the center frequency of a noise band having a width of 160 Hz; the y-axis is the level of noise required to mask the 1000 Hz tone presented 10 dB above threshold. Note that the lowest point on all three graphs (each for a separate listener) is located at 1000 Hz on the x-axis. This follows from the idea discussed above that the lowest level of noise energy required to make the 1000 Hz tone just inaudible is found when the noise band is centered at 1000 Hz. When the noise band is centered at frequencies

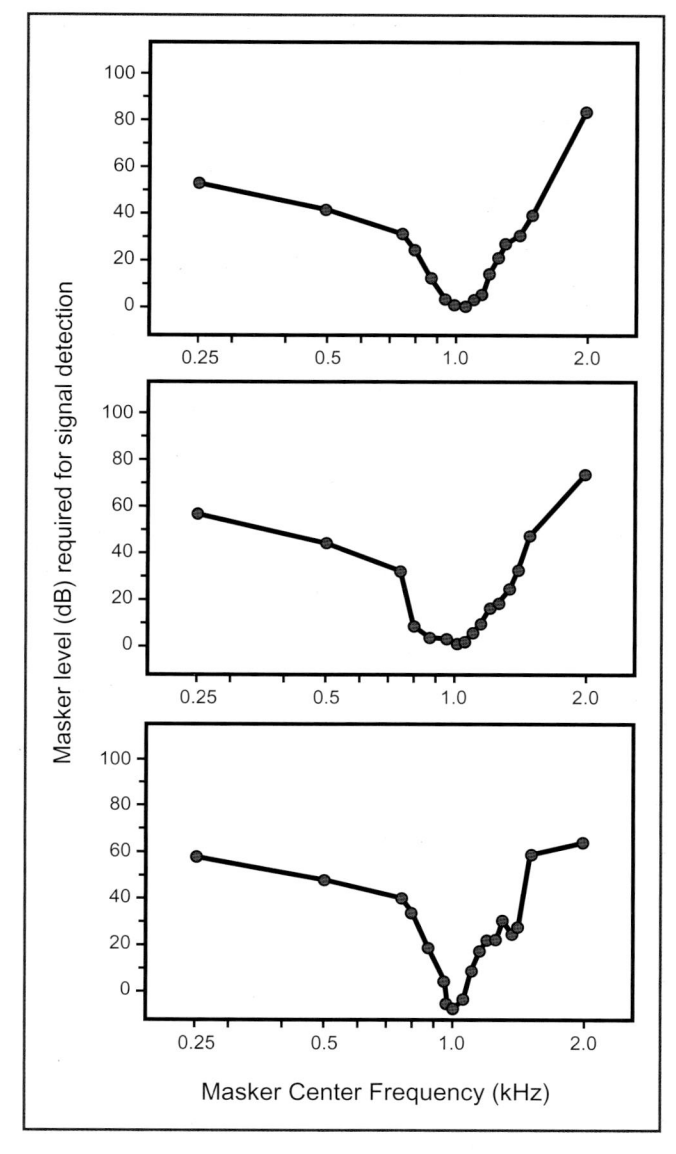

Figure 14–6. Psychophysical tuning curves (PTCs) from three listeners adapted from Kluk and Moore (2013). Each listener's data are plotted in separate panels (*top, middle, bottom*). The y-axis shows the masker level required to make the signal level of the tone just detectable. Center frequency of the noise band is on the x-axis, and the test tone is set at a constant frequency (in this case, 1000 Hz) and level approximately 10 dB above the level at quiet threshold. Even though the width of the masker noise is constant, as the center frequency of the noise band moves away from the sinusoid frequency, there is an increase in the level of the noise required to make the signal detectable.

> **Tuning Up Tuning Curves**
>
> The tuning curves described in the text are generated in humans using masked thresholds. Tuning curves can be generated in other ways, as well. In animal models of audition, scientists have inserted microelectrodes to individual nerve fibers attached to inner hair cells, and monitored their rate of firing in response to different input frequencies. Because nerve fibers generate action potentials spontaneously, with no input, a firing-rate threshold must be set to find the lowest level at which the nerve fiber is first responsive to whatever frequency and intensity is used as input. The theory of this experiment is that the characteristic frequency of a nerve fiber (that is, a frequency that can be predicted well, if not exactly, by the position of the nerve-bearing hair cell along the basilar membrane) will evoke the fastest rate of firing above this threshold. As input frequencies move away from the characteristic frequency, firing rates decline until a frequency is reached where the nerve fires at the spontaneous (i.e., no input signal) rate. A graph of firing rate on the y-axis and frequency on the x-axis shows a tuning curve for the selected auditory nerve fiber. Happily, the tuning curves obtained from animals appear to be similar to the ones obtained from humans.

below or above the 1000 Hz test tone, a higher level is required to make the 1000 Hz test tone just inaudible. For example, the level of the 160 Hz noise band centered at 500 Hz (the second plotted point from the left in each of the three panels) that just masks the 1000 Hz test tone is about 50 dB higher than the test signal. When the noise band is centered at 1000 Hz, the noise level required to mask the tone is nearly 50 dB lower, roughly equivalent or even a bit less than the level of the test tone.

Like neural tuning curves, these PTCs are upside-down representations of auditory filters. The "tip" of these curves occurs where the test tone matches the center frequency of the noise band; this is the frequency at which the filter allows the most energy through. The tails of the curves (the parts of the curves that rise from the characteristic frequencies) show how the filter blocks, to various degrees, the passage of acoustic energy at frequencies different from the "tip" frequencies. The "tip" frequencies are analogous to the "characteristic frequencies" discussed above and in Chapter 13 for neural tuning curves. Note in Figure 14–6 the consistency of the PTCs across the three listeners, including the asymmetry of the curves. At frequencies higher than the "tip" frequency the slope is quite steep, meaning that the amount of noise energy required to mask the test tone increases quickly as the distance from the "tip" frequency increases. In contrast, at frequencies lower than the "tip" frequency the slope is steep in the frequency range closest to the tip and then becomes shallower in the lower frequencies, with only small increases in level of the masking noise as the distance from the "tip" frequency becomes greater. What this means for the auditory filter centered at 1000 Hz is that energy at and immediately around 1000 Hz is passed with greatest amplitude, but energy at frequencies above 1000 Hz are blocked by rapidly increasing amounts as frequency becomes increasingly different from 1000 Hz. For frequencies immediately below 1000 Hz (to about 800 Hz) there is also a rapid decrease in energy passed by the filter, but at even lower frequencies the blocking of energy changes more gradually (see Figure 14–6).

PTCs for four "tip" frequencies are shown for a single listener in Figure 14–7. This plot is adapted from Carney and Nelson (1983) who used a slightly different method than the one presented above but serves to make two points. First, for each of the four test tones (500, 1000, 2000, and 4000 Hz, indicated by arrows in Figure 14–7), the shape of the PTCs is generally consistent with the PTCs shown in Figure 14–6 for 1000 Hz. For all four test frequencies, PTC shape is asymmetric in the same way: rapid and substantial blocking of energy above the "tip" frequency, shallower slopes below the "tip." By inference the shape of the auditory filters are consistent across these frequencies, at least between 500 and 4000 Hz. Second, parts of the PTCs for different frequencies overlap, suggesting that auditory filters are not sequenced from low to high frequency as independent passbands. This is an even more compelling observation given the sparse sampling in Figure 14–7 of all possible PTCs that could be determined, for every frequency, if an experimenter had sufficient time and listeners with enough patience and stamina.

Even though the general shape of PTCs shown in Figure 14–7 is similar across frequencies, the width of the filters is not (note for the PTC at 4000 Hz the greater difference between frequencies just above the tip frequency). Considerable research effort has been devoted to the identification of a mathematical expression that reflects the differing width of these filters as a function of frequency. Evidence from animals and humans shows convincingly that the filter widths increase as frequency increases (a technical review is available in Greenwood, 1990). Filter widths are much greater at, for example, 8000 Hz (width ~600 Hz) compared with 800 Hz (width ~90 Hz). These bands are often referred to as critical bandwidths (the concept

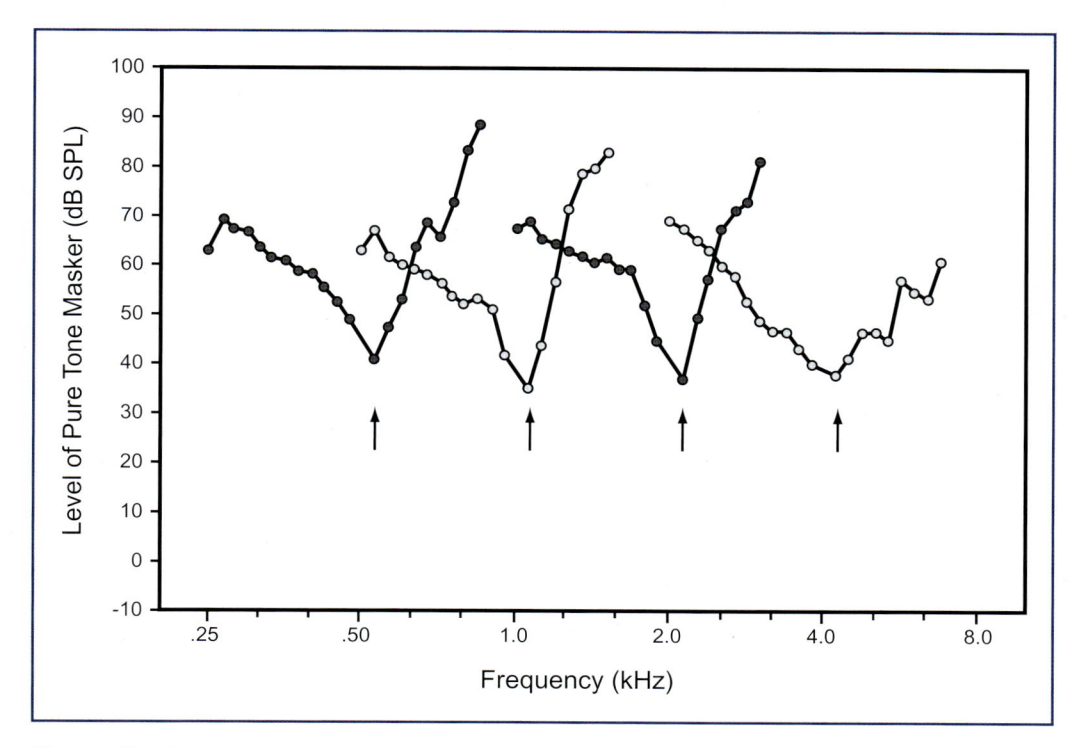

Figure 14–7. Psychophysical tuning curves (PTCs) for four different "tip" frequencies, adapted from human data reported by Carney and Nelson (1983). These tuning curves are from a single listener and used a slightly different method than the one used by Kluk and Moore (2004).

is also referred to as equivalent rectangular bands). Although the mathematical function that relates filter bandwidth to frequency is a continuous one, the frequency analysis capabilities of the basilar membrane are often partitioned into 35 critical bands. Each of the 35 bands is thought to correspond to a distance along the basilar membrane of roughly 1 mm (the human basilar membrane is 35 mm in length). The correspondence of a length along the basilar membrane with a critical band is not a linear function: a length of 1 mm

Auditory Filters: Do They Matter?

Is the concept of auditory filters relevant to the way we hear real-life signals, or simply a laboratory invention? This is a reasonable question that brings us back to the concept of the spectrum. Recall that a spectrum is a representation of amplitude variation across frequency. A spectrum is computed by Fourier analysis and displayed on a screen as a plot, with frequency (in Hz) on the x-axis and amplitude (in dB) on the y-axis. For many years scientists studied the acoustic characteristics of speech sounds by inspecting such spectra to understand the acoustic cues used by listeners to identify speech sounds. However, several researchers considered the possibility that the filtering characteristics of the auditory system meant that the speech-sound spectrum, transformed into neural signals after analysis by auditory filters, was not the same as the spectrum entering the ear canal. In the case of vowels, for example, the formant structure seen in a so-called linear-frequency spectrum (before auditory filtering) was likely to be substantially different from the auditory representation of the signal. Thus, the term "auditory spectrum" was coined to refer to the spectrum as processed by the auditory system. Scientists still debate whether the differences between linear and auditory spectra are critical to listeners' perception of vowels. See Syrdal and Gopal (1986); Adank, Smits, and van Hout (2004); and Moore (2008) for reviews of this issue.

of basilar membrane at the base of the cochlea covers a much greater range of frequencies than 1 mm of basilar membrane length at the apex.

The Critical Band Concept and the Loudness of Complex Sounds

What happens when the loudness of a sinusoid (pure tone) is matched to the loudness of a complex acoustic event having frequency components falling outside the critical bandwidth whose center (tip) frequency corresponds to the frequency of the sinusoid? The relevant experiments have been performed and published by several scientists, but the discussion here is confined to work reported by Florentine, Buus, and Bonding (1978). Florentine et al. asked listeners to adjust a control knob until the loudness of two signals was equivalent. The knob controlled the intensity of one of the signals while the other was held constant. We are specifically interested in two of their comparisons, one in which the loudness of a 1000 Hz tone was matched to the loudness of a two-tone (that is, two-sinusoid) complex, the other in which the loudness of a 1000 Hz tone was matched to a noise signal whose bandwidth had lower and upper frequency limits equivalent to the tone frequencies used in the two-tone match.

For the loudness match of the 1000 Hz tone to a two-tone (two-sinusoids) signal separated by 1592 Hz (one tone at 468 Hz, the other at 2060 Hz), the 1000 Hz signal had to be about 3 dB greater than the two-tone signal. Stated otherwise, when the intensities of the single tone and the two-tone signal were equal, the two-tone signal sounded louder than the single tone.

For the match of the 1000 Hz tone to a noise with the same bandwidth of 1592 Hz, the 1000 Hz tone had to be roughly 14 dB greater than the noise to achieve a loudness match. This finding led Florentine et al. (1978) to wonder if the difference between the two-tone and noise match was due to the noise signal's many frequency components (energy at every frequency from 468 to 2060 Hz) compared with the energy of the two sinusoids of the two-tone signal. They did a further experiment in which they added tones to the two-tone signal and found that additional tones made the tonal complex louder relative to the 1000 Hz sinusoid. Loudness seemed to be determined, at least to a significant degree, by the number of sinusoidal components in a signal. The limit of adding sinusoids to a multitone signal is adding equal energy at every frequency in the band, which is equivalent to creation of a bandpass, filtered white noise at 468 Hz on the low end and 2060 Hz on the high end.

What is the relationship between the findings of Florentine et al. (1978) and the concept of auditory filters? Hearing scientists estimate the size of the critical band centered around 1000 Hz to be roughly 150 to 160 Hz (see, for example, Figure 1 in Moore & Glasberg, 1983). This means that the target signal—the 1000 Hz sinusoid—is "competing" for loudness with a two-tone signal. The two-tone signal in this case has a frequency range that is far greater than the filter width around 1000 Hz. Because all signals are presented at the same SPL, it makes sense that the two-tone signal causes more widespread motion of the basilar membrane, and therefore more activation of nerve fibers attached to hair cells, compared with the motion and neural activation of the single component at 1000 Hz. It is as if the two-tone signal creates outputs of two auditory filters (where "output" means the energy "delivered" to the auditory nerve fibers), compared with the single output of the 1000 tone. With greater overall neural activation, it makes sense that the two-tone signal is louder even when the SPLs of the target and comparison signals are equivalent. Similarly, the loudness of a noise band centered at 1000 Hz but extending far below and above the critical bandwidth at 1000 Hz means even more motion and neural stimulation—more filter outputs—compared with that of a single sinusoid at 1000 Hz. Even when the noise signal has the same SPL as the 1000 Hz sinusoid, the former has much greater loudness than the latter. The energy of the noise signal is spread across several critical bands and produces a neural excitation pattern in excess of the excitation produced by a single tone.

Comparisons of loudness across different signals is notoriously tricky because it is affected by many factors. The description provided here provides the basics of the relationship between sound energy, perceived loudness, and the concept of the peripheral auditory system as a series of overlapping filters. The science of loudness is more than a sterile laboratory exercise: fitting of hearing aids, adjustments of the processors of cochlear implants, and design of speech recognition and synthesis programs all depend on an understanding of variables that determine the loudness of complex sounds.

Sensitivity of the Auditory System to Loudness Change

In the study of the senses (hearing, vision, taste, smell, touch) there has always been interest in the smallest change in a physical stimulus that can be detected reliably. These perceptual distinctions are known as difference limens (DLs) or just noticeable differences (JNDs). For this discussion, the term loudness DL is used.

According to the Acoustical Society of America Standards (ASA standard 11.35, June 2016, https://

asastandards.org/Terms/difference-limen-for-loudness/), the loudness DL is defined as follows:

> For an individual listener and a sound of specified frequency under specified conditions, the minimum change of sound pressure level and frequency that is just noticed as a change in loudness. Unit, decibel (dB).

Note how this definition includes variables likely to affect the DL for loudness. Some variables that can affect the loudness DL are not specified explicitly in the ASA standard ("under specified conditions"), but point to the complex nature of even a simple perceptual phenomenon such as detecting loudness change.

Loudness DLs have been investigated extensively. Most students get a first exposure to loudness DLs (and other aspects of audition) in an introductory course on experimental psychology, where Weber's law is introduced (the law is sometimes called the Weber–Fechner law, Fechner's law being derived from Weber's law). Even though Weber's experiments concerned perceived heaviness and brightness of light, the results were generalized as a rule for any sensory distinction. Simply stated, the loudness DL was thought to be a constant proportion of the reference SPL. The greater the reference SPL (and therefore loudness), the greater the change in SPL required for a listener to detect a change in loudness. The amount of this required change is assumed to be a constant fraction of the reference SPL. Listeners can therefore detect smaller changes in SPL as changes in loudness when the reference sound has low SPL. Increasingly larger SPL changes are required to detect a loudness change with increases in the reference SPL. Weber's law can be expressed this way:

$$DL_{loudness} = \Delta SPL / SPL_{standard}$$

and

$$\Delta I / SPL_{standard} = k$$

where ΔSPL (Δ being the Greek symbol indicating "change") is the change in SPL of a stimulus that allows the detection of loudness change relative to the SPL of the standard. $SPL_{standard}$ is the SPL of the standard, or reference stimulus. In other words, k is a constant regardless of $SPL_{standard}$.

A schematic illustration of a typical experiment designed to determine the loudness DL is shown in Figure 14–8 (after Florentine, Buus, & Mason, 1987). A listener hears two sinusoids in succession, each tone having a duration of 500 ms (half a second) and separated from each other by a silent interval of 250 ms (a quarter of a second, called the interstimulus interval). The black horizontal lines indicate the "on" interval for

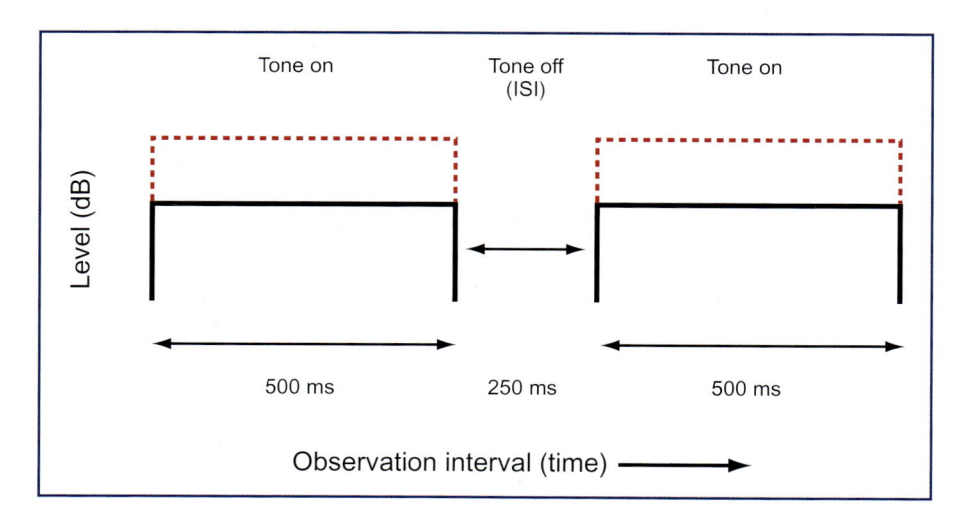

Figure 14–8. A schematic diagram of one version of an experiment investigating the difference limen for loudness. Two tones are shown, separated by a quiet, interstimulus interval. One tone is the standard SPL ($SPL_{standard}$) (indicated by the height [y-axis] of the *horizontal black line*), the other tone has a slightly higher intensity. The order of the standard tone and the tone with an intensity increment added to the standard (*indicated by the horizontal, red dashed line*) is randomized across the trials (one trial being the presentation of the two tones in the "observation interval" shown in this figure). The listener presses a button indicating whether the tone with greater loudness was the first or second of the two tones.

the standard tones (SPL$_{standard}$), whereas the red dashed lines show the level to which one or the other tone must be increased (the ΔSPL + SPL$_{standard}$) to determine whether a listener can detect a loudness difference. Both sequenced tones are shown as having a standard and increased level because on any given trial, either the first or second tone may have the increased level. In this way, potential order effects are controlled. During the experiment, the listener presses one of two buttons to indicate which of the two tones is louder.

Florentine et al. (1987) showed that the loudness DL was variable as a function of signal frequency and reference signal level. In addition, the six listeners studied by Florentine and colleagues often had different loudness DLs, even at the same frequency and SPL. For example, loudness DLs, for a 1000 Hz tone presented at a standard level of 40 dB SPL, were ranked across the six listeners from smallest to greatest, 1.29, 1.69, 2.03, 2.79, 2.98, and 3.30 dB. The differences across listeners are large. With this listener variability in mind, a summary of Florentine et al.'s findings can be summarized as follows: (1) loudness DLs cannot be said to follow the predictions of Weber's law (which claims that loudness DLs are a constant proportion of the reference SPL), although in some cases and across high frequencies (from 10.0–16.0 kHz), the prediction is *almost* upheld, (2) the loudness DL tends to decrease slowly with increased levels of the reference stimulus, especially at lower frequencies (e.g., 250, 500, and 1000 Hz) and to some extent at frequencies such as 2000 and 4000 Hz, and (3) at very high frequencies (8.0, 10.0, 12.0, 14.0 kHz) the loudness DL is larger than at lower frequencies and seems to be relatively independent of the standard level.

A broader view of the loudness DL is that at frequencies where the auditory system is most sensitive, say between 1000 and 4000 Hz, and at levels corresponding roughly to sounds that are not too soft or too loud (around 70 dB SPL), loudness DLs are very small, on average about 1 dB (estimate derived from Florentine et al., 1987, their Table 1). Loudness differences can be heard with very small differences in sound pressure level over the frequency region where those differences may have an important impact on perception (such as in speech or in music). The extension of these DL data from pure tones to the perception of more complex sounds is not direct, but they show the auditory system to have the capability for very fine distinctions of loudness.

PSYCHOPHYSICS OF PITCH

Just as loudness is a psychological phenomenon that is *related* to the physical magnitude of sound energy, pitch is a psychological phenomenon that is *related* to the frequency of sound. And just like loudness, pitch can be measured by listener report. The Acoustical Society of America standards define pitch as "the attribute of auditory sensation by which sounds are ordered on the scale used for melody in music" (standard 11.01, https://asastandards.org/Terms/pitch/).

Experiments with Sinusoids: Why?

It is fair to ask why so many auditory experiments use sinusoidal stimuli—the simplest acoustic event—when most sounds in the environment, and especially sounds such as speech and music, are so complex. The question might be answered with a different question, to wit, why study the structure and function of individual brain cells to understand behavior (which many scientists do)? This does not answer the original question directly, and is not meant as a textbook smirk. In fact, a careful understanding of the role of simple components of any process is likely to point in the direction of understanding complex behavior. A basic tenet of acoustics, as discussed in Chapter 7, is that any complex sound can be decomposed into its individual sinusoidal components. Complex acoustic events with multiple sinusoids can be analyzed as a spectrum (amplitude of sinusoidal components as a function of frequency) and a spectrum can be described by its shape. An area of research called auditory profile analysis (Green, 1988; Zera, Onsan, Nguyen, & Green, 1993) investigates the ability of listeners to detect changes in spectral shape of auditory signals that contain multiple frequency components. The results are complicated (as usual), but it appears that human listeners need no more than a 2 to 3 dB change of a single sinusoidal component within a multitone signal to detect a change in spectral shape. If you buy the idea that analysis of complex sounds is analysis of the individual components of the sound, the work on simple sinusoids makes sense.

Strike the keys on a piano keyboard in sequence from left to right and each successive key produces a sound that is higher in pitch than the previous key. It is also the case that each key strike brings a hammer down on a string that is shorter and less massive than the previous key. Hence the vibratory rate (frequency) of the strings increases as the key strikes move from left to right. Taken together, these observations suggest a fairly direct relationship between pitch and vibratory frequency. When one pitch is described as higher than another, it is almost certain that the higher pitch corresponds to a higher frequency.

Pitch of Sinusoids

Although the relationship between pitch and frequency is very strong, it is more complicated than a simple correspondence between the two. For example, the frequency range within the auditory capabilities of humans is generally said to be 20 to 20,000 Hz, yet the relationship between frequency and pitch observed below 5000 Hz is different from the relationship above 5000 Hz. This difference is so marked that listeners who easily reproduce a simple melody for a sequence of tones varying in frequency below 5000 Hz cannot do so when the sequence involves frequencies above 5000 Hz (Moore, 2013). Another complication is that pitches are associated with names, these being related to musical notes. Middle A (or "concert" A), which is by musical standards associated with 440 Hz (whether the vibration is sinusoidal or a complex harmonic vibration with a fundamental frequency of 440 Hz and harmonics at multiples of this frequency), sounds like the same note as the A one octave below (220 Hz) or one octave above (880 Hz), in other words like other A's along the musical scale. It is true that these various A's are clearly lower or higher in pitch than the other A's, but most people will identify them as the same note.

The relationship between frequency and the pitch of the musical note A is illustrated in Figure 14–9. The x-axis is frequency from 0 Hz to 3520 Hz, and the y-axis is marked in pitch by the succession of A notes from A_0 (the lowest A note humans can hear as a pitch) to A_7 (the highest A note humans hear in a reliable octave relationship with other A's). This graph could have been constructed with any other musical note (B, G, etc.). The frequency distance between adjacent octaves is always a ratio of 2:1 (for an octave higher than a reference tone) or 1:2 (for an octave lower than a reference tone).

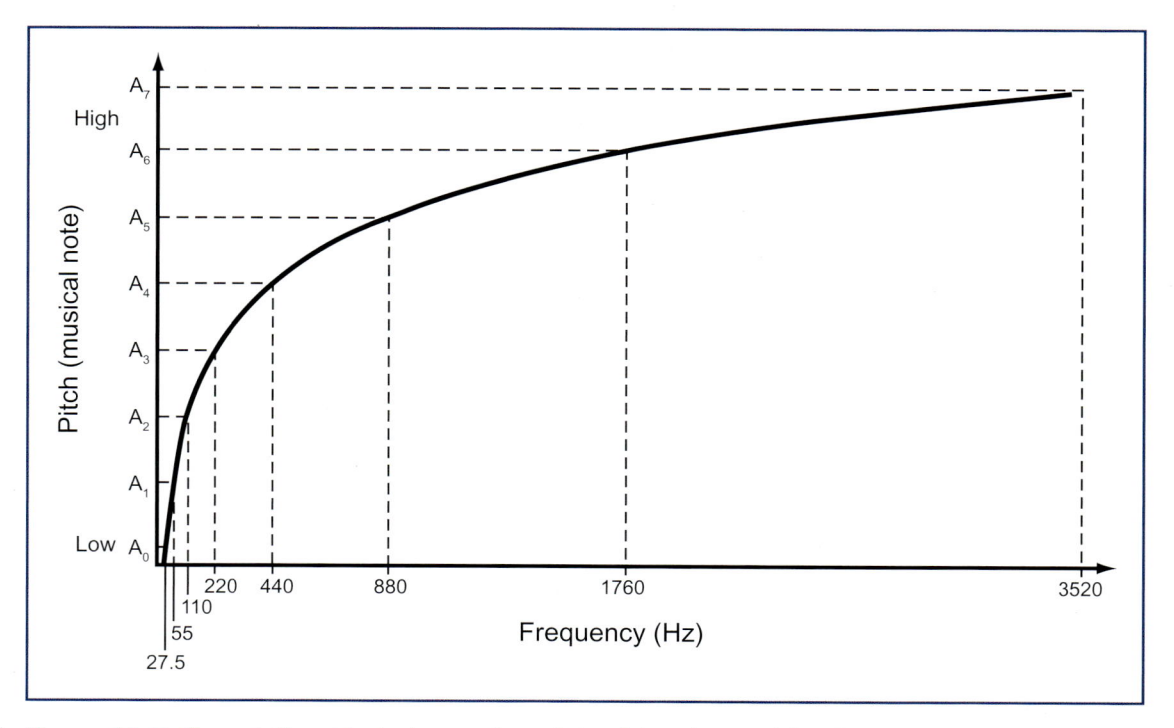

Figure 14-9. The relationship between the pitch of A notes and the frequency associated with those notes. The limits of the y-axis are the lowest (A_0) and highest (A_7) A notes for which listener can reliably determine octave relationships.

Figure 14–9 illustrates two important aspects of pitch and its relationship with frequency. First, the psychological distances between successive A's from low to high pitch are equivalent. This means that listeners judge the distance (in this case the pitch distance) between A_3 and A_4 to be the same as the distance between A_4 and A_5 or between A_5 and A_6. The perceived distance along the musical scale between any two adjacent notes with the same name is called an octave.

The second important feature of the graph in Figure 14–9 is the nonlinear relationship between pitch and frequency: increasingly larger frequency differences between consecutive octaves are associated with a doubling of pitch—equal pitch ratios (e.g., 2:1) are not associated with equivalent frequency differences. Within the frequency range shown in Figure 14–9, the change from a lower-pitch A to the immediately higher-pitched A—an octave change—is associated with relatively small frequency difference. Increasingly larger frequency differences are associated with a doubling of pitch as the notes get higher (e.g., A_3, A_4, A_5 ... etc.) For example, A_4 is associated with a frequency of 440 Hz, whereas A_5 has a frequency of 880 Hz, and A_6 has a frequency of 1760 Hz, and so on. The frequency differences for A4 to A5 and from A5 to A6 are different, but the listener regards the differences as the same pitch difference. This nonlinearity means that increasingly larger changes in frequency are required to evoke the same percept of pitch change when moving from low to high across the musical scale. As an extreme example of this nonlinear relationship, the frequency difference between A_6 and A_7, which is 1760 Hz, evokes a pitch change that is the same as the frequency difference of 110 Hz between A_2 and A_3. Experiments have shown that when listeners are presented with a reference tone (a reference frequency) and asked to adjust a comparison tone to one octave above the reference, they make the adjustment to a frequency very close to double the frequency of the reference tone (see summary in Moore, 2004).

Slightly different results for the relationship between sinusoidal frequency and perceived pitch have been obtained when magnitude estimation has been used (magnitude estimation is described above for studies of loudness and its relation to SPL). Miśkiewicz and Rakowski (2012) obtained magnitude estimates of pitch for frequencies ranging from 31.5 Hz to 12,500 Hz, in discrete steps (that is, frequencies were not varied continuously between the lowest and highest frequencies, but consisted of a series of individual tones at 31.5, 40, 50, 64 Hz . . . 12.5 kHz). A portion of their results is shown in Figure 14–10, where frequency (x-axis) and magnitude estimates (the y-axis, labeled "Pitch in arbitrary units"—i.e.,

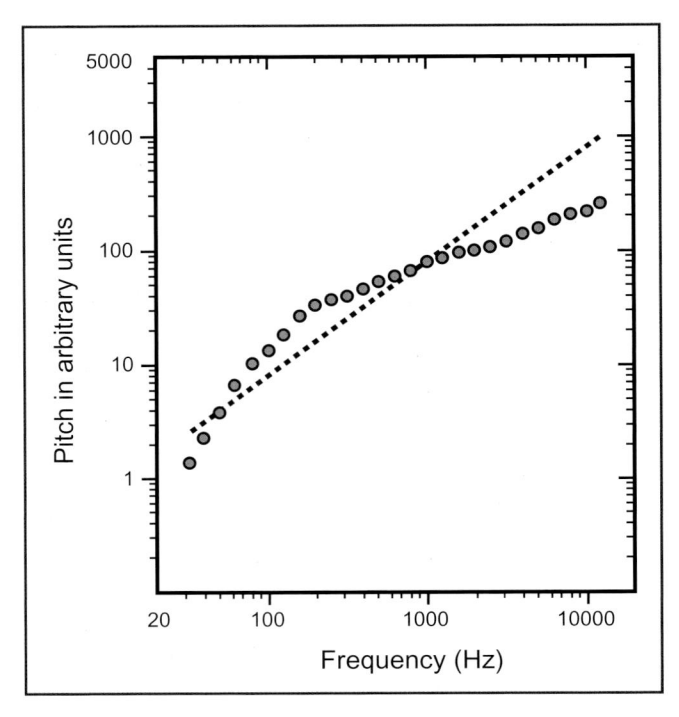

Figure 14–10. A plot of pitch versus frequency, adapted from Miśkiewicz and Rakowski (2012). Both axes are log-transformed. The straight line represents the results expected if a doubling of frequency always resulted in a doubling of pitch. The plotted points show average magnitude estimates of pitch from 30 listeners, for pure tones at each of 27 frequencies.

the magnitude estimates) are shown after logarithmic transformation of each axis. Each filled circle is the mean of 30 magnitude estimates (one judgment for each of the 30 listeners) at each of the 27 test frequencies. The straight, dotted line is the form the data *would* take if doubling of frequency resulted in the judgment of a doubling of pitch, an expectation based on octave relationships.

There are two notable features of these data. First, magnitude estimation clearly results in a plot showing increasing numbers with increasing signal frequency. The higher the frequency, the higher the perceived pitch.

Second, the curve of the plotted data points is not the straight line expected from a doubling of pitch with doubling of frequency. Below 200 Hz the curve is steeper than the straight line, indicating that perception of pitch change was very sensitive to frequency change. For the low frequency range, a doubling in frequency of the pure tones was associated with a mean pitch ratio of about 3.5:1. For the high-frequency range, a doubling in frequency of the pure tones was associated with a mean pitch ratio of roughly 1.4:1. The remainder of the frequency range, from 200 Hz to the highest frequency of 12,500 Hz, required a ratio of greater than 2:1 to evoke a perception of a doubling of pitch (Miśkiewicz & Rakowski, 2012).

This apparent difference in pitch perception across frequencies is related to how the cochlea and auditory nerve fibers code frequency, but there is not strict agreement on the exact mechanism. The *place theory* of frequency analysis, introduced in the previous chapter, depends on the tonotopic arrangement of frequency along the basilar membrane. The location of maximum displacement of the basilar membrane determines which hair cells and nerve fibers are stimulated by the sound-induced motion of the membrane. If the maximum displacement is toward the apex of the cochlea, low-frequency hair cells and nerve fibers are maximally excited. When the maximum displacement is toward the base of the cochlea, high frequency hair cells and nerve fiber are excited. Most scientists believe this theory accounts for cochlear frequency analysis, and by extension pitch perception, for frequencies above 300–500 Hz, and possibly up to the maximum limit of human frequency analysis of 20,000 Hz. This statement needs to be qualified by the observation that pitch perception is not very reliable above 5000 Hz.

The *timing theory* of frequency analysis and, by extension, pitch perception is based on the idea that for some frequencies, auditory nerve fibers produce firing rates, in synchrony, during every period of a puretone sinusoid. The nerve fibers are thought to "lock on" to one aspect of a sinusoid's repeating amplitude fluctuations—usually the peaks of the waveform—to produce a sequence of action potentials that mimics the temporal variation of the acoustic signal. In the timing theory, the code for frequency analysis (and hence pitch) is the number of times per second the auditory nerve fibers "fire" in response to the basilar membrane motion.

This view of how the cochlea and auditory nerve fibers analyze frequency is feasible only for relatively low frequencies. The refractory interval of auditory neurons appears to allow nerve fibers to produce distinct action potentials only for frequencies below 500 Hz. The refractory interval is the short time after depolarization when the nerve fibers are insensitive to another depolarization). At higher frequencies, individual action potentials are "smeared" in time, which does not permit a sufficiently fine count of the individual amplitude peaks of a sinusoid (see reviews by Miller, Abbas, & Robinson, 2001 and Oxenham, 2013). The data from Miśkiewicz and Rakowski (2012) shown in Figure 14–10 may therefore reflect the sensorineural analysis of frequency by a timing code for low frequencies, and a place code for high frequencies. Both mechanisms, place and timing, are likely relevant to frequency analysis in the cochlea and significantly related to pitch perception of both simple (sinusoidal) and complex (harmonic and inharmonic) acoustic events (see sidetrack on this page).

> **Of Place and Time**
>
> Place and timing theories of frequency analysis in the sensorineural component of the auditory system are not mutually exclusive views of how the business of pitch perception is accomplished. As pointed out by Oxenham (2014), many years of research have been devoted to identifying which of these mechanisms best explains pitch perception. Perhaps, as suggested by Miśkiewicz and Rakowski (2012), the mechanism depends on the frequency range over which pitch perception is studied. Most likely both mechanisms come into play for almost any pitch perception, at any frequency (or in the case of complex acoustic events, *frequencies*) but the precise mix of mechanisms remains unknown. Why are scientists so interested in this issue? One reason is that persons with cochlear and/or auditory nerve disorders that result in hearing loss, or persons with profound deafness who have received cochlear implants, have a notoriously difficult time placing the pitch of acoustic events along a reliable pitch scale. A full understanding of the mechanisms of sensorineural frequency analysis and pitch perception might lead to enhancements of the software used in the processors for hearing aids and cochlear implants.

Sensitivity of the Auditory System to Pitch Change

As in the case of the difference limen for loudness described above, there has been a long-standing interest in the limit of humans' ability to detect minimal difference in pitch. The Acoustical Society of America's standards define the difference limen for pitch as "the minimum fractional change of the frequency and sound pressure level that is just noticed as a change of pitch" (http://asastandards.org/Terms/difference-limen-for-pitch/). The inclusion of sound pressure level in this definition recognizes the possibility that a tone presented at a single frequency may have different pitches

> **Difference Limen for Loudness/ SLP Versus Difference Limen for Pitch/Frequency**
>
> There is a fine distinction here. The difference limens discussed in this chapter are for the perceptual variables loudness and pitch (loudness DL and pitch DL). The ASA standards for loudness DL and pitch DL are concerned with the minimal changes in SPL or frequency that can be detected as loudness or pitch changes, respectively, with fractional changes in a standard SPL or frequency. Difference limens for *intensity* or *frequency* (DLI and DLF, respectively) are technically different. For example, it is possible that different frequency tones with the same sound pressure may have different loudness; and the difference limen for frequency is the minimal difference in frequency between two tones that can be detected reliably regardless of whether the listener perceives the difference as a change in pitch (the detection of a frequency change may be based on any perceptual difference between the two tones, including but not limited to pitch). In the current text, the discussion is mainly focused on loudness and pitch DLs.

depending on its level of presentation. Great emphasis has been placed on the frequency-analysis capabilities of the peripheral auditory system, most specifically the sensorineural part of the mechanism. The pitch DL is basic to frequency analysis in the cochlea and auditory nerve and has implications for the design of devices such as hearing aids and cochlear implants. For this discussion the term "pitch DL" is used in the way stated above in the ASA standard.

A technical analysis of a dozen studies of the pitch DL was published by Micheyl, Xiao, and Oxenham (2012). Readers interested in a straightforward experiment on pitch DL are referred to the often-cited study by Wier, Jesteadt, and Green (1977). A typical experiment on pitch DL uses presentation of two sinusoids, one of which is a constant-frequency tone (the "standard" or reference) and another that varied in small frequency increments. This is a typical approach to determine the minimal frequency difference that can be detected as a change in pitch.

As is typical in research on human audition, the results of studies on the pitch DL are systematic but complicated. As illustrated by the results of Wier, Jesteadt, and Green (1977) and the review analysis by Micheyl, Xiao, and Oxenham (2012), there are three important aspects of the pitch DL. The first is that the typical pitch DL for pitch varies as a function of standard frequency, with pitch DL becoming increasingly larger with increasing standard frequency. For example, for tones presented 20 dB above threshold, average DLs for pitch increase across frequency in the following way, with DL for pitch in Hz and standard frequency in parentheses: 1.3 (200 Hz), 1.4 (400 Hz), 1.6 (600 Hz), 2.6 (800 Hz), 2.2 (1000 Hz), 5.8 (2000 Hz), 21.8 (4000 Hz), and 73.1 (8000 Hz) (Wier et al., 1977). This pattern was qualitatively similar at other presentation levels (e.g., when the tones were presented 40 or 80 dB above threshold).

These data show that, for frequencies up to 2000 Hz, the human auditory system is capable of very fine pitch discrimination (i.e., at 600 Hz a 0.27% change in frequency can be detected as a pitch change; at 1000 Hz a 0.22% change in frequency can be detected as a pitch change). In contrast, the DL for pitch is markedly larger (in absolute frequency) for frequencies above 2000 Hz. These data indicate that the auditory system has greater precision for pitch analysis at lower compared with higher frequencies.

The second important aspect is that DL for pitch becomes smaller (improves) with increases in the presentation level of the reference and comparison signals. For example, Wier et al. (1977) reported pitch DLs at 1000 Hz (presentation level in dB above threshold in parentheses) of 9.9 (5 dB), 4.3 (10 dB), 2.2 (20 dB), 1.9 (40 dB), and 1.3 (80 dB). This pattern of improved pitch DLs with increased presentation level was qualitatively similar for other reference frequencies, and is most notable at lower presentation levels, between 5 and 20 dB.

The third aspect of pitch DLs is that, for a given standard frequency, larger DLs are obtained when the signal frequencies are very brief. In the summary of relevant data from the published literature, Micheyl et al. (2012) concluded that pitch DLs were quite large (worse) at very brief durations (40 ms or less) and settled down to more typical values reported in the literature for signal durations of 100 ms or longer.

The data on DLs for pitch support the idea that the peripheral sensorineural mechanism of hearing is a precision frequency analyzer, but one with different sensitivities at different frequencies and dependent on the level and duration of input signals. This precision frequency analysis leads to precision ability in pitch discrimination, especially across certain frequency ranges. The dependence of pitch DLs on frequency is, at first glance, not all that surprising. Recall the discussion of the cochlear and auditory nerve mechanism as a series of filters, with bandwidths increasing from low characteristic frequencies (toward the apex of the basilar membrane) to high characteristic frequencies (at base of the basilar membrane). Presumably, the wider bandwidths with increasing characteristic frequency—the center frequency of the filter band—mean that frequency analysis (and pitch discrimination) should become less precise with increasing frequency. The low-frequency filters with smaller bandwidths can presumably perform a higher-precision frequency analysis of incoming signals because they are more narrowly tuned. Unfortunately, attempts to show that pitch DLs vary according to the bandwidth of the auditory analysis filter have not been successful (see Moore, 2013). In fact, the precision of frequency (and pitch) discrimination at higher frequencies seems *better* than predicted by the presumed, larger bandwidths of high-frequency filters. Researchers are still wrestling with this issue, and especially with the relationship of DL for pitch to the underlying mechanisms of frequency analysis.

Pitch of Complex Acoustic Events

As discussed in Chapter 7, complex acoustic events contain more than one frequency component. Complex *periodic* acoustic events have multiple frequency components that are harmonically related. Examples of complex periodic events are tones generated by wind instruments, piano notes, and the vibration of healthy human vocal folds. Complex *aperiodic* events also have multiple frequency components, but the relation between them is not harmonic. These are often referred to as noises, examples of which are white noise (equal average energy at all frequencies), narrowband noises (frequencies represented within a specified bandwidth,

---

Speaking of Difference Limens

Speech sounds have complex spectra, so it might be expected that characteristics of these spectra present tougher discrimination problems than the ones observed for sinusoids. Kewley-Port and Goodman (2005) reviewed the work on difference limens for steady (constant) formant frequencies of vowels and reported that they are about 10 times larger than difference limens for sinusoids of roughly the same frequency. When the formant frequencies change over time, as they often do during speech production, the difference limens are even larger, but not so large as to interfere with the distinction between steady vowel formants of different but closely related vowels (as in the English /i/ and /ɪ/) or between formant transitions of closely related semivowels (as in /r/ vs. /l/) or diphthongs (as in /aɪ/ vs /ɔɪ/). When it comes to speech, it looks like we are discriminating listeners for the task of phonetic perception.

Do Trained Musicians Have an Edge?

Most people probably believe that highly trained musicians have better auditory skills compared with "non-musical" listeners. There may be something to this. One study (Liang et al., 2016) of pitch DLs for sinusoids suggests that musicians detect pitch differences for smaller frequency differences compared with non-musicians, at least at a relatively low frequency (160 Hz). A similar comparison at 1200 Hz, however, failed to reveal a difference between musicians and non-musicians. Even at 160 Hz, the difference pitch DLs for between musicians (~6.7 Hz) and non-musicians (~11.5 Hz) was relatively small. Another study (Mandikal Vasuki, Sharma, Demuth, & Arciuli, 2016) showed that musicians were better at learning auditory patterns compared with non-musicians. Importantly, the same advantage for musicians was not observed when the patterns were visual. The researchers concluded that the musicians' advantage in the auditory, but not visual, task was related to their extensive auditory training, whether active (instructed) or simply through experience (performing music over a long period, getting a huge amount of auditory feedback). Mandikal Vasuki and colleagues noted, however, that the auditory advantages shown for the musician group were not consistent across tasks, including a speech task. Perhaps that is why the title of their study begins with "Musicians' edge," rather than something more definitive like "Musicians dominate." In any case, when studying auditory behavior it is probably a good idea to avoid mixing highly trained musicians with people who sing even simple melodies, like "Happy Birthday," on a single repeated note.

say 500–800 Hz), the frication noise associated with speech sounds such as /s/ and /f/, and the sound generated by a single hand clap (or any other very brief, impulse-like acoustic event).

Pitch of Complex Periodic Events

Figure 14–11 illustrates an acoustic signal composed of a series of frequency components with a lowest frequency (fundamental frequency or first harmonic) of 100 Hz and an infinite series of additional components at whole-number multiples of 100 Hz (i.e., 2, 3, 4, 5, 6 . . . *n* times the fundamental frequency). The first six harmonics decrease slightly in amplitude with increasing frequency (left panel, frequency domain), and the corresponding waveform (right panel, time domain) shows a sawtooth (not sinusoidal) waveform with a repeating pattern whose period is 10 ms (the waveform reflects the infinite series of harmonics, not just the six shown in Figure 14–11; see Chapter 7). Imagine that an experiment is conducted in which listeners match the pitch of this complex periodic sound to the pitch of a sinusoid. The frequency of the sinusoid is adjusted by the listener until he or she is satisfied that the pitches of the two sounds are the same. The result of this experiment is that listeners adjust the sinusoid to a frequency very close to the lowest frequency of the complex periodic sound. Listeners appear to assign primary importance to the pitch of the first harmonic (fundamental frequency) of complex periodic sounds when they are matched to the pitch of a sinusoid (Moore, 2013). Experiments have also shown that filtering out the lowest-frequency component of a complex periodic sound does not change this result: listeners still match the pitch of the "missing fundamental" complex tone to the pitch of the sinusoid eliminated from the

> **Operator, Will You Help Me Place This Call?**
>
> A friend calls you, maybe from South Philadelphia, you know who it is almost immediately after a syllable or two. You recognize the voice, you know the resonance characteristics of the friend's vocal tract, you know the pitch of the friend's voice. A remarkable phenomenon, considering landlines transmit acoustic signals, including speech, over a narrow bandpass filter of roughly 350 to 3400 Hz; cell phones have even narrower bandpass transmission (Byrne & Foulkes, 2004). Of great relevance to this chapter is the ability to recognize the friend's voice pitch even without the transmission of energy at the voice fundamental frequency, especially in adult males whose fundamental frequencies are 100 to 120 Hz and therefore excluded from the telephone transmission. Apparently just another case of the life and times of an auditory system, restoring the missing fundamental with its spectral analysis bag of tricks.

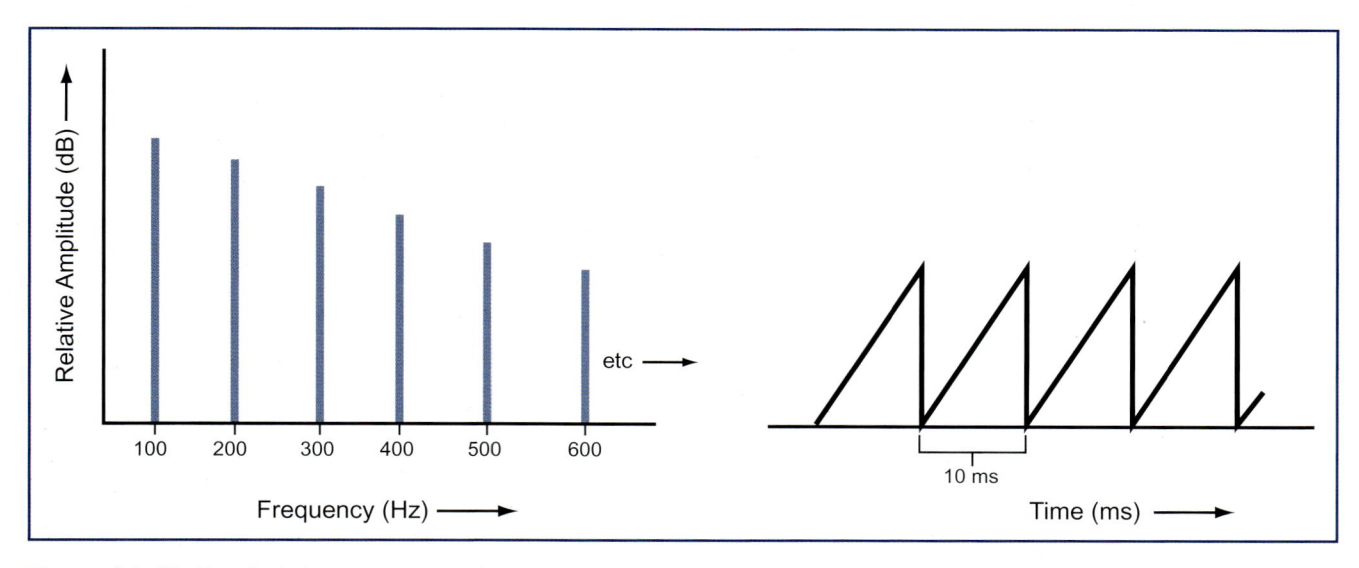

Figure 14–11. The first six harmonics of a complex periodic acoustic event (*left*) and the waveform of this spectrum with an infinite series of harmonics (not shown here to simplify the figure). The fundamental frequency of the complex acoustic event is 100 Hz, hence the period is 10 ms.

complex sound. Apparently, listeners are capable of "recovering" the missing fundamental, although the reasons for this ability remain a subject of debate (Moore, 2013). It should be noted, however, that the elimination of the fundamental frequency of a complex periodic tone may change the *timbre* (quality) of the sound even though the pitch remains the same as when the fundamental is present. Timbre is discussed in an upcoming section.

In theory, if the multiple frequency components in a complex periodic tone cause basilar membrane displacement at multiple locations in the cochlea, any of the harmonics could be heard well enough and serve as a match to the pitch of the adjusted sinusoid. Why, then, does the pitch of a complex periodic tone match the pitch of the sinusoid that is the lowest component of the complex sound? One explanation relates to the concept of the basilar membrane and auditory nerve fibers as a series of filters. As described earlier, the low-frequency filters, whose characteristic frequencies approximate the fundamental frequency of many complex periodic sounds, have a very narrow bandwidth. As the center frequency of the filters moves to higher frequencies, the bandwidths of the filters widen, meaning the frequency analysis of the filter becomes less precise. This view of auditory filters leads to the idea that the lowest-frequency filters, because of their narrow bandwidths, process only single frequencies —the ones close to their characteristic frequency. One example of this is the fundamental frequency of the complex acoustic event. This very precise processing presents the low-frequency components to further auditory analysis in a clear and prominent way. Listeners having access to such a clear frequency analysis base their estimate of pitch of the complex periodic sound on this prominent, clear output. On the other hand, the broad bandwidths of higher-frequency filters may include multiple harmonics within their analysis range which do not serve as a useful pitch cue for the complex acoustic event.

The idea of auditory filters and how they may contribute to the pitch of a complex periodic event is consistent with a place theory of frequency analysis and pitch perception. According to an alternate view, the poor frequency resolution of high-frequency auditory filters, within which two or more harmonics are analyzed together and not separated into their individual frequency components, may turn out to produce a cue to the period of the complex sound. When two adjacent harmonics (e.g., the twentieth and twenty-first harmonic of 100 Hz—2000 and 2100 Hz) are processed by the same high-frequency auditory filter, their respective amplitudes will go in and out of phase over time because of their frequency difference (see Chapter 7).

The phase variability is systematic with a repeating pattern of summating and canceling amplitudes of the two frequencies at the rate of the fundamental frequency waveform (which is also the frequency difference between the two higher frequency components, or any two adjacent harmonics in this spectrum). A timing code could measure the period of this complex waveform (e.g., 10 ms in Figure 14–11) and the pitch of the complex periodic event may be derived from a timing (not place) analysis of the output of high-frequency filters. This may also explain why the fundamental frequency can be filtered out during a pitch matching experiment but still yield a complex sound match to a sinusoid of the same frequency as the lowest component of the complex periodic sound.

Pitch of Complex Aperiodic Events

Noise signals can evoke a reliable perception of pitch, especially when the signals have a narrow bandwidth. Narrowband noises are created from white noise signals that are shaped by digital filters (see Chapter 7 for description of filters). An example of a narrowband noise created from filtered white noise is one with frequencies ranging from 900 to 1100 Hz. A high-pass filter removes frequencies below 900 Hz and a low-pass filter removes all frequencies above 1100 Hz. This narrowband noise, with a bandwidth of 200 Hz, evokes in listeners the perception of a noisy tonality. When an experiment is performed to determine how the pitch of the narrowband noise matches the pitch of a sinusoid, the best match is typically obtained for a sinusoid whose frequency is the center frequency of the noise. In the case of the narrowband noise with bandwidth 900 to 1100 Hz, the noise is matched in pitch to that of a 1000 Hz sinusoid (see review in Bilsen, 1977). Such pitch matches are reliable provided that the noise band is sufficiently narrow. As the noise bandwidth is widened, the tonality of the noise becomes increasingly ambiguous, as does the ability to match its pitch to that of a sinusoid.

These observations seem to be consistent with a place theory of pitch perception. Narrowband noises, such as the 200 Hz band described above, produce a localized traveling wave with maximum amplitude near the center of the noise band. This explains why the pitch of this noise signal is matched reliably to the pitch of the sinusoid whose frequency is at the center of the noise band. As a noise signal is widened, the maximum displacement of the traveling wave becomes more broadly distributed across the basilar membrane, the signal becomes less tonal, and the ability to reliably match the noise pitch to the pitch of a sinusoid is degraded.

PSYCHOPHYSICS OF TIMBRE

Timbre (pronounced /ˈtæmbɚ/) is the technical term that describes the quality of an auditory perception. ASA standard 11.09 defines timbre as "that multidimension attribute of auditory sensation which enables a listener to judge that two non-identical sounds, similarly presented and having the same loudness, pitch, spatial location, and duration, are dissimilar. Timbre is related to sound quality, often specified by qualitative adjectives (e.g., bright or dull)." An example of timbre differences, discussed above, is removal of the fundamental frequency from a harmonically rich, complex periodic sound, which does not change perceived pitch but may change the quality of the sound (the sound may be "brighter" or possibly "thinner" when the fundamental frequency is removed). Other examples of timbre differences from the musical world include the ability to differentiate the same note, at the same frequency, played by similar instruments, such as a middle C plucked on a guitar, mandolin, banjo, or lute. The plucks produce the same fundamental frequency, but the distribution of harmonic amplitudes as a function of frequency—the spectrum of the sound—results in timbre differences.

An in-depth treatment of timbre and its relationship to underlying physical stimuli is beyond the scope of this textbook, but two interesting aspects of this area of auditory psychophysics are worth mention. First, research on "profile analysis" (Green, 1988) aims to understand listeners' sensitivity to changes in spectral shape for multiple-component sounds. When the frequencies in a complex sound are held constant, how sensitive are listeners to modifications in the amplitude of one or more of these frequencies? Depending on the number of frequency components in a complex acoustic event, listeners are quite sensitive to small changes in the amplitude of a single frequency component within the multi-component signal (Green, 1988; Lentz, 2005). The ability of the human auditory system to detect these slight spectral variations is an important part of timbre sensitivity.

Second, profile analysis may provide a way to learn how listeners make use of acoustic information to know their environment. Listeners are quite good at using sound to identify, for example, the kind of plate (glass versus pottery versus metal) dropped on the floor, the force with which an iron bar has been struck by a wooden mallet as well as the composition of the bar (e.g., hollow or solid) and the likely material (thin versus thick) thumped by a drum stick (see reviews in Lutfi [2001] and Lutfi, Liu, & Stoelinga [2011]). Hearing scientists view this research as important because an understanding of how humans use variations in spectral and timing characteristics of complex sounds to identify auditory objects may have implications for the design of hearing aids and cochlear implants. Research to date demonstrates that listeners can make distinctions between auditory objects like the ones referred to above, but unfortunately (at least so far) different listeners seem to use different information to make these distinctions. Thus, there seem to be no general rules across individual listeners that relate the underlying acoustics to perceptual distinctions between closely related real-world auditory events.

PSYCHOPHYSICS OF TIME

This section deals with the relationship of objectively measured duration (or duration differences) to the perception of time. How does perceived time relate to measured duration and vice versa? For example, if the duration of a noise signal is varied in 50-ms steps from 100 ms (0.1 sec) to 5000 ms (5 sec) and listeners are asked to provide a magnitude estimate of signal time for each stimulus, what is the relationship between the physical and psychological variables? Stevens and Galanter (1957) summarized the available research on this issue by arguing that for signal durations between 250 ms and 4000 ms, magnitude estimates (i.e., the psychological estimate of time) were not a strictly linear function of actual signal duration. Stevens and Galanter also showed that the relationship between the physical and psychological variables depended on several experimental factors, including the distribution of signal durations throughout the experiment. Signal durations that were equally distributed from short to long resulted in functions different from signal durations with stimuli "loaded" at the short or long duration ends of the duration continuum. Just as in the case of pitch and loudness, the relationship of the psychological variable of time to physical durations is complicated and affected by how the experiment is conducted.

There are other ways to study the psychophysics of time. For example, simple discrimination experiments have been performed in which listeners are presented with two signals separated by a short time interval (e.g., 500 ms) and asked to indicate which signal is longer. With a very brief (10 ms) reference duration, a 3 to 4-ms difference in the comparison signal can be detected as longer. When the reference stimulus duration is increased to 100-ms, a 10 to 15 ms difference is required for a listener to reliably judge a difference. The required difference increases to about 60 ms when the standard signal duration is 1000 ms (estimated from

Figure 1 in Abel, 1972). This kind of two-alternative, forced-choice experiment (the listener must pick one of the two successive sounds as longer or shorter, even when they are perceived to have the same duration) and the results just described are illustrated in Figure 14–12. Reliable detection thresholds for duration —difference limens for duration (DLDs)—seem to increase with the duration of the standard signal. This result is found for both sinusoids and noise signals and is minimally affected by the level of the signals except at very low presentation levels (e.g., near threshold).

Auditory time perception can also be evaluated by studying the minimum time required to detect the onset difference between two signals. Zera and Green (1993) conducted a clever experiment in which listeners were asked to discriminate between two complex, periodic signals whose component frequencies and relative amplitudes were identical. The "standard" spectrum contained 20 harmonics and a fundamental frequency of 200 Hz. The comparison spectrum had the same characteristics with a single exception: the onset of one of the harmonics was very slightly delayed relative to the synchronous onset of all the other harmonics. The onset delay for the asynchronous (delayed) harmonic was equal to a half-period of the component sinusoid. Thus, the delay in time varied with the frequency of the delayed harmonic. For example, if a fundamental frequency was delayed, the time delay was 2.5 ms (because the period of a 200 Hz sinusoid is 5 ms, F = 1/T, 200 Hz = 1/.005 and half of .005 is .0025). If the fifth harmonic (1000 Hz) was delayed, the time delay was 0.5 ms (1000 Hz = 1/.001). Remarkably, listeners heard the difference between two 20-harmonic sounds in which one harmonic was delayed by 0.5 ms (half a millisecond!) relative to the onsets of the other components.

A different task for judgment of auditory timing is the identification of the order of two or more auditory events. Such judgments involve detection of asynchrony but also require listeners to identify which event occurred first (or second). A famous experiment by Hirsh (1959, p. 759) addressed the question of (in his own words) "how much time must intervene between the onsets of two sounds for their order to be reported correctly?" Hirsh used two sinusoids that differed in frequency (by a small, moderate, or large amount) and systematically changed their relative onsets from −60 ms to +60 ms in 10 ms steps. Listeners were asked to identify which tone—the lower pitched or higher

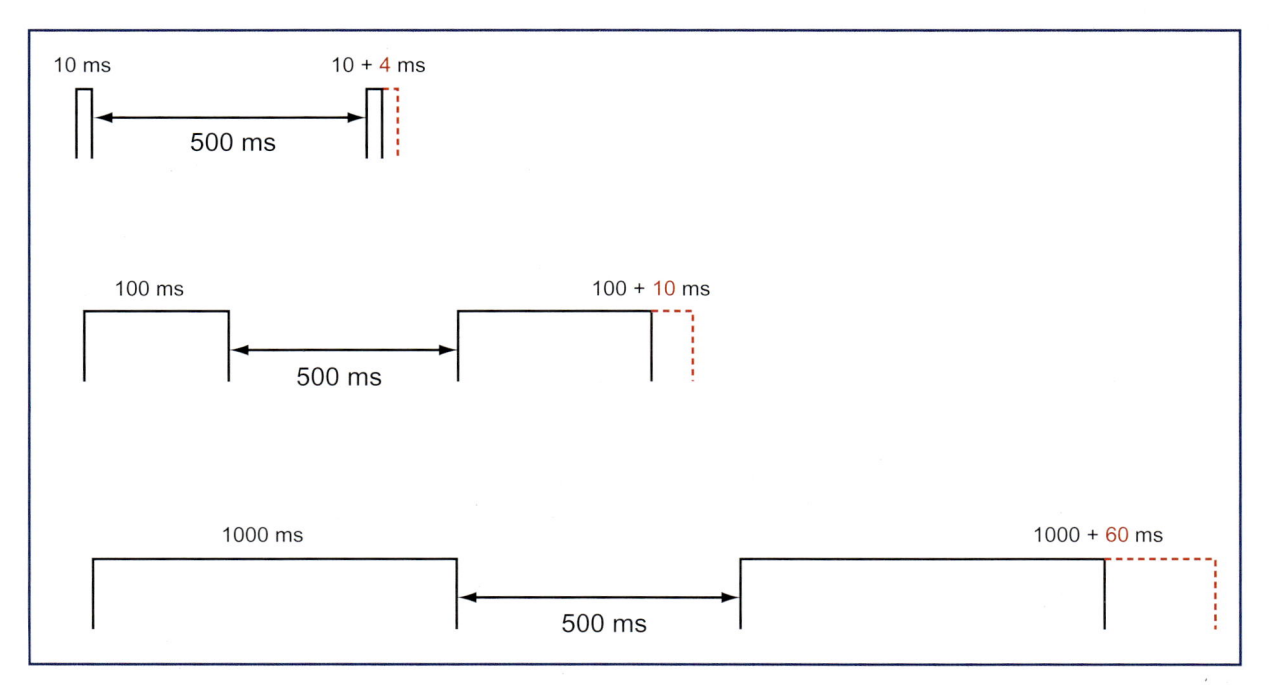

Figure 14–12. Schematic drawing of one approach to determining difference limens for duration (DLDs) as reported by Abel (1972). Each row shows two signals (length of *black rectangles*), an interstimulus interval fixed at 500 ms, and the increment in duration required for a listener to detect a duration difference between the two signals (*indicated by the red extensions of the second signal and the duration increment value*). The reference signal durations are 10 ms (*top row*), 100 ms (*middle row*), and 1000 ms (*bottom row*). The schematic is not drawn exactly to scale because of the wide range of signal durations.

pitched—occurred first. The results showed that an onset difference of just below 20 ms was required for reliable identification of the order (low frequency first, or high frequency first) of the two sinusoids. Presentation level of the two signals and the extent of frequency difference between the signals did not seem to change the time difference required for accurate identification of signal order. Hirsh pointed out that the question of identifying the order of successive acoustic events is different from the question of identifying whether one or two events has (have) occurred. At an onset separation of 2 ms, listeners can reliably identify the *presence* of two events (at separations of less than 2 ms listeners hear only a single event). The separation between the two events must be increased to close to 20 ms for a reliable report of the *order* of the events. Similar results for order identification of acoustic events have been reported by Pisoni (1977) and Pastore, Harris, and Kaplan (1982), although the estimates of the minimal time separation reported by the latter authors (a little more than 10 ms) is slightly better than the separation time reported by Hirsch (see sidetrack on this page).

PSYCHOPHYSICS OF SOUND LOCALIZATION

The study of binaural (two-ear) hearing is a very broad and complex area of research that has demonstrated repeatedly that having two ears is not simply a matter of redundancy. Binaural phenomena range from the simple observation that hearing sensitivity is greater (i.e., thresholds are lower) in binaural fields than in monaural (one ear) fields (Figure 14–1, above; and Sivian & White, 1933) to the impressive observation that people can identify the source of objects in the environment because auditory information is available to two separate ears. In the present chapter, binaural hearing is primarily discussed with consideration of localization of sound sources in space; other binaural topics are covered in Moore (2013) and Ahvenenin, Kopĉo, and Jääskeläinn (2014).

There are systematic acoustic effects at the two ears that result from different locations of sound sources relative to the head. The acoustic effects, as discussed below, include differences in time of arrival of sound wave information between the two ears, and differences in the level of the sound waves at the two ears (among other effects not discussed in this chapter). The perceptual response to these acoustic effects is the localization of the sound source in space. The physical and perceptual effects are separate but are discussed here together.

Localization is a psychoacoustical phenomenon that requires an explicit appreciation of central auditory mechanisms. The information provided above on loudness, pitch, timbre, and duration is presented as if peripheral mechanisms played the primary role in the relevant psychophysical phenomena. There may be a good bit of truth in this statement, but central auditory mechanisms, in the brainstem, thalamus, and cortex, also contribute to these perceptions. These mechanisms are not discussed in this text because they go beyond the scope of its presentation. Localization of sounds, one aspect of the spatial aspects of hearing (including

---

Auditory Mechanisms in Music and Speech Perception

Chapter 12 includes a section on "auditory theories" of speech perception. These theories are based on the idea that the perception of speech uses "general" auditory brain mechanisms, rather than brain mechanisms specialized in humans for encoding and comprehending sequences of speech sounds. Studies of the perception of temporal order such as those of Hirsh (1959), Pisoni (1977), and Pastore et al. (1982), as well as more contemporary battles in the literature concerning this issue (see Samuel [2011] and Carbonell & Lotto [2014] for reviews), are sometimes used to support or refute such theories. For example, Pisoni's demonstration of the necessity of a 20-ms separation between two auditory signals to identify order of the events, as well as the categorical perception of intervals with a boundary at 20 ms (below 20 ms was one category, above 20 ms was a different category) led him to conclude that there were basic auditory mechanisms to "measure" voice-onset time (VOT), an important acoustic variable in the voiced-voiceless distinction of stop consonants (see Chapter 9, Figure 9–16). At a more general level, speech is a sequence of rather brief sounds unfolding in time, so the order of these sounds must be established somewhere along the auditory pathways. The point is that the experiments described in the text may seem contrived with respect to reality, but one does not need to look far to find realistic phenomena similar to experimental manipulations such as those employed by Hirsh and other scientists.

distance estimation, object size estimation, and detection of movement in the environment), is presented here as a prominent example of binaural processing.

As described by Moore (2013), auditory localization skills are typically measured in two ways. The first measure is accuracy—the correspondence of a listener's identification of the location of a sound with its actual position in space. The second is very much like the difference limens discussed above; these include perceptual measures of the smallest detectable change of the position of a sound source in space. Both measures are expressed as angles within a coordinate system defined by the intersection of three anatomical planes through the head (coronal, mid-sagittal, horizontal). The three planes allow an expression of localization in the front to back (coronal), side to side (midsagittal), and up to down (horizontal) dimensions. There is also interest in the distance of a sound source from the listener. This is covered briefly below.

Figure 14–13 shows a representation of the human head through which lines are drawn extending directly forward from the center of the head ("in front of head") and through the ear at the level of the two external auditory meatuses ("side"). The location of a sound source from side to side can be expressed as an angle with 0° as a reference. A sound source position directly in front of the head is said be at 0° azimuth. For a sound source directly to the side of an ear, the angle is 90° azimuth. The location of any sound source on the horizontal plane can be described in terms of the angles between 0° and 90°. A right angle is also shown for elevation of a sound source relative to the horizontal plane. This is the case when the sound source is directly above the center of the head. Sound source locations for elevations are also expressed as angles between 0° and 90°. For example, a sound located halfway between the line extending from the center of the head and the top of the head is at 45° elevation. Azimuth and elevation can be combined to indicate a location. For example, a sound source located midway between a point extended in front of the horizontal plane (in front of the nose) and the ear would be at 45° azimuth. If the sound source is then raised halfway between the horizontal plane and the top of the head, the source is halfway between the nose and ear and raised halfway between the horizontal plane and head. The red arc in Figure 14–13 shows the arc of the 90° plane from nose to ear, and the black arc the angle between the nose and top of the head.

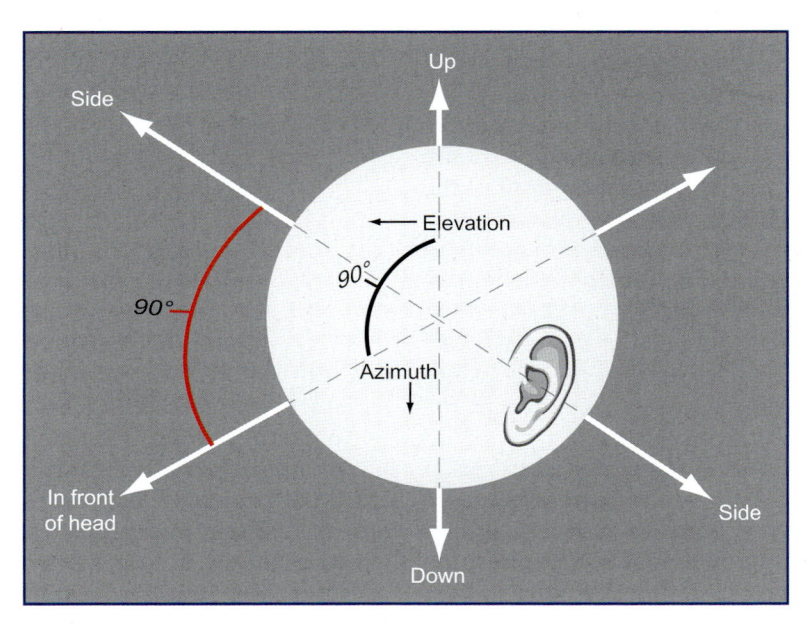

Figure 14–13. A schematic representation of the human head, showing anatomical reference planes and possible positions of a sound source, expressed in degrees within the coordinate system defined by these planes. The intersection of the horizontal (side-to-side) and midsagittal (up and down) planes is the origin of the coordinate system. A point projected along the center of the horizontal plane, outside the head, defines 0° azimuth, as well as 0° for sound sources located above and below the head.

Of course, this two-dimensional view cannot capture the three-dimensional spatial relationships of a sound source located relative to the two planes.

Interaural Cues to Sound Location

The term "interaural cues" refers to a comparison of sound wave properties at the two ears. Frequently studied interaural (between ears) cues include interaural time differences (ITDs) and interaural level differences (ILDs). ITD is the relative arrival, in time, of sound waves at the two ears; this measure is usually expressed in microseconds (μsec). ILD is the relative level of the sound waves at the two ears, usually expressed in dB. In "real" acoustic environments, ITDs and ILDs do not vary independently, but they can be manipulated separately in the laboratory to determine how time and level cues contribute to the localization of a sound source.

Figure 14–14 provides a schematic account of why ITD and ILD vary with the location of a sound source in the left-to-right plane. The view of the head is from above, with the nose at the bottom of the circle. The left ear is therefore at the right of the schematic drawing. The line projecting from the center of the head straight forward, representing 0° azimuth, lies along the horizontal plane. The red oval at the end of this is the location of a sound source at 0° azimuth. When a source at 0° azimuth produces sound waves, the distance between the sound source and the two ears is virtually the same because the source is centered in front of the head. In controlled conditions, the ITD is zero (or very close to it) for a sinusoidal sound source emanating in front of the head at 0° azimuth. For sinusoidal sources, the amplitude variation of the signal is in phase at the two ears—the instant of occurrence of the peak positive amplitude at the left ear is the same as the instant of occurrence of the peak positive amplitude at the right ear.

The time of arrival of the sinusoidal waveforms at the two ears is slightly altered when the sound source is moved 30° to the left of 0° azimuth, as shown in Figure 14–14. With the sound source at 30° azimuth the pathways to the two ears, represented by the dashed black lines, are unequal in length. The arrival of the sinusoidal waveform (or any waveform) at the left ear is slightly ahead of the arrival of the sinusoidal waveform at the right ear. More specifically, the first (and succeeding) peak amplitude(s) of the sinusoid arrives at the left ear very shortly before it arrives at the right ear. The ITD is the difference in time of arrival of these distinctive landmarks of the sinusoid at the two ears. In the case shown in Figure 14–14 of a sinusoid at 30°

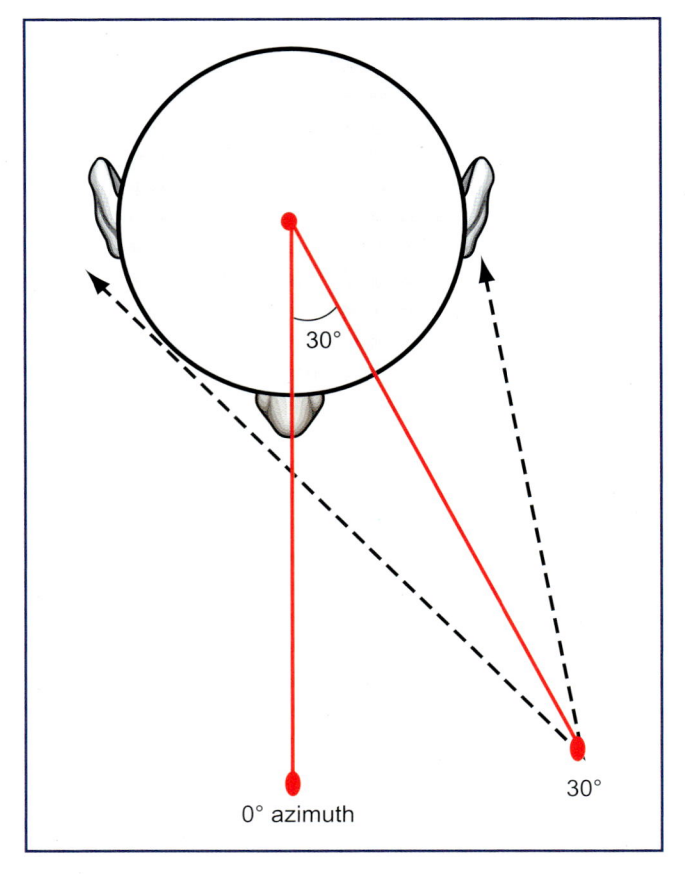

Figure 14–14. View of a head from above, showing 0° azimuth and a sound source located at 30° off azimuth to the left of the head. The dashed lines show for both source locations the distances that the sound waves must travel from the sound source to the left and right ears. At 0° azimuth the distances are the same, at 30° azimuth the distances are different.

azimuth, the ITD is roughly .25 ms, or 250 μsec (value extracted from Figure 1 of Fedderson, Sandel, Teas, & Jeffress, 1957). Binaural hearing capabilities in humans include the detection of this incredibly brief time difference to locate accurately a sound source in space.

The ITD for sinusoids increases from 0° to 90° azimuth, as the sound source position moves from directly in front of the head to directly opposite the ear canal. The variation in the ITD with this changing angle is the same whether the sound source is moved toward the left or right ear. At 90° azimuth the ITD for a sinusoid is roughly 650 μsec. Change of the sound source position around the back of the head are mirror images of the changes just described.

There is a limit to the ability of the auditory system to detect ITDs: the ability is dependent on the frequency of the sinusoidal source. For a single sinusoidal source, lower frequencies have longer periods, with recurring "landmarks" of the waveform (such as the periodically recurring maximum amplitudes) sufficiently separated in time to allow easy detection. At higher frequencies, the time difference between these "landmarks" are relatively short (because the period is short). This means that localization of sound sources using ITD depends on smaller and smaller ITDs as frequency increases. At some point, the time differences between the landmarks of high-frequency waveforms are sufficiently small to reduce their effectiveness for localization. For this reason, investigators have often reached the conclusion that ITDs are effective cues for localization of low-frequency sound sources, but less so for high-frequency sound sources. It has been estimated that the average threshold for detecting an interaural time difference is around 10 μs, although the sensitivity may vary with frequency (Brughera, Dunai, & Hartmann, 2013). Using this information, the binaural auditory system must be very good at estimates of sound-source locations.

ITD and ILD do not vary independently. In Figure 14–14, the longer path traveled by the sinusoidal wave to the right ear, compared with the left ear, results in a slightly less intense sound at the right ear as well as an ITD greater than zero. The ILD is explained partly by the fact that the level of a sound source decreases as the sound wave moves away from the source. The greater the distance from the source, the lower the level of the sound, and the left ear is closer than the right ear to the sound source at 30°, left of center. This is mainly true for sound sources relatively close to the head; the ILD effect is greatly reduced when the sound source is located more than a meter from the head. Fedderson et al. (1957, their Figure 2) reported that at an azimuth of 30° the ILD for a 1000 Hz tone was roughly 2 to 3 dB when the source was located 7 feet from head (less than 1 m). The ILDs at 30° azimuth for 3000, 4000, and 5000 Hz tones were approximately 8, 9, and 10 dB, respectively. Listeners are able to detect ILDs as small as 1 dB at most frequencies (Yost & Dye, 1988), especially when the "reference" ILD is zero (when there is no level difference between the two ears). Thus, ILDs greater than 1 dB are also potentially useful cues to sound source localization.

Why does the ILD increase with an increase in frequency at a particular azimuth? The answer can be found in the diffraction effect—the way sound waves bend (or do not bend) around objects along their path. When low-frequency sound waves are directed at the human head, their wavelengths are long relative to the diameter of the head and can bend around it. As a sound's frequency increases and its wavelength shortens, the pressure wave cannot bend around the head and is increasingly likely to "bounce off" it, interacting with the pressure fluctuations of the incoming wave. In addition, this "diffraction effect" (the pressures associated with short wavelengths bouncing off a surface much larger than the wavelength) prevents much energy from reaching the opposite ear. The reflections of a high-frequency sound wave may sum with the pressure fluctuations of the original wave, increasing the pressure at the ear canal above that associated solely with the incoming wave. The result is a sound level at the entrance to the ear canal that is more than that accounted for solely by the distance of the ear from the source. In Figure 14–14, the diffraction effect is greater at the left compared with the right ear. The ILD should increase with increasing frequency.

Sound localization in the horizontal plane almost certainly depends on a combination of ITD and ILD cues. A reasonable summary statement is that for sinusoids presented in the horizontal plane, ITDs are the primary cues for localization at low frequencies (below ~1500 Hz) and ILDs the primary cue at high frequencies (>1500 Hz). Using ITD and ILD cues, as well as others not discussed here, humans have been shown to detect changes of around 1 degree for a sound source

---

Kitty's Mobile Ears

Do you have an off-center uncle who can move his ears on command? Most humans cannot do this, but a few people, either by intense practice or personal aural anatomy, have a rudimentary ability to position their pinnae. Even among individuals who can move their pinnae, the movement is usually bilateral and does not result in a pinna point; rather the position of the pinna seems to ride up and down or back and forth relative to the skull. This is in great contrast to your cat, who can point a pinna precisely for localization of a sound in space. Cats have about 30 muscles in the external ear that can change the orientation of a pinna, compared with about 6 in humans. Pinna prowess in Persians and other felines extends to individual control of pinna pointing. One pinna may aim posteriorly while the other pinna remains in place. In fact, the cat pinna can rotate up to 180° from the preferred, pinna-forward position. So, in addition to using the interaural cues described in the text, your kitty's localization skills are pumped up by muscle power, pinpointing the location of interesting and possibly appetite-pleasing noises.

located on the horizontal plane (side-to-side), and about 3.5 degrees for sources on the vertical plane (up and down).

These incredibly precise localization skills demonstrate the effectiveness of binaural hearing for identification of a sound source's location. The experiments cited above used sinusoids as sound sources. As pointed out by Moore (2013), cues for source location and precision of localization skills are a good deal more complicated when the experimental stimuli are complex acoustic events.

Auditory Objects and Auditory Scene Analysis

Sound source localization is an exceedingly complicated aspect of audition in both humans and other mammals. The discussion of localization presented in this chapter omits a good deal of information relevant to binaural hearing in real environments. Some of this information, likely to be covered in advanced courses on auditory processing, includes the role of head movement in localization, the localization of complex and moving sound sources, the effect of echoes on sound localization (as in localizing a sound source in a closed room), and the use of binaural hearing capabilities in separating a single source from many simultaneous sound sources. There is also great interest in how the auditory system forms "objects" based on acoustic information. This is often referred to as auditory scene analysis, a brief discussion of which brings the current chapter to a close.

It is easy to think about the role of the visual system as seeking and identifying objects in the environment. The same is true for the sense of touch—seeking, manipulating, and identifying objects (the "seeking and manipulating" aspect of the tactile sense is called "haptics"). A little more thought is required to understand audition in the same way; it comes down to a willingness to broaden the concept of "objects of perception." Take, for example, the visual identification of a train, which is easy to understand (you see it, you know what it is). What about the auditory identification of the same object? The sound of steel wheels rolling continuously on steel tracks leads to the formation of the auditory object, "train" (see a related example in Bendixen, 2014). The auditory system provides cues to the category "train" just as the visual system employs cues to identify the same object. Many similar parallels between visual, auditory, and haptic object identification can be imagined—you see a round object made of some bounceable material, hold a rubber orb in your hand, bounce it, and hear a series of hollow, pop-like impacts with a surface. In each case the relevant sensory system identifies the object as a ball.

Despite these (apparently) straightforward examples, there are many scientific questions concerning what constitutes an "object of perception." More specifically, questions exist concerning the ability of the auditory mechanism to perform object perception in the same way as the visual system. In an essay on definitions of "auditory objects," Griffiths and Warren (2004, p. 887) stated, "the concept of objects in senses other than vision continues to pose both theoretical and experimental difficulties." The situation has still not been substantially clarified, but scientists remain very interested in the idea of auditory objects of perception.

One example of the theoretical difficulties posed by the idea of auditory objects is whether the auditory system can perform a version of "edge detection." Edge detection is a well-researched aspect of visual

---

Unpacking the Unfamiliar

Students who are assigned and struggle to understand a scientific paper often see their difficulties as a metric of their possibility of success in an academic field. Scientists are supposed to write clearly, after all, to communicate their reasoning and experiments and results, and their conclusions, in an accessible way. But the question is, accessible to who? When scientists write a paper, they do so for their peers. They expect these peers to have the foundational understanding of the jargon, familiarity with the methods, and judgment of the conclusions in a critical, constructive way. One of your authors remembers as a doctoral student being assigned an important paper, reading it, and not understanding *anything* written by the authors. He prepared to pack up, leave the Midwest, and find something else to do back East. When his mentor was told this news, and the reason for it, he said, "Tell you what, read it a second time, then a third, and let me know if rereading helps you; if it doesn't, go home." "Why read something multiple times?" the one of us in this story thought, but he did it and the meaning and relevance of the article came into focus. So much so that he read it a fourth and fifth time. The lesson was applied when reading the scientific literature in psychoacoustics, in preparation for writing this chapter. We hope it worked.

> ### The Difference in Your Ears May Be More Than Aesthetic
>
> How do hearing scientists use the difference between a sound spectrum measured just before it arrives at the pinna, and the spectrum measured at the tympanic membrane? The two spectra differ because of modifications imposed on the "outside" spectrum by the head, pinna, and external auditory canal; the signal reaching the tympanic membrane is changed by the anatomy of the external ear (possibly by other body parts, too). The transformation of the spectrum by external ear anatomy is called the head related transfer function (HRTF). Because the HRTF differs across individuals (due to varying anatomical features of ears), it has been speculated that the large differences across individuals in sound localization skills in the vertical (up-down) and sagittal (back-front) planes depend on cross-individual differences in HRTF, which are the result of cross-individual differences in pinna (and other) anatomy. To study this, scientists deliver a processed signal via headphones to the entrance of the external auditory meatus. The processed signal may be consistent with the anatomy of your pinna, or with someone else's! The hypothesis is that the filtering characteristics of your own pinna allow you to localize sound sources better than the simulated (processed) filtering of someone else's pinna. Does it work? Do listeners localize sound better when using their own HRTF than when using a simulated or other person's HRTF? The jury is still out. It seems there are other factors that determine localization of auditory sources, such as perceptual and attention ability. Andéol, Savel, and Guillaume (2015) review this very interesting work.

object perception, both behaviorally (e.g., the response of viewers to objects with different edge properties) and at the level of brain mechanisms (e.g., cells in the visual cortex which fire specifically in response to object edges). Evidence of edge detection—or even what an auditory "edge" might be—has been difficult to identify in auditory research. Perhaps the auditory system performs object perception as well as any other sense, but not by the same cognitive rules and brain mechanisms. Perhaps the rules and mechanisms are unique to audition.

The psychophysics of auditory object perception must deal with at least three challenging issues. First, humans are exceedingly skilled in the use of auditory information to identify objects. That skill, which most of us take for granted, can be disrupted or lost completely in cases of acquired neurological disease (as in stroke) or as a characteristic of a developmental disorder (as in so-called auditory processing disorders of unknown anatomical and/or physiological bases). Second, unlike most of the psychoacoustical phenomena presented above, auditory identification of objects involves multiple dimensions of sound, including change in acoustic properties as a function of time. Third, the auditory system is often presented with multiple sources of sound simultaneously, such as the many voices heard at a party or the street noise associated with traffic, construction, and other urban sounds. The "cocktail party effect" and the concept of auditory streams are phenomena that exemplify the complexity of the workings of the auditory system.

The cocktail party effect (Cherry, 1953) describes a human's ability to focus on and hear a single talker among many talkers speaking at the same time. The talker who is heard among many does not have to be alongside the listener; indeed, the listener may focus auditory *attention* on a talker several yards away without looking at him or her. The listener may even pretend to be listening to someone right next to him while focusing, auditorily, on the speech of the more distant person. In lay terms, the listener "locks on" to a person's speech and continues to monitor that person's speech as—now using more technical language—an integrated "stream" separate from all other speech streams. What are the auditory abilities responsible for this skill?

In a cocktail party situation, all the waveforms produced by many people talking at the same time are mixed together. The sound pressure waves reaching the listener's ears are the sum of the many sound pressure waves produced by each speaker. To understand what an individual talker is saying, the listener must separate and track the waveform produced by that speaker from the mix of pressure waves arriving at the tympanic membrane. Stated otherwise, the listener must identify and track the stream of that single talker's speech output.

The study of auditory streams extends the cocktail party effect to all sounds. The problem is the same as originally considered by Cherry (1953) for separation of one talker from many, but has been extended to the general case of how simultaneous and sequential sounds are grouped together or separated from one another. This auditory ability is often referred to as auditory scene analysis. Interested readers may want to consult the influential book on auditory scene analysis published by Bregman (1990), as well as his laboratory's website (http://webpages.mcgill.ca/staff/Group2/abregm1/web/).

An auditory stream has been defined as "a perceptually-bound collection of sounds that together constitute an event" (Griffiths & Warren, 2004, p. 889). The "perceptually bound" part of the definition implies some common feature of simultaneous or sequential sounds, or both, that suggest they originate from the same source. For example, in laboratory studies the manipulation of pitch, sound location, loudness, synchronous versus asynchronous onsets, and spectral content have been shown to cause integration of sound streams (belonging to the same event) or segregation of sound streams (belonging to different events). Imagine an experiment in which two harmonic spectra are played at the same time and the experimenter manipulates their frequency components to be either quite similar or quite different. Spectra that are similar and presented to listeners at the same time are likely to be heard as one event, or more specifically as fused—the listener does not hear two separate sounds. When the spectra are sufficiently different, they are heard as two different sounds; the two signals "segregate" into two unique events.

The case of a series of sinusoids played over time in which the manipulation is a regular change of frequency from one tone to the next illustrates the streaming aspect of auditory analysis. As the sequence alternates between lower and higher frequencies, the listener hears a single melody of repeating lower and higher pitches. This single melody is a unified auditory stream. When the frequencies are sufficiently different, the exact difference depending on the particular experiment, the sequence of higher frequencies segregate from the sequence of lower frequencies, and the listener hears two separate auditory streams, one high-pitched, the other low-pitched.

One claim is that the segregation of simultaneously presented sounds and the grouping of segregated sounds across time (streaming) is a built-in, automatic characteristic of auditory processing (Bendixen, 2014). This is not the same as a sophisticated processing mechanism that requires active searching on the part of the listener for different auditory events. Of course, some level of cognitive choice enters the process, as in a decision to listen to one speaker among many in a crowd. Once attention has been directed at a source, however, the built-in, automatic processes may be engaged.

Returning to the cocktail party effect, the segregation part of the analysis may be based on different fundamental frequencies among the many talkers, and even on different vocal tract lengths cued by different formant structures. Listeners seem able to lock on to these differences within the "babble" of many talkers and use the differences to "build up" and track a unique auditory stream (Bronkhorst, 2015). Details of precisely how this is done, how the multidimensional acoustic information in an environment is "broken down" to isolate an auditory stream of interest, is a high-level process of auditory psychophysics. This process is described as high level because it almost certainly requires extensive top-down, cognitive processes along with the analysis performed by the sensorineural apparatus (the peripheral auditory mechanism). Interestingly, and perhaps unsurprisingly, research has shown the importance of binaural processing in auditory scene analysis. Two ears are better than one in the extraction of an event of interest among many simultaneous events. A contemporary review of the cocktail party effect is available in Bronkhorst (2015).

The Breakdown of Auditory Scene Analysis

"Auditory scene analysis" is more than just a cool name coined by a hearing scientist to describe high-level auditory skills (although it is a cool term). There is a good deal of clinical relevance in the auditory skill of separating an auditory object of interest from other competing auditory objects, or of grouping a series of time-varying auditory objects as belonging together. Two examples make this clear. Young adults with normal hearing perform well when focusing on one talker whose speech is mixed with that of a group of talkers, or when listening to a talker in a good deal of nonspeech noise (such as street noise). Persons with hearing loss, even those who are young, have much more difficulty with these tasks. The second example is of a wide number of clients (e.g., young children with diagnosis of auditory processing problems, persons with certain kinds of brain injury) who cannot follow a sequence of auditory events. The ability to separate and sequence auditory events is an important auditory skill that can be degraded or lost in certain clinical populations, and the basic science described in the text is a first step to designing treatment approaches for those whose auditory scene analysis is less than optimal.

REVIEW

The relationship between the acoustic characteristics and the psychological response to them is often complicated, rather than (for example) a two-to-one change in an acoustic measure, such as sound level or frequency, resulting in a two-to-one change along a psychological scale such as loudness or pitch.

Auditory thresholds, or the minimal sound pressure level required to just hear (detect) a sinusoid, are very low sound pressures that vary across frequency.

Very low and very high frequency sinusoids (tones) require greater sound pressure levels to be detected than do mid-frequency sinusoids (~1000 to 5000 Hz).

Minimal audible field thresholds (threshold measured in a room, where both ears receive the signals) are better than thresholds obtained under inserts (or other types of headphones). They eliminate the resonance of the external auditory meatus; minimal audible field thresholds are also with two ears (binaural) compared with one ear (monaural).

Equal loudness curves across frequency, where the loudness of sinusoids at different frequencies is matched to the loudness of a standard tone (usually a 1000 Hz sinusoid), show that the SPL required to match the loudness of the standard varies across frequency; equal loudness curves flatten with increased SPL of the two tones.

The phon is a psychological unit of loudness, expressed as a loudness level and based on the matching of the loudness of two tones.

The phon scale uses the loudness level of a 1000 Hz sinusoid as its reference; the loudness of a 1000 Hz tone at 40 dB SPL has a loudness level of 40 phons, and so forth; a 1000 Hz sinusoid at 60 dB SPL has a loudness level of 60 phons, and so forth.

Phons allow tones of different frequency to be equated for loudness; the same loudness level in phons does not imply equal sound level.

Sones are also a psychological unit of loudness, based on the idea that listeners can, using numbers, quantify the loudness ratio of two tones presented at different levels; the numbers are called magnitude estimates.

Stevens formulated a power law for the relationship of sones to tone SPL, the law stating that when the logarithm of the magnitude estimates is plotted as a function of decibels (a logarithmic scale), the result is a single line relating loudness magnitude estimates to SPL.

When sinusoids are matched for loudness to complex acoustic events such as two-tone signals or noises, the sinusoid must be adjusted to a higher SPL to match the loudness of the complex events.

Loudness matches between sinusoids and two-tone acoustic or noise signals whose width exceeds the width of the auditory filter centered at (for example) 1000 Hz reflect the difference between the output of multiple auditory filters (the two-tone or noise signal) and the output of a single filter (the 1000 Hz tone).

More recent research indicates that a single line relating magnitude estimates to SPL may be more or less correct for midrange levels, but not for low-level (threshold to 20 dB) or high-level (90 dB and above) signals.

Frequency analysis by the sensorineural component of the hearing mechanism is analogous to a series of overlapping bandpass filters.

The characteristics of an auditory filter include a characteristic frequency (CF, the frequency at which the filter passes maximum energy) as well as a shape which shows that as frequencies move away from the CF, less and less energy is passed; this effect is more gradual for frequencies lower than the CF, and much steeper for frequencies above the CF.

Tuning curves, which show the shape of auditory filters that have a characteristic frequency that passes the greatest amount of energy, and surrounding frequencies that pass less energy in differing amounts as a function of distance from the characteristic frequency, have been obtained for auditory nerve fibers in animals, and in humans using non-invasive techniques such as noise masking of carefully chosen sinusoids.

There is good correspondence between tuning curves obtained from animals and those obtained for humans, as well as good correspondence in tuning curves across multiple human listeners.

Tuning curves, and by implication auditory filters, become "wider" (pass energy at a greater range of frequencies) as the CF increases.

The difference limen for loudness (loudness DL) is defined as the minimum change in SPL that is just noticed as a change in loudness.

Early research suggested that the loudness DLs was a constant proportion of the standard SPL, with an increasing DL with increases in the SPL of the standard; this is known as the Weber–Fechner law.

Loudness DLs are often quite small (1–3 dB at 1000 Hz), even though the range of for different listeners can vary, and are often close to 1 dB across the most sensitive frequency range in humans.

Pitch is the attribute of auditory sensation by which sounds are ordered on the scale used for melody in music.

Relative pitch judgments are made reliably by listeners for tone contrasts below 5000 Hz, but much less reliably for tones above 5000 Hz.

Musical notes serve listeners as categories and may complicate the investigation of the relationship between frequency, the relevant physical variable, and pitch, the relevant psychological variable.

Octaves are both a physical and psychological variable, the former representing a doubling or halving of frequency (for adjacent octaves); the latter is a psychological assignment of the same musical "note" name to tones that are doubled or halved in frequency.

In musical terms, the psychological distances between (as an example) the octave between A1 and A2 (where A1 is a low 'A' and A2 is the next 'A' up the musical scale) and A2 and A3 are equivalent, but the corresponding frequency differences are not equivalent (frequency range between A1 and A2 = 55 Hz, between A2 and A3 = 110 Hz).

When pitch is studied by means of magnitude estimates, the results deviate from the straight line expected if a doubling of pitch is always associated with a doubling of frequency.

Two major theories of pitch (and frequency analysis in the cochlea and auditory nerve) have been proposed, one in which the pitch is the result of which location along the basilar membrane (which hair cell with a specific characteristic frequency) has the maximum displacement (the "place theory"), the other involving a counting of synchronized nerve action potentials to determine the period between (and hence, the frequency of) the action potentials' firings (the "timing theory").

The "timing" theory is more consistent with analysis of low frequencies, the "place" theory with analysis of high frequencies, but pitch perception probably reflects both types of analysis.

The difference limen for pitch (pitch DL) is defined as the minimal fractional change of the frequency at a specific sound pressure level that is just noticed as a change of pitch.

Pitch DLs are a function of the standard frequency (the frequency to which a change is referred), with increasing pitch DL as the frequency of the standard increases.

Below 2000 Hz, pitch DLs range between 1 and 5 Hz (at 100 Hz the DLF is 2–3 Hz); above 2000 Hz, pitch DLs are larger, indicating that at low frequencies the auditory system is a very precise frequency analyzer.

For a given standard frequency, pitch DLs become increasingly smaller (better) as the presentation level is increased.

When the pitch of a sinusoid is matched to the pitch of a complex periodic sound, the match is typically to the pitch of the lowest frequency component (the fundamental frequency, or the first harmonic) of the complex periodic event.

When the fundamental frequency of a complex periodic event is removed by filtering, listeners still match the pitch of the complex event to that of a sinusoid at the removed fundamental frequency, indicating that the harmonic relationship of the other components to the "missing fundamental" allows listeners to "recover" the fundamental frequency.

The matching of the pitch of the sinusoid to the lowest component of a complex periodic sound can be understood within the framework of auditory filters, where the low-frequency filters process only a single, easily identified sinusoid because of the narrow bandwidth of low-frequency filters and very precise frequency analysis.

A single sinusoid can be matched to the pitch of a complex aperiodic event (a noise signal), provided the bandwidth of the noise signal is sufficiently narrow; the pitch match is usually to the center frequency of the narrowband noise.

Timbre is the term used to describe the quality of a sound, where "quality" is a perceptual variable (everything else that is not loudness, perceived duration, or pitch).

A good example of timbre and why it depends on the spectrum of a complex periodic event is the ability to hear the difference between plucked strings of a guitar, banjo, mandolin, and lute, even when the note has the same fundamental frequency.

Profile analysis, the study of listeners' ability to detect level differences between spectra with the same multiple frequency components, reveals that listeners are sensitive to small changes in intensity of components within a spectrum; this sensitivity contributes to timbre sensitivity.

Perception of increasing measured time (physical measurement) is accompanied by judgments of longer signals, but the relationship between the measured and judged time is not linear.

Determination of the difference limen for duration (duration DL), where two signals are presented in succession with one signal serving as the standard, shows that listeners are able to detect very small duration differences (10–15 ms) with relatively short duration standards (e.g., 100 ms) but require longer duration differences (60 ms) when the standard is relatively long (e.g., 1000 ms, or 1 sec).

The auditory system is sensitive to very small duration differences as determined by experiments that include the relative onset of harmonic components in a multi-component, harmonic signal, as well as the occurrence of one or two signals when two signals are presented with very small differences in onset time, or the order of two signals separated by small durations.

Humans localize sound sources in space in the horizontal plane by using the interaural (between ear) time and level differences at the two ears.

Localization of sound sources in the midsagittal plane (up versus down relative to the head) is based primarily on variation of sound spectra reaching the tympanic membrane, the spectral variation with different elevations depending on the shape of the pinna.

Auditory scene analysis is a complex aspect of auditory psychophysics that seeks to understand how multiple acoustic signals occurring at the same time are separated and grouped together by the auditory system, for perception of separate sources or objects.

A good example of auditory scene analysis is the cocktail party effect, in which a listener can focus on a single speaker—can extract the speaker's signal—when many speakers are talking simultaneously and the multi-talker speech acoustic waveforms reaching the listener's tympanic membranes are mixed together.

Auditory scene analysis is related to auditory analyses used to identify objects by their different acoustic characteristics.

REFERENCES

Abel, S. M. (1972). Duration discrimination of noise and tone bursts. *Journal of the Acoustic Society of America, 51*, 1219–1223.

Adank, P., Smits, R., & van Hout, R. (2004). A comparison of vowel normalization procedures for language variation research. *Journal of the Acoustical Society of America, 116*, 3099–3107.

Ahvenenin, J., Kopĉo, N., & Jääskeläinn, I. P. (2014). Psychophysics and neuronal bases of sound localization in humans. *Hearing Research, 307*, 86–97.

Andéol, G., Savel, S., & Guillaume, A. (2015). Perceptual factors contribute more than acoustical factors to sound localization with virtual sources. *Frontiers in Neuroscience, 8*, 1–17.

Bendixen, A. (2014). Predictability effects in auditory scene analysis: A review. *Frontiers in Neuroscience, 8*, 1–16.

Bilsen, F. A. (1977). Pitch of nose signals: Evidence for a "central" spectrum. *Journal of the Acoustic Society of America, 61*, 150–161.

Bregman, A. S. (1990). *Auditory scene analysis. The perceptual organization of sound.* Cambridge, MA: MIT Press.

Bronkhorst, A. W. (2015). The cocktail-party problem revisited: Early processing and selection of multi-talker speech. *Attention Perception & Psychophysics, 77*, 1465–1487.

Brughera, A., Dunai, L., & Hartmann, W. M. (2013). Human interaural time difference thresholds for sine tones: The high-frequency limit. *Journal of the Acoustic Society of America, 133*, 2839–2855.

Buus, S., & Florentine, M. (2001). Growth of loudness in listeners with cochlear hearing losses: Recruitment reconsidered. *Journal of the Association for Research in Otolaryngology, 3*, 120–139.

Byrne, C., & Foulkes, P. (2004). The 'mobile phone effect' on vowel formants. *Journal of Speech, Language, and the Law, 11*, 83–102.

Carbonell, K. M., & Lotto, A. J. (2014). Speech is not special ... again. *Frontiers in Psychology: Language Sciences, 5*, 1–4.

Carney, A. E., & Nelson, D. A. (1983). An analysis of psychophysical tuning curves in normal and pathological ears. *Journal of the Acoustic Society of America, 73*, 268–278.

Cherry, E. C. (1953). Some experiments on the recognition of speech, with one and with two ears. *Journal of the Acoustical Society of America, 25*, 975–979.

Fedderson, W. E., Sandel, T. T., Teas, D. C., & Jeffress, L. A. (1957). Localization of high frequency tones. *Journal of the Acoustic Society of America, 29*, 988–991.

Fletcher, H., & Munson, W. A. (1933). Loudness, its definition, measurement and calculation. *Journal of the Acoustic Society of America, 5*, 82–108.

Florentine, M., Buus, S., & Bonding, P. (1978). Loudness of complex sounds as a function of the standard stimulus and the number of components. *Journal of the Acoustical Society of America, 64*, 1036–1040.

Florentine, M., Buus, S., & Mason, C. R. (1987). Level discrimination as a function of level for tones from 0.25 to 16 kHz. *Journal of the Acoustical Society of America, 81*, 1528–1541.

Florentine, M., & Epstein, M. (2006). To honor Stevens and repeal his law (for the auditory system). *Proceedings of Fechner Day, 22*, 1–7.

Green, D. M. (1988). *Profile analysis: Auditory intensity discrimination.* Oxford, UK: Oxford University Press.

Greenwood, D. D. (1990). A cochlear frequency-position function for several species—29 years later. *Journal of the Acoustical Society of America, 87*, 2592–2605.

Griffiths, T. D., & Warren, J. D. (2004). What is an auditory object? *Nature Reviews: Neuroscience, 5*, 887–892.

Hirsh, I. J. (1959). Auditory perception of temporal order. *Journal of the Acoustical Society of America, 31*, 759–767.

Kewly-Port, D., & Goodman, S. S. (2005). Thresholds for second formant transitions in front vowels. *Journal of the Acoustical Society of America, 118*, 3252–3260.

Killion, M. C. (1978). Revised estimate of minimum audible pressure: Where is the "missing 6 dB"? *Journal of the Acoustical Society of America, 63*, 1501–1508.

Kluk, K., & Moore, B. C. J. (2004). Factors affecting psychophysical tuning curves for normally hearing subjects. *Hearing Research, 194*, 118–134.

Lentz, J. J. (2005). Profile analysis: The effect of rove on sparse spectra. *Journal of the Acoustical Society of America, 118*, 2794–2797.

Liang, C., Earl, B., Thompson, I., Whitaker, K., Cahn, S., Xiang, J., ... Zhang, F. (2016). Musicians are better than non-musicians in frequency change detection: Behavioral and electrophysiological evidence. *Frontiers in Neuroscience, 10*, 464. doi:10.3389/fnins.2016.00464

Lutfi, R. A. (2001). Auditory detection of hollowness. *Journal of the Acoustical Society of America, 110*, 1010–1019.

Lutfi, R. A., Liu, C-J., & Stoelinga, C. N. J. (2011). Auditory discrimination of force of impact. *Journal of the Acoustical Society of America, 129*, 2104–2111.

Mandikal Vasuki, P. R., Sharma, M., Demuth, K., & Arciuli, J. (2016). Musicians' edge: A comparison of auditory processing, cognitive abilities, and statistical learning. *Hearing Research, 342*, 112–123.

Marks, L. E., & Florentine, M. (2011). Measurement of loudness, Part I: Methods, problems, and pitfalls. In M. Florentine, A. N. Popper, & R. R. Fay (Eds.), *Loudness* (pp. 17–56). New York, NY: Springer-Verlag.

Micheyl, C., Xiao, L., & Oxenham, A. J. (2012). Characterizing the dependence of pure-tone frequency limens on frequency, duration, and level. *Hearing Research, 292*, 1–3.

Miller, C. A., Abbas, P. J., & Robinson, B. K. (2001). Response properties of the refractory auditory nerve fiber. *Journal of the Association for Research in Otolaryngology, 2*, 216–232.

Miśkiewicz, A., & Rakowski, A. (2012). A psychophysical pitch function determined by absolute magnitude estimation and its relation to the musical pitch scale. *Journal of the Acoustical Society of America, 131*, 987–992.

Moore, B. C. J. (2013). *An introduction to the psychology of hearing* (6th ed.). Bingley, UK: Emerald Group.

Moore, B. C. J. (2008). Basic auditory processes involved in the analysis of speech sounds. *Philosophical Transaction of the Royal Society of London B: Biological Sciences, 363*, 947–963.

Moore, B. C. J., & Glasberg, B. R. (1983). Suggested formulae for calculating auditory filter bandwidths and excitation patterns. *Journal of the Acoustical Society of America, 74*, 750–753.

Oxenham, A. J. (2013). Revisiting place and temporal theories of pitch. *Acoustical Science and Technology, 34*, 388–396.

Pastore, R. E., Harris, L. B., & Kaplan, J. K. (1982). Temporal order identification: Some parameter dependencies. *Journal of the Acoustical Society of America, 71*, 430–436.

Perrott, D. R., & Saberi, K. (1990). Minimum audible angle thresholds for sources varying in both elevation and azimuth. *Journal of the Acoustical Society of America, 87*, 1728–1731.

Pisoni, D. B. (1977). Identification and discrimination of the relative onset time of two-component tones: Implications for voicing perception in stops. *Journal of the Acoustical Society of America, 61*, 1352–1361.

Samuel, A. G. (2011). Speech perception. *Annual Review of Psychology, 62*, 49–72.

Schooneveldt, G. P., & Moore, B. C. J. (1989). Comodulation masking release (CMR) as a function of masker bandwidth, modulator bandwidth, and signal duration. *Journal of the Acoustical Society of America, 85*, 273–281.

Sivian, L. J., & White, S. D. (1933). On minimal audible sound fields. *Journal of the Acoustical Society of America, 4*, 288–321.

Stevens, S. S. (1955). On the measurement of loudness. *Journal of the Acoustical Society of America, 27*, 815–829.

Stevens, S. S., & Galanter, E. (1957). Ratio scales and category scales for a dozen perceptual continua. *Journal of Experimental Psychology, 54*, 377–411.

Syrdal, A. K., & Gopal, H. S. (1986). A perceptual model of vowel recognition based on the auditory representation of American English. *Journal of the Acoustical Society of America, 79*, 1086–1100.

Wier, C. C., Jesteadt, W., & Green, D. M. (1977). Frequency discrimination as a function of frequency and sensation level. *Journal of the Acoustical Society of America, 61*, 178–184.

Yost, W. A., & Dye, R. H., Jr. (1988). Discrimination of interaural differences of level as a function of frequency. *Journal of the Acoustic Society of America, 83*, 1846–1851.

Zera, J., & Green, D. M. (1993). Detecting temporal onset and offset asynchrony in multicomponent complexes. *Journal of the Acoustic Society of America, 93*, 1038–1052.

Zera, J., Onsan, A., Nguyen, Q. T., & Green, D. M. (1993). Auditory profile analysis of harmonic signals. *Journal of the Acoustical Society of America, 93*, 3431–3441.

15

Neural Structures and Mechanisms for Speech, Language, and Hearing

INTRODUCTION

This chapter introduces the role of the central and peripheral nervous systems in speech, language, and hearing. Although other chapters in this text are focused on the speech apparatus (Chapters 2–6), the speech signal it produces (Chapters 7–11), and the perception of that signal (Chapter 12), the perspective is broadened in the current chapter to include selected aspects of language as well as speech production and perception. This recognizes the role of the nervous system in all aspects of normal and disordered communication and emphasizes the likelihood of overlap and interactions among speech, language, and hearing functions of the brain. Reference is made to early studies of the brain and human communication. These were primarily concerned with aphasia, the loss of language performance and possibly competence resulting from damage to specific brain locations.

The chapter begins with an overview of major concepts. Next, gross neuroanatomy is presented for the cerebral hemispheres and cerebral white matter, subcortical nuclei (e.g, basal ganglia and thalamus), cerebellum, brainstem and cranial nerves, cortical innervation patterns, and the spinal cord and its peripheral nerves. Cells within the nervous system and selected aspects of their function are discussed, followed by descriptions of meninges, ventricles, and the blood supply to the brain. Aspects of neurophysiology are interwoven with neuroanatomy throughout the chapter, along with selected clinical implications for the speech-language pathologist and audiologist. The chapter concludes with a well-known model of speech production that shows how known anatomy and physiology of the brain can be translated to the understanding of communication disorders.

THE NERVOUS SYSTEM: AN OVERVIEW AND CONCEPTS

In this chapter, the term "brain structures" refers to the anatomy of the central nervous system. Coverage of nervous system anatomy is focused primarily on gross anatomy—structures easily observable when handling and dissecting a whole brain, or when viewed using modern imaging techniques. More limited information is provided on cellular and even molecular anatomical levels, to provide a foundation for understanding neurological diseases affecting these fine-structure components of the nervous system. The term "brain mechanisms" refers to the physiology of the brain, at the molecular, cellular, neurochemical, and system levels. "System" levels of brain function are presumably the ones associated with observable *behaviors*, such as producing a sentence or providing behavioral evidence for understanding spoken language (as in following an instruction).

The major concepts provide a framework and set of reference terms that can be consulted throughout the chapter. They include central versus peripheral nervous system, autonomic nervous system, anatomical planes and directions, white versus gray matter, tracts versus nuclei, nerves versus ganglia, efferent and afferent, and lateralization and specialization of function.

Central Versus Peripheral Nervous System

The concepts of *central nervous system* (CNS) and *peripheral nervous system* (PNS) are familiar to most readers of this textbook. The CNS includes the cerebral hemispheres and its contents, the cerebellum, and the brainstem and spinal cord. The PNS includes the nerves issued from the brainstem and spinal cord, plus clusters of sensory nerve cells, called ganglia, located in close proximity to, but outside, the brainstem and spinal cord. In Figure 15–1, the major components of the CNS are labeled, as are nerves of the PNS, extending from the brainstem and spinal cord. Ganglia, located close to the brainstem and spinal cord, are not shown here but are discussed below.

Later in this chapter the structure of nerve cells is presented in some detail. For the current discussion of CNS and PNS, nerve cells (neurons)—consist of a cell body and an axon. The axon conducts electrical impulses away from the cell body to its endpoint, where the electrical energy is converted into chemical energy. Neurons not only conduct electrical impulses that are converted to chemical energy, but also control contraction of voluntary (striated) and involuntary (smooth) muscle, as well as secretions of glands. Bundles of axons are found in abundance in both the CNS and PNS. A bundle of axons in the CNS is called a *tract*; a bundle of axons in the PNS is called a *nerve*.

Autonomic Nervous System

The autonomic nervous system (ANS) controls involuntary actions, sometimes called subconscious behaviors. Examples of these behaviors include control of heartbeat, vegetative breathing, taste, and contraction of smooth muscle of the heart, digestive system, and eye (for control of pupil size), as well as other systems. Secretions of glands are also controlled by the ANS. Selected aspects of ANS function are mentioned in the section on cranial nerves.

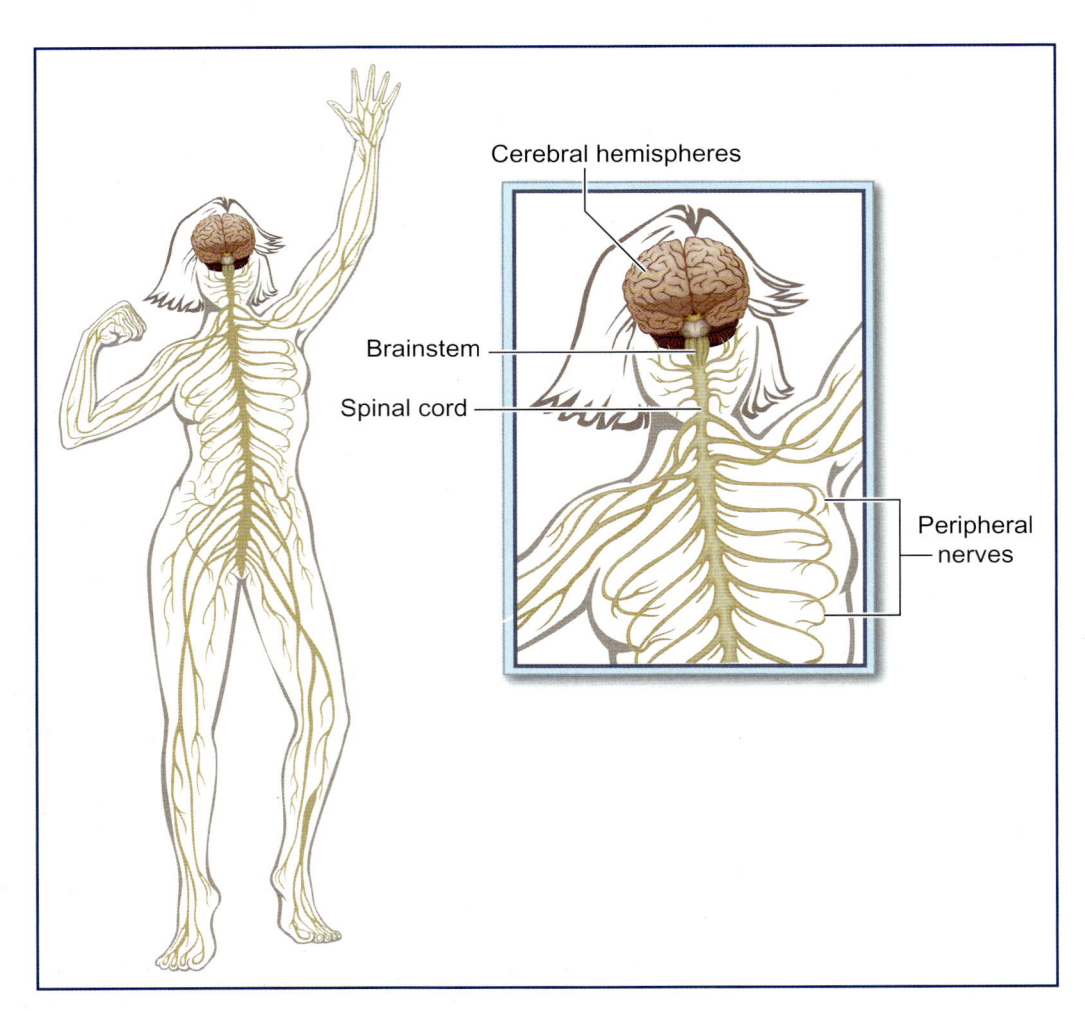

Figure 15–1. Major components of the nervous system, including four major subdivisions of the CNS (cerebral hemispheres, cerebellum, brainstem, spinal cord), and cranial and spinal nerves of the PNS.

Anatomical Planes and Directions

The terminology for planes and directions varies depending on the part of the CNS under discussion. The left part of Figure 15–2 shows an artist's rendition of three anatomical planes as they are applied to the cerebral hemispheres. The *coronal plane* cuts the cerebral hemispheres into front and back sections, the *sagittal plane* into left and right sections, and the *horizontal plane* (also called *axial* or *transverse*) into upper and lower sections. Each of these planes can be moved along an axis perpendicular to the plane to cut through the cerebral hemispheres at different locations. For example, the horizontal plane can be moved up or down to obtain higher or lower cuts through the hemispheres. Similarly, the sagittal plane can be moved left or right, away from the midline (called the midsagittal plane), which divides the brain into equal left and right halves. Sagittal cuts away from the midline are referred to as *parasagittal* planes.

Several structures within the cerebral hemispheres have complex, curved shapes. Some structures are buried within the cerebral hemispheres and are difficult to visualize without multiplane views. Views of the brain in all three of the "standard" planes—coronal, sagittal, horizontal—are necessary to appreciate the form and location of these curved structures. A good example of the varying appearance of a single structure, the corpus callosum, is shown on the right side of Figure 15–2. Coronal (top), midsagittal (middle), and horizontal (bottom) slices through the structure are shown in magnetic resonance images (MRI). The corpus callosum is a massive bundle of fibers (a tract) linking structures in the left and right cerebral hemispheres. The top image is a coronal slice, roughly at the midway point between the front and back of the cerebral hemispheres. The red arrow points to a gently concave, white band of tissue located above two black "horns." This coronal plane image intersects the corpus callosum at a single location, where the structure extends laterally from the

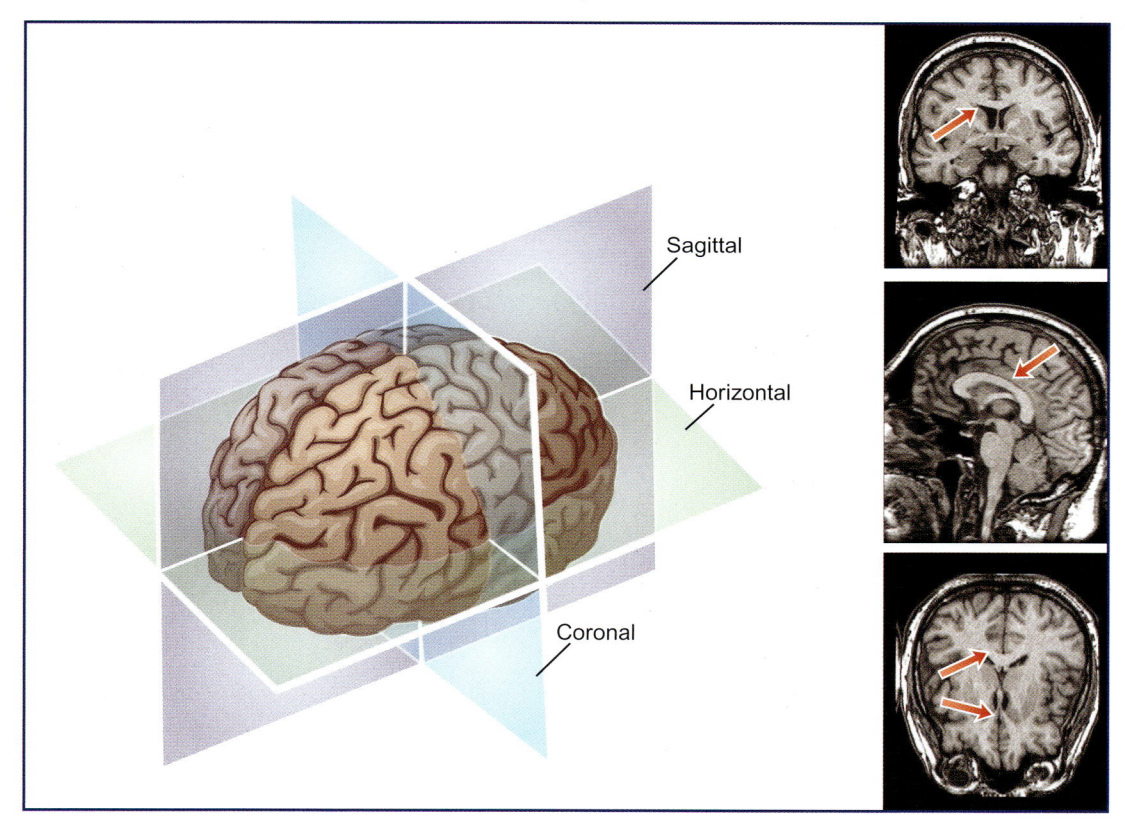

Figure 15–2. Left, major anatomical planes as seen in an anatomical drawing of the cerebral hemispheres, viewed from slightly above the hemispheres and from the side (coronal in light blue, sagittal in light purple, horizontal in light green); right, three MR images shown in the coronal (*top*), sagittal (*middle*), and horizontal (*bottom*) planes. In each of the MR images the red arrows point to the corpus callosum.

midline into the two hemispheres (the arrow is just off the midline, in the right hemisphere, which appears on the left from the reader's view). The appearance of the corpus callosum in the coronal plane varies depending on where the slice is located along the front-to-back extent of the hemispheres. This is better appreciated by examining the midsagittal plane image (see Figure 15–2, middle). The white band of callosal ("callosal" = of the corpus callosum) tissue extends along a good part of the front-to-back length of the brain, and has a flattened, archlike shape with relatively complex form at its front and back ends. The coronal slice shown above the sagittal slice was taken just in front of the red arrow on the sagittal slice; this slice interrupts the corpus callosum in the middle of the flattened arch. The bottom image in Figure 15–2 shows a horizontal slice in which the white bands of corpus callosum tissue are indicated by two red arrows, one toward the front (lower part of image) and one toward the back (upper part of image) of the hemispheres. Between these two regions of corpus callosum tissue, other callosal fibers are not apparent. This is because the horizontal slice is placed below the highest point of the arch seen in the midsagittal slice, which means it does not intersect this part of the corpus callosum. In fact, the horizontal slice cuts through two parts of the corpus callosum, as indicated by the two arrows in Figure 15–2.

Locations of brain structures are often identified relative to locations of other brain structures. Figure 15–3 shows an MR image in the coronal plane, slightly posterior to the halfway point between the anterior and posterior "poles" (the anterior and posterior tips of the cerebral hemispheres, seen in a midsagittal slice) of the cerebral hemispheres. Along the right-hand side of the image is a vertical dimension labeled *dorsal* at the top of the section, and *ventral* at the bottom; across the left-to-right extent of the image is a dimension labeled *lateral* (left), *medial* (center), and *lateral* (right). Within the cerebral hemispheres, dorsal means toward the top and ventral toward the bottom; therefore, the dorsal surface of the brain is the top surface and the ventral surface the underside of the brain. The side-to-side dimension within the cerebral hemispheres uses the term medial for the midline of the coronal view, and lateral for the sides of the brain, away from the midline.

The location of one structure relative to another is expressed by combinations of the ventral-dorsal and medial-lateral terms. In Figure 15–3, the cortex is the outermost tissue layer of the cerebral hemispheres, shown as a dark "rind" of tissue around the edge of the

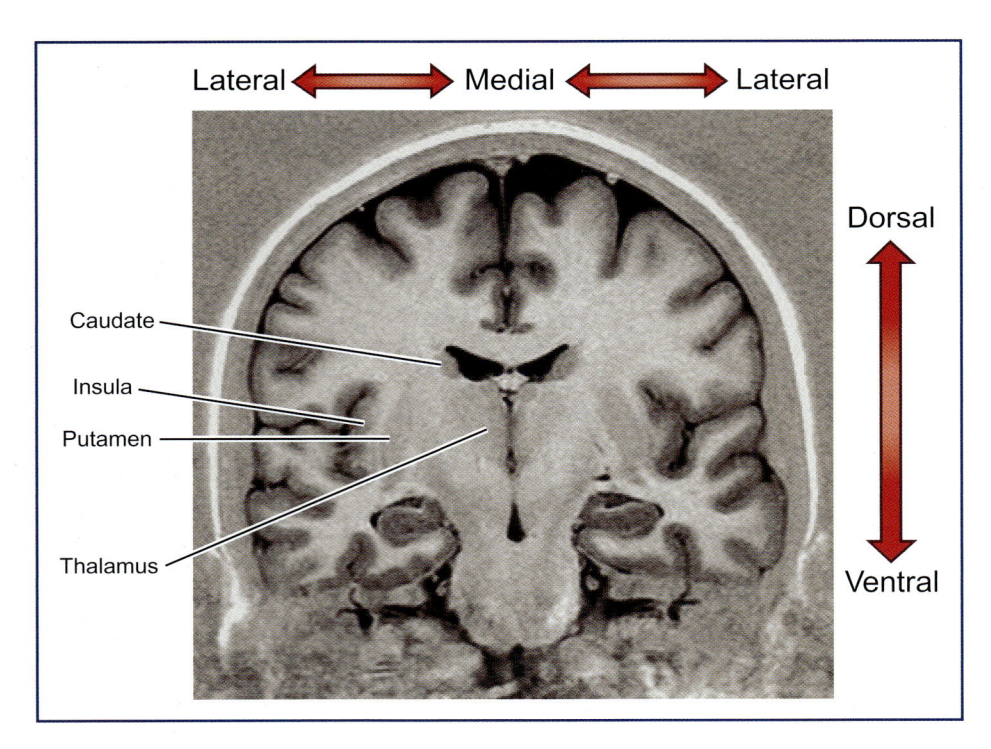

Figure 15–3. MR image in the coronal plane. Labels along the top and side axes of the image show directional terms. Selected structures within the cerebral hemispheres are labeled to illustrate the use of combined directional terms discussed in the text.

coronal image. Inside the cortical layer there is a good deal of white tissue, as well as several clusters of grayish tissue. Three of these grayish masses are labeled here: the *putamen*, *caudate*, and *thalamus*. In addition, the *insula*, a "hidden" part of the cortex beneath the lateral surface of either cerebral hemisphere, is labeled in the image (note how the insula is covered by two folds of the outer rind of cortex).

These four labeled structures are described more specifically below. They are included here to show how the terms *dorsal*, *ventral*, *medial*, and *lateral* are used to locate one structure relative to another within the cerebral hemispheres. For example, in the coronal section shown in Figure 15–3, the insula is lateral to the putamen, and the caudate is dorsal to both the putamen and the thalamus. The position of the caudate relative to the thalamus and putamen, however, is somewhat more complex than simply "dorsal." The caudate is dorsal to the putamen, but also medial to it (closer to the midline), so a more precise statement is that the caudate is dorsomedial to the putamen. Similarly, the caudate is not only dorsal to the thalamus, but somewhat lateral as well. The caudate is therefore dorsolateral to the thalamus (or, reversing the reference structure, the thalamus is ventromedial to the caudate). These combinations can also include the terms *anterior* and *posterior*, as in one structure being anterolateral to another (see horizontal slice in Figure 15–4). This directional terminology is important because of its frequent use in descriptions of neuroanatomical structures, both in basic anatomical study and in imaging studies performed for diagnostic purposes.

Figure 15–4 shows a horizontal MR image on the left, and a sagittal image on the right that includes the brainstem. Toward the top of the horizontal image—in this case, the front of the cerebral hemispheres—is the anterior direction, toward the bottom the posterior direction. The anterior-posterior dimension is also shown in the sagittal image on the right of Figure 15–4; here the directions are obvious because of the image of facial features.

The sagittal image, which includes the lateral aspect of one cerebral hemisphere and the brainstem, introduces an interesting change in the use of direction terms. In the cerebral hemispheres there is a distinction between the dorsal-ventral and anterior-posterior dimensions. For neuroanatomical structures from the top of the brainstem and below, however, the dorsal-ventral and posterior-anterior dimensions are one and the same. The top of the brainstem is indicated in the sagittal image by a horizontal dashed line. Below this line, dorsal and posterior indicate the same direction—toward the back of the body—and ventral and anterior indicate toward the front of the body. The identity between the terms *dorsal/posterior* and *ventral/anterior* applies to spinal cord structures as well.

The terms *deep* and *superficial* are also used to locate one structure relative to another. These terms are typically used to designate the relative locations of structures on a path from "outside to inside" (or the

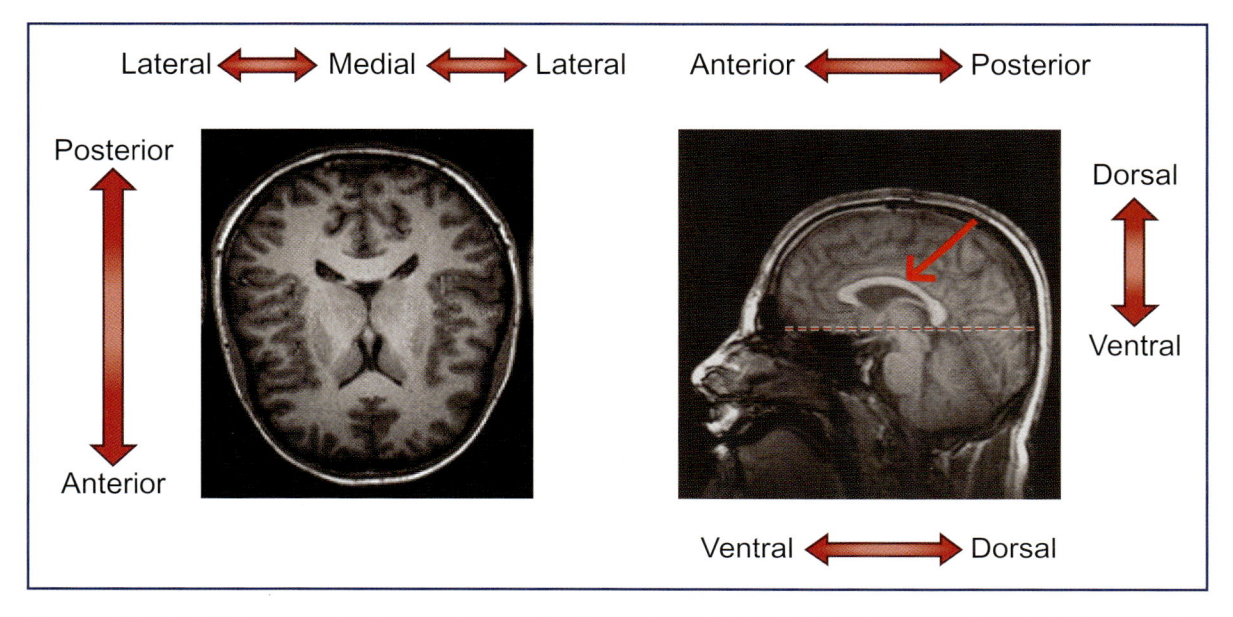

Figure 15–4. MR images in the horizontal (*left*) and sagittal (*right*) planes. In the right image, the dashed red line shows approximate location of the top of the brainstem and the red arrow points to the corpus callosum. See text for discussion of direction terminology above and below the brainstem.

reverse). The question, "What is beneath this surface?" is equivalent to asking, "What is deep to this surface?" For example, the white matter of the cerebral hemispheres is deep to the cortex (or the cortex is superficial to the white matter).

White and Gray Matter, Tracts and Nuclei, Nerves and Ganglia

When a brain is removed from the skull with the intention of preserving it for later study, it is "fixed" in a solution of formalin, a fluid that hardens biological tissue. A formalin-preserved brain shows certain regions having a grayish-brown appearance, and other regions with a pale, near-white appearance. Similarly, in conventional MR images of the brain, some regions appear grayish, and some appear whitish. The coronal plane MR images in Figures 15–2 through 15–4 show both *gray* and *white matter*. Gray matter consists of clusters of neuron cell bodies (*somata*, the plural of *soma*, which means cell body). White matter is formed from myelinated axons issued by those cell bodies. Bundles of axons are called tracts in the CNS, and nerves in the PNS.

Gray Matter and Nuclei

The cortex, the outermost thick covering of the cerebral hemispheres, consists of densely packed cell bodies; the cortex is a major part of gray matter in the cerebral hemispheres. Figure 15–3 shows the cortical "rind" of gray matter enclosing extensive white matter. Within this white matter are several regions of additional gray matter (e.g., the structures labeled "caudate," "putamen," and "thalamus"). A specific cluster of cell bodies inside the cerebral hemispheres, or within the brainstem or spinal cord, is referred to in the singular as a *nucleus* (as in "caudate nucleus") or in some cases as a group of nuclei (as in "cranial nerve nuclei," which are clusters of cell bodies within the brainstem). The clusters of cell bodies deep to the cortex but within the cerebral hemispheres, such as the caudate, putamen, and thalamus, are *subcortical nuclei*. Some subcortical nuclei, such as the thalamus, are collections of many smaller nuclei but are often referred to jointly as a single structure. The term *subcortical nuclei* does not include nuclei within the brainstem, cerebellum, and spinal cord, but is reserved for clusters of cell bodies within the cerebral hemispheres. Nuclei are also found in the cerebellum; these are referred to as cerebellar nuclei.[1]

Neuronal cell bodies, whether in the cortex, subcortical region, cerebellum, brainstem, or spinal cord, most often cluster together for a common purpose; they do not aggregate randomly. In a specific region of cortex, for example, cell bodies related to eye movements, or to auditory perception, are likely to cluster together. A region of cortex, or within a subcortical or brainstem nucleus in which cells have a common function, may have a more fine-grained, systematic grouping of cells. For example, the most posterior gyrus (where gyrus = a hill of tissue on the cortical surface, separated from other gyri by deep fissures, or sulci) of the frontal lobe is the primary motor cortex, containing cells that have direct control over the timing, force, and duration of muscle contractions. Within this primary motor cortex, cells associated with particular parts of the body aggregate together. As one example, hand and finger

---

Somatotopic Representation Is Not Always "Clean"

Many studies have demonstrated the "truth" of somatotopic representation in primary motor and sensory cortices. These studies include correlations between highly localized lesions and affected body parts, electrical stimulation of very discrete locations along the cortex and observation of the resulting movements or reported sensations, and functional MRI (fMRI) studies in which very local movements, as in raising of a single finger, result in the "lighting up" of a small region of the primary motor cortex. Somatotopy, however, is not always neat and clean. For example, fMRI studies of representation of speech apparatus structures in the primary motor cortex have revealed that cells for muscles of the pharynx, tongue, and lips "share" space close to the bottom of the central fissure, where the primary motor cortex meets the sylvian fissure (Takai, Brown, & Liotti, 2010). These cortical cells are not perfectly segregated by structure as might be expected by a strict somatotopy. Takai and colleagues call the mixing of cells for these three speech apparatus structures "somatotopy with overlap." As argued by these authors, the overlap makes functional sense for the control of coordinated behaviors such as swallowing and speaking.

---

[1] The terms "nucleus" and "nuclei" are not used when referring to clusters of cell bodies in the cortex; these organizations of cell bodies are referred to as cortex, cortical region, cortical tissue, and so forth. Similarly, the term "nucleus" is used only sparingly when referring to gray matter in the spinal cord.

cells are found in close proximity in the primary motor cortex. The cellular representation according to body parts within a specific cortical area is called *somatotopic organization*. Somatotopic organization is a maplike projection of the body plan onto the cortex as well as on subcortical nuclei, the cerebellum, the brainstem, and even in the organization of fiber tracts. Somatotopy is characteristic of both motor and sensory systems in the CNS (see below, Figure 15–6).

The concept of somatotopic representation is important not only for understanding brain anatomy, but also for gaining clinical perspectives on the effects of lesion location on function. For example, somatotopic organization explains (in part) how a stroke can affect a client's ability to walk but leave speech and language unaffected; or how a stroke can affect speech and language in the absence of other obvious problems.

White Matter and Fiber Tracts

Neurons have a cell body, an axon, and a terminal (end) structure. The primary function of a neuron is to conduct electrical impulses from the cell body along the axon to the terminal structure, also called the terminal segment or button. As discussed in more detail below, the majority of axons in the brain are wrapped in a fatty substance called *myelin*. Myelin insulates axons and in so doing makes neuronal conduction of electrical impulses faster and more efficient. Myelin gives axons the whitish appearance in fixed brains and brain images. The coronal section shown in Figure 15–3 shows a good deal of white matter, and therefore many, many myelinated axons.

Axons connect different areas of gray matter. These connections are referred to as pathways, fiber tracts, fiber bundles, fasciculi (singular = fasciculus), and lemnisci (singular = lemniscus). Bundles of axons connect different cortical regions to one another, cortical cells to subcortical and brainstem nuclei, spinal nuclei to brainstem and subcortical nuclei, cerebellar nuclei to many different nuclei in the brain—in short, myelinated pathways are everywhere in the brain, connecting and interconnecting different masses of gray matter. These pathways are typically organized somatotopically, in much the same way as the areas of gray matter they connect.

Ganglia

The term "ganglia" (singular = ganglion) is almost exclusively reserved for clusters of nerve cell bodies located *outside* the CNS. Ganglia are technically part of the PNS. They receive sensory fibers coming from receptors in the body (such as tactile receptors, or from receptors in the cochlea or retina) where a first synapse (connection with another neuron) is made prior to entry of the information into the CNS. For example, tactile receptors in the hand are special end organs of the PNS, embedded in skin or muscle and connected by a sensory fiber to the CNS. When the end organ is stimulated (e.g., by the compression of touch), it "fires," sending electrical impulses to the nervous system via the sensory fibers. These fibers make first contact—that is, make first synapses—with cells in a ganglion immediately outside the spinal cord. The ganglion cells receiving this information deliver it, via its own axons, to sensory cells in the spinal cord. Similar receptors are found in muscles of the speech apparatus, including muscles of the respiratory system, larynx, and upper airway (pharyngeal, oral, and nasal passageways).

The spinal cord is associated with a series of *dorsal root ganglia*, arranged from the top to bottom segments of the cord. These ganglia serve as first synapses for much of the sensory information delivered from the limbs and trunk to the CNS. There are also ganglia immediately outside the brainstem that serve as the first synapses for sensory information from head and neck structures. For example, the hair cells of the cochlea are the specialized sensory endings for hearing, and when they are deformed by motion of the basilar membrane they fire, sending impulses to the spiral ganglion, a bundle of nerve cells outside the brainstem. First synapses for auditory neurons are made in the spiral ganglion cells, which send axons into the brainstem to make synapses within the first set of nuclei along the auditory pathway (see Chapter 13).

Efferent and Afferent

The terms *efferent* and *afferent* are used in two different ways to describe information flow in the nervous system. The first use of the terms concerns overall information flow for production of muscular effort (efferent) in contrast to the information flow for the sensation of an environmental event (afferent). When motor commands are issued from cortical tissue and travel along descending pathways through one or more motor nuclei before eventually being directed by peripheral nerves to muscles, the pathways are referred to as efferent. Sometimes the term *efference* is equated with the basic components—brain-directed muscle contractions and their patterns in space and time—of motor control. In contrast, when a sensory receptor (such as a tactile receptor in a finger, or the hair cells of the cochlea) is stimulated and the resulting signal travels via peripheral nerves to the spinal cord or brainstem and then through ascending pathways to a final destination in the cortex, the pathways are said to be afferent. *Afference* is often taken to mean "sensory."

A second use of the terms *efferent* and *afferent* indicates the inputs and outputs of nuclei *within* the CNS. This usage does not imply a motor act or sensation to or from a body structure, but rather the flow of information from one nucleus to another, or from nuclei to cortex or cortex to nuclei. For example, the *substantia nigra* (SN) is a nucleus in the midbrain that sends a neurotransmitter called dopamine to several subcortical and brainstem cells. The cells of the SN send information via a fiber tract to the striatum, a subcortical nucleus group made up of the caudate and putamen. The output of the SN to the striatum is therefore referred to as an *efferent projection* of the SN. On the other hand, the SN receives efferent projections from the *subthalamic nucleus* (STN), another subcortical nucleus. These inputs to the SN from the STN are afferent projections. The SN, and many other cells in both subcortical nuclei and the cortex, issue efferent projections to other nuclei (or cortical cells) and receive afferent input from other cell groups.

For the present purposes, the specific nuclei sending information to, or receiving information from, other nuclei are not important. Rather, the concept of efferent and afferent projections within the CNS is crucial. Note the importance of a reference structure in naming the efferent and afferent projections of a nucleus: a nucleus' efferent projections are pathways sent to another nucleus (or the cortex), whereas the nucleus' afferent projections are pathways received from other nuclei (or the cortex). A single nucleus, such as the SN or STN, typically has both efferent and afferent projections—the nucleus influences other cell bodies, and is influenced by other cell bodies. Sometimes these influences are in a loop, so two nuclei may communicate with each other via both efferent and afferent projections.

Most nuclei, and cortical cells as well, receive and send information to multiple locations within the brain. Each cortical region or nucleus is likely to have multiple efferent and afferent projections. The dense and overlapping interconnections within the brain, including the efferent projections of a single nucleus (or cortical area) to many different nuclei (or areas), plus the variety of afferent inputs to a single nucleus (or cortical area), make the simple distinction of efferent versus afferent less useful than once thought. For example, motor systems are not isolated from, or independent of, sensory systems. In fact, motor and sensory systems are highly interdependent, with certain brain "circuits"—interconnected nuclei—performing sensorimotor integration for the most efficient and skilled actions. *Sensorimotor control* is often the preferred term to represent action such as the coordinated motions of the articulators (pharyngeal-oral and velopharyngeal-nasal structures), larynx, and breathing system to produce the acoustic signal we call speech.

Neurons and Synapses

Neurons are the "firing" cells of the CNS and PNS. Under the right circumstances, neurons generate electrical potentials that allow them to cause other neurons to "fire." A synapse includes the anatomical structures serving the transfer of information from one neuron to another. The transfer information across neurons is accomplished by the conversion of electrical energy to neurochemical energy, which in turn is converted back to electrical energy.

Lateralization and Specialization of Function

"Lateralization" and "specialization" may sometimes be used interchangeably, but the terms have different technical meanings. When a function is said to be "lateralized" in the brain, the function is primarily controlled by one hemisphere relative to the other. Lateralization is also referred to as "hemispheric asymmetry" for function and can be applied strictly to anatomical structure (as in the case of similar locations in the two hemispheres having different volumes of neural tissue). Good examples of lateralized functions include (of course) speech and language (thought to be controlled by left hemisphere structures in about 95% of the population), handedness (also controlled by the left hemisphere in about 95% of the population), and emotions (thought to be controlled primarily by right hemisphere structures). Lateralization of speech and language function to the left hemisphere has been demonstrated by clinical cases and research studies, including the common observation of disrupted speech and language function when a stroke affects the blood supply to the left hemisphere but not the right hemisphere. Lateralization of speech and language has also been shown by the ability to elicit speech and language behaviors during surgical procedures, when an electrical current stimulates regions of the left hemisphere's cortical surface. Stimulation in the same cortical regions of the right hemisphere does not typically elicit these speech and language behaviors.

A test of brain lateralization of speech and language functions is to inject a drug, called amobarbital, into either the left or right carotid artery so that the left or right hemisphere is anesthetized for a brief period of time. The carotid arteries are the main source of blood flowing from the heart to the cerebral hemispheres. An injection of amobarbital into the left carotid artery initially distributes the drug to the left hemisphere, leaving the right hemisphere unaffected for a short time. The drug temporarily blocks neural activity in the anesthetized cerebral hemisphere, and therefore provides a technique to determine which hemisphere is implicated for speech and language function. If injection into the left carotid artery results in speech and language deficits, but injection into the right carotid artery does not, this is good evidence for lateralization of speech and language functions to the left hemisphere.

The amobarbital test, called the *Wada test* after the Japanese-Canadian neurologist Juhn Wada, who developed the procedure in the late 1940s, is used in patients undergoing resection (extraction) of parts of the brain to relieve chronic, severe epilepsy. Before the Wada test, clinical cases of stroke affecting either the left or the right cerebral hemisphere led physicians and scientists to regard speech and language functions of the brain as lateralized to the left hemisphere. This suggested that the same lateralization of speech and language functions was typical of neurologically normal individuals. In epilepsy, however, there was (and is) the sense that a seizure-causing lesion in the left hemisphere may result in speech and language functions being "transferred" to the right hemisphere, or to be split more equally between the two hemispheres. The Wada test is used in these patients to identify the hemisphere to which speech and language function is lateralized, to indicate areas where surgical resection should be avoided or minimized for maximal preservation of communication ability.

Many studies using the Wada test have been reported in the clinical literature (for two good examples, both of which contain reviews of much of the pertinent literature, see Lee et al. [2008], and Springer et al. [1999]). Use of the Wada test in neurologically normal individuals to determine if laterality varies by handedness has been challenged by the difficulty of assembling a large enough group of left-handers to compare with more easily recruited right-handers. When the Wada test has been used to compare laterality of left- and right-handers, it is usually among presurgical patients with epilepsy. This work shows about 96% of right-handed people to have left hemisphere lateralization for speech and language, compared with 85% of left-handers (or "mixed" handers; see Rasmussen & Milner, 1977). When contemporary brain imaging methods are used to estimate lateralization of speech and language, estimates for right-handers almost match the data from Rasmussen and Milner, but more left-handers show lateralization of speech and language to the right hemisphere (Swanson, Sabsevitz, Hammeke, & Binder, 2007). Using an imaging technique similar to fMRI (see sidetrack on this page), Knecht et al. (2000) obtained results showing a relationship between degree of left-handedness and the likelihood of speech and language being lateralized to the *right* hemisphere. Hard-core righties were almost all left-lateralized (~96%), whereas only about 73% of hard-core "southpaws" were left-lateralized. The sample of people with various degrees of "mixed" handedness fell, as a group, between these two numbers.

This brief review of the literature on lateralization of speech and language function suggests at least two broad conclusions, as well as one additional thought concerning the concept of lateralization. First, most people, either left or right-handed, have speech and language lateralized to the left hemisphere. Second, there is a greater chance for language to be lateralized to the right hemisphere, or for its representation to be split between the hemispheres, in people who are clearly left-handed. Still, the majority of left-handers are "left-dominant" for speech and language, even though they are "right-dominant" for handedness.

---

fMRI

MR images are obtained by placing a body structure within a strong magnetic field and then, by application and withdrawal of a second magnetic field, causing cell nuclei to generate magnetic properties that are sensed by a coil. The coil detects different amounts of energy generated by the cells, depending on cell properties, cell locations, and other factors. Software processes the signals generated by the cells and assembles them into an image of the target structure (for example, see right side of Figure 15–2). Functional MRI (fMRI) makes use of the same general principle, but with a twist (that's a pun for those of you familiar with the magnetized behavior of brain cell nuclei). When neurons are active, the active region attracts blood flow from arteries; such arterial blood flow is oxygen rich, and oxygen-rich blood has different magnetic properties than run-of-the-mill blood. When an area of the brain is being used for a specific task, like speaking, that area generates a different signal than an area not being used for that task. The software is designed to make that active area "light up" because of increased blood flow. So, now you know that you can actually light up a room when you speak words of cheer!

> ### Genes, Hands, and Brains
>
> Scientists continue to be interested in the relationship between handedness and lateralization of speech and language function. In a recent study, Schmitz, Lor, Klose, Güntürkün, and Ocklenburg (2017) performed an analysis of the genetic overlap between handedness and lateralization of speech and language. In the past, handedness was thought to be determined by a single gene, but more recent research has demonstrated that it is more likely determined by a group of genes. Schmitz et al. found only a small overlap between sets of genes for handedness and sets for speech and language lateralization. In lay language, handedness and lateralization of speech and language do not develop solely as a result of common genetic mechanisms. Why is this important? In many studies of speech and language function, handedness is often used as a control variable to rule out possible messiness in the data due to different degrees of lateralization among participants. The work by Schmitz et al. suggests that restricting a participant sample to right-handers only may not guarantee the degree of left lateralization of speech and language skills.

Finally, the concept of lateralization for speech and language to one hemisphere or the other is not an absolute, either-or concept. Lateralization for speech and language appears to be a continuous phenomenon, not only because of the demonstration of greater likelihood for right-hemisphere dominance with increasing left-handedness (Knecht et al., 2000), but also because certain aspects of speech and language—such as prosody—have been shown to be represented primarily in the right hemisphere. Even though associations exist between handedness and lateralization of speech and language function, the association is not necessarily due to a common underlying mechanism; handedness and lateralization of speech and language function are related only partly in a causal way (Ocklenburg, Beste, Arning, Peterburs, & Güntürkün, 2014). When the term "dominant hemisphere for speech and language" is used, these qualifying thoughts should be kept in mind.

How is "specialization" different from "lateralization"? Although it may seem reasonable to say that the left hemisphere is specialized for speech and language (in the same way it is lateralized for speech and language), the term "specialization" is used in a more specific—pun intended—sense. Specialization means that certain brain regions have evolved to serve distinct functions, whether lateralized or not. For example, a well-known claim for specialization is that portions of the frontal lobe are specialized for executive function (see Alvarez & Emory, 2006 for a review of evidence for and against this claim). "Executive function" is, broadly speaking, the ability to organize behavior to achieve a goal or set of goals and to connect current behavior with future outcomes. If the brain is a movie in production, executive function is the director of the production. Executive function coordinates brain function, matches behaviors to desired outcomes, and regulates actions. In neurologically intact individuals, tasks requiring organization of complex material to achieve a certain outcome often cause parts of the frontal lobes to "light up" in fMRI studies. People with damage to the frontal lobes are likely to show impaired ability to deal with complex decision making and demonstrate poor regulation of behavior. Some scientists and clinicians regard the frontal lobes *of both hemispheres*, or at least certain parts of them, to be specialized for executive function. Here we have a case of specialization without obvious lateralization.

Another example of hypothesized specialization is in regions of the brain thought to be critical for the representation and programming of articulatory gestures for speech. Some scientists place these two processes in a very small portion of the posterior, ventral edge of the left frontal lobe (more is said about this below). The actual neural tissue for the *execution* of speech sounds—where execution means transforming the represented and programmed sounds into movements—is thought to be located slightly posterior to this programming tissue, but still in the frontal lobe. This is an example of specialization within lateralization: speech is left-lateralized, and within this lateralized function there are finer degrees of tissue specialization for the production of speech and language.

A popular view of specialization, one that takes the concept to a logical (but in some views, extreme) conclusion, is found in the idea of brain modules. Modules are thought to be regions of brain tissue that are specialized for particular tasks—"dedicated," in computer terminology—and in fact insulated from other tasks. Some scientists and clinicians believe, for example, that in humans a very specific region on the underside of the temporal lobe contains a module for human face recognition (matching a person's identity with his or her face; see Said, Haxby, & Todorov, 2011). This brain region is thought to be "insulated" from other tasks because it is not active for recognition of nonhuman/nonface objects such as cars, dogs, and so forth. Closer to home, some speech scientists believe there is a module for speech perception in the left hemisphere, a species-specific (human) collection of neural tissue activated only by human speech or simulations of it (i.e., computer generated speech) (see Chapter 12).

CEREBRAL HEMISPHERES AND WHITE MATTER

The cerebral hemispheres are part of the CNS (see Figure 15–1). Each hemisphere contains four lobes, each lobe having gray and white matter.

Cerebral Hemispheres

Figure 15–5 shows the cerebral hemispheres in four views. The top-left view is from above the brain, looking down to the dorsal surfaces of the two hemispheres. The front of the brain is toward the top of the image. This view shows the left and right cerebral hemispheres, separated by a long, front-to-back fissure called the *longitudinal fissure* (also called the *interhemispheric* or *sagittal fissure*). The visible surface tissue is *cortex*, regarded as the most complex and "sophisticated" part of the brain. The cortex covers the entire surface of the cerebral hemispheres. Note the ridges or "hills" of the cortex, and the "dips" between them. The

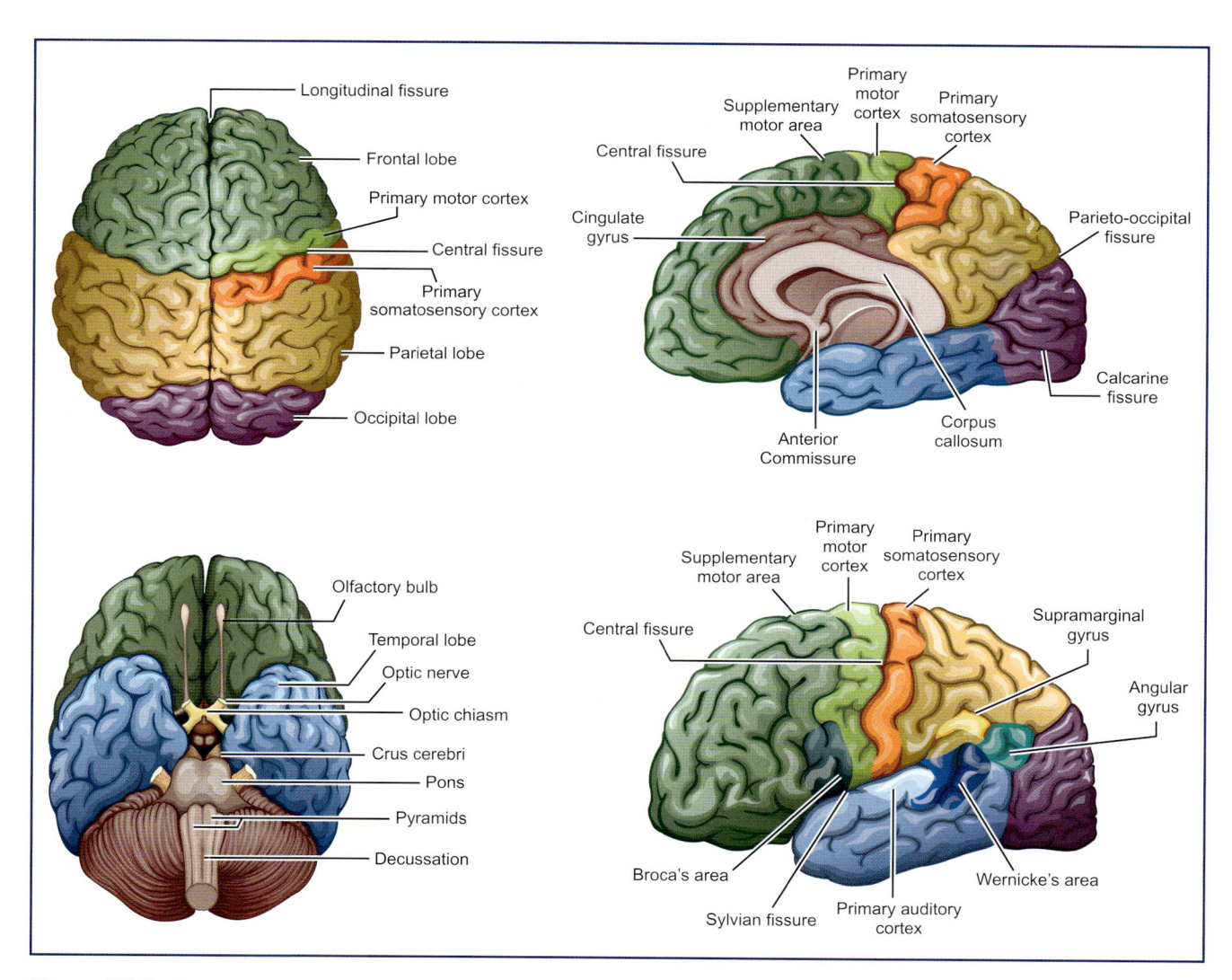

Figure 15–5. Four views of the cerebral hemispheres. *Top left*, dorsal surface of hemispheres; *bottom left*, ventral surface of hemispheres; *top right*, medial surface of right hemisphere, seen in midsagittal view; *bottom right*, sagittal view of lateral surface of left hemisphere.

ridges are called *gyri* (singular = *gyrus*) and the "dips" *sulci* (singular = *sulcus*) or *fissures* (the term "fissure" is typically used to mean a particularly deep sulcus, such as the longitudinal fissure). One notable difference between the human brain and the brain of animals such as sheep, cats, and dogs is that humans have relatively deep and numerous sulci defining the cortical surface. These deep sulci are infoldings of cortical surface forming unseen "walls" of tissue that contribute to a greater volume of cortical cells in the human brain relative to other animals. The hidden cortical surface area and its corresponding thickness add to the cognitive and performance power of humans. By gently separating any sulcus on the surface of a prepared (formalin-hardened) brain, the walls of hidden cortical tissue are revealed. Some authors have estimated that close to two-thirds of the human cortex is hidden inside sulcal walls (Zilles, Armstrong, Schleicher, & Kretschmann, 1988). This unique feature of the human brain appears to be an evolutionary solution to packing lots of cortical tissue into a container—the skull—of limited size.

A dramatic view of "hidden" cortical tissue can be gained by putting your thumbs inside the longitudinal fissure of a prepared brain, your two hands resting on the two hemispheres, and gently separating the hemispheres without tearing the tissue. This exposes the deep inside (medial) walls of the two hemispheres. The medial wall of the right cerebral hemisphere is shown in the top-right view of Figure 15–5. A prominent feature of this midsagittal view is the *corpus callosum*, the massive bundle of tissue that connects structures across the two hemispheres.

Figure 15–5, bottom-right, shows a side view of the left hemisphere of the brain. The front of the brain is toward the left of the image. This view shows the four lobes of the brain, their boundary landmarks, plus additional regions important to speech, language, and hearing. The image shows the frontal (green), parietal (light brown), temporal (blue), and occipital (purple) lobes. This color code is modified at specific locations to highlight important cortical regions within the hemisphere. What follows is a more detailed consideration of each of these lobes. The structure and function of two additional cerebral regions, the insula and limbic system, are also discussed.

Frontal Lobe

The frontal lobe is bounded posteriorly by the *central fissure* (also called the *fissure of Rolando*), and below by the anterior part of the *lateral sulcus* or *sylvian fissure* (see Figure 15–5, top left and right for central fissure, bottom right for sylvian fissure). The gyrus immediately in front of the central sulcus, and therefore within the frontal lobe, is the *primary motor cortex* (shown as a lighter shade of green in Figure 15–5). The primary motor cortex contains cells called motor neurons that send signals to motor neurons in the brainstem and spinal cord, which, in turn, send axons to muscles to control their contraction patterns. The pathway: primary motor cortex neurons → brainstem/spinal cord motor neurons → muscles can be thought of as the route of direct nervous system control of the timing, strength, and speed of muscle contractions for head, neck, limb, and torso structures. As discussed later in this chapter, this direct route to muscle control is modulated and fine-tuned by activity in several different parts of the CNS, including other cortical regions (such as the supplementary motor area, primary somatosensory cortex, and Broca's area, shown in Figure 15–5, top and bottom right), the basal ganglia and cerebellum to produce everyday movement as well as highly skilled, specialized movement.

Primary Motor Cortex. The somatotopic arrangement of cells (motor neurons) in the primary motor cortex is like an inverted map of the body. Figure 15–6 shows that the map extends from the top of the brain (at the longitudinal fissure), down the lateral surface of the hemisphere to the sylvian fissure. The map is found in both hemispheres. The map reflects not only *which* body parts are represented in a specific region of the primary motor cortex, but the *amount* of cortex devoted to the control of specific body parts, as shown in the bottom left image of Figure 15–6. A notable characteristic of the body map of the primary motor cortex is the upside-down representation of the body: cells that control muscles of the lower part of the body (such as muscles of the hip and knee) are at the top of the primary motor cortex (or even along the medial wall of the cortex—note the location of cells for muscles of the feet), whereas control of muscles of the face, tongue, and larynx are toward the bottom of the gyrus, just above the sylvian fissure. Larger representation of body parts on the map indicate a greater number of cells devoted to control of the body part. Note the very large size of the face and its associated structures (the tongue, lips, larynx) compared with the size of the feet or the trunk. A disproportionate number of cells in the primary motor cortex is associated with control of the structures of primary interest to speech-language pathologists. The auditory cortex, not represented here, has its own systematic plan for cells, arranged according to signal frequency (Chapter 13).

The disproportionate representation of cells that control movements of orofacial structures suggests

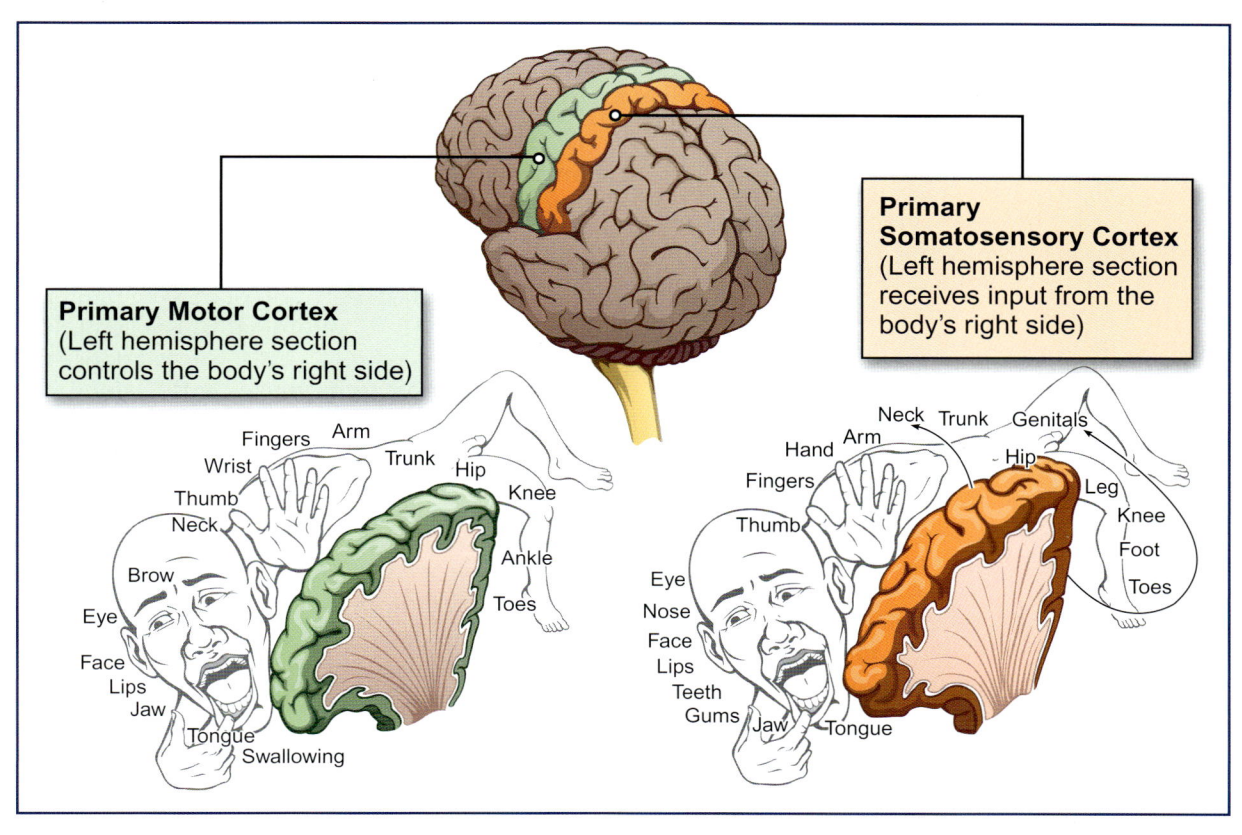

Figure 15–6. Somatotopic representations along the primary motor (*green*) and sensory (*orange*) cortices. In these slices the wall of cortex within the longitudinal fissure is at the back of each slice.

their great relevance to the lives of humans. Not much imagination is required to make the case for the centrality of eating and breathing in human function, and the need for sophisticated muscular control to support these behaviors. The same case can be made for any mammal, but the disproportionate representation of these structures within the primary motor cortex of humans is very much a function of our unique ability to generate spoken language. Notice the phrase "spoken *language*"; it is not just the production of sounds—many animals do this for simple communicative purposes —but the extensive use of a signal system (the acoustic signal emerging from the vocal tract) to give meaning to abstract, complex ideas, to convey the same idea in different ways, even to *create* ideas (Deacon, 1997).

The location of orofacial and laryngeal cells at the "bottom" (ventral aspect) of the primary motor cortex is of interest because they are close to Broca's area, a premotor cortical region located in the left hemisphere on the ventrolateral surface of the frontal lobe (Figure 15–5, bottom right). Broca's area is immediately adjacent to the primary motor cortical representation of orofacial and laryngeal control. Surely this is not a coincidence.

Broca's Area. The inferior frontal gyrus, on the lateral surface of the *left* frontal lobe and immediately above the anterior end of the sylvian fissure, is called *Broca's area*. Broca's area is shown in Figure 15–5, bottom right, as the frontal lobe region colored dark green. Broca's area (or at least some of it), along with several other related areas of the frontal lobe, is *premotor cortex*, the latter term indicating a role in motor control different from the direct control of muscles associated with cells in the primary motor cortex. Broca's area is believed to have a central role in the planning and organization of motor behavior required for speech production. This conclusion was first formulated by Paul Broca (1824–1880), the famous French physician who between 1861 and 1865 reported on a few patients with primarily expressive speech-language disorders resulting from neurological disease (usually a stroke). On autopsy, Broca noted lesions in and around the third frontal gyrus (the lower part of the inferior gyrus) of the left hemisphere. The patients examined by Broca had expressive speech problems but largely unaffected speech and language comprehension. Because the autopsy revealed damage in the lower, posterior frontal lobe, Broca concluded that this region of the brain was responsible for speech expression. The conclusion was reinforced by observations that lesions in the inferior gyrus of the *right* frontal lobe did not produce speech or language disorders. The emerging picture was of specialization for expressive control of speech and language in the left hemisphere, in the third frontal convolution of the frontal lobe. This brain region has since been known as "Broca's area."

We know now that historical and contemporary interpretations of Broca's observations are too simplistic. First, damage to the brains of people with expressive disorders like those described by Broca (often called "Broca's aphasia") typically extends to regions well beyond the third frontal gyrus (Keller, Crow, Foundas, Amunts, & Roberts, 2009). In fact, the actual brains autopsied by Broca were examined again almost 20 years ago with imaging techniques and shown to have widespread damage in addition to the obvious lesion to the inferior convolution of the left frontal lobe (Dronkers, Plaisant, Ibas-Zisen, & Cabanis, 2007). Second, there is evidence that Broca's area is involved in language *comprehension*, specifically of utterances with relatively complicated syntax (Grodzinsky & Santi, 2008) and semantics (Willems & Hagoort, 2009). Third, tissue in and around Broca's area has been shown to respond to non-linguistic events, two of which are *watching* finger and/or mouth movements. Broca's area "lights up" when participants *observe* these movements (Lindenberg, Fangerau, & Seitz 2007). Finally, for the great majority of people, speech and language control in Broca's area is both *lateralized* to one hemisphere and *specialized* by virtue of a specific area of left hemisphere cortex devoted to speech and language function. There is asymmetry of function among most people, but a small number of people have lateralization of speech and language function to the right hemisphere, or no lateralization at all. Lesions to the right hemisphere may produce the same speech and language signs as lesions to the left hemisphere, at least in a small number of people. *Broca's area* is the term used to designate a specialized region in the left hemisphere for speech expression, but in cases of right hemisphere lateralization for these functions, the relationship between anatomy and function is not so clear.

Broca's area is clearly important for speech and language behavior, but is not devoted exclusively to speech expression. Instead, Broca's area is part of a *network* involving extensive interconnections and shared functions, serving the complexity of all aspects of human communication. It is not productive to expect simple matches between damage to specific areas of the brain and specific functions.

Premotor and Supplementary Motor Area. The gyrus just forward of, and parallel to, the primary motor cortex is called *premotor cortex* (often called PMA, for "Premotor Area," not labeled in Figure 15–5; see the darker green gyrus immediately anterior to the lighter green gyrus in Figure 15–5, bottom right). The ventral part of premotor cortex is Broca's area, colored dark green in Figure 15–5, lower right image. In the lateral view of the left hemisphere, the dorsal limit of premotor cortex is the supplementary motor cortex (SMA) (Figure 15–5, lower right). The SMA also extends down the medial wall of the frontal lobe (Figure 15–5, upper right). PMA and SMA are thought be cortical areas in which action (motor acts) is *planned*; primary motor cortex is the cortical area from which commands are issued to *perform* movements. This distinction is important to the speech-language pathologist, who is often asked to make a diagnostic judgment of whether a speech motor control disorder is one of execution or planning (or both). Execution disorders of speech motor control are called *dysarthrias*; planning disorders are called *apraxias* or *dyspraxias*.

Prefrontal Cortex. The large mass of frontal lobe tissue anterior to the primary motor cortex and PMA/SMA is called *prefrontal cortex*. Many scientists (see, for example, Ridderinkhof, Ullsperger, Crone, & Nieuwenhuis, 2004) believe that this part of the frontal lobe, plus its ventral surface, performs *executive function* in the brain. Executive function is the guidance of all cognitive (and perhaps lower level) brain functions. Executive function is the brain's monitoring, selecting, and "tuning" of higher-level actions and behavioral goals. Executive function guides decisions such as when it is "okay" to use certain words or drink certain beverages, why it is not okay to employ violence as a reaction to situations, whether or not a certain behavior may have a profound effect on your own or someone else's life in the future, and how the tuning of your sensory systems (like hearing and vision) changes from situation to situation (among other things). This short list makes it is easy to understand why scientists have connected prefrontal cortex with aspects of personality. Lesions of the prefrontal cortex may have direct relevance to speech-language pathologists who work with patients with frontal lobe lesions and impaired executive function. Patients with traumatic brain injury, or with dementia, may show executive function problems due (in part) to frontal lobe lesions.

Parietal Lobe

The parietal lobe (shown in light brown in Figure 15–5 except for its most anterior gyrus, which is colored orange) is bounded at the front by the *central fissure* (or *sulcus*) or *fissure of Rolando*, below by the posterior part of the *sylvian fissure* (or *lateral sulcus*), and toward the back of the brain by the *parieto-occipital fissure*. The parieto-occipital fissure, which is the boundary between the parietal and occipital lobes, is easy to see on the medial wall of the cerebral hemisphere (see Figure 15–5, top right) but only partially visible when viewing the external surface of the hemisphere. The boundary shown between the parietal and occipital lobes in the bottom right view of Figure 15–5 is therefore approximate. Similarly, the boundary between the lower part of the parietal lobe and the back of the temporal lobe is not clearly marked in the bottom right view of Figure 15–5.

Primary Somatosensory Cortex. The gyrus immediately in back of the central (Rolandic) fissure—the most anterior gyrus of the parietal lobe—is the *primary somatosensory cortex*. The primary somatosensory cortex, colored orange in Figure 15–5, runs parallel to the primary motor cortex. Like the primary motor cortex, the primary somatosensory cortex is organized somatotopically, although not in precisely the same way as the motor cortex (see sidetrack on "Somatotopic Representation Is Not Always 'Clean,'" and Figure 15–6).

Stated broadly, cells in the primary somatosensory cortex respond to touch and pain stimuli from all body locations. The primary somatosensory cortex is, in fact, a good deal more complicated than this broad view. There are extensive interconnections among cell types within the somatosensory cortex and subcortical nuclei, as well as brainstem nuclei and the cerebellum. Some cortical cells receive basic touch information from subcortical and brainstem nuclei, some use this basic information to encode the texture or shape of touched objects, and some may respond to the magnitude and direction of a tactile stimulus (Bear, Connors, & Paradiso, 2007). Cells in the primary somatotopic cortex receive information about pain and temperature, and some cells are interconnected with cells in primary motor cortex.

Posterior Parietal Cortex. The parietal cortex posterior to the primary somatosensory cortex and anterior to the occipital lobe as well as the portion sharing a boundary with the temporal lobe is called the *posterior parietal cortex* (PPC). The PPC contains cell groups that integrate and process different sensory stimuli to create complex sensory experiences. These cells are also involved in the planning of complex motor acts such as reaching, grasping, and tool use (Culham & Valyear, 2006). Recall that primary somatosensory cortex receives information on touch and pain; what of other sensations and combinations of sensations we experience? For example, the experience of taking care to cross a street when hearing an ambulance siren and then seeing the rapidly approaching vehicle involves an integration of (at least) auditory and visual sensations with the action plan of stepping backward to the curb or sprinting across the street. Discussion of auditory and visual cortex follows below, but here it can be stated that the "primary" information on auditory and visual stimuli arrives in the temporal and occipital lobes, respectively. This information is sent to the PPC where it is analyzed and integrated into increasingly more complex perceptual and action forms. In this sense, the PPC functions as *association cortex*, literally associating different types of sensory stimuli and directing action plans based on this integration.

Two examples of the integrative function of PPC are noteworthy. First, object recognition by the hand requires the ability to identify size, shape, texture, hardness/softness, and other characteristics. Activity in primary somatosensory cortex related to these "simple" characteristics of an object is sent to PPC for association and integration, and ultimately recognition of the object. Recognition of an object requires an attachment of meaning to the object's properties. Individuals with damage to PPC may experience *agnosia*, which is the inability to recognize objects even though basic sensory skills (as revealed by a simple test of taction) appear to be normal. Agnosias may also occur in the visual and auditory modalities. Although basic tests of visual and auditory sensitivity reveal "normal" abilities, the person with damage to PPC may not be able to connect meaning to visual or auditory input.

The second example illustrates the complexity of PPC function in representing the sensations around us. The PPC is a major player in the creation of proper spatial relationships between our bodies and the world. The absence of such relationships can play havoc with our concept of body image and the ability to produce coordinated movements to negotiate or influence an environment. People with damage to PPC in one hemisphere experience a neurological symptom called *hemineglect*, where one side of the body or one-half of the environment is regarded as if it doesn't exist. People with hemineglect may dress themselves on only one side of the body, or even reject one of their limbs as belonging to their body. Clinical observations such as these, when a person is known to have brain damage in PPC, illustrate the complex role of the parietal lobe in the integration and even construction of perception and action.

Supramarginal Gyrus and Angular Gyrus. Two other landmarks on the parietal lobe are shown in Figure 15–5. These are specific regions of parietal association cortex involved in high-level language function. The *angular gyrus* is shown as the dark turquoise region immediately behind and slightly above the posterior end of the sylvian fissure (see Figure 15–5, lower right). Note the location of the angular gyrus at the boundaries of the parietal, occipital, and temporal lobes. Clinically, lesions to the angular gyrus result in complex language deficits, such as the understanding of metaphor, and difficulty with mathematical concepts and performance. An older theory of language and brain functioning imagined the angular gyrus as the site where written language was transformed into an auditory code for spoken language (Geschwind, 1965). Immediately above and slightly in front of the angular gyrus is the *supramarginal gyrus*, shown in Figure 15–5 (lower right) as a yellow region of PPC. The supramarginal gyrus is thought to be involved in word meaning, the relation of individual speech sounds to the formation of words, and the ability to connect word meanings with action patterns (i.e., to enable the performance of action on verbal command, such as, "Show me how you whistle").

Temporal Lobe

The temporal lobe, shown in blue in Figure 15–5, is located on the lower side of each cerebral hemisphere. Toward the front of each cerebral hemisphere, the sylvian fissure is the boundary between the temporal lobe and the frontal lobe above; toward the back the same fissure separates the temporal lobe from the parietal lobe. The upper part of the temporal lobe has a back boundary with the lower parietal lobe, and the lower parts of the temporal lobe have a posterior boundary with the occipital lobe.

Major Gyri. The surface of the temporal lobe visible from the side has three major gyri—superior, medial, and inferior. Immediately below the sylvian fissure is the superior temporal gyrus. As shown in the light blue area of Figure 15–5 (lower right), the upper lip and some surrounding tissue of the superior temporal gyrus is called *primary auditory cortex* or *Heschl's gyrus*. The primary auditory cortex is the first cortical location for processing of auditory signals. More complex processing follows when this initial analysis is forwarded to other locations within the temporal lobe.

Primary Auditory Cortex and Planum Temporale. The anatomy of primary auditory cortex—Heschl's gyrus—requires additional description with the assistance of a different view of the brain. Imagine drawing an oblique line parallel to and slightly above the sylvian fissure, as shown by the cut line in the upper image of Figure 15–7. Think of this line as one edge of a plane cutting through the cerebral hemispheres, dividing them into upper and lower halves. This horizontal (axial) section is angled to follow the "pitch" of the sylvian fissure. Looking down on the cerebral hemispheres from above after this cut is made and the

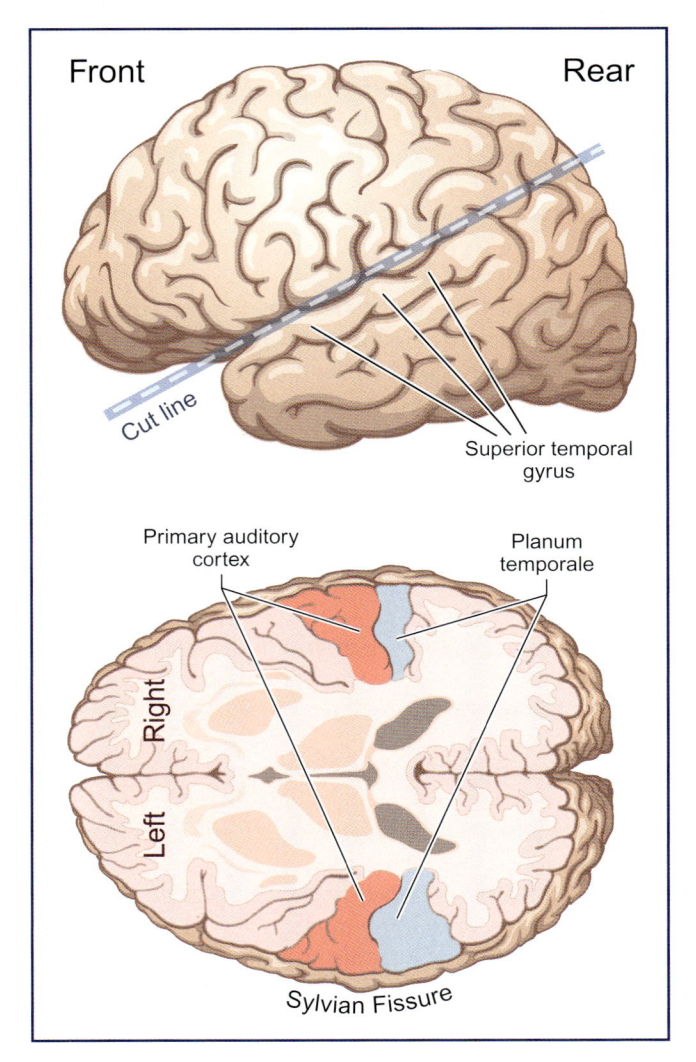

Figure 15–7. Top, lateral surface of left hemisphere, showing an oblique plane whose edge follows the upward tilt of the sylvian fissure; bottom, a view of the dorsal surface of the brain cut into upper and lower parts along this oblique plane. This section shows the "shelf" of auditory cortex inside the sylvian fissure, including the more anterior primary auditory cortex (*colored salmon*) and the more posterior planum temporale (*colored blue*). The planum temporale has more cortical area in the left, compared with right, hemisphere.

top half of the hemispheres removed, the top (dorsal) surfaces of the temporal lobes are visible. This view is shown in the bottom image of Figure 15–7. The superior temporal gyrus extends medially from its upper lip, like a shelf of cortex. This shelf, previously hidden inside the sylvian fissure, is an important part of the auditory cortex; it is a continuation of the superior temporal gyrus toward the center of the brain. Part of this surface is called the *planum temporale*. The lower image in Figure 15–7 shows, for both hemispheres, the primary auditory cortex (colored salmon) as well as the planum temporale (colored blue). In both hemispheres the primary auditory cortex is anterior to the planum temporale. Note the larger surface area of the planum temporale in the left as compared with the right hemisphere.

The primary auditory cortex and planum temporale have interesting features. First, the cells in primary auditory cortex are arranged systematically with respect to auditory signal frequency; this does not seem to be the case for the planum temporale (Langers, Backe, & van Dijk, 2007). A fundamental aspect of *peripheral* auditory anatomy is the systematic frequency map of sensory receptors embedded within the organ of Corti along the extent of the basilar membrane. The basilar membrane is a ribbonlike membrane housed inside the cochlea, the snail shell–like structure in the inner ear. The sensory receptors along the basilar membrane, and specifically within the organ of Corti, are called hair cells. The cochlea spirals from its base to its tip, and the basilar membrane follows this spiral. Along this systematic map, the highest frequencies (~20,000 cycles per second) heard by humans are sensed by hair cells at the base of the basilar membrane. Moving from the base toward the tip of the membrane the hair cells are sensitive to increasingly lower frequencies. At the tip of the basilar membrane the hair cells are sensitive to the lowest frequency (~20 cycles per second) heard by humans. This systematic frequency representation along the basilar membrane is referred to as *tonotopic representation*. More detailed information on cochlear anatomy is presented in Chapter 13.

The tonotopic representation of the basilar membrane is projected onto the primary auditory cortex. Research has shown that, moving in a roughly straight line across cell groups within the primary auditory cortex, cells change their responsiveness from very high frequencies to very low frequencies with the same orderly progression of base to tip of the basilar membrane. Note the conceptual similarity between tonotopic organization and somatotopic representation in primary motor and sensory cortex.

Kandel, Schwartz, and Jessel (2000) described the primary auditory cortex as a core of cells surrounded by cortical tissue devoted to increasingly higher-level processing of auditory information. This surrounding tissue is called secondary auditory cortex, and the planum temporale falls into this category. The basic characteristics of acoustic signals, such as frequency, intensity, and duration, are analyzed in primary auditory cortex. This analysis is sent to surrounding temporal lobe tissue (secondary auditory cortex) for higher-level analyses. A form of higher-level auditory analysis is that required for speech and language perception and understanding. The planum temporale is important to perceptual analysis of speech and language, and the evidence of anatomical asymmetries for this part of the temporal lobe has encouraged the view of this cortical region as important to the aptitude among humans to develop and use speech and language.

Wernicke's Area. Just posterior to the primary auditory cortex, along the back portion of the superior temporal gyrus, is a region of the temporal lobe (and perhaps the lateroventral portion of the parietal lobe) called *Wernicke's area* (see lower right image in Figure 15–5, dark blue area toward back of the sylvian

---

Planum Temporale

The planum temporale has a lofty sounding name (the *temporal plane*) and a scientific history as murky as lofty ideas tend to be. This wedge of brain tissue (see Figure 15–7) tends to be larger in the left than the right hemisphere, including in preverbal infants (Tervaniemi & Hugdahl, 2003). Unfortunately, at least for scientists who enjoy equating size differences with functional differences, chimps also have a larger left than right planum temporale. If only chimps communicated like humans, this would not be a theoretical problem. "Oh bother," as Winnie the Pooh might say, that is, if bears could talk. In fMRI studies the planum temporale tends to light up on the left side for speech sounds, and on the right side for tones. Some scientists argue that lateralization to the left hemisphere for *detection* of speech sounds can be found in the planum temporale, but that the broader needs of speech processing (extracting meaning from sound sequences) are accomplished bilaterally (Hickok, 2009). Maybe more chimp research can resolve the true role of the planum temporale in human communication: according to Winnie the Pooh, "Some people talk to animals. Not many listen though. That's the problem."

fissure). Wernicke's area was originally defined as the brain region associated with speech and language comprehension. Postmortem examination of the brains of several patients revealed a lesion in this area for those who were known in life to have comprehension impairment for spoken language, with little or no impairment of speech production. These patients had lesions at the very back of the sylvian fissure, in the superior temporal gyrus. Dr. Carl Wernicke, a Prussian physician, examined one famous patient when he was alive and on postmortem examination of the brain located the region known as Wernicke's area.

Recent imaging of the perisylvian (surrounding the sylvian fissure) language areas, and the temporal lobe specifically, during speech perception and language comprehension tasks supports the general ideas outlined above. The primary auditory cortex, roughly in the middle of the upper lip of the superior temporal gyrus, is active when a person is required to make decisions concerning individual speech sounds, and especially when these decisions do not require word, sentence, or discourse meaning. The task of detecting and identifying speech sounds activates the part of the auditory cortex devoted to analysis of basic signal characteristics. When a person is required to make language input decisions involving meaning, more widespread regions of the temporal lobe are activated. Single word meaning, meaning tied to different levels of grammatical complexity, and abstract meaning (as in metaphor) engage many different regions of the temporal lobe, as well as regions of the parietal, frontal, and occipital lobes (see Price, 2010 for an excellent review of brain imaging and speech and language perception/comprehension).

The anterior part of the temporal lobe and the middle and inferior temporal gyri also seem to play a role in *naming* of objects or actions. Almost certainly, the idea of Wernicke's area as the important location in the temporal lobe for speech and language understanding is an oversimplification.

Occipital Lobe

The occipital lobes (colored purple in Figure 15–5) comprise the posterior parts of the cerebral hemispheres; they are the smallest among the four lobes of the brain. The occipital lobes contain primary visual cortex, whose tissue processes information entering the brain through the eyes. Like the auditory cortex, the occipital lobes contain cells that perform basic analysis of visual signals, as well as cells that perform more abstract, elaborate visual processing. The top right image of Figure 15–5 shows the medial wall of one hemisphere, where the *calcarine fissure* divides the occipital lobe into an upper (*cuneus*) and lower (*lingual gyrus*) portion. Primary visual processing is performed by cortical tissue deep within the calcarine fissure. Extensive connections between cells in the calcarine fissure and other cells within the occipital cortex power more elaborate visual processing.

Insula

In Figure 15–8 the left cerebral hemisphere is shown with the lower "lips" of the frontal and parietal lobes and the upper lip of the temporal lobe pulled away to reveal underlying gyri and sulci. The retractable lips of the frontal, parietal, and temporal lobes are referred to as *opercula* (singular = *operculum*, from the Latin word for "lid"). The cortex revealed when the opercula are retracted is called the *insula* or *insular cortex*. The insula is sometimes described as part of a fifth hemispheric lobe, the *limbic lobe* (see below). In this chapter the terms *insula* and *insular cortex* are used to denote this cortical region without commitment to the notion of the insula as part of a fifth lobe.

Among other functions, the insula appears to be a critical part of cortical tissue engaged in speech and language functions (Ackermann & Riecker, 2010). Clinical cases (where patients with known lesions in and around the insula exhibit certain speech and lan-

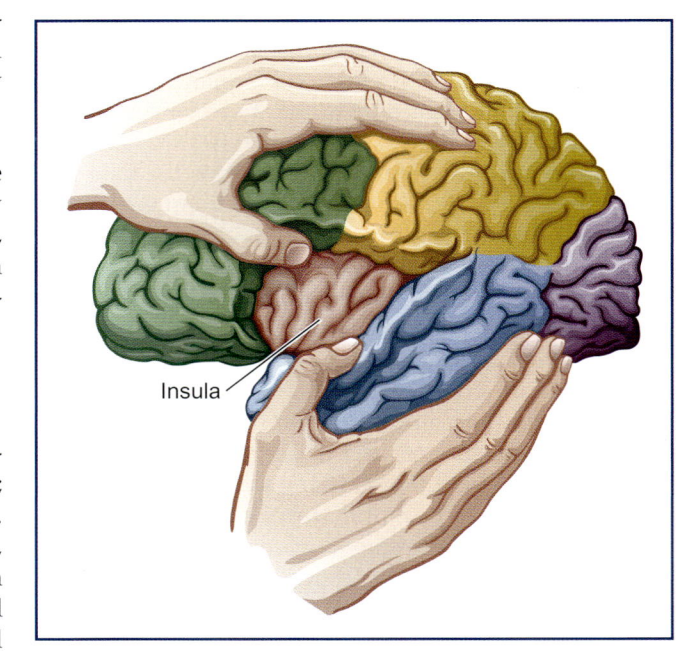

Figure 15–8. View in the sagittal plane of the left hemisphere, showing the opercula ("lips") of the frontal, parietal, and temporal lobes gently retracted to reveal the underlying insular cortex.

guage difficulties), surgical cases (brain tumors requiring resection of insular tissue), electrical stimulation of exposed brain (in patients undergoing brain resections for severe epileptic seizures), and fMRI studies of healthy individuals point to a role for the front part of the insula in speech motor control and possibly in speech perception. These speech functions of the insula appear to be lateralized to the left hemisphere, in much the same way as speech and language functions are lateralized to Broca's and Wernicke's regions in a majority of individuals. Note the proximity of the anterior insula to Broca's area in the frontal lobe.

The insula also seems to play a role in swallowing, self-awareness, control of heart rate, blood pressure, perception of pain and temperature, dyspnea (breathing discomfort), as well as other functions related to emotions and general body awareness. As pointed out by Ackermann and Riecker (2010), clinical cases involving isolated lesions of the insula are rare. Generally, when a stroke or surgical removal of brain tissue involves insular tissue, other nearby areas of the brain (such as regions in and around Broca's area, or parts of the primary auditory cortex, or even fiber tracts below the cortical tissue) are also affected.

Limbic System (Limbic Lobe)

Heimer and Van Hoesen (2006) recommend the term *limbic lobe* to designate the collection of structures within the cerebral hemispheres involved in emotions, motivation, memory, and adaptive functions. Not all authors assign limbic structures the status of a lobe of the cerebral hemispheres, at least in the same sense as the frontal, parietal, temporal, and occipital lobes. Some authors refer to a limbic *system* to reflect a collection of structures within the brain, all of which play an important role, broadly speaking, in emotional and motivational aspects of behavior. Even authors who have argued persuasively for the existence of a limbic lobe, based on similarities in anatomical characteristics and physiological functions of its component structures, say the "system" versus "lobe" debate is not likely to be settled soon (Heimer & Van Hoesen, 2006). For the following brief discussion, the term *limbic system* is used.

The most easily visualized structures of the limbic system are seen on the medial surface of a hemisphere (see Figure 15–5, top right). The *cingulate gyrus* forms an incomplete ring above and around the corpus callosum. The ring is partially completed on the lower side of the hemisphere by the upper gyrus of the medial temporal lobe, called the *parahippocampal gyrus* (unlabeled in Figure 15–5, top right: locate the most superior blue gyrus to identify the parahippocampal gyrus). The cingulate and parahippocampal gyri are part of the cortex, but their cell structure is different from cells in the primary motor, primary somatosensory, or association cortex (Heimer & Van Hoesen, 2006). The cell structure of limbic cortical areas in humans have been described as more primitive than the cell structure in other cortical areas.

Deep within the parahippocampal gyrus of the temporal lobe is a cell group called the *hippocampus*, and another cell cluster called the *amygdala*. These structures are part of the limbic system. In addition, parts of the insula and basal ganglia, as well as cortical structures related to olfaction (sense of smell), and the ventral gyri of the frontal lobe (shown in Figure 15–5, bottom left image) are considered components of the limbic system. These structures are interconnected and make connections with the more sophisticated parts of the cortex as well as with subcortical and brainstem structures.

The sketch presented here of structures and connections of and within the limbic system is complicated, and may seem far removed from the concerns of the speech-language pathologist. Nevertheless, its relevance becomes clear when considering disorders such as dementia, a behavioral syndrome characterized by memory loss, behavioral change, and communication impairment. Dementia has a neurobiological basis that largely originates in structures of the limbic system. In addition, limbic structures are often compromised by brain damage sustained in traumatic brain injury (TBI). Communication problems in persons with TBI often include difficulties with social communication (pragmatics) that can be traced at least partially if not largely to limbic system damage.

Cerebral White Matter

The surface of the cerebral hemispheres is made up of many gyri and sulci, some of which have been identified above. This surface topography is composed of gray matter, formed by densely packed clusters of neuronal cell bodies. Cut into the cerebral hemispheres, either by dividing them into left and right halves (a sagittal cut), front and back parts (a coronal cut), or top and bottom parts (a horizontal or transverse cut) and a tremendous volume of white matter is revealed. White matter consists of bundles of myelinated axons running from one group of cell bodies to another group of cell bodies. White matter connects nearby and distant cell groups within the CNS.

As described above, a coronal section of the cerebral hemispheres (see Figure 15–3) shows extensive white matter. At any location within the white matter, fibers run in many different directions, to and from different cell groups. Even though fiber tracts are typically "bundled" together, with a given bundle running from a specific group of cell bodies to another specific group of cell bodies, a selected volume of white matter contains an intermixing of several bundles. A relatively new brain imaging technique called diffusion tensor imaging (DTI) allows scientists to establish the origin, course, and termination of major fiber tracts in the human brain (see sidetrack on DTI). DTI research has established a detailed account of fiber bundles within the brain. Much of the following information, including an organizational scheme for classifying fiber bundles within the cerebral hemispheres, is adapted from a review article by Schmahmann, Smith, Eichler, and Filley (2008). Table 15–1 outlines this classification system. Smits, Jiskoot, and Papma (2014) provide a revew of DTI findings specific to speech and language behaviors.

Association Tracts

Association tracts connect one part of the cortex to another, *within the same hemisphere (intrahemispheric)*. These *ipsilateral* connections may consist of small groups of fibers running between adjacent gyri, or between more distantly separated gyri within the same lobe. Of greater importance for the current discussion are several tightly organized association tracts that connect cortical areas in one lobe to cortical areas in a different lobe. Table 15–2 lists some of these major ipsilateral, interlobe tracts; these tracts are found in both hemispheres, but may have slightly different forms depending on which hemisphere is examined (see below). The listing of these tracts highlights the extensive interconnectedness of lobes within a single hemisphere. The capability exists for a great deal of information to be shuttled between different cortical regions within a single hemisphere.

As discussed toward the end of the chapter, increasing knowledge of the interconnectedness of intrahemispheric lobes (as well as interhemispheric connections) is guiding scientists away from a "center" oriented view of human behavior (e.g., a focus on Broca's and Wernicke's areas in speech and language performance) to a "network" view, wherein multiple brain locations and pathways are organized as a system to generate complex human behaviors.

Arcuate Fasciculus and Speech and Language Functions. Further consideration of one association (intrahemispheric) tract is warranted because of its

Table 15–1. A Simple Organizational Scheme for Classifying Tracts (Fiber Bundles), and Their Principal Connections

FIBER BUNDLE TYPE	CONNECTIONS
Association tracts	*Intra*hemispheric, both within and between lobes
Striatal tracts	From cortex to basal ganglia (principally to caudate and putamen, but also to claustrum), and from cortex to subthalamic nucleus
Commissural tracts	*Inter*hemispheric, from area of one hemisphere to similar area of the other hemisphere
Descending projection tracts	
Corticobulbar	• Cortex to cell groups in brainstem
Corticospinal	• Cortex to cell groups in spinal cord
Corticothalamic	• Widepsread regions of the cortex to cell groups in the thalamus
Ascending projection tracts	
Posterior column medial lemniscal	• Spinal cord to brainstem nuclei and thalamus
Anterolateral	• Spinal cord to thalamus
Thalamocortical	• Cell groups in the thalamus to widespread regions of the cortex

Source: Adapted and modified from Schmahmann et al. (2008).

Table 15–2. Some Association Fiber Tracts and the Lobes They Connect

TRACT	CONNECTIONS
Middle longitudinal fasciculus	Parietal to temporal and frontal lobes Parietal, temporal, and frontal lobes to limbic areas
Inferior longitudinal fasciculus	Occipital to temporal and parietal lobes
Fronto-occipital fasciculus	Occipital and parietal lobes to frontal lobe
Uncinate fasciculus	Temporal to frontal lobes
Superior longitudinal fasciculus (arcuate fasciculus)	Parietal to frontal lobe (Wernicke-angular-supramarginal-Broca)

Note. In the "connections" column, a description such as "Parietal to Temporal Lobe" does not necessarily mean the fibers go in only one direction.

Dorsal and Ventral Streams

An association tract, the arcuate fasciculus (AF), has been known for many years to play a critical role in speech and language functions. The AF connects the posterior part of the superior temporal gyrus (Wernicke's area) and parts of the parietal cortex to the inferior frontal gyrus (Broca's area) as well as frontal lobe areas just anterior to Broca's area. The AF has an important role in phonological processing and complex syntactic structure, for both speech perception and production. Another tract, the uncinate fasciculus (UF), connects anterior portions of the temporal lobe to the inferior frontal gyrus and more anterior regions of the frontal lobe; the UF also has extensive connections with parts of the limbic system. The UF is thought to have a role in semantic processing—the extraction of meaning in language production and comprehension. These two pathways have been combined for a "dorsal stream" (the AF) and "ventral stream" (the UF) model of speech and language processing. The "dual stream" model of the brain basis of speech and language function is controversial but has generated interesting hypotheses for imaging studies and behavioral studies of patients with lesions to the AF and UF. Dick, Bernal, and Tremblay (2014) provide an excellent review of the presumed anatomy and function of the dual-stream hypothesis.

historical and contemporary importance in speech and language functions of the brain. Table 15–2 lists a tract called the *superior longitudinal fasciculus*, the main part of which is the *arcuate fasciculus* (AF) (see Bernal & Ardila, 2009). Figure 15–9 is a DTI reconstruction of the AF, as well as of the inferior longitudinal fasciculus and uncinate fasciculus (compare the course of these latter two tracts to the information provided in Table 15–2). The AF is the arched pathway (hence "arcuate") with one leg of the "bottom" of the arch in the temporal lobe, from which fibers run slightly back and up into the parietal lobe before turning forward to end as the other leg of the arch in the back part of the frontal lobe. Table 15–2 lists four cortical areas connected by the AF, including Wernicke's area (temporal lobe), the angular and supramarginal gyri (parietal lobe), and Broca's area (frontal lobe). This is a standard way to describe the AF, as a fiber tract connecting the receptive language areas (Wernicke's area and possibly parts of the angular and supramarginal gyri) to the expressive area (Broca's area). In a structural and functional study of the AF, Takaya, Kuperberg, Liu, Greve, Makris, and Stufflebeam (2015) reported that in semantic tasks, activity in the AF connections in the left hemisphere (the cortical gray matter) were correlated during a semantic task; the connected cortical areas "lit up" together. The right hemisphere regions connected by the AF were not correlated during the semantic task. These functional differences are accompanied by structural differences when the left and right

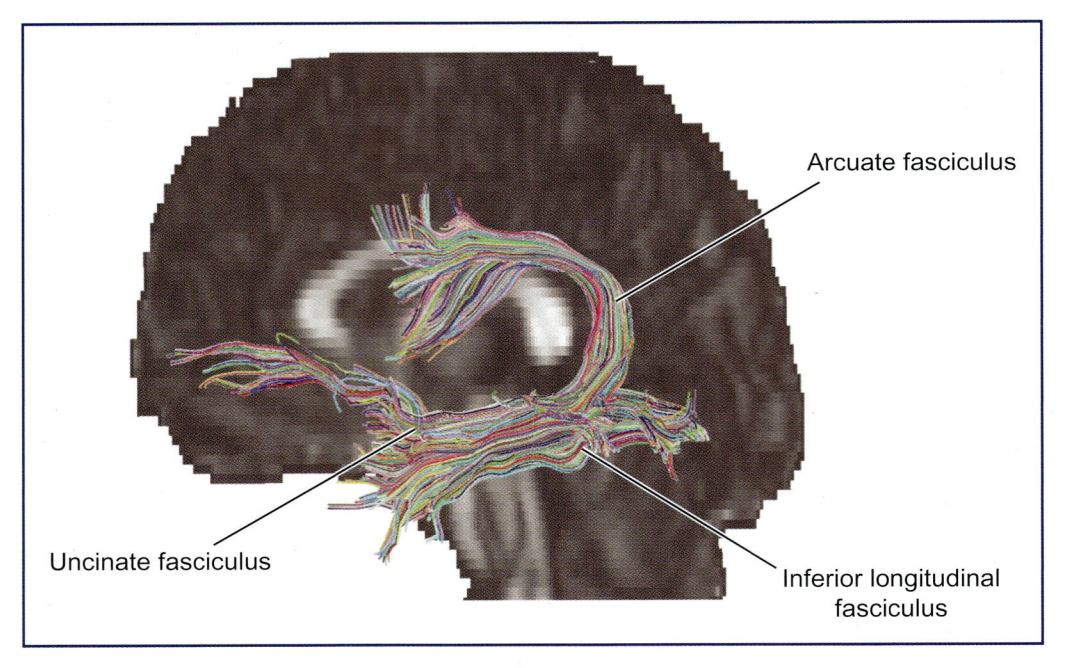

Figure 15–9. DTI image showing the arcuate fasciculus (the "arched" fiber tract contained within the superior longitudinal fasciculus, which runs from the parietal to the frontal lobe), inferior longitudinal fasciculus (which runs from the occipital to the temporal to the parietal lobe), and the uncinate fasciculus (which runs from the temporal to the frontal lobe).

DTI

Because fiber tracts within the cerebral hemispheres are intermixed and so densely packed, it is difficult to establish the origins, pathways, and destinations of connections between cell groups. Techniques used in animal research, such as introducing certain chemicals into the brain which "label" specific fiber tracts are mostly not usable in human research. Fortunately, a technique called diffusion tensor imaging (DTI) as well as other related techniques make it possible to monitor selected pathways without posing danger to humans. Water molecules move along specific pathways (fiber tracts) in ways that can be identified by proper computer settings of a brain scanner. In region-of-interest techniques, the brain-scanning instrument is directed at the presumed location of specific pathways, and computer reconstructions of the pathways show their extent, volume, and orientation. Conturo et al. (2008) provide an explanation of the DTI technique, and Saur et al. (2008) and Smits, Jiskoot, and Papma (2014) show how it can be used to understand speech and language connectivity of the brain.

hemispheres are compared. Dick, Bernal, and Tremblay (2014) and Takaya et al. argue that the AF is lateralized to the left hemisphere for speech and language function.

The AF is emphasized because of its prominent role in theories of speech and language functions in healthy and diseased brains. The most prominent and influential of these theories has been referred to as the Wernicke-Geschwind model (Geschwind, 1965), in which the comprehension area of the brain (Wernicke's area) is connected to the expressive region (Broca's area) by means of the AF. In this model, acoustic properties of spoken words are first analyzed by the listener in the primary auditory cortex, then sent to Wernicke's area to convert this "raw" auditory analysis into meaning. The meaningful phonetic sequences thus identified—the words—can be transferred to Broca's area for production via the AF. In the Wernicke-Geschwind model, the processing centers (cortical cell bodies) and pathways (fiber tracts) are fully engaged when a person is asked to repeat a word or series of words. The neurologically intact individual has no problem with this task, because she can comprehend meaning (has a healthy primary auditory cortex and Wernicke's area) and transfer the comprehended phonetic information via the AF to the brain region specialized for speech production. Within the context of the repetition task, the model predicts that damage to Wernicke's area impairs repetition due to failure to comprehend. The patient cannot generate a proper, phonetically based "word image" to repeat, even though her brain center for production is intact. This is so even if the primary auditory cortex performs an accurate analysis of the acoustic properties of the incoming speech. A patient with damage to Wernicke's area who is asked to repeat a simple, short sentence may have normal-sounding articulation (consistent with a "healthy" Broca's area) but may exchange sounds ("take" instead of "cake" or "burzday" for "birthday") and even make sentences more complex by adding words and/or additional phrases not included in the target sentence. These errors and complications are recognized by the patient. On the other hand, the limitation on repetition ability in patients with damage to Broca's area is explained strictly on the basis of impaired production skills. Asked to repeat a short sentence including words such as "cake" and "birthday," the patient may struggle to produce the words with hesitations, labored dysfluencies, and an unusually slow speaking rate, as evidenced by abnormally long speech sounds. Despite this poor production in the repetition task, the patient demonstrates through comprehension tasks that she knows the words she is supposed to produce.

What are the repetition problems in a patient with a damaged AF but undamaged Wernicke's and Broca's areas? This patient can, according to the Wernicke–Geschwind model, comprehend and produce speech in a nearly normal way, but cannot transfer the comprehended message between these two cortical centers. The patient can be shown to have normal comprehension, using nonverbal comprehension tasks such as, "Point to the picture of a dog." This simple task is challenging for the patient with damage to Wernicke's area. The patient with damage isolated to the AF has fluent speech, but within this fluent stream may have numerous sound exchange errors ("take" for "cake") recognized by the patient as mistakes, as revealed by successive attempts to repeat the target utterance to "get it right." What is unique about the patient's repetition performance is her inability to repeat, on command, words and sentences when intact comprehension skills are demonstrated. The patient's spontaneous, conversational speech is likely to be better than her repetition performance.

The performance problems in conduction aphasia are said to be the result of a *disconnection syndrome*, which in this case is the disconnection of Wernicke's area from Broca's area due to an AF lesion. Some have argued that the AF is responsible for transmitting the order of sounds in a word from the comprehension to production areas of the brain (Papagno et. al, 2017).

Other disconnection syndromes have been discussed in the literature for their potential to disrupt speech and spoken or written language performance. For example, disconnection of the occipital from temporal and parietal cortex, resulting from damage to the inferior longitudinal fasciculus (see Table 15–2, Figure 15–9), may impair the ability to read words even though the cortical tissue is healthy (Epelbaum et al., 2008). More generally, a wide range of white matter diseases, in which fiber tracts are damaged but cortical regions are spared, appears to play a significant role in dementia (Schmahmann et al., 2008). Dementia, a disorder of cognition and more specifically of memory and its use in complex tasks such as speech and language, has a high prevalence within the aging population. With respect to speech and language function, white matter clearly matters.

Striatal Tracts

Deep within the cerebral hemispheres there are several clusters of cell bodies, collectively referred to as subcortical nuclei. One group of these nuclei comprises components of the *basal ganglia* (sometimes called *basal nuclei*). The *thalamus*, itself a collection of many nuclei, is another major subcortical nucleus. Beneath the cortical rind of gray matter, these nuclei appear as collections of gray matter within the extensive white matter of the cerebral hemispheres. *Striatal tracts* are fiber tracts connecting the cortical gray matter and these subcortical nuclei. Many of these connections form a loop between cortical and subcortical gray matter structures. This loop plays an important role in motor control, including speech motor control and possibly language production. There are also fiber tracts that connect individual nuclei of the basal ganglia, as well as components of the basal ganglia and the thalamus. These connections also fall under the general category of striatal tracts. Additional detail on the cortical-basal ganglia-thalamus-cortical loop is provided below.

Commissural Tracts

Commissural tracts typically connect a specific region of one hemisphere with its similar topographical region in the other hemisphere. The wording of this description is purposely careful, because of the notion of *lateralization of function*. Brain regions having the same locations in the two hemispheres most likely do not have the same function. For example, Broca's area has a sister region in the right hemisphere, but it is not called Broca's area. The lateralization of speech and language function to the left hemisphere in most people suggests that the same topographical regions in the two hemispheres do not share the same functions. Nevertheless, the third frontal convolutions are connected across the hemispheres by fibers running in the corpus callosum. The same can be said for the other cortical regions described above—they are connected across the hemispheres by the corpus callosum, but the connection does not imply connection for identical function.

Corpus Callosum. The corpus callosum is a massive and complex bundle of fibers. A classic view of the corpus callosum is viewed in the midsagittal plane (see Figure 15–5, top right), where the front-to-back extent of the tract appears as a thick length of arched white matter, shaped somewhat like a flattened letter "C" turned on its right side. The frontmost and backmost parts of the corpus callosum are the *genu* and *splenium*, respectively. Between the genu and splenium is the central, main bulk of the corpus callosum, called the *body*. At the genu, the corpus callosum has a curl of fibers (one end of the "C") pointing slightly downward and toward the back of the cerebral hemispheres; this backward-directed curl is called the *rostrum*.

The most anterior and most posterior extensions of the corpus callosum do not extend to the front and back "poles" (end points) of the hemispheres (see Figure 15–5, upper right). Nevertheless, fiber tracts extend from the corpus callosum forward and backward into the most anterior regions of the frontal lobe and most posterior regions of the occipital lobes, connecting these regions across the hemispheres. Finally, although in the midsagittal plane the body of the corpus callosum is beneath cortical tissue, the connecting fibers project upward to reach cortical layers at the top of the hemispheres. The extension of corpus callosum fibers into the front and back parts of the hemispheres, as well as to the top of the cortex, is shown in the sagittal plane (DTI image in Figure 15–10). The "flat" part of the tract, corresponding to the view in Figure 15–5 of the medial part of the corpus callosum, is seen in the middle of the tract in Figure 15–10, and the upcurled fibers reaching to cortical layers are seen all along the length of the tract.

The many millions of fibers (about 200,000,000) in the corpus callosum have a topographical arrangement. The term *topographical* in this context implies both somatotopicity and systematic fiber arrangement for external signal properties (as in audition and vision).

As shown in Figure 15–5, top right, the rostrum of the corpus callosum terminates its backward path immediately in front of a structure identified as the *anterior commissure*. The anterior commissure is an interhemispheric (commissural) pathway that connects the orbital cortex (frontal lobe) and parts of the temporal lobe cortex across the two hemispheres. If a pencil point is placed on the anterior commissure and moved

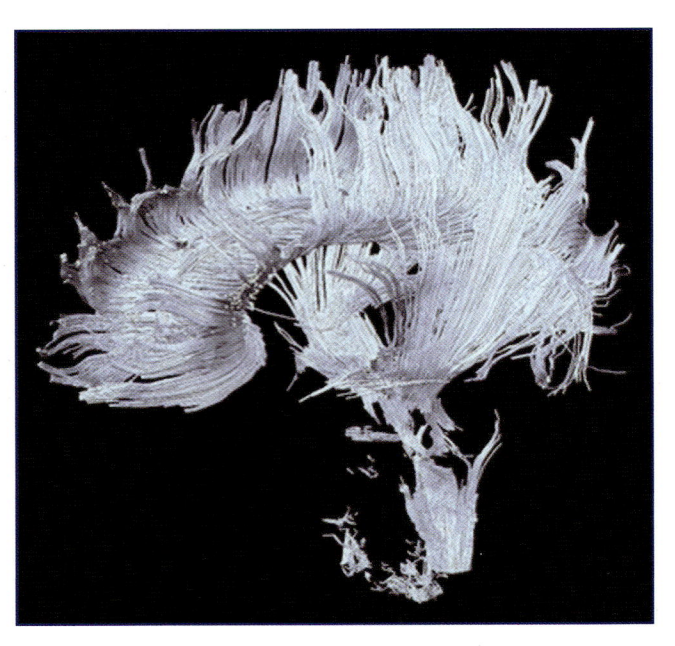

Figure 15–10. DTI image of the corpus callosum, showing the fibers extending up toward the dorsal surface of the hemispheres as well as into anterior and posterior parts of the hemispheres.

toward the back of the brain along a straight line angled slightly downward, the pencil line intersects the *posterior commissure* (not shown in Figure 15–5). The posterior commissure is an interhemispheric (commissural) pathway connecting parts of the brain involved in the reflex response of the eye's pupil to light. The line connecting the anterior and posterior commissures is often used to define a surgical reference plane, especially for the therapeutic placement of intracranial electrodes.

The corpus callosum plays a storied role in the history of disconnection syndromes. As reviewed by Gazzaniga (2000) and Doron and Gazzaniga (2008), various parts of the corpus callosum, and in many cases the entire corpus callosum, have been surgically cut to relieve chronic epileptic seizures that cannot be controlled by drugs. Many of these "split-brain" patients, when tested under controlled laboratory conditions, have provided evidence of the different functions of the two hemispheres and the consequences of not having communication between the hemispheres. In some cases, one side of the brain literally does not know what is going on in the other side of the brain.

Descending Projection Tracts

Descending projection tracts include the corticobulbar and corticospinal tracts, as well as tracts running from many cortical regions to the thalamus (corticothalamic tracts, see Table 15–1). Figure 15–11 shows in a schematic coronal view the corticobulbar and corticospinal fiber tracts. The corticobulbar tract ("bulbar" is a term used to indicate the brainstem, and more specifically the pons and medulla), represented in Figure 15–11 by the solid pinkish-red and orange lines, includes fibers originating in cortical cell bodies that make a first synapse in one of the several brainstem motor nuclei. The corticospinal tract, represented in Figure 15–11 by the dashed blue lines, includes fibers originating in the cortex and making a first synapse in motor cells of the ventral spinal cord. Motor nuclei in the brainstem and spinal cord axons leave the CNS to innervate muscles of head and neck structures and the limbs and torso.

As the corticobulbar and corticospinal tracts descend from the cortex to lower regions of the CNS, their *location* within the brain is designated by different terms. For example, fibers of the two tracts are issued from cell bodies all over the cortex and form a fanlike pattern called the *corona radiata*. The fibers of the corona radiata contribute to a good portion of the white matter immediately below the cortex. The corona radiata are represented schematically in Figure 15–11, and in the more anatomically correct image of Figure 15–12. As fibers in the corona radiata descend, they gather into a relatively tight bundle that passes between subcortical nuclei to reach the more inferior brainstem. The sagittal view in Figure 15–12 shows the corona radiata merging into this tight bundle. This part of the descending tracts, where the corticobulbar and corticospinal tracts are lateral to the medial thalamus and medial to the caudate nucleus and lateral lentiform (globus pallidus and putamen) nuclei is called the *internal capsule* (see Figures 15–11 and 15–12).

Internal Capsule. The coronal slices in previous figures show the internal capsule at a single location along the front-to-back extent of the cerebral hemispheres (e.g., see top right of Figures 15–2 and 15–3, slice location not labeled in the figures). A greater appreciation for the distribution of these fiber tracts is gained from careful examination of Figure 15–12 (upper left), where the front of the head is toward the left of the image. Here the cortical tissue has been stripped away

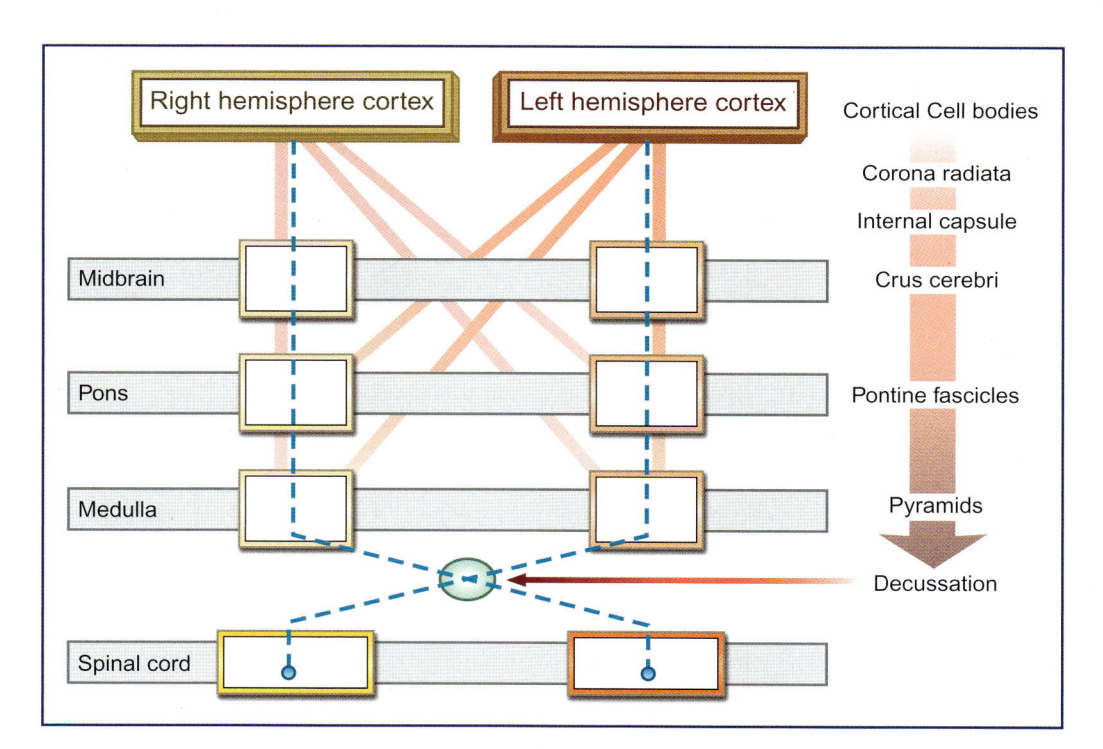

Figure 15–11. Schematic coronal view of the descending corticobulbar (*thicker pink and orange lines*) and corticospinal (*dashed blue lines*) tracts. The corticobulbar tracts are both ipsilateral and contralateral, sending axons to brainstem nuclei on the same and opposite side as their cortical origin. The ipsilateral and contralateral connections depend on which brainstem motor nucleus is under discussion. The corticospinal tract is primarily contralateral, crossing at the decussation of the pyramids and sending axons to ventral horn nuclei in the spinal cord on the side opposite the cortical origin.

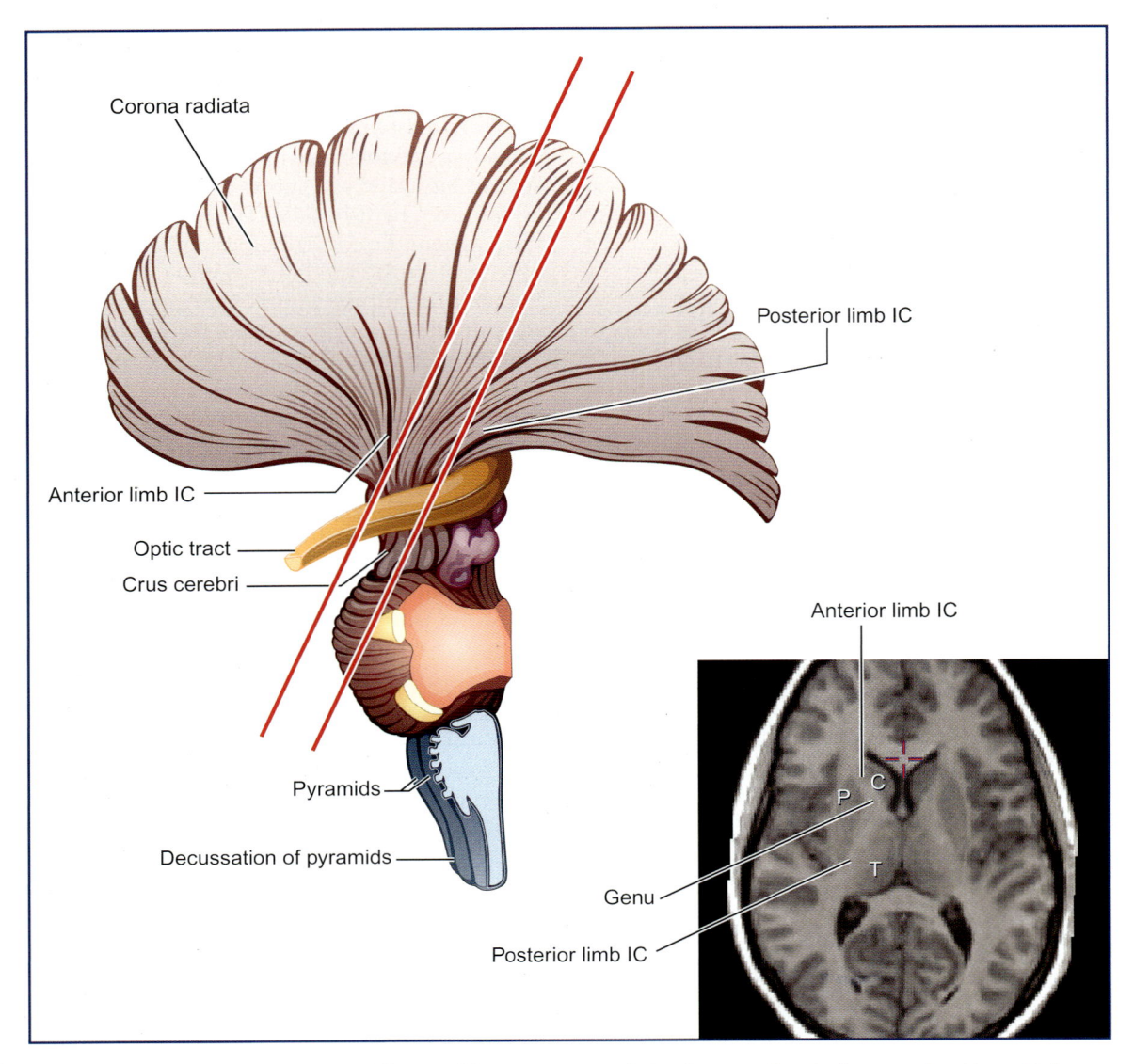

Figure 15–12. *Upper left,* view of fibers of the corona radiata descending in the cerebral hemispheres and gathering into a narrow bundle called the internal capsule (IC), which passes between several subcortical nuclei en route to the brainstem. *Lower right,* horizontal section of cerebral hemispheres showing the "boomerang" shape of the internal capsule. The anterior and posterior limbs plus the genu of the internal capsule are labeled. C = caudate nucleus; P = putamen; T = thalamus.

to reveal the fibers of the corona radiata and internal capsule. Even though the internal capsule is the tightly gathered merger of the many fibers of the corona radiata, the internal capsule has an anterior, middle, and posterior part (IC = internal capsule in Figure 15–12, upper image). The precise location of a coronal slice therefore determines which part of the internal capsule is displayed. Like so many other parts of the brain, the internal capsule is not a random jumble of fibers, but is arranged systematically based on the cortical origin of the fibers. In a horizontal (axial) slice (inset, lower right of Figure 15–12; the anterior part of the brain is toward the top of the image) the internal capsule in each hemisphere has a boomerang shape with the "angle" of the boomerang most medial and the two arms extending away from this angle anterolaterally and posterolaterally. To provide a rough idea of the systematic arrangement of fibers within the internal capsule, most corticobulbar fibers associated with control of facial, jaw, tongue, velopharyngeal, and laryngeal muscles run through a compact bundle close to or within the angle (called the genu) of the internal capsule. Fibers descending to motor neurons in the spinal cord are mostly located in the posterior arm (called the "posterior limb") of the internal capsule, and within that limb the fibers for the legs are most posterior, and those for the arms are closer to the angle. These are illustrations of the systematic arrangement of fibers within the internal capsule, and are not meant to be exhaustive. For example, fibers running to the cortex from the thalamus also form parts of the internal capsule (see section below on Ascending Projection Tracts).

Descending fibers leave the internal capsule and continue their downward path in the *cerebral peduncles*, a tract in the central part of the midbrain. The largest portion of these fibers runs in the *crus cerebri*, an anterior part of the cerebral peduncles (the terms "cerebral peduncles" and "crus cerebri" are occasionally used interchangeably; see Figure 15–12). The fibers continue through the pons in small bundles, or fascicles, and are gathered back together in the medulla as the pyramids. Some descending fibers in the cerebral peduncles, pontine fascicles, and medulla leave the descending tract to make synapses with motor nuclei in the midbrain, pons, and medulla. These fibers belong to the corticobulbar tract, and the synapses they make within the brainstem define the termination of the tract for those fibers. The fibers continuing into the spinal cord belong to the corticospinal tract; these make synapses in the ventral (anterior) gray matter of the spinal cord, where spinal motor neurons are found.

The general routes of the corticobulbar and corticospinal tracts are summarized in the right column of Figure 15–11. A slightly more detailed representation of the corticobulbar tract is provided in Figure 15–13. For the sake of simplicity, Figure 15–13 shows connections originating from only the right hemisphere. The left corticobulbar and corticospinal tracts are a mirror image of the tracts issued from the right hemisphere. The view is as if you were looking at the ventral surface of the brainstem and spinal cord. The lines are shown terminating at each of the three levels of the brainstem (midbrain, pons, medulla), indicating the presence of motor nuclei at each level (see section below on Cranial Nerves and Associated Brainstem Nuclei).

Innervation of Brainstem and Spinal Motor Neurons. In Figure 15–13, the solid pink lines represent *bilateral* innervation of cell bodies in the brainstem by cortical cell bodies. In other words, cells in the cortex of one

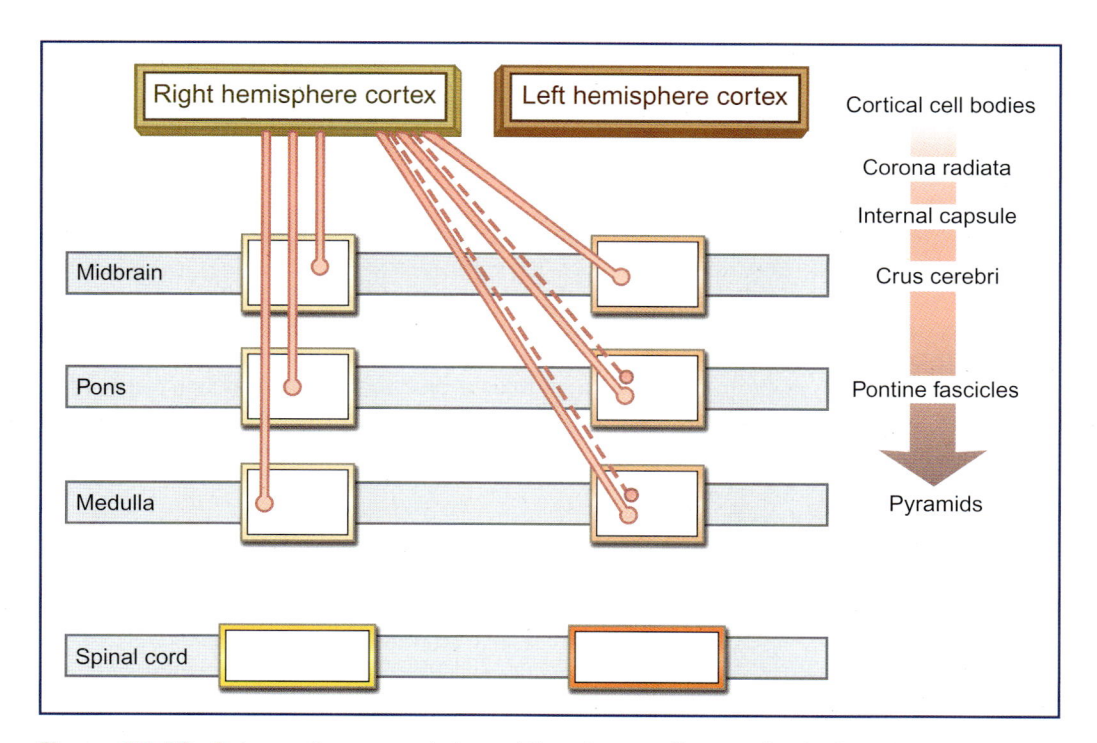

Figure 15–13. Schematic coronal view of the descending corticobulbar tracts, showing patterns of ipsilateral and contralateral connections from cortex to levels of the brainstem. Connections are shown only from the right hemisphere; connections from the left hemisphere are mirror images of these. Bilateral connections (both ipsilateral and contralateral connections) are indicated by the solid pink lines; these are made from the cortex to all three levels of the brainstem (midbrain, pons, medulla). Exclusively contralateral connections are indicated by the dashed lines; these are made from the cortex to nuclei in the pons and medulla. See Table 15–4 for specific details.

hemisphere—say, those controlling contraction of the *palatal levator* muscle, the muscle that lifts the soft palate and pulls it back toward the posterior pharyngeal wall—are connected by corticobulbar fibers to the nucleus containing palatal levator motor neurons on *both* sides of the brainstem. Bilateral innervation means that there is an ipsilateral (same side) and contralateral (opposite side) connection. This is shown in Figure 15–13 by solid lines extending from the right hemisphere to the right (ipsilateral) and left (contralateral) sides of the brainstem, at all three levels.

The overall innervation pattern of brainstem motor nuclei by corticobulbar fibers is mostly, but not exclusively, bilateral. Figure 15–13 shows by dashed lines exclusively contralateral connections between cortical cells in the right hemisphere and motor nuclei in the pons and medulla levels of the *left* brainstem. Certain brainstem nuclei, or parts of nuclei, are innervated only by fibers arising in the cortex of the opposite hemisphere. These facts concerning the connection patterns in the corticobulbar tract are considered in greater detail below in the section on cranial nerves. As explained in that section, knowledge of the bilateral and contralateral connection patterns in the corticobulbar tract has substantial value to the practicing speech-language pathologist.

The path of the corticospinal tract is shown in Figure 15–14 for one side of the brain. Fibers from each hemisphere run down their respective sides until the majority of fibers from one side (about 80%) cross to the other side at the decussation of the pyramids, a landmark on the ventral surface of the medulla created by the crossing fibers (see below, Figure 15–20). The fact that so many fibers from one cerebral hemisphere eventually travel in the spinal cord on the side opposite to their cortical origin accounts for the well-known fact that the left hemisphere controls limbs on the right side, and the right hemisphere controls limbs on the left side. In Figure 15–14, the descent of the corticospinal tract through the internal capsule and to its crossover point within the inferior medulla is summarized by the pathway of the green line.

Ascending Projection Tracts

Ascending fiber tracts are typically associated with sensory pathways, which are projection tracts from points below to points above. Sensory events begin in an end organ of the body, which may include touch, pressure, limb position and velocity, vibration, pain, temperature, taste, odor, light, and sound receptors. When these receptors are stimulated, an impulse is, in most cases, sent from them to a ganglion. Ganglia contain first synapses along a sensory pathway located

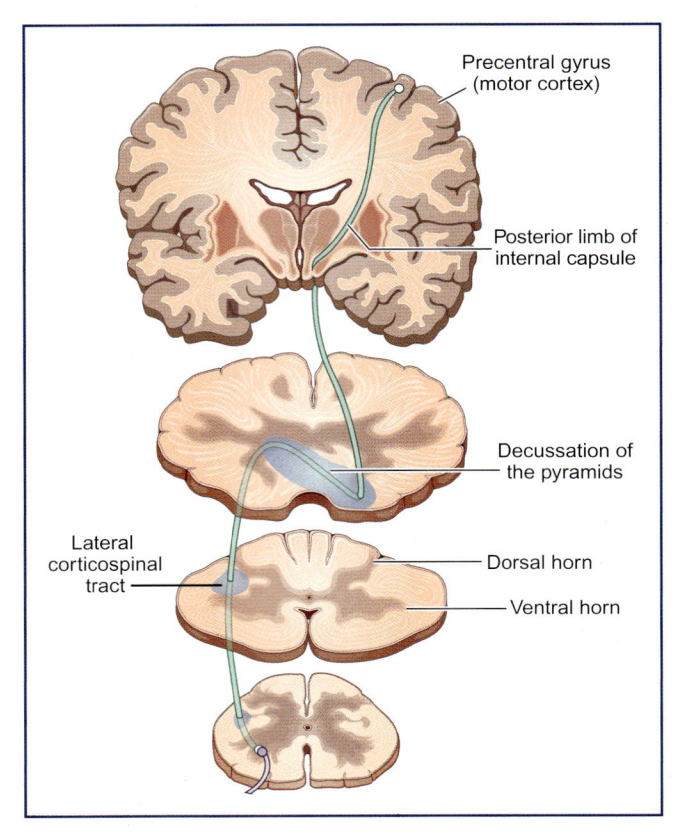

Figure 15–14. Pathway of corticospinal tract. The green pathway shows the tract originating in the cortex of one hemisphere and descending on the same side until it reaches the medulla where about 80% of the fibers cross over to the opposite side to descend in the lateral corticospinal tract. The pathway on the other side of the hemisphere is a mirror image of the one shown. Descending fibers leave the corticospinal tract at all segments of the spinal cord to make synapses with ventral horn cells (spinal motor neurons). The purple fiber shown leaving the spinal cord at the lowest level represents axons sent via peripheral nerves to muscles.

outside the CNS but close to the entry point near the spinal cord or brainstem.

Somatosensory Pathways. Somatosensory pathways constitute a major portion of the ascending projection tracts. These tracts run in the opposite direction from the descending projection tracts. The "points below" are the end organs, where stimuli are sensed, and the "points above" include several synapses along the ascending pathway with a final destination in the cortex.

Posterior Columns. There are two major somatosensory pathways for stimuli sensed below the neck (that is, on the torso or limbs). One of these, the posterior column-medial lemniscal tract (Blumenfeld, 2010), carries sensory information from one side of the body. This sensory information enters the spinal cord after making a first synapse in a dorsal root ganglion. The fibers entering the spinal cord run up the same side of the body until reaching the dorsal part of the medulla (the lowest part of the brainstem, at the top of the spinal cord), where the fibers make a synapse and cross to the opposite side to run up through the brainstem and thalamus before terminating in the primary sensory cortex and surrounding areas. This means that sensation from one side of the body is processed in the cortex on the opposite side of the brain. Note the parallel to the corticospinal tract, one of the major descending projection tracts described above. The descending corticospinal tract crosses over on the ventral surface of the medulla, whereas the ascending posterior column-medial lemniscus tract crosses over in the dorsal (posterior) part of the medulla. This ascending tract carries information on fine touch, vibration, and joint position.

Pain, Temperature, Crude Touch. A second ascending pathway for sensory stimuli entering the spinal cord is called the anterolateral tract. This tract carries information on pain, temperature, and "crude" touch (Blumenfeld, 2010). Like the posterior column-medial lemniscus tract, the anterolateral tract conveys information to the cortex on the side opposite to the stimulation. An important difference from the posterior column-medial lemniscus tract is the crossover point—the decussation—for pain/temperature/crude touch fibers entering the spinal cord. The latter fibers cross over to the other side of the spinal cord almost immediately after entering the cord, roughly at the level of entry. The fibers then ascend in the anterolateral tract on the side opposite their entry point. Recall that the posterior column-medial lemniscus fibers ascend in the spinal cord on the *same* side of entry before crossing over in the posterior medulla. The difference in decussation points for these two major ascending tracts has important clinical implications when a neurologist administers a set of tests to localize a lesion.

Both the posterior column-medial lemniscus and anterolateral tracts send their information to the thalamus, where synapses are made and fibers are sent to the cortex. In addition, visual and auditory ascending fibers, carrying information from the retina (vision) and hair cells (audition), make synapses in the thalamus before projecting to the visual and auditory cortical areas. This mass of thalamocortical fibers, or projections, constitute a significant volume of the white matter of the cerebral hemispheres. The internal capsule and corona radiata include these ascending fibers. Typically, any region of white matter in the cerebral hemispheres includes a mix of descending and ascending pathways as well as fibers running to and from the cortex and striatum, and cortex and cerebellum. The intertwined, dense, multimillion-fiber nature of the white matter requires special techniques to determine where fibers originate and where they end (see sidetrack on "DTI"). This mixing of so many fiber types within any given region of white matter also means that white matter disease, as in certain dementias, is likely to produce multiple symptoms associated with multiple systems within the brain that send and receive axon bundles for transmission of important information.

SUBCORTICAL NUCLEI AND CEREBELLUM

The subcortical nuclei include the various structures of the basal ganglia (also referred to as the basal nuclei), the thalamus, the hypothalamus, and other structures of the limbic system (such as the amygdala and septal nuclei). The cerebellum is subcortical but is typically discussed separately from subcortical structures. In this section the focus is on the basal ganglia, thalamus, and cerebellum.

Basal Ganglia

The basal ganglia include the caudate and putamen nuclei (which together constitute the striatum), the globus pallidus (which paired with the putamen is referred to as the lenticular or lentiform nucleus), the subthalamic nucleus, and the substantia nigra. Technically, the substantia nigra is not a subcortical nucleus (that is, below the cortex but within the cerebral hemispheres) but rather a brainstem nucleus, located in the ventral midbrain (see below, Figure 15–23). The substantia nigra is included here as a subcortical nucleus because of its close anatomical and functional connections with the striatum and subthalamic nucleus.

The gross anatomy of the basal ganglia is best appreciated in two views, one coronal and the other sagittal. Figure 15–15 shows coronal slices of the cerebral hemispheres and the top of the brainstem, roughly midway between the front and back of the brain. In these artist's renditions, nuclei are shown as darker areas, tracts as lighter areas. The caudate, putamen, globus pallidus, substantia nigra, and subthalamic nucleus are labeled on the left and right images; the left image is a "zoom" view of the full slice on the right. The thalamus is not a basal ganglia structure but is shown here for orientation purposes and because of its role in the processing of basal ganglia information (see below). Note the location of the putamen, deep to the insula; in this coronal slice the putamen is the most

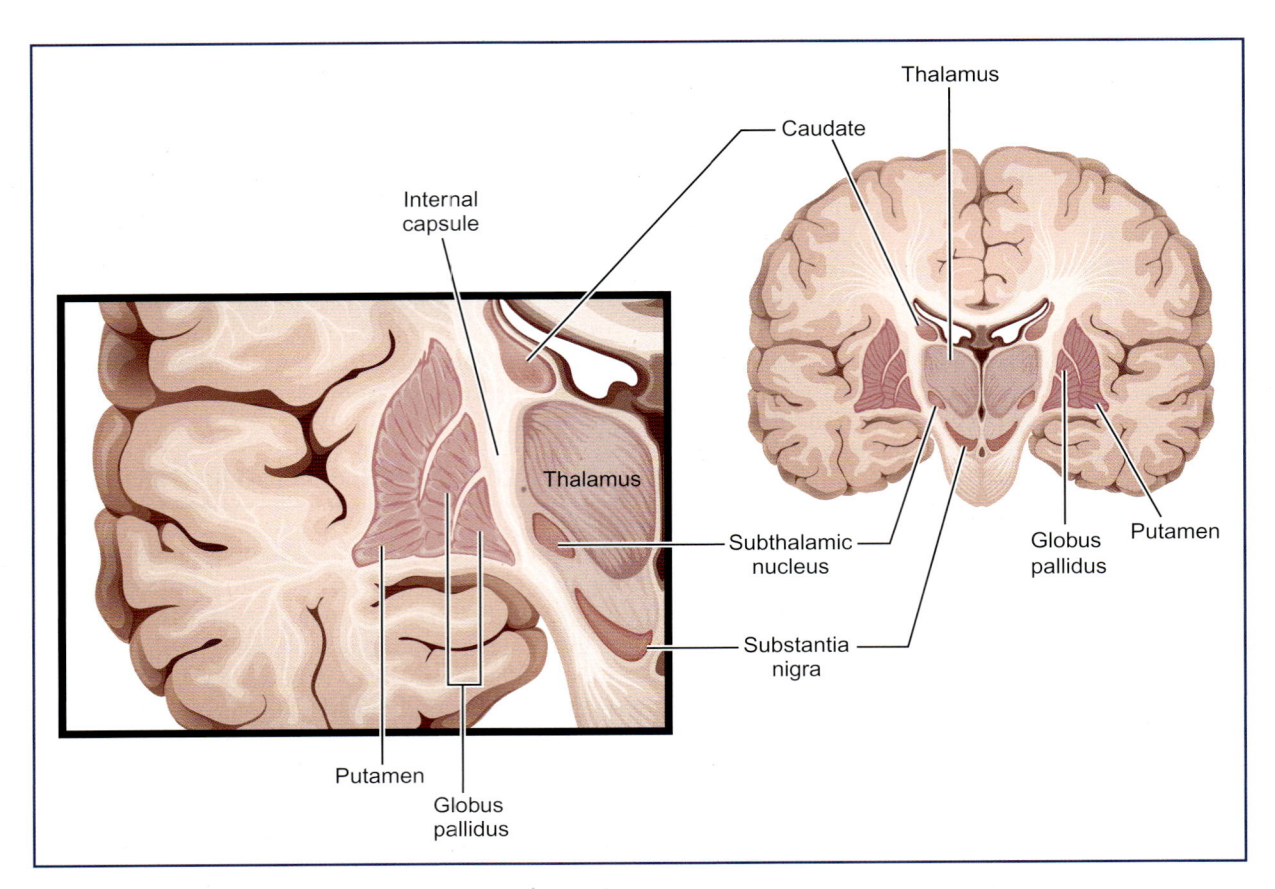

Figure 15–15. Structures of the basal ganglia shown in a coronal slice of a fixed human brain.

lateral of the basal ganglia structures. Just medial to the putamen is the globus pallidus, and together these two structures form a curved, lens-like mass of cells, explaining why the combined nuclei are called the lentiform or lenticular nucleus. Superior and medial to the lentiform nucleus and just lateral to the lateral ventricle is the caudate nucleus, which appears in this slice as a small, oval mass. Recall that the caudate and putamen are together called the striatum—note how the superior tip of the putamen is "pointing" toward the caudate. The significance of the caudate-putamen proximity is explained in the next paragraph. Inferior and medial to the lentiform nucleus is the aptly named subthalamic nucleus (note its position relative to the massive thalamus). Inferior to the subthalamic nucleus, the relatively long, oblique strip of darkened tissue is the substantia nigra, located ventrally in the superior part of the midbrain.

Also labeled in Figure 15–15 is a pale white strip of tissue—a fiber tract—separating the lentiform nucleus from the more medial caudate, thalamus, subthalamic nucleus, and substantia nigra. Much of this fiber tract is composed of the corticospinal and corticobulbar tracts, as well as striatal tracts. The tract also includes fibers carrying sensory information from the thalamus to the cortex, and from brainstem structures to structures of the basal ganglia. The part of this tract running through the basal ganglia structures is the internal capsule (see Figure 15–12). The internal capsule is an important anatomical landmark and often figures prominently in deficits resulting from stroke.

The specific appearance of basal ganglia structures, and in some cases the presence of a structure in a single coronal slice depends substantially on the location of the slice along the anteroposterior axis of the cerebral hemispheres. An appreciation for this dependency can be gained by studying Figure 15–16 (the front of the brain is to the left), a sagittal-view drawing of the complex configuration of basal ganglia structures. The cerebral cortex and cerebral white matter have been eliminated from the figure, leaving the structures of the basal ganglia "floating" free from their moorings within the cerebral hemispheres. Note the "C"-shaped form of the caudate nucleus, which is massive

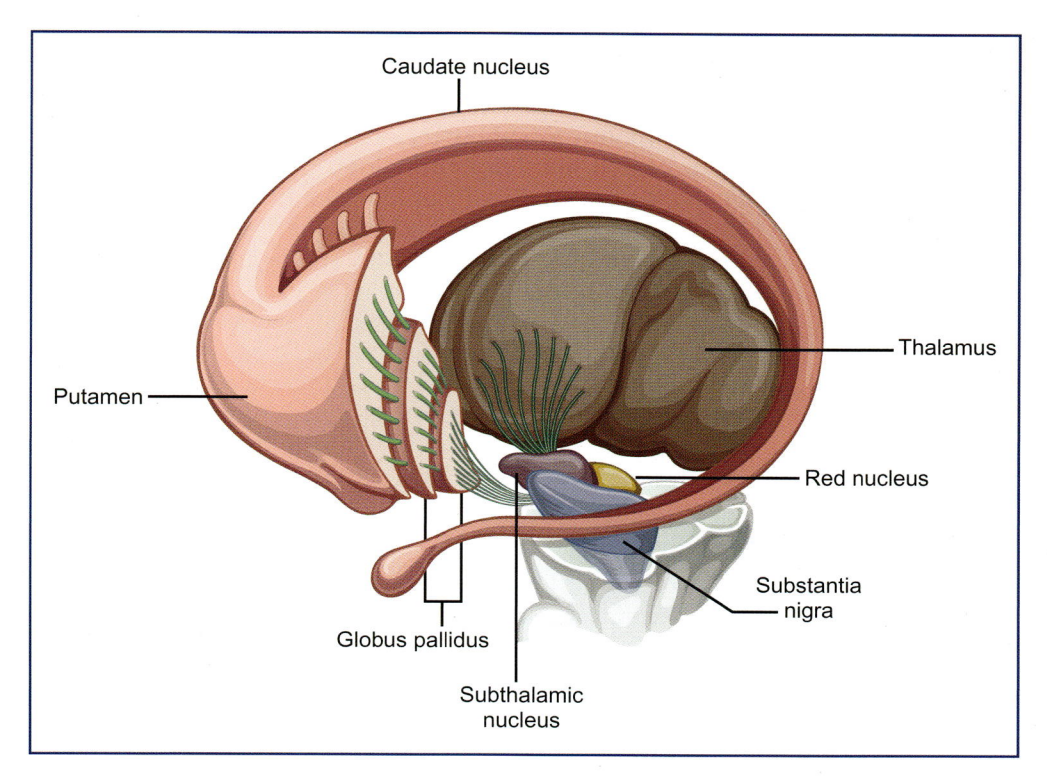

Figure 15–16. Sagittal-view drawing of the complex configuration of basal ganglia and adjacent structures. Front (anterior) is to the left. Green lines show fiber tracts running between the nuclei. The light pink strands toward the front of the basal ganglia structures show cell body connections between the anterior caudate and putamen.

Basal Ganglia or Basal Nuclei?

Language usage is *conventional*. If a sufficient number of people agree on the meaning of a word or phrase, its meaning is established, and technical analysis of language is, well, meaningless. A prominent part of this textbook is about speech, but "speech" is just a way to convey the concept in English. In German, speech is *sprache*, in French *parle*, in Mandarin Chinese *yanyu*, in Korean *mal*, in Russian *rech*. No one of these words captures the idea of "speech" more accurately than any other, no one of the words is intrinsically "right." The words mean "speech" because speakers of the languages agree on the meaning. So it is with the term "basal ganglia." "Basal ganglia" is technically a misnomer because a ganglion is a cluster of cell bodies just outside the CNS, and the components of the basal ganglia (caudate, putamen, and so forth) are within the CNS. In a grave statement issued in 1998, the International Federation of Associations of Anatomists (IFAA) declared that the term basal *nuclei* should be used for this collection of structures due to the obvious error of referring to these cell groups as *ganglia* (Sarikcioglu, Altun, Suzen, & Oguz, 2008). Unfortunately for the IFAA, most scientists do not seem to be paying attention. A PubMed search done by one of your authors on September 14, 2017, using the keywords "basal ganglia" and restricting the search from 2007 to the present, giving the scientific community close to two decades to respect the 1998 proclamation by IFAA, registered 12,411 "hits." In contrast, the keywords "basal nuclei" produced only 111 hits. These numbers are similar to the search conducted for the previous edition of this textbook (12, 956 for basal ganglia, 180 for basal nuclei). In this text, we side with the majority, choosing convention over technical accuracy. We choose the term "basal ganglia."

toward the front of the hemispheres and increasingly narrow as it curls toward the back of the brain and turns around to point forward. The tail of the caudate nucleus points so far forward it terminates ventral to the globus pallidus. The caudate and putamen are joined at the anterior end of the nuclei and split apart as the image is viewed from left to right (that is, from anterior to posterior within the cerebral hemispheres). The channel between the caudate and putamen, created as they separate, is filled by fibers of the internal capsule. The strands of light pink tissue "bridge" the spaces between the caudate and putamen at their most anterior location. This streaked or striated appearance of the internal capsule gives the name "striatum" to the putamen and caudate nuclei. The sagittal view also shows the globus pallidus in relation to the more lateral putamen, and the complex spatial configurations of the other nuclei discussed above.

Cortico-Striatal-Cortical Loop

The complexity of basal ganglia structures extends to their interconnections, as well as their connections to other parts of the CNS. The major connections are shown schematically in Figure 15–17. Boxes containing structure names represent nuclei (clusters of cell bodies) and arrows represent fiber tracts connecting nuclei or cell groups in the cortex to basal ganglia nuclei or other cortical cell groups. The thick purple arrows show the main loop by which information is delivered from the cortex to the striatum, and then to the globus pallidus. The globus pallidus is the primary "output" of the basal ganglia, integrating all the processing done in the basal ganglia and sending it to the thalamus. The thalamus returns the information received from the globus pallidus to the cortical areas from which the input to the striatum was derived, completing what is referred to as the cortico-striatal-cortical loop.

Cortical input to the striatum includes not only motor areas of the frontal cortex (both primary and premotor cortex, as well as the supplementary motor area), but also limbic cortex and occipital cortex. Note also in Figure 15–17 the direct connection between the cortex and the subthalamic nucleus. An interesting feature of the basal ganglia is that there are no direct projections—that is, no direct pathways—connecting these subcortical nuclei to the motor nuclei of the brainstem or spinal cord. The role of the basal ganglia in motor behavior is best thought of as one of modifying the eventual code issued from the motor cortex to the motor neurons of the brainstem and spinal cord, via the corticobulbar and corticospinal tracts.

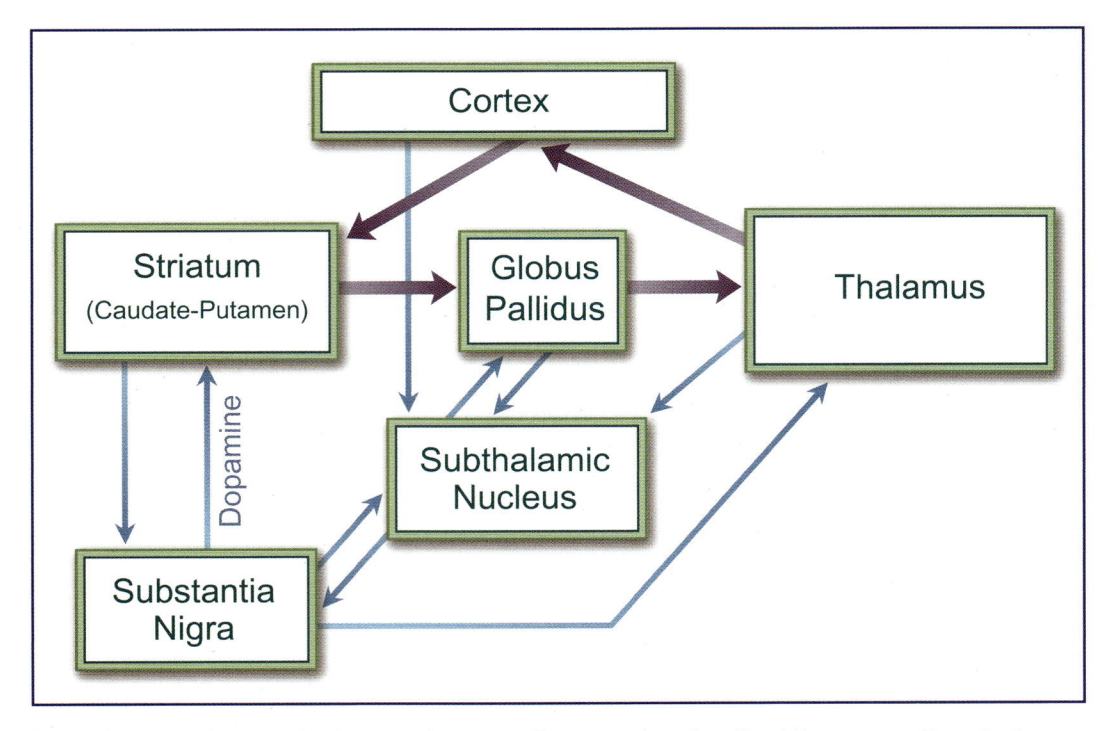

Figure 15–17. Schematic box-and-arrows diagram showing the interconnections between the cortex, basal ganglia structures, and thalamus. Boxes represent cortical cells and subcortical nuclei, arrows represent fiber tracts. The cortico-striatal-cortical loop is shown by structures connected by thick, purple arrows.

Role of Basal Ganglia

Several basic statements can be made to clarify the anatomical facts and functional roles of the basal ganglia in both limb and speech motor control. First, the cortico-striatal-cortical loop provides a pathway to "cycle" movement information between the cortex and basal ganglia, and in so doing refines the selection, activation, and timing of motor programs and direct commands from cells in the primary motor cortex. The concept of a "motor program" is of a *plan* for the activation of muscles, both over time and space and in terms of force of activation. Such a plan or program (much like computer code) can exist without being put into action. The idea of activity in the loop refining a motor program, and especially a program with a fair degree of complexity, is important because many authors have argued for the critical role of the basal ganglia in learning skilled movement and in packaging these skills as efficient units to be "turned on" or "turned off" at appropriate times (Nambu, 2008). In fact, a very broad description of the role of the basal ganglia in motor control is to facilitate or inhibit motor activity, depending on the nature of neuronal activity in the loop (Obeso & Lanciego, 2011).

Second, there are several bidirectional connections between nuclei of the basal ganglia, including two-way connections between the subthalamic nucleus and substantia nigra, the striatum and substantia nigra, and globus pallidus and subthalamic nucleus. Moreover, information not only flows from the basal ganglia to the thalamus and then to the cortex, but from the thalamus to the basal ganglia via the subthalamic nucleus (see Figure 15–17). The bidirectionality of connections is therefore not only found within the basal ganglia, but between the basal ganglia and its main output "target" (that is, the thalamus). The extensive, bidirectional connections within the basal ganglia and the potential influence of the thalamus on basal ganglia activity emphasize the difficulty of assigning a specific function to individual structures within the basal ganglia. It is difficult to say that a lesion in one structure of the basal ganglia results in a specific and unique motor deficit. The basal ganglia are a highly integrated system in which different lesion locations may produce similar symptoms and signs. A good example of this is the difficulty of isolating separate lesion correlates for diseases such as dystonia, athetosis, tics, and myoclonic jerks, all of which involve involuntary movements that have been attributed to basal ganglia disease.

Third, several neurotransmitters are important for normal basal ganglia function, the best-known of which is dopamine. Dopamine is manufactured by cells in the substantia nigra and conveyed to the striatum via the nigrostriatal pathway (in Figure 15–17 this pathway is labeled "Dopamine"). The neuropathology of Parkinson's disease includes, as a major component, the death of dopamine-producing cells in the substantia nigra. The loss of dopamine production results in a deficit of usable dopamine in the striatum. Interestingly, more than half of the dopamine-producing cells of the substantia nigra can be lost before the appearance of the early signs and symptoms of Parkinson's disease. The signs include tremor, slowness and reduction of movement, and stiff limbs (in Parkinson's disease the stiffness is referred to by the term "rigidity," a type of elevated muscle tone). The loss of dopamine is connected with these signs, but the precise effect of dopamine reduction on the occurrence and severity of the signs is not fully understood. Generally, the presence of dopamine in the striatum is thought to control the excitability of striatal neurons—how easily they are depolarized by connections from the cortex. A deficit in this excitability makes the striatum less "active," which may partially explain why people with Parkinson's disease move less and more slowly, and why dopamine-replacement therapy reduces these signs.

Fourth and finally, much is known about the basal ganglia and its role in motor behavior, but much is unknown as well. For example, in Figure 15–17, the *direct* projection from the motor cortex to the subthalamic nucleus is poorly understood. Scientists are very interested in this connection because the subthalamic nucleus is the preferred insertion target for electrodes used in deep brain stimulation (DBS), a surgical approach to relieving some of the signs and symptoms of Parkinson's disease. Obeso and Lanciego (2011), Nambu (2008), and Postuma and Dagher (2006) provide excellent reviews of the anatomical and functional connections of basal ganglia structures.

Lesions of basal ganglia structures are known to produce speech disorders. These disorders are included under the larger category of "motor speech disorders." Basal ganglia damage may result in hypokinetic dysarthria, a dysarthria thought to be the result of small and slow movements of speech structures, such as the tongue, lips, and jaw, as well as the vocal folds and respiratory apparatus. Hypokinetic dysarthria is usually associated with Parkinson's disease. Also connected with basal ganglia disease are (1) hyperkinetic dysarthria, thought to be the result of uncontrolled muscle tone or excessive, sudden, and/or rhythmic contraction of muscle groups within the speech apparatus, and (2) apraxia of speech (also resulting from cortical damage), a disorder in which the programming of speech sequences is disturbed even though the speech muscles are able to perform normally in oromotor, nonverbal tasks such as maximum strength efforts. Textbooks, including Duffy (2013) and Weismer (2006a), provide full introductions to motor speech

Deep Brain Stimulation

Deep brain stimulation (DBS) is a therapeutic approach to relieving the symptoms and signs of Parkinson's disease. Neurosurgeons implant an electrode in a selected basal ganglia structure and attach the electrode to an external stimulator that is under the control of the doctor and patient. In Parkinson's disease, the typical (but certainly not the only) sites for implantation of the electrode are the subthalamic nucleus and globus pallidus (see Figure 15–17). The idea is that these normally inhibitory nuclei are overactive in Parkinson's disease, producing a heightened inhibitory effect on the output of the basal ganglia. This increased inhibition results in the slow, small movements associated with the disease. Electrical stimulation of an implanted electrode acts like a lesion, calming down the activity of the cells and reducing the amount of inhibition of motor behavior. The good news is that there is ample evidence that DBS improves limb function in Parkinson's disease. The not-so-good news is that DBS comes with a host of negative side effects, including (possibly) depression, cognitive decline, sleep problems, anxiety, and *worsening* of the dysarthria associated with Parkinson's disease. See Fasano, Daniele, and Albanese (2012) for an excellent review of all these issues.

---

disorders, including those associated with basal ganglia lesions.

Thalamus

Figure 15–15 shows the thalamus as a massive group of nuclei on either side of the midline of the hemispheres (the two thalami surround the third ventricle, as described below). In the sagittal plane (see Figure 15–16) the thalamus appears as an egg-shaped structure. The thalamus is a collection of specialized nuclei, many of which relay a specific type of sensory information from lower parts of the brain to cortical areas. For example, auditory and visual nuclei within the brainstem send information to specialized nuclei within the thalamus, which in turn relay the information to auditory and visual cortical areas. Similarly, tactile information from the limbs and torso is relayed through the thalamus to somatosensory regions of the cortex. Tactile information from the head and neck travels via brainstem nuclei to the thalamus before delivery to appropriate cortical areas. Taste information (but not smell) is also relayed through the thalamus.

The thalamus is the main sensory relay of the brain. All sensory roads with the exception of olfaction connect the outside world to the cortex via the thalamus.

Cerebellum

The cerebellum is located below the occipital lobe and posterior to the brainstem. The cerebellum has two lobes, and is easily distinguished from other parts of the brain due to its unique appearance, which has been likened to a cauliflower (Figure 15–18, lower image).

The surface of the cerebellum is composed of a series of very slim tissue slabs, separated from each other by parallel, narrow fissures. In a prepared (fixed) brain, these tissue slabs, or *folia* (folium = a thin layer, or leaf), can be separated from one another with the careful use of dissecting instruments. Cerebellar folia are much more tightly packed than the gyri and sulci of the cortex.

Like the cerebral hemispheres, the cerebellar lobes have an outer cortex (gray matter), as well as white matter and nuclei deep within the cortical mantle. The structure and function of the cerebellum are exceedingly complex. For the purposes of this chapter, several general observations are presented for relevance to general and speech motor control.

First, the cerebellum is connected via fiber tracts to the spinal cord, brainstem, and cortex. The cerebellar peduncles, massive bundles of axons on the ventral and lateral surfaces of the brainstem (see Figures 15–20 and 15–21, below), serve as connections between the cerebellum and the rest of the CNS.

The inferior cerebellar peduncle contains fibers running to and from the cerebellum. In general, fibers running to the cerebellum in the inferior cerebellar peduncle carry sensory information on position and movement of body structures. Fibers running from the cerebellum to brainstem nuclei, in the inferior cerebellar peduncle, are associated with balance mechanisms. The middle cerebellar peduncle, the most massive of these fiber tracts, conveys information from the pontine nuclei to the cerebellum. Finally, the superior cerebellar peduncle carries fibers from the deep cerebellar nuclei to nuclei in the midbrain and pons, and most importantly (for the current purposes) to a nucleus in the thalamus. This thalamic nucleus relays cerebellar information to the cortex.

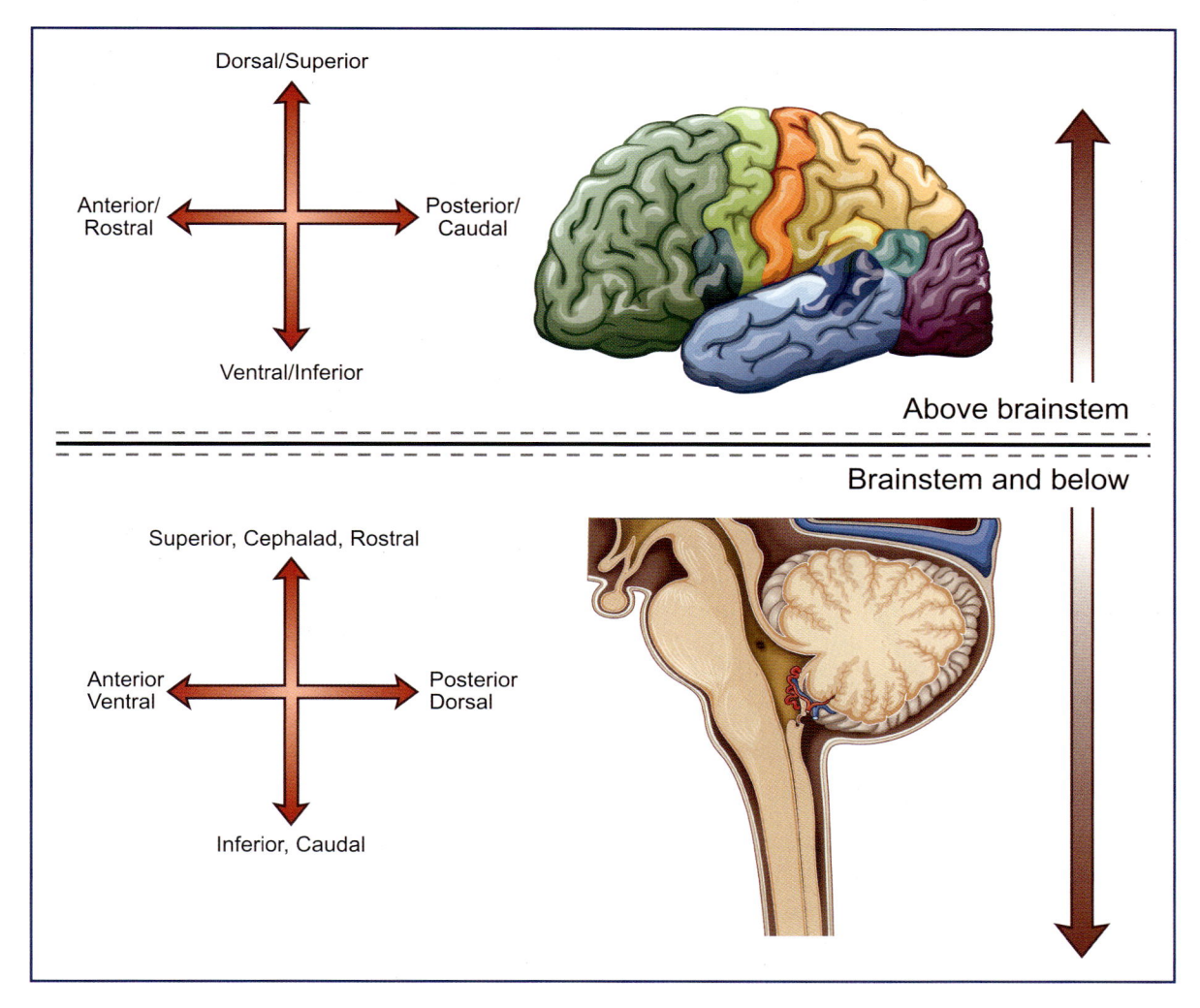

Figure 15–18. Artist's rendition of the cerebral hemispheres (*top image*) and the brainstem, cerebellum, and upper part of spinal cord (*bottom image*). Both images are shown in the sagittal plane.

Cortico-Cerebellar-Cortical Loop

Second, the cerebellum, like the basal ganglia, is connected to the cortex by means of a loop that runs from cortex to cerebellum and back to the cortex as illustrated schematically in Figure 15–19. Corticobulbar fibers from many areas of the cortex travel to the pontine nuclei, where synapses are made and information is forwarded to the cerebellum via the middle cerebellar peduncle. This information crosses the midline and enters the cerebellar cortex on the side opposite the cortical origin of this part of the loop. That is, the corticobulbar tract on the right side of the brain makes synapses with pontine cells whose output is directed to the left cerebellar hemisphere, and vice versa. The input to the cerebellum, delivered by the middle cerebellar peduncle, is directed to cells of the cerebellar cortex and then the dentate nuclei, which are clusters of cell bodies deep within the lateral cerebellar hemispheres. The dentate nuclei send processed information out of the lateral cerebellum to the thalamus on the opposite side of the brain, via the superior cerebellar peduncle. This fiber tract crosses the midline in the midbrain. The cortico-cerebellar-cortical loop therefore crosses once on the way down from cortex to cerebellum, and then again on the way up from cerebellum to cortex. Finally, information received in the thalamus is processed and returned, via thalamocortical fibers in the internal capsule and corona radiata, to the cortical areas where the information originated.

Role of Cerebellum

Because the cerebellum is connected via the cortico-cerebellar-cortical loop to so many parts of the cerebral cortex, as well as to the brainstem and

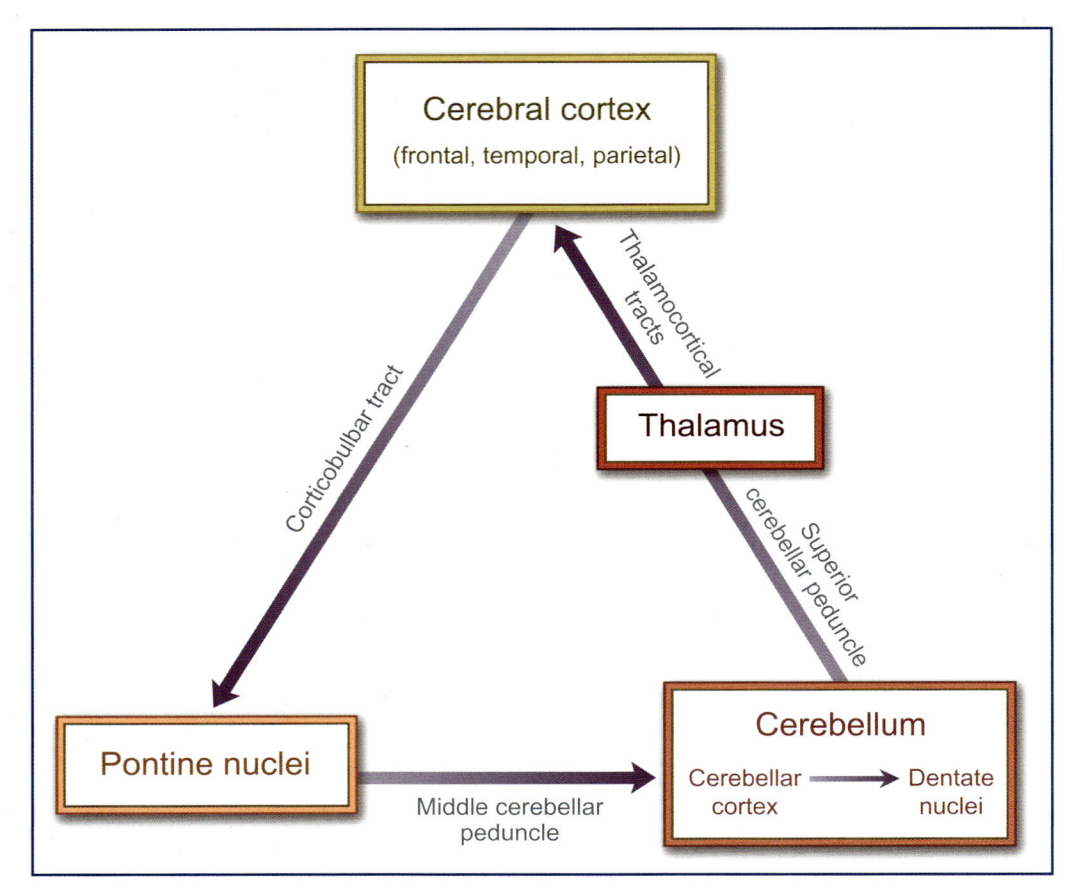

Figure 15–19. Schematic box-and-arrows diagram showing the interconnections between the cortex and the cerebellum. The cortico-cerebellar-cortical loop shown here is simplified by not depicting the two fiber tract crossovers in this loop. One crossover is in the pons as fibers descend from cortex to cerebellum, the other is in the midbrain as fibers ascend from the cerebellum on their way to the cortex via the thalamus.

spinal cord, it serves many functions. Traditionally the cerebellum has been regarded as critical to motor control, and specifically to coordination of the many muscles involved in skilled action, including speech production. People with cerebellar lesions, which may occur as a result of stroke, tumors, degenerative disease, and penetrating head injuries, often demonstrate coordination difficulties. People with cerebellar lesions produce jerky movements, lacking the smooth and integrated motions of the neurologically healthy individual. Patients have difficulty controlling the precision and force of muscular efforts, as evidenced by (for example) an inability to point to a target or generate a specific degree of effort (such as lifting a weight to a prespecified height). In the traditional neurological test of "close your eyes and touch your nose with your index finger," people with cerebellar lesions may miss the tip of their nose and hit their face with too much (or too little) force. Finally, a cerebellar lesion may result in disproportionately impaired movement deficits as task complexity is increased. Tasks requiring very carefully coordinated movements are likely to be performed with a dramatic degree of impairment compared with the performance of more simple tasks.

Cerebellum and Basal Ganglia: New Concepts

A traditional view of the cortico-striatal-cortical loop (see Figure 15–17) and cortico-cerebellar-cortical loop (see Figure 15–19) is one in which the output of cortical cells in the primary motor cortex is modulated by their circulating information. The idea has been that both loops deliver information to the cortex via the thalamus; the globus pallidus is the basal ganglia output to the thalamus, and the dentate nucleus is the cerebellar output to the thalamus. The thalamic information, already modulated by processing in both the basal ganglia and cerebellum, is sent back to the cortex.

In recent years, the role of these loops in brain function has been rethought to include not only aspects of motor control, but more global cognitive functions such as the planning of actions and learning of skilled behavior. As reviewed by Middleton and Strick (2000) and Bostan and Strick (2010), both loops send distinct projections to the *prefrontal* cortex via the thalamus, not just to the primary motor cortex. The anatomical connections between the two loops and the prefrontal cortex implicate the basal ganglia and cerebellum in prefrontal functions such as cognitive aspects of motor control, action planning, and learning. It is relevant to note that diseases of the basal ganglia, such as Parkinson's disease and Huntington disease, as well as cerebellar disease, are known to include deficits of action sequence planning and action learning.

The complex connections in the CNS and their role in behavior emphasize the challenges of regarding the brain as a segregated group of structures, each having separate and possibly exclusive functions. "Programming disorders," for example, which are quite popular as an explanation for the speech disorder called "apraxia of speech," cannot easily be assigned to a single brain location (however, see Graff-Radford et al., 2014). Many brain structures may play a role in the same function, and when damaged may produce the same signs and symptoms, even with varying lesion locations.

BRAINSTEM AND CRANIAL NERVES

The brainstem can be thought of as a stalk of nervous system tissue, connected above to the cerebral hemispheres and its contents, and below to the spinal cord. The top part of the brainstem stalk is surrounded by overhanging tissue of the hemispheres. Refer again to Figure 15–4, where the midsagittal MR image (right image) shows a dotted red line separating the top of the brainstem from the bulk of the cerebral hemispheres. In this midsagittal view, identification of the major components of the brainstem is made easy by the bulging, middle part of the brainstem called the *pons*. A horizontal line drawn lower and parallel to the red dotted line in Figure 15–4, through the nose of the imaged person, intersects the pons in the middle of its bulge. The smaller, narrower structure above the pons, the midbrain (mesencephalon), is the most superior component of the brainstem. The most superior edge of the midbrain extends to the dotted red line. Below the pons is a short, narrow length of tissue called the *medulla* (also called the *medulla oblongata*). The medulla is the most inferior component of the brainstem and its lower border is continuous with the superior boundary of the spinal cord.

An artist's rendition of the brainstem and nearby structures in the sagittal plane is shown in the lower part of Figure 15–18. Note the location of the cerebellum, posterior to the pons and medulla and beneath the occipital lobe of the cerebral hemispheres. At the top of the brainstem is a narrow canal (colored dark brown) running through the midbrain, posterior to the superior part of the pons. This canal expands into a larger cavity separating the cerebellum from the pons and medulla. The narrow canal is the *cerebral aqueduct* and the cavity into which it expands is the *fourth ventricle*. These cavities are part of the ventricular system through which cerebrospinal fluid (CSF) flows.

The brainstem is small in comparison to the cerebral hemispheres but contains cells and tracts critical to a wide variety of sensorimotor behaviors, as well as to consciousness, mood, and vegetative functions. A great deal of nervous system tissue with a broad range of functions is packed into the small volume of the brainstem, and it is precisely these close quarters that explain why blood deprivation to the brainstem—as in the case of brainstem strokes—can have such devastating consequences. Of special interest to the speech-language pathologist and audiologist are the nuclei and fiber tracts of the brainstem associated with a subset of the 12 paired cranial nerves. These brainstem structures and the nerves associated with them control muscles of the head and neck, and sensation (including hearing) from the same structures. Speech, swallowing, and hearing function are very much dependent on the integrity of brainstem structures and the cranial nerves.

In this section, surface features of the brainstem are reviewed first, followed by consideration of each of the 12 cranial nerves and their associated brainstem nuclei. The cranial nerves are introduced as surface features of the brainstem, and later, their anatomy within the brainstem, and their functions are presented, with special emphasis given to those nerves serving motor and sensory functions of head and neck structures important for speech, swallowing, and hearing.

The landmarks of cranial nerve attachments to the brainstem are often referred to as "roots." For example, "Cranial nerve V emerges as a large root about halfway between the top and bottom of the pons, on its ventrolateral aspect" refers to the attachment of cranial nerve V to the pons just as it enters (or exits) the brainstem.

Surface Features of the Brainstem: Ventral View

A ventral view of the brainstem, plus the thalamus above it, is shown in Figure 15–20. Recall that "ventral" and "anterior" imply the same direction or surface when referring to structures from the top of the brainstem down through the spinal cord. The view in Figure 15–20 is obtained if the midsagittal views of Fig-

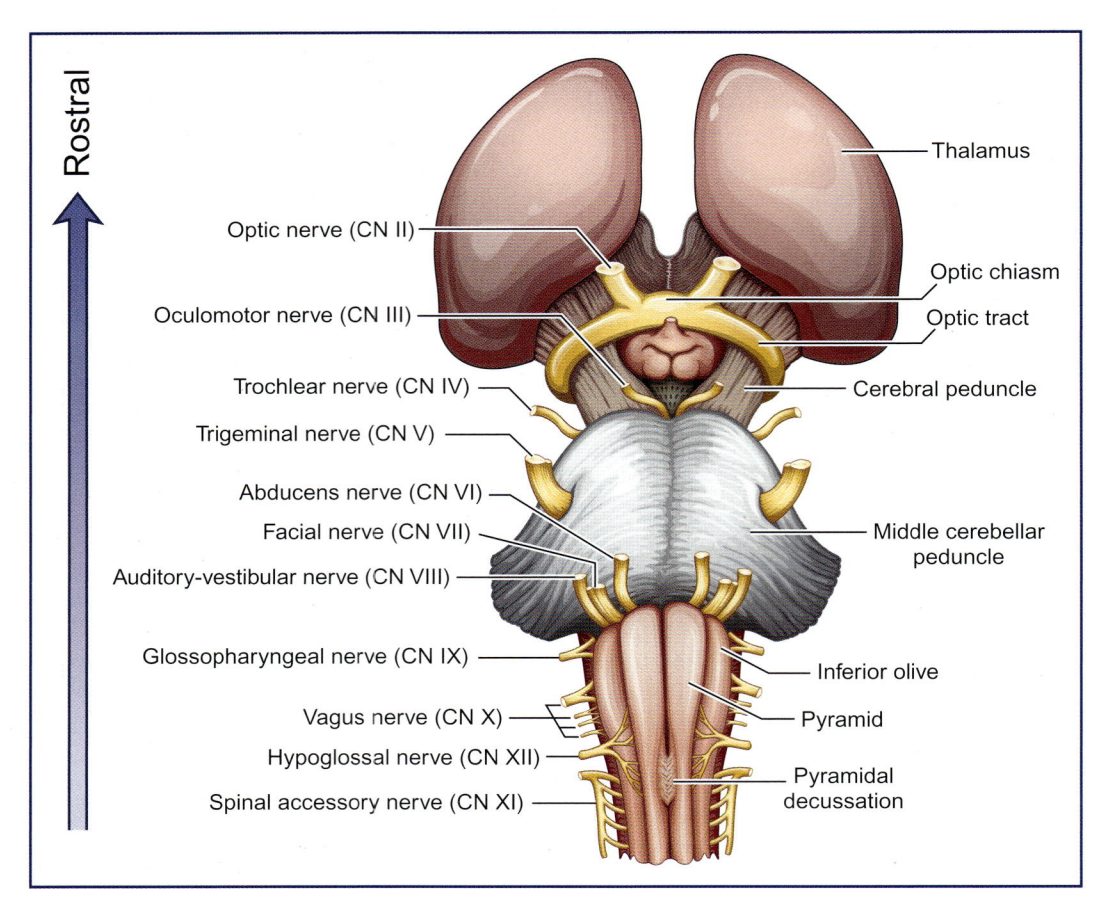

Figure 15–20. Ventral surface of the brainstem, showing major landmarks.

ures 15–4 and 15–18 are rotated counterclockwise 90 degrees. In these figures the observer views the front, or ventral/anterior surface, of the brainstem.

Ventral Surface of Midbrain

Prominent surface features of the ventral midbrain include the *cerebral peduncles* (often called the *crus cerebri*, even if this term is not technically equivalent to the cerebral peduncles). The cerebral peduncles are the midbrain component of the massive, long fiber tract running from cortical motor cells to motor nuclei in both the brainstem (corticobulbar tract) and spinal cord (corticospinal tract). Figure 15–20 labels the cerebral peduncle on the left side of the midbrain (right side from the reader's point of view). The matching cerebral peduncle on the right side of the brain is a mirror image of the left-side tract. The cerebral peduncles continue through the pons below its ventral surface.

The *optic chiasm* is located at the midline of the ventral surface of the midbrain. The optic chiasm is the location where the two optic nerves (paired cranial nerve II) meet before continuing into the cerebral hemispheres as the optic tracts. In Figure 15–20 the optic nerves have been cut because this view of the brainstem is drawn with more anterior structures—principally the face and neck—removed. The optic nerves originate at the retinas, and the destination of the optic tracts is the occipital lobes of the cerebral hemispheres. Figure 15–20 shows the optic nerves entering the chiasm, where about half the fibers from each eye continue to the hemisphere on the same side as the eye, and the other half crosses over to the opposite hemisphere. Each optic tract therefore carries fibers from both eyes, and a visual "field" from each eye is represented in both hemispheres.

Two additional landmarks on or near the ventral surface of the midbrain are cranial nerve III (oculomotor nerve) and the appearance of IV (trochlear nerve). The oculomotor nerve emerges from the midbrain at its junction with the pons, and the trochlear nerve exits the brainstem on its dorsal surface and circles around to be visible on the ventrolateral aspect of the brainstem, as shown in Figure 15–20. These cranial nerves are critical to the control of eye movements.

Ventral Surface of Pons

The ventral surface of the pons is dominated by thick bands of fibers running across this surface (see Figure 15–20). These fiber tracts create the "bulge" of the pons, and consist of three separate tracts called the superior, middle, and inferior *cerebellar* peduncles. The middle cerebellar peduncle (labeled in Figure 15–20) is the largest of these tracts and forms the bulk of the ventral surface of the pons. Collectively the three cerebellar peduncles connect the cerebellum to the spinal cord, brainstem, and thalamus, as described above. Pons is a word meaning "bridge," an apt name because it serves as a bridge from the cerebellum to each major part of the CNS.

Other landmarks on the ventral surface of the pons include the roots of four cranial nerves. Figure 15–20 shows these four nerves cut shortly after emerging from the brainstem. They include cranial nerves V (trigeminal), VI (abducens), VII (facial), and VIII (auditory-vestibular). Cranial nerve V emerges as a large root about halfway between the top and bottom of the pons, on its ventrolateral aspect. Cranial nerves VI, VII, and VIII emerge between the lower edge of the pons and upper edge of the medulla, in a medial-to-lateral order with VI being most medial and VIII most lateral. The roots of these three cranial nerves are included as surface features of the ventral pons because the nuclei to which they are attached are completely (VI, VII) or partially (VIII) within the pons (see Figure 15–22, below).

Ventral Surface of Medulla

The ventral surface of the medulla shows two pairs of prominent columns. The two most medial columns are the *pyramids*; Figure 15–20 labels the left medullary pyramid. The pyramids are the continuation into the medulla of the corticobulbar and corticospinal tracts. As noted above, these tracts descend in the midbrain as the crus cerebri (cerebral peduncles) and in the pons below its ventral surface (inside the pons) as pontine fascicles (not visible in Figure 15–20). The pyramids are formed from the corticobulbar and corticospinal fibers emerging from inside the pons and organized in the medulla as the relatively long, medial columns on its ventral surface. Toward the inferior border of the medulla, Figure 15–20 shows a landmark labeled "Pyramidal decussation." This is where the majority of corticospinal fibers (roughly 80%) from one pyramid cross over to the other pyramid before continuing their descent into the spinal cord. Fibers originating in the left cerebral hemisphere descend in the brain on the left side until crossing to the other side via the pyramidal decussation. Fibers from the right hemisphere descend in the brain on the right side, before crossing to the left side via the decussation. The fibers from both hemispheres form an "X"-like pattern as they cross at the bottom of the medulla. The word "decussate" means a crossing pattern that forms an "X." The boundary between the medulla and the spinal cord is at the inferior edge of the pyramidal decussation.

Just lateral to each pyramid, and separated from it by a groove or fissure (called the anterolateral fissure, not labeled in Figure 15–20), is a swelling of the ventral medulla due to an underlying nucleus called the *inferior olive*. The inferior olive delivers information coming from the spinal cord to the cerebellum. For the current purposes it is important to recognize these columns lateral to the pyramids as landmarks on the ventrolateral surface of the medulla, and especially for locating the four cranial nerves attached to the medulla.

These four cranial nerves attach to the medulla on its ventral and ventrolateral surface. The most superior of these is cranial nerve IX (glossopharyngeal), shown exiting the right side of the medulla just lateral to the olive. Just inferior to the exit point of cranial nerve IX is cranial nerve X (vagus), attached in the groove lateral to the olive as a group of rootlets. Cranial nerve XII (hypoglossal) is inferior to the exit point of cranial nerve X, but more medial, exiting the medulla in the anterolateral fissure that separates the pyramid from the olive. Finally, the most inferior of the nerves exiting the ventral surface of the medulla is cranial nerve XI (spinal accessory nerve, sometimes called the accessory nerve), which like cranial nerves IX and X emerges lateral to the olive.

Surface Features of the Brainstem: Dorsal View

A dorsal view of the brainstem, plus the thalamus above it, is shown in Figure 15–21. Recall that "dorsal" and "posterior" imply the same direction or surface when referring to structures from the top of the brainstem down through the spinal cord. The view in Figure 15–21 is obtained if the midsagittal views of Figures 15–4 and 15–5 are rotated clockwise 90 degrees, so that the back—the dorsal/posterior surface—of the brainstem is facing the observer. The cerebellum has been removed from this figure, as the clockwise rotation of the intact brain with the cerebellum in place blocks a clear view of the dorsal surface of the brainstem. The cranial nerves attached to the medulla can also be seen in this dorsal view (as well the attachment point of cranial nerve IV; see the next section, "Dorsal Surface of Midbrain"), but these are described above as ventral surface features.

Dorsal Surface of Midbrain

Prominent surface features of the dorsal midbrain include the *superior* and *inferior colliculi* and the root of cranial nerve IV (trochlear) (see Figure 15–21). The super-

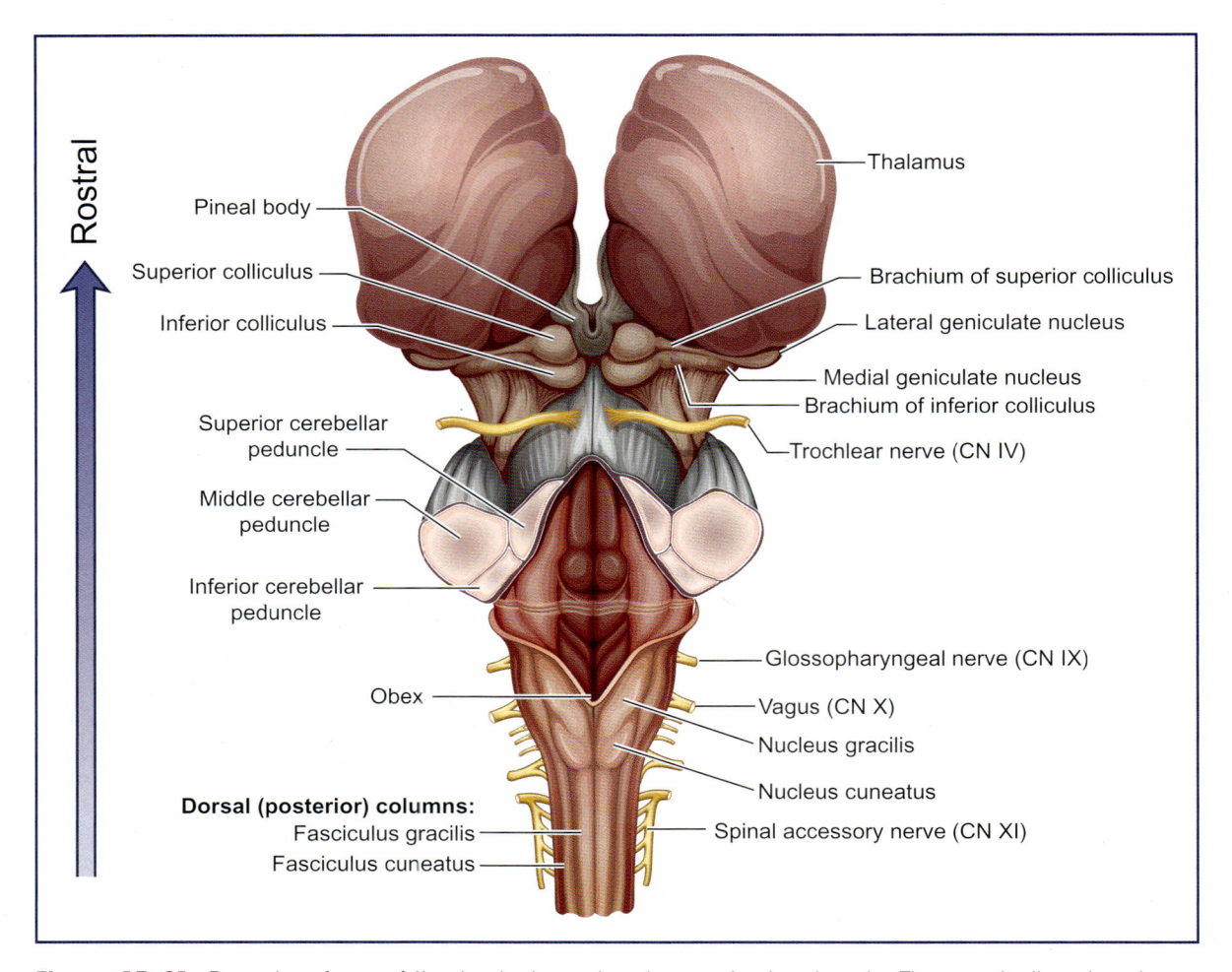

Figure 15–21. Dorsal surface of the brainstem, showing major landmarks. The cerebellum has been removed for this view and the cerebellar peduncles are shown with cuts prior to their entry point to the cerebellum.

What's Your Peduncle's Name?

Brain anatomy is complicated. It is made more complicated (and confusing!) by the naming of some of its parts. Particularly confusing is when the same term is used for different parts or when the same part is given different names. For example, the terms *crus cerebri* and *cerebral peduncles* are often used interchangeably to denote the portion of the corticobulbar and corticospinal tracts that passes through the midbrain and makes up a good deal of the midbrain's ventral surface. The term peduncle is also used to refer to *cerebellar* peduncles, which connect the cerebellum to various parts of the brain. "Peduncle" means stalk or stem, and is used widely in anatomy, botany, and any other field in which objects are attached to other objects by means of a short stalk, stem, or base. To keep the brain anatomy structures straight, focus on the adjectives: the *cerebral* peduncles connect the cerebrum (cerebral hemispheres) with structures in the brainstem and spinal cord, whereas the *cerebellar* peduncles connect the cerebellum with parts of the spinal cord, brainstem, and thalamus.

ior and inferior colliculi are paired "bumps" forming the roof of the midbrain. These four bumps are collectively referred to as the *corpora quadrigemina*. Re-examination of Figure 15–4 (right image) shows these "bumps" on the small island of tissue that is separated from, and dorsal to, the bulk of the midbrain. The narrow channel separating the bulk of the midbrain from these dorsal bumps is the cerebral aqueduct, one of the series of cavities in the brain through which CSF is circulated.

The superior and inferior colliculi are nuclei along the visual and auditory pathways of the brain, respectively. These nuclei relay visual (superior colliculus) and auditory (inferior colliculus) information from more inferior nuclei in the brainstem to nuclei in the thalamus. Note the pathways labeled "Brachium of superior colliculus" and "Brachium of inferior colliculus" in Figure 15–21. These are fiber bundles that emerge from the colliculi and terminate in thalamic nuclei. These nuclei are the lateral geniculate nucleus (vision) and the medial geniculate nucleus (audition). The lateral geniculate nucleus sends its output to the visual auditory cortex on the same side. The medial geniculate nucleus sends its output to the auditory cortex, also on the same side.

The root of cranial nerve IV (trochlear) emerges from the inferior border of the dorsal midbrain, close to the midline. Figure 15–21 shows the paired nerves running laterally from their roots. The nerves wrap around the brainstem and are seen in the ventral view as well (see Figure 15–20). Cranial nerve IV is distinct among the 12 cranial nerves as the only one with a root emerging from the dorsal surface of the brainstem.

Dorsal Surface of Pons

Recall that the ventral surface of the pons is formed by fibers of the three cerebellar peduncles, which connect regions of the cerebral hemispheres, the brainstem, and the spinal cord to the cerebellum. These fiber tracts wrap around the brainstem to enter or exit the cerebellum. The dorsal view of the brainstem in Figure 15–21 shows the peduncles cut, because the cerebellum has been removed from this view. The superior cerebellar peduncle primarily connects the cerebellum to the thalamus, the middle cerebellar peduncle connects the brainstem to the cerebellum, and the inferior cerebellar peduncle connects the cerebellum to the spinal cord. The diamond-shaped cavity surrounded superiorly and laterally by the cerebellar peduncles and laterally and inferiorly by the medulla is the *fourth ventricle*, which is also seen in the midsagittal images of Figure 15–18. The obex, at the inferior edge of the fourth ventricle, is where the fourth ventricle narrows down to continue as the central canal of the spinal cord, the spinal conduit for CSF.

Dorsal Surface of Medulla

Several bumps and bands of tissue can be seen in the "floor" of the fourth ventricle (colored dark brown in Figure 15–21), especially below the cut level of the inferior cerebellar peduncle. The floor of the fourth ventricle is its ventral wall, as seen from the dorsal view of Figure 15–21. The "roof" of the fourth ventricle is its dorsal wall, formed largely by the cerebellum, especially along or close to the midline. The bumps and bands are swellings of nuclei and fiber tracts that give the floor of the fourth ventricle its distinctive topography. Similar topographical features are also seen in the floor of the fourth ventricle at the level of the pons.

At the bottom of the dorsal surface of the medulla two pairs of columnlike landmarks can be seen rising superiorly to the fourth ventricle. The columns on either side of the midline are called the *fasciculi gracilis*, the columns just lateral to them are the *fasciculi cuneatus*. Collectively, these four columns are called the posterior columns, which are fiber tracts carrying sensory information on touch, vibration, and proprioception (position and movement sensation of body parts relative to each other) up the spinal cord to the medulla, where they synapse in the paired *nucleus gracilis* and *nucleus cuneatus*. These two nuclei, shown as slight swellings in the caudal medulla along its dorsal border, receive information from the ascending posterior columns (see Figure 15–21). Fibers leaving the nucleus gracilis and nucleus cuneatus cross to the other side and ascend to make synapses with thalamic nuclei before traveling in fiber tracts to the cortex.

Cranial Nerves and Associated Brainstem Nuclei

Table 15–3 lists the 12 cranial nerves, their associated nuclei, and their major function(s). Figure 15–22 is a dorsal view of the brainstem showing the medio-lateral and superior-inferior locations of the cranial nerve nuclei. The drawing does not indicate the position of the nuclei along the ventral-to-dorsal (anterior-to-posterior) dimension of the brainstem, as would be seen in a transverse section. Each cranial nerve and its associated nucleus (or nuclei) is (are) discussed below, but emphasis is given to cranial nerves V, VII, VIII, IX, X, XI, and XII because of their relevance for speech and hearing. Table 15–3 and Figure 15–22 should be consulted frequently throughout this discussion.

Some of the cranial nerves have purely sensory functions, some purely motor functions, and some have both sensory and motor functions. In Table 15–3, cranial nerves with purely sensory function (CN I, II, VIII) are listed in normal font and those with purely motor

Table 15-3. Cranial Nerves, Their Associated Brainstem Nuclei and Location(s) and General Function(s)

NERVE (NAME)	NUCLEI	LOCATION	FUNCTION(S)
I (Olfactory)	Olfactory bulb[a]	Ventral surface of brain	Olfaction
II (Optic)	Midbrain[b]	Retinal ganglion cells	Vision
III (Oculomotor)	**Oculomotor; Edinger–Westphal**	**Midbrain**	**Eye movement, pupil size, and accommodation**
IV (Trochlear)	**Trochlear**	**Midbrain**	**Eye movement (one muscle)**
V (Trigeminal)	Motor n. of V	Pons	Control of jaw muscles (closers and opener), **mylohyoid** m., **tensor veli palatine** m., **tensor tympani** m.
	Sensory n. of V		Sensation from entire face, teeth, palate, gums, anterior two-thirds of tongue
VI (Abducens)	**Abducens**	**Pons**	**Eye movement (single muscle)**
VII (Facial)	Facial motor n.	Pons	Control of muscles of facial expression and **stapedius** m.
	Sup. salivatory n.		Control of salivatory glands
	Sensory n. of V		Possible sensation from parts of external ear and parts of tonsils
	n. solitarius		Taste from anterior two-thirds of tongue
VIII (Auditory-vestibular)	Cochlear n.	Pons and medulla	Audition
	Vestibular n.		Balance
IX (Glossopharyngeal)	n. ambiguus	Medulla	Control of **stylopharyngeus** m.
	Sensory n. of V		Sensation from parts of external ear, medial surface of eardrum, upper pharynx, posterior one-third of tongue
	Salivatory n.		Control of salivatory glands
	n. solitarius		Detection of chemical and pressure changes in blood; taste to posterior one-third of tongue
X (Vagus)	n. ambiguus	Medulla	Control of velopharyngeal, pharyngeal, and laryngeal muscles, and one tongue muscle
	Sensory n. of V		Sensation from meninges, parts of external ear and ear canal, external surface of eardrum, pharynx and larynx
	Dorsal motor n.		Control of smooth muscle and glands of pharynx, larynx, heart, and digestive system
	n. solitarius		Sensation from heart, digestive system, esophagus, and trachea
XI (Accessory)	Accessory spinal n. (upper cervical cord)	Upper cervical (spinal cord)	Control of **sternocleidomastoid** and **trapezius** m.

Table 15–3. *continued*

| XII (Hypoglossal) | Hypoglossal n. | Medulla | Control of three of the four muscles of the tongue and all intrinsic muscles of tongue |

Note. Nerves that are purely sensory are in regular font, nerves that are purely motor are in bold font, and mixed nerves (with both sensory and motor function) are in italicized font.

[a]The olfactory nerve has sensory receptors embedded within the cribriform plate of the ethmoid bone, and the "nuclei" are in the olfactory bulbs (see Figure 15–5, lower left image) which are located on the base of the frontal lobe, external to the brainstem. The olfactory "nerve" is therefore really the olfactory "tract" but is typically called a "nerve" (see text).

[b]The optic nerve does not make connections with brainstem nuclei in the sense of cranial nerves III–XII, but rather sends fibers from the retina (the sensory receptors) to the lateral geniculate nucleus of the thalamus, which forwards this information to the visual cortex. Some optic nerve fibers go to the midbrain, where information is used by cranial nerves III, IV, and VI to control eye movements.

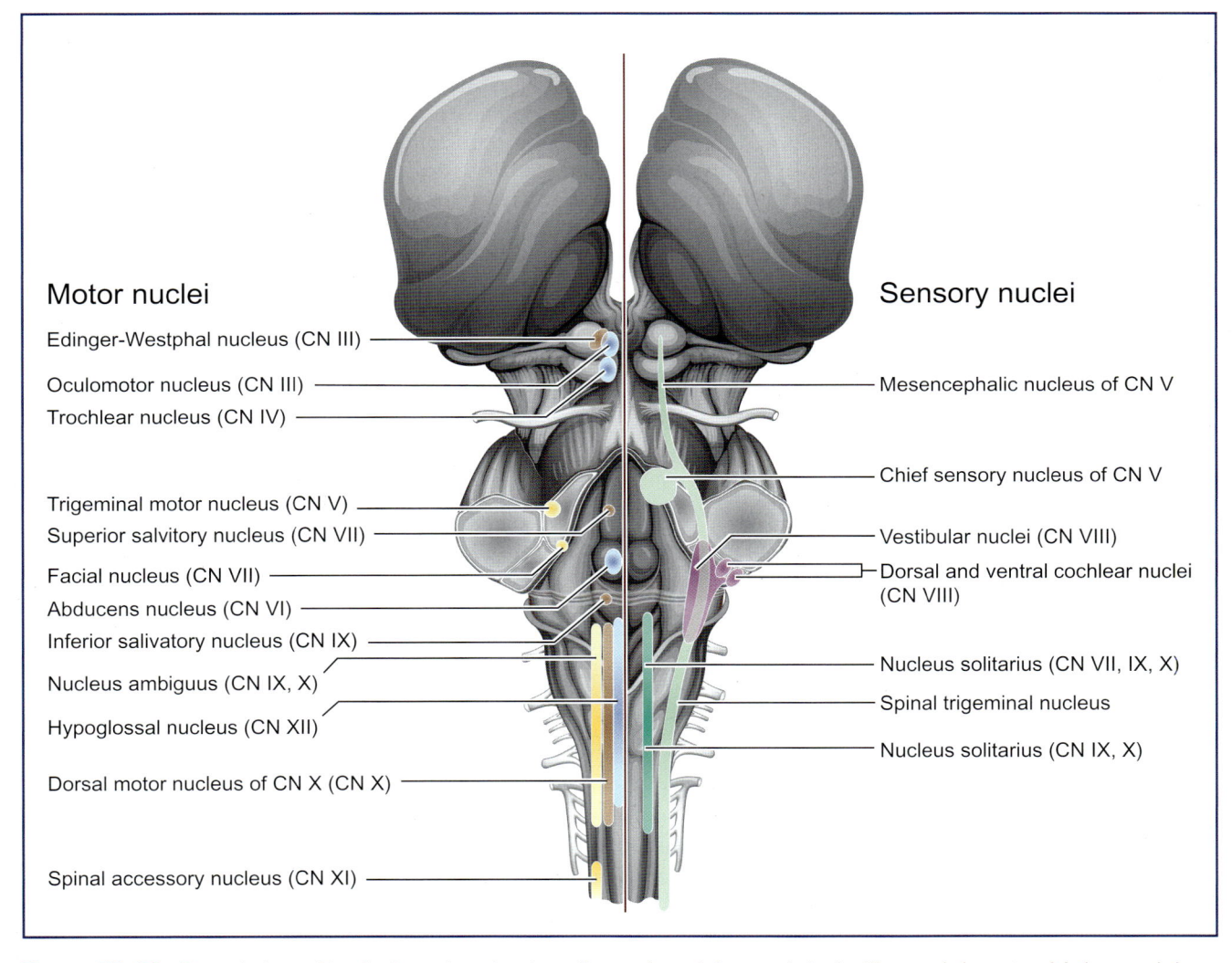

Figure 15–22. Dorsal view of brainstem showing locations of nuclei associated with cranial nerves. Motor nuclei are shown on the left side of the brainstem, sensory nuclei on the right side. This view allows an estimate of the location of nuclei along the medial-to-lateral plane of the brainstem, as well as the length of nuclei along the inferior-superior dimension of the brainstem, but does not provide information on nuclei location along the anterior-posterior (that is, ventral-dorsal) dimension.

function (CN III, IV, VI, XI, XII) in bold font. Those having both motor and sensory function are called mixed nerves and are listed in italicized font.

Two of the cranial nerves (I and II) are not directly associated with nuclei in the brainstem. Cranial nerves I and II are both sensory, and have their cell bodies in ganglia outside the brainstem, close to their specialized receptors. One cranial nerve with purely motor function, cranial nerve XI, has its nuclei in the upper part of the cervical spinal cord. The remaining cranial nerves all have motor nuclei within the brainstem, or in the case of sensory components, ganglia whose projections are to nuclei within the brainstem.

Cranial Nerve I (Olfactory)

The sensory receptors for olfaction are embedded within a bony structure at the top of the ethmoid bone (see Figure 4–1) called the cribriform plate. These receptors send axons to the olfactory bulbs, where they make a first synapse in what is essentially an olfactory nucleus. As seen in the lower left image of Figure 15–5, the olfactory bulbs are located on the base of the frontal lobes. These bulbs (typically intact and available for naked-eye inspection in a fixed brain when it is turned upside down for examination of the ventral surface of the cerebral hemispheres) are swellings at the end of long, thin bands of tissue that disappear into the cortex close to the adjacent boundaries of the frontal and temporal lobes. The thin bands of tissue running posteriorly, into the cortex, are called the olfactory nerves, or the paired cranial nerve I. Most fibers from the olfactory nerves enter the cortex and other parts of the temporal lobes. The ventromedial portions that serve olfaction in the temporal lobe are closely associated with memory mechanisms in the same lobe.

Cranial Nerve II (Optic)

The sensory receptors associated with the optic nerves are the rods and cones in the retina. Rods and cones are the photocells of the retina, sensitive to light and color. When light strikes the photocells, they transform the photon energy to electrical impulses. These impulses are sent to ganglia within the retina where the first synapse is made. Axons emerging from the ganglia form the optic nerves, which exit each retina and run posteriorly and medially, toward the optic chiasm.

The bottom, left image of Figure 15–5 shows the cut optic nerves entering the optic chiasm. The continuation of the optic pathway beyond the chiasm is called the optic tract (see Figure 15–20). Fibers from both retinas travel through the optic chiasm and continue via the optic tracts to visual cortex in the occipital lobes.

The mapping from the external world to retina, and from retina to cerebral hemispheres is orderly, but complex. For example, fibers of the optic nerve are arranged retinotopically: the retina is arranged so its rods and cones respond to specific regions of the visual field. As stated above, both retinas are represented in both hemispheres. Because of the way images from the external world are projected onto the retina, the left visual field is represented in the right visual cortex, and the right visual field is represented in the left visual cortex.

Cranial Nerve III (Oculomotor)

Figure 15–22 shows two motor nuclei (left side of figure) near the midline of the midbrain, one the oculomotor nucleus (blue), the other the Edinger–Westphal nucleus (brown). These nuclei are roughly at the level of the superior colliculus along the inferior-superior axis of the brainstem. When the nuclei are viewed in a transverse section they are ventral to the colliculi, just anterior to the cerebral aqueduct. Two types of motor fibers arise from the nuclei associated with cranial nerve III. The oculomotor nucleus contributes fibers to innervate four extrinsic muscles that move the eyeball up, down, and toward the nose, as well as fibers to the muscle that raises the eyelid. The muscles that attach to the eyeball have their origin outside the eyeball, from a ring of tendinous tissue surrounding the inner eye socket. The Edinger–Westphal nucleus innervates intrinsic muscles of the eye that control the size of the pupil and the shape of the lens. The oculomotor nucleus and nerve exert "voluntary" control over muscles that control eye position, whereas the Edinger–Westphal nucleus controls the involuntary muscles of the pupil and lens. As shown in Figure 15–20, fibers from both the oculomotor and Edinger–Westphal nuclei run together and exit the brainstem as the oculomotor nerve at the inferior edge of the ventral surface of the midbrain.

Cranial Nerve IV (Trochlear)

In Figure 15–22 the trochlear nucleus is shown slightly inferior to the oculomotor nucleus, roughly at the level of the inferior colliculus. In a horizontal section of the midbrain through the level of the inferior colliculus the trochlear nucleus is seen ventral to the cerebral aqueduct (Figure 15–23, left and right images: the slice on the left was prepared with a process that stains fiber tracts dark [note the crus cerebri at the anterior, ventral edge of the slice] and nuclei light [note the substantia nigra, just posterior to the crus cerebri]). An artist's rendition reproduces the slice features except with the dark and light areas reversed to show the nuclei as gray

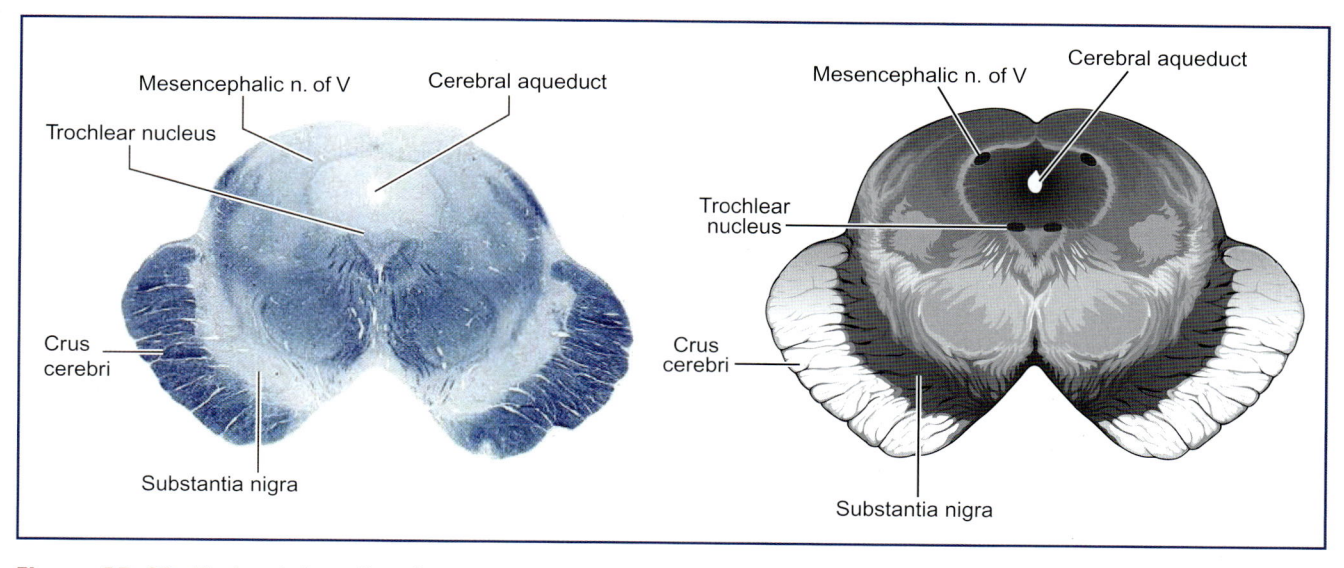

Figure 15–23. Horizontal section through a human midbrain, roughly halfway between its superior and inferior boundaries. Left slice prepared by a process that stains nuclei white and fiber tracts dark; right slice shows artist's rendition of the same slice with light and dark areas reversed so that dark areas = nuclei, light areas = fiber tracts.

areas and fiber tracts as white areas, in the more traditional way. Figures 15–24 to 15–27 (below) are an artist's renditions drawn in the same way as the right side of Figure 15–23. The small hole in the center and somewhat posterior part of the section is the cerebral aqueduct, the passageway through which CSF flows from the third to fourth ventricles (see Figure 15–37, below). The trochlear nucleus is the origin of cranial nerve IV, and serves a purely motor function by innervating a single, extrinsic muscle of the eye that produces upward, downward, rotary, and side-to-side movements of the eyeball. The eye movements produced by this muscle are complex and depend on the position of the eyeball when the muscle contracts.

Cranial nerve IV is unique among the cranial nerves for two reasons. First, the trochlear nerve is the only cranial nerve that emerges from the dorsal surface of the brainstem. As described above, these paired nerves exit the dorsal surface of the midbrain and curl around the cerebral peduncles to run anteriorly in the cranial cavity, on their way to the eyes. Second, fibers emerging from the trochlear nuclei run dorsomedially within the midbrain and cross at the midline before exiting as cranial nerve IV. The trochlear nerve emerging from the right side of the brainstem (and innervating the muscle in the right eye) is therefore from the left trochlear nucleus (and the left trochlear nerve is from the right trochlear nucleus). All other motor nuclei in the brainstem, including the ones associated with cranial nerve III, emerge on the same side of the brainstem as their originating nuclei.

Cranial Nerve V (Trigeminal)

Cranial nerve V is a mixed nerve (both sensory and motor function) with three major divisions—ophthalmic, maxillary, and mandibular. The trigeminal nerve emerges from the ventrolateral surface of the pons as a large root (see Figure 15–20) containing sensory and motor fibers. A short distance away from the brainstem, the root separates into three major branches. The ophthalmic and maxillary divisions are purely sensory, carrying information on touch, pressure, and pain from the mid and upper face including the forehead, front part of the scalp, and eyeball, maxillary teeth, sinuses, and meninges of the anterior and middle cranial fossa. The anterior and middle cranial fossa are the front and middle depressions in the base of the skull that house ventral and lateral parts of the cerebral hemispheres.

The mandibular division of cranial nerve V contains both sensory and motor fibers. The sensory fibers carry information on touch, pressure, and pain from the lower teeth, the skin of the lower face, the anterior two-thirds of the tongue, the external auditory meatus, and parts of the external ear. The sensory division also carries information from specialized organs in the jaw-closing muscles to a sensory nucleus in the brainstem. These specialized organs are called muscle spindles and are an important component of the jaw-jerk reflex. The motor part of the mandibular division innervates the jaw closing muscles and the single jaw-opener (anterior belly of the *digastric* muscle), the *palatal tensor* muscle, the ***tensor tympani*** muscle, and the ***mylohyoid*** muscle (see Chapters 3, 4, and 5).

The motor fibers of cranial nerve V are derived from the trigeminal motor nucleus (also called the motor nucleus of V), located in the pons roughly midway between its superior and inferior borders (see Figure 15–22, left side). In a transverse section of the pons, the trigeminal motor nuclei are found ventral to the floor of the fourth ventricle and lateral to the midline (Figure 15–24). The motor fibers from the trigeminal motor nucleus make ipsilateral connections (i.e., same side as the nucleus and nerve) with the muscles of the jaw, velopharynx, and middle ear cavity.

As shown in light green on the right side of Figure 15–22, the sensory nucleus of V runs the entire length of the brainstem, from midbrain to medulla and has three parts. The parts are the mesencephalic-nucleus of V in the midbrain, the chief (or principal) sensory nucleus in the pons, and the spinal trigeminal nucleus in the lower pons and throughout the length of the medulla. Figure 15–24 shows the principal sensory nucleus of V just lateral to the motor nucleus of V.

A simple account of the functions of the three parts of the sensory nucleus of V is as follows. The chief (principal) sensory nucleus in the pons receives information on touch and pressure from the face, tongue, teeth, and other facial structures whose sensory function is served by the trigeminal nerve. The spinal trigeminal nucleus receives information on pain and temperature from these same areas, as well as touch and pressure information from small regions of the head and neck. The mesencephalic nucleus of V, in the midbrain, is specialized to receive fibers originating in the muscle spindles of the jaw closing muscles. Muscle spindles issue sensory fibers that are directed to the brainstem and spinal cord and are part of the stretch reflex of the jaw (see Internet document on clinical evaluation of the cranial nerves, as well as a detailed explanation of the stretch reflex).

Cranial Nerve VI (Abducens)

The abducens nerve originates in the abducens nucleus, which, as shown in Figure 15–22, is close to the midline of the brainstem, roughly midway between the superior and inferior borders of the pons. The abducens nucleus and nerve control the ***lateral rectus*** muscle of the eye. This muscle attaches to the side of the eyeball and, when it contracts, causes movement consistent with the name of the nucleus and nerve—it abducts the eyeball, turning it away from the nose toward the lateral surface of the head.

A transverse section of the pons at the level of the abducens nucleus shows the paired nuclei close to the midline and in the floor of the upper part of the fourth ventricle (Figure 15–25). The two light, round structures at the ventral edge of the image, just lateral to

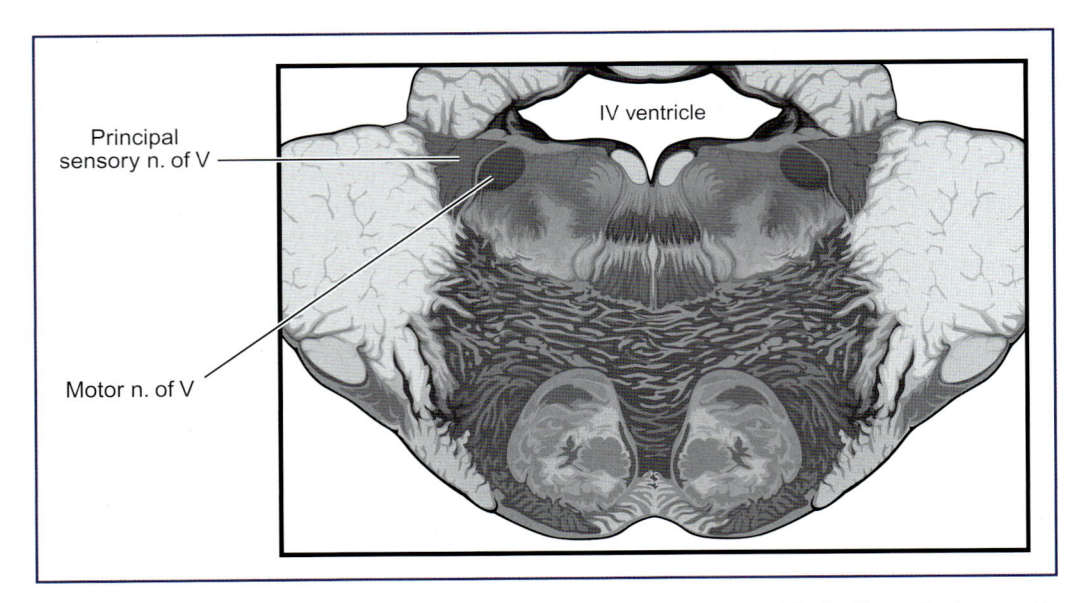

Figure 15–24. Horizontal section through a human pons, roughly halfway between its superior and inferior boundaries. The section was made to intersect the motor nucleus of V, roughly between the superior and inferior borders of the pons (see relative inferior-superior location of motor nucleus of V in Figure 15–22).

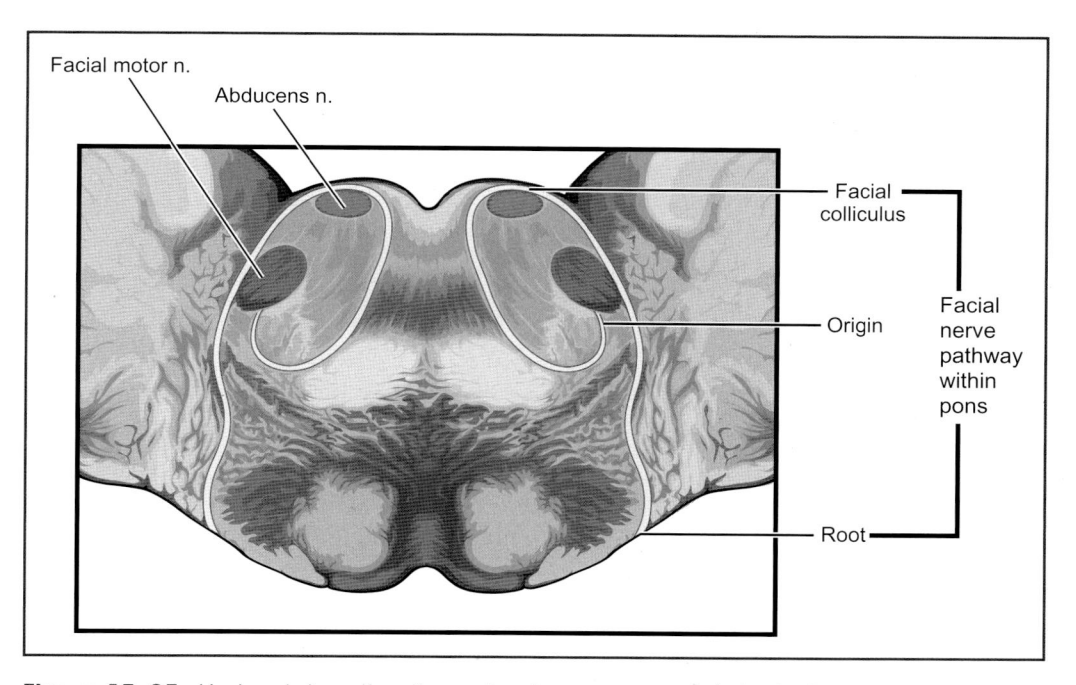

Figure 15–25. Horizontal section through a human pons, inferior to the cut shown in Figure 15–24. The section was made to intersect the facial motor nuclei and the abducens nuclei (see relative inferior-superior location of these two motor nuclei in Figure 15–22). The right side of the section shows the pathway of the tract leading from the facial motor nucleus to the exit of cranial nerve VII on the ventral surface of the brainstem, at the junction between the medulla and pons. Note the "looping" of the pathway around the abducens nucleus, in the floor of the fourth ventricle, before the tract turns ventrally toward its exit point from the brainstem.

the midline, show the corticospinal tract as it passes through this level of the pons. Axons exit the nuclei, run ventrally and slightly laterally to emerge from the ventral surface of the brainstem at the junction of the pons and medulla (see Figure 15–20).

Cranial nerve VI is often considered together with cranial nerves III (oculomotor) and IV (trochlear), because all three nerves control eye movements. In Figure 15–22, note how the motor nuclei for the extrinsic muscles of the eye (colored blue on the left side of the brainstem) line up along the midline. The two nuclei in the midbrain and the one in the pons are derived from the same embryonic cells and are interconnected to produce the complex and rapid motions of the eyeballs.

Cranial Nerve VII (Facial)

The facial nerve is a mixed nerve. The facial nerve originates in the facial motor nucleus, located in the mid-pons, just inferior to the motor nucleus of V. The nucleus is slightly ventral and lateral to the abducens nucleus, as labeled on the left side of Figure 15–22. The facial nerve emerges from the brainstem between cranial nerves VI and VIII, at the junction of the lower pons and upper medulla

The tract issuing from the facial motor nucleus follows an interesting course within the pons before emerging from the brainstem. This tract has been outlined and labeled in three locations on both sides of the pons, as shown in Figure 15–25. The origin of the tract is where axons emerge from the facial motor nucleus. The tract runs dorsally, toward the floor of the fourth ventricle, and loops around the abducens nucleus before heading ventrally to exit the brainstem. The exit point, immediately lateral to the exit point for cranial nerve VI, is labeled "root" in Figure 15–25. Within the pons, the loop of fibers around the abducens nucleus is called the *internal genu* of the facial nerve. The bump created in the floor of the fourth ventricle by the genu and the immediately ventral abducens nucleus is the *facial colliculus*.

Virtually all muscles of facial expression (see Chapter 5) are innervated by the voluntary motor component of the facial nerve, issued from the facial motor nucleus. The facial nerve also innervates the *stapedius* muscle, which attaches to the neck of the stapes in the middle ear and pulls on it reflexively, in response to acoustic events having extremely high sound energy (Chapter 13). The acoustic (stapedius) reflex protects hair cells in the cochlea, the end organ of hearing, from extremely loud sounds. The innervation of the stapedius muscle from the same pool of fibers supplying muscles of facial expression is a useful anatomical datum when a clinical profile includes both facial paralysis and absence of the acoustic reflex.

Cranial nerve VII also carries autonomic motor fibers to glands that secrete tears and saliva. The term "autonomic" is reserved for nervous system function that is not voluntary (such as production of saliva, regulation of blood pressure, sweat glands, and so forth). The motor cells for this part of the nerve are found in the superior salivatory nucleus (see Figure 15–22, left side, small nucleus colored brown in pons, superior to the abducens nucleus). The salivatory axons exit the brainstem with the rest of the facial nerve fibers.

The sensory component of cranial nerve VII includes general touch and pressure, and taste. Sensory innervation for touch and pressure is limited to small regions of the external ear, including the ear canal and the external surface of the eardrum. These sensory fibers make an initial synapse in a ganglion outside the brainstem, within the skull, and enter the brainstem through the root of cranial nerve VII. The fibers terminate in the chief sensory nucleus of V (see Figure 15–22, right side). Taste fibers innervate the anterior two-thirds of the tongue, have an initial synapse in the same ganglion as the other sensory fibers, and enter the brainstem with the root of cranial nerve VII, terminating in the upper part of the nucleus solitarius (see Figure 15–22, right side).

The voluntary motor function of cranial nerve VII is of obvious importance to the speech-language pathologist. As one example, the motor component of cranial nerve VII controls the *orbicularis oris* muscles and the associated muscle complex (including muscles such as the *mentalis, levator anguli oris*, etc., see Chapter 5). These muscles are critical to the production of vowel contrasts that depend on labial configuration, as well as labial motions and configurations for consonants such as /p/, /b/, /f/, and /v/. These muscles, as well as muscles of the cheeks, also have an important role in swallowing (Chapter 16).

Cranial Nerve VIII (Auditory-Vestibular Nerve)

The auditory-vestibular nerve is sensory. The nerve has a double name because it carries information to the brainstem from both the cochlea and the vestibular apparatus of the inner ear. The cochlea contains the end organ cells for hearing, and the vestibular apparatus the end organs for balance and movement coordination of the eyes, head, and trunk (see Chapter 13).

The cochlea and vestibular apparatus are related structures, containing fluid-filled chambers embedded within the temporal bone of the skull. Within these fluid-filled chambers are hair cells whose position and shape are changed by displacement of the fluid. In the case of the cochlea the fluid displacement and resulting effect on the hair cells is typically due to sound energy entering the external ear canal, vibrating the eardrum and the three ossicles (bones) of the middle ear, causing the ossicle coupled to the cochlea (the stapes) to move in and out of one of the fluid-filled chambers. In the case of the vestibular apparatus, the hairs cells are displaced with changes in head position. The hair cells of both structures are connected to sensory fibers that are depolarized or hyperpolarized when the hair cells are displaced by fluid motion. These sensory fibers make a first synapse in ganglia outside the brainstem (the spiral ganglion in the case of the cochlea; vestibular [Scarpa's] ganglion in the case of the vestibular apparatus). The sensory fibers exiting these ganglia run together as the two parts of cranial nerve VIII—the auditory (cochlear) nerve and the vestibular nerve—to their respective nuclei in the brainstem.

The two nerve bundles of cranial nerve VIII approach and enter the dorsolateral aspect of the brainstem close to the junction of the medulla and pons (the pontomedullary junction). Figure 15–26 shows a transverse section of the brainstem in the upper medulla, slightly inferior to the pontomedullary junction. Note the entry point of the auditory portion of cranial nerve VIII, and the close proximity of the cerebellum to the inferior, dorsolateral surfaces of the pons. The narrow space between the pons and cerebellum is referred to as the *cerebellopontine angle*. Cerebellopontine angle tumors are a class of tumors in which a mass at or within the angle presses on the ventral and ventrolateral surface of the brainstem and (most commonly) affects the function of cranial nerves V, VII, and VIII.

Fibers of the cochlear (auditory) division of cranial nerve VIII synapse on cells in the cochlear nuclei (two on each side), located just below the dorsolateral surface of the pontomedullary junction (see Figure 15–26). Fibers from the vestibular division of the nerve make synapses on cells of the vestibular nuclei (four on each side), located dorsally, facing the ventral surface of the cerebellum. In the inferior-superior dimension shown

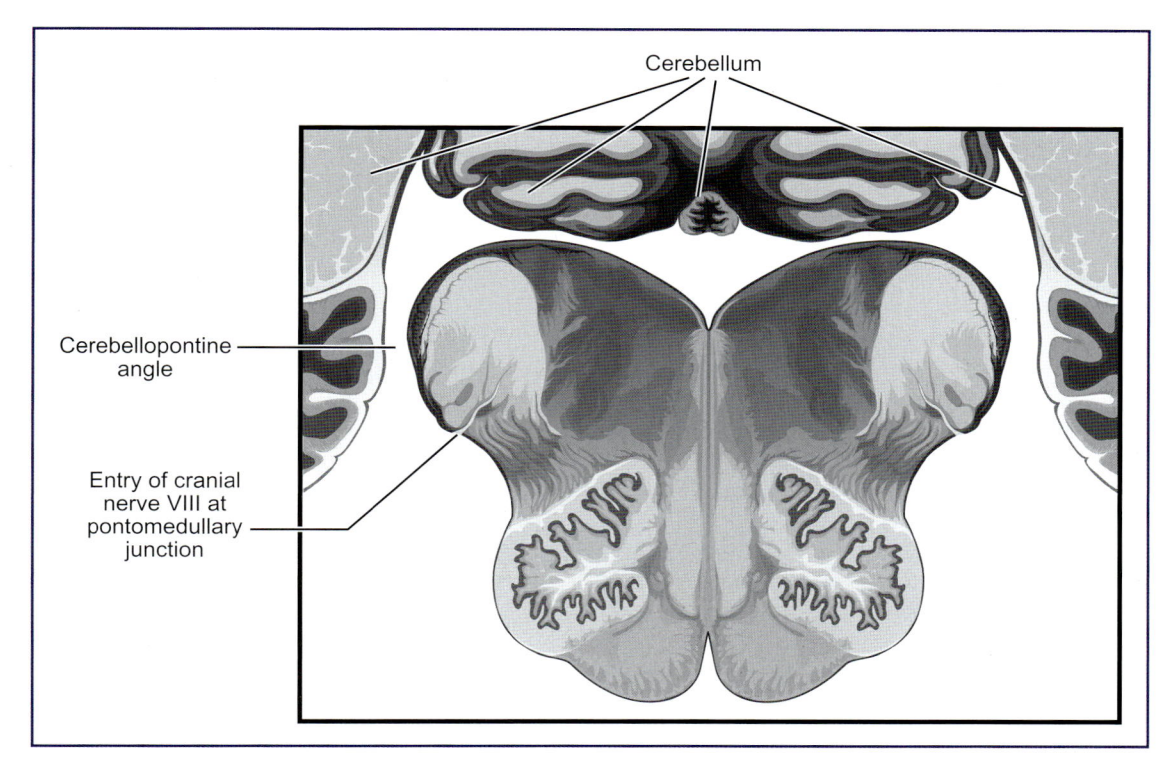

Figure 15–26. Horizontal section through a human brainstem, in the high medulla just below its junction with the pons. The section shows brainstem tissue surrounded by cerebellar tissue (note the small white space at the midline, between the posterior edge of the brainstem and the more posterior cerebellum; the white space is part of the fourth ventricle). The section shows the entry point of cranial nerve VIII to the brainstem, as well as the small, lateral space between the lower pons and the surrounding cerebellar tissue. This space is the cerebellopontine angle. The "coiled" nuclei in the ventrolateral part of the brainstem section are the inferior olivary nuclei (also see Figure 15–27) whose lateral-most "bend" forms the inferior olive landmark on the ventral surface of the brainstem (see Figure 15–20).

on the right side of Figure 15–22 (in purple), the vestibular nuclei extend above and below the pontomedullary junction.

The *central auditory pathways* consist of fiber tracts and several intervening nuclei connecting the cochlear nuclei to the primary auditory cortex. A signal moves along the auditory pathway from the cochlea to the auditory nerve, from the auditory nerve to the cochlear nuclei, from the cochlear nuclei to several other nuclei in the brainstem, the last of which are the inferior colliculi in the midbrain, then to the medial geniculate bodies of the thalamus and finally to the primary auditory cortex. Signals are processed from the auditory nerve through the brainstem very, very quickly, with a 5 to 6 ms lag between the firing of auditory nerve fibers and firing of cells in the inferior colliculus.

The vestibular nuclei send information received from the vestibular component of cranial nerve VIII up the brainstem to the oculomotor, trochlear, and abducens nuclei for coordination of head and eye movements. The nuclei also send information down the spinal cord and to the cerebellum for coordination of head and trunk movement.

Cranial Nerve IX (Glossopharyngeal)

The glossopharyngeal is a mixed nerve. As seen in Figure 15–20, the nerve is attached to the upper, ventral medulla in the groove just lateral to the swelling of the inferior olive. Motor fibers to a single voluntary muscle originate in the superior portion of the nucleus ambiguus (a long column of motor neuron cells located (in cross section) about midway between the ventral and dorsal surfaces of the medulla, and well lateral to the midline. Figure 15–27 shows a horizontal cut of the medulla taken between its superior and inferior

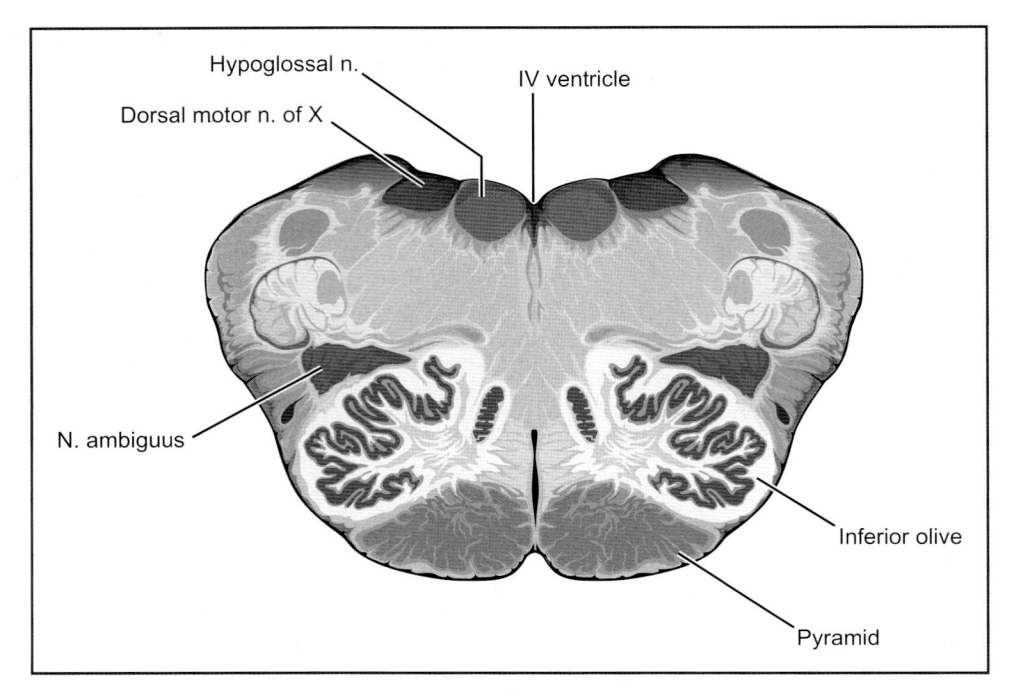

Figure 15-27. Horizontal cross-section of the medulla, roughly midway between its superior and inferior boundaries. Note the positions of the nucleus ambiguus, the hypoglossal nucleus, and the pyramids.

borders. In this cross-section, the nucleus ambiguus is seen just dorsal to the inferior olive. The nucleus ambiguus extends throughout the entire superior-inferior length of the medulla (see Figure 15–22, left side, in yellow). The motor component of cranial nerve IX innervates the *stylopharyngeus* muscle. As described in Chapter 4, contraction of the paired *stylopharyngeus* muscles may lift and widen the pharyngeal tube. The specific role of this muscle in speech production is unknown, but it almost certainly plays a role in swallowing by shortening the pharyngeal tube (Meng, Murakami, Suzuki, & Miyamoto, 2008; see also Chapters 4 and 16).

The glossopharyngeal nerve also has an autonomic motor component. The inferior salivatory nucleus (see Figure 15–22, left side of brainstem, nucleus in upper medulla, close to the midline) gives off fibers that exit the brainstem along with the voluntary motor fibers derived from the nucleus ambiguus. The autonomic fibers separate from the fibers en route to the *stylopharyngeus* muscle to innervate the parotid gland. The parotid, the largest salivary gland of the head and neck, is wrapped around the ramus of the mandible. When stimulated by the autonomic fibers of cranial nerve IX, the gland secretes saliva into the oral and pharyngeal cavities.

The sensory component of the glossopharyngeal nerve transmits information on touch, temperature, and pressure from the posterior one third of the tongue, parts of the pharynx, and the external ear and surface of the eardrum facing the middle ear cavity. The various sensory fibers serving these regions make first synapses in a pair of ganglia, then enter the brainstem together at the root of cranial nerve IX (see Figure 15–20) and terminate in the brainstem, within the spinal part of the sensory trigeminal nucleus (see Figure 15–22, right side of brainstem, lower part of light green nucleus). Cranial nerve IX also has an autonomic, sensory component, part of which carries taste information from the posterior one-third of the tongue to cells at the top of the column-like nucleus solitarius. Another autonomic sensory component of cranial nerve IX conveys information on blood gases and blood pressure from receptors near the split of the common carotid artery into the internal and external carotid arteries. Fibers from these receptors go to cells at the bottom of the nucleus solitarius column.

Cranial Nerve X (Vagus)

Cranial nerve X is a mixed nerve. The nerve is attached to the brainstem as a series of roots in the groove just lateral to the inferior olive, immediately inferior to the point of attachment of cranial nerve IX (see Figure 15–20). Like cranial nerve IX, the voluntary motor fibers of the vagus nerve originate in cells of the nucleus ambiguus (see Figures 15–22 and 15–27). These cells and the fibers they give rise to innervate the pharyngeal constrictor muscles, the *palatal levator*, the *salpingopharyngeus*, the *palatopharyngeus* and *palatoglossus* muscles, and the intrinsic muscles of the larynx (*cricothyroid, thryoarytenoid, posterior cricoarytenoid, lateral cricoarytenoid*, and *arytenoid*) (see Chapters 3 through 5). The voluntary muscle component of cranial nerve X plays an important role in speech and swallowing, given its control of muscles that adjust the dimensions of the velopharyngeal port, the pharyngeal lumen, aspects of tongue motion, and the tension and configuration of the vocal folds.

Cranial nerve X also has an autonomic motor component. Most of these fibers arise from the dorsal motor nucleus of X, which like the nucleus ambiguus forms a column throughout the medulla. The dorsal motor nucleus of X is medial and dorsal to the nucleus ambiguus; the location of the dorsal motor nucleus of X, in the floor of the fourth ventricle, gives the nucleus its name (see Figure 15–27). Fibers arising from cells in the dorsal motor nucleus of X (and possibly from a small region of the nucleus ambiguus as well) stimulate mucous glands within the pharynx and larynx, and glands within the gut and other organs. Autonomic motor fibers derived from the dorsal motor nucleus of X also control smooth (involuntary) muscle of the heart and gut.

Information on touch, pressure, and temperature is carried by sensory fibers of cranial nerve X from the pharynx, larynx, parts of the external ear and eardrum, and the meninges from the posterior part of the cerebral hemispheres. Like touch, pressure and temperature information traveling in any cranial nerve (see information above on cranial nerves V, VII, IX), the sensory fibers of cranial nerve X make initial synapses in ganglia outside the brainstem, enter the brainstem where the nerve roots for cranial nerve X are indicated in Figure 15–20, and travel to the chief and lower part of the sensory nucleus of V (see Figure 15–22, right side of brainstem, light green column).

Cranial nerve X includes an autonomic sensory component that carries sensation from the gut. These sensations are not conscious, as in the case of touch or pressure, but may result in a sense of "feeling good" or "feeling bad" (Wilson-Pauwels et al., 2002). Autonomic fibers also arise from chemoreceptors and the mucosal surface of the larynx. This information makes a first synapse in a pair of ganglia, which send fibers into the brainstem at the point of attachment of the vagus roots and subsequently make synapses in the nucleus solitarius (see Figure 15–22, right side, dark green column).

Cranial Nerve XI (Spinal Accessory Nerve)

Cranial nerve XI, which only has motor fibers, is called the spinal accessory nerve because its motor neurons are in the ventral horn of upper segments of the cervical spinal cord. Figure 15–22 (left side) shows the approximate location of this column of spinal cells, called the spinal accessory nucleus, extending from the junction of the medulla and spinal cord four or five segments down into the cervical spinal cord. Note how the spinal accessory nucleus is in line with the columnar nucleus ambiguus.

Why is a nerve with cells of origin in the spinal cord considered a cranial nerve? First, the nerve supplies motor innervation to two muscles of the head and neck, the *sternocleidomastoid* muscle and the *trapezius* muscle. The former muscle turns the head and lifts the chin toward the side opposite the contraction (when the right *sternocleidomastoid* contracts with its sternum end fixed, the head is turned and lifted toward the left side, and vice versa), and the latter muscle produces rotation of the scapula and raises the arm above the shoulder. Second, many authors regard the accessory nucleus as a continuation of the nucleus ambiguus. Both columns seem to be derived from the same embryological tissue. In fact, as reviewed in Chapter 3, some authors believe the spinal accessory nucleus may innervate muscles of the larynx along with branches of cranial nerve X. Third, the fibers issued from the accessory nucleus emerge from the spinal cord and ascend into the skull to travel with fibers of cranial nerves IX and X. Note in Figure 15–20 how the several rootlets of the accessory nerve emerge lateral to the inferior olive, like the rootlets of cranial nerves IX and X, and travel superiorly along the edge of the spinal cord. Cranial nerves IX, X, and XI exit (or, in the case of the sensory components of IX and X, *enter*) the skull through the same opening (the jugular foramen, a large opening in the base of the skull through which nerves pass).

Cranial Nerve XII (Hypoglossal)

Cranial nerve XII is regarded as strictly a motor nerve, innervating all the intrinsic muscles and all but one of the extrinsic muscles of the tongue (the exception being the *palatoglossus* muscle, innervated by cranial nerve X). The fibers of cranial nerve XII originate in the hypoglossal nucleus, a column of motor cells near the midline of the medulla (see Figure 15–22, left side). A horizontal section through the medulla, halfway between its upper and lower borders, shows the hypoglossal nuclei in the floor of the fourth ventricle, on either side of the midline (see Figure 15–27). Axons from these cells run ventrally and laterally to emerge as

The Final Common Pathway, Part I

What is this? The last path we will all travel? No, it is a term used when referring to a certain part of the motor system, the part containing nuclei of cell bodies whose axons go directly to muscles. The term "motor neuron" is typically reserved for the cells in these nuclei, which receive information primarily from descending fiber tracts coming from the cortex. They are the last stop before motor commands are sent via cranial and spinal nerves to muscles in the jaw, lips, rib cage wall, and other parts of the speech apparatus and body. The idea of a final common pathway recognizes that a particular motor nucleus in the brainstem or spinal cord may receive input from several different sources and be subject to a "net effect" of all those different inputs. The idea of a final common pathway in motor systems was originally formulated by the famous neurophysiologist Charles Sherrington, and described in his then revolutionary 1906 text, *The Integrative Action of the Nervous System*.

The Final Common Pathway, Part II

Think about the complex difference between the precision of tongue configuration for a fricative such as /ʃ/ and the rhotic /r/. Now consider the corticobulbar pathways that descend and make synapses with cells in the hypoglossal nucleus. The hypoglossal nucleus issues motor fibers that exit the brainstem as cranial nerve XII—the hypoglossal nerve—the final common pathway for fibers that control movements, configurations, and positions of the tongue. Brainstem nuclei and their associated nerves are often thought of as low-level but well-meaning cells, ensuring proper execution of motor commands to their target muscles. But somehow, cells within a motor nucleus "know" a lot about the kind of precision motor behavior required for articulatory behavior; the final common pathway is a lot more than common. How is this done? Are these cells "trained" by the cortex to issue commands for the complex behaviors of the tongue? Are there specific motor cells in the hypoglossal nucleus for configuration, speed, and so forth? Stay tuned, hints abound in the animal literature on tongue control, as well as in the control of, yes, the human hand.

cranial nerve XII on the ventral surface of the medulla, in the sulcus between the pyramid and the inferior olive (see Figure 15–20).

The control of both intrinsic and extrinsic tongue muscles by cranial nerve XII means that virtually any lingual behavior relevant to speech production is vested in the integrity of this nerve and its brainstem nuclei. Tongue positions, movements, and configurations include fine adjustments to create the precision configurations required for the grooved tongue of fricatives such as /s/ and /sh/, the gross adjustments of tongue position and configuration associated with distinctions between (for example) front and back vowels, and the speed and placement of the tongue as it moves within the vocal tract. Although some older theories of lingual muscle function and speech production viewed the intrinsic muscles as mostly associated with consonant production and the extrinsic muscle with vowel production, both muscle groups work together to produce tongue configurations and gestures for intelligible speech.

CORTICAL INNERVATION PATTERNS

This section describes the innervation of brainstem motor nuclei by cortical cells, and specifically of the motor nuclei associated with speech-related muscles of the head and neck. These nuclei include the motor nucleus of V (trigeminal), the facial motor nucleus, the nucleus ambiguus, the spinal accessory nucleus, and the hypoglossal nucleus. The cortical innervation of the oculomotor nuclei (oculomotor, trochlear, and abducens nuclei) is not discussed here, nor is the innervation of nuclei associated with outflow of the autonomic system (salivatory nuclei, dorsal motor nucleus of X).

Table 15–4 summarizes the innervation patterns for the five paired brainstem motor nuclei that control speech musculature of the head and neck. When both members of a specific motor nucleus pair receive input from the left and right motor cortices (from the primary motor cells in both the left and right hemispheres), the nuclei are bilaterally innervated. Table 15–4 classifies

Table 15–4. Cortical Innervation Patterns of the Brainstem Motor Nuclei for Speech Musculature

MOTOR NUCLEUS	INNERVATION
Motor nucleus of V (V)	Bilateral
Facial motor nucleus (VII)	Bilateral (upper face)
	Contralateral (lower face)
Nucleus ambiguus (IX, X, XI)	Bilateral
Accessory nucleus (XI)	Bilateral (*sternocleidomastoid* muscle)
	Contralateral (*trapezius* muscle)
Hypoglossal nucleus (XII)	Contralateral

Note. The cranial nerves associated with these motor nuclei are indicated in parentheses.

the motor nucleus of V, part of the facial motor nucleus, the nucleus ambiguus, and the accessory nucleus as receiving bilateral innervation. For example, both motor nuclei of V—on the left and right sides of the pons—receive corticobulbar projections from both the left and right hemispheres. Stated in another way, the left motor nucleus of V receives an ipsilateral projection from the left hemisphere and a contralateral projection from the right hemisphere. The mirror-image innervation pattern applies to the right motor nucleus of V.

Table 15–4 describes both contralateral and bilateral innervation of cells in the facial motor nucleus. The facial motor nucleus contains cells specific to muscles of the upper face and different cells specific to muscles of the lower face. Cells for control of the lower facial muscles receive only contralateral innervation from the cortex, whereas cells for control of the upper facial muscles receive bilateral innervation from the motor cortex. Raising your eyebrows in surprise, for example, involves commands from both sides of the motor cortex to both facial motor nuclei, whereas movement of the corner of your right lower lip is produced by commands from the left motor cortex to the right facial motor nucleus.

Like the facial motor nucleus, the accessory nucleus has both contralateral and bilateral innervation from the motor cortex. There is some dispute about the pathways from the motor cortex to the upper regions of the cervical spinal cord, where the accessory nucleus is located. The most conservative view is that the *sternocleidomastoid* muscle is innervated bilaterally, and the *trapezius* muscle contralaterally (DeToledo & David, 2001). Some authors (Wilson-Pauwels et al., 2002) claim that the *sternocleidomastoid* muscle is innervated only ipsilaterally—that is, the left motor cortex innervates only the left accessory nucleus, the right motor cortex only the right accessory nucleus. Because these muscles have relevance to speech performance only under high-effort conditions, further description of the innervation patterns of the accessory motor nucleus is not pursued here.

The hypoglossal nucleus, which controls muscles of the tongue, is the only motor nucleus of the brainstem with strictly contralateral innervation from the motor cortex. Tongue cells in the left motor cortex innervate cells in the right hypoglossal nucleus, and vice versa.

Why Innervation Patterns Matter

These innervation patterns have significance for clinical signs of neurological disease. Because the brainstem motor nuclei innervate the muscles of the speech apparatus ipsilaterally—that is, motor nuclei on the left and right sides of the brainstem innervate muscles on the left and right sides of the head and neck, respectively—knowledge of the innervation of the brainstem nuclei by cortical structures can lead to important clues concerning lesion location. These clues are based on the appearance of head and neck structures at rest, or their performance during voluntary maneuvers. For example, a unilateral, cortical lesion of cells that control muscles of the face should not result in a deficit of upper face control, but may result in a loss of lower face control on the side opposite the lesion. The unilateral cortical lesion will cause loss of input to facial motor nucleus cells that control the upper face on the same side (ipsilateral to the lesion) and to the facial motor nucleus for upper face control on the opposite side (contralateral to the lesion). In the case of an ipsilateral cortical lesion these facial motor nuclei still receive healthy ipsilateral and contralateral input from the undamaged motor cortex on the other side of the brain. This allows for more or less normal appearance and functional contraction of muscles of the upper face. The unilateral cortical damage does, however, result in a deficit in appearance and control of the lower face contralateral to the lesion. This is because the cells in the facial motor nucleus that control lower face muscles receive cortical input only from the contralateral hemisphere.

Consider several hypothetical clinical presentations. One person appears to have impairment of *all* facial muscles (upper and lower) on one side of the face, with normal-appearing muscles on the other side. With the face at rest, the impaired side might show, in varying degrees, a smoothed forehead (as opposed to the furrows created by normal tone in the muscles of the forehead), reduced depth or complete absence of the nasolabial fold (the fold of skin forming a line between the side of the nose and the corner of the mouth), and/or a drooping lower lip. Based on the innervation patterns described above, the presence of both upper and lower facial paralysis on one side but normal-appearing facial characteristics on the other side suggests a unilateral lesion in the facial motor nucleus in the pons, or in cranial nerve VII close to its exit from the brainstem and the skull, before it splits into various "local" nerves that supply individual muscles of the face (this is called a lower motor neuron lesion; see sidetrack on "Upper Versus Lower Motor Neuron Lesions"). Because brainstem motor nuclei innervate head and neck muscles ipsilaterally, the lesion in the brainstem or the cranial nerve is on the same side as the observed paralysis.

Why is it relatively easy to rule out a *cortical* lesion in the case of this half-face pattern of weakness/paralysis? The explanation is the bilateral innervation of the facial motor nuclei for muscles of the upper face, which means that a unilateral cortical lesion does not produce noticeable impairment of the upper face at rest. Only a unilateral, lower motor neuron lesion produces this set of signs. Bilateral cortical lesions result in paralysis on *both* sides of the face, as do bilateral lesions of the facial motor nucleus or cranial nerve VII close to its exit point from the brainstem. When both sides of the face are paralyzed, the distinction between bilateral cortical versus bilateral brainstem/cranial nerve lesions is not so difficult because a brainstem lesion large enough to affect both sides of the pons also produces marked effects on other behaviors, a description of which is beyond the scope of this chapter.

Similar reasoning applies to apparent paralysis of the velopharyngeal muscles or the larynx. The brainstem motor nucleus for the majority of velopharyngeal and laryngeal muscles is the nucleus ambiguus, which is innervated bilaterally from the motor cortex (see Table 15–4). If you ask a neurologically normal individual to open her mouth and observe the motion of the velum when she says "ah," the upward motion of the velar tissue flap is rapid and symmetrical when the velopharyngeal port is closed for the vowel production. A unilateral cortical lesion in cells associated with velopharyngeal muscles does not affect this rapid and symmetrical motion to a significant degree, because the nucleus ambiguus receives bilateral innervation from the cortex. A unilateral lesion in the nucleus ambiguus or in cranial nerve X, however, results in weakness on the same side of the lesion. When the patient says "ah," the upward movement of the velum is asymmetrical, with rapid elevation on the side of the healthy nucleus ambiguus and weak or no movement on the side of the brainstem/cranial nerve lesion. Similarly, a unilateral cortical lesion among laryngeal motor cells has little or no effect on normal vibration of the vocal folds, whereas a unilateral lesion in the nucleus ambiguus or cranial nerve X results in vocal fold paralysis on the same side as the lesion, which in many cases affects voice quality.

Unlike the cases of bilateral innervation reviewed above, a unilateral lesion of tongue cells in the motor cortex results in an observable deficit. The contralateral-only innervation of the hypoglossal nuclei suggests this expectation. For example, a unilateral lesion among tongue motor neurons in the right motor cortex affects the strength of muscles on the left side of the muscular complex of the tongue. The several muscles of the tongue are capable of very complex tongue motions and configurations, but a simple test of the integrity of tongue motion is to request an individual to protrude his tongue, in a straight line. In the neurologically healthy individual, the tongue is centered as it is protruded. The centering is the result of the equivalent strength of the musculature on either side of the tongue midline (primarily the *genioglossus* muscle) producing the protrusion. In a person with a unilateral cortical lesion in tongue cells, the tongue muscles on the side opposite the lesion are weak. When the tongue is protruded, the healthy side pushes the tongue "away from the lesion." For example, a lesion in the left motor cortex results in weakness of the *genioglossus* muscle on the right side of the tongue, which causes the tongue to deviate rightward when protruded from the mouth. The tongue deviates toward the weak side during a protrusion gesture because the "strong" *genioglossus* on the left side of the tongue is not balanced by an equally strong *genioglossus* on the right side of the tongue.

This scenario makes sense for a unilateral cortical lesion because of the exclusively contralateral innervation of the hypoglossal nuclei from the motor cortex. Deviation of the tongue on protrusion to one side or the other, however, is also symptomatic of a lesion to the

> ### Upper Versus Lower Motor Neuron Lesions
>
> There are motor neurons in the cortex, the brainstem, and the spinal cord. Cortical motor neurons send long axons to cells in both the brainstem and the spinal cord, which in turn send axons into the peripheral nervous system to end on muscles. Muscle control problems can result from damage anywhere along this path from cortex to muscle fiber. Neuroscientists and neurologists have a professional jargon to refer to sites of lesions along these motor pathways. "Upper motor neuron" lesions are those occurring in the cortical motor neurons or in the axons they issue, *before those axons make synapses with the motor neurons in the brainstem or spinal cord*. "Lower motor neuron" lesions are those occurring in the nuclei of the brainstem or motor cells of the spinal cord, or in the axons they issue and the peripheral nerves in which those axons travel. "Upper" motor neuron lesions result in muscles with excessive resting tone (stiff muscles) and hypersensitive reflexes. "Lower" motor neuron lesions result in loss of muscle mass (wasting, or atrophy), small muscle twitches visible to the naked eye (called fasciculations), and in some cases insufficient resting tone. In both upper and lower motor neuron lesions the involved muscles tend to be weak for tasks requiring strength.

hypoglossal nucleus or hypoglossal nerve on the *same side* as the lesion (and therefore, the same side of the weakness). Recall that the muscles of the head and neck are innervated *ipsilaterally* from the brainstem motor nuclei. A lesion in the right hypoglossal nucleus, or to the hypoglossal nerve exiting the right side of the brainstem, produces weakness of the muscles on the right side of the tongue. In the case of such a lesion, the tongue deviates to the right (weak) side when protruded, just as it does when there is contralateral cortical lesion.

In both cases described above, the tongue deviates to the side with weak muscles. In one case the weakness is the result of a contralateral, upper motor neuron lesion, in the other the result of an ipsilateral, lower motor neuron lesion (see sidetrack on Upper Versus Lower Motor Neuron Lesions). Because the clinical sign—deviation to the weak side—is the same for both lesion locations, is it possible to use other signs to identify the site of lesion? Lower motor neuron lesions typically produce fasciculations (small muscle twitches) and muscle wasting (atrophy), so a combination of tongue deviation to one side on protrusion with loss of muscle mass and fasciculations on the half of the tongue to which the deviation occurs suggests that the lesion is in the hypoglossal nucleus and/or cranial nerve XII. Conversely, tongue deviation to one side with no loss of muscle mass and no fasciculations is suggestive of an upper motor lesion on the side opposite the deviation.

The Cranial Nerve Exam and Speech Production

Table 15–4 and the summary provided in the Internet document "Cranial Nerve Tests" and the preceding section are guides to interpretation of lesion location when orofacial and laryngeal gestures deviate from expectations for the healthy brain. The tests described here, and especially those to distinguish upper from lower motor neuron damage, are conducted primarily with nonspeech (e.g., lifting the eyebrows versus lateralizing the corner of the mouth; protrusion of the tongue) or speechlike (saying /a/ quickly, or phonating an extended vowel) tasks. The value in understanding these tasks is partly in appreciating the "wiring" of the craniofacial apparatus, in knowing what a speech-language pathologist is looking for when she asks a client to protrude the tongue or examines the appearance of the face at rest, and in grasping an important part of the standard neurological examination. The results of these evaluations do not predict, with any degree of precision, actual speech production performance. A client may have some deviation of the tongue and some obvious facial weakness yet still have intelligible speech. Conversely, a client whose cranial nerve exam appears to be within normal limits may have obvious problems with conversational speech. The cranial nerve exam yields valuable information, but this information is specific to the tasks used in the clinical evaluation. Speech motor control, like general motor control, has been shown to be *task specific* (Weismer, 2006). A speech-language pathologist should not assume the results of the cranial nerve exam tell her all she needs to know about a client's *speech* motor control abilities. Additional reasons for caution in interpreting these standard neurological tests in terms of speech motor control are discussed in the concluding section of this chapter.

SPINAL CORD AND SPINAL NERVES

Spinal Cord

The spinal cord includes gray and white matter and extends as a long column of tissue from the first cervical vertebrae (C1) to the first or second lumbar vertebrae (L1, L2). The superior edge of the spinal cord is continuous with the inferior edge of the medulla. The inferior edge of the spinal cord terminates at L1 or L2, but the protective coverings of the brain (including the dura and arachnoid mater, labeled in Figure 15–28; see section below, "Meninges, Ventricles, Blood Supply") extend to nearly the bottom of the sacral vertebrae. Spinal nerves from the bottom of the spinal cord run inferiorly and exit below the inferior termination of spinal cord tissue.

A vertical segment of spinal cord tissue, plus its protective coverings and nerves exiting and entering the cord, is shown in Figure 15–28. The view is from the front and slightly above and to the right of a horizontal (transverse) slice across the cord. The roughly H-shaped, darker part seen in this transverse slice are clusters of cell bodies of neurons (gray matter). The whitish area surrounding these cells (white matter) are axons.

The size and form of the H-shaped cluster of cell bodies varies according to the level of the spinal cord at which a horizontal slice is made. The location of the cut in Figure 15–28 is at the lower end of the cervical cord, but the anatomical facts described in the next paragraphs apply to any level of the cord.

The anterior (ventral) midline of the spinal cord is defined by the *anterior median fissure*. The midline groove on the posterior (dorsal) aspect of the spinal cord is called the *posterior median septum*. At any level of the spinal cord, the H-shaped cluster of cell bodies is nearly symmetrical with respect to these anterior and posterior median landmarks. As labeled in Figure 15–28, the spinal cord gray matter has paired posterior horns and paired anterior horns. The "horns" are the clusters of cell bodies in the ventral (anterior) or dorsal (posterior) halves of a given transverse section. Dorsal horn cells are typically sensory, receiving input from axons traveling from peripheral body structures to the spinal cord, and ventral horn cells issue axons that exit the spinal cord to provide motor innervation to muscles.

The cells in the ventral horn gray matter are largely motorneurons. For the most part, the cells

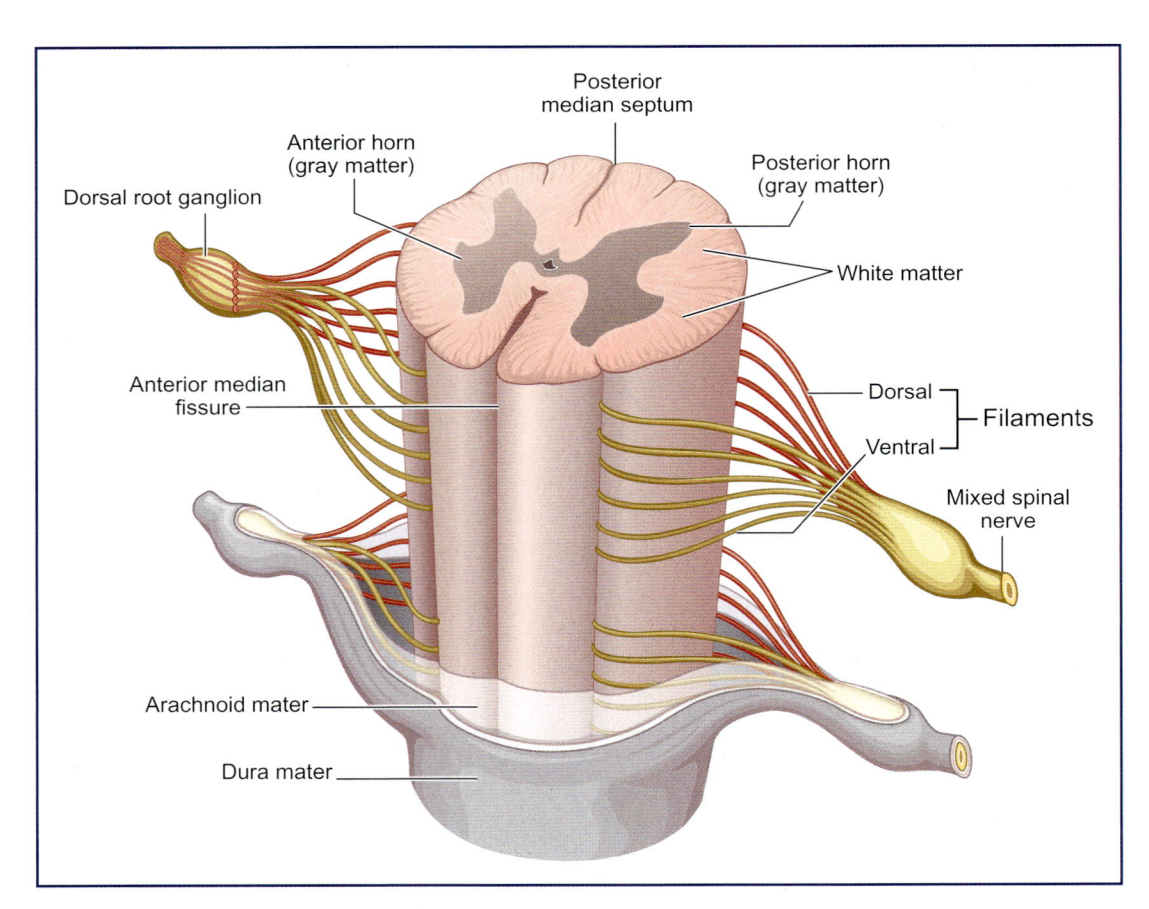

Figure 15–28. View of a section of the spinal cord from the front and slightly above a horizontal cut through the lower cervical cord. The horizontal cut shows the central gray matter in an H-shaped pattern and the white matter surrounding it. The dorsal and ventral root filaments entering and leaving the spinal cord, respectively, are also shown, as are the meningeal coverings.

issue axons that emerge from the spinal cord as spinal nerves, which innervate muscles. These motorneurons are the final common pathway in the transmission of information from the cortex to muscles of the limbs and torso. Some of the cell bodies in the ventral horn are connected to other ventral horns by short axons.

The white matter of the spinal cord is a dense composition of axons running in many different directions. In any transverse section, spinal cord white matter includes axons entering and leaving the cord, ascending and descending in the cord, and even traveling between cell bodies within the cord. The details of each of these fiber tracts are outside the scope of this text, but like the white matter in the cerebral hemispheres, fibers tracts within any section of the spinal cord are arranged systematically. For example, the corticospinal tract descends as a tight bundle in the lateral part of the spinal cord. This bundle is called the lateral corticospinal tract. At each level of the spinal cord, the lateral corticospinal tract issues axons to the anterior horn cells on the same side. Recall that a small proportion (about 20%) of motor fibers originating in the motor cortex do not decussate in the medulla, but continue into the spinal cord on the same side as their cortical origin. These fibers form the anterior corticospinal tract, which runs in the anterior (ventral) part of the spinal cord, just lateral to the anterior median fissure. Other motor tracts in the spinal cord are not discussed here.

Sensory fibers, primarily ascending in the spinal cord from posterior (dorsal) horn cells, run through several synapses in the brainstem and thalamus and terminate in cortical cells, many of which are located in the primary sensory cortex. In the spinal cord, these tracts run primarily in the posterior (dorsal) white matter columns lateral to the posterior median septum. These fibers carry information on touch, pain, and temperature from peripheral body structures.

Spinal Nerves

Spinal nerves are attached to each segment of the spinal cord (see Figure 15–28). The general organizational scheme for spinal nerves is as follows. Motor and sensory fibers are attached at different locations for a given segment of the spinal cord. Dorsal root filaments, which carry sensory information, enter the spinal cord close to the most posterior (dorsal) tip of the spinal gray matter. Ventral root filaments exit the spinal cord lateral to the anterior median fissure, close to the most anterior border of the anterior (ventral) horns. Note the use of the term "filaments": at each segment of the spinal cord, an entering or exiting nerve gives off several separate nerves. Figure 15–28 shows the sensory (dorsal) filaments as red fibers entering the spinal cord, and the motor (ventral) filaments as yellow fibers exiting the spinal cord.

At a very short distance from the entrance or exit of these nerves into or from the spinal cord there is a series of ganglia extending from the top to bottom of the cord. They are called dorsal root ganglia (see Figure 15–28) because they contain the first synapses for sensory fibers from peripheral structures en route to the spinal cord. On the left side of Figure 15–28, the sensory cells of one ganglion are represented by small red circles through which fibers run from the periphery to the dorsal horn of the spinal cord. When sensory fibers enter the spinal cord, the synapse made in a posterior horn cell is the *second* synapse in the sequence of information transfer from periphery to cortex. This is generally true for all sensory information in transit through the spinal cord, with the exception of sensory information derived from muscle spindles in voluntary muscles of the jaw, limbs, and trunk (see Internet document "Clinical Evaluation of Cranial Nerve Function"). Muscle spindles from the limbs, trunk, and jaw issue fibers that bypass ganglion cells and travel directly to either a sensory nucleus in the brainstem (jaw) or a dorsal horn segment in the spinal cord (limbs, trunk). In the case of muscle spindles in the jaw, the sensory fibers make a first synapse in the mesencephalic nucleus of V (see Figure 15–22, right side). The muscle spindles in jaw muscles are the basis of the jaw-jerk reflex, described in the Internet document "Clinical Evaluation of Cranial Nerve Function." By bypassing a synapse in a ganglion and making a first synapse in the spinal cord (limb and trunk) and mesencephalic nucleus of V (jaw), the speed of limb and jaw reflexes is increased.

Figure 15–28 shows motor nerves derived from anterior (ventral) horn cells exiting the spinal cord and running *through* a ganglion. These motor filaments do not make synapses within ganglia, but run through them and exit each ganglion "bundled" together with sensory fibers. Beyond the ganglia, toward the periphery, motor and sensory fibers run together in spinal nerves. Spinal nerves are therefore mixed (both sensory and motor) nerves. For example, the spinal nerves associated with the **internal intercostal** and **external intercostal** muscles are derived from from the first (T1) through eleventh (T11) thoracic segments (see Chapter 2). Sensory fibers from receptors in these muscles carry information back to the spinal cord concerning touch, pressure, and stretch (the latter via muscle spindles). Motor fibers in these nerves control the contraction properties of the muscles.

In general, the level at which a spinal nerve exits the spinal cord is consistent with the body level of the structures innervated by the nerves. Thus, arm and hand muscles are innervated by spinal nerves from cervical segments of the cord, rib cage wall muscles by spinal nerves from thoracic segments, and abdominal wall muscles from lumbar segments. Two well-known exceptions to this general rule are the diaphragm, which corresponds in position to the lower level of the thoracic cord but is innervated from the third through fifth cervical segments of the spinal cord, and the feet and legs, which are innervated from lumbar segments of the spinal cord.

NERVOUS SYSTEM CELLS

The CNS is composed of fluids, blood vessels, and several cell types. The cell types can be divided into the two major categories of *neurons* and *glia*. Imagine all the cells of the nervous system sitting in fluids—in the *extracellular spaces*—with very precise, yet changeable, chemistry. This chemistry is regularly changed on a short-term basis—in fact, millions of times per second—and on a long-term basis as well. Interactions between neurons and glial cells contribute to both the precision and changeability of the chemical profile. The traditional understanding of the difference between the two major types of cells is that neurons are the signaling cells in the brain, whereas glial cells do not transmit signals but provide support and nourishment for neurons. Signaling cells send information to other cells and receive information from one or many cells. This idea is familiar to students who have studied synaptic transmission in the brain (discussed more fully below). According to recent research, some glial cells may also receive and send signals, but in this chapter the traditional distinction between neurons and glial cells is emphasized.

Depending on the source, the human brain is said to contain roughly 80 to 95 billion neurons and either the same number or many more glial cells. Whatever numbers one chooses to accept, the brain contains a lot of cells packed into the relatively small container of the skull. The signaling cells send and receive an enormous amount of information per unit time, and in doing so generate and expend a tremendous amount of energy.

There is practical value in understanding the structure and physiology of nervous system cells, because many neurological diseases that have consequences for speech, language, and hearing behavior are explained partly or largely in terms of dysfunction of basic cellular anatomy and physiology. In addition, pharmacological and other treatments for these diseases often target aspects of basic cellular physiology. The following sections cover the structure and function of glial cells and neurons, the nature of the neuronal potentials (resting and action), synaptic transmission and neurotransmitters, and the neuromuscular junction.

Glial Cells

Figure 15–29 shows a neuron and some glial cells with which it shares brain space. The primary role of glial cells, according to present understanding, is to support the integrity of the signaling cells—the neurons—in several ways. Glial cells come in several forms, including *astrocytes, oligodendrocytes*, and others, as listed in Table 15–5.

The most numerous glial cells are *astrocytes*, shown in Figure 15–29 as star-shaped cells with appendage-like projections from a central body (other subtypes of astrocyte may have different forms). At one time astrocytes were thought of as not much more than biological filler material between neurons, but recent research suggests a much more important role for these cells. This role includes a contribution to the control of the chemical makeup of the extracellular (outside the cell) environment, including regulation of the molecules permitted to pass from the blood supply of the brain to the extracellular fluid (i.e., through the blood–brain barrier, see below). In addition, astrocytes form protective barriers around synapses, apparently to ensure that neurotransmitters released at a synapse do not spread to other locations where they are not needed or where they might interfere with other transmissions. Astrocytes also play a role in the removal of excess neurotransmitter after it has been released. Finally, astrocytes provide "anchors" for neurons, almost as if they were the skeletal framework on which neurons are hung.

Another type of glial cell lays down myelin on axons. Axons are the slim projections that carry electrical impulses from the cell body of a neuron to its terminus. Glial cells that wrap axons in myelin are called *oligodendrocytes* (in the PNS the analogous glia are *Schwann cells*). The oligodendrocytes in Figure 15–29 are shown extending short "arms" to the axon. These arms wrap the axon with the fatty substance myelin, described in greater detail below.

Other glial cells include those responsible for "cleaning up" dead material in the brain; these are called *microglia*. Finally, the fluid-filled ventricles of the brain contain ependymal cells along their walls. These cells generate the fluid (CSF) inside the ventricles. Ependymal cells are not technically glia because their embryological origin is different from the origins of astrocytes and oligodendrocytes. They are included here because they are not neurons.

Neurons

The structure of the neuron is critical to understanding its normal physiology, and how this physiology is affected by disease. Figure 15–30 is a schematic image

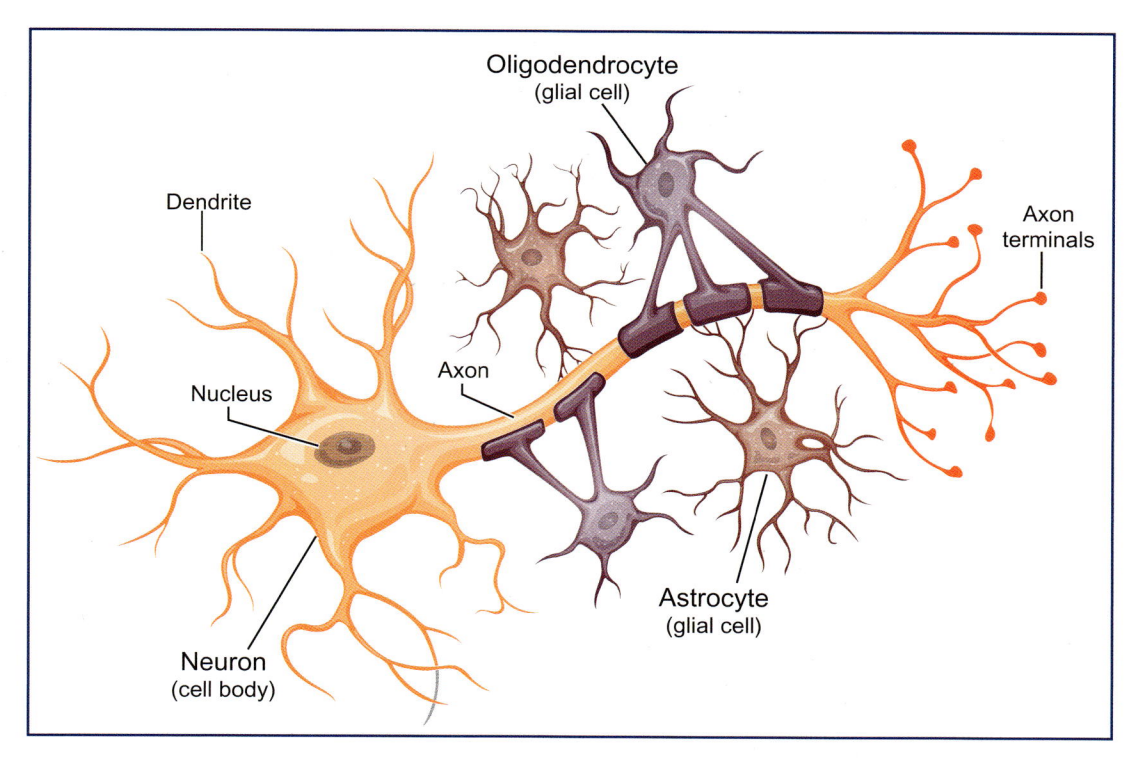

Figure 15–29. Neuron and glial cells.

Table 15–5. Types and General Functions of Neurons and Glial Cells

TYPE	FUNCTION
Glial	Nonsignaling
Astrocytes	"Anchor" neurons to blood supply. Regulate neuron extracellular environment.
Oligodendrocytes (Schwann cells in PNS)	Myelin-forming
Microglia	Clean up dead material
Ependymal	Produce cerebrospinal fluid
Neurons	Signaling
Many types	

of a neuron and several of its component structures. Neurons differ in size, shape, and complexity, dependent on their location and function within the brain. Table 15–5 therefore lists "many types" under the general heading of "neurons." All neurons, however, have a cell body (soma), dendrites, axon, and axon terminal called a terminal button (also referred to as a terminal segment or terminal *bouton*). Neurons reside in a fluid medium, or extracellular environment (shaded blue area in Figure 15–30). The structures inside the neuron are its intracellular components. The intracellular components of a neuron are separated from the extracellular environment by a membrane with special properties. The membrane is impermeable to various molecule types, but can change permeability to certain molecules by the action of substances manufactured within the cell body.

Cell Body (Soma)

The cell body or *soma* is typically a relatively large, spherical structure. To call the cell body "relatively

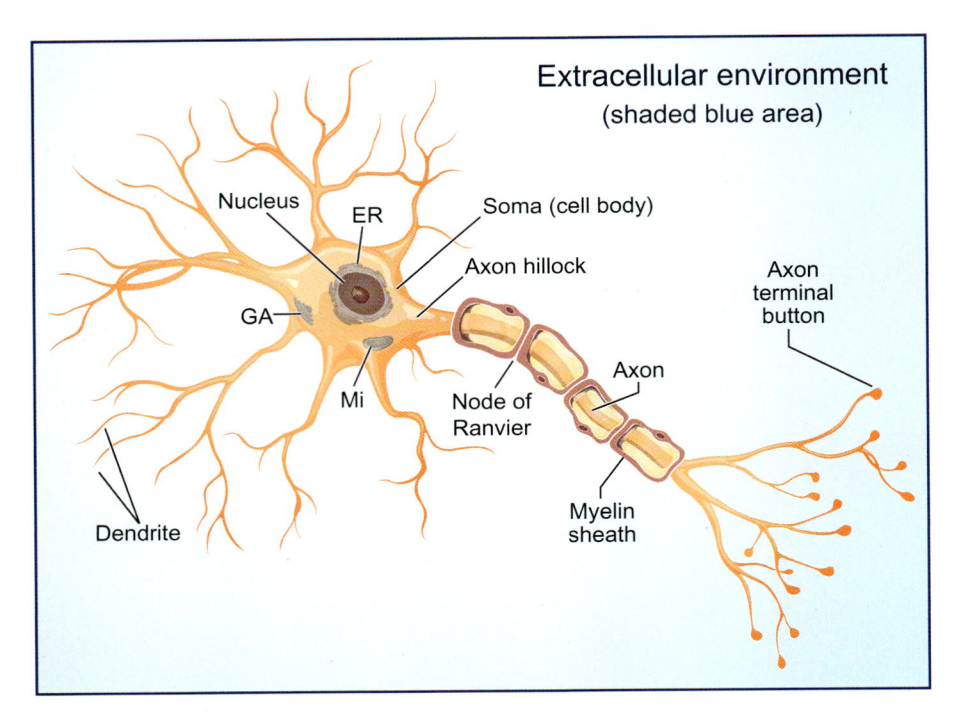

Figure 15–30. Neuron showing structures within the soma (ER = endoplasmic reticulum; Mi = mitochondria; GA = golgi apparatus) that manufacture proteins and neurotransmitters. The myelin sheath is not continuous down the entire length of the axon; the small gaps between adjacent myelin wraps are called nodes of Ranvier. Note the many dendrites associated with the soma, and the many terminal buttons of the axon.

large" is to describe the size of a tiny structure in a brain-world of other tiny structures. A typical soma is about 20 μm in diameter (0.000020 meters, perhaps 100 times smaller than the diameter of a poppyseed). Inside the cell body is the nucleus, as well as critical structures called *organelles*. Among the organelles shown schematically in Figure 15–30 are mitochondria (Mi), endoplasmic reticula (ER, where reticulum is the singular), Golgi apparatus (GA), and ribosomes (protein-synthesizing organelles, not labeled in the figure). These organelles serve the neuron's metabolic functions, generate proteins that affect the cell membrane's properties, and manufacture and transport neurotransmitters used to signal from one neuron to another.

The cell body and its contents are separated from the extracellular environment by a membrane composed of lipids (fatty and/or oily substances that are insoluble in water) in which numerous protein molecules are embedded. The membrane's permeability to various molecules can change very rapidly by the action of these proteins. These changes in permeability are critical to understanding the neuron's basic function of conducting electrical impulses.

The nucleus of a neuron, like the nucleus of almost any cell in the body, contains deoxyribonucleic acid (DNA). Information in the DNA is transported out of the nucleus by messenger ribonucleic acid (mRNA), into the main fluid of the cell body where the organelles are located. The function of mRNA is to link up with organelles such as the endoplasmic reticula and ribosomes to enable the synthesis of proteins. The newly synthesized proteins serve critical functions, one of which is to allow the cell body membrane to make very brief changes in its permeability to specific molecules. Changes in the membrane's permeability allow molecules to pass from the extracellular environment into the cell body, or from the cell body to the extracellular environment. Additional details of the process of protein synthesis in neurons are outside the scope of this chapter; the interested reader is referred to one of several outstanding neuroscience and general biology textbooks in which this information is presented in a highly readable form (Bear et al., 2016; Kandel et al., 2013).

The cell body contains microtubules which extend down the axon. These miniature tubes are like railway tracks extending from the cell body to the end of the axon. Proteins and other substances synthesized in the cell body are transported across these tracks, down the axon to its terminal button.

Finally, as shown in Figure 15–30, many branch-like projections from the cell body extend into the extracellular space. These projections are called *dendrites*, and the entire set of them extending from the cell body is called a *dendritic tree*. The surface of dendrite membranes is studded with protein molecules called *receptors*. Receptors detect specific neurotransmitters. The section below on "Synaptic Transmission and Neurotransmitters" provides information on how the terminal buttons of one neuron interact with the dendritic tree of a different, nearby neuron.

Axon and Terminal Button

Axons are cablelike projections that arise from the cell body at a location called the axon hillock. The axon ends at the terminal buttons. Axons can be very short in length (less than a millimeter) or very long (close to a meter). The axon is the means by which a neuron transmits an electrical impulse from the cell body to the terminal button(s).

The intracellular content of axons is distinct from that of the cell body of a neuron. The microtubules that extend from the boundary between the cell body and initial part of an axon (the axon hillock) extend to the terminal buttons where neurotransmitters are stored in vesicles. The protein-synthesizing organelles (the ribosomes) do the work of synthesizing and packaging neurotransmitters in the soma. The main function of the microtubules is to carry proteins to the terminal buttons. The intracellular contents of the terminal button(s) of an axon, which may include just a few or many buttons (Figure 15–30 shows about a dozen buttons), include numerous small "packets" called synaptic vesicles. These vesicles are tiny, membrane-encased packets of neurotransmitter. The terminal buttons also include many mitochondria, which indicates a high level of energy expenditure within this part of an axon.

The length of axon between the axon hillock and the terminal buttons has a wrapping-like covering called *myelin*, the fatty substance produced by oligodendrocytes. The oligodendrocytes wrap the axon with multiple, concentric rings of myelin. Figure 15–30 shows the myelin wrapping to be discontinuous from the axon hillock to terminal buttons. Intervals of myelin-covered axon are interrupted by very small breaks. The small breaks in the myelin wrapping are called *nodes of Ranvier*. As explained below, the myelin wrapping and nodes of Ranvier have great importance to the conduction of electrical impulses from the cell body to terminal *boutons*. Most axons in the CNS and PNS are myelinated, but certain functional systems (such as the pathways responsible for pain perception) have a fair number of unmyelinated axons.

Synapses

Figure 15–31 illustrates the essential features of a synapse. The typical synapse is the terminal button-to-dendrite synapse, but other synapse types—such as terminal button-to-soma, or even terminal button-to-axon—are also found in the CNS. Attention is focused here on the terminal-button-to-dendrite synapse. The inclusion of synapses under the general heading of "neurons" may be slightly misleading, because a synapse involves a collection of structures, including the extracellular environment. The collection of structures comprising a synapse includes a neuron's *presynaptic membrane* (membrane of the terminal buttons), the *postsynaptic membrane* (most typically the membrane covering a branch of the dendritic tree arising from the soma of a second, nearby neuron), and the extracellular substance separating and even *joining* the two membranes, called the *synaptic cleft*.

Presynaptic Membrane. The presynaptic membrane is the cell wall at the end of the axon and encases the synaptic vesicles within the terminal buttons. Embedded within the presynaptic membrane are special proteins which enable synaptic vesicles, under the right conditions, to attach and subsequently "dump" their neurotransmitter contents into the synaptic cleft. A single terminal button may contain synaptic vesicles storing different kinds of neurotransmitters; individual neurons are not limited to a single neurotransmitter. The presynaptic membrane can be thought of as the component of a synapse from which neural signals are sent.

Postsynaptic Membrane. The postsynaptic membrane is the receiving part of a synapse. This is where signals sent from the presynaptic membrane of one neuron are "picked up" for processing by another neuron. Like the presynaptic membrane, the postsynaptic membrane is partly composed of protein molecules that serve the specialized purpose of receiving these signals. These molecules form receptors designed not only to pick up neuronal signals in general, but to capture specific neurotransmitters. A postsynaptic membrane of a single neuron may contain receptors specialized for a variety of neurotransmitters, and even for subvarieties of one neurotransmitter.

Synaptic Cleft. The synaptic cleft is the "space" between the presynaptic and postsynaptic membranes. The scare quotes around the word "space" emphasize its miniature width (between 20 and 50 millionths of a millimeter). This cleft consists of a meshwork of proteins which not only serves as the medium through which a neurotransmitter is conveyed from the presynaptic (sending) to postsynaptic (receiving) membranes,

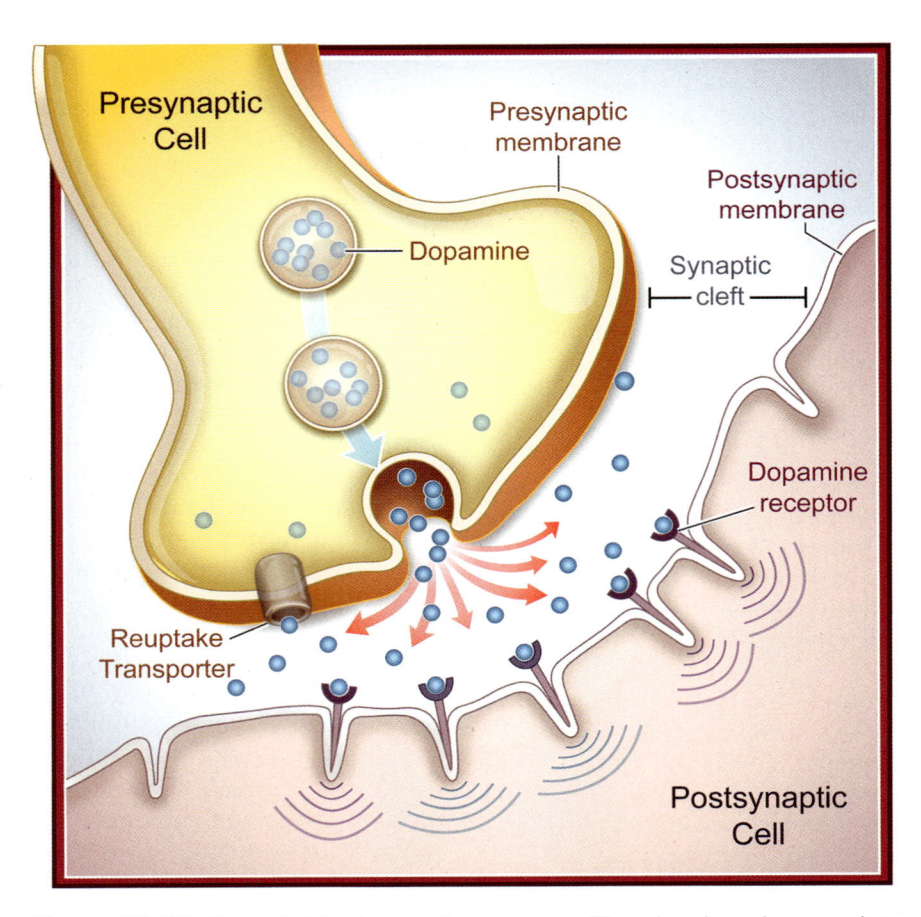

Figure 15–31. Essential features of a synapse. The drawing shows a terminal button, whose covering is called the presynaptic membrane. Inside the button are packets containing neurotransmitter molecules, illustrated in this drawing by dopamine molecules. The postsynaptic membrane, associated with a different neuron, is shown in light purple and separated from the presynaptic membrane by a small gap of extracellular fluid called the synaptic cleft. Embedded within the postsynaptic membrane are receptors specialized for a particular neurotransmitter; the receptors shown are dopamine receptors. The dopamine released from the presynaptic membrane "binds" to the dopamine receptors on the postsynaptic membrane. Excess neurotransmitter is usually released into the synaptic cleft, so a mechanism called the reuptake transporter brings the excess molecules back into the terminal button and repackages them for later use.

but also to attach the two membranes to each other. The presynaptic membrane, synaptic cleft, and postsynaptic membranes are bound together as an anatomical unit.

Resting Potential, Action Potential, and Neurotransmitters

Information is transmitted in the nervous system largely by the conversion of electrical energy into neurochemical energy, which is then transformed back into electrical energy. A key to understanding how neurons send electrical signals from the soma to the terminal buttons is an appreciation of the changeable characteristics of cell membranes. The following paragraphs present a brief, simplified introduction to this signaling process.

Resting Potential

Figure 15–32 shows a schematic neuron with a focus on the chemical, ionic environment of the soma and extracellular fluid when the neuron is at rest (not stimulated). Some of these ions have a positive electrical charge, whereas others have a negative electrical charge. The two most important, positively charged ions are potassium (K+) and sodium (Na+). The concentration of NA+ is much greater outside the cell body compared with inside the cell body, and the concentration of K+ is slightly greater inside the cell body as compared with outside the cell body. Within the cell body, in the intracellular fluid, a group of unspecified, negatively charged ions are shown. Keep in mind the schematic nature of this drawing: the depiction of K+ and Na+ ions does not mean these ions are exclusively outside or inside the cell body; it is the relative concentration that is important.

At rest, the membrane of a neuron cell body is relatively permeable—allows passage—to K+ molecules from inside the cell body to the extracellular fluid. On the other hand, the membrane is not permeable to Na+ molecules or the negatively charged ions concentrated inside the soma. The selective membrane permeability to K+ is the result of selectively "tuned" K+ openings within the cell membrane. These special openings are a relatively constant characteristic of the cell membrane. The presence of these openings helps explain how "ionic equilibrium," the equal and opposite electrical forces across the cell membrane that define the rest state of the cell, is achieved.

Before ionic equilibrium is established, K+ molecules are "naturally" concentrated *inside* the soma— their numbers inside the soma are greater than in the extracellular fluids. Ions with unequal concentrations in two locations always seek to establish equilibrium of concentration between these locations, which in the present case are the intracellular and extracellular regions. Because of the unequal concentration of K+ inside and outside the soma, the permanent openings to K+ within the cell membrane result in more K+ traffic outward to the extracellular fluid, compared with traffic inward to the intracellular fluid. When more K+ molecules pass out of the soma than move into it, the result is a more negative charge within the soma (intra-

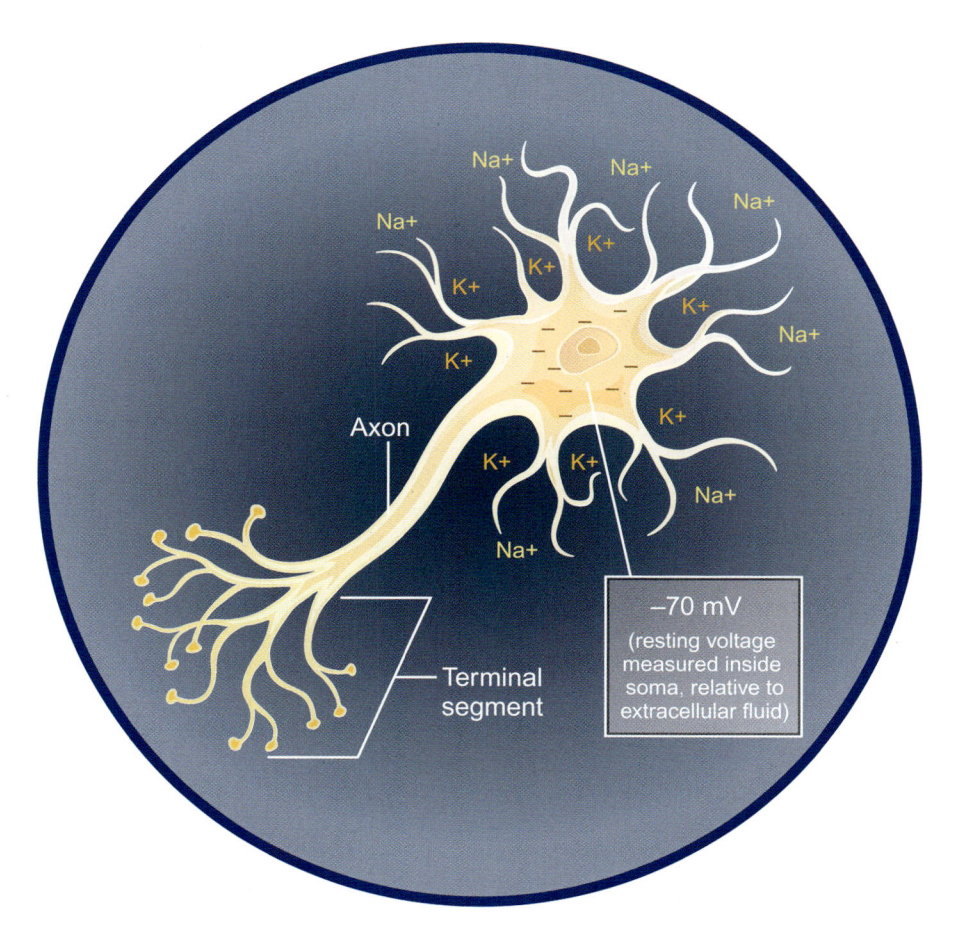

Figure 15–32. Drawing of a neuron showing the relative distribution of negative and positive ions inside the soma versus the extracellular fluid.

cellular fluid) relative to outside the soma (extracellular fluid.) The negative charge is also related to the high concentration of Na+ in the extracellular fluid: at rest, the cell membrane is not permeable to Na+. A critical phase in this process of net K+ movement to the extracellular fluid is when the tendency of the positively charged ions to leave the soma is exactly balanced by the negative electrical charge inside the soma. When this occurs, equilibrium is reached and stops the movement of K+ ions. This can be likened to two forces pulling with identical magnitudes in opposite directions. The K+ molecules exert a force to "run down" its concentration gradient from inside to outside the cell to establish K+ equilibrium. At the same time, the K+ ions are attracted back to the intracellular fluid as a result of loss of positive charges inside the cell. The loss of positive charge is due to the K+ ions running down its concentration gradient to the extracellular fluid. The negative charge inside the soma tries to "pull back" the positively charged ions. The movement of K+ ions leaving the soma and their simultaneous attraction back into the soma produces an electrical resting state. This, paired with the heavy concentration of Na+ outside the cell body comprises the ionic balance across the cell membrane at rest. Neither K+ or Na+ moves across the cell membrane at rest.

At rest, the neuron membrane is said to be *polarized*. Potentials refer to voltage differences between two points, and the electrical potential difference between the inside and outside of the cell body is roughly 70 millivolts (mV) (0.070 volts). Because the voltage inside the soma is negative relative to outside the soma, the resting potential of a neuron is expressed with a negative sign. In this electrical state, the neuron does not fire impulses down its axon.

Action Potential

An action potential is the change of the negative resting potential to a positive value, and the subsequent return of the potential to the negative resting value. These changes in membrane potential occur in response to stimulation of a sensory organ (induced by an external stimulus such as a change in shape of an end organ resulting from touch, or exposure of an organ to light, as in vision), or due to exposure of the neuron's membrane to neurotransmitters released by another, nearby neuron. The action potential occurs very rapidly (on the order of 1/1000th of a second, or 1 ms), and propagates down the entire length of the axon to its terminal button. The arrival of the action potential at the terminal button causes packets of neurotransmitter to be "dumped" into the synaptic cleft between the terminal button and the dendrites of an adjacent neuron (or neurons). The more detailed description of the action potential presented below is highly schematic; for greater detail on the molecular basis of the action potential, Kandel et al. (2013) is an excellent source.

Figure 15–33 shows a schematic action potential. The *x*-axis is time (units = ms), the *y*-axis voltage (units = mV). The red trace shows the voltage measured inside the soma relative to the voltage of the surrounding extracellular fluid as a function of time. The narrow, blue-shaded rectangle extending across the time axis shows a small range of membrane potentials (between −60 mV and −80 mV) consistent with the typical resting potential of about −70 mV. In this drawing, the action potential trace begins within this range. Less than half a millisecond after the beginning of the trace, the potential begins to move in the positive direction, toward zero, indicating that the neuron has been stimulated. The potential begins to change in the positive direction when the stimulation causes the membrane

---

Faster Than the Speed Of . . .

Nerves conduct action potentials very, very quickly. A general rule is that myelinated nerves conduct impulses faster than unmyelinated nerves, and within the class of myelinated nerves, those with larger axonal diameters conduct impulses faster than those with smaller diameters. How quick is quick? The ulnar nerve, a mixed (motor and sensory) nerve that exits the spinal cord around the first thoracic (T1) segment of the spinal cord, carries motor impulses to muscles of the forearm and pinky finger at a speed of at least 60 m/sec. For those of you who do not like metric, that's about 134 miles per hour. Closer to home, the facial nerve conducts motor impulses at a speed of roughly 50 m/sec, and the motor part of the trigeminal nerve (to jaw muscles) conducts at a rate of about 55 m/sec. Some nerve fibers conduct at slower speeds, such as those that lack a myelin wrapping or have just a thin myelin sheath; these are primarily fibers that carry the sensations of pain and temperature, and their conduction speeds may be no more than 20 m/sec. Everyone has had the experience of touching something hot and realizing it only after what seems to be a long time. This experience reflects the relatively slow conduction speed of thin or unmyelinated neural pathways. The time between stimulation of the temperature receptors and recognition of the heat seems relatively long.

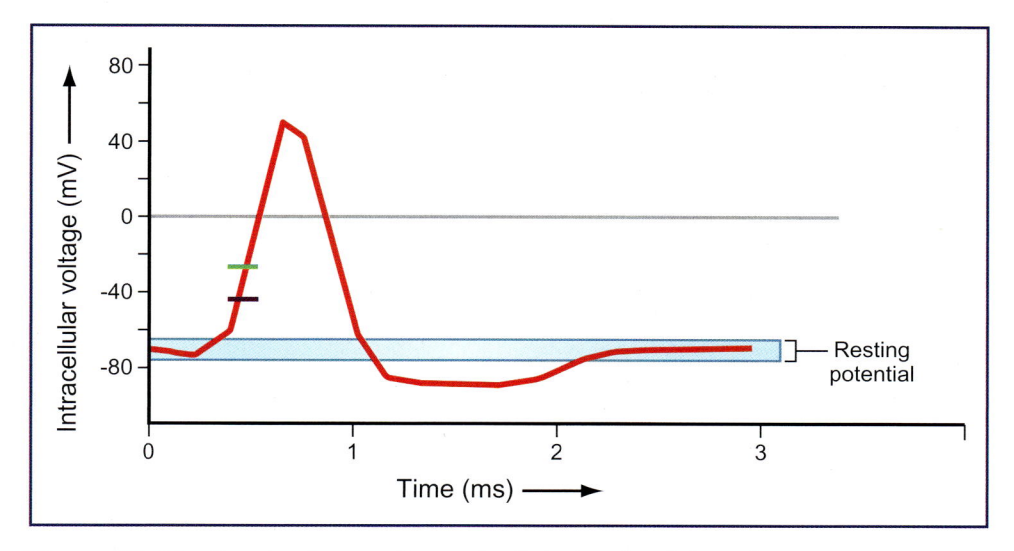

Figure 15–33. Graph of an action potential, showing intracellular voltage (in mV, relative to the voltage of the extracellular fluid) on the *y*-axis and time (in ms) on the *x*-axis. The range of resting potential values is shown by the blue rectangle centered on an intracellular voltage around −70 mV. The dark purple, horizontal line shows the voltage change that must be reached to produce the "all-or-none" action potential, and the green horizontal line shows the cell potential at which the K+ channels are opened to reestablish the resting potential, as described in the text. Both events are examples of voltage-gated membrane permeabilities to specific ion flows.

to become moderately permeable to Na+ ions, which at rest were concentrated in the extracellular fluid relative to the inside of the soma. When the membrane becomes permeable to Na+ the ions move down their concentration gradient to the inside of the cell body. The initial stimulation of the neuron, by an external event or neurotransmitter, causes *some* Na+-specific channels in the soma membrane to open, allowing a modest flow down the concentration gradient, into the cell body. The membrane potential therefore begins to change in a positive direction.

The real action in the action potential begins when the changing membrane potential reaches a value of roughly −45 mV. At this voltage level, a "threshold effect" occurs and a huge number of Na+ channels in the membrane are instantly opened, allowing a rush of Na+ into the cell body. This threshold is indicated in Figure 15–33 by the short, horizontal, dark purple bar that crosses the rising action potential trace. The term "voltage-gated sodium channel" refers to a special membrane pore that is switched on, like flipping a switch, when a specific membrane potential (voltage) is reached. Considering the thousands and thousands of voltage-gated channels on each neuron membrane, their simultaneous opening at the threshold voltage allows the rush of Na+ into the soma. As seen in Figure 15–33, this causes the potential to shoot up past zero and perhaps as high as +40 mV, *depolarizing* the membrane in less than 1 ms. A depolarized membrane is one in which the normal (resting) negative potential is "flipped" into the positive region for a very brief interval. The depolarized membrane initiates the conduction of electrical impulses down the axon, to the terminal button.

As shown in Figure 15–33, the action potential is not only defined by the rapid increase from a negative to a positive membrane potential, but also by the reversal of this process and a return to a negative potential. The return to a negative potential is, for a brief time, to a value slightly *more negative* than the resting potential of −70 mV. Why does this happen? First, when the action potential approaches its peak positive value, the Na+ channels are closed as suddenly as they were opened; this is another voltage-gated channel effect. The cessation of Na+ ions rushing into the soma initiates the process of repolarizing the cell membrane. But another mechanism is equally if not more important in repolarizing the membrane potential, and this is the result of the large number of voltage-gated K+ channels in the cell membrane. Very shortly after the threshold voltage has been reached and the Na+ channels have been instantly opened (see Figure 15–33, purple bar), the depolarization triggers a relatively slow (relatively slow on a "neuron-time" scale, that is) opening of K+ channels. The voltage at which this occurs is indicated by the green bar on the action potential trace. Keep in mind, when the membrane is strongly depolarized—when positive ions inside the membrane are more concentrated than outside the membrane—there should be a strong gradient for K+ to flow from inside to outside the membrane (the reverse of the gradient direction during the resting potential). When the voltage-gated K+ channels are turned on shortly after depolarization, by the time the action potential has reached its maximum value the K+ channels are wide open and allow positive ions to rush out of the soma into the extracellular fluid. For a short period of time this drives the membrane potential into the negative range, to a value more negative than the resting potential of around −70 mV. This is shown in Figure 15–33 where the potential dips below the resting potential rectangle, between 1 and 2 ms along the time scale, before returning to a typical resting potential value. The time period during which the soma potential is more negative than the resting potential is called the refractory period; the neuron is said to be *hyperpolarized*. The refractory period makes the neuron relatively unresponsive to stimulation—the neuron's ability to be depolarized is reduced.

When the cell membrane is depolarized, the change in electrical potential from negative to positive propagates down the axon, to the terminal buttons where neurotransmitter is stored in tiny packets. One way to think about the conduction of the action potential down the axon is like a fuse that, when lit at the end, continuously ignites along the extent of the burning material until reaching its destination, where the effect produced is, say, an explosion. This analogy is not a bad one, but is a bit off the mark for two reasons. First, the end effect of the propagating action potential, when it reaches the terminal button, is not to initiate an explosion but rather a set of complicated processes designed to unload neurotransmitter into the synaptic cleft. Second, the fuse analogy is explicitly one of continuous depolarization down the axon, but for the great majority of neurons the propagation is not continuous, but rather "jumps" from section to section of the axon.

The explanation for the action potential jumping down the axon, rather than propagating continuously, is revealed by the anatomy of a typical neuron, as shown in Figure 15–30. The myelinated wrap around the axon functions as an electrical insulator for the flow of current through the axon that results from depolarization of the soma. The nodes of Ranvier, the regular interruptions in the myelin sheath, are shown in Figure 15–30. The lengths of myelin wrapping are represented by the purple rectangles. The axons are visible inside the myelin wrapping by the artist's trick of making the wrapping transparent. The action potential appears to jump down the axon from one node of Ranvier to the next. The jumping action potential is referred to as *saltatory transmission* (the word "saltatory" having a Latin origin meaning leaping, or dancing). The net effect of the myelin wrapping and the jumping action potential is to make transmission of electrical impulses from soma to terminal button very fast. Healthy myelin wrapping is critical to an efficiently and effectively functioning nervous system; demyelinating diseases such as multiple sclerosis slow neural transmission and may cause a range of sensory and motor problems.

Synaptic Transmission and Neurotransmitters

A good grasp of the concepts of resting potential, depolarization, and hyperpolarization is important to understand how signaling is accomplished in the nervous system. The following discussion focuses on action potentials in the CNS, where the properties of neuron membranes and their ability to change polarity (electrical charge) are largely dictated by the chemicals to which they are exposed. Signaling in the nervous system—sending messages from one brain region to another—is largely a recurring process of conversion of energy forms. The most typical of these energy conversions is from an electrical to a chemical form, and then back to an electrical form. When the action potential (electrical energy) reaches the terminal button of the axon, processes are initiated that cause neurotransmitter (chemical energy) to be released into the synaptic cleft. In the synaptic cleft these chemicals bathe the membrane of an adjacent neuron's dendrites, and in so doing affect the membrane properties. The effect on the membrane properties is to open or close ion channels, which may result in a change in the membrane's polarity. The membrane is either depolarized or hyperpolarized. The electrical-chemical-electrical pattern of energy conversion recurs constantly over time and space (that is, in different brain regions at the same time, or the same brain region at different times). This constant demand for energy conversion and consumption in the brain explains why the metabolic requirements of brain function are disproportionately large relative to the weight of the organ.

The terminal button of a neuron contains packets of neurotransmitter, shown in Figure 15–31 as blue dots that represent neurotransmitter molecules. The neurotransmitter and their packets are manufactured and packaged in the cell soma (or in certain cases in other parts of the neuron) and transported down the axon to the terminal button. When an action potential propagates down an axon and reaches the terminal button, a series of chemical reactions (not described here) cause some of these packets to dump their neurotransmitter contents into the synaptic cleft, represented in Figure 15–31 as the very light blue "medium" between the terminal button and the curved, purplish surface depicted "across the way" from the end of the terminal button.

This curved surface represents the membrane of a dendrite extending from the soma of a postsynaptic neuron; this surface is adjacent to the terminal button of the presynaptic neuron. The dendritic membrane is studded with special organs, shown here as small spikes with semicircular receptacles reaching into the synaptic cleft. These special organs are neurotransmitter receptors, typically "tuned" for specific neurotransmitter types. When the action potential moving down the presynaptic axon reaches the terminal button, causing the neurotransmitter molecules to be dumped into the synaptic cleft, some of these molecules "bind" to the dendritic receptors that are tuned for their chemical properties. The binding of neurotransmitter molecules to these receptor sites is shown by the blue dots sitting within the semicircular receptacles.

The neurotransmitters that bind to these receptors modify the permeability of the dendrite membrane. Some neurotransmitters make the membrane more permeable to Na+, resulting in an inflow of positive ions to the cell body and the generation of an action potential. This neurochemical gating of ion channels is directly analogous to the voltage-dependent gating described above; the difference is in what causes the channels to open. A neurotransmitter that causes Na+ channels to open and flips the negative resting potential to a positive one is referred as an *excitatory* effect, because it causes the postsynaptic neuron to fire. Other neurotransmitters close membrane channels that permit positive ions to flow into the cell body. This makes the membrane potential more negative (hyperpolarized), which inhibits the production of an action potential. The neurotransmitters that hyperpolarize membrane potentials are called *inhibitory*.

One of the many interesting aspects of brain neurochemistry is that the clinical effect on human behavior of drugs that block or amplify a neurotransmitter depends on which part of the synapse the drug acts upon. Clinical effects are likely to be different for drugs that affect the presynaptic release of a given neurotransmitter than those that affect the postsynaptic uptake of the same neurotransmitter.

The discussion to this point has used a single neuron (see Figure 15–30), or a zoom view of parts of two neurons separated by a synaptic cleft (see Figure 15–31), to illustrate the action potential and the signaling capability of neurons by electrical-chemical-electrical conversion across synapses. In reality, each neuron in the CNS receives input from many neurons and delivers output to many neurons. The dendritic tree is extensive, as are the multiple terminal buttons projecting from the axon. This allows the brain to receive and send neural information from and to many other neurons. The situation is even more complex because many neurons are not specialized for a specific neurotransmitter; they have receptors on dendrites for multiple neurotransmitters, and may package more than one neurotransmitter in their terminal buttons. The receptors on the dendrites may be tuned to both excitatory and inhibitory neurotransmitters, and the terminal buttons may contain packages of both types. How does this work?

Think of the many inputs converging on the dendrites of a single neuron as summing their effects on the dendritic membrane, with the net effect determining the dendritic membrane potential. The dendrites of a given neuron may receive thousands of excitatory inputs (neurotransmitter baths from multiple neurons) that open ion channels, and thousands of inhibitory inputs that close these same channels and perhaps also allow negatively charged ions into the cell. If there are more excitatory inputs than inhibitory inputs, the net effect is excitatory and an action potential is generated in the neuron receiving the multiple inputs. The opposite situation hyperpolarizes the cell, maintaining or exaggerating the negative membrane potential. Summed over millions and millions of neurons, the state of brain activity at any given moment is very much a statistical process involving net inputs and outputs.

Neurochemically gated ion channels involve a large range of neurotransmitter types. Some well-known (and well-studied) neurotransmitters are listed in Table 15–6, together with their primary function (excitatory or inhibitory) and primary role in behavior. It is important to understand the use of the term "primary" function. A neurotransmitter may have a primary excitatory function (such as acetylcholine) but still be able to produce inhibitory effects when binding to specialized, inhibitory receptors. Similarly, a neurotransmitter may play a primary role in motor control (such as dopamine or acetylcholine), yet also have major involvement in functions such as memory and attention. This summary table is not only a simplification of the complex functions and roles of the selected entries, but also omits a good number of other neurochemicals known to affect signaling in the nervous system.

Neuromuscular Junction

The neuromuscular junction is a special type of synapse in the PNS. It is the location at which the terminal

Table 15-6. Well-Studied Neurotransmitters in the Human Brain, Their Primary Function, and Some Behaviors with Which They Have Been Linked

NEUROTRANSMITTER	PRIMARY FUNCTION	BEHAVIORS
Glutamate	Excitatory	Widespread (memory, learning)
GABA	Inhibitory	Widespread (muscle tone)
Dopamine	Excitatory	Motor, mood, reward
Norepinephrine	Excitatory	Mood, attention, sleep, pain
Epinephrine	Excitatory, inhibitory	Blood pressure, airway diameter
Serotonin	Excitatory, inhibitory	Mood, arousal
Acetylcholine	Excitatory	Muscle contraction (sk)
	Inhibitory	Muscle contraction (ht)

Note. GABA = gamma aminobutyric acid; sk = skeletal; ht = heart.

buttons of motor axons make contact with specialized receptors on the surface of muscle tissue. A schematic drawing of a neuromuscular junction is shown in Figure 15–34, where a terminal button of a motor axon is shown adjacent to a motor endplate on muscle tissue. A motor endplate contains specialized receptors sensitive to the neurotransmitter acetylcholine. As shown in Figure 15–34, packets of acetylcholine are stored in the terminal buttons of motor nerve axons. When an action potential travels down a motor nerve axon and reaches the terminal button, acetylcholine is released into the synaptic cleft separating the terminal button from the motor endplate. The terminal button at a neuromuscular junction is the presynaptic membrane, and the motor endplate is the postsynaptic membrane. The release of acetylcholine into the synaptic cleft results in binding of the neurotransmitter to specialized acetylcholine receptors embedded in the motor endplate. This binding opens Na+ channels in the muscle tissue membrane, resulting in a postsynaptic potential that causes the underlying muscle fibers to slide across each other.

This is the microview of what happens when a motor endplate is depolarized. The macroview is that the summed effect of the bathing of acetylcholine receptors on the many motor endplates within a whole muscle causes many individual muscle fibers to slide across each other and produce a contraction in the entire muscle.

Voluntary (skeletal) muscles have many motor end plates, but as a general rule muscles involved in more precise movements (such as those of the fingers or larynx) have many more motor endplates per unit area of muscle tissue compared with muscles that produce gross movements (such as muscles of the trunk). Motor endplate distributions have been studied in limb and trunk muscles, but not so much in orofacial muscles.

A disease called *mysasthenia gravis* (MG) is specifically associated with neuromuscular junction disease. In MG the immune system attacks the acetylcholine receptors, rendering many of them nonfunctional. This results in muscle weakness and rapid fatigue of muscular effort. The weakness and fatigue may affect the speech apparatus and result in a speech motor control disorder.

On the presynaptic side of the neuromuscular junction, the release of acetylcholine from storage packets in the terminal button can be inhibited by administration of botulinum toxin, more commonly known as Botox®. The drug works by preventing the packets from attaching to the presynaptic membrane, an important first step in the "dumping" of a neurotransmitter into the synaptic cleft. Botox® is perhaps best known as a cosmetic drug, used to offset the effects of aging on muscles of the facial area (e.g., to eliminate wrinkles). Botox® is also used to treat certain neuromuscular disorders in which excessive amounts of muscle contraction cause disruption of movement. For example, Botox® may be used to inhibit the excessive muscle contractions in the basal ganglia disorder called *dystonia*. Dystonia causes initiation of a purposeful action (such as turning the head to look to the left or right) to evolve into sustained and excessive muscle contractions. A voice and speech disorder called spasmodic dysphonia (SD) is thought to be a dystonia focused in the larynx and surrounding structures (Ludlow, 2011). Botox®, injected directly into the vocal folds, can relieve spasms in the laryngeal muscles and the resulting interruptions

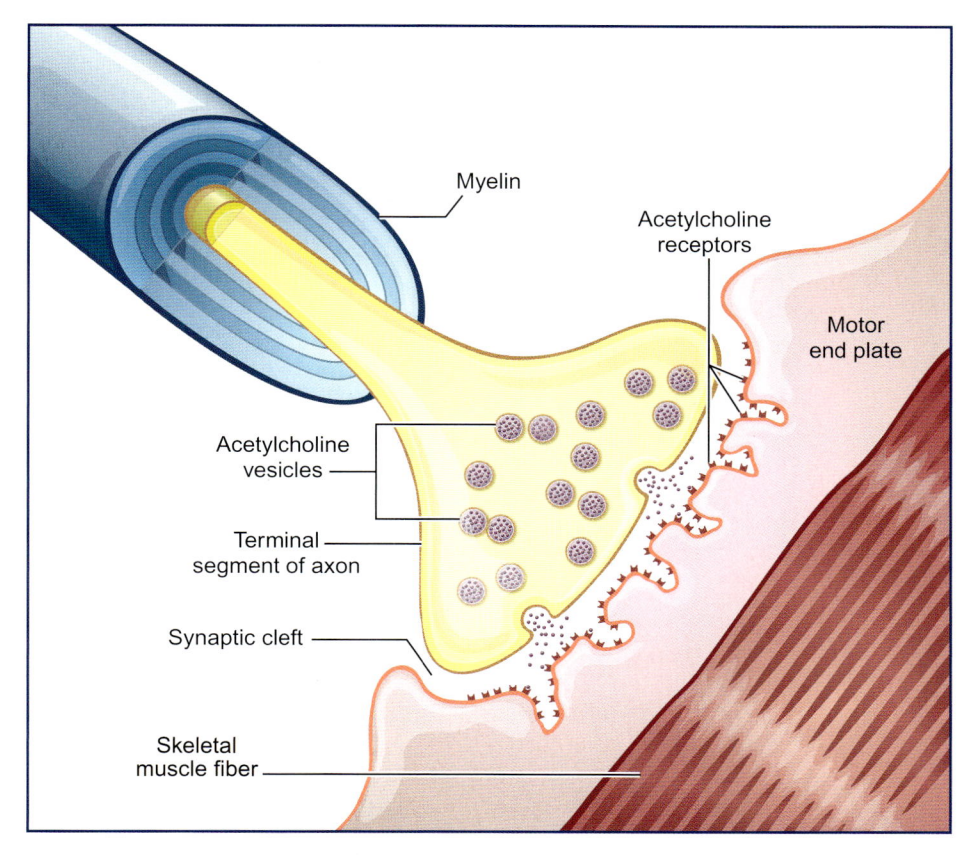

Figure 15–34. A neuromuscular junction, the specialized synapse at the junction between a peripheral motor nerve and muscle tissue. The terminal button containing packets of the neurotransmitter acetylcholine is the presynaptic component of the synapse, and the motor endplate is the postsynaptic component. Embedded within the motor endplate are specialized receptors for acetylcholine. When acetylcholine released by the presynaptic membrane binds to receptors in the motor endplate, the muscle fibers are depolarized and contract.

of phonation characteristic of this disorder (van Esch, Wegner, & Stegeman, 2017). The presumed therapeutic mechanism, both in SD specifically and dystonia more generally, is the reduction of acetylcholine released at the neuromuscular junction and therefore less powerful muscle contractions.

MENINGES, VENTRICLES, BLOOD SUPPLY

In this section the coverings of the brain, the cavities within the CNS that produce, contain, and transport CSF, and the brain's blood supply are described. These three major areas of brain anatomy and physiology are considered together because they have interrelated functions.

Meninges

The cerebral hemispheres, the brainstem, and spinal cord are masses of cells and fiber tracts encased by layers of nonneural tissue. These casings serve a protective function, as well as other functions related to metabolic activities of neural tissue. The brain "floats" inside this protective housing. The layers of tissue providing this protective function are collectively called the meninges (the plural of the Greek word *meninx*, meaning "membrane").

An artist's rendition of the relationship of the cortex and its underlying white matter to the meningeal covering layers is shown in Figure 15–35 (bottom image). Imagine this rectangular slab of multilayered tissue shown in the coronal plane to be extracted from the top part of the head, a centimeter or two posterior

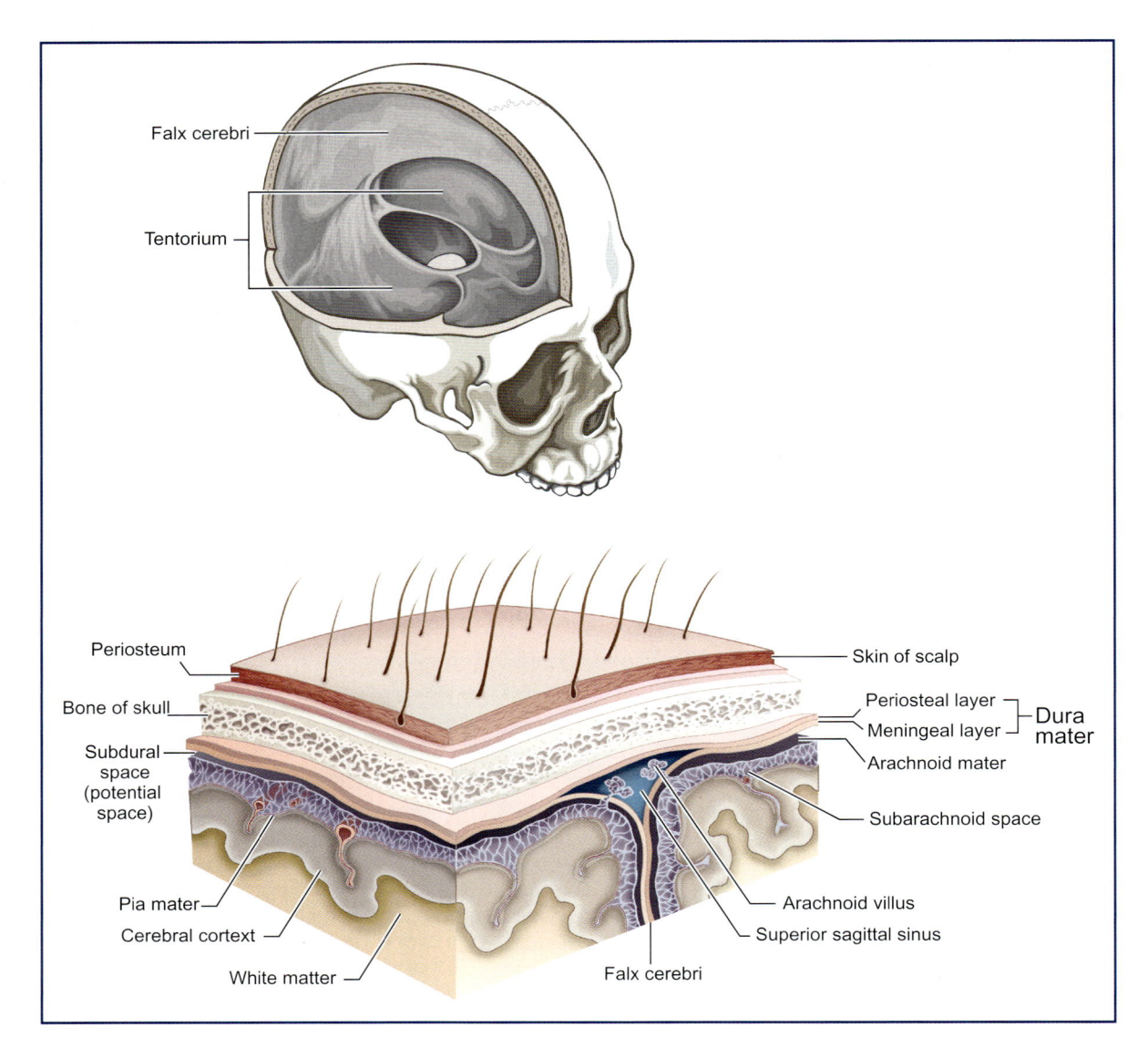

Figure 15–35. Rectangular slab of skull plus part of cerebral hemisphere (*bottom image*), showing the meningeal layers and associated spaces relative to the underlying nervous system tissues. The various folds of the dura mater are shown (*top image*) with all brain tissue removed; note the falx cerebri and the tentlike covering—the tentorium cerebelli—of the brainstem and cerebellum created by the infoldings of the dura mater.

to the top of the forehead. This view shows white matter toward the inferior edge of the slab, and the cortical layer of gyri and sulci above it. The labels for white matter and cerebral cortex are shown in the sagittal plane view, on the left side of the slab.

Above the cortex and its underlying white matter are multiple layers of tissue. The top layer is the skin of the scalp (with hairs protruding from it), beneath which is a relatively thick, bony layer, the skull. Immediately beneath the skull is the most superficial layer of the meninges, the dura mater. Deep to this layer is the arachnoid mater, followed by the pia mater, the deepest layer of the meninges. The dura, arachnoid, and pia mater form the meninges of the brain.

Dura Mater

The term "dura mater" means "tough mother," an appropriate term because the tissue has a leathery, hidelike texture. Figure 15–35 (bottom image) shows the dura mater as tissue in two layers, the more superficial of which is called the periosteal layer, the deeper one the meningeal layer. The periosteal layer of the dura mater adheres to the underside of the bony skull, whereas the meningeal layer is in contact with the arachnoid mater. These two layers of the dura mater are labeled toward the upper right edge of the coronal plane "wall" of the slab. The dura mater also continues inferiorly to encircle the spinal cord.

As shown on the coronal face of the slab (see Figure 15–35, bottom image), the meningeal layer separates from the periosteal layer toward the midline, to form a barrier between the left and right hemispheres. The bilayered dura mater approaches the midline, and the meningeal layers on either side dip inferiorly and form a nearly vertical separation between the tissues of the two hemispheres. This partition is called the falx cerebri; it runs from the front to the back of the hemispheres. When viewed in the sagittal plane, the falx cerebri forms a sheet having the shape of the letter C rotated 90 degrees clockwise. The anterior-to-posterior extent of the falx cerebri is roughly the same as the anterior-posterior extent of the corpus callosum, which sits immediately ventral to the inferior edge of the falx. The falx cerebri is shown in a separate image at the top of Figure 15–35, an image drawn with all brain tissue removed from the contents of the skull cavity. In this image, the darker gray folds depict "infoldings" of the meningeal layer of the dura mater.

The tentorium cerebelli is formed from another separation of the meningeal layer of the dura mater from the periosteal layer. This part of the dura mater is like a tent (hence, "tentorium") draped over the brainstem, separating it from the cerebral hemispheres. The tentorium cerebelli also forms a boundary between the cerebellum and the ventral surface of the occipital lobes. Although the configuration of the tentorium cerebelli is difficult to appreciate in a two-dimensional drawing, Figure 15–35, top image, shows the tentlike structure with an opening in the middle, formed by the infoldings of the meningeal layers of the dura. The cerebral hemispheres are above this opening, the brainstem and cerebellum below it. The posterior edge of the opening is the midline of the dural covering that separates the cerebellum from the ventral surfaces of the occipital lobes. When you hear the term "supratentorial," reference is made to a structure or disease process (such as a stroke or tumor) above the opening between the cerebral hemispheres and brainstem. "Infratentorial" refers to structures or disease processes below this opening, in the brainstem and/or cerebellum. In clinical settings, the term "transtentorial herniation" refers to a pathological process in which parts of the cerebral hemispheres—most typically medial structures of the temporal lobes—are pushed through the tentorial opening shown in Figure 15–35, into the "compartment" normally occupied by the brainstem. This may happen when there is excessive pressure in the cerebral hemispheres, forcing the contents of the cerebral hemispheres inferiorly. The excessive pressure can be one result of a stroke, or nonpenetrating brain injury from a blow to the head, or even a large tumor in one of the hemispheres. Transtentorial herniation is an extremely serious condition.

The dura mater serves a protective function for the neural tissue of the CNS. The dura "holds in" the CSF in which the cerebral hemispheres and brainstem float. As discussed in the next section, CSF circulates throughout the CNS. One prominent region of CSF circulation is immediately below the second layer of the meninges, which is the arachnoid mater.

Arachnoid Mater

The arachnoid mater is a thin membrane attached to the underside of the dura mater. Below this membrane is a small space in which CSF circulates. As shown in the bottom image of Figure 15–35, the subarachnoid space appears as a honeycombed chamber. The typical thickness of this space, extending from the arachnoid membrane to the pia mater below, is roughly 5 to 6 mm but varies depending on where the measurement is taken. The honeycombed appearance results from delicate membranes extending from the arachnoid layer adhered to the underside of the dura, down to the pia mater. These membranes, together with the CSF circulating in the subarachnoid space, create a spongy cushion that protects neural tissue against damage.

Although not shown in Figure 15–35, arteries enter and veins exit brain tissue via the subarachnoid space. Arteries distribute blood to brain tissue via smaller vessels that penetrate the deepest layer of the meninges (the pia mater). Veins in the arachnoid space carry blood away from the brain by sending smaller veins into sinuses created by the separation of the two layers of the dura mater. The major venous return of blood to the heart is via these sinuses. A cross-section of one such sinus, the superior sagittal sinus, is shown in Figure 15–35.

Pia Mater

The pia mater, the deepest layer of the meninges, is an extremely thin membrane that adheres closely to the surface of the cerebral hemispheres, following the topography of its gyri and sulci. In a fixed brain prepared for dissection, in which the dura and arachnoid have been removed, the pia is often intact and appears as a filmy, milky-colored membrane that can be "pinched" away from the gyri and sulci. The pia mater is so closely adherent to the cortical surface it is sometimes not immediately apparent, on casual inspection by eye, that there is a membrane investing the surface of the hemispheres.

Meninges and Clinically Relevant Spaces

Clinically, the meninges are often referenced when a case involves bleeding in one of the spaces between the layers of these protective coverings. These are "potential spaces" in the sense of not having any measurable volume until something causes them to expand and create a "real" space. For example, the undersurface of the skull and the top surface of the dura are normally tightly bound to one another, but the potential space between them, called the epidural space, may be filled by blood when an artery bleeds. Similarly, the potential space between the dura and arachnoid layers can be filled by blood when an artery or vein bleeds. The term "subdural hematoma" refers to pooled blood in the space between the dura and arachnoid layers of the meninges. Any collection of blood within the meningeal spaces can exert pressure on the underlying brain tissue and cause behavior deficits, including deterioration or loss of speech and/or language function.

Ventricles

The meningeal layers, as described above, include the honeycombed subarachnoid space filled with CSF. CSF is produced, circulated, and delivered back to the venous system (the drainage of blood from brain to heart) within a system of ventricles, which are chambers deep within the cerebral hemispheres and brainstem. CSF also flows through a central conduit in the spinal cord.

The ventricular system and associated conduits are shown in Figure 15–36. This sagittal view of the hemispheres and brainstem is transparent for better appreciation of the location and configuration of the ventricular system. The lateral ventricle is the complexly shaped, green structure, the third ventricle is shown in light blue, the cerebral aqueduct in purple, and the fourth ventricle in reddish orange. Below the fourth ventri-

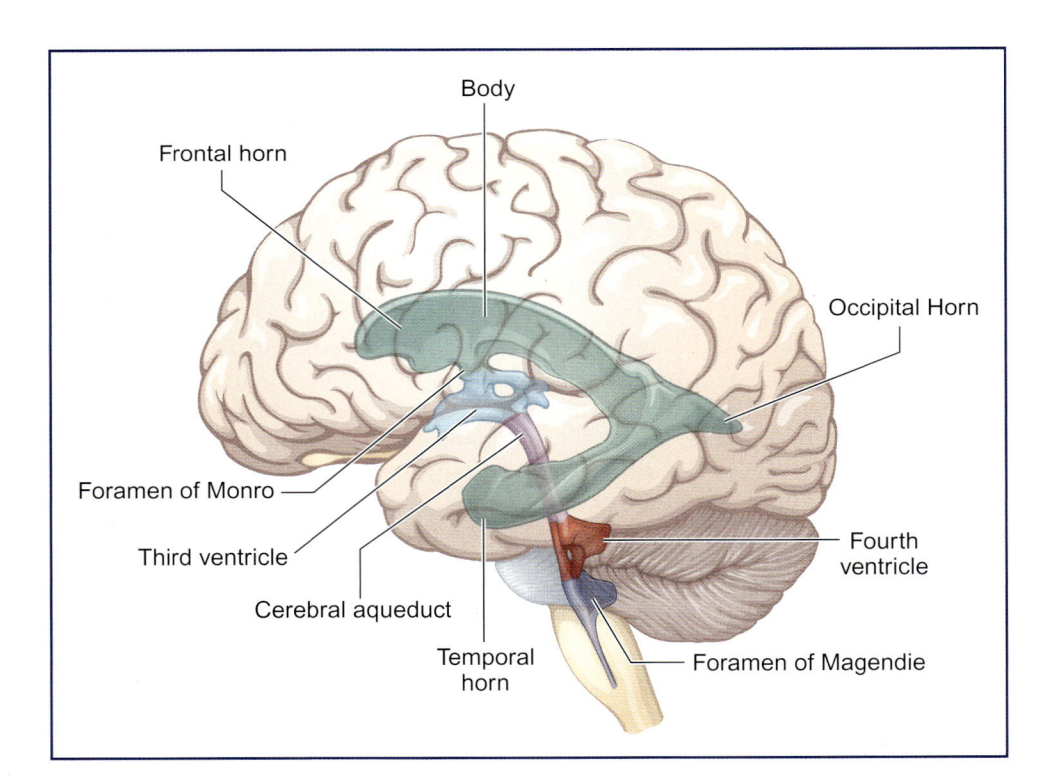

Figure 15–36. Sagittal view of the cerebral hemispheres, brainstem, and cerebellum, drawn to show the location and configuration of the ventricles. Lateral ventricles in green, third ventricle in light blue, cerebral aqueduct in purple, and fourth ventricle in reddish orange. The dark blue part of the ventricular system, inferior to the fourth ventricle, includes the beginning of the central canal of the spinal cord as well as other conduits through which CSF flows to the subarachnoid spaces in the cerebral hemispheres.

cle, in darker blue, is the foramen of Magendie and a downward projection that leads into the central canal of the spinal cord. Figure 15–37 shows these structures in a coronal view, looking from the front of the cerebral hemispheres toward the occipital lobes, and color-coded in the same way as in Figure 15–36. This view shows the lateral ventricles (green) to be paired, symmetrical structures in the two hemispheres, and the third ventricle and cerebral aqueduct to be midline (axial) structures. The fourth ventricle is a chamber between the brainstem and cerebellum, and is symmetrical with respect to both halves of the brainstem.

Lateral Ventricles

The sagittal view of Figure 15–36 shows the lateral ventricle to be a large, reversed C-shaped chamber occupying deep locations in all four lobes of the brain. The frontal horn of the lateral ventricle is in the frontal lobe, the body is in both the frontal and parietal lobes, and an occipital horn extends into the occipital lobe. The lower part of the reversed-C shape is the temporal horn of the lateral ventricle, which extends anterolaterally into the temporal lobe, from the junction of the body and occipital horn.

Notable landmarks are associated with the complex shape of the lateral ventricle. For example, the corpus callosum, the massive fiber tract that connects cells in one hemisphere to cells in the other hemisphere, is located just superior to the upper edge of the frontal horn and body of the lateral ventricle (see Figure 15–5, upper right). The caudate nucleus, a component of the basal ganglia (see Figure 15–3), is the lateral boundary of the lateral ventricle and follows its inverted-C shape (see Figure 15–16) from the frontal lobe to its curl into the temporal lobe. Immediately below the temporal horn of the lateral ventricle, in the temporal lobe, is the hippocampus.

Third Ventricle

In the sagittal view of Figure 15–36, the third ventricle is shown in blue as a flattened, complexly shaped cavity. The coronal view of Figure 15–37 shows the lateral ventricles connected to the third ventricle by narrow conduits which join in the midline and form a single channel, the *foramen of Monro*. The foramen of Monro drains CSF from the lateral ventricles into the third ventricle. In addition to its role in the transport of CSF throughout the CNS, the third ventricle is an important

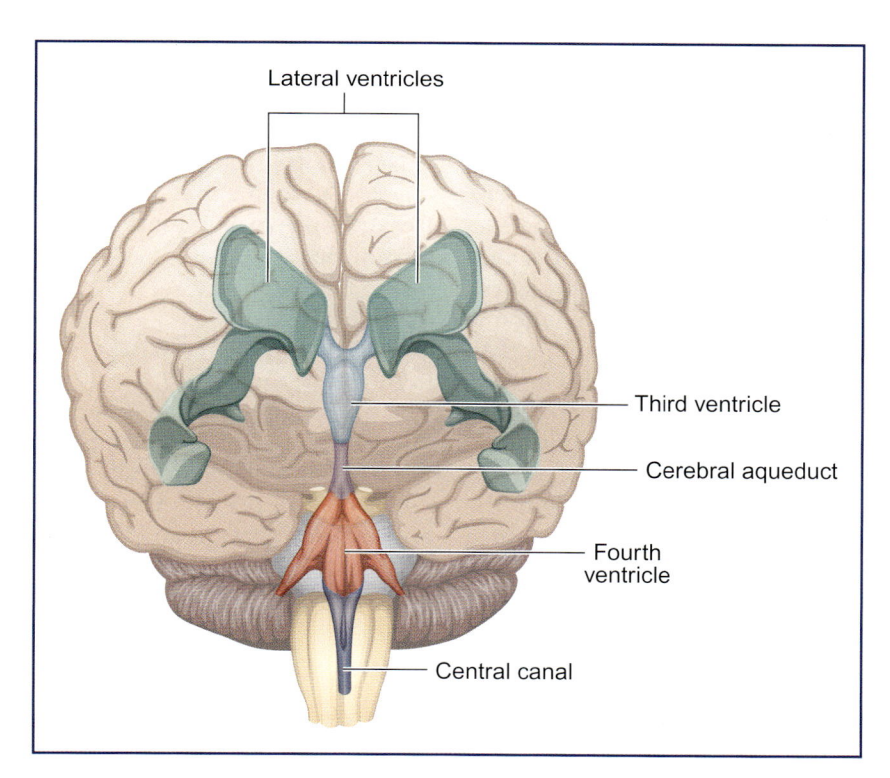

Figure 15–37. Coronal view of the cerebral hemispheres, brainstem, and cerebellum, looking from the front of the hemispheres to the back, drawn to show the configuration of the ventricles. Color coding of the ventricles is the same as in Figure 15–36.

anatomical landmark because it is the medial boundary of the two thalami (see the coronal view of Figure 15–3, in which the lateral ventricles are the two winglike cavities next to the caudate nuclei, and the third ventricle is the narrow "slit" between the thalami). There is often a connection between the left and right thalami, *through* the third ventricle. This is shown in Figure 15–36 as the circular opening in the third ventricle depicted in the same color as the brain tissue. This connection is called the interthalamic adhesion.

Cerebral Aqueduct, Fourth Ventricle, and Other Passageways for CSF

At the posterior, inferior end of the third ventricle, roughly at the top of the midbrain, the cavity narrows down and forms the cerebral aqueduct, shown in purple in Figures 15–36 and 15–37. This narrow channel courses through the midbrain and expands in the pons and medulla as a diamond-shaped cavity called the fourth ventricle. The fourth ventricle is just posterior to much of the pons and medulla, and anterior to the cerebellum. This fluid-filled cavity can be thought of as a boundary between the cerebellum and the lower two parts of the brainstem. The cerebellum is often referred to as the "roof" of the fourth ventricle, and the pons and medulla the "floor" of the fourth ventricle.

The fourth ventricle has several outlets that deliver CSF to the spinal cord and the subarachnoid space. In Figures 15–36 and 15–37 the thin blue passageway extending down from the fourth ventricle is the beginning of the central canal of the spinal cord. In horizontal cross sections of the spinal cord (such as Figure 15–28), this canal is the small circle in the center of the section, surrounded by gray matter. CSF flows through the canal and collects toward the bottom of the spinal cord in a small cavity below the inferior termination of spinal cord tissue, which is a few segments higher than the termination of the vertebral column. This inferior cavity is the insertion point for a spinal tap, when a suspected medical condition requires the withdrawal of a small amount of CSF for laboratory analysis.

Two additional conduits projecting from the fourth ventricle in posterolateral directions are seen in Figure 15–37. These are passageways from the fourth ventricle into the subarachnoid space that covers the cerebral hemispheres.

Production, Composition, and Circulation of CSF

CSF is generated primarily by cells in the lateral ventricles. These cells, collectively called the choroid plexus, are derived from embryological ependymal cells (see Table 15–5). The choroid plexus cells are suspended from the roof of the lateral ventricles and generate roughly half a quart of CSF every 24 hours. As CSF circulates through the ventricles, some fluid from the fourth ventricle continues inferiorly into the central canal of the spinal cord, and some exits via the lateral passageways shown in Figure 15–37 to circulate in the subarachnoid space surrounding the cerebral hemispheres. Because the subarachnoid space can hold only about one-third of the volume of CSF produced by the choroid plexus, a mechanism exists to drain CSF from the brain into the bloodstream. Figure 15–35 (bottom image showing a slab of skull and underlying meningeal and neural tissue) includes a small structure labeled "arachnoid villus," also called arachnoid granulations. These structures extend from the subarachnoid space into the sinuses created by separation of the two layers of the dura mater. The arachnoid villi return circulating CSF from the subarachnoid space into the venous system, effectively draining off excess CSF and maintaining a healthy pressure inside the ventricles and subarachnoid spaces. The draining of CSF into the venous system also serves the purpose of carrying neural waste products—the brain "trash" generated as neural and glial cells perform their metabolic tasks—away from the brain to be dissolved harmlessly in blood returning to the heart.

CSF is a clear fluid containing many different kinds of molecules, including proteins, chemical elements such as magnesium, chloride, potassium, and sodium, and other substances such as glucose, urea, and carbon dioxide. Normal values are available for each of these substances, and may be used as reference data when spinal tap fluid is analyzed as part of a diagnostic workup for diseases such as meningitis or certain cancers.

Blood Supply of Brain

The blood supply to the brain is often separated into anterior versus posterior circulation. This broad principle is illustrated in Figure 15–38, where the anterior circulatory components of the arterial supply to the brain are shown in brown and the posterior components in red. Both anterior and posterior circulations originate in major arteries emerging from the heart.

Anterior Circulation

For this part of the discussion, the reader should make frequent reference to the labeled arteries on the left side of Figure 15–38. The aorta, the largest artery in the body, emerges from the heart and ascends in the thorax before turning around and descending toward

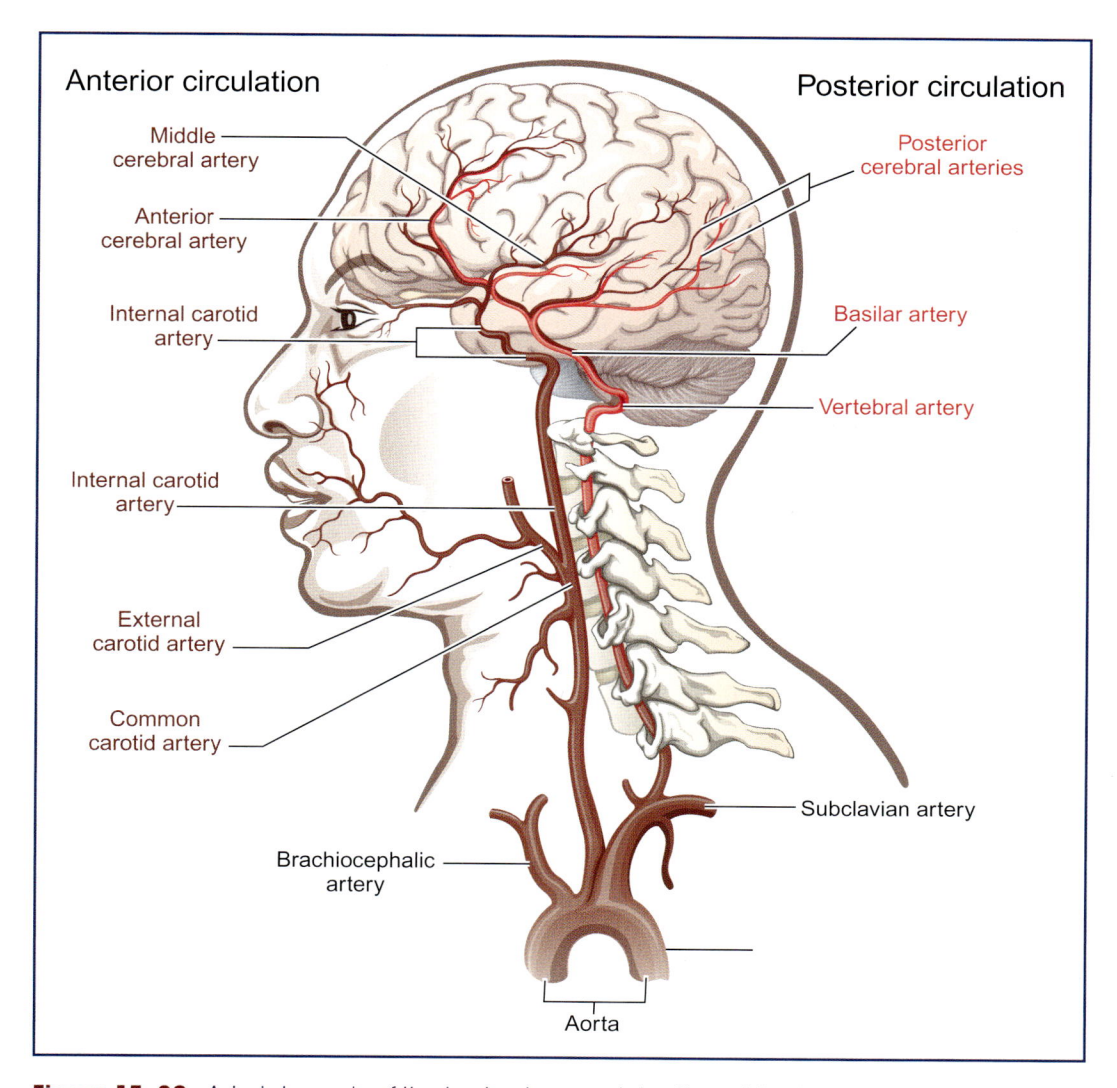

Figure 15–38. Arterial supply of the brain, shown originating at the heart. The anterior supply is shown as the brown arteries, the posterior supply as the red arteries.

the abdomen. At the top of the aortic arch, two major arteries arise and move blood toward the head. These are the common carotid arteries, one being the left common carotid artery (supplying the left side of the face and the left hemisphere of the brain) and the other the right common carotid artery. For the sake of clarity, Figure 15–38 shows only the left common carotid artery and the left hemisphere. The anatomy of the blood supply to the brain on the right side is identical to the description in the next paragraph.

As the common carotid artery ascends in the neck it bifurcates (gives off two branches) roughly at the level of the mandible. One of these branches is the external carotid artery, which provides blood to structures such as the pharynx, tongue, face, and eyes. The other branch appears as a continuation of the common carotid artery. This is the internal carotid artery, a main source of blood supply to the brain. Note how the internal carotid artery makes several sharp turns when it reaches the ventral surface of the temporal lobe. One of these is shown in Figure 15–38 as a hard right turn, along the line of the sylvian fissure. This branch of the internal carotid artery is called the middle cerebral artery (MCA). The MCA supplies most of the lateral cortical surface as well as the anterior temporal lobe, insula, and parts of the internal capsule and basal ganglia. Another branch of the internal carotid artery is the anterior cerebral artery (ACA), shown in Figure 15–38 as a leftward turn off the main path of the internal carotid artery. The ACA supplies blood to medial portions of the frontal and parietal lobes, much of the corpus callosum, and small portions of basal ganglia structures. The importance of the MCA in speech, language, and hearing function is discussed below.

Posterior Circulation

The posterior circulation is shown on the right side of Figure 15–38. The subclavian artery is a major branch of the aortic arch, supplying blood to the arm on the same side as the artery. The vertebral artery arises from the subclavian artery and ascends the neck within small openings in the ventral portions of the cervical vertebrae. When it reaches the base of the skull, the vertebral artery courses through the foramen magnum and continues to ascend on the ventral surface of the medulla until it joins with the vertebral artery from the other side, at the junction of the medulla and pons. When the two vertebral arteries join, they form the basilar artery. Before the vertebral arteries join at the junction of the medulla and pons, they deliver blood to one part of the cerebellum and the lateral part of the medulla via the posterior inferior cerebellar artery (PICA). The PICA is shown in Figure 15–39, a view of the ventral surface of the cerebral hemispheres, the cerebellum, and the medulla and pons, as well as an illustration of the joining of the two vertebral arteries to form the basilar artery. As the basilar artery ascends the pons it issues two more branches, the anterior inferior cerebellar artery (AICA) and the superior cerebellar artery (SCA). The AICA supplies blood to parts of the pons and the central part of the cerebellum, whereas the SCA serves the upper part of the cerebellum and parts of the midbrain.

The basilar artery provides the posterior circulation for the cerebral hemispheres, by issuing the posterior cerebral artery (PCA; see Figures 15–38 and 15–39). The PCA provides blood to the posterior parts of the cerebral hemispheres, including the occipital lobes, and parts of the thalamus and corpus callosum.

Circle of Willis

A view of the arterial anatomy on the base of the brain shows the ACA and MCA, both major branches of the internal carotid artery, and the PCA, the main branch of the basilar artery. These arteries form a circular pas-

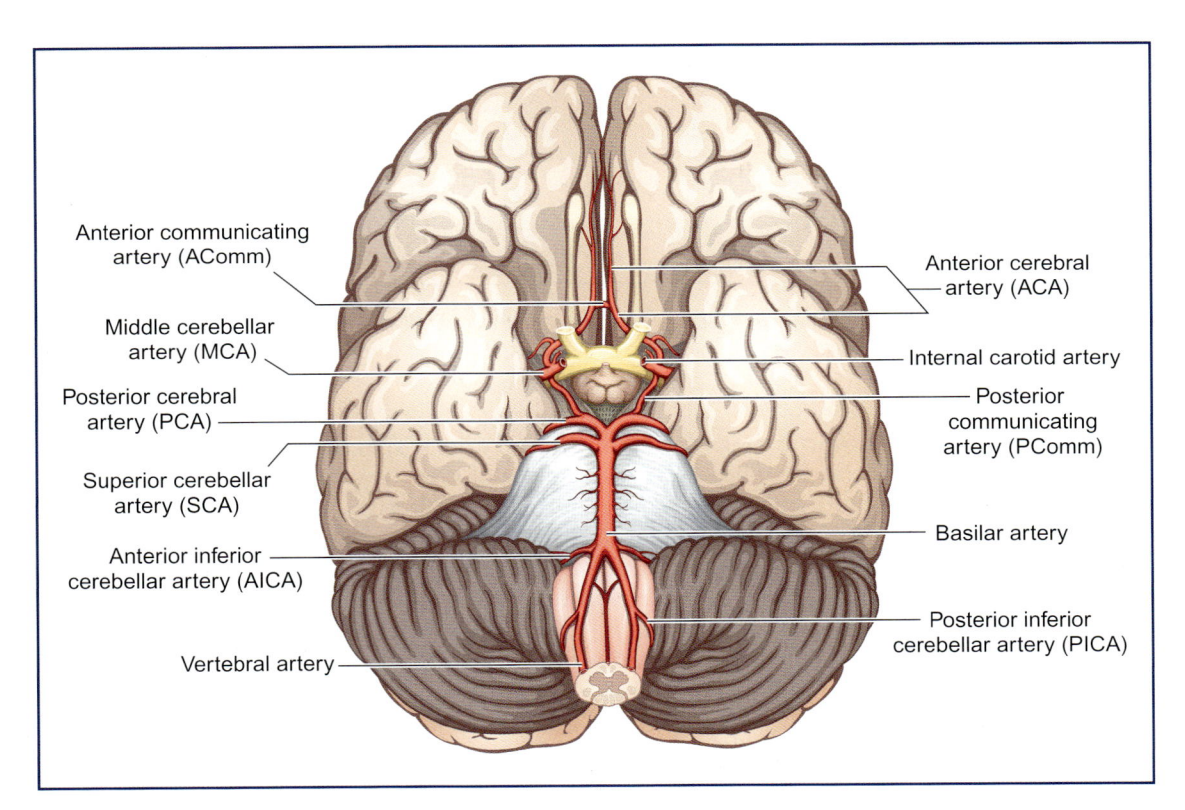

Figure 15–39. Ventral surface of the cerebral hemispheres, showing the paired vertebral arteries ascending the medulla, their junction to form the basilar artery at the base of the pons, and important branches into the brainstem and cerebellum. The circle of Willis can also be seen in this drawing (see also Figure 15–40).

sageway called the *circle of Willis*. (Figure 15–40). Follow the basilar artery up the pons and note where the PCA branches off into the left and right hemispheres. The PCA on both sides give off a branch called the posterior communicating artery (PComm), which links to the MCA. The MCA, labeled on the left side of Figure 15–40, is a continuation of the internal carotid artery (see below). The MCA is not included in the circle of Willis; the internal carotid artery, just as it gives off the MCA, is part of the circle of Willis. The ACA connects from the internal carotid artery to the anterior part of the brain, and the two ACAs are connected via the anterior communicating artery (AComm).

Blood at the base of the brain flows in a circular pattern because the two main, paired branches of the carotid artery (ACA, MCA) and the one main, paired branch of the basilar artery (PCA) are connected by communicating arteries. The circular blood flow pattern created by the circle of Willis can compensate for loss of blood flow from one of the main blood supplies to the brain. For example, blockage of the internal carotid on one side of the circle of Willis may be compensated for by increased flow from the basilar artery to the PCA, because both main arteries contribute to the circular blood flow pattern. This is especially important in cases of temporary blockage of one of the arteries. This classic description of circle of Willis anatomy must be taken with a grain of salt because there is a good deal of variation across individuals in the components of this circular arrangement. Some scientists believe this anatomical variation across individuals may help explain racial and ethnic differences in stroke risk (Eftekhar et al., 2006).

MCA and Blood Supply to the Dominant Hemisphere

The MCA is of interest to the speech-language pathologist and audiologist because it supplies blood to most of the lateral aspect of the cerebral hemispheres. More

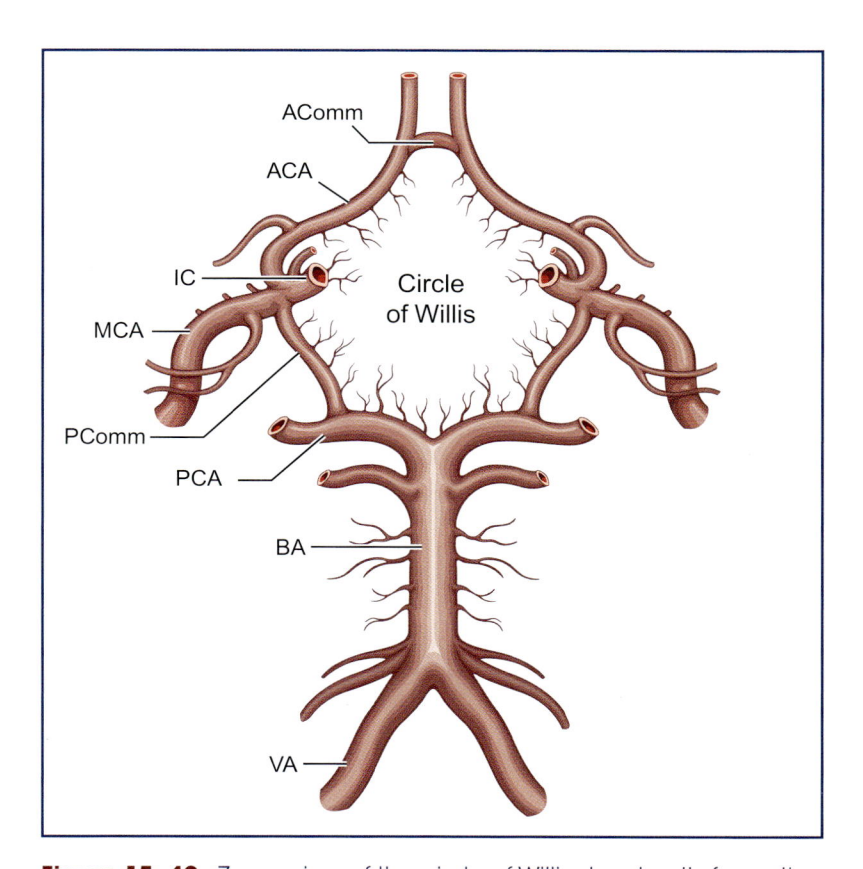

Figure 15–40. Zoom view of the circle of Willis showing its formation from the main blood supply sources to the brain: the basilar artery (*posterior supply;* BA) and middle cerebral arteries (*anterior supply;* MCA). The circle is completed by linking arteries (*posterior cerebral artery,* PCA; *posterior communicating artery,* PComm; *anterior cerebral artery,* ACA; *and anterior communicating artery,* AComm).

specifically, the MCA is the source of blood for the perisylvian speech, language, and hearing areas of the dominant hemisphere (the left hemisphere, in about 95% of the population). Blockage of the left MCA, or of one of its more local branches or associated small vessels deeper in the brain, has the potential to affect brain tissue critical to normal communication function. Many strokes associated with speech and language deficits are the result of loss of blood flow in the left MCA or its branches.

Figure 15–41 shows how the MCA gives off branches across the lateral surface of the left hemisphere; the same pattern applies to the right hemisphere. Note how the MCA emerges on the surface of the hemisphere near the anterior tip of the temporal lobe and the lower surface of the frontal lobe. The MCA courses along the sylvian fissure, posteriorly and superiorly, giving off an upper branch and a lower branch. The upper branch supplies blood primarily to frontal lobe tissue, whereas the lower branch distributes blood to parietal lobe tissue. Note also the offshoots from the main trunk of the MCA to the temporal lobe.

In theory, a blockage to blood flow can occur at any point along the course of the MCA and its branches. Blockages at the sharp right-angle turn from the internal carotid artery to the MCA are not uncommon, and affect the entire distribution of blood to the lateral surface of the hemisphere. Blockages can also occur in the turn to the upper or lower branches of the MCA, or in the offshoots into the temporal lobe.

A simplified, but in many cases clinically useful, way to correlate these blockage possibilities with functional consequences is as follows. A blockage at the turn from the internal carotid artery to the MCA deprives the anterior and posterior parts of the left hemisphere of blood and therefore affects both expressive (anterior lesions) and receptive (posterior lesions) speech and language functions. Loss of blood supply to both the anterior and posterior perisylvian regions may result in a communication disorder called global aphasia. Blockage at the junction of the MCA and the offshoot labeled "MCA upper branch" (see Figure 15–41) might be expected to have a primary influence on expressive ability, whereas blockage at the junction of the MCA and the offshoot labeled "MCA lower branch" might be associated with a primary receptive problem. This is consistent with the idea of anterior and posterior lesions in the dominant hemisphere serving expressive and comprehension abilities, respectively. This simplified view of speech and language functions of the brain is consistent with certain diagnostic categories of communication function following stroke and left hemisphere damage. More is said about the issue of brain structures and specific speech and language functions

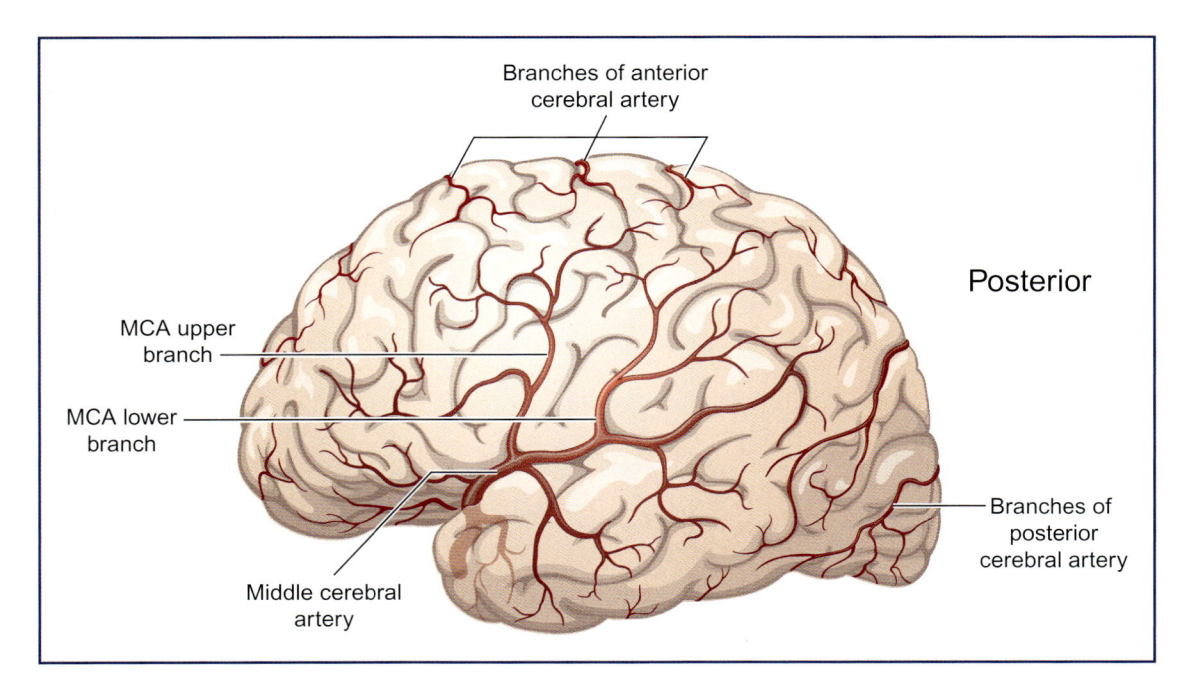

Figure 15–41. Distribution of middle cerebral artery (MCA) branches across the lateral surface of the left hemisphere. As the MCA emerges on the surface of the hemisphere between the anterior tip of the temporal lobe and lower, posterior lip of the frontal lobe, it gives off upper and lower branches as labeled in the figure. Branches of the anterior cerebral artery (ACA) and posterior cerebral artery (PCA) are also shown.

in the section titled "Speech and Language Functions of the Brain: Possible Sites and Mechanisms."

The MCA also is a significant source of blood for structures deep within the cerebral hemispheres. A view of the distribution of MCA blood to the contents of the cerebral hemispheres is given in Figure 15–42, which is an artist's rendition of a coronal section roughly midway between the front and back of the hemispheres. The left side of the section shows labeled brain structures, and the right side shows the source of blood supply to these structures from the main components of the circle of Willis (MCA, ACA, PCA). The purple shaded regions indicate the areas of the hemispheres supplied by the upper and lower branches of the MCA, including the cortical regions on the lateral surface of the hemisphere and the underlying white matter of the coronal radiata. Deep branches of the MCA (light bluish gray) also provide blood to the caudate, putamen, parts of the globus pallidus, and parts of the internal capsule.

Speech and language problems plus limb deficits on the right side of the body, a frequently seen combination in stroke clinics, are explained by interruptions of MCA blood flow which affect the perisylvian areas (speech and language) and the internal capsule (limbs). Figure 15–42 also shows regions of the internal capsule, caudate, and globus pallidus to be supplied by the anterior choroidal artery (ACha), an offshoot of the internal carotid artery close to the branching of the MCA at the base of the brain.

The PCA supplies the ventral part of the temporal lobe, with deeper branches supplying the thalamus and hypothalamus. The most dorsal and medial aspects of the cerebral hemispheres are supplied by the ACA.

The major arteries supplying the brain with blood are summarized in Table 15–7. The advantage of knowing the blood supply of the brain is the ability to understand the co-occurrence of symptoms and signs, such as the speech-language and limb problems mentioned

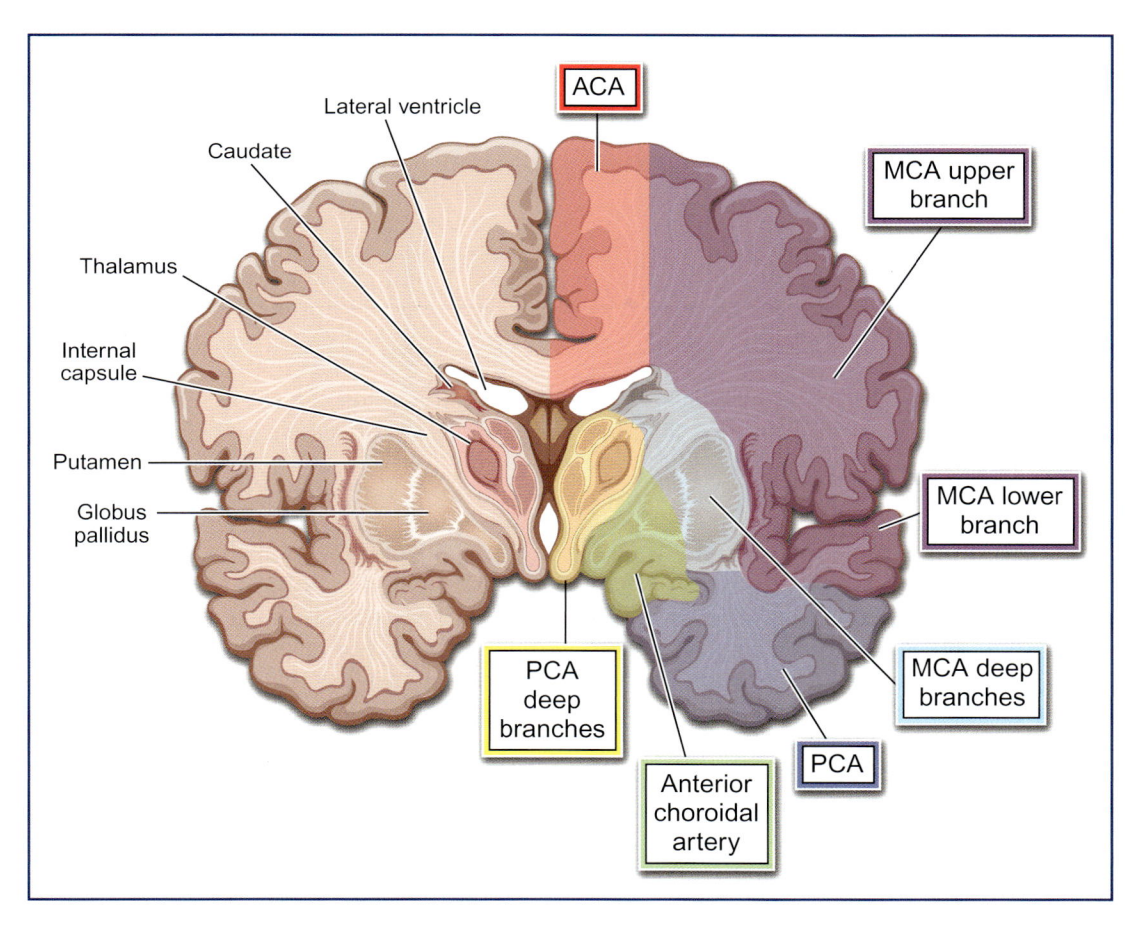

Figure 15–42. Distribution of cerebral artery supply to both surface and deep components of the cerebral hemispheres, shown in a coronal slice made roughly midway between the anterior and posterior ends of the hemispheres. The left side of the slice shows labels for subcortical structures. The right side of the slice identifies the arteries supplying different regions. MCA = middle cerebral artery; PCA = posterior cerebral artery; ACA = anterior cerebral artery.

Table 15-7. Arteries Supplying the Brain

CAROTID ARTERY	MAIN DISTRIBUTION
Internal Carotid	Source of blood for cerebral hemispheres and contents
Anterior Circulation	
Middle cerebral artery	Blood to most of lateral cortex; anterior temporal lobe and insula; parts of internal capsule and basal ganglia
Anterior cerebral artery	Medial surfaces of frontal and parietal lobes, corpus callosum, small portion of basal ganglia
Subclavian Artery	
Posterior Circulation	
Vertebral artery	Part of cerebellum; lateral medulla via posterior inferior cerebellar artery
Basilar artery	Posterior circulation for cerebral hemispheres; part of pons and central medulla via anterior inferior cerebellar artery; upper parts of cerebellum and parts of midbrain via superior cerebellar artery; occipital lobes and parts of thalamus
Circle of Willis	
Posterior cerebral artery	
Posterior communicating artery	
Anterior cerebral artery	
Anterior communicating artery	
Internal carotid artery	

above. Neurologists often use such co-occurrences to make preliminary, educated estimates of where a stroke has occurred (that is, the location of blood flow interruption). These estimates may or may not be confirmed by imaging studies.

Not all strokes produce obvious problems at first. The very small vessels that penetrate to the deep structures of the hemispheres, such as the basal ganglia and internal capsule, may be blocked with a resulting loss of blood to very local regions of brain tissue. Eventually, a sufficient number of these small infarcts (loss of blood flow) can produce personality changes and dementia. Indeed, one category of dementia, broadly referred to as vascular dementia, seems to be the result of multiple small regions of damage. On autopsy, the brain tissue sometimes has a "pin-cushion" appearance, with many small holes in the brain tissue.

Blood-Brain Barrier

In most parts of the body, substances flowing in the bloodstream can be transferred to tissue by passing through the walls of the vessels, directly into the tissue. The walls of vessels in the brain are different than walls of vessels in other parts of the body. Brain blood vessels have a structure that forms a protective barrier against chemicals or toxins that have the potential to destabilize the neurochemistry of the brain. This *blood–brain barrier* is especially relevant when certain drugs are administered to alleviate symptoms and signs of a CNS disease. For example, it is well known that Parkinson's disease is at least partly a result of reduction of the neurotransmitter dopamine in the brain. Dopamine is manufactured by cells in the substantia nigra and plays an important role in the normal functioning of basal ganglia structures such as the striatum. To address the reduction of dopamine in the brain, why not administer a drug, orally, with the molecular composition of dopamine? As it turns out, dopamine molecules are blocked by the blood–brain barrier. In the 1960s, scientists figured out that a precursor of dopamine—a chemical compound that is one of the steps in the neuronal synthesis of dopamine—was able to cross the blood–brain barrier. Patients were given this precursor, called L-dOPA. Once in the brain, L-dOPA was converted into dopamine by "normal" neuronal processes. In this case, knowledge of the blood–brain barrier and the chemical transformations in the synthesis of dopamine permitted an effective treatment for many of the problems associated with Parkinson's disease.

SPEECH AND LANGUAGE FUNCTIONS OF THE BRAIN: POSSIBLE SITES AND MECHANISMS

Scientists have considered models of speech and language functions of the brain for well over a century. The models typically highlight sites (locations in the brain where certain functions are accomplished) and pathways connecting these sites. The models may also include mechanisms, which are accounts of how nuclei and tracts produce sensations, perceptions, and behavior, among other aspects of human function. Early on, simple models of speech and language sites and functions of the brain were offered by Broca and Wernicke, who interpreted postmortem regions of brain damage in relation to speech and language performance of the patients prior to their death. According to these models, speech-language expression and comprehension were vested in tissue around Broca's and Wernicke's areas, respectively. A parallel, "site-based" development occurred in models of motor speech disorders, a group of speech disorders caused by neurological damage to several different locations within the CNS and PNS. Motor *speech* disorders are typically separated from neurologically based *language* disorders (the type considered by Broca and Wernicke), because the former are assumed to reflect damage only to motor control systems, with language representations completely (or nearly so)[2] intact. The dominant model of motor speech disorders (Darley, Aronson, & Brown, 1975; Duffy, 2013) makes explicit associations between specific sites of damage (such as in the cerebellum, versus the corticobulbar tracts) and specific speech problems. Early models of aphasia and motor speech disorders were therefore very much concerned with anatomical sites of damage, and somewhat less with mechanisms causing the speech disorders.

Network View of Brain Function

Over the last 20 years there has been an explosion of research on speech and language functions of the brain, especially due to the widespread use and increasing sophistication of brain imaging techniques. This research has brought us to a point where the strict idea of sites matching up with specific speech and language functions does not seem reasonable. The general notion of a link between sites and function is probably still viable—posterior lesions in the dominant hemisphere are more likely to result in comprehension problems compared with anterior lesions. Similarly, damage to the cerebellum is more likely to make a person's speech sound slightly drunk as compared with the damage associated with Parkinson's disease, which is likely to make a patient sound soft, mumbly, and dysfluent. With the addition of imaging techniques designed to trace *connections* in the brain (see sidetrack on "DTI" p. 600), as well as accumulating evidence of certain neurological diseases having a major influence on these connections (in addition to, or rather than, major influence on the connected *sites*), clinicians and scientists are beginning to consider the brain as a network in which multiple sites and their connections are devoted to integrated functions. This is a *system* view, as compared with a site view, of speech-language functions of the brain. A system view might explain, for example, why different sites of brain damage can produce very similar motor speech signs/symptoms, or very similar comprehension problems.

DIVA

A recent approach to understanding brain systems is to combine brain imaging findings in healthy people and persons with brain diseases with computer simulations of brain processes. The computer simulations are implemented by software written to mimic brain locations, their presumed functions, and the way in which information is transferred between specific cortical regions or subcortical nuclei. This kind of model can be used to run elegant simulation experiments. The simulations can include hypothetical lesions in specific cortical regions or along the pathways connecting these regions. Selected speech and language components (phonemes, syllables, words) can serve as input to the model to see how it "performs" under varied conditions of damage. This simulated performance can be compared with the performance of humans with documented lesions in the areas "damaged" in the simulation. If human performance matches the simulation performance, a tentative conclusion is that the region of simulated damage, whether in nuclei or tracts, is responsible for the speech and

---

[2] An example of a motor speech disorder that may be associated with developmental language delays is found in many cases of cerebral palsy, which often has dysarthria as a sign. Some cases of Parkinson's disease may also have cognitive decline that affects language capabilities.

language performance matched between the human and computer.

A well-known model of this sort is called DIVA (**D**irections **i**nto **V**elocities of **A**rticulators), developed by Dr. Frank Guenther of Boston University and under continuous development (see Bohland et al., 2010; Guenther, 1995, 2006; Guenther, Ghosh, & Tourville, 2006; Guenther & Hickok, 2015; Peeva et al., 2010). DIVA is a neural network model of speech motor control that includes the programming of articulatory movements as well as direct commands to guide the articulators after the programming has been done. DIVA, a neural network model, is a computer simulation of speech motor control. DIVA has been used to test the effects of simulated lesions in components of its speech motor control network, and the results have been compared with speech production signs reported in persons with documented lesions matching those tested in the simulations. The neural network is connected to a speech synthesizer, which "talks" based on the settings of the simulations. A fitting way to end this chapter is to consider DIVA in a moderate amount of detail, and to ask how an understanding of such a model may be useful to speech-language pathologists who want to use their knowledge of brain function to diagnose and treat clients from an evidence-based, anatomico-physiological perspective.

A simplified adaptation of the DIVA model is shown in Figure 15–43. Three of the boxes represent cortical regions; arrows represent fiber tracts connecting these regions.

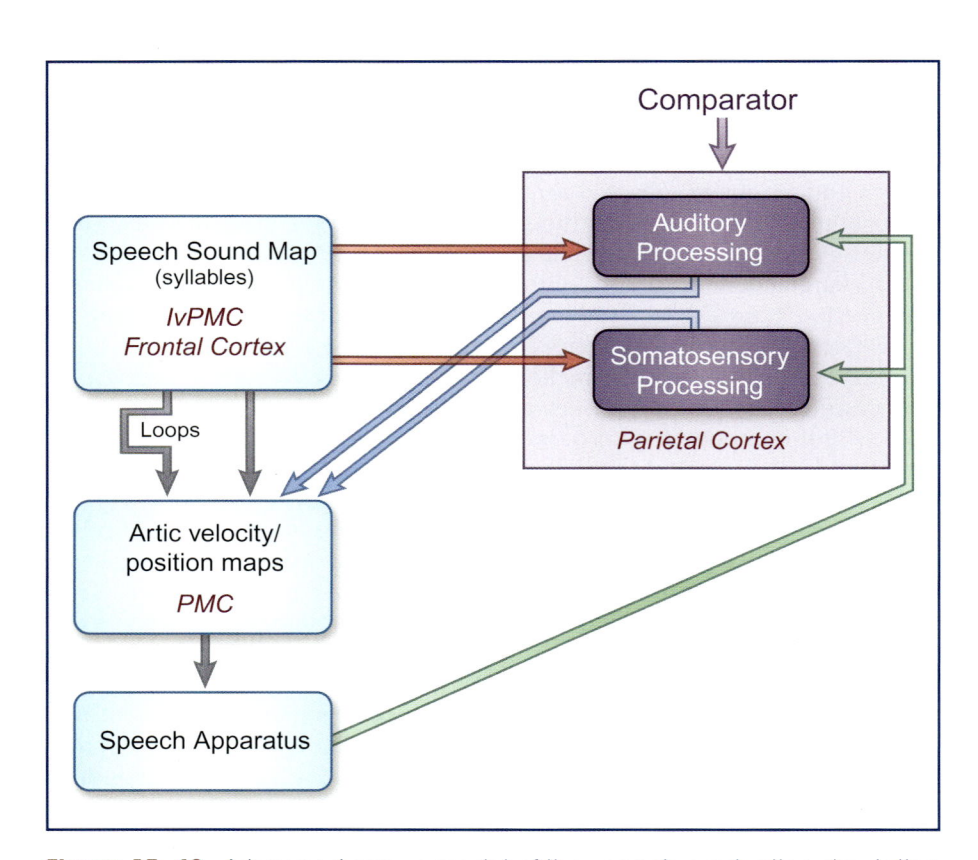

Figure 15–43. A box-and-arrows model of the speech production simulation called DIVA. The model shown here is adapted and simplified from Guenther (2006), Peeva et al. (2010), Guenther and Hickok (2015), and other publications from Professor Guenther's laboratory. Boxes represent cortical areas for speech motor control (and the speech apparatus), arrows represent tracts connecting these areas (or the apparatus to these areas). The speech sound map, where syllables are represented, is presumed to be in the lateral ventral premotor cortex (lvPMC), close to or including what is regarded as Broca's area. Articulatory velocity and position maps are located in the primary motor cortex (PMC). Auditory and somatosensory processing and comparisons are thought to take place in the ventral parietal cortex (close to the posterior sylvian fissure) and the angular gyrus.

Apraxia of ... Speech

The term "apraxia" was borrowed for application to speech from the general neurological literature. Following a stroke, some people cannot produce certain behaviors on command (e.g., "Show me how you use this pencil") but spontaneously produce the behavior (e.g., signing a document), demonstrating the ability to use the muscles to produce the action. This disorder—the inability to produce action on command—is called apraxia (meaning, "without action") to distinguish it from action disorders explained by obvious muscle weakness or sensory disturbance. Frederick Darley apparently was the first to graft the idea of apraxia onto post-stroke speech problems in adults. He used the term "apraxia of speech" in a 1969 paper presented at the annual convention of what was then the American Speech and Hearing Association (see Ogar, Slama, Dronkers, Amici, & Gorno-Tempini, 2005). Fifteen years earlier, Morley, Court, and Miller (1954) employed the term "articulatory dyspraxia" to mean precisely what Darley wanted to capture with the term "apraxia of speech." Morley et al. (1954, p. 9) said, when referring to case studies of children who seemed to have neurologically based developmental speech disorders, "In the remaining six children . . . movements of the lips, tongue, and palate appeared normal on voluntary movements carried out at the examiner's request, but clumsy and awkward when the children attempted the more complex and rapid movements of articulation. We have regarded such cases as possible examples of 'dyspraxic dysarthria' or 'articulatory dyspraxia." Today, childhood apraxia of speech (CAS) is regarded by many clinicians and scientists as a neurologically based speech sound disorder in some children. See https://www.apraxia-kids.org/ for information on this controversial disorder

DIVA: Speech Sound Map (lvPMC)

The box titled "Speech Sound Map" represents an area of the frontal lobe, the *lateral ventral premotor cortex* (lvPMC), where basic units of speech production are represented. In DIVA, the basic units are consonant-vowel (CV) syllables. The lvPMC is a region of the premotor cortex just anterior to the face area of primary motor cortex. Some scientists say it is adjacent to Broca's area, others may include portions of it *in* Broca's area. This region is thought to be important in the planning of action—it is considered an area of the brain involved in the assembly and preparation of motor programs. The lvPMC is not necessarily a speech-specific region, but plays a role in action production in general and may contain cells specialized for observing action ("mirror neurons") as well. An assumption of DIVA is that the representation of syllables is always "correct." This means that prior to programming, the syllabic chunks that are ready to be programmed are correctly represented. The representation of "sigh," for example, is the syllable /saɪ/, not /s/ and /aɪ/ individually.

It is possible that frequently used syllables, such as "the," and "neh" in words like "never," are tightly packaged in lvPMC almost like indivisible units, for easier access and assembly for production. Syllables having a lower frequency of occurrence (such as "wah" and "tih," as in "wash" and "tip") may have to be assembled from individual sounds (that is, from phonemes) when producing a word containing the syllable.

The lvPMC plays an important role in the way DIVA accounts for certain "normal" speech phenomena, as well as for speech production deficits following strokes or other brain injuries that affect this area. For example, if lvPMC is the site for syllable selection and/or assembly, and more generally the programming of a speech sequence, the more complex the programming requirements, the greater the expected activity in this brain region. Similarly, damage to lvPMC is expected to result in speech production behaviors that reflect programming problems.

How do scientists manipulate speech motor programming requirements, and what speech behaviors suggest a speech programming problem? Speech motor programming requirements are varied by manipulating the phonetic complexity of a speech task. These variations take two primary forms. One is to vary the number of syllables in a speech production task. Comparisons are made between conditions in which a speaker is required to produce single-syllable, two-syllable, and three-syllable utterances. Two-syllable utterances are thought to require more programming resources than one-syllable utterances, three-syllable utterances more resources than two-syllable utterances. In fMRI studies, the expected outcome for neurologically normal individuals is for greater lvPMC activity with increasing number of syllables (that is, with increasing programming demands). Some studies have supported this outcome, although the results are not uniformly consistent with this prediction (for a review, see Peeva et al., 2010).

Another way to vary phonetic complexity is to change the structure of a syllable while holding constant the number of syllables in an utterance. For example, the syllables /sɑ/, /stɑ/, and /strɑ/ are thought to require increasingly complex speech motor programming as the utterance is changed from a consonant-vowel (CV) (/sɑ/), to a CCV (/stɑ/), to a CCCV (/strɑ/) syllable (see Wright et al., 2009). In experiments with neurologically normal speakers, participants are asked to say one of these syllable forms as quickly as possible when given a "go" signal (such as a brief tone). A frequent finding is for reaction time (RT: time from the onset of the "go" signal to the onset of the syllable) to increase as the syllable complexity increases (i.e., RTs for /strɑ/ are reliably longer than RTs for /sɑ/). The interpretation of the increasing RT across CV, CCV, and CCCV syllable forms is that programming a complex syllable such as /strɑ/ requires more time than a simple syllable such as /sɑ/. In a sense, the longer RT for /strɑ/ is the extra time required for processing in the lvPMC to "prepare" the utterance for production.

The hypothesis of increasing programming requirements with increasing utterance complexity is relevant to the disorder called apraxia of speech (AOS; see sidetrack on "Apraxia of . . . Speech"). In adults, AOS is almost always associated with a known lesion, and is thought to be a speech motor programming disorder independent of weakness or paralysis of muscles in the speech apparatus (Darley et al., 1975; McNeil, Robin, & Schmidt, 2009). Many authors have noted the presence of a lesion in or around lvPMC when signs of AOS are documented clinically (interested students are encouraged to read a classic paper by Mohr et al. [1978]).

Of greatest interest is the frequent claim that a diagnostic feature of AOS is an increase in articulatory errors with increasing phonetic complexity of utterances. Whether the phonetic complexity is in the form of multiple-syllable utterances or single syllables with complex forms, adults with AOS are said to have a disproportionately difficult time producing words such as "statistical" and "Mississippi" compared with "sat" and "miss" (Rosenbek, Kent, & LaPointe, 1984).

DIVA can be programmed to evaluate how a simulated lesion in lvPMC affects utterances having different numbers of syllables, or different syllable complexity. The speech synthesizer that is the output of DIVA's settings is used to determine how the model "produces" the utterances. Does the model hesitate longer before producing utterances with increased phonetic complexity, and is this hesitation exaggerated when the model contains a lesion in lvPMC? Does the model produce a greater number of articulatory errors under conditions of greater articulatory complexity when a lesion is simulated in lvPMC? These are examples of how a model such as DIVA can be manipulated and compared with data from humans with lesions in lvPMC. A match of simulated data to human data supports the idea of lvPMC as a brain region for programming articulatory behavior.

Despite the value of DIVA in addressing the role of lvPMC in speech production, computer models have some limitations in their ability to explain human speech and language behavior. For example, children with a diagnosis of childhood apraxia of speech (often abbreviated CAS) may have signs similar to those observed in adults (such as slower RT or more errors with increasing phonetic complexity), but the underlying cause is not the same as in adults. The lesion often seen in adults with AOS is not seen in children with diagnoses of CAS. In fact, it is almost always the case that brain scans *fail* to show the presence of a lesion in children with CAS. The presence of abnormal speech signs in CAS, with no known lesion, suggests other brain mechanisms or deficits (or immaturities) in the mechanisms associated with programming behavior. In addition, brain lesions in locations other than the lvPMC, both cortical and subcortical, may produce signs consistent with a speech motor programming disorder (see Ogar et al., 2005; and Pramstaller & Marsden, 1996). This suggests either that multiple locations in the speech motor control network can program articulatory behavior or that the network functions as an integrated system of many brain areas and connections. This idea is different from attaching specific articulatory behaviors with specific brain regions.

DIVA: Articulatory Velocity/ Position Maps (PMC)

The primary motor cortex (PMC) contains cells connected to brainstem and spinal motor neurons via the corticobulbar and corticospinal tracts, respectively. These PMC cells are the primary command cells for specification of muscle contraction characteristics—how forceful, how fast, how short or long, and so forth. In DIVA, the PMC cells of interest are the ones associated with head and neck (corticobulbar) and respiratory (corticospinal) muscles. These cells receive programmed instructions from the lvPMC via a fiber tract connecting the two areas. This is represented in Figure 15–43 by the unlabeled arrow from the "Speech Sound Map" to the PMC. Activity in PMC is presumed to be devoted strictly to execution. Cells in the PMC are thought to be insensitive to phonetic complexity, unlike cells in the complexity-sensitive lvPMC. Damage to PMC cells presumably results in dysarthria, an execution (not programming) disorder, and there is good clinical evidence to support this expectation (Urban et al., 2003, 2006).

As shown in Figure 15–43, however, the input to the PMC is not restricted to the hypothesized programs constructed in the lvPMC. The arrow labeled "loops" in Figure 15–43 represents the potential modification of PMC cell activity by information circulating in the two cerebral sensorimotor loops described above: the cortico-striatal-cortical loop and the cortico-cerebellar-cortical loop. Both the basal ganglia and cerebellum have been identified as brain structures involved in aspects of motor programs, meaning that loops between these structures and the PMC must have something to do with "direct" motor activity in PMC cells. As stated eloquently by Terband and Maassen (2010), the dense interconnectedness of the many and widespread motor components of the brain makes it exceedingly difficult to use speech data of any single kind or from a single task to make clean distinctions between programming (i.e., apraxia) and execution (i.e., dysarthria) problems. The effect of these loops on the execution cells in the PMC also emphasizes the concept of *sensorimotor control* noted in this chapter. "Speech motor control" is more properly referred to as "speech sensorimotor control."

DIVA: Auditory and Somatosensory Processing: Parietal Cortex and Frontal-Parietal Association Tracts

Figure 15–43 shows projections (association fiber tracts; see Table 15–2) from the lvPMC to the auditory and somatosensory parietal cortex (red arrows) and projections from the auditory and somatosensory cortices to the PMC (blue arrows). The model also shows connections, indicated by green arrows, from the speech apparatus to somatosensory and auditory cortices. This group of connections within the CNS (red and blue arrows), and from the peripheral apparatus back to the CNS (green arrows), play a critical role in the uniqueness of DIVA as a model of speech sensorimotor control.

Consider first the intrahemispheric association tracts, connecting cortical areas in the frontal, temporal, and parietal lobes. The anatomical evidence for these connections is firm, and includes the arcuate fasciculus (to account at least for auditory information) as well as other fibers connecting the region near the lvPMC with the parietal lobe (to account at least for somatosensory information; see Martino et al. [2011]). Information in these association tracts flows in both directions—temporal and parietal to frontal lobe, and frontal to temporal and parietal lobe (Hickok & Poeppel, 2007).

Consider next the red arrows projecting from lvPMC to the parietal auditory and sensory association areas. For a syllable stored in lvPMC (or assembled from smaller, phonemic "parts" in the case of a low-frequency syllable), this projection tract carries a data-based model of the expected sensory consequences of the articulatory gestures required to produce that syllable. In the production of the word "sigh," for example, there are tactile and motion consequences of moving the front of the tongue from the tight, slightly leaking contact with the alveolar ridge required for the fricative /s/ to the constantly changing vocalic configurations required for the diphthong /ɑɪ/. Similarly, there are acoustic consequences of these movements—the frication noise for the voiceless /s/ and the rapid formant transitions (reflecting the rapid changes in vocal tract configuration) of /ɑɪ/. Over many repetitions of this syllable, from the time a child first starts to produce speech and throughout the thousands and perhaps millions of "sigh" syllables in many different words, humans build up a data-based model, or calibration, of how these particular movements should "feel" (tactile, motion sense, and so forth) and sound (acoustic) when the syllable is produced correctly. These calibrations are established by means of the connections between the speech apparatus and somatosensory and auditory association areas in parietal cortex. As the structures of the speech apparatus move during speech production, tactile receptors, baroreceptors (receptors sensitive to air pressure), and receptors sensitive to parameters of muscle contraction (such as speed of contraction and force exerted by the contraction) send information to somatosensory cortex, just like information that is sent to auditory cortex from sensory receptors in the cochlea and through the auditory pathways of the CNS. This information is encoded in the association cortex as a set of expectations for correct productions. It is as if the motor commands issued from the brain to the speech apparatus are linked, as a critical part of speech motor control, with the sensory movement consequences of those commands. The two-way pathways between the parietal and frontal lobes allow these expectations to be transferred to the lvPMC, where the programming of syllables is combined with the sensory consequences of their production. When a syllable is being programmed and delivered to PMC, the set of sensory expectations for the syllable is sent to the somatosensory and auditory association areas in the parietal lobe. The idea of a calibration of results *expected* from a syllable plan and the comparison of that plan to the actual feedback received from sensory receptors in the vocal tract and in the ear are novel concepts in DIVA. The use of this feedback in speech motor control is consistent with the idea of speech sensorimotor control.

Do the sensory expectations for a given syllable *match* the incoming somatosensory and acoustic data? This question is evaluated by the Comparator, shown in Figure 15–43 as the shaded box around the somatosensory and auditory processing boxes. If the incoming data match the sensory expectations, as they typically do in a person with a normal speech apparatus and a healthy cortex, the process of speech production continues without the need for adjustments. But if the sensory input from the speech apparatus does not match the expected calibration signals, the comparator detects an error and corrections are sent, via the blue lines, to PMC for modification of the motor commands in PMC. Although not shown in Figure 15–43, comparisons that indicate a consistent error over many repetitions also send information back to the lvPMC where the calibration, or expectations, can be updated for future productions of the syllable. The model can learn from its mistakes.

Why is this process of calibration, error detection, and correction of the calibration important to speech-language pathologists? The primary reason is that the integration of sensory consequences, and especially those related to the auditory channel, are critical to the concept of *speech* sensorimotor control. Note the avoidance of the term *tongue* motor control, or *jaw* motor control, but rather the focus on *speech* sensorimotor control. As suggested by DIVA, an important part of the speech sensorimotor control network is the comparison of expected and actual sensory consequences, and a major component of sensory consequences is the acoustic speech signal. Therefore, diagnostic or therapeutic efforts aimed at (for example) tongue or velar strength, jaw wags, and speed of lateral tongue motions are inappropriate. These oromotor, nonspeech motions certainly have sensory consequences, but an acoustic signal generated by the vocal tract for purposes of communication is not among them. Nor are the sensory consequences from sensory receptors from the speech apparatus and ear the same as those associated with, for example, maximum strength contractions of the tongue or jaw. The mounting evidence against the relevance of oromotor, nonverbal tasks for understanding speech sensorimotor control is consistent with DIVA's incorporation of the acoustic speech signal and somatosensory signals specific to speech gestures into the concept of speech sensorimotor control. (Relevant readings, showing divergent views on this topic, include Ballard, Robin, & Folkins, 2003; Forrest, 2002; Kent, 2015; Maas, 2017; Ruscello, 2008; Weismer, 2006b; and Ziegler, 2003; among others).

DIVA: Where Is Aphasia, Where Are Dysarthria Types?

As noted above, DIVA assumes the "correctness" of syllabic representations in the brain. Also, in DIVA the primary command cells in PMC are apparently not sensitive to the phonetic complexity issues inherent in cells of the lvPMC. Recently, a role of PMC in syllable complexity has been proposed (Guenther & Hickok, 2015), but theoretical details of this hypothesized mechanism have not been worked out.

There are different types of dysarthria. For example, a lesion in either the corticobulbar tract or cerebellum may result in dysarthria, but the speech signs are very different for the two neuromotor disorders. Simulated lesions in DIVA have not been explored to compare the model results across the various dysarthrias. Simulations for each of the lesions known to be associated with dysarthria are needed to determine if the model produces the lesion-dependent speech signs that are well described in the literature (Duffy, 2013). The simulations must include variation in severity, because the speech characteristics in a single dysarthria vary with severity.

Presently, PMC handles the act of producing sequences planned in lvPMC. These plans are delivered to PMC and adjusted by information circulating in the cortico-striatal-cortical and cortico-cerebellar-cortical loops (see Figures 15–17 and 15–18). One motor speech disorder that has been simulated by DIVA is ataxic dysarthria, which is usually the result of damage to the cerebellum. The speech characteristics of ataxic dysarthria include syllable timing abnormalities, difficulty with prosody (the control of speech rate, pitch, and intensity contours), and rhythmic abnormalities, which may be a function of abnormal syllable timing. DIVA includes a simulation of the cortico-cerebellar-cortical loop, which refines the motor commands issued by the PMC to brainstem and spinal cord motor neurons. The DIVA simulation of cerebellar lesions results in speech output with abnormal timing, which is one of the characteristics of ataxic dysarthria. The match of the simulation to one of the "real" speech characteristics in ataxic dysarthria is an interesting start on modeling motor speech disorders with models like DIVA.

Finally, DIVA and the related "dual-stream" model of speech and language perception and production (Hickok, 2012) regard conduction aphasia as a result of damage to the cortical regions associated with the integration of perceptual and motor processing for speech motor control. People with conduction aphasia often have normal speech fluency but make frequent phonetic errors; they also have good comprehension. They apparently recognize their production errors but are unable to correct them, even with multiple attempts to do so. So where is the lesion that results in conduction aphasia? One possibility is a cortical lesion in the region where auditory and motor information are put together for the smooth and accurate production of speech. Damage to the planum temporale and/or the posterior, superior temporal gyrus has been proposed as the lesion site for conduction aphasia. This is the site where auditory control of planned articulatory behavior is thought to reside. The damage does not affect the fluency of speech motor behavior, nor does it interfere with comprehension. Because of the lesion location, incoming auditory information that is part of the calibration between vocal tract movements and expected auditory consequences cannot function to correct inaccurate speech motor commands. The result is conduction aphasia, in which fluency and comprehension are preserved but ability to correct production errors is impaired.

Auditory processes are therefore critical to speech motor control. This is a very different view compared with the frontal lobe being the region of speech motor control and the posterior part of the superior temporal gyrus the region of speech and language perception.

DIVA is a remarkable achievement and has produced new and important insights to speech production and its disruption by brain lesions. Future developments are likely to include new simulations of aphasia, and new simulations of the execution functions of the model. The fact that a model cannot explain everything about a process as complicated as speech and language, and even makes mistakes or produces difficult-to-interpret results concerning the processes it is designed to explain, does not make it less valuable. It is, in effect, a highly structured guide to future theoretical (modeling) and clinical investigations of the nervous system basis of human communication.

REVIEW

The chapter is initiated with a summary of general concepts including central versus peripheral nervous system (CNS vs. PNS), anatomical planes and directions, white versus gray matter, tracts versus nuclei, nerves versus ganglia, afferent and efferent, and lateralization and specialization of function.

The cerebral hemispheres include cortical tissue (gray matter), fiber tracts (white matter), and subcortical nuclei (gray matter), and the surface of the cerebral hemispheres is defined by gyri (hills) and sulci (valleys).

Each cerebral hemisphere has four lobes, including the frontal, parietal, temporal, and occipital lobes, and regions within these lobes that have been proposed as serving specialized roles in speech, language, and hearing.

Two other areas of cortical tissue—the insula and components of the limbic system—may play important roles in speech, language, and hearing.

Cerebral white matter is composed of many types of tracts (association, striatal, commissural, descending, and ascending) that connect different cortical cells and nuclei of the CNS to each other, one of the most important of which for speech and language is the arcuate fasciculus.

Descending tracts from the cortex to the brainstem (corticobulbar tract) and spinal cord (corticospinal tract) innervate lower motor neurons that represent the final common pathway to muscles of the speech apparatus.

Ascending tracts are primarily associated with sensory pathways and carry information about touch, pain, temperature, hearing, vision, vibration, and proprioception.

The basal ganglia are a group of subcortical nuclei (nuclei within the cerebral hemispheres and above the brainstem) that connect to the cortex via loops and are important in aspects of speech sensorimotor control such as the refinement and programming of motor behavior.

The thalamus is the major relay for all sensory information (except smell) ascending in the CNS to the cortex and is also an output target to the cortex, via the globus pallidus, for information processed in the basal ganglia.

The cerebellum is connected to the spinal cord, brainstem, and cerebral hemispheres by the cerebellar peduncles, and to the cortex (via loops, like the basal ganglia) and contributes to the coordination of complex motor behavior, and balance, and possibly plays a role in programming motor sequences such as successive articulatory gestures.

The brainstem, a stalk of tissue connecting the spinal cord to the cerebral hemispheres and cerebellum, has three levels, including (from superior to inferior) the midbrain (mesencephalon), pons, and medulla, each containing sensory and motor nuclei, as well as descending, ascending, and crossing fiber tracts.

Prominent features on the ventral and dorsal surfaces of the brainstem are entrance and exit locations of most of the cranial nerves, including those associated with control of head and neck muscles (cranial nerves V, VII, IX, X, XI, XII).

The 12 cranial nerves have names and numbers (olfactory [I], optic [II], oculomotor [III], trochlear [IV], trigeminal [V], abducens [VI], facial [VII], auditory-vestibular [VIII], glossopharyngeal [IX], vagus [X], spinal accessory [XI], and hypoglossal [XII]) and are composed of motor, sensory, or both motor and sensory fibers that transmit information between the CNS and the body.

The spinal cord, which is continuous with the inferior border of the medulla and extends from the first cervical vertebrae to the upper lumbar vertebrae, contains central gray matter consisting of neuron cell bodies (sensory cells in the dorsal part of the cord, motor cells in the ventral part) and surrounding white matter consisting of axons that supply the muscles of the breathing apparatus as well as other voluntary musculature of the limbs and torso.

Cells in the nervous system include signaling cells (neurons); glial cells (astrocytes, oligodendrocytes, Schwann cells), which provide metabolic and protective support to the neurons; and ependymal cells, which secrete CSF.

Neurons, or signaling cells, are composed of a cell body (soma), dendrites, an axon, and a terminal button or buttons, and communicate with each other by conversion of electrical-to-neurochemical energy, which is then converted back to electrical energy.

An action potential is initiated at the dendrites, which depolarizes the soma, causing electrical energy to be propagated down the axon to the terminal buttons, which are encased by a presynaptic membrane and where neurotransmitter is released into the cleft between the terminal button and the dendrites of an adjacent neuron (postsynaptic membrane).

The presynaptic/synaptic cleft/postsynaptic structures and conversion of electrical to chemical to electrical energy is called a synapse.

The neuromuscular junction is where a motor nerve makes contact with a motor endplate attached to muscle fiber; the neurotransmitter acetylcholine is released by the terminal buttons of the peripheral nerve to bind to special receptors embedded in the motor endplate, thereby causing an action potential to be generated in the muscle fiber and the muscle fiber to shorten (contract).

The meninges are protective coverings of the cerebral hemispheres, brainstem, and spinal cord and include the dura mater, arachnoid mater, and pia mater.

CSF flows throughout the ventricular system, which includes the lateral ventricles, third ventricle, fourth ventricle, and central canal of the spinal cord.

The blood supply of the brain originates from arteries emerging from the heart and includes an anterior and posterior supply, with one of the most important anterior arteries for speech, language, and hearing function being the middle cerebral artery.

The computer simulation model called DIVA makes certain predictions about how damage to regions of the frontal lobe affect speech output, as well as damage to parts of the parietal lobe and the effect on a speaker's ability to produce articulatory gestures with known acoustic results.

REFERENCES

Ackermann, H., & Riecker, A. (2010). The contributions(s) of the insula to speech production: A review of the clinical and functional imaging literature. *Brain Structure and Function, 214,* 419–433.

Alvarez, J. A., & Emory, E. (2006). Executive function and the frontal lobes: A meta-analytic review. *Neuropsychology Review, 16,* 17–42.

Ballard, K. J., Robin, D. A., & Folkins, J. W. (2003). An integrative model of speech motor control: A response to Ziegler. *Aphasiology, 17,* 37–48.

Bear, M. F., Connors, B. W., & Paradiso, M. A. (2016). *Neuroscience: Exploring the brain* (4th ed.). Philadelphia, PA: Wolters Kluwer.

Bernal, B., & Ardila, A. (2009). The role of the arcuate fasciculus in conduction aphasia. *Brain, 132,* 2309–2316.

Bohland, J. W., Bullock, D., & Guenther, F. H. (2010). Neural representations and mechanisms for the performance of simple speech sequences. *Journal of Cognitive Neuroscience, 22,* 1504–1529.

Blumenfeld, H. (2010). *Neuroanatomy through clinical cases* (2nd ed.). Sunderland, MA: Sinauer Associates.

Bostan, A. C., & Strick, P. L. (2010). The cerebellum and basal ganglia are interconnected. *Neuropsychology Review, 20,* 261–270.

Catani, M., & Mesulam, M. (2008). The arcuate fasciculus and the disconnection theme in language and aphasia: History and current state. *Cortex, 44,* 953–961.

Conturo, T. E., Lori, N. F., Cull, T. S., Akbudak, E., Snyder, A. Z., Shimony, J. S., . . . Raichle, M. E. (2008). Tracking neuronal fiber pathways in the living human brain. *Proceedings of the National Academy of Sciences USA, 96,* 10422–10427.

Culham, J. C., & Valyear, K. F. (2006). Human parietal cortex in action. *Current Opinion in Neurobiology, 16,* 205–212.

Darley, F. L., Aronson, A. E., & Brown, J. R. (1975). *Motor speech disorders.* Philadelphia, PA: W. B. Saunders.

Deacon, T. W. (1997). *The symbolic species: The co-evolution of language and the brain.* New York, NY: W. W. Norton.

DeToledo, J. C., & David, N. J. (2001). Innervation of the sternocleidomastoid and trapezius muscles by the accessory nucleus. *Journal of Neuro-Ophthalmology, 21,* 214–216.

Dick, A. S., Bernal, B., & Tremblay, P. (2014). The language connectome: New pathways, new concepts. *The Neuroscientist, 20,* 453–467.

Dronkers, N. F., Plaisant, O., Ibas-Zisen, M. T., & Cabanis, E. A. (2007). Paul Broca's historic cases: High-resolution MR imaging of the brains of LeBorgne and Lelong. *Brain, 129,* 1164–1176.

Duffy, J. D. (2013). *Motor speech disorders: Substrates, differential diagnosis, and management.* St. Louis, MO: Elsevier Mosby.

Eftekhar, B., Dadmehr, M., Ansari, S., Ghodsi, M., Nazparvar, B., & Ketabchi, E. (2006). Are the distributions of variations of circle of Willis different in different populations? Results of an anatomical study and review of literature. *BMC Neurology, 6,* 22. Retrieved from http://www.biomedcentral.com/1471-2377/6/22

Epelbaum, S., Pinel, P., Gaillard, R., Delmaire, C., Perrin, M., Dupont, S., . . . Cohen L. (2008). Pure alexia as a disconnection syndrome: New diffusion imaging evidence for an old concept. *Cortex, 44*, 962–974.

Fasano, A., Daniele, A., & Albanese, A. (2012). Treatment of motor and non-motor features of Parkinson's disease with deep brain stimulation. *Lancet Neurology, 11*, 429–442.

Forrest, K. (2002). Are oral-motor exercises useful in the treatment of phonological/articulatory disorders? *Seminars in Speech and Language, 23*, 15–26.

Gazzaniga, M. (2000). Cerebral specialization and interhemispheric communication: Does the corpus callosum enable the human condition? *Brain, 123*, 1293–1326.

Geschwind, N. (1965). Disconnection syndromes in animals and man. *Brain, 88*, 237–294.

Graff-Radford, J., Jones, D. T., Strand, E. A., Rabinstein, A. A., Duffy, J. R., & Josephs, K. A. (2014). The neuroanatomy of pure apraxia of speech in stroke. *Brain & Language, 129*, 43–46.

Grodzinsky, Y., & Santi, A. (2008). The battle for Broca's region. *Trends in Cognitive Sciences, 12*, 474–480.

Guenther, F. H. (1995). Speech sound acquisition, coarticulation, and rate effects in a neural network model of speech production. *Psychological Review, 102*, 594–621.

Guenther, F. H. (2006). Cortical interaction underlying the production of speech sounds. *Journal of Communication Disorders, 39*, 350–365.

Guenther, F. H., Ghosh, S. S., & Tourville, J. A. (2006). Neural modeling and imaging of the cortical interactions underlying syllable production. *Brain and Language, 96*, 280–301.

Guenther, F. H., & Hickok, G. (2015). Role of the auditory system in speech production. *Handbook of Clinical Neurology, 129*, 161–175.

Heimer, L., & Van Hoesen, G. W. (2006). The limbic lobe and its output channels: Implications for emotional functions and adaptive behavior. *Neuroscience and Biobehavioral Reviews, 30*, 126–147.

Hickok, G. (2009). The functional neuroanatomy of language. *Physics of Life Reviews, 6*, 121–143.

Hickok, G., & Poeppel, D. (2007). The cortical organization of speech processing. *Nature Reviews: Neuroscience, 8*, 393–402.

Ito, T., & Gomi, H. (2007). Cutaneous mechanoreceptors contribute to the generation of a cortical reflex in speech. *NeuroReport, 18*, 907–910.

Kandel, E. R., Schwartz, J. H., Jessel, T. M., Siegelbaum, S. A., & Hudspeth, A. J. (2013). *Principles of neural science* (5th ed.). New York, NY: McGraw-Hill.

Keller, S. S., Crow, T., Foundas, A., Amunts, K., & Roberts, N. (2009). Broca's area: Nomenclature, anatomy, typology, and asymmetry. *Brain and Language, 109*, 29–48.

Kent, R. D. (2015). Nonspeech oral movements and oral motor disorders: A narrative review. *American Journal of Speech Language Pathology, 24*, 763–789.

Kent, R. D., Martin, R. E., & Sufit, R. L. (1990). Oral sensation: A review and clinical perspective. In H. Winitz (Ed.), *Human communication and its disorders* (Vol. 3, pp. 135–191). Norwood, NJ: Ablex.

Knecht, S., Dräger, B., Deppe, M., Bobe, L., Lohmann, H., Flöell, A., . . . Henningsen, H. (2000). Handedness and hemispheric language dominance in healthy humans. *Brain, 123*, 2512–2518.

Kuehn, D. P., Templeton, P. J., & Maynard, J. A. (1990). Muscle spindles in the velopharyngeal musculature of humans. *Journal of Speech and Hearing Research, 33*, 488–493.

Langers, D. R. M., Backe, W. H., & van Dijk, P. (2007). Representation of lateralization and tonotopicity in primary versus secondary human auditory cortex. *NeuroImage, 34*, 264–273.

Lee, D., Swanson, S. J., Sabsevitz, D. S., Hammeke, T. A., Winstanley, F. S., Possing, E. T., & Binder, J. R. (2008). Functional MRI and Wada studies in patients with interhemispheric dissociation of language functions. *Epilepsy and Behavior, 13*, 350–356.

Lindenberg, R., Fangerau, H., & Seitz, R. J. (2007)."Broca's area" as a collective term? *Brain and Language, 102*, 22–29.

Ludlow, C. L. (2011). Spasmodic dysphonia: A laryngeal control disorder specific to speech. *Journal of Neuroscience, 19*, 793–797.

Maas, E. (2017). Speech and nonspeech: What are we talking about? *International Journal of Speech Language Pathology, 19*, 345-359.

Martino, J., De Witt Hamer, P. C., Vergani, F., Brogna, C., de Lucas, E. M., Vázquez-Barquero, A., . . . Duffau, H. (2011). Cortex-sparing fiber dissection: An improved method for the study of white matter anatomy in the human brain. *Journal of Anatomy, 219*, 531–541.

McNeil, M. R., Robin, D. A., & Schmidt, R. A. (2009). Apraxia of speech. In M. R. McNeil (Ed.), *Clinical management of sensorimotor speech disorders* (2nd ed., pp. 249–268). New York, NY: Thieme.

Meng, H., Murakami, G., Suzuki, D., & Miyamoto, S. (2008). Anatomical variations in stylopharyngeus muscle insertions suggest interindividual and left/right differences in pharyngeal clearance function of elderly patients: A cadaveric study. *Dysphagia, 23*, 251–257.

Middleton, F. A., & Strick, P. L. (2000). Basal ganglia and cerebellar loops: Motor and cognitive circuits. *Brain Research Reviews, 31*, 236–250.

Mohr, J. P., Pessin, M. S., Finkelstein, S., Funkenstein, H. H., Duncan, G. W., & Davis, K. R. (1978). Broca aphasia: Pathologic and clinical. *Neurology, 28*, 311–324.

Morley, M., Court, D., & Miller, H. (1954). Developmental dysarthria. *British Medical Journal, 1*, 8–10.

Nambu, A. (2008). Several problems on the basal ganglia. *Current Opinion in Neurobiology, 18*, 595–604.

Obeso, J. A., & Lanciego, J. L. (2011). Past, present, and future of the pathophysiological model of the basal ganglia. *Frontiers in Neuroanatomy, 5*, 1–6.

Ocklenburg, S., Beste C., Arning, L., Peterburs, J., & Güntürkün, O. (2014). The ontogenesis of language lateralization and its relation to handedness. *Neuroscience and Biobehavioral Reviews, 43*, 191–198.

Ogar, J., Slama, H., Dronkers, N., Amici, S., & Gorno-Tempini, M. L. (2005). Apraxia of speech: An overview. *Neurocase, 11*, 427–432.

Papagno, C., Comi, A., Riva, M., Bizzi, A., Vernice, M., Casarotti, A., Fava, E., & Bello, L. (2017). Mapping the brain network of the phonological loop. *Human Brain Mapping, 38*, 3011–3024.

Peeva, M. G., Guenther, F. H., Tourville, J. A., Nieto-Castanon, A., Anton, J-L., Nazarian, B., & Alario, F-X. (2010). Distinct representation of phonemes, syllables, and suprasyllabic sequences in the speech production network. *NeuroImage, 50,* 626–638.

Picton, T. (2010). *Human auditory evoked potentials.* San Diego, CA: Plural.

Postuma, R. B., & Dagher, A. (2006). Basal ganglia functional connectivity based on a meta-analysis of 126 positron emission tomography and functional magnetic resonance imaging publications. *Cerebral Cortex, 16,* 1508–1521.

Pramstaller, P. O., & Marsden, C. D. (1996). The basal ganglia and apraxia. *Brain, 119,* 319–340.

Price, C. J. (2010). The anatomy of language: A review of 100 fMRI studies published in 2009. *Annals of the New York Academy of Sciences, 1191,* 62–88.

Rasmussen, T., & Milner, B. (1977). The role of early left-brain injury in determining lateralization of cerebral speech functions. *Annals of the New York Academy of Sciences, 299,* 355–369.

Ridderinkhof, K. R., Ullsperger, M., Crone, E. A., & Nieuwenhuis, S. (2004). The role of the medial frontal cortex in cognitive control. *Science, 306,* 443–447.

Rosenbek, J. C., Kent, R. D., & LaPointe, L. L. (1984). Apraxia of speech: An overview and some perspectives. In J. C. Rosenbek, M. R. McNeil, & A. E. Aronson (Eds.), *Apraxia of speech* (pp. 1–72). San Diego, CA: College-Hill Press.

Ruscello, D. M. (2008). An examination of non-speech oromotor exercises in children with velopharyngeal inadequacy. *Seminars in Speech and Language, 29,* 294–303.

Said, C. P., Haxby, J. V., & Todorov, A. (2011). Brain systems for assessing the affective value of faces. *Philosophical Transactions of the Royal Society B, 366,* 1660–1670.

Saigusa, H., Yamashita, K., Tanuma, K., Saigusa, M., & Niimi, S. (2004). Morphological studies for retrusive movement of the human adult tongue. *Clinical Anatomy, 17,* 93–98.

Sanders, I., Han, Y., Wang, J., & Biller, H. (1998). Muscle spindles are concentrated in the superior vocalis subcompartment of the human thyroarytenoid muscle. *Journal of Voice, 12,* 7–16.

Sarikcioglu, L., Altun, U., Suzen, B., & Oguz, N. (2008). The evolution of the terminology of the basal ganglia, or are they nuclei? *Journal of the History of the Neurosciences: Basic and Clinical Perspectives, 17,* 226–229.

Saur, D., Kreher, B. W., Schnell, S., Kümmerer, D., Kellmeyer, P., Vry, M. S., . . . Weiller, C. (2008). Ventral and dorsal pathways for language. *Proceedings of the National Academy of Sciences of the United States, 18,* 18035–18040.

Schmahmann, J. D., Smith, E. E., Eichler, F. S., & Filley, C. M. (2008). Cerebral white matter: Neuroanatomy, clinical neurology, and neurobehavioral correlates. *Annals of the New York Academy of Sciences, 1142,* 266–309.

Schmitz, J., Lor, S., Klose, R., Güntürkün, O., & Ocklenburg, S. (2107). Functional genetics of handedness and language lateralization: Insights from gene ontology, pathway and disease association analyses. *Frontiers in Psychology, 8.* doi:10.3389/fpsyg.2017.01144

Smits, M., Jiskoot, L.C., & Papma (2014). White matter tracts of speech and language. *Seminars in Ultrasounds, CT, and MRI, 35,* 504-516.

Springer, J. A., Binder, J. R., Hammeke, T. A., Swanson, S. J., Frost, J. A., Bellgowan, P. S. F., . . . Mueller, W. M. (1999). Language dominance in neurologically normal and epilepsy subjects: A functional MRI study. *Brain, 122,* 2033–2046.

Takai, O., Brown, S., & Liotti, M. (2010). Representation of the speech effectors in the human motor cortex: Somatotopy or overlap? *Brain and Language, 113,* 39–44.

Takaya, S., Kuperberg, G. R., Liu, H., Greve, D. N., Makris, N., & Stufflebeam, S. M. (2015). Asymmetric projections of the arcuate fasciculus to the temporal cortex underlie lateralized language function in the human brain. *Frontiers in Neuroanatomy, 9,* 119. doi:10.3389/fnana.2015.00119

Terband, H., & Maassen, B. (2010). Speech motor development in childhood apraxia of speech: Generating testable hypotheses by neurocomputational modeling. *Folia Phoniatrica et Logopaedica, 62,* 134–142.

Tervaniemi, M., & Hugdahl, K. (2003). Lateralization of auditory-cortex functions. *Brain Research Reviews, 43,* 231–246.

Urban, P. P., Marx, J., Hunsche, S., Gawehn, J., Vucurevic, G., Wicht, S., . . . Hopf, H. C. (2003). Cerebellar speech representation: Lesion topography in dysarthria as derived from cerebellar ischemia and functional magnetic resonance imaging. *Archives of Neurology, 60,* 965–972.

Urban, P. P., Rolke, R., Wicht, S., Keilmann, A., Stoeter, P., Hopf, H. C., & Dieterich, M. (2006). Left hemispheric dominance for articulation: A prospective study on acute ischaemic dysarthria at different localizations. *Brain, 129,* 767–777.

van Esch, B. F., Wegner, I., & Stegeman, I. (2017). Effect of botulinum toxin and surgery among spasmodic dysphonia patients: A systematic review. *Otolaryngology-Head and Neck Surgery, 156,* 238–254.

Weismer, G. (2006a) (Ed.). *Motor speech disorders.* San Diego, CA: Plural.

Weismer, G. (2006b). Philosophy of research in motor speech disorders. *Clinical Linguistics and Phonetics, 20,* 315–349.

Willems, R. M., & Hagoort, P. (2009). Broca's region: Battles are not won by ignoring half of the facts. *Trends in Cognitive Sciences, 13,* 101.

Wilson-Pauwels, L., Akesson, E. J., Stewart, P. A., & Spacey, S. D. (2002). *Cranial nerves in health and disease.* Hamilton, Ontario: B. C. Decker.

Wright, D. L., Robin, D. A., Rhee J., Vaculin, A., Jacks, A., Guenther, F. H., & Fox, P. T. (2009). Using the self-select paradigm to delineate the nature of speech motor programming. *Journal of Speech, Language, and Hearing Research, 52,* 755–765.

Ziegler, W. (2003). Speech motor control is task-specific: Evidence from dysarthria and apraxia of speech. *Aphasiology, 17,* 3–36.

Zilles, K., Armstrong, E., Schleicher, A., & Kretschmann, H. J. (1988). The human pattern of gyrification in the cerebral cortex. *Anatomy and Embryology, 179,* 173–179.

16

Swallowing

INTRODUCTION

Some of the most enjoyable activities of daily living involve eating and drinking. These include meals (where eating and drinking are the purpose of the activity), special events such as receptions (where eating and drinking enhance the celebration), and relaxation activities such as going to the movies (where eating popcorn and drinking soda are an integral part of the experience for some people). Figure 16–1 is a cartoon that depicts the anticipation of a good meal and the social context in which it is enjoyed.

The ease of eating and drinking is deceptive. These are complicated activities that require intricately coordinated actions of the lips, mandible, tongue, velum, pharynx, larynx, esophagus, and other structures. Because eating and drinking engage many of the same structures and much of the same airway as those used for speaking and breathing, it is not uncommon for there to be competition between these activities or for tradeoffs to occur when trying to do them simultaneously. For example, chewing must stop to be able to speak clearly and breathing must stop to be able to swallow safely.

The entire act of placing liquid or solid substance in the oral cavity, moving it backward to the pharynx, propelling it into the esophagus, and allowing it to make its way to the stomach is called *deglutition*. Although the word *swallowing* is sometimes used as a synonym for deglutition, swallowing actually includes only certain phases of deglutition. Nevertheless, to simplify the explanations that follow, the term *swallowing* is used in place of deglutition and is meant to include all phases of deglutition.

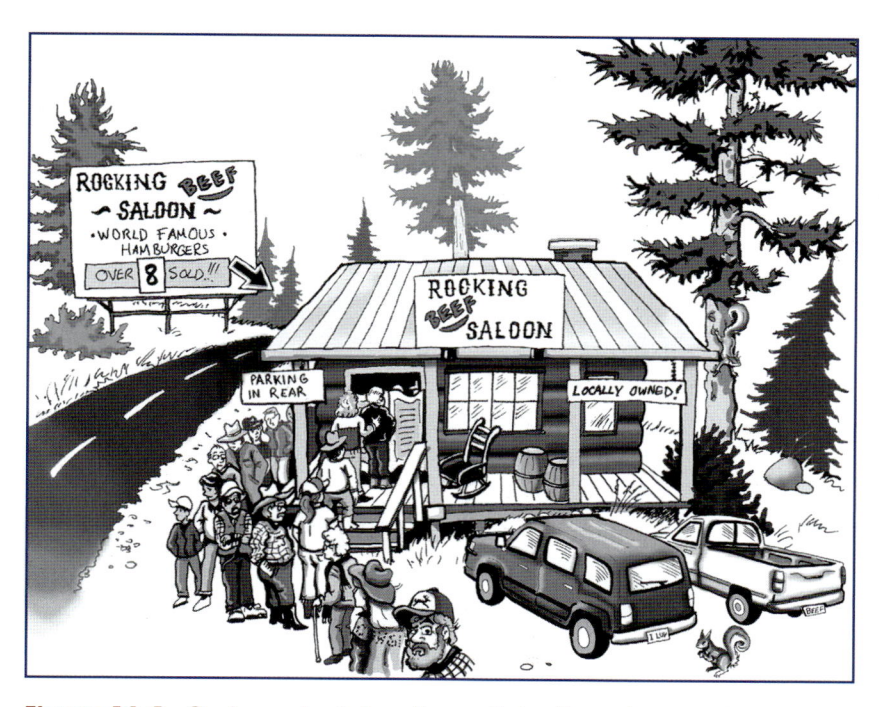

Figure 16–1. Cartoon depicting the anticipation of a good meal and the social context in which it is enjoyed.

669

This chapter begins with discussion of the anatomy of swallowing, its forces and movements, the coordination of breathing with swallowing, and the neural control of swallowing. Discussion then moves to variables that influence swallowing, measurement and analysis of swallowing, and health care professionals involved in the evaluation and management of clients with swallowing disorders.

ANATOMY

Figure 16–2 shows the structures that participate in swallowing. These structures extend from the lips to the stomach. Most of these same structures also participate in speech production; notable exceptions are the esophagus and stomach.

Breathing, Laryngeal, Velopharyngeal-Nasal, and Pharyngeal-Oral Structures

Structures within the breathing, laryngeal, velopharyngeal-nasal, and pharyngeal-oral subsystems participate in swallowing. These include the chest wall, vocal folds, ventricular folds, epiglottis, pharynx (laryngopharynx, oropharynx, nasopharynx), velum, tongue, mandible, and lips. Their anatomy is described in Chapters 2, 3, 4, and 5, and their functions during swallowing are

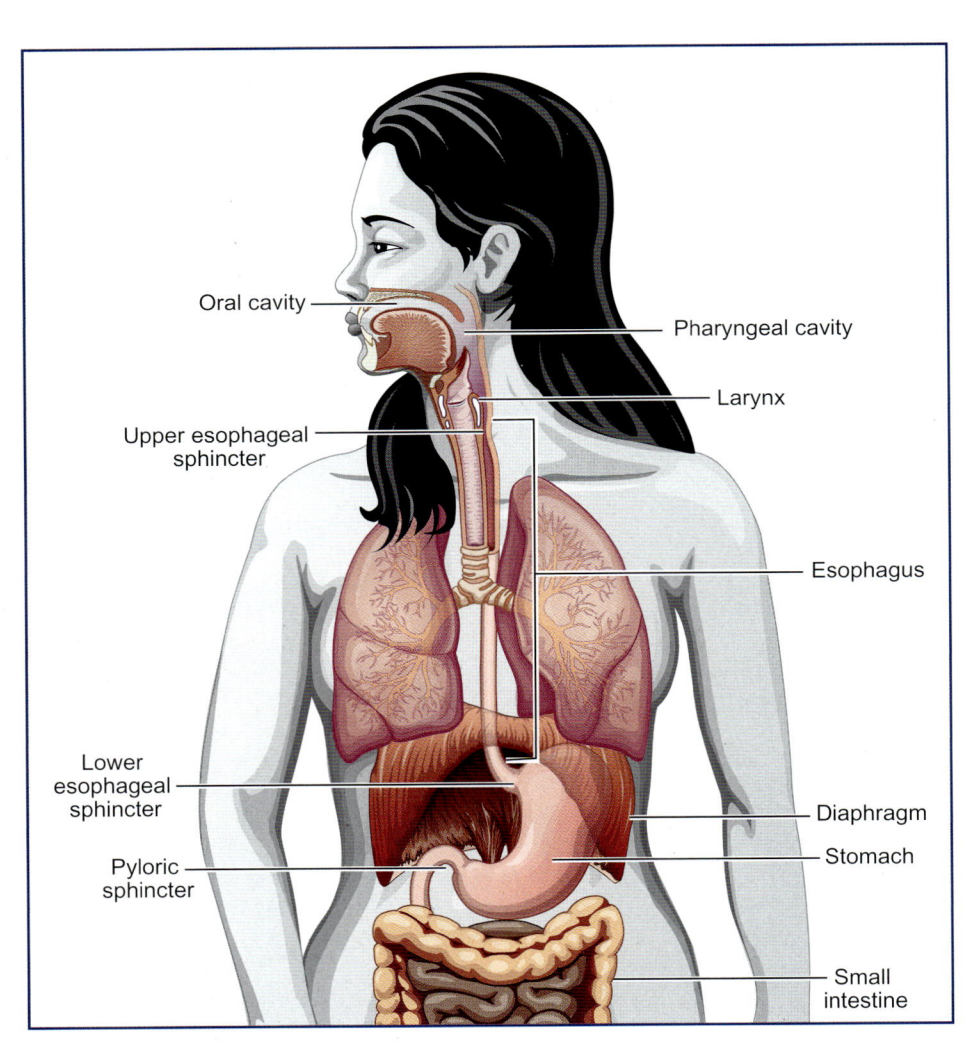

Figure 16-2. Structures of the swallowing apparatus. These include structures that participate in speech production (see Chapters 2, 3, 4, and 5 for detailed descriptions), as well as structures that do not (esophagus, stomach, and intestines and their associated sphincters).

described below. The anatomy of the esophagus and stomach is not covered in the other chapters and warrants attention here.

Esophagus

The esophagus is a flexible tube, about 20 to 25 cm long in adults, which extends from the lower part of the pharynx to the stomach. The esophagus begins below the base of the larynx and runs behind the trachea, pulmonary apparatus, and heart. It courses through the diaphragm (see Figure 2–6) and enters the abdominal cavity, where it connects to the stomach. The esophagus is usually in a flattened state, but can stretch to accommodate substances passing through it. The cervical (upper) esophagus consists of striated (voluntary) muscle, whereas the thoracic (middle) esophagus comprises a mixture of striated and smooth (involuntary) muscle in its upper region and purely smooth muscle in its lower region. The abdominal (lower) esophagus is composed of only smooth muscle. The esophagus is lined with a thick layer of mucosa, beneath which lies connective tissue and glands that secrete mucus to aid in the movement of substances through it.

The esophagus is bounded at its upper end by the upper esophageal sphincter (sometimes called the pharyngoesophageal segment, or PE segment) and at its lower end by the lower esophageal sphincter. These sphincters mark the entrance and exit of the esophagus and are operationally defined as zones of high pressure, rather than as precise anatomical entities. It is uncertain which structures are responsible for creating these high-pressure zones. Nevertheless, indirect evidence suggests that the *cricopharyngeus* muscles of the pharynx (considered by some to be part of the *inferior constrictor* muscles) are the primary contributors to the contraction–relaxation pattern of the upper esophageal sphincter (Hila, Castell, & Castell, 2001).

The upper end of the esophagus is positioned among several of the pharyngeal and laryngeal structures discussed in Chapters 3, 4, and 5. These structures are depicted in two different views in Figure 16–3. Figure 16–3A depicts the laryngeal area and the top of the esophagus (in its closed state) as viewed from above. Of particular interest in the context of swallowing are the pyriform sinuses and the epiglottic valleculae. The pyriform sinuses are cavities that are located near the back of the larynx and lateral to the aryepiglottic folds. The epiglottic valleculae (one vallecula on each side) are depressions located toward the front of the larynx on the lingual (tongue) side of the epiglottis and just behind the root of the tongue. Figure 16–3B shows the pharyngeal, laryngeal, and upper esophageal areas as viewed from the back, with the pharyngeal muscles intact (left side) and with those muscles removed and the pharynx open at the back (right side). The *cricopharyngeus* muscle (lower part of the *inferior constrictor* muscle) is shown to surround the region of the upper esophagus. Also shown in Figure 16–3B is the relationship of the esophagus to one pyriform sinus and one epiglottic vallecula, as well as the epiglottis, tongue, and velum.

Stomach

The stomach is a large, saclike structure made up of smooth muscle, mucosa, and other tissue. It is on the left side of the abdominal cavity, against the undersurface of the diaphragm (see Figure 16–2). The stomach connects to the esophagus via the lower esophageal sphincter and to the small intestine via the pyloric sphincter. After a typical meal, the stomach holds about a liter of solid and/or liquid substance, although it can stretch to hold much more if necessary. Gastric juices in the stomach break up ingested substances so that they can be absorbed into the body through the stomach lining.

America Regains the Mustard Yellow Belt

Holy stomach full! Japan's Takeru Kobayashi was the six-time hot-dog-eating world champion and ate 63 hot dogs and buns (6 more than his personal best) on July 4, 2007, at Coney Island, New York. With more than 50,000 people in attendance and in the glare of national television cameras, Kobayashi lost his crown to Joey Chestnut of San Jose, California. Sanctioned by Major League Eating, the world governing body of all stomach-centric sport, Nathan's Famous International Fourth of July Hot Dog Eating Championship has been held each year on the 4th of July since 1916. In 2007, Chestnut put down an astounding 66 hot dogs and buns to set a new world's record. On July 4, 2018, with ten wins already under his belt, Chestnut once again exceeded his personal best by ingesting 74 dogs and buns in just 10 minutes. And, yes, there is a women's competition too. The women's 2018 winner was Miki Sudo, who ingested 37 hot dogs to take home her fifth Nathan's title in a row.

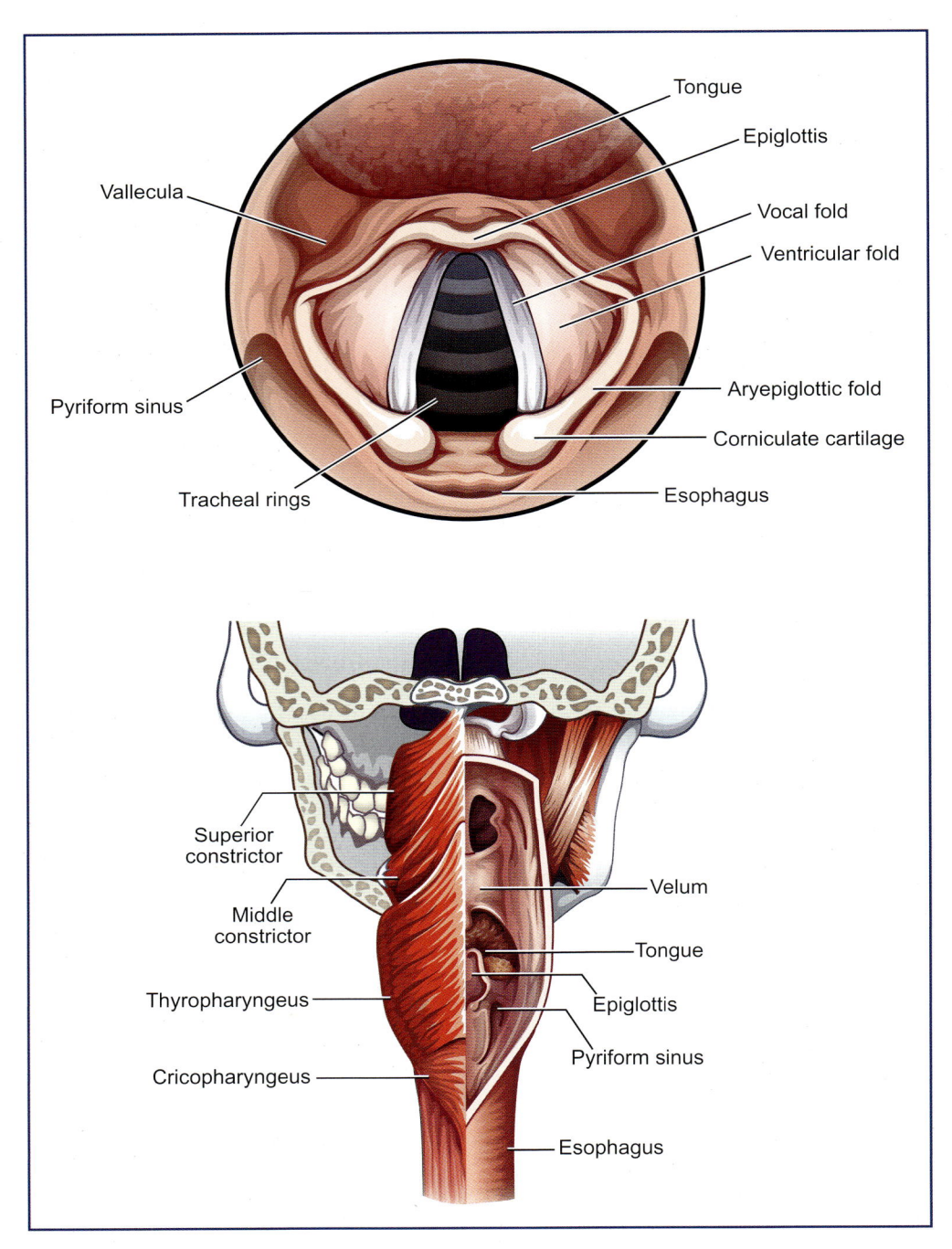

Figure 16–3. Two views of laryngeal and pharyngeal structures. The top figure (**A**) depicts the laryngeal area viewed from above. In particular, note the location of the pyriform sinuses (toward the back), esophagus (behind the larynx), and the epiglottic valleculae (toward the front, near the tongue root). The bottom figure (**B**) is a view from the back. Its left side shows the **superior**, **middle**, and **inferior** (**thyropharyngeus** and **cricopharyngeus** divisions) **constrictor** muscles intact. Its right side shows these muscles removed to reveal the pharyngeal and laryngeal regions (again, note the location of the pyriform sinus).

FORCES AND MOVEMENTS OF SWALLOWING

Although many of the structures that participate in swallowing are the same as those that are used for speaking, the forces and movements for the two activities are very different. In general, the forces are greater and many of the movements are slower during swallowing than during speech production.

To set the stage for understanding the forces and movements of swallowing, it is useful to begin by considering certain pressures associated with the resting state of the swallowing apparatus. These pressures, pointed out in Figure 16–4, are shown with the swallowing apparatus at rest at the end of a tidal expiration. As expected, the pressure in the oral cavity, which is coupled to the outside via the velopharyngeal-nasal airway, is zero (equal to atmospheric pressure) at rest. The other pressures are not zero and their values as shown in Figure 16–4 are approximations; some of them can range substantially.

The pressure within the esophagus is below atmospheric pressure (approximately −5 centimeters of water [cmH_2O]). This pressure is negative because of pleural linkage—the link between a pulmonary apparatus that "wants" to contract and a chest wall

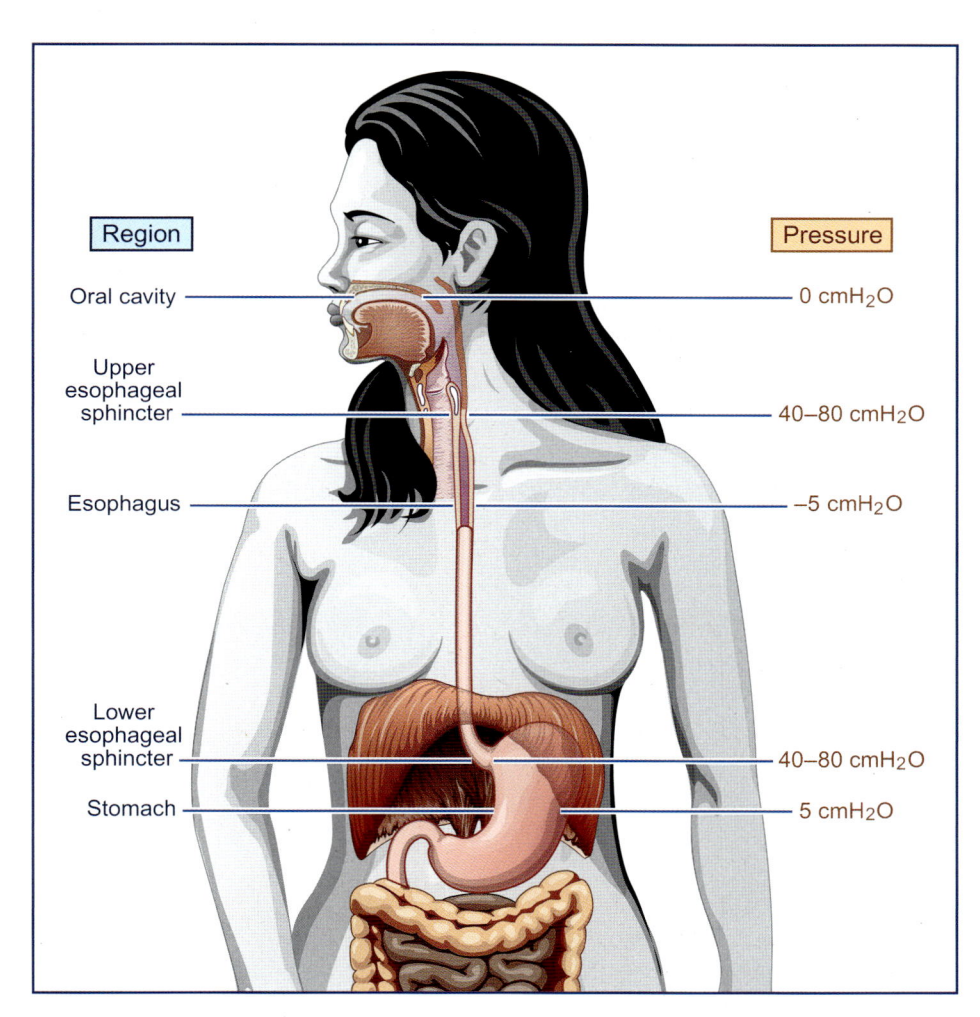

Region	Pressure
Oral cavity	0 cmH_2O
Upper esophageal sphincter	40–80 cmH_2O
Esophagus	−5 cmH_2O
Lower esophageal sphincter	40–80 cmH_2O
Stomach	5 cmH_2O

Figure 16-4. Relevant pressures associated with the resting state of the swallowing apparatus. Oral pressure is zero (atmospheric), esophageal pressure is slightly negative, and stomach (gastric) pressure is slightly positive. Both the upper and lower esophageal sphincters exert high pressure that can range considerably in magnitude. It is especially important that the lower esophageal sphincter pressure remain higher than the pressure within the stomach (gastric pressure) so that the contents of the stomach do not reflux.

that "wants" to expand (recall the spring analogy in Figure 2–4 representing the linked pulmonary apparatus and chest wall). This creates a negative pressure between the pleura (called pleural pressure; see Chapter 2), and that negative pressure is transmitted across the dividing wall to the esophagus.

The pressure in the stomach (gastric pressure) is slightly above atmospheric pressure (approximately 5 cmH$_2$O). This positive pressure is, in part, the result of the muscle tone exerted by the wall of the stomach. This pressure is also attributed to the hydrostatic properties of the abdomen.

In contrast to these relatively low esophageal and gastric pressures, the pressures within the upper and lower esophageal sphincters are high. These high pressures are attributable to the high tissue forces exerted by the sphincters. Although a typical range is 40 to 80 cmH$_2$O in the resting state, their absolute magnitudes depend on the measurement approach used as well as a variety of physiological factors (Goyal & Cobb, 1981; Linden, Hogosta, & Norlander, 2007). Because the upper and lower esophageal sphincters exert such high pressures, these regions function like forcefully closed valves while at rest. In particular, it is important that the pressure in the lower esophageal sphincter be substantially higher than the pressure in the stomach. Otherwise, substances from the stomach may reflux (flow back) into the esophagus.

The act of swallowing is driven by both passive and active forces. Passive force comes from many sources, including: (a) the natural recoil of connective tissues (ligaments and membranes), cartilages, and bones, (b) the surface tension between structures in apposition, (c) the pull of gravity, and (d) aeromechanical factors. Active force results from the activation of breathing, laryngeal, velopharyngeal-nasal, and pharyngeal-oral muscles in various combinations. Their contributions to active force are described in Chapters 2, 3, 4, and 5, and are discussed here as they relate to swallowing, as are the forces exerted by the esophagus.

Forces and movements of swallowing can be described as they pertain to four phases of swallowing. These phases, illustrated in Figure 16–5, are the oral preparatory phase, oral transport phase (sometimes called the oral propulsive phase or oral transit phase), pharyngeal phase, and esophageal phase. They are used to describe the movement of a bolus (shown in green in Figure 16–5) through the oral, pharyngeal, and esophageal regions of the swallowing apparatus. *Bolus* is the word used to refer to the volume of liquid or the mass of solid substance being swallowed. The physiological events associated with each of these phases are described in the text below and summarized in Table 16–1.

Oral Preparatory Phase

The oral preparatory phase is depicted in the first panel of Figure 16–5. This phase begins as a solid or liquid substance makes contact with the structures of the anterior oral vestibule. The mandible has already

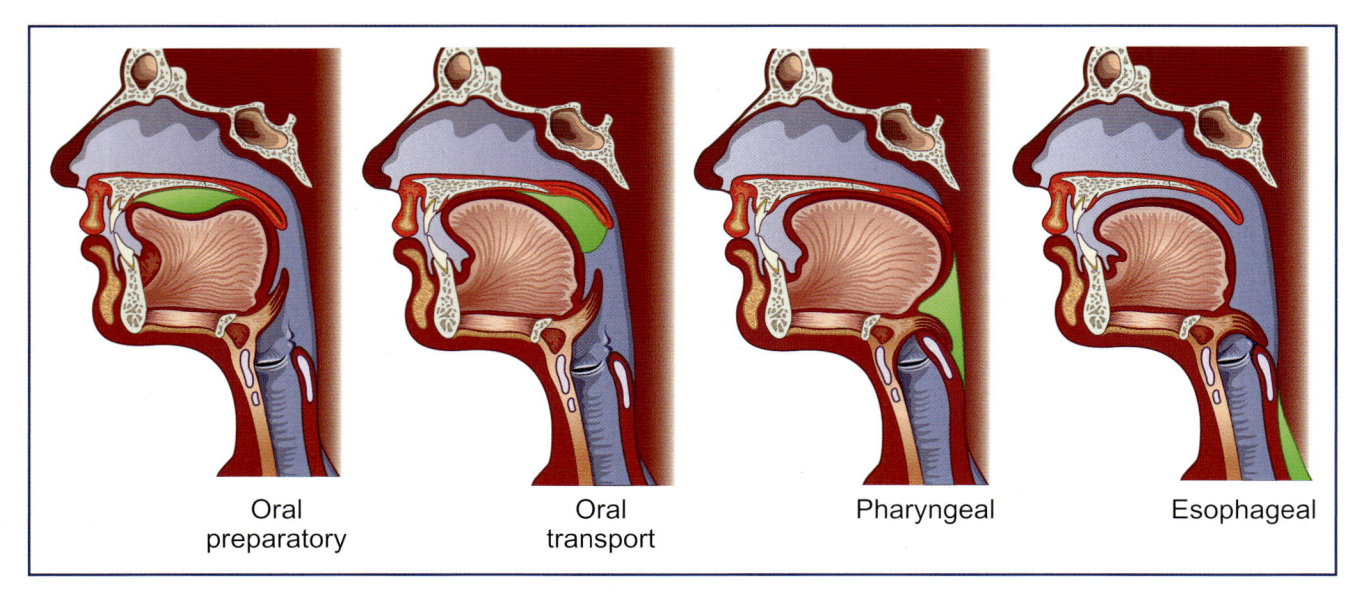

Figure 16–5. Depiction of the oral preparatory, oral transport, pharyngeal, and esophageal phases of swallowing. The actions associated with each phase are summarized in Table 16–1.

Table 16–1. Summary of the Actions Associated with the Four Phases of Swallowing

SWALLOWING PHASE	ACTIONS
Oral preparatory	This phase begins as the liquid or solid substance comes in contact with the oral vestibule and ends with the bolus held in the oral cavity with the back of the tongue elevated to contact the velum and create an impenetrable wall. This phase can be as short as 1 second when ingesting liquid and as long as 20 seconds when chewing (preparing) a solid food.
Oral transport	During this phase, sometimes called the oral propulsive or oral transit phase, the bolus is transported back through the oral cavity to the pharynx. To do so, the tongue elevates in progressively more posterior regions to push the bolus back toward the pharynx, the velum begins to elevate, and the upper esophageal sphincter begins to relax. This phase lasts less than 1 second.
Pharyngeal	During this phase, the bolus usually divides to run through the right and left valleculae and is transported through the pharynx to the upper esophageal sphincter. This phase is "triggered" automatically once the bolus passes the anterior faucial pillars (though the exact location can vary) and is associated with numerous and rapid events: the velopharynx closes, the tongue pushes the bolus backward, the pharynx constricts segmentally, the hyoid bone and larynx move upward and forward, the arytenoids move medially and tilt forward toward the epiglottis, the larynx closes at multiple levels (vocal folds, ventricular folds, and epiglottis), and the upper esophageal sphincter opens. This phase lasts less than 1 second.
Esophageal	This phase begins when the bolus enters the upper esophageal sphincter. At the same time, the lower esophageal sphincter relaxes. The bolus is moved through the esophagus by peristaltic contractions that alternately raise and lower the pressure regionally. This phase ends when the bolus enters the stomach and can last from 8 to 20 seconds.

lowered and the lips have abducted in anticipation of the swallow (Shune, Moon, & Goodman, 2016). What happens next largely depends on the nature of the substance to be swallowed.

If the substance is liquid, the mandible elevates and the lips adduct, forming an anterior seal to contain the bolus. The bolus is contained in the anterior region of the oral cavity by actions of the tongue and other structures, and held there momentarily (usually on the order of 1 second). The anterior tongue depresses and the sides of the tongue elevate to form a cup for the bolus. The bolus may be cupped in one of two ways, depending on the person. Some people hold the bolus with the tongue tip elevated and contacting the back surface of the maxillary incisors, and other people hold the bolus on the floor of the oral cavity in front of the tongue (dubbed "dipper" and "tipper" type swallows, respectively; Dodds et al., 1989). The back of the tongue elevates to make contact with the velum to form a back wall that separates the oral from the pharyngeal cavity and helps ensure that no substance can slip by and into the pulmonary airways. The velopharynx is open so that breathing can continue. Nevertheless, many people stop breathing momentarily at this point in the swallow (this is called the apneic interval) or even before the glass or straw reaches the lips (Martin, Logemann, Shaker, & Dodds, 1994; Martin-Harris, Brodsky, Price, Michel, & Walters, 2003; Martin-Harris, Michel, & Castell, 2005b). This apneic interval serves to reduce the risk of aspiration (defined as invasion of substances below the vocal folds).

These initial events are quite different when the substance to be swallowed is solid rather than liquid, primarily because solid substances need to be masticated (chewed) into smaller pieces and mixed with saliva before being transported toward the esophagus. Saliva is an important ingredient in this process because it moistens the solid substance to facilitate its transport; saliva also introduces enzymes that begin to break down the substance for digestion. Actions of the mandible (and teeth), lips, tongue, and cheeks grind and manipulate the solid substance into a cohe-

> **Mmm Mmm Good!**
>
> "Mmm, mmm, good!" Does this make you think of steamy, chunky soup? Or, better yet, freshly baked cookies just out of the oven? Maybe your imagination is so good that your mouth actually starts to water, which brings us to the point of this sidetrack: saliva. Saliva is produced by salivary glands and is critical to our ability to swallow and digest. Most saliva is swallowed alone (these are called "dry swallows"). During eating, saliva mixes with the food to moisten it for easier transport through oral, pharyngeal, and esophageal parts of the digestive tract and introduces enzymes that begin the digestive process. Do you have any idea how much saliva we produce? The answer is an amazing 1 to 2 liters of saliva every 24 hours! Although saliva production is continuous, its volume and content vary rhythmically; that is, saliva production has a circadian rhythm. Much less saliva is produced during sleep than during wakefulness. That's good. Best to save that saliva for the cookie-eating waking hours.

sive bolus and position it on the surface of the anterior tongue. The lips may adduct (though this is not necessary) while the mandible moves to grind the bolus. During chewing, the mandible moves up and down, forward and backward, and side to side. This is in contrast to speech production, during which the mandible moves primarily up and down. The velum makes contact with the back part of the tongue to seal off the oral from the pharyngeal cavity and prevent the bolus from moving into the pharynx and larynx. The velopharynx is open during preparation of the bolus, and breathing may either continue or be interrupted by apnea (McFarland & Lund, 1995; Palmer & Hiiemae, 2003). The duration of the oral preparatory phase for solid substances may last from as short as 3 seconds, when chewing a soft cookie, to as long as 20 seconds, when chewing a tough piece of steak.

At the end of the oral preparatory phase, the substance in the oral cavity is ready for consumption. Usually it is immediately transported back toward the pharynx (oral transport phase). There are choices at this point, however, including that the substance can be: (a) savored for a while by continued manipulation, (b) squirreled in the cheeks, or (c) expelled. The expulsion option is used when performing a sham feeding test to study the actions of the stomach in anticipation of receiving food.

Oral Transport Phase

The oral transport phase, also called the oral propulsion phase or oral transit phase, is shown in the second panel of Figure 16–5. From the ready position (either the "dipper" or "tipper" position for liquids), the bolus is transported back through the oral cavity. This is done by using the tongue tip to squeeze the bolus against the hard palate; then progressively more posterior regions of the tongue elevate and squeeze the bolus against the palate, moving the bolus back toward the pharynx. The tongue is an especially effective structure for moving and clearing the bolus because it behaves like a muscular hydrostat and can move and change shape in an almost infinite number of ways (see Chapter 5). The force needed to propel the bolus varies with bolus viscosity (the resistance offered by a fluid to flowing). The lips usually press together firmly (although this is not necessary) and the cheeks are pulled inward slightly to keep the bolus positioned over the tongue. At the same time, the velum begins to elevate and the upper esophageal sphincter is relaxing. The oral transport phase is short, lasting less than a second (Cook et al., 1994; Tracy et al., 1989).

Pharyngeal Phase

The pharyngeal phase of the swallow is "triggered" once the bolus passes the anterior faucial pillars; however, the exact location of the trigger varies, depending on the bolus type and the age of the individual. During this phase, depicted in the third panel of Figure 16–5, several events occur rapidly and nearly simultaneously to move the bolus quickly through the pharynx while protecting the airway. This phase is under "automatic" neural control, so that once triggered, it proceeds as a relatively fixed set of events that cannot be altered voluntarily (except in the magnitude and duration of the pressures generated). These events occur within about half a second (Cook et al., 1994; Tracy et al., 1989) and include velopharyngeal closure, elevation of the hyoid bone and larynx, laryngeal closure, pharyngeal constriction, and opening of the upper esophageal sphincter, as described below.

During the pharyngeal phase, the velopharynx closes like a flap-sphincter valve by elevation of the velum and constriction of the pharyngeal walls. This closure is forceful (more forceful than for speech production) so as to prohibit substances from passing through the nasopharynx into the nose.

The hyoid bone and larynx move upward and forward as a result of contraction of extrinsic tongue muscles, with major contributions from the *geniohy-*

oid muscles to upward movement and the *mylohyoid* muscles to forward movement (Pearson, Langmore, & Zumwalt, 2011). (Recall from Chapters 3 and 5 that several extrinsic muscles of the tongue attach to the hyoid bone.) As the hyoid bone is pulled upward and forward, the larynx is pulled along with it by its muscular and nonmuscular connections to the hyoid bone. In fact, this group of structures is often called the *hyolaryngeal complex* because of these anatomical connections and the tendency for them to move as a unit. Elevation of the larynx also causes the pharynx to shorten.

Closure of the larynx for swallowing has been described as a folding of the laryngeal apparatus (Fink & Demarest, 1978) that forms a seal to the entrance of the trachea to protect the pulmonary airways. Closure occurs at multiple levels, which include the vocal folds, the ventricular folds, and the aryepiglottic folds and epiglottis. The arytenoid cartilages move medially and then tilt forward to touch the epiglottis and both the vocal folds and ventricular folds adduct firmly. The epiglottis is forced down over the laryngeal aditus like a trap door and serves as a first line of defense against substances entering the larynx and pulmonary airways. Both passive and active forces appear to be responsible for downward movement of the epiglottis during swallowing (Ekberg & Sigurjonsson, 1982; Fink & Demarest, 1978; VanDaele, Perlman, & Cassell, 1995). The passive force derives from backward movement of the tongue and upward and forward movement of the hyoid bone and larynx, which mechanically deflect the epiglottis backward and downward. Upward and forward movement of the larynx simultaneously contributes to airway protection by tucking the larynx against the root of the tongue and deflecting the trachea away from the digestive pathway. The active force is somewhat less certain (Fink, Martin, & Rohrmann, 1979; Ramsey, Watson, Gramiak, & Weinberg, 1955; VanDaele et al., 1995), but is argued to derive from contraction of the *aryepiglottic* muscles (and possibly from vertically ascending lateral fibers of the *thyroarytenoid* muscles), which purportedly pull the epiglottis downward to complete the seal of the laryngeal aditus (Ekberg & Sigurjonsson, 1982).

As the tongue propels the bolus into the pharynx, the pharynx undergoes segmental contraction (from top to bottom). The tongue root moves backward and the pharyngeal walls constrict to squeeze the bolus toward the esophagus. The bolus often divides at the epiglottis as it passes through the left and right epiglottic valleculae (lateral channels between the root of the tongue and the epiglottis) and into the left and right pyriform sinuses (recesses bounded by the pharynx and larynx), or it flows down one side or through the midline of the covered laryngeal aditus (Dua, Ren, Bardan, Xie, & Shaker, 1997; Logemann, Kahrilas, Kobara, & Vakil, 1989).

As all of these events are playing out, the upper esophageal sphincter is opening to allow the bolus to pass into the esophagus. Two sets of actions appear to contribute to its opening: (a) stretching of the upper esophageal sphincter by forward and upward movement of the hyolaryngeal complex (likely accomplished by activity of the *mylohyoid*, *geniohyoid*, and *anterior* belly of the *digastric* muscles), and (b) relaxing of the *cricopharyngeus* muscles (Omari et al., 2016).

The bolus is propelled through the pharynx to the esophagus during the pharyngeal phase by a combination of mechanical (structural) forces and aeromechanical forces. The mechanical forces consist of the tongue pushing the bolus back into the pharynx and the pharynx contracting segmentally against the tongue root, as just described. The aeromechanical forces are in the form of regional pressure changes that help to move the bolus along. Specifically, backward movement of the tongue and constriction of the pharyngeal walls serve to narrow the airway and reduce the airway volume, thereby causing the pressure to rise in that region. At the same time, elevation of the larynx and dilation of the upper esophageal sphincter lowers the pressure below the bolus. The pressure differential (higher pressure behind the bolus than in front of it) helps to drive the bolus toward its destination.

It is also relevant to mention that the pharyngeal phase of swallowing can be stimulated by pooling of saliva in the pharynx and can be initiated in the absence of oral preparatory and oral transport phases (Logemann, 1998). These swallows occur regularly throughout the day and night and are called nonbolus swallows, dry swallows, or saliva swallows.

Esophageal Phase

The esophageal phase, the initial part of which is illustrated in the last panel of Figure 16–5, begins when the bolus enters the upper esophageal sphincter and ends when it passes into the stomach through the lower esophageal sphincter. This phase may last anywhere from 8 to 20 seconds (Dodds, Hogan, Reid, Stewart, & Arndorfer, 1973). At the same time the upper esophageal sphincter opens to allow the bolus to pass into the esophagus, the lower esophageal sphincter relaxes. The bolus is propelled through the esophagus by peristaltic actions (alternating waves of contraction and relaxation) of the esophageal walls. Peristaltic contraction raises pressure behind the bolus and relaxation lowers pressure in front of the bolus, creating the pressure differential needed to propel it toward the stomach. The nature of the peristaltic action varies somewhat depending on the nature of the bolus (liquid or solid), body position (relation of esophagus and bolus to gravity), and other factors. When a substance is left behind following the primary peristalsis, it is cleared by subsequent peristaltic action (called secondary peristalsis). Although the esophagus usually transports substances toward the stomach, it can also transport substances or gas away from the stomach (as in the case of vomiting or burping).

Overlap of Phases

Although the phases of swallowing are described above as though they are discrete and occur one after the other, in fact they overlap substantially. When a person is eating a solid substance, for example, preparation of part of the bolus in the oral cavity may continue while another part of the bolus moves into the pharyngeal area, as illustrated in Figure 16–6. This partial bolus may remain in the epiglottic valleculae as long as 10 seconds before it merges with the rest of the bolus and the pharyngeal transport phase of the swallow is triggered (Hiiemae & Palmer, 1999).

Overlap of phases is also apparent if swallowing is viewed in relation to the actions of individual structures, rather than in relation to the status of the bolus. Whereas the traditional description of swallowing (used in this chapter) focuses on preparation and transport of the bolus to define the phases of swallowing, there are schema that try to segment physiological events along somewhat different conceptual lines and to categorize them across different levels of observation (Martin-Harris et al., 2005b). This view of the swallowing process focuses on coordination of temporal events across structures. Figure 16–7 is an example of this type of conceptualization. Starting at the left side of the figure, the lips are abducted and the mandible and tongue tip are depressed to allow the bolus to enter the oral vestibule. Moving rightward from there, many structures (not an exhaustive list) take action to move the bolus back toward the esophagus and to protect the airways. Note that this figure presents a general representation of the sequence and relative time of the onsets of various events; actual measures of these events reveal substantial variability within and across people (Molfenter & Steele, 2012). Schema such as these that are based on cross-structure analyses reveal the overlapping elements of swallowing behavior and interactions among its components and hold promise for developing a better understanding of the swallowing process.

BREATHING AND SWALLOWING

Protection of the pulmonary airways during swallowing depends, in large part, on the coordination of breathing and swallowing. Without such coordination,

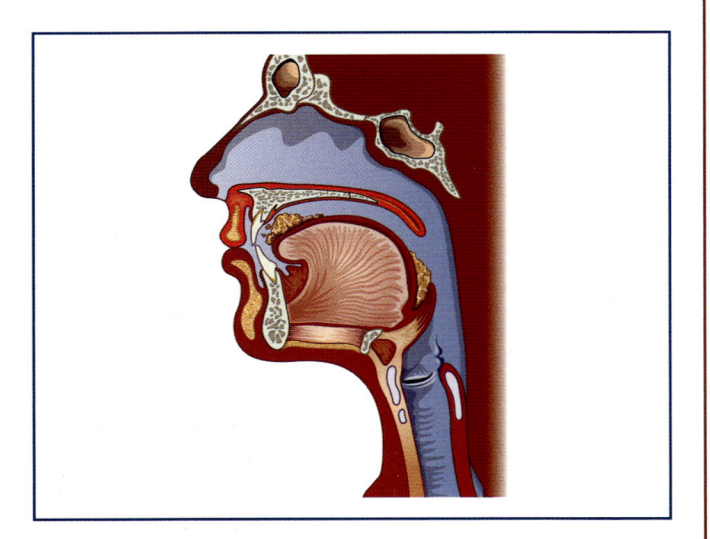

Figure 16–6. An illustration of eating, in which part of the bolus continues to be chewed while another part moves into the epiglottic valleculae, where it may remain for many seconds. This is an example of why the conceptualization of swallowing as comprising discrete phases can be problematic.

One Tug and Two Consequences

Breathing and swallowing cooperate in healthy individuals to prevent unwanted substances from entering the pulmonary airways. This cooperation can be more difficult with certain diseases. Chronic obstructive pulmonary disease (COPD) is one of these. When advanced, COPD expands the pulmonary apparatus, and the diaphragm rides low and flat because air is trapped in the alveoli and airways. The abnormal positioning of the diaphragm has two potential consequences for swallowing. One is that a downward tug is placed on the larynx that tends to abduct the vocal folds and diminish their ability to protect the pulmonary airways. A second possible consequence is that the same downward tug lowers the laryngeal housing and tethers it from below. This means that the larynx may have difficulty moving up during a swallow because it has farther to go and because it must work against the downward pull of the diaphragm. It's no wonder that many people with advanced COPD also have problems with their swallowing.

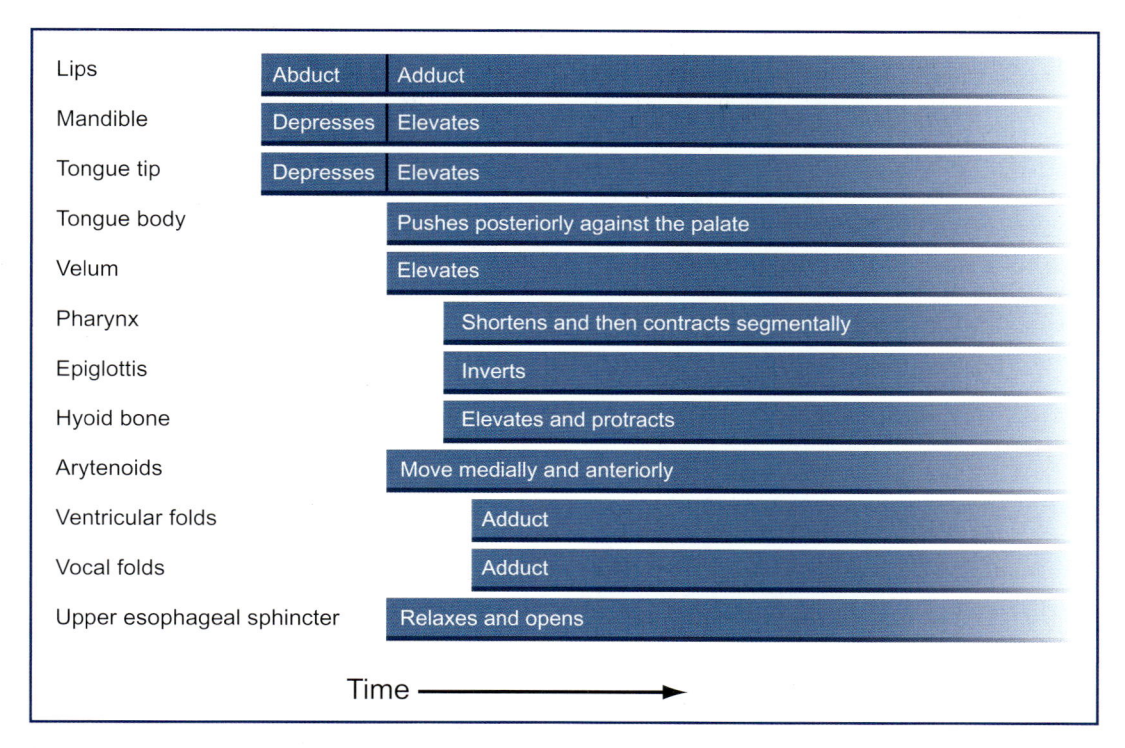

Figure 16–7. Schematic representation of the initiation of actions of several structures during a swallow. This is not meant to represent a fixed sequence or timing of actions (because they can differ across swallows and individuals, depending on many variables), but, rather, to illustrate that swallowing is a continuous physiological process that cannot be divided into a strict set of phases. Figure designed in collaboration with Rosemary Lester-Smith, PhD, CCC-SLP and based on Langmore (2001).

inspiration might occur at the same time a substance is being transported through the pharynx and that substance might be "sucked" through the larynx into the pulmonary airways (aspiration). This is avoided by closing the larynx (at multiple levels, as described above), an action that arrests breathing for a brief period during the swallow.

The risk of aspiration appears to be further reduced by timing the swallow to occur during the expiratory phase of the breathing cycle. During single swallows, the most common pattern is expiration-swallow-expiration; that is, expiration begins, the swallow occurs (accompanied by apnea), and then expiration continues (Martin et al., 1994; Martin-Harris, 2006; Nishino, Yonezawa, & Honda, 1985; Perlman, Ettema, & Barkmeier, 2000; Selley, Flack, Ellis, & Brooks, 1989; Smith, Wolkove, Colacone, & Kreisman, 1989). This pattern, illustrated in Figure 16–8, is the predominant one for swallowing over a broad range of bolus volumes and consistencies and under a variety of serving conditions, such as presenting a liquid bolus with a syringe, drinking water from a cup or straw, or eating a solid substance (Preiksaitis & Mills, 1996; Wheeler-Hegland, Huber, Pitts, & Sapienza, 2009). This appears to be a protective mechanism for potentially "blowing" any foreign substance away from the pulmonary airways. Swallowing during expiration is associated with a reduced risk of

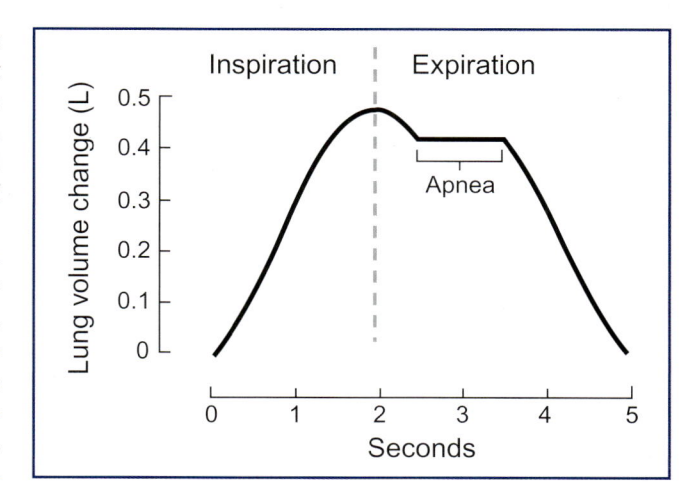

Figure 16–8. Typical breathing pattern during a single swallow, featuring a period of apnea (cessation of breathing). This pattern is described as expiration–swallow (accompanied by apnea)–expiration.

aspiration in people with various impairments (Steele & Cichero, 2014) and is the basis for part of a training protocol used to improve breathing-swallowing coordination for clients at risk for aspiration (Martin-Harris, Garand, & McFarland, 2017). Nevertheless, it is interesting to note that, even in healthy people, not every swallow is followed by expiration, and that some healthy individuals occasionally inspire immediately after a swallow. This is particularly prevalent in people over age 65 years (Martin-Harris et al., 2005a). It is also possible for healthy individuals to swallow voluntarily during the inspiratory phase of the breathing cycle (Ulysal, Kizilay, Ünal, Güngor, & Ertekin, 2013).

Although the apneic interval during swallowing typically lasts about 1 second, it can range from less than a second to several seconds (Klaun & Perlman, 1999; Martin et al., 1994; Martin-Harris et al., 2003, 2005a; Palmer & Hiiemae, 2003; Perlman et al., 2000; Preiksaitis & Mills, 1996). In some people, the duration of the apneic interval is influenced by variables such as bolus volume (Preiksaitis, Mayrand, Robins, & Diamant, 1992). Nevertheless, most of the variability in apnea duration can be attributed to variability in the onset of apnea relative to the eating or drinking event. For example, one person may stop breathing as the food or drink is approaching the mouth, whereas another person may continue to breathe until immediately before the larynx begins to elevate for the pharyngeal transport phase of the swallow (Martin et al., 1994).

The apnea associated with swallowing can cause dyspnea (breathing discomfort) and a subsequent increase in ventilation, even in healthy people (Lederle, Hoit, & Barkmeier-Kraemer, 2012) and can be particularly uncomfortable and challenging in people with pulmonary disease (Hoit, Lansing, Dean, Yarkosky, & Lederle, 2011). When healthy people experience high respiratory drive (such as might occur during exercise or at high elevations), they tend to shorten the apneic interval during swallowing (Hårdemark Cedborg et al., 2010; in this study, high respiratory drive was created by breathing gas with a greater-than-usual amount of carbon dioxide). Shortening apnea in this way likely helps to minimize dyspnea. Another way that people apparently minimize dyspnea is to breathe frequently during a series of swallows, such as when drinking a glass of water without stopping (Gürgor et al., 2013; Lederle et al., 2012).

Swallowing occurs at lung volumes that are almost always larger than the resting expiratory level (that is, the end-expiratory lung volume associated with resting tidal breathing), usually on the order of 10% to 20% larger (Lederle et al., 2012; McFarland et al., 2016; Wheeler-Hegland et al., 2009; Wheeler-Hegland, Huber, Pitts, & Davenport, 2011). This lung volume range is one in which the passive (recoil) pressure of the breathing apparatus is positive, on the order of 5 to 10 cmH$_2$O (see relaxation characteristic in Figure 2–18), and the tracheal pressures associated with swallowing generally fall in this recoil pressure range (Gross et al., 2012). The fact that swallowing occurs at lung volumes that are larger than the resting size of the breathing apparatus, but still within the midrange of the vital capacity, appears to have several advantages. To begin, because swallows are produced at lung volumes where the alveolar pressure is positive, post-swallow expirations are easily driven by the recoil pressure of the breathing apparatus. Also, because swallows are produced at lung volumes that are only moderately large, there is no need to exert inspiratory muscular pressure to brake excessive positive recoil pressure that prevails at large lung volumes. Finally, by avoiding larger-than-necessary lung volumes, the abductory force exerted on the vocal folds by the descent of the diaphragm is minimized (i.e., "tracheal tug," see Chapter 3). This optimal lung volume range has been incorporated as a component of a training protocol for clients with abnormal breathing-swallowing patterns who are at risk for aspiration (Martin-Harris et al., 2017).

Hungry for Air

People with chronic obstructive pulmonary disease (COPD) have other problems besides the expanded pulmonary apparatus and flattened diaphragm described in the previous sidetrack. One particularly troublesome problem is dyspnea (breathing discomfort), a condition that causes people with COPD to avoid activities that compete with their already strong drive to breathe. Perhaps surprisingly, eating is one of those activities. Most healthy people have no idea that they hold their breath when they swallow. But for people with severe COPD, it's quite a different story. They are often acutely aware of the competition that goes on between eating and breathing. The need to breath hold during the swallow causes "air hunger" and makes eating and drinking unpleasant chores rather than pleasurable pastimes. Do everything you can to avoid COPD and your life will be happier. Have you quit smoking yet?

NEURAL CONTROL OF SWALLOWING

The neural control of swallowing is complex and not completely understood. Nevertheless, studies of humans and animals have offered important insights into how swallowing is controlled by the nervous system. Some of the salient features of that control are discussed below as they relate to the participation of the peripheral and central nervous systems.

Role of the Peripheral Nervous System

Nearly all the structures involved in swallowing are the same as those involved in speech production (the most notable exceptions being the esophagus and stomach). Those structures that participate in both swallowing and speech production are innervated by the spinal nerves and cranial nerves described in previous chapters, as summarized in Table 16–2. As can be seen in the table, half of the cranial nerves (6 of 12) and most of the spinal nerves (22 of 31) are potential participants in swallowing (and speech production). The cranial nerves are involved in swallowing through their innervation of the lips, mandible, tongue, velum, pharynx, and larynx, whereas the spinal nerves are primarily involved in breathing and its cessation as they relate to swallowing.

Peripheral innervation of the esophagus differs along its length. The upper (cervical) region is made up of striated muscle, the type of muscle found in other structures of the swallowing apparatus (lips, mandible, tongue, velum, pharynx, larynx, and breathing structures). The cervical region, which includes the upper esophageal sphincter, is innervated by the recurrent branch of the vagus nerve (cranial nerve X), the same branch that innervates most of the intrinsic muscles of the larynx. Thus, the same peripheral nerve is responsible for the simultaneous actions of closing the larynx and opening the upper esophageal sphincter. This means that there is a strong neural link between actions that serve to protect the airway and actions that allow substances to pass into the esophagus. This strong link has obvious advantages for the coordination of the normal swallow, but also has the disadvantage that damage to the recurrent branch of the vagus nerve can have serious consequences for both voice production and swallowing (Corbin-Lewis & Liss, 2015).

In lower regions of the esophagus, where smooth muscle intermingles with striated muscle (thoracic esophagus) and where smooth muscle is the only type of muscle present (abdominal esophagus), a different form of neural control operates. This control comes from the autonomic nervous system, which is generally considered to be under automatic (as opposed to voluntary) control. The autonomic nervous system has two parts, the parasympathetic and sympathetic subdivisions. The parasympathetic subdivision is important for maintaining gastrointestinal motility so that a swallowed substance moves through the esophagus easily and quickly. In contrast, the sympathetic subdivision, best known for its importance in fight-or-flight responses to stressful situations, tends to inhibit gastrointestinal motility. This is one reason why gastrointestinal problems are associated with physical and emotional stress. Many of the nerve fibers of the autonomic nervous system travel with the vagus nerve.

Table 16–2. Summary of Motor and Sensory Nerve Supply to the Breathing Apparatus, Laryngeal Apparatus, Velopharyngeal-Nasal Apparatus, and Pharyngeal-Oral Apparatus

APPARATUS	INNERVATION MOTOR	INNERVATION SENSORY
Breathing	C1–C8, T1–T12, L1–L2	C1–C8, T1–T12, L1–L2
Laryngeal[a]	V, VII, X, XII, C1–C3	X[b]
Velopharyngeal-nasal	V, VII, IX, X, (XI)	V, VII, IX, X
Pharyngeal-oral	V, VII, IX, X, (XI), XII, C1	V, VII, IX, X

Note. Spinal nerves are designated by their segmental origins (C = cervical, T = thoracic, L = lumbar). Cranial nerves are V (trigeminal), VII (facial), IX (glossopharyngeal), X (vagus), XI (accessory), and XII (hypoglossal). This information is also available in Tables 2–2, 3–1, 4–1, and 5–2.
[a]Includes intrinsic, extrinsic, and supplementary laryngeal muscles
[b]Sensory innervation of extrinsic and supplementary laryngeal muscles includes other cranial nerves, such as V and VII.

Role of the Central Nervous System

Although swallowing and speech production are executed using many of the same peripheral nerves, central nervous system control of these two activities is quite different. This means that a given structure, such as the tongue, is under one form of neural control during swallowing and under another form of neural control during speech production. Because of this, it is possible to have central nervous system damage that impairs the function of a structure for speech production but not swallowing, and vice versa. There are two major regions within the central nervous system that are responsible for the control of swallowing. One is in the brainstem and the other is in cortical and subcortical areas.

The brainstem center is located primarily in the medulla, the part of the brainstem that is contiguous with the uppermost part of the spinal cord. Two main groups of brainstem neurons participate in swallowing: one group that appears to be primarily responsible for triggering the swallow and shaping its temporal pattern and another group that appears to allocate neural drive to the various motor nerves that participate in swallowing (Jean, 2001). This brainstem center has primary control over the more automatic phases of swallowing (pharyngeal and esophageal phases).

Many cortical and subcortical regions contribute to the generation and shaping of swallowing behaviors. The most consistent findings point to contributions of the primary motor and sensory areas of the cortex, anterior cingulate cortex, and insular cortex, with probable contributions from basal ganglia, thalamus, and cerebellum (Humbert & Robbins, 2007). Activity in these areas has a strong influence over the control and modulation of the more voluntary phases of swallowing (oral preparatory phase, including mastication, and oral transport phase). However, studies of people with cortical damage from strokes indicate that the cortex may also exert influence over what have traditionally been thought of as the automatic phases (pharyngeal and esophageal phases) of swallowing (Martin & Sessle, 1993).

Afferent input is critical to the generation of a normal swallow. The sources of afferent input are many and include, but are not limited to, information related to: (a) muscle length and rate of length change, (b) muscle tension, (c) joint position and movement, (d) surface and deep pressures, (e) surface deformation, (f) temperature, (g) taste, and (h) noxious stimuli. Afferent activity is generated by receptors in the swallowing apparatus and sent to the brainstem, where such activity may trigger the motor output required to elicit the pharyngeal phase of the swallow or it may modulate the motor output to accommodate a larger-than-expected bolus. Afferent activity may also be sent on to subcortical regions (such as the thalamus) or cortical regions (such as the sensorimotor cortex) where it may be consciously perceived. Often the perception is a pleasant experience, such as savoring the flavor and texture of ice cream, or it may be unpleasant (see sidetrack "Sphenopalatine Ganglioneuralgia" and Figure 16–9).

Sphenopalatine Ganglioneuralgia

Boy, that sounds like something you wouldn't want to meet in the dark. But it comes from something really good. As a child (or even as an adult) you may have said the phrase, "I scream, you scream, we all scream for ice cream." Scream has a meaning of anticipation in this context, but it can also have a meaning of hurting. You know the feeling. You take a bite of ice cream and momentarily hold it against the roof of your mouth before you swallow it. Then suddenly you get an intense, stabbing pain in your forehead. What's up? The pain is caused as your hard palate warms up after you made it cold. Cold causes vasoconstriction (reduction in blood vessel diameter) in the region, which is followed by rapid vasodilation (increase in blood vessel diameter). It's the rapid vasodilation that hurts and gets your attention. The technical term for this pain is *sphenopalatine ganglioneuralgia*. The common term (and the one more easily pronounced) is "brain freeze." Fortunately, the pain lasts only a few seconds. Be thankful. There's all that ice cream still waiting to be eaten.

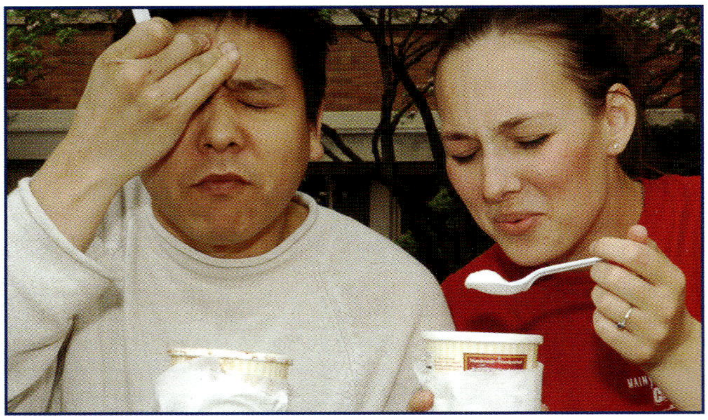

Figure 16–9. Sphenopalatine ganglioneuralgia (or so-called brain freeze) caused by placing something cold against the roof of the mouth. Image provided courtesy of the University of Cincinnati. Reproduced with permission.

VARIABLES THAT INFLUENCE SWALLOWING

A number of variables influence swallowing, including characteristics of the bolus, the swallowing mode, and body position. There are also developmental and aging effects on swallowing, but essentially no influence of sex.

Bolus Characteristics

Although the act of swallowing occurs generally as described near the beginning of this chapter, the precise nature of the swallow is determined, in part, by what exactly is being swallowed. Bolus consistency and texture, volume, and taste are variables that have been found to influence the act of swallowing.

Consistency and Texture

One of the most important contrasts that determines swallowing behavior is the difference between liquids and solids. Whereas a liquid bolus is usually held briefly in the front of the oral cavity before being propelled to the pharynx, a solid bolus may be moved to the pharynx and left there for several seconds while the remainder of the bolus continues to be chewed (Hiiemae & Palmer, 1999; Palmer, Rudin, Lara, & Crompton, 1992; see Figure 16–6). Although something similar can also happen with liquids (Linden, Tippett, Johnston, Siebens, & French, 1989), it is much less common, except in cases where a combined liquid/solid bolus is chewed and swallowed (Saitoh et al., 2007), such as what might occur during mealtime eating (Dua et al., 1997). Even when not combined, the consistency of liquids and the textures of solid food influence swallowing behavior.

Liquid substances can be characterized according to consistency, ranging from thin as water (low viscosity) to thick as pudding (high viscosity), and differences in consistency have been shown to influence swallowing. Specifically, thick liquids or puree consistencies tend to take longer to swallow than thin liquids (Chi-Fishman & Sonies, 2002; Im, Kim, Oommen, Kim, & Ko, 2012). This slowing is due to longer oral and pharyngeal phase events and longer upper esophageal sphincter opening durations (Dantas et al., 1990; Im et al., 2012). Tongue forces are higher when swallowing thick substances compared with thin liquids (Chi-Fishman & Sonies, 2002; Miller & Watkin, 1996; Steele & van Lieshout, 2004). As might be predicted, it is more difficult to maintain a cohesive (single) bolus when swallowing thinner liquids compared with thicker liquids. As a result, laryngeal penetration (where part of the bolus moves into the laryngeal vestibule but remains above the vocal folds; Robbins, Hamilton, Lof, & Kempster, 1992) is more common when swallowing thin liquids than when swallowing thicker substances (Daggett, Logemann, Rademaker, & Pauloski, 2006; Steele et al., 2015). The fact that vocal fold closure starts earlier and lasts longer with thinner compared with thicker liquids (Inamoto et al., 2013) is likely a mechanism to protect against this risk of aspiration.

The textures of solid substances can also influence the swallow (Steele et al., 2015). For example, the harder and drier the substance, the greater the number of chewing cycles (Engelen, Fontijn-Tekamp, & van der Bilt, 2005), the longer the duration of the initial transport of the bolus from the anterior oral cavity to the postcanine region (Mikushi, Seki, Brodsky, Matsuo, & Palmer, 2014), and the greater number of times the tongue squeezes the bolus back toward the pharynx (Hiraoka et al., 2017).

Many different terms have been used to refer to liquids of different thicknesses and substances of different textures, making it difficult to communicate clearly across clinical settings and within the research community. One proposed framework incorporates standardized terminology and rating scales for substances that are used in the evaluation and management of swallowing disorders (International Dysphagia Diet Standardization Initiative [IDDSI]; Cichero et al., 2017). In this framework, the two major categories are Drinks and Foods. Drinks are described as thin, slightly thick, mildly thick, moderately thick, and extremely thick, and Foods are described as liquidized, pureed, minced & moist, soft & bite-sized, and regular.

Volume

It seems intuitive that the volume (size) of the bolus might affect the swallow, and most studies indicate that, in fact, it does (Chi-Fishman & Sonies, 2002; Cook et al., 1989; Kahrilas & Logemann, 1993; Logemann et al., 2000; Logemann, Pauloski, Rademaker, & Kahrilas, 2002; Perlman, Palmer, McCulloch, & VanDaele, 1999; Perlman, Schultz, & VanDaele, 1993; Tasko, Kent, & Westbury, 2002). When a person is swallowing a larger bolus compared with a smaller bolus, tongue movements are generally larger and faster, hyoid bone movements begin earlier and are more extensive, pharyngeal wall movements and laryngeal movements are larger, and the upper esophageal sphincter relaxes and opens earlier and stays open longer (Cock, Jones, Hammer, Omari, & McCulloch, 2017; Kahrilas & Logemann, 1993; Lin et al., 2014). This means that events related to tongue propulsion of the bolus, closing of the velopharynx, protection of the pulmonary airways, and opening of the upper esophageal sphincter are conditioned by bolus volume in ways that are more sustained and more vigorous for larger boluses than smaller boluses. Whether or not apnea is longer during the swallowing of larger (versus smaller) boluses has yet to be convincingly determined (Martin-Harris, 2006).

Despite the success of the adjustments made to accommodate a larger bolus, there tends to be a greater frequency of laryngeal penetration as bolus size increases, at least for liquid boluses. For example, part of the bolus penetrates the laryngeal vestibule more than twice as often when swallowing a 10 mL bolus than when swallowing a 1 mL bolus (Daggett et al., 2006). Nevertheless, when laryngeal penetration occurs in healthy individuals, the substance is almost always pushed away from the larynx and transported to the esophagus without being aspirated (going below the vocal folds).

Taste

Taste contributes enormously to the enjoyment of the eating and drinking experience. Imagine, for a moment, eating a hot fudge sundae with some salty nuts on top, then think about biting into a lemon slice. Although the hot fudge sundae may be more enticing, there is evidence that the lemon elicits a more vigorous swallow response.

Tastes include sweet, salty, sour, bitter, and other tastes (such as umami, meaning meaty or savory), and how something tastes can influence certain features of the swallow. For example, substances with taste (sweet, salty, sour), compared with tasteless substances, are generally associated with higher peak tongue pressures (Pelletier & Dhanaraj, 2006; Pelletier & Steele, 2014), especially at higher taste intensities (Nagy, Steele, & Pelletier, 2014), and faster and greater activation of selected swallow-related muscle regions (Ding, Logemann, Larson, & Rademaker, 2003). Sour tastes, in particular, appear to elicit more effortful swallows (greater amplitude muscle activity) than other tastes (Leow, Huckabee, Sharma, & Tooley, 2007; Palmer, McCulloch, Jaffe, & Neel, 2005), as well as more frequent swallows (Mulheren, Kamarunas, & Ludlow, 2016). These behavioral effects are associated with taste-related differences in brain function. For example, the ingestion of tasty liquids stimulates significantly more activity in certain cortical regions compared with ingestion of unflavored water (Babael et al., 2010; Mulheren et al., 2016). Of course, it should also be recognized that tastes are accompanied by their associated smells, so that both the gustatory (taste) and olfactory (smell) senses are nearly always stimulated simultaneously.

Swallowing Mode

Much of the research on swallowing has focused on single swallows that either were cued ("Swallow now") or in which the bolus was introduced directly into the oral cavity with a syringe. Clearly, this is not how swallowing usually occurs. As the research base expands, there is growing evidence that sequential swallows differ from single swallows and that spontaneously initiated swallows differ from those that are elicited with an external cue, including the cue to swallow with greater-than-usual effort.

Single Versus Sequential Swallows

During eating and drinking, there are times when a swallow occurs in isolation. There are also times when swallows occur sequentially, one immediately after the other.

A swallow is characterized by the same major events whether it is produced singly or as part of a sequence—that is, the bolus is pushed back by the tongue, the velopharynx closes, the hyoid bone and larynx rise and close off the airway, the bolus is moved through the pharynx, and the upper esophageal sphincter opens to admit the bolus into the esophagus. Never-

---

Gutsy Stuff

Taste receptors in the tongue get all the press and all the credit for making things taste sweet—not surprising, given that there are about 10,000 of them. Put a little sugar or artificial sweetener in your mouth and the taste receptors in your tongue will come to attention and tell your brain about it. But the taste of sweetness is not just limited to your mouth. Receptors that sense sugar and artificial sweetener have also been found in the gut (Margolskee et al., 2007). These gut receptors taste glucose in the same way that taste cells in your tongue signal sweetness to the brain. They've been found to influence the secretion of insulin and hormones that regulate blood-sugar level and influence appetite. Those are two very important responsibilities. This is all very gutsy stuff and is touted by its discoverers as possibly leading to new treatment options for obesity and diabetes. Let's hope they're right.

theless, there are some subtle, yet important, differences between single swallows and sequential swallows that involve the relative timing of certain events and the nature of certain movements.

During both single and sequential swallows, the tongue moves upward to the palate (front to back) to push the bolus backward; however, certain aspects of these movements differ under these two conditions (Chi-Fishman, Stone, & McCall, 1998). To begin with, swallow time is shorter during sequential swallows compared with single swallows, something that may be accounted for by shorter contact times, faster movements, shorter movement distances, or some combination of these. Also, certain movements that usually follow one another during a single swallow, such as tongue tip lowering and tongue body raising, may occur simultaneously during sequential swallows. During a single swallow, the hyolaryngeal complex rises and then falls back to its original (resting) position. In contrast, during sequential swallows, the hyolaryngeal complex rises for the first swallow and then falls, but only part way toward the resting position, before rising again for the next swallow (Chi-Fishman & Sonies, 2000; Daniels et al., 2004; Daniels & Foundas, 2001). The velum rises and falls in synchrony with the hyolaryngeal complex during sequential swallowing (Chi-Fishman & Sonies, 2000). The epiglottis either moves in synchrony with the hyolaryngeal complex or it remains down over the laryngeal airway throughout swallow cycles with the hyolaryngeal complex maintained in a partially elevated position (Daniels et al., 2004).

During sequential swallowing, successive boluses often merge in the epiglottic valleculae before the pharyngeal phase is triggered (Dua et al., 1997; Hiiemae & Palmer, 1999). When this happens, the airway tends to stay closed for liquid substances, but not for solid substances (Chi-Fishman & Sonies, 2000). Unsurprisingly, laryngeal penetration is more common during sequential swallows than for single swallows, but in healthy individuals, the penetrated substance is almost always cleared on the next swallow. As is the case with single swallows, the swallow apnea associated with sequential swallows is usually followed by expiration; nevertheless, it is more common for inspiration to follow the apneic interval during sequential swallows than during single swallows (Lederle et al., 2012; Preiksaitis & Mills, 1996). During sequential swallows, the average size of the bolus is larger when drinking from a cup than when drinking from a straw (Veiga, Fonseca, & Bianchini, 2014).

Esophageal behavior is also different for sequential versus single swallows. For example, during sequential drinking of water, the pressure associated with esophageal peristalsis is lower and the frequency of peristalsis is lower than during single swallows (Meyer, Gerhardt, & Castell, 1981).

Cued Versus Uncued Swallows

The majority of swallowing studies, including those performed for both research and clinical purposes, have been conducted using external cues to swallow (Daniels, Schroeder, DeGeorge, Corey, & Rosenbek, 2007). These are usually verbal cues ("Swallow now"), but they can also be visual or tactile cues. In contrast, the swallowing associated with eating and drinking in daily life is seldom accompanied by such cuing (unless you are a child whose caregiver is saying, "Hurry up and drink your milk"). So, the question arises as to whether or not cuing alters the swallow. Studies that have addressed this question directly (Daniels et al., 2007; Nagy et al., 2013) have shown that under a cued condition, the substance (a single liquid bolus) is loaded into the anterior oral cavity and then moved somewhat back and held between the midline of the tongue and the hard palate in preparation for the cue, whereas in the noncued condition the bolus is moved immediately out of the anterior oral cavity as soon as loading is complete. This affects the timing measures associated with each of the phases of swallowing and has implications for how certain measures are obtained.

Sword Throats

Sword swallowing is an ancient art that continues to be practiced. There is even a Sword Swallowers Association International with both professional and amateur members from all over the world. The practice and ill effects of sword swallowing were discussed in an article in the prestigious *British Medical Journal* (Witcombe & Meyer, 2006). Major complications from sword swallowing are more likely when the swallower is distracted or when swallowing unusual swords. Sequelae can include perforation of the pharynx or esophagus, gastrointestinal bleeding, pneumothorax (collapsed lung), and chest pain. (All of this is little wonder, we think.) Novice sword swallowers must learn to desensitize the gag reflex, align the upper esophageal sphincter with the neck hyperextended, open the upper esophageal sphincter, and control retching as the blade is moved on toward the cardia. All in all it doesn't sound like fun to us. It also makes for a very long bolus.

Another form of cuing involves having a person voluntarily change the nature of the swallow. For example, an instruction such as "Squeeze hard when you swallow" tends to elicit higher tongue and/or pharyngeal pressures (depending, in part, on the precise wording of the instruction), greater muscle activation levels, and longer pharyngeal closure compared with swallows produced with usual effort (Fritz et al., 2014; Fukuoka et al., 2013; Steele & Huckabee, 2007; Wheeler-Hegland, Rosenbek, & Sapienza, 2008; Yeates, Steele, & Pelletier, 2010). Interestingly, effortful swallow maneuvers also appear to increase amplitudes of peristaltic pressure waves in regions of the esophagus containing smooth muscle, especially the region near the lower esophageal sphincter (Lever et al., 2007; O'Rourke et al., 2014). Effortful swallow maneuvers, and other forms of conscious maneuvers, are often used as behavioral strategies to help clients with swallowing disorders (Leonard, Kendall, McKenzie, & Goodrich, 2008; Logemann, 1998) and those with weak muscles due to normal aging (Park & Kim, 2016).

Body Position

Certain details of swallowing change with body position. For example, whether a person is in an upright body position or on "all fours" (on hands and knees, facing terra firma), swallowing usually occurs during the expiratory phase of the breathing cycle (McFarland, Lund, & Gagner, 1994). Nevertheless, there can be subtle changes in the onset time of the swallow within the expiratory phase. In an upright body position, the swallow usually occurs late in the expiratory phase, whereas when a person is on "all fours," the swallow is more apt to occur earlier in the expiratory phase. It is unclear why this happens, but it may be related to the pull of gravity on the abdominal content, which, in turn, is transmitted to the larynx via its mechanical connections through the diaphragm and pulmonary apparatus (McFarland et al., 1994). In addition, a liquid bolus tends to arrive in the pharynx earlier during swallows produced in an upright body position than during swallows produced in a facedown position (Saitoh et al., 2007), although this position-related timing difference does not appear to occur when a person is swallowing a solid bolus (Palmer, 1998; Saitoh et al., 2007).

There are also differences between swallows produced in supine versus upright body positions. For example, in the supine body position (compared with an upright body position): (a) the hyoid bone moves a greater distance anteriorly, the velum moves a smaller distance posteriorly, and the pharyngeal transport phase of the swallow is longer (Perry, Bae, & Kuehn, 2012), (b) pharyngeal pressure is more positive (Dejaeger, Pelemans, Ponette, & VanTrappen, 1994; Johnson, Shaw, Gabb, Dent, & Cook, 1995), (c) the upper esophageal sphincter pressure reaches its nadir (most subatmospheric pressure) slightly earlier (Castell, Dalton, & Castell, 1990), (d) bolus flow through the upper esophageal sphincter is faster (Johnson et al., 1995), (e) peristaltic waves in the esophagus (particularly in its distal region) are slower and stronger, and (f) the pressure in the lower esophageal sphincter is higher (Sears, Castell, & Castell, 1990). In addition, pressure in the nasopharyngeal region is higher in more supine compared with more upright positions (Rosen, Abdelhalim, Jones, & McCulloch, 2017). This is likely a compensatory neural mechanism to ensure that the velopharynx remains closed during the swallow so as to prevent nasal regurgitation. It is not clear whether or not the timing of pharyngeal events is influenced by body position (Castell et al., 1990; Ingervall & Lantz, 1973; Johnson et al., 1995; Su et al., 2015). Similarly, the timing of sensory and motor events related to vocal fold activation before, during, and after the swallow appears to be unaffected by a change from upright to supine position (Barkmeier, Bielamowicz, Takeda, & Ludlow, 2002).

Development

Infancy and childhood are times of significant anatomical and physiological development. Many of these developmental changes have been described in previous chapters (see Chapters 2, 3, 4, and 5). The focus here is on those changes that pertain to the development of feeding and swallowing.

There are many important anatomical changes that influence swallowing during the period from infancy through childhood. Some of these include the following (Arvedson & Brodsky, 2002): (a) the infant's tongue goes from nearly filling the oral cavity to filling only the floor of the oral cavity due to differential growth of oral structures; (b) the infant's oral cavity goes from being edentulous to having a full set of deciduous teeth; (c) the cheeks of the infant have fatty pads (sometimes called sucking pads) that eventually disappear, to be replaced with muscle; (d) the infant goes from having essentially no oropharynx to having a distinct one as the larynx descends; and (e) the infant's larynx goes from being one-third adult size, with relatively large arytenoid cartilages and a high position within the neck, to the adult configuration and position. It is interesting to note that although anatomical changes influence swallowing, the opposite is also true. That is, because the forces exerted during swallowing and chewing are quite large, they have a profound influence on molding the oral and pharyngeal anatomy of the infant and young child.

Swallowing (of amniotic fluid) begins well before birth, as early as 12.5 weeks gestation (Humphrey, 1970). Interestingly, although many of the components of swallowing are in place before birth, velopharyngeal closure during swallowing is not (Miller, Sonies, & Macedonia, 2003). Perhaps this is related to the fact that the entire digestive tract is infused with amniotic fluid so that there is little consequence of having an open velopharynx; that is, the amniotic fluid would infuse the nasal passages whether the velopharynx is open or closed. Immediately after birth, the velopharynx closes for swallowing and the infant exhibits a suckling pattern characterized by forward and backward (horizontal) movements of the tongue (Bosma, 1986; Bosma, Truby, & Lind, 1965). These tongue movements are accompanied by large vertical movements of the mandible and serve to draw liquid into the oral cavity. Around the age of 6 months, this suckling pattern converts to a sucking pattern which is characterized by raising and lowering (vertical) movements of the tongue, firm approximation of the lips, and less pronounced vertical movements of the mandible. Sucking is stronger than suckling and allows the infant to pull thicker substances into the oral cavity and to begin the ingestion of soft food (Arvedson & Brodsky, 2002).

During the first few months of life, the infant relies on breast feeding (or nipple feeding from a bottle) for all nutritional intake. This form of feeding consists of suck-swallow or suck-swallow-breathe sequences, typically repeated several times (8 to 12 times) and followed by a rest period (several seconds). It was once thought that infants swallow and breathe at the same time; however, they do not. Although infants can continue breathing during the suck, like adults, they stop breathing during the swallow (Wilson, Thach, Brouillette, & Abu-Osba, 1981) and their ventilation decreases as a result (Koenig, Davies, & Thach, 1990). During this period, several oral reflexes that aid in early feeding are active. These disappear around 6 months of age, with the exception of the gag reflex, which remains active throughout childhood and adulthood. Knowledge of the neural interactions among feeding, swallowing, and airway protection is essential for providing quality care for infants with impairments in any of these functions (Jadcherla, 2017).

By about 6 months of age, infants are ready to begin eating solid foods and being fed by spoon. Foods such as crackers and soft fruits and vegetables are introduced during the next few months. The basic patterns for chewing are in place by 9 months and continue to develop over the next few years of life (Green et al., 1997; Steeve, Moore, Green, Reilly, & Ruark McMurtrey, 2008). By 2 to 3 years of age, the child is able to eat regular table food.

Positive interactions between the infant and caregiver during feeding periods are critical to development (Arvedson & Brodsky, 2002; Pitcher, Crandall, & Goodrich, 2008) and are associated with physical and emotional pleasure that can lead to healthy bonding and communication. As an infant grows, mealtimes should continue to be pleasurable experiences that provide needed nutrition and, when shared with others, also provide social stimulation.

Aging

As with most physiological functions, swallowing changes with age across adulthood. The most robust age-related change is that swallowing becomes slower, particularly after age 60 years (Leonard & McKenzie, 2006; Logemann et al., 2002; Robbins et al., 1992; Sonies, Parent, Morrish, & Baum, 1988). Certain individual components of the swallow also tend to be delayed in older compared with younger adults. For example, the trigger for the pharyngeal phase is located closer to the esophagus in older adults (Robbins et al., 1992; Tracy et al., 1989) than in younger adults (Logemann, 1998). Also, it takes longer for the bolus to move through the pharynx and for the upper esophageal sphincter to open in older adults (Logemann et al., 2002; Mendell & Logemann, 2007; Nishikubo et al., 2015; Robbins et al., 1992). The apneic interval during the swallow is generally longer in older adults than younger adults (Hirst, Ford, Gibson & Wilson, 2002; Wang et al., 2015) and the offset of the apneic interval occurs later (Martin-Harris et al., 2005a). There is a greater tendency for older adults to initiate the swallow during inspiration (Yamada et al., 2017) or to inspire immediately after the swallow (Martin-Harris et al., 2005a). Tongue movements during swallowing are slower in older than younger adults (Steele & van Lieshout, 2009), though tongue pressures do not seem to change with age (Fei et al., 2013; Youmans, Youmans, & Stierwalt, 2009).

An outcome of the age-related slowing of the swallow (combined with age-related reductions in sensory function; for example, see Malandraki, Perlman, Karampinos, & Sutton, 2011) is that the frequency of laryngeal penetration increases with age (Daniels et al., 2004; Robbins et al., 1992). Laryngeal penetration occurs in people over 50 years about twice as often as it occurs in adults under 50 years, and more frequently when swallowing liquids than when swallowing solids (Daggett et al., 2006). Although this appears to be a dangerous situation and a possible precursor to aspiration, in healthy individuals the substance is moved out of the vestibule to be rejoined with the rest of the bolus (Daggett et al., 2006). Nevertheless, the risk of aspiration may be higher in senescent adults, compared with younger adults, because of their greater tendency to inspire immediately after swallowing (Martin-Harris et al., 2005a).

Sex

Several studies of swallowing have included participants of both sexes and some of these have revealed statistically significant differences in selected measures. Nevertheless, there do not appear to be consistent findings across studies that would lead to the conclusion that swallowing is different in men and women. Sex-related differences that have been reported are likely to be attributable to chance (such as that related to participant selection or statistical chance) or to variables other than sex (such as size and strength). Thus, given the current knowledge base, it seems safe to conclude that swallowing does not differ between the sexes in any consistent or important way and does not need to be taken into account in clinical endeavors (except in the absolute values of certain measures).

Chicken Dinner

Cancer had taken his tongue. He had no teeth. And signs of a stroke were on his face. His speech was remarkably good and arrangements were made to travel out of state with him to use special x-ray equipment to study his speaking and swallowing. The trip was by car and went well until a snowstorm forced an overnight stay. Dinner was instructive. To propel food toward his pharynx, he threw his head back in the way a chicken tosses its head when eating. Having no teeth helped him because he could touch his mandible to his maxilla and create a downward and backward sloping floor to his mouth. He poured liquids down this slope. When motion picture x-rays from his study were developed, they were enlightening. When he swallowed water, his epiglottis stood fully erect, as if at military attention, while liquid cascaded around it. He apparently hadn't read textbooks telling him how the epiglottis is always forced down over the larynx during swallowing.

MEASUREMENT AND ANALYSIS OF SWALLOWING

Measurement and analysis of swallowing is not only critical to research endeavors, but has also become essential to clinical practice and to the diagnosis and management of dysphagia (meaning swallowing disorders and pronounced dis-FAY-juh). Instrumental measurement of swallowing is especially important when considering that as many as half of the clients who aspirate do so "silently" without any signs of coughing or other signs of visible or audible struggle (Logemann, 1998). In such cases, aspiration can only be detected through instrumental examination.

There are many approaches to measuring and analyzing swallowing. Seven of them are highlighted here—videofluoroscopy, endoscopy, manometry, surface electromyography, ultrasonography, aeromechanical observations, and client self-report—because they have proven useful for both research and clinical applications and have direct relevance to the practice of speech-language pathology.

Videofluoroscopy

As described in Chapter 6, videofluoroscopy uses x-rays to image the movements of speech production. Videofluoroscopy can also be used to image movements associated with swallowing. In fact, videofluoroscopy is used routinely in clinical settings to evaluate swallowing in clients with suspected dysphagia. When used for this purpose, the substance to be swallowed is mixed with barium sulfate. Barium is a contrast material that allows the bolus to be tracked visually as it travels through the oral, pharyngeal, and esophageal regions.

The videofluoroscopic swallow examination, sometimes called a modified barium swallow (MBS) study, was first described by Logemann, Boshes, Blonsky, and Fisher (1977). The adjective "modified" is used to differentiate this study from a barium swallow study, which is conducted by a gastroenterologist to evaluate esophageal structure and function. A videofluoroscopic examination is usually conducted with the client seated in a specially designed chair. The examination is performed in a radiology laboratory, with a radiologist (or radiology technician) running the x-ray equipment and a speech-language pathologist directing the swallowing protocol. The examination protocol typically consists of the swallowing of a series of liquid and solid substances (mixed with barium or accompanied by ingestion of a barium capsule to provide contrast) that vary in volume and consistency or texture. For example, the protocol might include the swallowing of thin liquid, nectar, and pudding in small and large servings and the chewing and swallowing of a cookie or cracker. The drinking of the thin liquid might be from a spoon, cup, straw, or a combination of these. The exact protocol depends on the nature of the client's swallowing complaint (in a clinical setting) or the nature of the research question (in a research setting).

Figure 16–10 contains an example of a videofluoroscopic image of the oral preparatory phase of swallowing. Although only one still frame is displayed there, the actual image is a moving image that can be viewed in real time, recorded, and played back at normal speed, slow speed, or even frame by frame. Images can be obtained using a lateral view (as in this figure) and a frontal view (not shown). Each view offers different advantages for capturing certain swallowing events.

A variety of temporal and spatial measurements can be made from the videofluoroscopic images. Temporal measurements are generally in the form of objective values; for example, the time from the beginning of bolus movement from the oral cavity to its arrival at the upper esophageal sphincter. Spatial measurements may also be in the form of objective values, or they may be in the form of judgments or ratings. For example, ratings can be made of the extent of velar elevation (on a scale of none to fully elevated) or extent of hyoid bone excursion (on a scale of none to normal). One of the most popular assessment tools, the Penetration-Aspiration Scale (Rosenbek, Robbins, Roecker, Coyle, & Wood, 1996), is an eight-point categorical rating scale that provides descriptions of events that indicate laryngeal penetration or aspiration (ranging from "Material does not enter the airway" to "Material enters the airway, passes below the vocal folds, and no effort is made to eject").

It is generally agreed that videofluoroscopy provides the most comprehensive evaluation of swallowing, and for many it is considered the "gold standard" of measurement. It has several advantages over other measurement approaches, including the following: (a) it provides relatively clear views of nearly all the important structures involved in swallowing and their movements, with the exception of the vocal folds; (b) it is possible to visualize barium-laced substances through the oral preparatory, oral transport, pharyngeal, and esophageal phases; (c) it is possible to view swallowing events from at least two different perspectives (lateral and frontal); and (d) it is possible to identify penetration and aspiration events. The major disadvantages of videofluoroscopy are that it requires exposure to radiation, it must be coordinated with radiology, and it cannot be conducted at bedside.

Endoscopy

Another way to visualize swallowing is with endoscopy. First described by Langmore, Schatz, and Olson (1988), this approach requires the use of a flexible fiberoptic endoscope, like the one used for visualizing the larynx and velopharynx (see lower part of Figure 6–8 in Chapter 6). To view the swallowing apparatus, the endoscope is inserted through one of the nares (following the administration of topical anesthesia and decongestant), routed through the velopharyngeal port, and guided until its tip is positioned in the laryngopharynx. This approach has come to be known by the name of Flexible Endoscopic Evaluation of Swallowing (FEES). A FEES station is shown in Figure 16–11.

The examination usually includes a preliminary viewing of the velopharyngeal region, pharyngeal walls, back part of the tongue, epiglottis, aryepiglottic folds, epiglottic valleculae, pyriform sinuses, laryngeal

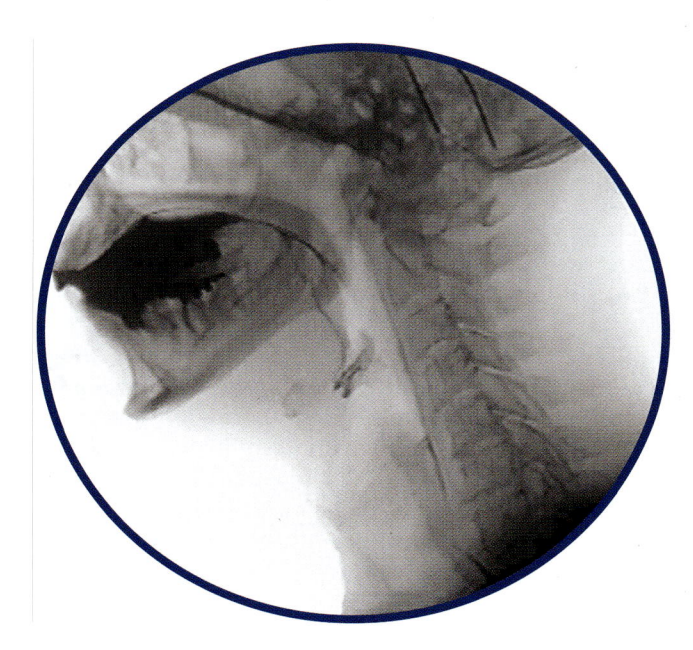

Figure 16–10. Videofluorosocopic image showing the oral preparatory phase of a swallow. The large, dark area in the oral region is the bolus. The thin, dark line that runs along the tongue to the epiglottal vallecula indicates that there may be some trace residue from a previous swallow or that there has been some premature spillage during the oral hold. From "Dynamic swallow studies: measurement techniques," by R. Leonard and S. McKenzie in *Dysphagia assessment and treatment planning: A team approach* (2nd ed., p. 273). Edited by R. Leonard and K. Kendall, 2008, San Diego, CA: Plural Publishing, Inc. Copyright 2008 by Plural Publishing, Inc. Modified and reproduced with permission.

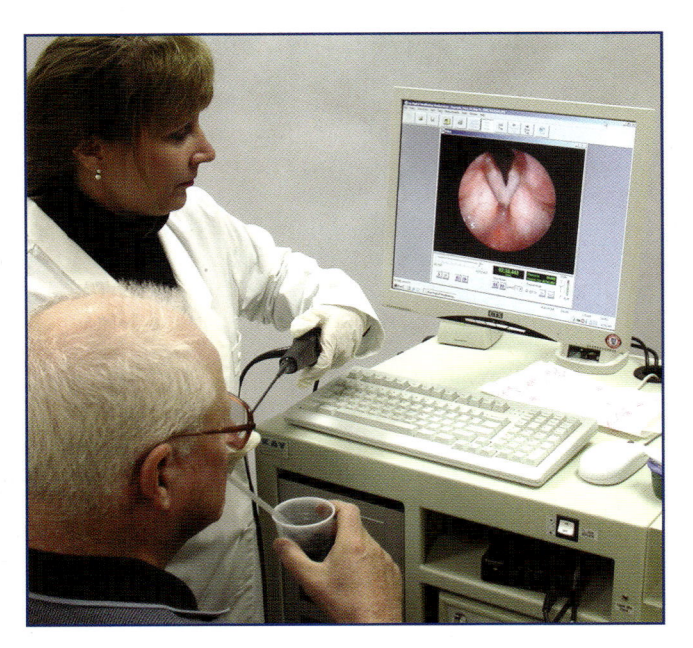

Figure 16–11. Fiberoptic endoscope used for evaluation of swallowing. Image provided courtesy of KayPENTAX, Montvale, NJ. Reproduced with permission.

vestibule, ventricular folds, and vocal folds. Abnormalities in structure or color are noted and are used to help interpret abnormal swallow behaviors. The evaluation protocol is similar to that used for videofluoroscopic examination, using liquid and solid substances of different consistencies, textures, and volumes, with the major difference being that no barium is required. Descriptions provided by the speech-language pathologist might include the presence of substance remaining in the epiglottic valleculae or pyriform sinuses following the pharyngeal phase of swallowing, whether or not substance invaded the laryngeal vestibule (laryngeal penetration), and whether or not there is evidence that substance traveled below the vocal folds (aspiration).

Endoscopy offers certain advantages over other approaches to evaluating swallowing. To begin with, the equipment is easily portable so that the examination can be done at bedside in a hospital, there is no exposure to x-rays and no need to use barium products, and it is possible to see structural and color abnormalities. In addition, the procedure can often be performed by a speech-language pathologist without the direct oversight of a physician or the aid of other health care professionals. Finally, the speech-language pathologist can observe the client eat an entire meal at the client's usual pace.

The major disadvantage of an endoscopic approach is that, during the pharyngeal phase of the swallow, there is a moment when the endoscopic view is blocked as the tongue and pharynx approximate (called the moment of "white out"). Also, there are some clients who cannot tolerate the procedure, including those with structural abnormalities such as a deviated nasal septum, hyperkinetic movement disorders, bleeding disorders, and certain cardiac conditions. Furthermore, it is sometimes difficult to detect penetration and aspiration with endoscopy. One way to improve such detection is to infuse the swallowed substance with blue dye. In this way, the endoscope can be directed into the laryngeal vestibule immediately following the swallow to look for any blue substance that may have been deposited near or below the vocal folds.

When FEES is accompanied by sensory testing, it is called Flexible Endoscopic Evaluation of Swallowing with Sensory Testing (FEESST) (Aviv et al., 1998). Sensory testing involves the delivery of brief air pressure pulses through the endoscope to the anterior wall of the pyriform sinus or the aryepiglottic folds, regions innervated by the superior laryngeal nerve (a sensory branch of cranial nerve X, vagus). In a healthy person, this air pressure pulse elicits the laryngeal adductor reflex, a brainstem-mediated reflex that results in adduction of the vocal folds. This reflex is an important mechanism for protecting the lower airways from aspiration.

Manometry

Manometry, as discussed in Chapter 6, refers to the measurement of pressure. In the context of swallowing, the type of manometer of interest is one that consists of multiple sensors that transduce pressure change at different locations along the swallowing pathway. Older manometer systems, which have provided much of the seminal data on pharyngeal and esophageal pressures during swallowing, typically included no more than three sensors. In contrast, present-day "high resolution" systems typically include three dozen miniature, closely spaced sensors. High-resolution manometry is used routinely by gastroenterologists to evaluate esophageal function (see section on "Health Care Professionals" below) and has more recently been applied to research on pharyngeal function during swallowing and clinical evaluation of swallowing by speech-language pathologists (Knigge, Thibeault, & McCulloch, 2014).

Figure 16–12 contains videofluoroscopic images showing a high-resolution manometer in situ (right side of figure) and high-resolution pressure data recorded during a swallow (left side of figure) for a healthy individual (upper images) and for someone with a swallowing disorder (lower images). The catheter containing the sensors (black rectangles in the videofluoroscopic images) has been inserted through the nose

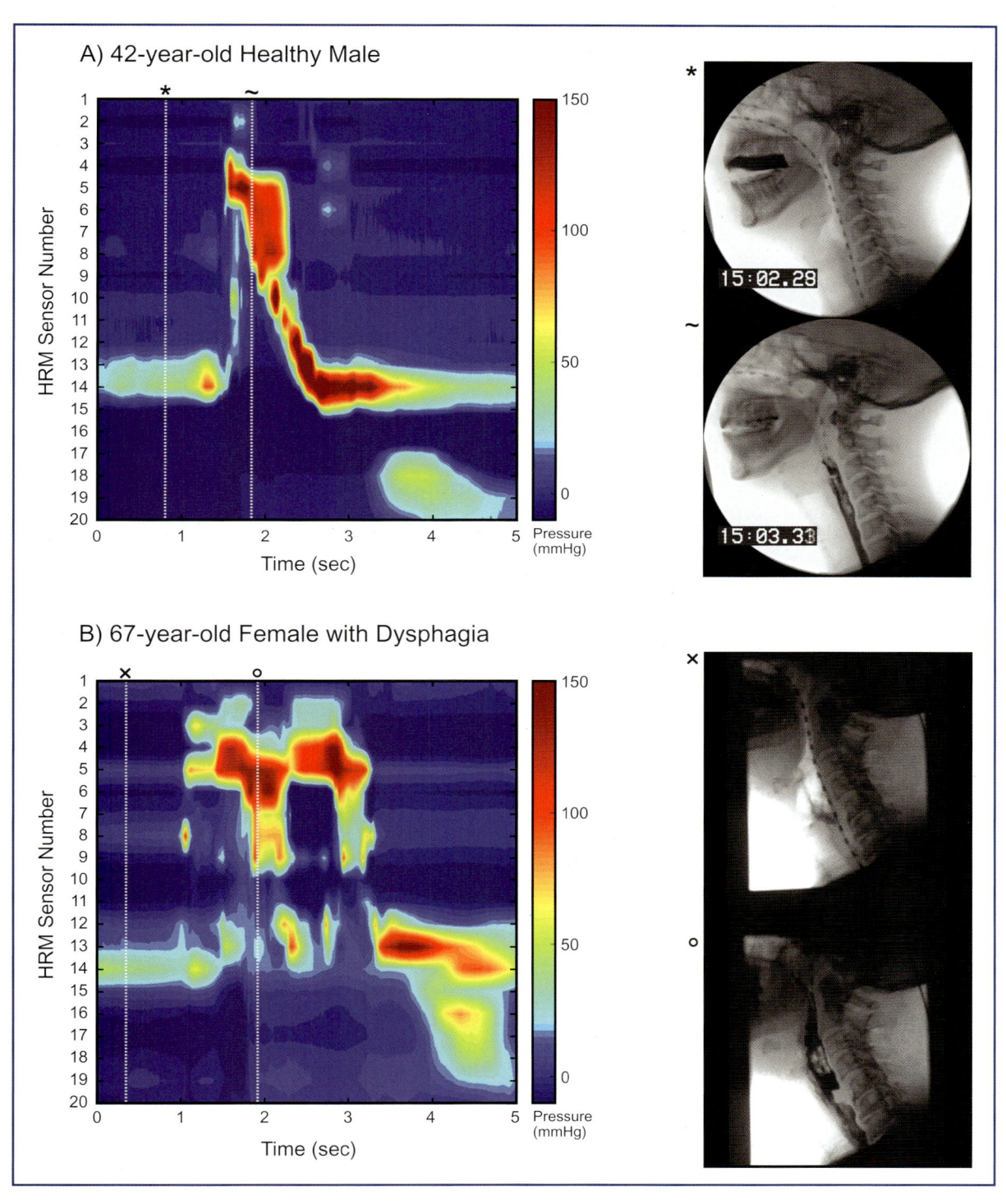

Figure 16–12. Simultaneous videofluoroscopy and pharyngeal high-resolution manometry of a 10 cc thin barium swallow from a 42-year-old healthy man (**A**) and a 67-year-old woman with dysphagia (**B**). High-resolution manometry sensors appear as black rectangles on the videofluoroscopy stills. Videofluoroscopy still images correspond to the time indicated by the vertical lines on the manometry plot with the same symbol at the top. In the data from the healthy man, pressures in the pharynx are low at rest (sensors 4–12: *dark blue*), whereas pressure is higher in the upper esophageal sphincter (sensors 13–14: light *blue/green*). During swallowing, the pharynx constricts, creating high pressures (*orange/red*) at the same time the upper esophageal sphincter relaxes (*dark blue*). The data from the woman with dysphagia reveals that she swallowed twice to clear the bolus, as indicated by the gap in the pressure wave (sensors 10–11: dark blue). Also note the area of elevated pressure in the upper esophageal sphincter (sensor 13: *light blue/green*) during opening. Courtesy of Timothy McCulloch, MD, and Corinne Jones, PhD, CCC-SLP.

(following lidocaine application) and routed through the pharynx and upper esophageal sphincter into the cervical esophagus. The output signals from the sensors reflect pressure changes generated during the swallow at a series of locations. The upper left image shows that in a healthy person at rest (during the first second of the data recording), the pressures in the pharynx are very low (sensors 4–12; dark blue), whereas the pressure in the region of the upper esophageal sphincter is somewhat higher (sensors 13–14; light blue/green). As the swallow begins (at around 1.5 seconds into the recording), the pressure in the pharynx increases substantially (orange/red) from top to bottom during the next second or so and then returns to rest. The lower left image contains data from someone with dysphagia. Several abnormalities are apparent in this image; for example, some areas of the pharynx are generating abnormally low pressure and the upper esophageal sphincter is generating abnormally high pressure during the swallow, both of which were likely contributors to the fact that the client had to swallow twice to clear the bolus.

Surface Electromyography

Although videofluoroscopy, endoscopy, and manometry offer extremely valuable information about swallowing, there are times when less invasive measurement approaches are preferred and when less detailed information about the swallow is required. Surface electromyography (EMG), which provides a way to record underlying muscle activity from the skin's surface, is one such approach. In the case of swallowing, it is common to record muscle activity from the region "under the chin" (between the hyoid bone and the mandible). This is often referred to as submental surface electromyography (sEMG) and is believed to reflect a combination of muscle activities that originate primarily from the ***mylohyoid, geniohyoid,*** and ***digastric*** (***anterior*** belly) muscles (Palmer, Luschei, Jaffe, & McCulloch, 1999). Recall that these are suprahyoid muscles that attach to the hyoid bone and when contracted, pull the hyoid bone (and the rest of the larynx along with it) upward and forward (see Chapter 3). Activation of these muscles can signal the onset of the pharyngeal phase of the swallow, and the amplitude of the activation can provide an indication of the muscle forces involved in the swallow.

Figure 16–13 contains an example of submental sEMG activity during a swallow. The upper tracing contains the raw EMG signal (just as it was recorded) and the lower tracing contains the same signal displayed in rectified form (that is, with all the negative EMG values "flipped" to positive values). During the first second of the tracings, the muscle activity is low and constant and is considered to be the resting baseline activity level. The initial rise in activity (which begins slightly after 1 second) can be used to demark the onset of the swallow; the peak amplitude of the activity (at about 1.6 seconds) can be interpreted to reflect the relative force being exerted by the muscles of interest. Although interpretation of sEMG can be problematic, submental sEMG recordings can provide valuable information regarding the swallow, especially if it is recorded along with other types of swallowing-related data (e.g., Cock et al., 2017).

Ultrasonography

Another way to visualize swallowing events is with ultrasonography. The use of ultrasonography as it applies to the measurement of speech production is discussed in Chapter 6 (and illustrated in Figure 6–18), and similar procedures can be applied to the measurement of swallowing. Briefly, ultrasonography requires the use of a transducer that generates and receives a high-frequency signal (sound waves). The transducer is pressed against the skin (usually on the undersurface of the mandible) and the signal is transmitted through the tissue toward the airway. When the signal encounters air, it reflects back. The receiver senses the returning sound waves, and the resultant signal is processed to provide an image of the outline of the proximal border of the airway.

Ultrasonography is applied to the measurement of swallowing much less frequently than are other forms of measurement, such as videofluoroscopy and flexible endoscopy. Nevertheless, it provides a noninvasive approach to characterizing behavior of the tongue (Stone & Shawker, 1986), lateral pharyngeal walls (Miller & Watkin, 1997), and other structures by way of images obtained in sagittal, frontal, and transverse planes. It may also be a useful biofeedback tool in the management of oral preparatory phase behavior (Blyth, McCabe, Madill, & Ballard, 2017; Shawker & Sonies, 1985).

Aeromechanical Observations

Another noninvasive measurement approach used in swallowing evaluation is nasal air pressure (or airflow). This measurement involves sensing pressure near the anterior nares using a small, double-barreled catheter connected to a pressure transducer, such as that described in Chapter 6 (and illustrated in Figure 6–14).

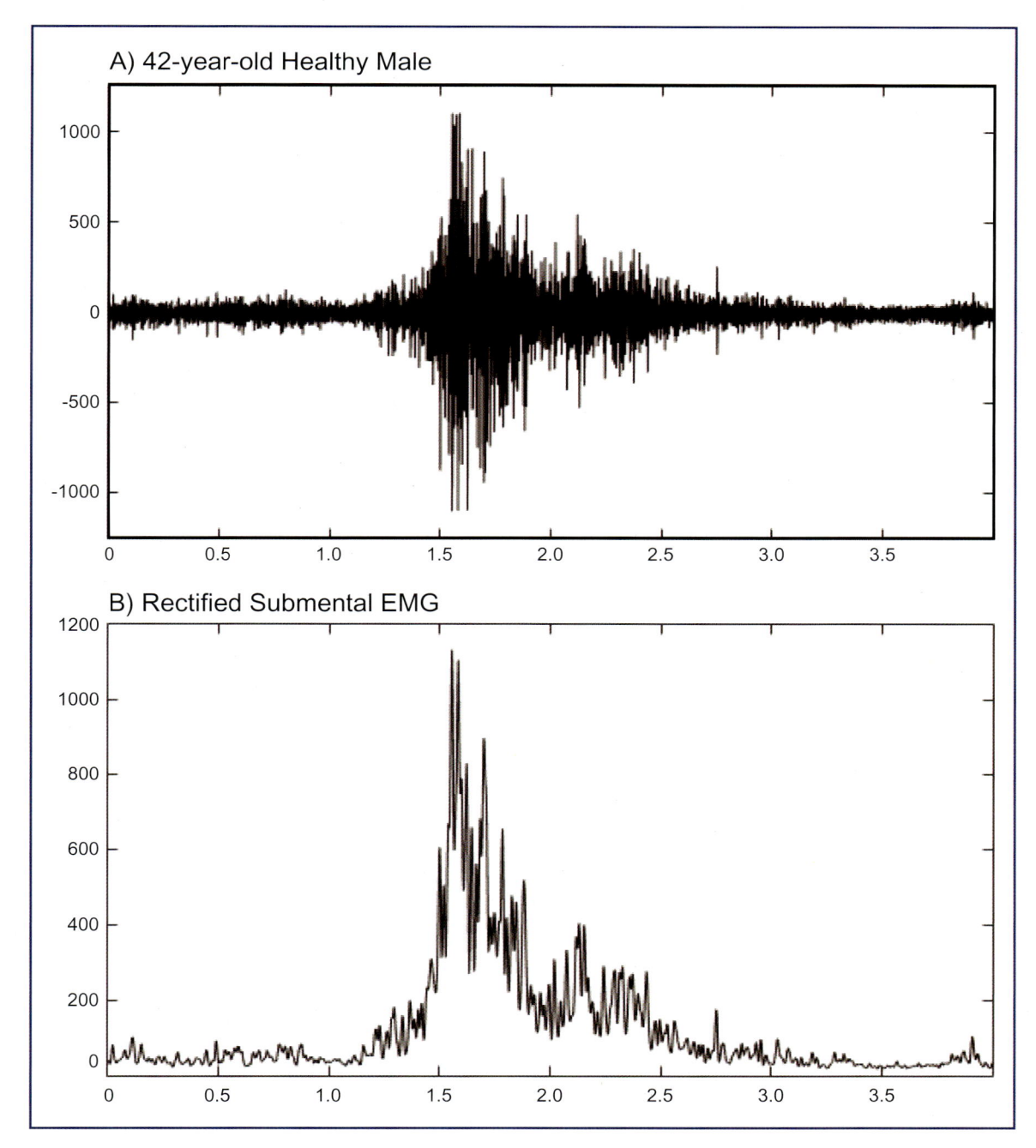

Figure 16–13. Raw (**A**) and rectified (**B**) surface electromyography (EMG) of the submental musculature during a 10-cc water swallow from a healthy 22-year-old man. EMG was rectified using root-mean-square. Courtesy of Timothy McCulloch, MD, and Corinne Jones, PhD, CCC-SLP.

During nasal breathing, this pressure is below atmospheric for inspiration and above atmospheric for expiration. When nasal pressure is recorded simultaneously with videofluoroscopic imaging, it is possible to infer the temporal relationships among certain swallowing events and the inspiratory, expiratory, and apneic phases of breathing (Martin-Harris et al., 2005a; Perlman, He, Barkmeier, & Van Leer, 2005). A nasal pressure signal can also be used as a form of biofeedback when training a client to modify breathing-swallowing coordination (Martin-Harris et al., 2015). It is interesting to note that a brief negative nasal pressure is routinely observed during swallowing; this has been interpreted to reflect a pressure drop associated with a widening of the pharynx near the end of the pharyngeal phase of the swallow (and, therefore, is not a breathing-related event) (Brodsky, McFarland, Michel, Orr, & Martin-Harris, 2012).

Client Self-Report

An important form of measurement, especially in clinical settings, is the client self-report. The client self-report can reveal symptoms (e.g., pain during swallowing, lump in the throat, difficulty swallowing certain foods) that indicate the need to perform instrumental evaluation of swallowing using measurement procedures such as those described above. One way to glean information about the client's perspective of the swallowing problem is by using an unstructured interview. An alternative or complementary approach is to use a more formal, symptom-specific assessment tool. There are several to choose from, one of which is called the Eating Assessment Tool-10 (EAT-10; Belafsky et al., 2008). The EAT-10 contains several statements, such as, "My swallowing problem has caused me to lose weight" and "I become short of breath when I eat," that the client rates on a scale ranging from "No problem" to "Severe problem." Research has shown a good correspondence between the symptoms reported on the EAT-10 and the identification of dysphagia-related signs obtained from physiologic measures (Arrese, Carrau, & Plowman, 2017; Plowman et al., 2015).

HEALTH CARE PROFESSIONALS

Evaluation and management of dysphagia (swallowing disorder) is a large part of the clinical practice of speech-language pathology. Although there are cases of functional dysphagia (wherein there is no known physical reason for the dysphagia) (Baumann & Katz, 2016), dysphagia usually has an identifiable structural, neurogenic, and/or systemic cause. Structural causes include tumors (malignant or benign), diverticula (abnormal pouches in the wall of a structure), osteophytes (bone spurs on the spine that can press on the esophagus), deformation caused by surgical removal of tissue or trauma, congenital malformations, and tracheostomy (a surgically created opening at the front of the neck), among others. Dysphagia can also have neurogenic causes such as stroke, degenerative diseases (such as Parkinson's disease), and traumatic brain injury. Systemic or other causes of dysphagia might include scleroderma (causing weakening of the esophageal tissue), immune deficiency disease, pulmonary disease, drug-induced or radiation-induced xerostomia (dry mouth), or gastroesophageal reflux disease (see sidetrack on GERD and LPR).

GERD and LPR

Your stomach is rich with chemicals that have about the same acidity as the battery acid in your car. That's right, that's the same battery acid that will burn a hole in your clothes if you splash some of it on you. Gastroesophageal reflux disease (GERD), is a chronic condition in which acid from the stomach backs up into the esophagus when the lower esophageal sphincter (the valve that separates the esophagus and stomach) fails to do its job properly. Although a certain amount of reflux (backflow) from the stomach into the esophagus is considered normal, too much can cause heartburn and the need to see a gastroenterologist (GI doctor). When stomach acid travels all the way through the esophagus and spills onto the larynx it is called laryngopharyngeal reflux (LPR). LPR can irritate and erode laryngeal tissue. LPR can cause a hoarse voice, chronic cough, frequent throat clearing, and other problems that may lead to the need to seek help from an otolaryngologist (ENT doctor). Some helpful hints for avoiding GERD and LPR: don't stuff yourself before you go to bed, lay off foods that make it worse, and sleep with your body inclined so that your head is higher than your feet.

Accurate evaluation and appropriate management of dysphagia is critical to quality of life, and sometimes to life itself. Dysphagia can be accompanied by pain (called odynophagia) that requires treatment to bring relief. Even more importantly, dysphagia can result in malnutrition and dehydration from inadequate ingestion of food and liquid. It can also cause pneumonia when unwanted substance is aspirated into the pulmonary apparatus. When dysphagia is so severe as to pose such risks, it may be necessary to use a non-oral (tube-feeding) approach to sustain life. Evaluation and management of swallowing disorders often require a team of health care professionals, including a speech-language pathologist, radiologist, gastroenterologist, otolaryngologist, dietitian, occupational therapist, and others, depending on the nature of the swallowing disorder.

The speech-language pathologist is responsible for the evaluation and behavioral management of oropharyngeal dysphagia (swallowing disorders involving the oral preparatory, oral transport, and pharyngeal phases). Usually the speech-language pathologist is asked by a physician to evaluate a client with a potential swallowing disorder. The speech-language pathologist may begin by performing a bedside swallowing evaluation, which includes a case history interview, a physical examination of the swallowing structures, and visual, auditory, and tactile observation of the client during swallowing of water and possibly other substances. If a problem is suspected, the speech-language pathologist will perform a videofluoroscopic swallowing examination in collaboration with a radiologist. During the swallow study, the speech-language pathologist may screen for esophageal problems, and if any are noted, a gastroenterologist is notified. Alternatively, a fiberoptic endoscopic evaluation of swallowing may be conducted, a procedure that can usually be performed by the speech-language pathologist independently. Behavioral management might include the teaching of postural strategies to improve swallowing, diet (consistency) recommendations, therapeutic exercises (to improve strength and coordination of swallow-related structures), and counseling regarding the swallowing disorder.

The radiologist has a limited, but critical, role in the evaluation of swallowing. Specifically, the radiologist is responsible for the instrumental aspects of videofluoroscopic swallow (modified barium swallow) studies and barium swallow studies and, in some instances, may help in their interpretation.

Although the speech-language pathologist can screen for esophageal disorders, it is the gastroenterologist who diagnoses and treats disorders of the esophagus. Evaluation approaches used by the gastroenterologist include barium swallow studies, esophageal endoscopy, esophageal manometry, and other procedures that provide information about the structure and function of the esophagus and stomach. The gastroenterologist is responsible for the management of gastroesophageal reflux disease (GERD) and for placement of a feeding tube into the stomach (called a percutaneous endoscopic gastrostomy tube, or a PEG tube) of the client whose swallow is so dysfunctional as to cause risk of aspiration. Management approaches used by gastroenterologists are usually pharmaceutical or surgical.

An otolaryngologist (also called an ear, nose, and throat physician, or ENT) is responsible for evaluating oral, pharyngeal, nasal, and laryngeal structures for pathology. An otolaryngologist may diagnose pharyngeal cancer and surgically remove it or diagnose vocal fold paralysis, a condition sometimes associated with aspiration, and treat it by surgical medialization (by inserting a substance in the vocal fold to move it toward the midline of the airway). The otolaryngologist may also perform the surgical placement of a tracheostomy tube. Tracheostomy tubes can cause or contribute to dysphagia, in part because they tend to tether the larynx and thereby restrict its elevation during the swallow.

A dietitian is often critical in developing menus that meet the caloric and nutritional needs of clients with swallowing disorders. Whereas the speech-language pathologist recommends the best consistencies, textures, and volumes of the liquid and solid substances for a client, the dietitian helps determine whether or not the client is able to meet nutritional needs solely through oral ingestion or whether nonoral supplementation (tube feeding) should be requested. It falls to the client and the client's physician to decide whether or not nonoral feeding will be used.

Many clients, particularly infants and children, require the expertise of an occupational therapist. An occupational therapist can provide devices, compensatory strategies, and behavioral therapy to improve the ability to self-feed. For example, the occupational therapist might provide special utensils and cups that make it possible for the client to eat and drink independently.

There are many other health care professionals who may be involved in the evaluation and management of a client with a swallowing disorder. For example, if the cause of the dysphagia is neural, a neurologist will be a critical member of the team. Similarly, if dysphagia is associated with pulmonary disease, a pulmonologist and respiratory therapist will be involved in the client's management. A dentist or prosthodontist participates in the care of clients with swallowing disorders if dental or other oral structural problems are contributing factors, such as in cases of oral cancer, cleft palate, or structural abnormalities associated with a congenital syndrome. A physical therapist might be needed to help the client achieve the best posture for eating and drinking. Nurses and nurses' aides often screen for swallowing problems, alerting the physician of any problem noted, and helping to carry out the management plan. Clearly, it is critical that health care professionals representing many disciplines collaborate to determine the nature of a swallowing problem and how best to manage it.

REVIEW

Eating and drinking involve intricately coordinated actions of the lips, mandible, tongue, velum, pharynx, larynx, esophagus, and other structures.

The act of placing liquid or solid substances in the oral cavity, moving it backward to the pharynx, propelling it into the esophagus, and allowing it to make its way to the stomach is called *deglutition*.

The term *swallowing* is ingrained as a synonym for deglutition and is used as such in this chapter, although swallowing technically involves only part of the deglutition process.

Many of the important anatomical and physiological components of the speech production apparatus, discussed in Chapters 2 through 5 of this text, are also important anatomical and physiological components of the swallowing apparatus.

The esophagus is a muscular tube that extends from the lower border of the pharynx to the stomach and is bounded at its two ends by high-pressure valves (the upper and lower esophageal sphincters) that govern the passage of liquid and solid substances into and out of the structure.

The stomach is a liter-sized sac whose upper end connects to the esophagus through the lower esophageal sphincter and whose lower end connects to the small intestine through the pyloric sphincter.

The forces of swallowing are greater and the movements of swallowing are generally slower than those associated with speech production.

Passive forces of swallowing come from the natural recoil of structures, surface tension between structures in apposition, gravity, and aeromechanical factors, whereas active forces result from the activation of breathing, laryngeal, velopharyngeal-nasal, pharyngeal-oral, and esophageal muscles in various combinations.

Different pressure gradients are critical to the swallowing process and are influenced by pressures existing within the oral cavity, the upper esophageal sphincter, the esophagus, the lower esophageal sphincter, and the stomach.

The forces and movements associated with the act of swallowing can be categorized in four phases, which include an oral preparatory phase, oral transport phase, pharyngeal phase, and esophageal phase.

The oral preparatory phase involves taking liquid or solid substance in through the oral vestibule and manipulating it within the oral cavity to prepare the bolus (liquid volume or lump of solid) for passage.

The oral transport phase involves moving the bolus (or a part of it) through the oral cavity toward the pharynx by rearward propulsion.

The pharyngeal phase is usually "triggered" when the bolus passes the anterior faucial pillars or beyond, and consists of a combination of compressive actions that force the bolus downward toward the esophagus while at the same time protecting the lower airways.

The esophageal phase begins when the bolus enters the esophagus and continues as the bolus is moved toward the stomach by a series of peristaltic waves of muscular contraction and relaxation that progress down the muscular tube and are followed by secondary waves that clear the esophagus.

Although it is convenient to describe swallowing as four discrete phases, the reality is that there is enormous overlap among the phases, and more physiologic schemes may offer better ways to characterize the swallowing process.

Swallowing usually occurs during expiration at lung volumes that are somewhat larger than the resting expiratory level and is associated with a brief apneic interval (cessation of breathing).

The neural control of swallowing is vested in the brainstem and in other higher brain centers that oversee automatic and voluntary aspects of the different phases of swallowing.

Characteristics of the bolus can influence the swallowing pattern, including bolus consistency and texture, volume, and taste.

The mode of swallowing has an impact on the swallowing process, with differences observed for single swallows versus sequential swallows, cued swallows versus spontaneous swallows, with dependencies on how the substance is presented and what instructions are given.

Details of the swallowing pattern may change with changes in body position, including when swallowing occurs during the breathing cycle, the timing of certain swallowing events, and the magnitudes of certain pressures.

The development of swallowing from infancy is rapid and complex and moves through different sucking and chewing patterns toward adult-like eating and drinking behaviors, and carries with it important developmental processes related to social and emotional development.

The effect of aging on the swallow is an overall slowing and a subtle deterioration in the spatial and temporal coordination among certain structures of the swallowing apparatus.

The sex of the individual makes little difference to the nature of swallowing.

Several ways to measure and analyze swallowing are available and include videofluoroscopy (which uses x-rays to image all phases of swallowing), endoscopy (which uses a flexible endoscope to image the pharyngeal and laryngeal regions), manometry (which uses pressure transducers to sense pressure change in the pharynx and esophagus), surface electromyography (which records activity from muscles underlying the skin), ultrasonography (which uses ultrasound to image selected structures), aeromechanical observations (such as air pressure that can signal certain breathing events related to the swallow), and client self-report (which provides insight into the client's experiences with swallowing).

Some of the more important health care professionals who work with clients with dysphagia (impaired swallowing) include speech-language pathologists, radiologists, gastroenterologists, otolaryngologists, dietitians, and occupational therapists.

REFERENCES

Arrese, L., Carrau, R., & Plowman, E. (2017). Relationship between the Eating Assessment Tool-10 and objective clinical ratings of swallowing function in individuals with head and neck cancer. *Dysphagia, 32,* 83–89.

Arvedson, J., & Brodsky, L. (2002). *Pediatric swallowing and feeding: Assessment and management* (2nd ed.). Clifton Park, NY: Thomson Learning (Singular).

Aviv, J., Kim, T., Thomson, J., Sunshine, S., Kaplan, S., & Close, L. (1998). Fiberoptic endoscopic evaluation of swallowing with sensory testing (FEESST) in healthy controls. *Dysphagia, 13,* 87–92.

Babael, A., Kern, M., Antonik, S., Mepant, R., Ward, B., Li, S-J., . . . Shaker, R. (2010). Enhancing effects of flavored nutritive stimuli on cortical swallowing network activity. *American Journal of Physiology: Gastrointestinal and Liver Physiology, 299,* G422–G429.

Barkmeier, J., Bielamowicz, S., Takeda, N., & Ludlow, C. (2002). Laryngeal activity during upright vs. supine swallowing. *Journal of Applied Physiology, 93,* 740–745.

Baumann, A., & Katz, P. (2016). Functional disorders of swallowing. *Handbook of Clinical Neurology, 139,* 483–488.

Belafsky, P., Mouadeb, D., Rees, C., Pryor, J., Postma, G., Allen, J., & Leonard, R. (2008). Validity and reliability of the Eating Assessment Tool (EAT-10). *Annals of Otology, Rhinology & Laryngology, 117,* 919–924.

Blyth, K., McCabe, P., Madill, C., & Ballard, K. (2017). Ultrasound in dysphagia rehabilitation: A novel approach following partial glossectomy. *Disability and Rehabilitation, 39,* 2215–2227.

Bosma, J. (1986). Development of feeding. *Clinical Nutrition, 5,* 210–218.

Bosma, J., Truby, H., & Lind, J. (1965). Cry motions of the newborn infant. *Acta Paediatrica Scandinavica, 163,* 63–91.

Brodsky, M., McFarland, D., Michel, Y., Orr, S., & Martin-Harris, B. (2012). Significance of nonrespiratory airflow during swallowing. *Dysphagia, 27,* 178–184.

Castell, J., Dalton, C., & Castell, D. (1990). Effects of body position and bolus consistency on the manometric parameters and coordination of the upper esophageal sphincter and pharynx. *Dysphagia, 5,* 179–186.

Chi-Fishman, G., & Sonies, B. (2000). Motor strategy in rapid sequential swallowing: New insights. *Journal of Speech, Language, and Hearing Research, 43,* 1481–1492.

Chi-Fishman, G., & Sonies, B. (2002). Effects of systematic bolus viscosity and volume changes on hyoid movement kinematics. *Dysphagia, 17,* 278–287.

Chi-Fishman, G., Stone, M., & McCall, G. (1998). Lingual action in normal sequential swallowing. *Journal of Speech, Language, and Hearing Research, 41,* 771–785.

Cichero, J., Lam, P., Steele, C., Hanson, B., Chen, J., Dantas, R., . . . Stanschus, S. (2017). Development of international terminology and definitions for texture-modified foods and thickened fluids used in dysphagia management: The IDDSI framework. *Dysphagia, 32,* 293–314.

Cock, C., Jones, C., Hammer, M., Omari, T., & McCulloch, T. (2017). Modulation of upper esophageal sphincter (UES) relaxation and opening during volume swallowing. *Dysphagia, 32,* 216–224.

Cook, I., Dodds, W., Dantas, R., Kern, M., Massey, B., Shaker, R., & Hogan, W. (1989). Timing of videofluoroscopic, manometric events, and bolus transit during the oral and pharyngeal phases of swallowing. *Dysphagia, 4,* 8–15.

Cook, I., Weltman, M., Wallace, K., Shaw, D., McKay, E., Smart, R., & Butler, S. (1994). Influence of aging on oral-pharyngeal bolus transit and clearance during swallowing: Scintigraphic study. *American Journal of Physiology, 266,* G972–G977.

Corbin-Lewis, K., & Liss, J. (2015). *Clinical anatomy and physiology of the swallow mechanism*. Independence, KY: Cengage Learning.

Daggett, A., Logemann, J., Rademaker, A., & Pauloski, B. (2006). Laryngeal penetration during deglutition in normal subjects of various ages. *Dysphagia, 21,* 270–274.

Daniels, S., Corey, D., Hadskey, L., Legendre, C., Priestly, D., Rosenbek, J., & Foundas, A. (2004). Mechanism of sequential swallowing during straw drinking in healthy young and older adults. *Journal of Speech, Language, and Hearing Research, 47,* 33–45.

Daniels, S., & Foundas, A. (2001). Swallowing physiology of sequential straw drinking. *Dysphagia, 16,* 176–182.

Daniels, S., Schroeder, M., DeGeorge, P., Corey, D., & Rosenbek, J. (2007). Effects of verbal cue on bolus flow during swallowing. *American Journal of Speech-Language Pathology, 16,* 140–147.

Dantas, R., Kern, M., Massey, B., Dodds, W., Kahrilas, P., Brasseur, J., Cook, I., & Lang, I. (1990). Effect of swallowed bolus variables on oral and pharyngeal phases of swallowing. *American Journal of Physiology, 258,* G675–G681.

Dejaeger, E., Pelemans, W., Ponette, E., & VanTrappen, G. (1994). Effect of body position on deglutition. *Digestive Diseases and Sciences, 39,* 762–765.

Ding, R., Logemann, J., Larson, C., & Rademaker, A. (2003). The effects of taste and consistency on swallow physiology in younger and older healthy individuals: A surface electromyographic study. *Journal of Speech, Language, and Hearing Research, 46,* 977–989.

Dodds, W., Hogan, W., Reid, D., Stewart, E., & Arndorfer, R. (1973). A comparison between primary esophageal peristalsis following wet and dry swallows. *Journal of Applied Physiology, 35,* 851–857.

Dodds, W., Taylor, A., Stewart, E., Kern, M., Logemann, J., & Cook, I. (1989). Tipper and dipper types of oral swallows. *American Journal of Roentgenology, 153,* 1197–1199.

Dua, K., Ren, J., Bardan, E., Xie, P., & Shaker, R. (1997). Coordination of deglutitive glottal function and pharyngeal bolus transit during normal eating. *Gastroenterology, 112,* 73–83.

Ekberg, O., & Sigurjonsson, S. (1982). Movement of epiglottis during deglutition: A cineradiographic study. *Gastrointestinal Radiology, 7*, 101–107.

Engelen, L., Fontijn-Tekamp, & van der Bilt, A. (2005). The influence of product and oral characteristics on swallowing. *Archives of Oral Biology, 50*, 739–746.

Fei, T., Polacco, R., Hori, S., Molfenter, S., Peladeau-Pigeon, M., Tsang, C., & Steele, C. (2013). Age-related differences in tongue-palate pressures for strength and swallowing tasks. *Dysphagia, 28*, 575–581.

Fink, B., & Demarest, R. (1978). *Laryngeal biomechanics*. Cambridge, MA: Harvard University Press.

Fink, B., Martin, R., & Rohrmann, C. (1979). Biomechanics of the human epiglottis. *Acta Otolaryngologica, 87*, 554–559.

Fritz, M., Cerrati, E., Fang, Y., Verma, A., Achiatis, S., Lazarus, C., Branski, R., & Amin, M. (2014). Magnetic resonance imaging of the effortful swallow. *Annals of Otology, Rhinology & Laryngology, 123*, 786–790.

Fukuoka, T., Ono, T., Hori, K., Tamine, K., Nozaki, S., Shimada, K., . . . Domen, K. (2013). Effect of the effortful swallow and the Mendelsohn maneuver on tongue pressure production against the hard palate. *Dysphagia, 28*, 539–547.

Goyal, R., & Cobb, B. (1981). Motility of the pharynx, esophagus, and esophageal sphincters. In L. Johnson (Ed.), *Physiology of the gastrointestinal tract* (pp. 359–390). New York, NY: Raven Press.

Green, J., Moore, C., Ruark, J., Rodda, P., Morvee, W., & VanWitzenburg, M. (1997). Development of chewing in children from 12 to 48 months: Longitudinal study of EMG patterns. *Journal of Neurophysiology, 77*, 2704–2716.

Gross, R., Carrau, R., Slivka, W., Gisser, R., Smith, L., Zajac, D., & Sciurba, F. (2012). Deglutitive subglottic air pressure and respiratory system recoil. *Dysphagia, 27*, 452–459.

Gürgor, N., Arici, S., Incesu, T. Seçil, Y., Tokuçoglu, F., & Ertekin, C. (2013). An electrophysiological study of the sequential water swallowing. *Journal of Electromyography and Kinesiology, 23*, 619–626.

Hårdemark Cedborg, A., Bodén, K., Witt Hedström, H., Kuylenstierna, R., Ekberg, O., Eriksson, L., & Sundman, E. (2010). Breathing and swallowing in normal man: Effects of changes in body position, bolus types, and respiratory drive. *Neurogastroenterology and Motility, 22*, 1201–1208.

Hiiemae, K., & Palmer, J. (1999). Food transport and bolus formation during complete feeding sequences on foods of different initial consistency. *Dysphagia, 14*, 31–42.

Hila, A., Castell, J., & Castell, D. (2001). Pharyngeal and upper esophageal sphincter manometry in the evaluation of dysphagia. *Journal of Clinical Gastroenterology, 33*, 355–361.

Hiraoka, T., Palmer, J., Brodsky, M., Yoda, M., Inokuchi, H., & Tsubahara, A. (2017). Food transit duration is associated with the number of stage II transport cycles when eating solid food. *Archives of Oral Biology, 81*, 186–191.

Hirst, L., Ford, G., Gibson, G., & Wilson, J. (2002). Swallow-induced alterations in breathing in normal older people. *Dysphagia, 17*, 152–161.

Hoit, J., Lansing, R., Dean, K., Yarkosky, M., & Lederle, A. (2011). Nature and evaluation of dyspnea in speaking and swallowing. *Seminars in Speech and Language, 32*, 5–20.

Humber, I., & German, R. (2013). New directions for understanding neural control in swallowing: The potential and promise of motor learning. *Dysphagia, 28*, 1–10.

Humbert, I., & Robbins, J. (2007). Normal swallowing and functional magnetic resonance imaging: A systematic review. *Dysphagia, 22*, 266–275.

Humphrey, T. (1970). Reflex activity in the oral and facial area of the human fetus. In J. Bosma (Ed.), *Second symposium on oral sensation and perception* (pp. 195–233). Springfield, IL: Charles C. Thomas.

Im, I., Kim, Y., Oommen, E., Kim, H., & Ko, M. (2012). The effects of bolus consistency in pharyngeal transit duration during normal swallowing. *Annals of Rehabilitation Medicine, 36*, 220–225.

Inamoto, Y., Saitoh, E., Okada, S., Kagaya, H., Shibata, S., Ota, K., . . . Palmer, J. (2013). The effect of bolus viscosity on laryngeal closure in swallowing: Kinematic analysis using 320-row area detector CT. *Dysphagia, 28*, 33–42.

Ingervall, B., & Lantz, B. (1973). Significance of gravity on the passage of bolus through the human pharynx. *Archives of Oral Biology, 18*, 351–356.

Jadcherla, S. (2017). Advances with neonatal aerodigestive science in the pursuit of safe swallowing in infants: Invited review. *Dysphagia, 32*, 15–26.

Jean, A. (2001). Brain stem control of swallowing: Neuronal network and cellular mechanisms. *Physiological Reviews, 81*, 929–969.

Johnson, F., Shaw, D., Gabb, M., Dent, J., & Cook, I. (1995). Influence of gravity and body position on normal oropharyngeal swallowing. *American Journal of Physiology, 269*, G653–G658.

Kahrilas, P., & Logemann, J. (1993). Volume accommodation during swallowing. *Dysphagia, 8*, 259–265.

Klaun, M., & Perlman, A. (1999). Temporal and durational patterns associating respiration and swallowing. *Dysphagia, 14*, 131–138.

Knigge, M., Thibeault, S., & McCulloch, T. (2014). Implementation of high-resolution manometry in the clinical practice of speech language pathology. *Dysphagia, 29*, 2–16.

Koenig, J., Davies, A., & Thach, B. (1990). Coordination of breathing, sucking, and swallowing during bottle feedings in human infants. *Journal of Applied Physiology, 69*, 1623–1629.

Langmore, S. (2001). *Endoscopic evaluation and treatment of swallowing disorders*. New York, NY: Thieme Medical.

Langmore, S., Schatz, K., & Olson, N. (1988). Fiberoptic endoscopic evaluation of swallowing safety: A new procedure. *Dysphagia, 2*, 216–219.

Lederle, A., Hoit, J., & Barkmeier-Kraemer, J. (2012). Effects of sequential swallowing on drive to breathe in young, healthy adults. *Dysphagia, 27*, 221–227.

Leonard, R., Kendall, K., McKenzie, S., & Goodrich, S. (2008). The treatment plan. In R. Leonard & K. Kendall (Eds.), *Dysphagia assessment and treatment planning: A team approach* (2nd ed., pp. 295–336). San Diego, CA: Plural.

Leonard, R., & McKenzie, S. (2006). Hyoid-bolus transit latencies in normal swallow. *Dysphagia, 21*, 183–190.

Leow, L., Huckabee, M., Sharma, S., & Tooley, T. (2007). The influence of taste on swallowing apnea, oral preparation time, and duration and amplitude of submental muscle contraction. *Chemical Senses, 32,* 119–128.

Lever, T., Cox, K., Holbert, D., Shahrier, M., Hough, M., & Kelley-Salamon, K. (2007). The effect of effortful swallow on the normal adult esophagus. *Dysphagia, 22,* 312–325.

Lin, T., Xu, G., Dou, Z, Lan, Y., Yu, F., & Jiang, L. (2014). Effect of bolus volume on pharyngeal swallowing assessed by high-resolution manometry. *Physiology & Behavior, 128,* 46–51.

Linden, M., Hogosta, S., & Norlander, T. (2007). Monitoring of pharyngeal and upper esophageal sphincter activity with an arterial dilation balloon catheter. *Dysphagia, 22,* 81–88.

Linden, P., Tippett, D., Johnston, J., Siebens, A., & French, J. (1989). Bolus position at swallow onset in normal adults: Preliminary observations. *Dysphagia, 4,* 146–150.

Logemann, J. (1998). *Evaluation and treatment of swallowing disorders* (2nd ed.). Austin, TX: Pro-Ed.

Logemann, J., Boshes, B., Blonsky, E., & Fisher, H. (1977). Speech and swallowing evaluation in the differential diagnosis of neurologic disease. *Neurologia, Neurocirugia, and Psiquiatria, 18*(2–3 Suppl.), 71–78.

Logemann, J., Kahrilas, P., Kobara, M., & Vakil, N. (1989). The benefit of head rotation on pharyngo-esophageal dysphagia. *Archives of Physical Medicine and Rehabilitation, 70,* 767–771.

Logemann, J., Pauloski, B., Rademaker, A., Colangelo, L., Kahrilas, P., & Smith, C. (2000). Temporal and biomechanical characteristics of oropharyngeal swallow in younger and older men. *Journal of Speech, Language, and Hearing Research, 43,* 1264–1274.

Logemann, J., Pauloski, B., Rademaker, A., & Kahrilas, P. (2002). Oropharyngeal swallow in younger and older women: Videofluoroscopic analysis. *Journal of Speech, Language, and Hearing Research, 45,* 434–445.

Malandraki, G., Perlman, A., Karampinos, D., & Sutton, B. (2011). Reduced somatosensory activations in swallowing with age. *Human Brain Mapping, 32,* 730–743.

Margolskee, R., Dyer, J., Kokrashvili, Z., Salmon, K., Ilegems, E., Daly, K., . . . Shirazi-Beechey, S. (2007). T1R3 and gustducin in gut sense sugars to regulate expression of Na+-glucose cotransporter 1. *Proceedings of the National Academy of Sciences, 104,* 15075–15080.

Martin, B., Logemann, J., Shaker, R., & Dodds, W. (1994). Coordination between respiration and swallowing: Respiratory phase relationships and temporal integration. *Journal of Applied Physiology, 76,* 714–723.

Martin, R., & Sessle, B. (1993). The role of the cerebral cortex in swallowing. *Dysphagia, 8,* 195–202.

Martin-Harris, B. (2006, May 16). Coordination of respiration and swallowing. *GI Motility Online.* doi:10.1038/gimo10

Martin-Harris, B., Brodsky, M., Michel, Y., Ford, C., Walters, B., & Heffner, J. (2005a). Breathing and swallowing dynamics across the adult lifespan. *Archives of Otolaryngology–Head and Neck Surgery, 131,* 762–770.

Martin-Harris, B., Brodsky, M., Price, C., Michel, Y., & Walters, B. (2003). Temporal coordination of pharyngeal and laryngeal dynamics with breathing during swallowing: Single liquid swallows. *Journal of Applied Physiology, 94,* 1735–1743.

Martin-Harris, B., Garand, K., & McFarland, D. (2017). Optimizing respiratory-swallowing coordination in patients with oropharyngeal head and neck cancer. *Perspectives of the ASHA Special Interest Groups, 2,* 103–110.

Martin-Harris, B., McFarland, D., Hill, E., Strange, C., Focht, K., Wan, Z., Blair, J., & McGrattan, K. (2015). Respiratory-swallow training in patients with head and neck cancer. *Archives of Physical Medicine and Rehabilitation, 96,* 885–893.

Martin-Harris, B., Michel, Y., & Castell, D. (2005b). Physiologic model of oropharyngeal swallowing revisited. *Otolaryngology–Head and Neck Surgery, 133,* 234–240.

McFarland, D., & Lund, J. (1995). Modification of mastication and respiration during swallowing in the adult human. *Journal of Neurophysiology, 74,* 1509–1517.

McFarland, D., Lund, J., & Gagner, M. (1994). Effects of posture on the coordination of respiration and swallowing. *Journal of Neurophysiology, 72,* 2431–2437.

McFarland, D., Martin-Harris, B., Fortin, A., Humphries, K., Hill, E., & Armeson, K. (2016). Respiratory-swallowing coordination in normal subjects: Lung volume at swallowing initiation. *Respiratory Physiology & Neurobiology, 234,* 89–96.

Mendell, D., & Logemann, J. (2007). Temporal sequence of swallow events during the oropharyngeal swallow. *Journal of Speech, Language, and Hearing Research, 50,* 1256–1271.

Meyer, G., Gerhardt, D., & Castell, D. (1981). Human esophageal response to rapid swallowing: Muscle refractory period or neural inhibition? *American Journal of Physiology, 241,* G129–G136.

Mikushi, S., Seki, S., Brodsky, M., Matsuo, K., & Palmer, J. (2014). Stage I intraoral food transport: Effects of food consistency and initial bolus size. *Archives of Oral Biology, 59,* 379–385.

Miller, J., Sonies, B., & Macedonia, C. (2003). Emergence of oropharyngeal, laryngeal and swallowing activity in the developing fetal upper aerodigestive tract: An ultrasound evaluation. *Early Human Development, 71,* 61–87.

Miller, J., & Watkin, K. (1996). The influence of bolus volume and viscosity on anterior lingual force during the oral stage of swallowing. *Dysphagia, 11,* 117–124.

Miller, J., & Watkin, K. (1997). Lateral pharyngeal wall motion during swallowing using real time ultrasound. *Dysphagia, 12,* 125–132.

Molfenter, S., & Steele, C. (2012). Temporal variability in the deglutition literature. *Dysphagia, 27,* 162–177.

Mulheren, R., Kamarunas, E., & Ludlow, C. (2016). Sour taste increases swallowing and prolongs hemodynamic responses in the cortical swallowing network. *Journal of Neurophysiology, 116,* 2033–2042.

Nagy, A., Steele, C., & Pelletier, C. (2014). Differences in swallowing between high and low concentration taste stimuli. *BioMed Research International.* doi:10.1155/2014/813084

Nishikubo, K., Mise, K., Ameya, M., Hirose, K., Kobayashi, T., & Hyodo, M. (2015). Quantitative evaluation of age-related alteration of swallowing function: Videofluoroscopic and manometric studies. *Auris Nasus Larynx, 42,* 134–138.

Nishino, T., Yonezawa, T., & Honda, Y. (1985). Effects of swallowing on the pattern of continuous respiration in human adults. *American Review of Respiratory Disease, 132,* 1219–1222.

Omari, T., Jones, C., Hammer, M., Cock, C., Dinning, P., Wiklendt, L., Costa, M., & McCulloch, T. (2016). Predicting the activation states of the muscles governing upper esophageal sphincter relaxation and opening. *American Journal of Physiology–Gastrointestinal and Liver Physiology, 310,* G359–G366.

O'Rourke, A., Morgan, L., Coss-Adame, E., Morrison, M., Weinberger, P., & Postma, G. (2014). The effect of voluntary pharyngeal swallowing maneuvers on esophageal swallowing physiology. *Dysphagia, 29,* 262–268.

Palmer, J. (1998). Bolus aggregation in the oropharynx does not depend on gravity. *Archives of Physical Medicine and Rehabilitation, 79,* 691–696.

Palmer, J., & Hiiemae, K. (2003). Eating and breathing: Interactions between respiration and feeding on solid food. *Dysphagia, 18,* 169–178.

Palmer, J., Luschei, E., Jaffe, D., & McCulloch, T. (1999). Contributions of individual muscles to the submental surface electromyogram during swallowing. *Journal of Speech, Language, and Hearing Research, 42,* 1378–1391.

Palmer, P., McCulloch, T., Jaffe, D., & Neel, A. (2005). Effects of a sour bolus on the intramuscular electromyographic (EMG) activity of muscles in the submental region. *Dysphagia, 20,* 210–217.

Palmer, J., Rudin, N., Lara, G., & Crompton, A. (1992). Coordination of mastication and swallowing. *Dysphagia, 7,* 187–200.

Park, T., & Kim, Y. (2016). Effects of tongue pressing effortful swallow in older healthy individuals. *Archives of Gerontology and Geriatrics, 66,* 127–133.

Pearson, W., Langmore, S., & Zumwalt, A. (2011). Evaluating the structural properties of suprahyoid muscles and their potential for moving the hyoid. *Dysphagia, 26,* 345–351.

Pelletier, C., & Dhanaraj, G. (2006). The effect of taste and palatability on lingual swallowing pressure. *Dysphagia, 21,* 121–128.

Pelletier, C., & Steele, C. (2014). Influence of the perceived taste intensity of chemesthetic stimuli on swallowing parameters given age and genetic taste differences in healthy adult women. *Journal of Speech, Language, and Hearing Research, 57,* 46–56.

Perlman, A., Ettema, S., & Barkmeier, J. (2000). Respiratory and acoustic signals associated with bolus passage during swallowing. *Dysphagia, 15,* 89–94.

Perlman, A., He, X., Barkmeier, J., & Van Leer, E. (2005). Bolus location associated with videofluoroscopic and respirode glutometric events. *Journal of Speech, Language, and Hearing Research, 48,* 21–33.

Perlman, A., Palmer, P., McCulloch, T., & VanDaele, D. (1999). Electromyographic activity from human laryngeal, pharyngeal, and submental muscles during swallowing. *Journal of Applied Physiology, 86,* 1663–1669.

Perlman, A., Schultz, J., & VanDaele, D. (1993). Effects of age, gender, bolus volume, and bolus viscosity on oropharyngeal pressure during swallowing. *Journal of Applied Physiology, 75,* 33–37.

Perry, J., Bae, Y., & Kuehn, D. (2012). Effect of posture on deglutitive biomechanics in healthy individuals. *Dysphagia, 27,* 70–80.

Pitcher, J., Crandall, M., & Goodrich, S. (2008). Pediatric clinical feeding assessment. In R. Leonard & K. Kendall (Eds.), *Dysphagia assessment and treatment planning: A team approach* (2nd ed., pp. 117–136). San Diego, CA: Plural.

Plowman, E., Tabor, L., Robison, R., Gaziano, J., Dion, C., Watts, S., . . . Gooch, C. (2015). Discriminant ability of the Eating Assessment Tool-10 to detect aspiration in individuals with amyotrophic lateral sclerosis. *Neurogastroenterology & Motility, 28,* 85–90.

Preiksaitis, H., Mayrand, S., Robins, K., & Diamant, N. (1992). Coordination of respiration and swallowing: Effect of bolus volume in normal adults. *American Journal of Physiology, 263,* R624–R630.

Preiksaitis, H., & Mills, C. (1996). Coordination of respiration and swallowing: Effects of bolus consistency and presentation in normal adults. *Journal of Applied Physiology, 81,* 1707–1714.

Ramsey, G., Watson, J., Gramiak, R., & Weinberg, S. (1955). Cinefluorographic analysis of the mechanism of swallowing. *Radiology, 64,* 498–518.

Robbins, J., Hamilton, J., Lof, G., & Kempster, G. (1992). Oropharyngeal swallowing in normal adults of different ages. *Gastroenterology, 103,* 823–829.

Rosen, S., Abdelhalim, S., Jones, C., & McCulloch, T. (2017). Effect of body position on pharyngeal swallowing pressures using high-resolution manometry. *Dysphagia.* doi:10.1007/s00455-017-9866-3

Rosenbek, J., Robbins, J., Roecker, E., Coyle, J., & Wood, J. (1996) A penetration-aspiration scale. *Dysphagia, 11,* 93–98.

Saitoh, E., Shibata, S., Matsuo, K., Baba, M., Fujii, W., & Palmer, J. (2007). Chewing and food consistency: Effects on bolus transport and swallow initiation. *Dysphagia, 22,* 100–107.

Sears, V., Castell, J., & Castell, D. (1990). Comparison of effects of upright versus supine body position and liquid versus solid bolus on esophageal pressures in normal humans. *Digestive Diseases and Sciences, 35,* 857–864.

Selley, W., Flack, F., Ellis, R., & Brooks, W. (1989). Respiratory patterns associated with swallowing: Part I. The normal adult pattern and changes with age. *Age and Ageing, 18,* 168–172.

Shawker, T., & Sonies, B. (1985). Ultrasound biofeedback for speech training. *Investigative Radiology, 20,* 90–93.

Shune, S., Moon, J., & Goodman, S. (2016). The effects of age and preoral sensorimotor cues on anticipatory mouth movement during swallowing. *Journal of Speech, Language, and Hearing Research, 59,* 195–205.

Smith, J., Wolkove, N., Colacone, A., & Kreisman, H. (1989). Coordination of eating, drinking, and breathing in adults. *Chest, 96,* 578–582.

Sonies, B., Parent, L., Morrish, K., & Baum, B. (1988). Durational aspects of the oral-pharyngeal phase of swallow in normal adults. *Dysphagia, 3,* 1–10.

Steele, C., Alsanei, W., Ayanikalath, S., Barbon, C., Chen, J., Cichero, J., . . . Lam, P. (2015). The influence of food texture and liquid consistency modification on swallowing physiology and function: A systematic review. *Dysphagia, 30,* 2–26.

Steele, C., & Cichero, J. (2014). Physiological factors related to aspiration risk: A systematic review. *Dysphagia, 29,* 295–304.

Steele, C., & Huckabee, M. (2007). The influence of orolingual pressure on the timing of pharyngeal pressure events. *Dysphagia, 22,* 30–36.

Steele, C., & van Lieshout, P. (2004). Influence of bolus consistency on lingual behaviors in sequential swallowing. *Dysphagia, 19,* 192–206.

Steele, C., & van Lieshout, P. (2009). Tongue movements during water swallowing in healthy young and older adults. *Journal of Speech, Language, and Hearing Research, 52,* 1255–1267.

Steeve, R., Moore, C., Green, J., Reilly, K., & Ruark McMurtrey, J. (2008). Babbling, chewing, and sucking: Oromandibular coordination at nine months. *Journal of Speech, Language, and Hearing Research, 51,* 1390–1404.

Stone, M., & Shawker, T. (1986). An ultrasound examination of tongue movement during swallowing. *Dysphagia, 1,* 78–83.

Su, H., Khorsandi, A., Silberzweig, J., Kobren, A., Urken, M., Amin, M., Branski, R., & Lazarus, C. (2015). Temporal and physiologic measurements of deglutition in the upright and supine position with videofluoroscopy (VFS) in healthy subjects. *Dysphagia, 30,* 438–444.

Tasko, S., Kent, R., & Westbury, J. (2002). Variability in tongue movement kinematics during normal liquid swallow. *Dysphagia, 17,* 126–138.

Tracy, J., Logemann, J., Kahrilas, P., Jacob, P., Kobara, M., & Krugler, C. (1989). Preliminary observations on the effects of age on oropharyngeal deglutition. *Dysphagia, 4,* 90–94.

Ulysal, H., Kizilay, F., Ünal, A., Güngor, H., & Ertekin, C. (2013). The interaction between breathing and swallowing in healthy individuals. *Journal of Electromyography and Kinesiology, 23,* 659–663.

VanDaele, D., Perlman, A., & Cassell, M. (1995). Intrinsic fibre architecture attachments of the human epiglottis and their contributions to the mechanism of deglutition. *Journal of Anatomy, 186,* 1–15.

Veiga, H., Fonseca, H., & Bianchini, E. (2014). Sequential swallowing of liquid in elderly adults: Cup or straw? *Dysphagia, 29,* 249–255.

Wang, C-M., Chen, J-Y., Chuang, C-C., Tseng, W-C., Wong, A., & Pei, Y-C. (2015). Age-related changes in swallowing, and in the coordination of swallowing and respiration determined by novel non-invasive measurement techniques. *Geriatrics & Gerontology International, 15,* 736–744.

Wheeler-Hegland, K., Huber, J., Pitts, T., & Davenport, P. (2011). Lung volume measured during sequential swallowing in healthy young adults. *Journal of Speech, Language, and Hearing Research, 54,* 777–786.

Wheeler-Hegland, K., Huber, J., Pitts, T., & Sapienza, C. (2009). Lung volume during swallowing: Single bolus swallows in healthy young adults. *Journal of Speech, Language, and Hearing Research, 52,* 178–187.

Wheeler-Hegland, K., Rosenbek, J., & Sapienza, C. (2008). Submental sEMG and hyoid movement during Mendelsohn maneuver, effortful swallow, and expiratory muscle strength training. *Journal of Speech, Language, and Hearing Research, 51,* 1072–1087.

Wilson, S., Thach, B., Brouillette, R., & Abu-Osba, Y. (1981). Coordination of breathing and swallowing in human infants. *Journal of Applied Physiology, 50,* 851–858.

Witcombe, B., & Meyer, D. (2006). Sword swallowing and its side effects. *British Medical Journal, 333,* 1285–1287.

Yamada, T., Matsuo, K., Izawa, M., Yamada, S., Masuda, Y., & Ogasawara, T. (2017). Effects of age and viscosity on food transport and breathing-swallowing coordination during eating of two-phase food in nursing home residents. *Geriatrics & Gerontology International, 17,* 2171–2177.

Yeates, E., Steele, C., & Pelletier, C. (2010). Tongue pressure and submental surface electromyography measures during non-effortful and effortful saliva swallows in healthy women. *American Journal of Speech-Language Pathology, 19,* 274–281.

Youmans, S., Youmans, G., & Stierwalt, J. (2009). Differences in tongue strength across age and gender: Is there a diminished strength reserve? *Dysphagia, 24,* 57–65.

Name Index

A

Abbas, P. J., 561
Abbott, K., 113
Abdelhalim, S/, 696
Abd-El-Malek, S., 177
Abel, H., 57
Abel, S. M., 567
Abele, T. A., 505
Abramson, A., 113, 442
Abu-Osba, Y., 687
Ackermann, H., 458, 596
Adams, L., 159
Adams, R., 58
Adank, P., 555
Adler, C., 500
Afshan, A., 234
Ahmad, K., 118
Ahvenenin, J., 568
Akita, M., 73
Alameda-Pineda, X., 232
Albanese, A., 612
Alessio, H., 58
Allen, E., 109
Allen, G., 237
Alperin, N., 159
Altman, M., 56
Altun, U., 609
Alvarez, J. A., 588
Alwan, A. A., 339, 423, 423n9
Amerman, J., 205
Amici, S., 661
Amunts, K., 592
Andoni, S., 474
Andreassen, M., 158, 159
Andrews, G., 441
Antonelli, P. J., 505
Aoba, T., 153
Arai, T., 323
Arciuli, J., 563
Ardila, A., 599
Ardran, G., 70
Arias, C., 234
Arkebauer, H., 236
Armstrong, e., 590
Arndorfer, R., 677

Arnold, G., 82
Aronson, A., 114, 115, 459, 497, 659
Arrese, L., 694
Arvedson, J., 686, 687
Assman, P. F., 395, 404, 489
Astheimer, L. B., 500
Atal, B., 387
Atkinson, J., 106, 111
Austin, D., 116, 205
Auzou, P., 442
Aviv, J., 158, 205, 690
Awan, S., 117, 420
Azzam, N., 141

B

Babael, A., 684
Babu, S., 205
Backe, W. H., 595
Badin, P., 232, 331, 332, 414, 419
Bae, Y., 156, 157, 159, 232, 686
Baer, T., 435, 436
Baggett, H., 178
Bailey, E., 58
Baken, R., 104, 106, 221, 222, 391
Baker, B., 408
Baker, S., 58
Ballard, K. J., 664, 692
Ballraj, A., 205
Banal, I., 117
Banzett, R., 217
Bänziger, T., 455
Bardan, E., 677
Baribeau, L., 115
Barin, K., 505
Barkmeier, J., 679, 686, 693
Barkmeier-Kraemer, J., 113, 680
Barlow, S., 206
Barnes, M., 149
Barney, H., 391, 392, 392n1, 393, 394, 395, 400
Barnwell, Y., 178
Barry, R., 235
Barsoumian, R., 140
Bartlett, D., 152
Basek, M., 71

Bauer, H., 385
Baum, B., 205, 687
Baum, S., 433, 434
Baumann, A., 694
Baylis, A. L., 228
Bear, M. F., 593, 638
Beaumont, K., 149
Beckford, N., 115
Behlau, M., 115
Behrens, S., 426, 433, 434
Behrman, A., 113, 118
Békésy, G. v., 530
Bell, J., 115
Bell, K., 493
Bell-Berti, F., 150, 153, 337
Benchetrit, G., 36, 39
Bendixen, A., 572
Beneragama, T., 96
Benes, F., 204
Benjamin, B., 115, 117
Bennett, K., 146
Benventano, T., 158, 204
Beranek, L., 247
Berger, D., 69
Berger, G., 158
Berisha, V., 396
Berke, G., 102
Bernal, B., 599, 600
Bernthal, J., 56
Berry, D., 103
Berry, J. J., 322
Best, C., 480
Bettens, K., 420
Beukelman, D., 56, 493, 495
Beyer, R., 247
Bianchini, E., 685
Bielamowicz, S., 686
Biever, D., 115, 118
Biller, H. F., 79, 96, 97
Bilodeau-Mercure, M., 205, 206
Bilsen, F. A., 564
Bilston, L., 184
Blackstock, D. T., 247
Bladon, A., 316, 418
Blake, M., 458
Bless, D., 115, 118, 222

Blonsky, E., 688
Blumstein, S., 359, 416, 418, 426, 433, 434, 443, 445, 447, 448, 449, 450, 452, 453, 479, 482
Blythk, K., 692
Bodanis, D., 192
Bohland, J. W., 660
Boliek, C., 55, 56, 57
Bona, J., 206
Bonding, P., 550, 556
Boorman, J., 139
Borg, E., 538
Borkan, G., 205
Boshes, B., 688
Bosma, J., 113, 157, 687
Bostan, A. C., 615
Bowling, D., 224
Boyce, S. E., 424
Bradlow, A., 396, 399, 408, 443
Braida, L., 397, 408, 443, 444
Breare, R., 430
Breen, G., 430
Bregman, A. S., 574
Bressman, T., 232, 420
Bridger, G., 151
Broad, D., 78, 79, 99, 105, 106
Brocaar, M., 222
Brodsky, L., 686, 687
Brodsky, M., 675, 683, 694
Bronkhorst, A. W., 574
Brooks, W., 679
Brouillette, R., 687
Browman, C., 201
Brown, J., 459, 497, 659
Brown, R., 217
Brown, S., 584
Brown, T., 117
Brown, W., 109
Bruns, T., 149
Buchwald, A., 430
Buder, E., 56
Buhr, R., 157
Bunn, J., 57, 58
Bunton, K., 153, 157, 228, 233, 289, 449, 450, 498
Burdumy, M., 232
Burk, F., 232
Burkard, R., 206
Burke, P., 203
Burnham, J., 430
Butchart, S., 474
Butcher, A., 430
Butler, J., 184
Buus, S., 549, 550, 556, 557
Byrd, D., 201, 354, 439, 441, 445
Byrne, C., 564

Byun, T., 235, 424, 430
Bzoch, K., 152, 153, 159

C

Cabanis, E., 592
Calandruccio, L., 408
Canady, J., 140, 146, 156
Canetta, R., 205
Cappella, J., 58
Carbonell, K. M., 568
Cardell, E., 408
Carney, P., 144
Carrau, R., 694
Carroll, R., 496
Caspar, M., 458
Casper, J., 222
Cassell, M., 139, 149, 677
Castell, D., 671, 675, 685, 686
Castell, J., 671, 686
Castelli, E., 419
Catford, J. C., 344
Catten, M., 73
Caulfield, T., 56
Cavagna, G., 106
Caviness, J. N., 459, 500
Cesari, U., 222
Chan, J., 396
Chaney, C., 424
Chang, Y., 200
Chapple, E., 59
Charles-Luce, J., 439, 440
Charpied, G., 82
Chauncey, H., 205
Chen, M., 419
Chen, T. H., 486, 487
Chen, W., 200
Chen, Y., 400, 437
Cheng, S., 184
Cherry, E. C., 573
Cheverud, J., 203
Chi, L-Y., 396
Chiba, T., 289
Chi-Fishman, G., 683, 685
Childers, D., 222
Cho, T., 442, 445
Chuang, H-F., 396, 397
Ciccia, A., 112
Cichero, J., 680, 683
Ciocca, V., 396
Clark, C., 235
Clark, M. J., 388, 392, 393, 401
Clark, R., 58, 498
Cleary, M., 486
Cleland, J., 235
Clopper, C., 394, 404

Clouse, S., 430
Cobb, B., 674
Cobb, R., 79
Cock, C., 683
Coffey-Corina, S., 489
Cohen, A., 203
Cohen, M. H., 322
Colacone, A., 679
Cole, P., 151, 152
Cole, R., 380, 467
Coleman, J., 457
Coleman, R., 106, 107, 109
Collins, M., 58
Colton, R., 109, 111, 222
Conboy, B. T., 489
Connaghan, K., 55
Connors, B. W., 593
Conrad, B., 58
Conture, E., 222
Conturo, T. E., 600
Conway, C., 159, 232
Cook, I., 676, 686
Cooke, P., 58
Cooper, D., 115
Cooper, F., 113, 417, 449, 469, 472
Cooper, N. P., 534, 535
Cooper, R., 157
Coppens, A. B., 247
Coppess, E., 488
Corbin-Lewis, K., 681
Corey, D., 685
Corfield, D., 36
Counter, S. A., 538
Court, D., 661
Coyle, J., 689
Craig, H., 430n14
Crandall, M., 687
Crelin, E., 113, 157, 203
Cristà, A., 491
Croft, C., 149, 150
Crompton, A., 683
Crone, E. A., 592
Crossman, E., 204
Crow, T., 592
Crystal, T., 407, 439, 445
Culham, J. C., 593
Cullen, K. E., 522
Curry, E., 115
Curtis, J., 109, 153
Cutler, A., 500
Cutting, C., 150

D

Dacakis, G., 117
Daggett, A., 683

Dagher, A., 611
Dahan, D., 492, 493, 500
Dailey, S., 222
Dallos, P., 505
Dalston, E., 149, 159
Dalston, R., 149, 421, 422, 424
Dalton, C., 686
Damste, H., 107, 109
Dang, J., 331, 332, 333, 333n2, 335, 417n7
Danhauer, J., 206
Daniele, A., 612
Daniels, S., 685, 687
Daniloff, R., 106, 112, 155, 196, 199, 424
Dantas, R., 683
D'Antonio, L., 224, 227
Darley, F., 459, 497, 659, 662
Darling, M., 56, 58
Darling-White, M., 56, 217
Davenport, P., 680
Davidsen-Nielsen, N., 444
Davidson, L., 232
Davies, N., 474
Davis, A., 687
Davis, J., 152, 237
Davis, P., 58, 80
Deacon, T. W., 591
Dean, K., 680
De Bodt, M., 205, 420
DeBrul, 168
Debruyne, C., 205
Decoster, W., 205
DeGeorge, P., 685
Dejaeger, E., 686
de Jong, K., 394, 404
Delaney, A., 456
Delano, P. H., 534
Delattre, P., 417
Deliyski, D., 222
Demarest, R., 677
de Melo, E., 73
DeMerit, J. L., 408
Demuth, K., 563
Denny, M., 58
Dent, J., 686
Dhanaraj, G., 684
Dhar, S., 408
Diamont, N., 680
Dick, A. S., 599, 600
Dickson, D., 68, 70, 79, 96, 97, 114, 149, 150, 152n1, 167, 172, 175, 178
Dickson, W., 152n1
Diehl, R., 445n17, 479, 484, 485, 487
Ding, R., 684

Dingus, N., 235
Dinnsen, D., 424n10
Di Puccio, F., 505
Dodds, W., 675, 677
Dolan, K., 230
Doornenbal, P., 93, 224
Doran, G., 178
Dougall, R., 429
Douglas, N., 206
Doust, J., 58
Drake, A., 152
Drettner, B., 151
Dromey, C., 107
Dronkers, N. F., 592, 661
Drucker, D., 104
Druker, D., 225
Dua, K., 677, 685
Duany, L., 230
DuBois, A., 155, 228
Duffy, J., 97, 455, 456, 611, 659, 664
Duifhuis, H., 505
Dupoux, E., 491
Durlach, N., 397, 408, 444
Dutka-Souza, J., 227

E

Eberle, L., 159
Echternach, M., 232
Edwards, B., 500
Edwards, J., 424n10
Eichhorn, J., 116, 117, 205, 206
Eimas, P., 474
Ekberg, O., 677
Elbert, M., 424n10
Elen, R., 205
Elgoyhen, A. B., 505
Elkadi, H., 139, 149
Ellis, E., 58
Ellis, R., 679
Emory, E., 588
Engelen, L., 683
Engelke, W., 149
Epanchin, V., 71
Epelbaum, S., 601
Epstein, M., 232, 550
Ertekin, C., 680
Eshghi, M., 228
Eskenazi, L., 222
Espy-Wilson, C. Y., 332, 334, 335n3, 337, 338, 414, 419, 422, 423
Ettema, S., 159, 679
Evison, G., 115
Ewanowski, S., 232
Eyal, A., 116
Eyzaguirre, C., 97

F

Fabre, D., 232
Fairbanks, G., 104, 107, 111, 112, 115, 171, 193, 410, 456
Fang, X., 158, 159
Fangerau, H., 592
Fant, G., 99, 107, 108, 207, 290, 301, 302, 308, 309, 314, 316, 324, 330, 332, 334, 335, 336, 340, 346, 354, 356, 419
Farnetani, E., 196, 198
Farnsworth, D., 290
Farol, P., 204
Fasano, A., 612
Faver, K., 227
Fedderson, W. E., 570
Fei, T., 687
Feldman, N. H., 488
Feller, R., 205
Feng, G., 419
Ferguson, S., 453
Ferreri, G., 115, 117, 204, 205
Fiddes, P., 206
Finch, E., 408
Fink, B., 71, 89, 677
Finkelstein, Y., 149, 158
Fischer, N., 230
Fisher, D., 232
Fisher, H., 117, 204, 205, 688
Fisher, K., 227
Fitch, W., 159, 206
Fizardm J., 205
Flack, F., 679
Flanagan, J., 107, 289
Fletcher, A. R., 396, 420
Fletcher, H., 188, 547
Fletcher, S., 157, 454
Flipsen, P., Jr., 458
Florentine, M., 546, 547, 549, 550, 556, 557, 558
Flores, A., 117
Fogel, A., 157
Folkard, C., 108
Folkins, J., 141, 150, 204
Folkins, J. W., 664
Foly, L., 153
Fonseca, H., 685
Fontijn-Tekamp, A., 683
Ford, G., 687
Ford, M., 231
Forner, L., 204
Forrest, K., 424n10, 429, 430, 449, 664
Forte, P., 505
Fosset, T., 200
Foster, T., 151

Foulkes, P., 564
Foundas, A., 592, 685
Fourakis, M., 399, 401, 403
Fourcin, A., 222
Fowler, C., 477, 478, 479, 486, 487, 487n5, 499
Fox, R. A., 395, 404, 412, 430
Frable, M., 70
Francis, E., 56
Francis, N., 155
Frank, J., 204
Fremont, A., 158, 205
French, J., 683
Frey, A. R., 247
Fridland, V., 318n6
Fritz, M., 686
Fritzell, B., 141, 150, 153
Fromm, D., 204, 206
Fruchter, D., 483
Fruchtman, D., 450
Fry, D., 457
Fuamenya, N., 114
Fuchs, S., 59
Fujimura, O., 232, 307, 308, 334, 414, 416, 417n7
Fukuoka, T., 686
Furr, M., 149

G

Gabb, M., 686
Gagner, M., 686
Galanter, E., 566
Galantucci, B., 486
Gallagher, K., 228
Gamage, J., 159
Gandevia, S., 184
Ganong, W. F., III, 492
Garabieta, I., 322
Garand, K., 680
Gardner, W., 36
Gareth Gaskell, M., 493
Gartian, M., 141
Gates, G., 117
Gauffin, J., 100, 219
Gautier, H., 151
Gay, T., 111, 410, 411
Gaza, C., 80
Gazzaniga, M., 602
Geddes, D., 203
Geibel, J., 458
Gerhardt, D., 685
Gerratt, B., 102, 113
Gerstman, L., 417
Geschwind, N., 594, 600
Getty, L. A., 388, 392, 393

Gherson, S., 100
Ghosh, P., 234
Ghosh, S. S., 660
Gibbon, F., 235, 498
Gibson, G., 687
Gibson, J. J., 486, 487
Gick, B., 155
Giedd, J., 159, 206
Gießing, S., 496
Gilbert, H., 237, 400
Girdany, B., 231
Girin, L., 232
Glasberg, B. R., 556
Glaze, L., 115
Glikson, E., 116
Goberman, A. M., 398, 408
Goffman, L., 204, 235, 485
Goldberg, J. M., 505
Golding-Kushner, K., 227, 231
Goldman, M., 40, 41n1, 47, 112, 217
Goldman-Eisler, F., 58
Goldstein, L., 201, 206, 232
Golman, M., 39
Gomez-Casti, M. E., 505
Goodman, S. S., 563, 675
Goodrich, S., 686, 687
Gopal, H. S., 412, 555
Gorno-Tempini, M. L., 661
Gotto, T., 153
Gould, W., 102
Goutman, J. D., 505
Goyal, R., 674
Grabe, E., 457, 459
Graber, T., 153
Graff-Radford, J., 615
Gramiak, R., 677
Gramming, P., 107
Granlund, S., 408
Graves, D., 225
Gray, S., 73
Gray, W., 100
Grayson, L., 204
Green, D. M., 558, 566, 567
Green, J., 56, 58, 204, 234, 235, 687
Green, R., 115
Greene, J., 58
Greilick, K., 412
Greve, D. N., 599
Griffith, B., 470
Griffiths, T. D., 572, 574
Grigos, M., 204
Grosjean, F., 58, 493
Gross, R., 680
Guenther, F. H., 660
Guinan, J. J., Jr., 534, 535
Güngor, H., 680

Guns, C., 205
Güntürkün, O., 588
Gürgor, N., 680
Guyette, T., 159
Guz, A., 36, 39

H

Hackett, A., 158
Hagedorn, C., 232
Hairfield, W., 151, 152
Haker, K., 339, 423, 423n9
Hale, M., 58
Haley, K., 430
Hall, A., 79
Hall, D., 237
Halle, M., 429, 445, 448
Hamdan, A-L., 117
Hamilton, A., 204
Hamilton, R., 36
Hammarberg, R., 196, 199
Hammer, M., 683
Hammilton, J., 683
Hammond, E., 73
Hammond, J., 115
Hammond, T., 73
Hammons, J., 115
Han, Y., 79, 97
Hanauer, S., 387
Hancock, P., 205
Hao, G., 205
Harada, H., 152n1
Hardcastle, W., 235
Hårdemark Cedborg, A., 680
Hardy, J., 236
Haritaa, Y., 152n1
Harrington, J., 411, 416, 418
Harrington, R., 153
Harris, K., 431, 458, 470
Harris, L. B., 568
Hartman, D., 206
Hartnick, C., 114
Hasegawa-Johnson, M., 397
Hasek, C., 115
Hashi, M., 490
Hately, B., 115
Havel, M., 335
Hawkins, B., 204
Hawkins, S., 335, 336, 419
Haxby, J. V., 588
Hazan, V., 408
He, X., 693
Heil, P., 535
Heimer, L., 596
Heise, G. A., 494, 495
Henderson, A., 58

Henke, W., 199
Henrich, J., 459
Herbert, E., 115
Herbst, C., 224
Herman, J., 117
Hertegård, S., 86, 219
Hertrich, I., 458
Hess, M., 100
Heuber, T., 232
Hickock, G., 595, 660, 663, 664
Hicks, D., 222
Higashakawa, M., 55
Higashikawa, M., 204
Hiiemae, K., 676, 678, 680, 683, 685
Hilak, A., 671
Hilbert, J., 450, 483
Hillenbrand, J., 388, 392, 392n1, 393, 394, 395, 396, 400, 401, 404, 405, 407, 410, 489
Hillman, R., 107, 109, 113, 222, 225
Hinkle, K., 149
Hinson, J., 106
Hinton, V., 151, 152
Hipp, J., 58
Hirano, M., 72, 73, 102, 104, 111, 112, 114, 115, 117, 118, 222
Hirose, H., 58, 73, 106, 111, 113, 435
Hirsh, I., 484, 567, 568
Hirst, L., 687
Hitcock, E., 235
Hixon, T., 15, 19, 20, 24, 36, 39, 40, 41, 41n1, 42, 42n1, 44, 47, 55, 56, 57, 58, 59, 92, 99, 100, 105, 106, 112, 115, 153, 154, 157, 158, 159, 183, 206, 214, 217, 219, 224, 225, 227, 232, 234, 236, 237
Hiyama, S., 157
Hodge, M., 57, 58, 59, 424n10
Hoffman, E., 206
Hoffman, G., 335
Hoffman, H., 470
Hoffman, P., 424
Hogan, J., 404
Hogan, W., 677
Hogen, T., 204
Hogosta, S., 674
Hoit, J., 15, 19, 20, 24, 36, 40, 41, 41n1, 42, 44, 55, 56, 57, 58, 59, 100, 115, 146, 153, 154, 156, 157, 159, 206, 214, 217, 228, 680
Holbrook, A., 410
Hollien, H., 105, 109, 111, 115, 116
Holliien, K., 109
Holmberg, E., 107, 109, 225
Holmes, L., 115
Holt, L., 479, 483, 485, 487, 490

Honda, K., 69, 82, 105, 106, 233, 331, 332, 333, 333n2, 417n7
Honda, Y., 679
Honjo, I., 115, 116, 117, 152n1
Hoole, P., 322
Hoops, R., 205
Horii, Y., 58
House, A., 313, 314, 316, 316n5, 317, 318, 319, 320, 321, 322, 323, 324, 326, 400, 407, 439, 445
Howell, P., 407, 455, 457, 458
Howie, P., 441
Hoyland, J., 158, 205
Hsu, H., 157
Huang, J., 205
Huang, Z., 141, 152
Huber, J., 56, 58, 116, 217, 680
Huckabee, M., 684, 686
Hudpseth, A. J., 505
Hugdahl, K., 595
Hughes, G., 429
Huisman, J., 153
Humbert, I., 682
Humphrey, T., 687
Hunt, F., 247
Hutchinson, J., 159
Hüttenbrink, K-B., 505, 517, 520
Huttenlocher, P., 204

I

Ibas-Zisen, M. T., 592
Iengo, G., 222
Iglesias, A., 153, 153n1, 154, 159
Illa, A., 234
Im, I., 683
Ingervall, B., 686
Ingrisano, D., 407
Irwin, J. R., 424
Isaakian, D., 114
Ishii, K., 73
Ishiwata, Y., 157
Iskarous, K., 200, 431
Israel, H., 205
Isshiki, N., 106, 111, 115, 116, 117, 152n1, 224, 237
Itoh, K., 232
Iuzzini-Seigel, J., 204
Iwata, S., 109

J

Jääskeläomm. I. P., 568
Jacewicz, W., 395, 404, 412
Jackson, M. T., 322
Jackson, R., 151

Jadcherla, S., 687
Jaffe, D., 684, 692
Jankovskaya, N., 97
Jaw, T., 158
Jeffress, L. A., 570
Jeng, J-Y., 396
Jessel, T. M., 595
Jiang, J., 104
Jiskoot, L. C., 598, 600
Johnson, C., 153
Johnson, F., 686
Johnson, K., 403, 445, 489, 490
Johnson, N., 205
Johnston, J., 683
Jones, C., 683, 686
Jones, K., 204
Jones, P., 55
Jongman, A., 349, 397n2, 399, 407n4, 426, 427, 427n11, 429, 429n13, 430, 431, 433, 434, 455, 457, 458
Jordan, H., 159
Jotz, G., 116
Jun, S-A., 445
Jusczyk, P., 474, 475

K

Kahane, J., 79, 97, 109, 113, 114, 115, 116, 117, 132, 139, 141, 159, 204, 206
Kahn, A., 114, 115
Kahrilas, P., 677, 683
Kajiyama, M., 289
Kakita, Y., 102
Kaltenborn, A., 153
Kamarunas, E., 684
Kandel, E. R., 595, 638, 642
Kang, A., 231
Kaplan, J. K., 568
Kapoor, K., 79
Kapur, K., 205
Karampinos, D., 687
Katto, Y., 97
Katz, P., 694
Kawano, M., 152n1
Kawasaki, H., 102
Kazarrian, A./, 114
Kazlin, M., 157
Keen, E., 70
Keleman, G., 115
Keller, S. S., 592
Kelly, J., 203
Kelsey, C., 183, 232
Kemp, F., 70
Kempster, G., 113, 683
Kendall, K., 222, 686
Kent, J., 58, 396, 494

Kent, R., 58, 114, 115, 116, 144, 154, 157, 171, 198, 201, 203, 204, 205, 206, 231, 233, 292, 385, 396, 455, 456, 488, 493, 494, 495, 496, 662, 664, 683
Kerr, W., 203
Kessinger, R., 443, 445
Kewley-Port, D., 449, 453, 499, 563
Khan, Y., 204
Kiefte, M., 485
Kier, W., 184
Killion, M. C., 544
Kim, H., 683
Kim, H-H., 397
Kim, Y., 683, 686
Kimble, C., 457
Kimura, D., 206
King, T., 232
Kingston, J., 445n17, 479
Kinsella-Shaw, J., 58
Kinsler, L. E., 247
Kirby, V. M., 499
Kirchner, J., 97
Kiritani, S., 232
Kitzing, P., 222
Kiyokawa, K., 115, 118
Kizilay, F., 680
Klaiman, G., 232
Klatt, D., 105, 346, 381n5, 407, 412, 481, 486
Klaun, M., 680
Klein, D., 205
Klenin, A., 155
Klich, R., 56, 57, 58
Klose, R., 588
Klubendorf, D., 57
Klueber, K., 178
Kluender, K., 485, 487
Kluk, K., 553
Knecht, S., 588
Knigge, M., 690
Ko, M., 683
Kobara, M., 677
Kobatake, H., 449
Kochanski, G., 457, 458
Koenig, J., 687
Koepchen, H., 57
Koepp-Baker, H., 158
Koike, Y., 111
Konig, W., 97
Konnai, R., 100
Kop o, N., 568
Koprowski, S., 146
Kowalski, C., 203
Kraljic, T., 493
Krause, J., 443

Kreisman, H., 679
Kretschmann, H., 590
Krishnamurthy, A., 222
Kronauer, R., 57
Kronrod, Y., 488
Kskarous, K., 232
Kubilis, P. S., 505
Kuchai, R., 79
Kucinski, P., 82
Kuehn, D., 132, 133, 139, 140, 141, 142, 149, 150, 153, 153n1, 154, 156, 158, 159, 230, 233, 335n3, 338, 339, 417n7, 419, 686
Kuhl, P., 396, 397, 475, 489
Kulkarni, G., 232
Kumazasa, T., 152n1
Kumazawa, T., 158
Kuo, C., 397, 398, 403
Kuperberg, G. R., 599
Kurita, S., 115, 117, 118
Kuroda, T., 157
Kurowski, K., 416, 418

L

Labov, W., 399
Ladefoged, P., 106, 316, 338, 403, 436, 438, 442, 445, 490
LaFerriere, M., 440
LaFortuna, C., 152
Laing, E. J. C., 485, 490
Laitman, J., 113, 157, 203
Lalwani, A., 222
Lam, D., 231
Lam, J., 396, 408
Lambiase, A., 102
Lammert, A. C., 289
Lanciego, J. L., 611
Lander-Portnoy, M., 232
Langdon, H., 178
Langers, D. R. M., 595
Langmore, S., 677, 679, 689
Lansford, K. L., 396, 397, 459
Lansing, R., 58, 680
Lantz, B., 686
LaPointe, L. L., 662
Lara, G., 683
Large, J., 109
Lassman, F., 115
Laures, J., 396
Laver, J., 108
Lay, C., 58
Lazarus, R., 235
Lea, W., 455, 457
Lecluse, F., 222
Lecours, A., 204

Lederle, A., 680, 685
Lee, A., 235
Lee, C. Y., 430
Lee, D., 587
Lee, D. J., 538
Lee, J., 184, 396
Lee, S., 141, 292, 410, 412
Leeper, H., 115, 158, 159, 225
LeGendre, S., 459
Lehet, M., 485
Lehiste, I., 410, 437, 454, 455, 459
Lemke, J., 141
Lemmerling, M. J., 505
Lenden, J., 458
Lenicone, R., 153n1
Leonard, R., 222, 686, 687
Leow, L., 684
Lerman, J., 400
Lester, R., 112, 156
Leung, K. K., 397n2
Leungj, 407n4
Lever, T., 686
Levin, P., 113
Levine, W., 70, 157
Levitt, A., 455
Li, N., 474
Liang, C., 563
Liberman, A., 417, 449, 450, 470, 472, 473, 475, 476, 477, 478, 479, 480, 482, 491
Lichten, W., 494, 495
Lieberman, P., 207, 437
Lin, T., 683
Lin, W., 158
Lind, J., 157, 687
Lindau, M., 403, 490
Lindblom, B., 403, 450, 452, 453, 482
Linden, M., 674, 683
Lindenberg, R., 592
Lindestad, P-Å., 219
Lindqvist, J., 307, 308
Lindstrom, M., 234, 490
Linville, R., 141
Linville, S., 115, 117, 118, 204, 205
Liotti, M., 584
Lisker, L., 113, 439, 440, 441, 442
Liss, J., 149, 206, 396, 397, 457, 459, 496, 498, 500, 681
Littlejohn, M. A., 396
Liu, C-J., 566
Liu, G., 158
Liu, H., 599
Liu, H-M., 396, 397
Liu, R., 485, 490
Liu, Y., 204
Lively, S. E., 489

Lof, G., 683
Löfqvist, A., 113, 435, 436
Logemann, J., 675, 677, 683, 684, 686, 687, 688
Lohmeier, H., 57
Long, S., 204
Lor, S., 588
Loring, S., 39, 217
Losee, J., 231
Lotto, A. J., 459, 479, 483, 485, 487, 490, 568
Lotz, W., 56, 224
Low, L., 459
Lowit, A., 459
Lubker, J., 150, 152, 153, 154
Luce, P., 439, 440
Ludlow, C., 70, 646, 684, 686
Luers, J. C., 505, 517, 520
Lund, J., 676, 686
Luschei, E., 104, 692
Lutfi, R. A., 566
Luytn, A., 420

M

Maas, E., 664
Mabis, J., 106
Macedonia, C., 687
MacNeilage, P., 196
MacPherson, M., 235
MacRae, D., 158
Madden, J., 474
Maddieson, I., 338, 438
Madill, C., 692
Mador, J., 36
Magen, H., 231
Magnuson, J., 492
Mahshie, J., 222
Makris, N., 599
Malandraki, G., 687
Malick, D., 146
Malinowski, A., 116
Mancuso, A. A., 505
Mandikal Vasuki, P. R., 563
Mandulak, K. C., 430
Maner, K., 204
Manetti, S., 505
Mann, V., 475, 476, 477, 479
Margaria, R., 106
Margolskee, R., 684
Marino, V., 227
Markl, M., 232
Marks, L. E., 546, 547
Marquardt, T., 441
Marsden, C. D., 662
Marsh, J., 227

Martel-Sauvageau, V., 430
Martin, B., 675, 679, 680
Martin, F. N., 493
Martin, R., 404, 494, 496, 498, 677, 682
Martin-Harris, B., 675, 678, 679, 680, 683, 687, 693, 694
Martino, J., 663
Marx, D., 235
Maryn, Y., 420
Mason, C. R., 557
Massaro, D. W., 486, 487
Massey, K., 115
Matsuo, K., 683
Matthews, S., 450, 452
Matthies, M. L., 322
Mattingly, I., 473, 479, 480, 482, 491
Mattys, S. L., 457, 459, 459nf16
Maue-Dickson, W., 68, 70, 79, 96, 97, 114, 167, 172, 175, 178
Maurer, R., 114
Mauszycki, S., 235
Mayet, A., 69, 79
Mayo, C., 498
Mayo, R., 152, 159
Mayrand, S., 680
McAllister, B. T., 424, 430
McAuliffe, M. J., 396
McCabe, P., 692
McCaffrey, H., 450, 452
McCall, G., 100, 149, 153n1, 685
McClean, M., 155
McClean, P., 58
McCormick, M., 146, 418
McCulloch, T., 683, 684, 686, 690, 692
McFarland, D., 58, 59, 676, 680, 686, 694
McGarr, N., 435
McGlone, R., 104, 109
McKenzie, S., 686, 687
McKerns, D., 159
McKinney, N., 106
McLean-Muse, A., 204
McMahon, P., 153
McMurtrey, J., 204, 687
McNeil, M., 200, 661
McRoberts, G., 455
McWhorter, J., 399n3
McWilliams, B., 160, 231
Mead, J., 39, 40, 41n1, 47, 57, 58, 105, 112, 217, 346
Meanock, C., 57, 58
Mefferd, A., 234
Mehta, D., 222
Melcon, C., 56, 115
Melsen, B., 203

Melsen, F., 203
Mendell, D., 687
Meng, H., 628
Menn, L., 204
Mennen, I., 459
Metz, D., 404
Meyer, D., 685
Meyer, G., 685
Meyer-Kress, G., 204
Michel, Y., 675, 694
Micheyl, C., 562
Middleton, F. A., 615
Mielke, J., 437
Mikushi, S., 683
Milenkovic, P., 115, 429, 432
Miller, C. A., 561
Miller, G. A., 494, 495
Miller, H., 661
Miller, J., 232, 474, 475, 499, 683, 687, 692
Miller, M., 157
Miller, N., 458
Mills, C., 679, 680, 685
Milner, B., 587
Minagawa-Kawai, Y., 491
Minifie, F., 59, 92, 99, 100, 106, 107, 113, 183, 201, 232
Mintz, S., 152
Miron, M., 112, 456
Miśkiewicz, A., 560, 561
Mitchell, H., 58–59, 59
Mitterer, H., 493
Miyamoto, S., 628
Miyawaki, K., 177, 178
Mizoguchi, A., 430
Mizrahi, E., 155
Modarresi, G., 450
Mognoni, P., 152
Mohr, J. P., 662
Molfenter, S., 678
Molinari, L., 159
Moll, J., 79
Moll, K., 152, 153, 155, 231
Monoson, P., 100
Monsen, R., 494, 496
Moon, J., 133, 139, 140, 141, 142, 146, 149, 150, 153, 153n1, 156, 453, 675
Moore, B. C. J., 543, 550, 551, 552, 553, 555, 556, 559, 563, 564, 568, 569, 572
Moore, C., 55, 56, 204, 687
Moore, G., 222
Moore, P., 70, 72, 102, 109, 111
Morgan, W., 55, 56
Morii, S., 158
Morita, K., 234

Morley, M., 661
Morr, K., 152
Morris, H., 153, 158, 160
Morrish, K., 687
Morrissey, P., 109
Morrongiello, B., 480
Mortimore, I., 206
Motta,G., 222
Mottau, B., 57
Moyer, C., 100
Mu, Y., 96
Mueller, P., 115, 116, 117
Muendnich, K., 69
Mukerji, S., 538
Mulheren, R., 684
Muller, F., 100
Munhall, K., 158, 196, 201
Munson, B., 424n10
Munson, W. A., 547
Muntz, H., 227
Murakami, G., 628
Mürbe, D., 335
Murphy, K., 36, 39
Murray, A., 157
Murry, T., 109, 115

N

Nachmani, A., 158
Nagy, A., 684
Nakajima, H. H., 515
Nakashima, T., 115
Nambu, A., 611
Naran, S., 231
Narayanan, S., 232, 289, 292, 339, 410, 423, 423n9, 427
Nearey, T., 395, 401, 404, 489
Neel, A., 684
Nelson, R., 206
Nelson, T., 489
Nerbonne, M., 159
Netsell, R., 56, 107, 111, 112, 149, 204, 219, 224, 231
Newell, K., 204
Newman, R., 430
Newport, E. L., 485
Nguyen, Q. T., 558
Nicholls, A., 57, 58
Nicholson, I., 115, 158
Nicholson, K., 206
Nieuwenhuis, S., 592
Niinimaa, V., 152
Nip, I., 58, 234, 235
Nishikubo, K., 687
Nishino,T., 679
Nissan, S., 430

Nittrouer, S., 204, 234
Nolan, F., 459
Nooteboom, S., 492
Norlander, T., 674
Norman, L., 437
Nossair, Z., 449
Nusbaum, E., 153

O

Oates, J., 117
Obeso, J. A., 611
Obrebowski, A., 74
Obrebowski-Karsznia, Z., 74
Ocklenburg, S., 588
Ogar, J., 661, 662
Oguz, N., 609
Ohala, J., 105, 106, 111
Ohde, R., 455
Ohtani, S., 449
Ohyama, G., 58
Okada, R., 141, 517
Okamura, H., 97
Okrazewska, E., 82
Oller, D. K., 56, 157
Olson, E. S., 505
Olson, N., 689
Omari, T., 677, 683
Ono, T., 157
Onsan, A., 558
Oommen, E., 683
Oommen, N., 205
Ophir, D., 158
Orlikoff, R., 79, 97, 104, 106, 109, 113, 221, 222, 391
O'Rourke, A., 686
Orr, S., 694
Otis, A., 58
Oxenham, A. J., 561, 562
Ozenberger, J., 152
Özyurt, J., 496

P

Padden, D., 475, 489
Paivio, A., 58
Palmer, J., 676, 678, 680, 683, 684, 685, 686, 692
Papagno, C., 601
Paradiso, M. A., 593
Pardo, J., 487
Parent, L., 687
Parham, D., 56
Park, S., 408
Park, T., 686
Parnell, M., 205

Pastore, R. E., 568
Patel, R., 222
Patrick, J., 58
Pattern, A., 234
Patterson, D., 475
Pauloski, B., 683
Paus, T., 204, 473
Pearson, W., 677
Peeva, M. G., 660, 661
Pegoraro-Krook, M., 227
Peladeau-Pigeon, M., 205, 206
Pelemans, W., 686
Pelletier, C., 684, 686
Pelley, C., 36
Pemberton, C., 117
Penner, H., 458
Penny, L., 117
Peplinski, A., 100
Peppelreuter, S., 149
Pepperberg, I., 475
Perkell, J., 107, 109, 225, 234, 322
Perlman, A., 159, 397, 677, 679, 680, 683, 687, 693
Perlmutter, N., 157
Perona, G., 58
Perry, J., 149, 156, 157, 158, 159, 686
Person, J. L., 424
Peters, J., 56
Peterson, A. J., 535
Peterson, G., 391, 392, 392n1, 393, 394, 395, 400, 410
Peterson, H., 441
Petrosino, L., 205
Petroski, R., 270
Pham Dinh, T., 39
Phillips, C., 227
Phillipson, E., 58
Picheny, M., 397, 401, 408, 443, 444
Pickles, J. O., 505, 525, 533
Pisoni, D., 58, 394, 396, 404, 483, 484, 485, 486, 489, 568
Piszcz, W., 82
Pitcher, J., 687
Pitts, T., 679, 680
Plaisant, O., 592
Platt, L., 441
Plexico, L., 227
Plowman, E., 694
Poburka, B., 222, 420
Poeppel, D., 663
Pollak, G., 474
Pols, L. C. W., 488
Ponette, E., 686
Pontes, P., 115, 118
Popper, K., 474
Port, R., 459n16

Postuma, R. B., 611
Potamianos, A., 292, 410
Potter, S., 430n14
Pramstaller, P. O., 662
Praneetvataku, V., 100
Pratt, S., 200
Preiksaitis, H., 679, 680, 685
Preisser, J. S., 228
Pressman, J., 72, 115
Preston, J., 206, 232
PriceC., 675
Primov-Fever, A., 116
Prince, J., 184
Principato, J., 152
Proctor, D., 151, 431
Province, M., 227
Pruthi, T., 331, 334, 335n3, 337, 338, 414, 419
Puschmann, S., 496

Q

Quilter, R., 205
Quinn, J., 204

R

Rademaker, A., 683, 684
Radovanovic, B., 232
Rai, S., 79
Rajendran, K., 141
Rakoff, S., 149
Rakowski, A., 560, 561
Ramig, L., 116
Ramsey, G., 677
Rand, T., 479
Raol, N., 114
Raphael, L., 458
Rasmussen, T., 587
Rath, E., 206
Recasens, D., 196, 198
Reid, D., 677
Reidenbach, M., 89
Reilly, K., 204, 687
Reinhart, J., 441
Reinisch, E., 493
Remez, R., 487
Remmers, J., 152
Ren, J., 677
Rens, R., 205
Repp, B., 416, 417, 418, 482, 488
Reynolds, A., 58
Reynolds, S., 205
Richardson, H., 234
Richstmeier, P. T., 485
Richter, B., 232

Richtsmeier, J., 203
Ridderinkhof, K. R., 592
Riecker, A., 596
Ringel, R., 116, 237
Rivera-Gaxiola, M., 489
Robb, M., 114, 400, 437
Robbins, J., 682, 683, 687, 689
Roberts, N., 592
Robin, D. A., 661, 664
Robins, K., 680
Robinson, B. K., 561
Robinson, K., 159
Robson, R., 480
Rochester, S., 58, 59
Rochet, A., 57, 58, 152
Rochet-Capellan, A., 59
Rodenstein, D., 157
Roecker, E., 689
Rogers, D., 114
Rohrmann, C., 677
Romeo, R., 408
Rong, P., 204, 335n3, 338, 339, 417n7, 419
Rosemann, S., 496
Rosen, K., 456
Rosen, S., 686
Rosenbek, J., 206, 456, 494, 662, 685, 686, 689
Rosenblum, L., 477, 478, 479
Rösler, G., 538
Rosner, B., 457
Rothenberg, M., 99, 100, 222
Roy, N., 420
Rubin, H., 100, 105
Rubin, J., 232
Rudin, N., 683
Rudnicky, A., 467
Ruscello, D., 149, 664
Russell, A., 117
Ryalls, J., 207
Ryan, K., 100
Ryan, W., 206

S

Saffran, J., 485
Sagiv, D., 116
Saibene, F., 152
Said, C. P., 588
Saitoh, E., 683, 686
Sakaguchi, S., 117
Saltzman, E., 201, 486
Samar, V., 404
Samman, N., 396
Sampson, S., 97
Samuel, A. G., 493, 568

Samuel, E., 115
Sandage, M., 227
Sandel, T. T., 570
Sanders, I., 79, 96, 97
Sanders, J. V., 247
Sanders, L. D., 500
Sandhu, G., 79
Sandoval, S., 396
Sanudo, J., 96
Sapienza, C., 56, 107, 679, 686
Sarikcioglu, L., 609
Sarkissian, L., 114
Sasaki, C., 94, 113, 157
Sato, K., 72, 73, 114, 115, 118
Saur, D., 600
Sawashima, M., 111, 113
Schalling, E., 459
Schatz, K., 689
Schellinger, S. K., 424n10
Scherer, K., 455
Scherer, R., 100
Schiavetti, N., 404, 498
Schinzel, A., 159
Schleicher, A., 590
Schmahmann, J. D., 601
Schmidt, R., 204, 662
Schmitz, J., 588
Schonharl, E., 102
Schönle, P., 58, 234
Schoonveveldt, G. P., 551, 552
Schroeder, M., 685
Schulte, L., 56
Schultz, J., 683
Schulze-Florey, A., 146
Schumm, F., 458
Schutte, H., 222, 224
Schwab, B., 146
Schwartz, J. H., 595
Schwartz, M., 206
Scott, J., 203
Scukanec, G., 205
Sears, V., 686
Seaton, D., 151, 152
Seaver, E., 150, 159
Sebastian, S., 205
Seelinger, E., 430
Seery, C., 204
Segre, R., 115, 117
Seidel, S., 457
Seitz, P., 418
Seitz, R. J., 592
Seki, S., 683
Sekizawa, K., 94
Selbie, W., 70
Sell, D., 420
Sellars, I., 70

Selley, W., 679
Sereno, J. A., 397n2, 399, 407n4, 455, 457, 458
Serpell, J., 96
Serrurier, A., 331, 332, 414, 419
Sessle, B., 682
Setlur, J., 114
Severeid, L., 144
Shadle, C., 343, 344, 431
Shaker, R., 675, 677
Shankweiler, D., 449, 455, 472, 473, 486, 499
Shapshay, S., 82
Sharkey, S., 204
Sharma, M., 563
Sharma, S., 684
Sharp, H., 420
Shaw, D., 686
Shawker, T., 205, 692
Shea, S., 36, 39
Shelton, R., 149, 160
Sherrington, C., 630
Shervanian, C., 69
Sheu, R., 158
Shipp, T., 104, 109, 116
Shprintzen, R., 149, 153n1, 158
Shriberg, L., 456, 458
Shriner, T., 155
Shune, S., 675
Sicher, H., 168
Siebens, A., 683
Siegel-Sadewitz, V., 158
Sigurjonsson, S., 677
Silverman, K., 455
Simberg, S., 222
Simmons, Z., 396
Simpson, A., 206, 395
Singh, S., 115
Sirosh, J., 450, 483
Sitler, R., 404
Sivian, L. J., 543, 544, 568
Skarbek, A., 58
Skolnick, L., 153n1, 231
Skolnick, M., 153n1
Skolnik, M., 149
Slama, H., 661
SMILJANIC, R., 408, 443
Smith, A., 58, 141, 157, 204, 206, 222, 228, 235
Smith, B., 159, 204, 206
Smith, H., 237
Smith, J., 679
Smith, K., 184
Smith, L., 152
Smitheran, J., 224, 225

Smits, M., 598, 600
Smits, R., 555
Smits-Engelsman, B., 204
Soderberg, G., 206
Soli, S. D., 499
Solomon, N., 100, 217
Solzhenitsyn, A., 369
Sommerlad, B., 139
Sonesson, B., 70
Sonies, B., 205, 683, 685, 687, 692
Spanias, A., 396
Sperry, E., 56, 57, 58
Spitzer, S. M., 459, 500
Springer, J. A., 587
Squibb, K., 205
Squire, C., 205
Stadlin, J., 115
Stager, S., 424
Stambuk, H. E., 505
Stanescu, D., 157
Stathopoulos, E., 56, 100, 107, 116, 439
Steele, C., 205, 206, 678, 680, 683, 684, 686, 687
Steele, C. R., 505
Steeve, R., 204, 687
Stegeman, I., 647
Stelmach, G., 204
Stephens, S., 206
Stepp, C. E., 512
Stevens, K., 99, 104, 107, 108, 112, 113, 313, 314, 316, 316n5, 317, 318, 319, 320, 321, 322, 323, 324, 326, 335, 336, 338, 343, 346, 354, 357, 359, 400, 419, 436, 445, 447, 448, 449, 450, 452, 453, 457, 479, 482, 483, 486
Stevens, S. S., 547, 548, 549, 566
Stewart, E., 677
Stierwalt, J., 206, 687
Stoelinga, C. N. J., 566
Stoicheff, M., 117
Stoksted, P., 152
Stone, M., 184, 205, 232, 685, 692
Story, B., 102, 103, 105, 112, 153, 206, 207, 289, 301, 332, 335n3, 337, 338, 419, 449, 450
Story, R., 435
Strand, E., 493
Strick, P. L., 615
Strocchi, R., 74
Strome, M., 111
Studdert-Kennedy, M., 449, 455, 472, 473, 486, 499
Stufflebeam, S. M., 599

Sturm, J., 204
Subtelny, J., 158
Sugarman, M., 204
Sugito, M., 58
Sullivan, C., 58
Summerfield, Q., 443
Sundberg, J., 100, 222, 335
Susser, R., 115
Sussman, H. M., 450, 452, 483, 488
Sussman, J., 117
Sutton, B., 158, 159, 232, 687
Suzen, B., 609
Suzuki, D., 628
Suzuki, H., 331
Suzuki, M., 97
Svec, J., 222, 224
Svirsky, M. A., 322
Swank, P., 227
Swartz, M., 235
Sweeney, R., 115
Sweeney, T., 420
Syrdal, A. K., 555
Szafran, J., 204

T

Tabain, M., 200, 430, 431n15, 434
Tait, C., 100
Takai, O., 584
Takano, S., 69, 82
Takaya, S., 599
Takeda, N., 686
Takishima, T., 94
Talacker, S., 58
Tan, T., 105
Tanaka, S., 102
Tasko, S. M., 412, 683
Taylor, I., 58
Teas, D. C., 570
Terreros, G., 534
Tervaniemi, M., 595
Thach, B., 687
Theodoros, D., 408
Thibeault, S., 690
Thiel, C. M., 496
Thiessen, E., 485
Thom, S., 157, 228
Thomas, J., 204, 455
Thomas, K., 204
Thompson, A., 153, 154, 158, 159, 227
Thompson, C., 430n14
Tiede, M., 231, 424
Timcke, R., 102
Timmins, C., 235

Tippett, D., 683
Tissington, M., 158
Titze, I., 69, 71, 79, 94, 102, 103, 104, 105, 106, 107, 108, 109, 111, 112, 206, 222, 225, 391
Tjaden, K., 396, 398, 408, 430
Tobin, M., 36
Todorov, A., 588
Tohkura, Y., 196
Tom, D., 155
Tomoda, T., 158
Tooley, T., 684
Torretta, G., 396
Tourne, L., 203
Tourville, J. A., 660
Toutios, A., 232
Tracy, J., 676
Traser, L., 232
Tremblay, P., 205, 206, 599, 600
Trier, W., 149
Trosset, M., 100
Truby, H., 157, 687
Tsao, F-M., 396, 397, 408
Tucker, G., 114
Tucker, J., 114
Tucker, L., 107
Tuomainen, O., 408
Turcio, J., 424
Turner, G. S., 396, 398, 430, 498
Turtle, M., 203

U

Ullsperger, M., 592
Ulysal, H., 680
Umeda, N., 381n5, 407, 412, 433, 434, 435, 439, 440, 443, 444
Ünal, A., 680
Urban, P. P., 662
Urbsheit, M., 206
Utianski, R., 396

V

Vadlamudi, J., 430
Vakil, N., 677
Vallino, L. D., 228
Valyear, K. F., 593
VanDaele, D., 677, 683
van den Berg, J., 69, 79, 82, 89, 93, 101, 105, 106, 109, 111, 224
van der Bilt, A., 683
van der Giet, G., 234
Vanderwegen, J., 205
Van de Vlugt, M., 492–493
van Dijk, P., 595
van Donselaar, W., 500
Van Engen, K., 408
van Esch, B. F., 647
Van Galen, G., 204
Van Hoesen, G. W., 596
van Hout, R., 555
Van Leer, E., 693
Van Lierde, K. M., 420
van Lieshout, P., 683, 687
VanLue, M., 146
Van Nuffelen, G., 205
Van Santen, J., 407
van Son, R. H. H., 488
Van Tassel, D. J., 499
VanTrappen, G., 686
Vatikiiotis-Bateson, E., 196
Veiga, H., 685
Vennard, W., 69, 111
Vercruyssen, M., 205
Verdolini-Marston, K., 225
Verschuure, J., 222
Vick, J., 204
Vig, P., 152, 203
Volandri, G., 505, 515, 521
von Leden, H., 70, 72, 97, 102, 109, 224
Vorperian, H., 113, 115, 116, 157, 159, 203, 205, 206
Voss, S. E., 512

W

Waggener, T., 57
Walker, G., 203
Walsh, B., 204
Walter, J., 36, 39
Walters, B., 675
Wambaugh, J., 235
Wang, J., 97
Wang, R., 72
Wang, Y., 234, 397n2, 407n4, 455
Wang, Y-T., 58, 396
Warner, R., 57, 59
Warren, D., 149, 151, 152, 155, 228, 230, 236, 237
Warren, J. D., 572, 574
Washington, J., 430n14
Wasowicz, J., 206
Watkin, K., 204, 232, 683, 692
Watkins, K., 473
Watson, C., 411
Watson, I., 418
Watson, J., 677
Watson, P., 55, 56, 59, 100, 112, 153
Watts, C., 420
Wayland, R., 349, 426
Wayler, A., 205
Webb, R., 59
Weber, A., 493
Wegner, I., 647
Weinberg, S., 677
Weismer, G., 40, 42n1, 56, 112, 206, 233, 234, 396, 397, 398, 403, 404, 408, 424n10, 429, 434, 439, 442, 443, 493, 494, 496, 498, 611, 633, 664
Welford, A., 204, 205
Wells, C., 153
Wemke, K., 114
Wendahl, R., 109
Westbury, J., 233, 234, 405, 490, 683
Whalen, D., 58, 231, 455, 475, 477, 478, 479
Wheeler, K., 388, 392, 393
Wheeler-Hegland, K., 679, 680, 686
White, L., 459, 459n16
White, S. D., 543, 544, 568
Whitehead, R., 404
Whitehill, T., 396
Whitfield, J. A., 398, 408
Widen, G. P., 499
Wier, C. C., 562
Wiggins, R. H., 505
Wilder, C., 58
Wilding, G., 408
Wiley, J., 115
Williams, D. R., 488
Williams, F., 59
Wilson, J., 687
Wilson, S., 687
Wilson-Pauwels, L., 628
Wind, J., 115, 204
Windsor, A. M., 538
Winkworth, A., 58
Wistbacka, G., 222
Witcombe, B., 685
Wohlert, A., 205, 206
Wojnowski, W., 74
Wolf, M., 116
Wolkove, N., 679
Wolpert, D., 204
Wong, S., 349, 426
Woo, J., 184
Wood, J., 689
Wood, S., 233, 235
Woodhouse, R., 183, 232
Wright, D. L., 662
Wright, S., 235
Wu, L., 96
Wustrow, F., 79

Wuytz, F. L., 420
Wyke, B., 97

X

Xiao, L., 562
Xie, P., 677
Xing, F., 184
Xu, L., 430
Xue, S., 205

Y

Yamada, T., 687
Yamashita, T., 158
Yamaski, R., 115
Yamauchi, A., 115, 222
Yan, J., 204
Yan, Y., 118
Yanagihara, N., 111
Yang, C-C., 396
Yang, J., 430
Yarkovsky, M., 680
Yeates, E., 686
Yin, Z., 430
Yonezawa, T., 679
Yorkston, K. M., 493, 495
Yoshida, T., 102
Yoshioka, H., 113
Yoshioka, Y., 436
Youmans, G., 687
Youmans, S., 206, 687
Yuen, I., 235
Yunusova, Y., 234, 498

Z

Zagzebski, J., 232
Zahorian, S., 449
Zaino, C., 158, 204
Zajac, D., 152, 158, 159, 228, 430
Zamel, N., 58
Zankl, A., 159
Zantema, J., 93, 224
Zelaznik, H., 204
Zemlin, W., 68, 69, 70, 78, 79, 80, 82, 83, 89, 100, 106, 114, 115, 170, 175, 178, 203, 205, 206
Zenker, W., 86
Zera, J., 558, 567
Zhai, W., 73
Zhang, D., 56
Zhang, L., 70
Zhou, R., 73
Ziegler, W., 664
Zierdt, A., 322
Zilles, K., 590
Zue, V., 380, 440
Zumwalt, A., 677

Subject Index

Note: Page numbers in **bold** reference non-text material.

A

Abdominal content, 12
Abdominal wall, 12, 21, 25, 48, 59
Abdominal wall muscles, 17–20, **19**
Abducens nerve (*See* Cranial nerves)
Acoustical Society of America (ASA), **247**
Acoustic invariance, 446–447, 449–450
    At interface of speech production and perception, 452–453
    Locus equation, 450–452
Acoustics phonetic data, 391
Acoustic theory of speech production, 329–330
Acoustic theory of vowel production
    Confirmation of the theory, 324–326
    Resonator
        Formant determinants, 307–308
        tube closed at one end, 297–303
        Tube constricted at given location, 309–319
    Source
        Frequency domain, 293–297
        Time domain, 290–293
    Summary of, 308–309
    Three-parameter model of vowel articulation, 313–324
Action potential, 642–644
Adam's apple, 64
Aeroacoustics, **276**
Aeromechanical observations, 235–237
    Laryngeal function, 224–227
    Velopharyngeal-nasal apparatus, 227–230
AF (arcuate fasciculus), 598–601
Afferent, 585–586
Affricate acoustics, defined, 360
Affricates, 453–454
Age effects
    Breathing apparatus, 55–57
    Laryngeal apparatus, 113–116
    Pharyngeal-oral apparatus, 202–206
    Swallowing and, 687
    Velopharyngeal-nasal apparatus, 157–159
Air pressure (*see* Pressure)
Airway resistance
    Laryngeal, 92–93, 227
    Velopharyngeal-nasal, 145

Alveolar air pressure, 352
Alveolar (lingua-alveolar) consonants (*see* Consonants)
Alveolar pressure, 28–31, 41, 46, 48, 60, **106,** 195
Anatomy of swallowing
    Breathing, laryngeal, velopharyngeal-nasal, and pharyngeal-oral structures, 670–671
    Esophagus, 671
    Stomach, 671
Anatomy of the auditory system, 505
    Auditory nerve and auditory pathways, 533–540
    Inner ear, 521–533
        Cochlea, 525–533
        Traveling wave is transformed to action potentials, 533
        Vestibular system, 522–525
    Middle ear, 512–521
        Auditory (eustachian) tube, 517–518
        Chambers, 512–513
        Ligaments, 515
        Medial and lateral wall views, 518–519
        Ossicles and associated structures, 513–515
        Transmission of sound energy by the conductive mechanism, 519–521
    Muscles (*see* Muscles of the middle ear)
    Outer ear, 508–512
        External auditory meatus, 509–511
        Pinna (auricle), 508–509
        Tympanic membrane (eardrum), 511–512
    Peripheral, 507–508
    Temporal bone, 505–507
Anatomy of the breathing apparatus
    Abdominal content, 12
    Abdominal wall, 12
    Chest wall, 12
    Diaphragm, 12
    Lungs, 12
    Pulmonary airways, 10–11
    Pulmonary apparatus, 10–12
    Pulmonary apparatus-chest wall unit, 12–13
    Rib cage wall, 12
    Skeletal framework, 9–10
Anatomy of the laryngeal apparatus
    Cartilages, 63–66
    Joints, 66–72

Anatomy of the laryngeal apparatus *(continued)*
  Laryngeal cavity, 72
  Laryngeal ventricles, 75
  Ligaments and membranes, 75–77
  Mucous membrane, 77
  Vocal folds, 72–75
Anatomy of the pharyngeal-oral apparatus
  Buccal cavity, 172
  Mandible, 166–167
  Maxilla, 165–166
  Mucous lining, 172
  Muscles (*see* Muscles of the pharyngeal-oral apparatus)
  Oral cavity, 170–171
  Pharyngeal cavity, 170
  Temporomandibular joints, 167–169
Anatomy of the velopharyngeal-nasal apparatus
  Muscles (*see* Muscles of the velopharyngeal-nasal apparatus)
  Nasal cavities, 133–134
  Outer nose, 134–135
  Pharynx, 130–132
  Skeletal framework, 127–130
  Velum, 132–244
Angular gyrus, 594
Anterior cerebral artery (ACA), 653–654, 657
Anterior commissure, 602
Anterior inferior cerebellar artery (AICA), 654
Anterior median fissure, 634
Anterior nasal dilator muscle, 160
Antiresonances, 331
Apraxias, 592
Arachnoid mater, 649
Arcuate fasciculus (AF), 598–601
Armygdala, 597
Articulation, 113
  nasal place of, 415–418
Articulatory phonology, 200–202
Articulatory tracking, 232–235
  Electromagnetic sensing (articulography), 234
  Electropalatographic monitoring, 235
  Optoelectronic tracking, 234–235
  X-ray microbeam imaging, 232–234
Articulography, 234
Aryepiglottic muscle, 82, 91
Arygepiglottic muscle, 677
Arytenoid cartilages, 65, 112
Arytenoid muscle, 78, 80–82, 88, 89, 94, 96, 100, 106, 629
Ascending auditory pathways, 536–540
Ascending projection tracts, 606–607
Aspiration intervals, 356
Aspiration noise, 356
Association cortex, 593
Association tracts, 598
Astrocytes, 636
Auditor filters, 551

Auditory bandpass filters, 551
Auditory (eustachian) tube, 517–518
Auditory psychoacoustics (*see* Psychoacoustics)
Auditory scene analysis, 574, **574**
Auditory streams, defined, 547
Auditory-vestibular nerve (*see* Cranial nerves)
Auricle (pinna), 508–509
Autonomic nervous system (ANS), 580
Axial plane, 581
Axons, 585, 639

B

/ba/-/da/-/ga/ experiment, 468–471
Bandwidth, 280
Basal ganglia, 607–610, **609,** 611–612, 614–615
Bell, Alexander Graham, **366**
Bell's palsy, **190**
Blood-brain barrier, 658–659
Blue boaters, **38**
Body position
  Breathing apparatus, 49–54
  Swallowing and, 686
  Velopharyngeal-nasal apparatus, 156–157
Body type, 58, 60
Boone, Daniel R., **88**
Botox®, 646
Boutons, terminal, 639
Brain
  Blood supply, 652–659
  Speech and language functions, 659
Brain freeze, **682**
Brainstem, 615–630
  Cranial nerves and, 615
  Dorsal view, 617–619
  Innervation of, 605–606
  Medulla, 617
  Midbrain, 616
  Pons, 617
  Ventral view, 615–616
Breathing and swallowing, 678–680
Breathing apparatus and speech production, 60
  Age, 55–57
  Body position, 49–54
  Body type, 58
  Cognitive-linguistic variables, 58–59
  Conversational interchange, 59
  Extended steady utterances, 40–44
  Extended steady utterances, supine, 50–52
  Running speech activities, 44–49
  Running speech activities, supine, 52–54
  Running speech activities, upright, 48
  Sex, 57
  Special acts of, 36–37
  Ventilation, 57–58
Broca's area, 591–592

Bronchial pressure, **106**
Brownian motion, 248, **531**
Burst (release) intervals, 354
Bursts, 445–449

C

Calcarine fissure, 596
Cell body (soma), 637–639
Central auditory pathways, 627
Central nervous system (CNS), 579–580, 651–652, 682
Central system fluid (CSF), 636, 649–650, 651–652
Cerebellopontine angle, 626
Cerebellum, 607–615
Cerebral aqueduct, 615
Cerebral hemispheres, 589–597
    Frontal lobe, 590–592
    Insula, 596–597
    Limbic system (limbic lobe), 597
    Occipital lobe, 596
    Parietal lobe, 593–594
    Temporal lobe, 594–596
Cerebral peduncles, 605, 616, 617
Cerebral white matter, 597–607
    Arcuate fasciculus (AF), 598–601
    Ascending projection tracts, 606–607
    Association tracts, 598, **599**
    Commissural tracts, 601–602
    Descending project tracts, 602–606
    Striatal tracts, 601
Chemoreceptors, 35
Chest wall, 34
    muscles, 12, **21,** 21–22
    shape, 31–33
    surface tracking, 215–217
Chewing, 191
Chronic obstructive pulmonary disease (COPD), **678, 680**
Cinefluorographic studies, 231, **231**
Cingulate gyrus, 597
Circle of Willis, 654–655
Clear speech, 408
Client self-report, 694
Clinical professionals
    Measurements and, 237–240
    Swallowing disorders, 694–695
Closure (silent) intervals, 353–354, 376, 439–440, 441
CNS (*see* Central nervous system (CNS))
Coarticulation, 196–200
Cochlea, 525–533
Cochlear amplifier, 541
Cocktail party effect, 573–574
Coding schemes, vowel, 192–194
Commissural tracts, 601–602
Comparative acoustic phonetics, 398–401
Complex acoustic events
    Aperiodic, 264
    Periodic, 259–261
    Pitch of, 563–565
    Summary, 264–266
Complex sounds, loudness of, 550–556
Compliance, 13
Consonants
    Affricate, 195
    Coupled (shunt) resonators, 330–340
    Dimensions of, 194–195
    Fricative, 195
    Nasal, 195
    Semivowels, 195
    Stop-plosive, 195
Consonant voicing, 407
Control variables of breathing apparatus (*see* Output variables of breathing apparatus)
Control variables of the laryngeal apparatus, 91
    Glottal size and configuration, 93–94
    Laryngeal airway resistance, 92–93
    Laryngeal opposing pressure, 92
Control variables of the pharyngeal-oral apparatus
    Pharyngeal-oral acoustic impedance, 189–190
    Pharyngeal-oral airway resistance, 188–189
    Pharyngeal-oral lumen size and configuration, 186–188
    Pharyngeal-oral structural contact pressure, 188
Control variables of the velopharyngeal-nasal apparatus
    Velopharyngeal-nasal acoustic impedance, 147–158
    Velopharyngeal-nasal airway resistance, 145
    Velopharyngeal sphincter compression, 146–147
COPD (chronic obstructive pulmonarry disease), **678**
Coronal plane, 581
Corona radiata, 603
Corpora quadrigemina, 619
Corpus callosum, 602
Cortical innervation patterns of cranial nerves (*see* Cranial nerves)
Cortico-cerebellar-cortical loop, 613
Cortico-striatal-cortical loop, 610
Coupled (shunt) resonators, 330–340
Cranial nerves (and associated brainstem nuclei), 619
    Cortical innervation patterns, 630–633
    Cranial nerve III (Oculomotor), **620,** 622
    Cranial nerve II (Optic), **620,** 622
    Cranial nerve I (Olfactory), **620,** 622
    Cranial nerve IV (Trochlear), **620,** 622–623
    Cranial nerve IX (Glossopharyngeal), **620,** 627–628
    Cranial nerve VI (Abducens), **620,** 624–625
    Cranial nerve VII (Facial), **620,** 625–626
    Cranial nerve VIII (Auditory-vestibular), **620,** 626–627
    Cranial nerve V (Trigeminal), **620,** 623–624
    Cranial nerve XII (Hypoglossal), **621,** 629–630
    Cranial nerve XI (Spinal Accessory), **620,** 629
    Cranial nerve X (Vagus), **620,** 628–629
Cricoarytenoid joints, 69–72

Cricoarytenoid muscle, 78
Cricoid cartilage, 64–65
Cricopharyngeus muscle, 671, 677
Cricothyroid joints, 68–69
Cricothyroid muscle, 82, 89, 94, 96, 104, 105, 111, 629
Crude touch, 607
Crus cerebri, 605
CSF (*see* Central system fluid (CSF))

D

Damping, 277–280
Decibel scale, 284–287
Deep brain stimulation (DBS), **612**
Deglutition, 669
Degree of major constriction, 194
Dementia, 597
Dental, 195
Dentists, 240
Deoxyribonucleic acid (DNA), 638
Depressor alae nasa muscle, 160
Descending projection tracts, 602–603
Development, swallowing and, 686–687
Diachronic sound change, **348**
Diaphragm, 12, 21, 23–25, 25, 59
Diaphragm muscle, 17, **18**
Difference limens (DLs), 556–558, **563**
Diffusion tensor imaging (DTI), 598, **600**
Digastric muscle, 85, 91, 96, 97, 623, 677
Digital spectrograms, 373
Diphthongs, 194, 409–412
Directions, terminology for, 581–584
DIVA (Directions into Velocities of Articulators) model, 659–665
DLs (*see* Difference limens (DLs))
DNA (deoxyribonucleic acid), 638
Dorsal root ganglia, 585
DTI (*see* Diffusion tensor imaging (DTI))
Duplex perception, 475–479
Dura mater, 648–649
Dynamic analogy, **319**
Dysarthrias, 592

E

Eardrum (tympanic membrane), 511
Efferent, 585–586
Electroglottography, 222–224
Electromagnetic sensing, 234
Electropalatographic monitoring, 235
Endoscopy, 219–222, 689–690
Epiglottis, 66, 91
Eustachian (auditory) tube, 517–518
Expiratory reserve volume (ERV), 27
Extended steady utterances, 40–44
External auditory meatus, 509–511

External intercostal muscles, 16, 17, 35, 59, 635
External oblique muscle, 19, 59

F

Facial colliculus, 625
Facial nerve (*see* Cranial nerves)
Fairbanks, Grant, **171**
Fant, Gunnar, **289**
Fasciculi cuneatus, 619
Fasciculi gracilis, 619
F-contours, 454–456
F0 declination, 454–455
Fechner's law, 557
FEES (*See* Flexible Endoscopic Evaluation of Swallowing (FEES))
FEESST (*See* Flexible Endoscopic Evaluation of Swallowing with Sensory Testing (FEESST))
First harmonic (H1), 293
Flap closures, 440–441
Flexible Endoscopic Evaluation of Swallowing (FEES), 689–690
Flexible Endoscopic Evaluation of Swallowing with Sensory Testing (FEESST), 690
Foramen of Monro, 651
Forces of swallowing, 673–678
Forces of the breathing apparatus
    Abdominal wall muscles, 17–20
    Active, 14–22
    Diaphragm muscle, 17, **18, 19**
    Passive, 13–14, 20–22
Forces of the laryngeal apparatus, 77
    Extrinsic muscles, 82–83
    Intrinsic muscles, 78–82
    Supplementary muscles (infrahyoid and suprahhyoid), 83–85
Formant bandwidths, 307–308
Formant frequencies
    Formant trajectories vs., 404–405
    Summary of, 403–404
    Within-speaker variability in, 401–403
Formant transitions, 368, **412**, 431
    Fricative distinctions and, 431
Format frequencies, 401–404
Fourier analysis, **266**
Fourth ventricle, 615
F-pattern of vowels, 307
FRC (functional residual capacity), 27
Frequency domain, 293–297
Frication interval, 355
Frication intervals, 355–356
Frication noise, 356
Frication source, 343
Fricative acoustics, theory of, 341–351
    Fluid flow in pipes and source types, 341–345
    Measurement of, 349–351

Mixed sources, 346
Shaping of sources by vocal tract resonators, 346–349
Summary of, 351
Typical wave form and its aeromechanical correlates, 345–346
Fricatives, 425, **433**
Duration, 432–436
Formant transitions, 431
Quantification of fricative spectra, 426–431
Siblants vs. nonsibilants, 425–426
Functional MRI (fMRI), **587**
Functional residual capacity (FRC), 27
Functions of the pharyngeal-oral apparatus
Chewing and swallowing, 191
Degree of coupling between oral cavity and atmosphere, 191
Sound generation and filtering, 191–192
Fundamental frequency (F0), 104–106, 293

G

Ganglia, 585
Gastroesophageal reflux disease (GERD), **694**
Genioglossus muscle, 85, 91, 96, 632
Geniohyoid muscle, 85, 91, 96, 677
Gesture theory, 200–202
Glial cells, 636
Globus pallidus, 610
Glossopalatine muscle, 160
Glossopharyngeal nerve (*see* Cranial nerves)
Glottal, 195
Glottal area function, 290, **292**
Glottal flow function (VG), 291, **292**
Glottal source signal, 292
Glottal source spectrum, 293
Glottis, 93–94
Gray matter, 584–585

H

/h/ acoustics, 436–438
Head related transfer function (HRTF), **573**
Health care professionals (*see* Clinical professionals)
Helmholtz resonators, 270–273
Hemineglect, 593
Heschl's gyrus, 594
Hippocampus, 597
H1 (first harmonic), 293
Hollien, Harry, **91**
Horizontal plane, 581
Hyoglossus muscle, 91, 96
Hyoid bone, 66
Hyperfunctional voice disorders, 296
Hyperpolarized neuron, 644
Hypofunctional voice disorders, 296
Hypoglossal nerve (*see* Cranial nerves)

Hypoglossus muscle, 85
Hypokinetic dysarthria, 611–612

I

Impulse-like events, 357
Inferior colliculi, 617–619
Inferior constrictor muscle, 82, 83, 91, 96, 160, 183, 671
Inferior laryngeal branch, 96
Inferior olive, 617
Infrahyoid muscles, 83–85
Input signals
Frequency domain, 293–297
Time domain, 290–293
Inspiratory capacity (IC), 27
Inspiratory reserve volume (IRV), 27
Insula, 596–597
Intelligibility
Speech, 493–499
Intensity level, 284–285, 286
Interarytenoid muscle, 435
Interaural cues, 570
Interaural level differences (ILDs), 570–571
Interaural time differences (ITDs), 570–571
Intercartilaginous internal intercostal muscles, 16
Interior intercostal muscles, 16
Internal capsule, 603–605
Internal genu of the facial nerve, 625
Internal intercostal muscles, 635
Internal oblique muscle, 19, 59
Interosseous internal intercostal muscles, 16
Inverse filtering, 292
Ipsilaterally, 633
Isochrony, 459

J

Just noticeable differences (JNDs), 558

K

Kent, Raymond D., **200**
König, W., 365–366

L

Labial, 195
Labiodental, 195
Laryngeal apparatus and speech production
Age effects, 113–116
Articulation, 113
Fundamental frequency, 111–112
Fundamental frequency-sound pressure level profiles (voice range), 107
Running speech activities, 111–113
Sex effects, 116–118

Laryngeal apparatus and speech production *(continued)*
   Sound pressure level, 112
   Spectrum, 107–108, 113
   Sustained turbulent utterances, 99–100
   Sustained voice production, 100–111
   Transient utterances, 99
   Voice registers, 108–111
Laryngeal cavity, 72
Laryngeal control, 95–97
Laryngeal devoicing gesture (LDG), 441–442
Laryngeal functions
   Containment of the pulmonary air supply, 98
   Degree of coupling between the trachea and pharynx, 97
   Protection of the pulmonary airways, 98
   Sound generation, 98
   Sound production (*see* Laryngeal apparatus and speech production)
Laryngeal opposing pressure, 92
Laryngeal ventricles, 75
Laryngologists, 240
Laryngopharyngeal reflux (LPR), **694**
Larynx, 113
Lateral cricoarytenoid muscle, 78, 80, 88, 89, 94, 95, 96, 100, 105, 106, 112, 435, 629
Lateral iliocostalis cervicis muscle, 17, 59
Lateral iliocostalis lumborum muscle, 17, 20, 55–59, 59
Lateral iliocostalis muscle group, 17
Lateral iliocostalis thoracis muscle, 17, 59
Lateralization of function, 586–589
Lateral rectus muscle, 624
Latissimus dorsi muscle, 16, 20, 59
LDG (laryngeal devoice gesture), 441–442
Levator anguli oris muscle, 626
Levatores costarum muscles, 17, 59
Levator labii superioris alaeque nasi muscle, 160
Levator veli palatini muscle, 517
Lexical activation, 493
Lexical stress, 607
Limbic system (limbic lobe), 597
Linear predictive coding (LPC), 387, **420**
Lip rounding, 194
Localization, 568–574
Loft voice register, 109–111
LPC (linear predictive coding), 387, **420**
LPR (laryngopharyngeal reflux), **694**
Lubker Bumps, **228**, 377
Lung capacities, 27–28
Lungs, 12
Lung volumes, 27–28, 41, 45, 60

M

Magnetic resonance imaging (MRI), 231–232
Major gyri, 594

Malleus, 513–514
Manner of production, 195
Manometry, 218–219, 690–692
MBS (modified barium swallow) study, 688
Measurement
   Acoustic (*see* Sound analysis and measurement)
   Breathing
     Chest wall surface tracking, 215–217
     Manometry, 218–219
     Spirometry, 213–215
   clinical professionals and, 237–240
   Of fricative acoustics, 349–351
   Laryngeal function
     Aeromechanical observations, 224–227
     Electroglottography, 222–224
     Endoscopy, 219–222
   Reducing the dimensionality of, 350
   Sound analysis and
     Digital techniques, 384–388
     History, 363–369
   Spectral, 359
   Of stop acoustics, 358–359
   Swallowing
     Aeromechanical observations, 692–694
     Client self-report, 694
     Endoscopy, 689–690
     Manometry, 690–692
     Surface electromyography, 692
     Ultrasonography, 692
     Videofluorscopy, 688–689
   Temporal, 350, 359
   Velopharyngeal-nasal apparatus
     Aeromechanical, 227–230
     Nasendoscopy, 227
   Velopharyngeal-nasal function
     Aeromechanical observations, 227–230
     Nasendoscopy, 227
Mechanical resonance, 267–270
Mechanoreceptors, 35, 96–97
Medulla
   dorsal surface, 619
   ventral surface, 617
Meninges, 647–650
   Arachnoid mater, 649
   Clinically relevant spaces and, 650
   Dura mater, 648–649
   Pia mater, 649–650
Mentalis muscle, 626
Microglia, 636
Middle cerebral artery (MCA), 653, 655–658
Middle constrictor muscle, 160, 183
Milenkovic, Paul, 373
Minimal audible field (MAF), 543
Modal voice register, 109
Modified barium swallow (MBS) study, 688

Motorboat, **78**
Motor program, 611
Movements of the breathing apparatus, 22–27
Movements of the laryngeal apparatus, 86–91
Movements of the laryngeal housing, 91
Movements of the pharyngeal-oral apparatus, 182
    Lips, 184–186
    Mandible, 183–184
    Pharynx, 183
    Tongue, 184
Movements of the velopharyngeal-nasal apparatus, 143–145
MRI (magnetic resonance imaging), 231–232
Murmurs (*See* Nasal murmurs)
Muscles of the auditory system
    Stapedius muscle, 538, 539, **539**, 541
    Tensor tympani muscle, 538
Muscles of the breathing apparatus
    Abdominal wall
        External oblique, 19
        Internal oblique, 19
        Lateral iliocostalis lumborum, 20
        Latissimus dorsi, 20
        Quadratus lumborum, 20
        Rectus abdominisu, 17
        Transversus abdominis, 19
    Diaphragm, 17
    Rib cage wall
        External intercostal, 16
        Internal intercostal, 16
        Lateral iliocostalis cervicis, 17
        Lateral iliocostalis lumborum, 17
        Lateral iliocostalis thoracis, 17
        Latissimus dorsi, 16
        Levatores costarum, 17
        Pectoralis major, 14–16
        Pectoralis minor, 16
        Quadratus lumborum, 17
        Scalenus anterior, 14
        Scalenus medius, 14
        Scalenus posterior, 14
        Serratus anterior, 16
        Serratus posterior inferior, 17
        Serratus posterior superior, 16–17
        Sternocleidomastoid, 14
        Subclavius, 16
        Transversus thoracis, 16
Muscles of the middle ear
    Stapedius, 516
    Tensor tympani, 516
Muscles of the pharyngeal-oral apparatus
    Lips
        Buccinator, 178, 179–180
        Depressor anguli oris, 178, 181
        Depressor labii inferioris, 178, 181
        Incisivus labii inferioris, 178, 181
        Incisivus labii superioris, 178, 181
        Levator anguli oris, 178, 181
        Levator labii superioris, 178, 180–181
        Levator labii superioris alaeque nasi, 178, 181
        Masseter, 180
        Mentalis, 178, 181
        Orbicularis oris, 178, 179
        Platysma, 178, 179, 181–182
        Risorius, 178, 179, 180
        Zygomatic major, 178, 181
        Zygomatic minor, 178, 181
    Mandible
        Digastric, 173, 175
        External pterygoid, 173, 175
        Geniohyoid, 173, 175
        Internal pterygoid, 173–175
        Masseter, 173
        Mylohyoid, 173, 175
        Temporalis, 173
    Pharynx
        Inferior constrictor, 172–173
        Middle constrictor, 173
        Stylopharyngeus, 173
    Tongue
        Extrinsic
            Genioglossus, 177, 178
            Hyoglossus, 177, 178
            Palatoglossus, 177–178
            Syloglossus, 177
        Intrinsic
            Inferior longitudinal, 175, 176, 177
            Superior longitudinal, 175–178
            Transverse, 175, 177
            Vertical, 175, 176–177
Muscles of the velopharyngeal-nasal apparatus
    Outer nose
        Anterior nasal dilator, 142
        Depressor alae nasi, 143
        Levator labii superioris alaeque nasi, 142
        Nasalis, 143
        Posterior nasal dilator, 142–143
    Pharynx
        Inferior constrictor, 135, 138
        Middle constrictor, 135, 137–138
        Palatopharyngeus, 135, 138–139
        Salpingopharyngeus, 135, 138
        Stylopharyngeus, 135
        Superior constrictor, 135–137, 138, 139
    Velum
        Glossopalatine, 139, 141
        Palatal levator, 139–140, 141
        Palatal tensor, 139, 140–141
        Pharyngopalatine, 139, 141–142
        Uvulus, 139, 141

Myasthenia gravis (MG), 646
Myelin, 585, 639
Mylohyoid muscle, 85, 91, 96, 97, 624, 677

N

Nasalance, 420
Nasalis muscle, 160
Nasalization, 330, 335–339, 418–420
Nasal murmurs, 330–335, 412–414
Nasal place of articulation, 415–418
Nasal septum, 133
Nasoendoscopy, 227
Nasometry, 420
Nervous system cells, 636
    Glial cells, 636
    Neurons, 636–637
Neural control (motor and sensory)
    Breathing apparatus, 34–40
    Swallowing, 681–682
    Velopharyngeal-nasal apparatus, 148–149
Neural tuning curves, 551
Neurologists, 239
Neuron cell bodies, 584–585
Neurons, 586, 636–637
    Axon, 639
    Cell body (soma), 637–639
    Postsynaptic membrane, 639
    Presynaptic membrane, 639
    Synapses, 639
    Terminal button, 639
Neurosmuscular junction, 645–647
Neurotransmitters, 644–645
Nodes of Ranview, 639
Noise waveform, 345
Nonsibilants, 425–426
Nucleus cuneatus, 619
Nucleus gracilis, 619
Null context vowels, 401

O

Oblique arytenoid muscle, 80–81, 82
Occipital lobes, 596
Oculomotor nerve (*see* Cranial nerves)
Ohala, John, **398**
Olfactory nerve (*see* Cranial nerves)
Oligodendrocytes, 636
Omohyoid muscle, 83, 84–85, 91, 96
Optic chiasm, 616
Optic nerve (*see* Cranial nerves)
Optoelectronic tracking, 234–235
Oral air pressure, 351
Oral pressure, 346
Orbicularis oris muscles, 626
Organelles, 510–511, 638

Oscillation, **101**
Ossicles, 513–515
Ossification, 115
Otorhinolaryngologists, 239–240
Outer ear, 508–512
    External auditory meaus, 509–511
    Pina (auricle), 508–509
    Tympanic membrane (eardrum), 511–512
Outer nose, 145
Output spectrum, 303
Output variables of the breathing apparatus, 27–33
    Pressure, 28–31
    Shape, 31–33
    Volume, 27–28

P

Pain, 607
Pairwise Variability Index (PVI), 459
Palatal levator muscle, 148, 160, 195, 606, 629
Palatal tensor muscle, 148, 160, 624
Palatoglossus muscle, 629
Palatopharyngeus muscle, 160, 629
Parahippocampal gyrus, 597
Paralinguistics, 455, **457**
Parasagittal planes, 581
Par rectus, 82
Pars media, 82
Pars oblique, 82, 89
Pattern-playback machine, 467, **468**
Pectoralis major muscle, 14–16, 59
Pectoralis minor muscle, 16, 59
Peduncle, 618
Peripheral nervous system (PNS), 579–580, 681
    Of breathing, 37
Peterson-Falzone, Sally, **238**
Pharyngeal flaps, **145**
Pharyngopalatine muscle, 160
Pharynx, 97, 143–144
Phases of swallowing
    Esophageal, **675**
    Oral preparatory, 674–676, **675**
    Oral transport, **675,** 676
    Pharyngeal, **675,** 676–677
Phoneme specific emission, 239
Phonetic transcription, 498–499
Phons, **545,** 547
Physical therapists, 239
Pia mater, 649–650
Ping puffers, **38**
Pinna (auricle), 508–509
Pipe organs, 280
Pitch, 558–559
    Complex acoustic events, 563–565
    Of sinusoids, 559–561
Place of major constriction, 192

Place of production, 195
Planes, terminology for, 581–584
Planum temporale, 595
Plastic surgeons, 240
Pleural pressure, 674
PNS (see Peripheral nervous system (PNS))
Pons
    dorsal surface, 619
    ventral surface, 617
Post cerebral artery (PCA), 654, 657
Posterior columns, 606–607
Posterior commissure, 602
Posterior cricoarytenoid muscle, 78, 79–80, 86, **87**, 89, 94, 96, 111, 435, 629
Posterior inferior cerebellar artery (PICA), 654
Posterior median septum, 634
Posterior nasal dilator muscle, 160
Posterior parietal cortex (PPC), 593
Postsynaptic membrane, 639, **640**
    Synaptic cleft, 639–640
Preclinical hearing science, 4–7
    Applications of data, 6–7
    Domain, 4, **5**
    Levels of observation, 4–5
    Subsystems, 5–6
Preclinical speech science, 1–4
    Applications of data, 4
    Domain, 1, **1**
    Levels of observation, 1–3
    Subsystems, 3–4
Prefrontal cortex, 592
Premoto cortex (PMA), 592
Pressure
    Alveolar, **106,** 28–31
    Bronchial, **106**
    Tracheal, **106**
Pressure waves, 247–255
Presynaptic membrane, 639
Primary auditory cortex, 594–595
Primary motor cortex, 590–591
Primary somatosensory cortex, 593
Prosody, acoustic characteristics of. *see also* Suprasegmentals
    defined, 454
    Phrase-level F0 contours, 454–456
    Phrase-level intensity contours, 456–457
    Rhythm, 458–459
    Stress, 457–458
Prosthodontists, 240
Psychoacoustical tuning curves (PTCs), **553,** 553–555, **554**
Psychoacoustics
    Loudness, 543–558
        Auditory thresholds, 543–546
        Equal loudness contours for sinusoids, 546
        Psychophysical function relating SPL to scaled loudness of sinusoids, 546–550

Psychologists, 239
Psychophysics, 543
    Loudness
        Auditory thresholds, 543–546
        Complex sounds, 550–556
        Equal-loudness contours, 546
        Sensitivity of the auditory system to loudness change, 556–558
        Sensitivity to change in, 556–558
    Pitch, 558–565
    Sound localization, 568–574
    Timbre, 566
    Time, 566–568
Pulmonary air supply, 98
Pulmonary airways, 10–11, 98
Pulmonary apparatus, 10, 12–13, 20
Pulmonologists, 239
Pulse voice register, 109
Pyramids, 617
Pythagoras, **247**

Q

Quadratus lumborum muscle, 17, 20, 59
Quasi-periodic, 294

R

Radiologists, 239
Raspberries, **194**
Rectus abdominis muscle, 17, 59
Recurrent laryngeal nerve, 96
Reference pressure, 286–287
References
    Chapter 2, 60–62
    Chapter 3, 119–125
    Chapter 4, 161–164
    Chapter 5, 208–212
    Chapter 6, 241–245
    Chapter 7, 283
    Chapter 8, 326–327
    Chapter 9, 361–362
    Chapter 10, 388–389
    Chapter 11, 460–465
    Chapter 12, 501–504
    Chapter 13, 541–542
    Chapter 14, 577–578
    Chapter 15, 666–668
    Chapter 16, 697–701
Release (burst) intervals, 354
Residual volume (RV), 27
Resonance, 266
    Acoustic
        Helmholtz resonators, 270–273
        Tube resonators, 273–277
    Mechanical, 267–270

Resonance *(continued)*
   Spring-mass model of, 267–269
Resonance curves, 277–282
Resonators
   Coupled (shunt), 339–340
Respiratory therapists, 239
Resting potential, 640—642
Reviews
   Chapter 1, 7
   Chapter 2, 59–60
   Chapter 3, 118–119
   Chapter 4, 160
   Chapter 5, 207–208
   Chapter 6, 240–241
   Chapter 7, 282–283
   Chapter 8, 326
   Chapter 9, 361
   Chapter 10, 388
   Chapter 11, 459
   Chapter 12, 501
   Chapter 13, 540–541
   Chapter 14, 575–577
   Chapter 15, 665–666
   Chapter 16, 695–697
Rhotics, **453**
Rib cage wall, 12, 21, 22, 25, 35, 39, 46, 59
Rib torque, **15**
Rostrum, 602
Running speech activities, 44–49

S

Sagittal plane, 581
Salpingopharyngeus muscle, 160, 629
Scalenus anterior muscle, 14, 59
Scalenus medius muscle, 14, 59
Scalenus posterior muscle, 14, 59
Secret Acoustical Society?, **247**
Semivowels, 421
   Acoustic and speech development, 423–424
   Constriction interval, 421–422
   Durations, 424
   Formant transitions, 422–423
Septum, nasal, 133
Serratus anterior muscle, 16, 59
Serratus posterior inferior muscle, 17, 59
Serratus posterior superior muscle, 16–17, 59
Sex effects
   Breathing apparatus, 57–58
   Pharyngeal-oral apparatus, 206–207
   Velopharyngeal-nasal apparatus, 159–160
Shunt (coupled) resonators, 330–340
Sibilants, 425–426
Sidetracks
   About, 7
   Air Molecules Do Not Rest, **531**

All /i/'s and /u/'s Are Not Creating Equal, **307**
Always Under Pressure, **29**
America Regains the Mustard Yellow Belt, **671**
Are We Wired for Rate?, **408**
Articulatory and Acoustic Phonetics, **405**
Auditory Filters: Do They Matter?, **555**
Auditory Mechanisms in Music and Speech
   Perception, **568**
Basal Ganglia or Basal Nuclei?, **609**
Beer and Flutes, **276**
Of Beer Bottles and Vocal Tracts, **299**
Being One with Your Larynx, **72**
A Bone to Pick, **517**
The Breakdown of Auditory Scene Analysis, **574**
Breathing as a Laughing Matter, **37**
Bringing the Bird to Auditory Threshold Testing, **544**
Calm Yourself with Dissonance, **267**
Can Unlabeled Spectrograms Be Segmented and
   Labeled?, **380**
The Cattle Are Lowing, **108**
Chicken Dinner, **688**
The Cold War, **186**
Coming and Going, **205**
Coming to Terms, **9**
Computers Are Not Smarter Than Humans, **363**
Corner Vowels?, **387**
Cornstarch, **235**
Counteracting Pop, **357**
Dancing in the Moonlight, **172**
Daniel R. Boone, **88**
Deep Brain Stimulation, **612**
The Difference in Your Ears May Be More Than
   Aesthetic, **573**
Difference Limen for Loudness/SLP vs. Differennce
   Liment for Pitch/Frequency, **562**
Digital Speech Samples and the Aural Flip Book, **385**
Disposing of Things, **135**
Donald Duck, **113**
Donation and a Growing Cause, **86**
Don't Put Things in Your Ears, **231**
Doral and Ventral Streams, **599**
Do Trained Musicians Have an Edge?, **563**
DTI, **600**
Duane C. Spriesterbach (1916–2011), **130**
Duck and Cover, **192**
Duplex perception, **475–479**
Dynamic Analogies, **319**
Early X-Games, **183**
Energy Present, Phonetic Utility Not, **385**
Experiments with Sinusoids: Why?, **558**
Eye Eye Eye Eye Eye, **202**
Faster than a Herd of Turtles, **207**
Faster Than the Speed of . . ., **642**
Fathers of Speech Acoustics, **289**
The Final Common Pathway, Part I and Part II, **630**
The Flap Flap, **145**

The Fluidity of Language, **522**
fMRI, **587**
Fourier Analysis Was Hot in the Nineteenth Century, **266**
Genes, Hands, and Brains, **588**
GERD and LPR, **694**
Get Thee Out, **98**
Getting a Boost, **510**
Gone but Not Forgotten, **176**
Good Dental Health = Nice Fricatives, **344**
Good Things Come in Small Packages, **355**
Grant Fairbanks (1910-1964), **171**
Growing Up in the 1950s and Speech Perception, **487**
Gutsy Stuff, **684**
Hardheaded Speech Acoustics, **304**
Harry Hollien, **91**
Having an Effect, **492**
Having It Both Ways, **138**
He Said–She Said, **117**
He's an Old Smoothie, **159**
How Sound Points, **257**
Hungry for Air, **680**
The Idiomatic Toolbox: Speech Phrases, **323**
Imperfect Perfection, **297**
Intelligibility in the Ear, **496**
It's Never That Simple, Even When It's Complex to Begin With, **395**
Kitty's Mobile Ears, **571**
Laundry Starch, **13**
Listen My Children and You Shall Hear, **108**
Locus Pocus, **452**
Low Energy Physics, **188**
Lubker Bumps, **228**
The Many Dimensions of Speech Perception, **397**
Mirror, Mirror, in the Brain, **473**
Mmm Mmm Good!, **676**
More than One Way to . . ., **49**
Motorboat, **78**
Of Mufflers, Heating Systems, and Nasals, **332**
Myth Conceptions, **191**
Needling the Teacher, **93**
No Ossicles??, **520**
Not Doing What Comes Naturally, **23**
One Tug and Two Consequences, **678**
Open Wide, **186**
Operator, Will You Help Me Place This Call?, **564**
To or Fro and To and Fro, **101**
Organic Music-Making Hats Off to Tube Resonators, **280**
Out Your Nose Like a Garden Hose, **230**
Paralinguistics, **457**
Pending Further Notice, **263**
Phonatory Turbulence, **356**
Pink Puffers and Blue Boaters, **38**
Of Place and Time, **561**
Planum Temporale, **595**

Playing by Her Own Rule, **154**
Raspberries, **194**
Raymond D. Kent, **200**
Rest in Peace, **106**
Ribbit, Ribbit, **12**
Rib Torque, **14**
Sally Peterson-Falzaone, Clinician-Scientist Extraordinaire, **238**
Secret Acoustical Society?, **247**
Seeking Phonic Clarity, **444**
Shouting at Early Microphones, **366**
Show Me Your Hand, **133**
The Sinuses Are Helmholtz Resonators, Part I, **333**
The Sinuses Are Helmholtz Resonators, Part II, **337**
Sizing Things Up, **60**
Slowly Released Slops, **361**
Somatotopic Representation Is Not Always "Clean," **584**
Some Things Are Not Quite What They Seem, **146**
Sonar in a Teacup, **144**
Sound Change, **348**
Sound Speed, **247**
Speaking of Difference Limens, **563**
Spectrographic Challenges, **420**
Speech Acoustics and Your Smile, **398**
Speech Perception: A Lost Soul in Clinical Training Programs, **500**
Speech Synthesis and Speech Perception, **481**
Sphenopalatine Ganglioneuralgia, **682**
Stops (Still) Win the Prize, **453**
Street Talk About Talking, **178**
Survival of the Phonetic Fittest, **437–438**
Sword Throats, **685**
Tacoma Narrows Bridge, **270**
Ten-Four, Good Buddy, **190**
That Cute Cuddly Infant Is Really a Statistical Model-Builder, **486**
They Didn't Quite Get It, **84**
Thomas J. Hixon (1940-2009), **40**
Three Shakers and Movers, **274**
Tick Tock, **98**
Tuning Up Tuning Curves, **554**
Two Worlds, **77**
The Ultimate Social Consequence, **431**
The Umbo and Its Tiny Ways, **521**
The Unknown Vocal Tract, **310**
Unpacking the Unfamiliar, **572**
Waving It to a More Advanced Course, **533**
What About Talking Birds?, **475**
What Did You Say?, **540**
What's Up with 1/10th Second?, **539**
What's Your Peduncle's Name?, **618**
When Is a Bad Nose Good and a Good Nose Bad?, **159**
Where Did That Come From?, **27**
Where's the Border?, **218**
Which Hunt, **146**

Sidetracks *(continued)*
    The World of Fricatives and Other Fricative-Centric
        Matters, **433**
    Writing from Experience, **371**
    The Young(er) and the Reckless, **38**
Silent (closure) intervals, 353–354, 376
Sinusoidal function, 258–259
Sinusoidal motion, 256–259
Sinusoids
    Experiments with, **558**
    Pitch of, 559–561
Solzhenitsyn, Alexander I, 369, **371**
Soma (cell body), 637–639
Somatosensory pathways, 606
Sones, 547–550
Soomatotopic organization, 585
Sound analysis and measurement
    Digital techniques, 384–388
    History, 363–369
Sound generation, 98
Sound location, psychophysics of, 568–574
Sound pressure level (SPL), 106–107, 285–286, 543, 544–545, 547
Sound spectrograms, 373, 388
    Aperiodic intervals, 378–379
    Axes, 373–375
    Digital, 373
    Formant frequencies, 375–376
    Glottal pulses, 375
    Segmentation, 379–382
    Silent intervals and stop bursts, 376–378
Sound spectrograph, 369–382
Spasmodic dysphonia (SD), 646–647
Speaking style, 408
Spearing rate, 407
Specialization of function, 586–589
Spectral measurements, 359
Spectral moments, 350
Spectrograph (*See* Sound spectrograph)
Spectrum, 107–108, 113
Spectrum analyzers, 367
Speech breathing (*see* Breathing apparatus and speech production)
Speech intelligibility, 493–499
    Scaled, 496–498
Speech intelligibility tests, **496**
    Explanatory, 495–496
Speech-language pathologists, 238–239
Speech perception, 467
    Acoustic invariance, 479–482
    Animals, 485
    Auditory theories, 488–489
    Categorical perception, 467–474
    Direct realism, 486–488, 490, 499
    General auditory explanation, 482–483
    Growing up in 1950s and, **487**
    Infants, 485
    Intelligibility (*see* Intelligibility)
    Motor theory, 474–482, 488
    Nonspeech sound perception, 483–485
    Normalization, 489–490
    Speech-language pathologists/audiologists and, 499–501
    Speech Synthesis and, **481**
    Summary of theories, 490–493
    Word recognition, 491–493
Speech production models (*See* DIVA)
Speech sound segments, 391
Sphenopalatine ganglioneuralgia, 682
Spinal accessory nerve (*see* Cranial nerves)
Spinal cord, 633–635
Spinal motor neurons, 605–606
Spinal nerves, 635–636
Spirometry, 213–215
Spriesterbach, Duane C., **130**
Spring-mass model of resonance, 267–269
Stages of swallowing (*see* Phases of swallowing)
Standing waves, 274
Stapedius muscle, 518, 626
Stapes, 626
Starting frequency (F2), 468–469
Sternocleidomastoid muscle, 14, 37, 59, 629
Sternohyoid muscle, 83–84, 91, 96, 106
Sternothyroid muscle, 82–83, 91, 106
Stevens, Kenneth, **289**
Stop acoustics
    measurement of, 358–359
    theory of, 351–358
Stop bursts, **355**, 376, 381n5
Stop consonants, 359–360
Stop consonant voice, 441–445
Stop duration, 381n5
Stop gaps, 376
Stops, 438–453
    Acoustic invariance, 449–450, 452–453
    Bursts, 445–449
    Closure interval, 439–441
    Locus equations, 450–452
    Voicing, 441–445
Stop segment, 381n5
Stop sources, 356–358
Stress, lexical, 407
Striatal tracts, 601
Structural and functional imaging
    Magnetic resonance imaging, 231–232
    Ultrasonic imaging, 232
    X-ray imaging, 230–231
Stylohyoid muscle, 85, 91, 96, 97
Stylopharyngeus muscle, 160
Stylopharyngeus muscle, 628
Subclavius muscle, 16, 59
Subcortical nuclei, 584, 607–617

Subcostal muscles, 17
Superior cerebellar artery (SCA), 654
Superior colliculi, 617
Superior constrictor muscle, 160, 517
Superior longitudinal fasciculus, 599
Supplementary motor cortex (SMA), 592
Suprahyoid muscles, 85
Supramarginal gyrus, 594
Suprasegmentals, 382–384
Surface electromyography, 692
Sustained turbulence noise production, 99–100
Sustained voice production, 100–111
Swallow apnea, 680
Swallowing. *see also* Anatomy of swallowing
    Apnea (*see* Swallow apnea)
    Breathing (*see* Breathing and swallowing)
    Forces (*see* Forces of swallowing)
    Measurement (*see* Measurement)
    Neural control (*see* Neural control)
    Phases (*see* Phases of swallowing)
    Variables (*see* Swallowing variables)
Swallowing disorders, clinical professionals and, 694–695
Swallowing variables
    Bolus characteristics
        Consistency and texture, 683
        Taste, 684
        Volume, 683–684
    Swallowing mode
        Cued vs. uncued, 685–686
        Single vs. sequential, 684–685
Sword swallowing, **685**
Synapses, 586, 639
Synaptic cleft, 639–640
Synaptic transmission, 644–645

T

Temperature, 607
Temporal bone, 505–507
Temporal measurements, 350–351, 359
Tensor tympani muscle, 624
Tensor veli muscle, 517
TF32 computer program, 373
Thalamus, 612–614
Three-parameter model of vowel articulation (Stevens and House), 313–324
Thyroarytenoid muscle, 78–79, 80, 86, 88, 89, 96, 104, 105, 106, 111, 112, 629, 677
Thyrohyoid muscle, 82, 83, 91, 96, 105
Thyroid cartilage, 63–64
Thyromuscularis muscle, 89, 94, 106
Thyrovocalis muscle, 88, 94, 104
Tibet Singing Bowls, **267**
Tidal breathing, 34–36, 38–40
Tidal volume (TV), 27

Timbre, psychophyics of, 566
Time, psychophysics of, 566
Time domain, 290–293
Tongue advancement, 316–318
Tongue height, 316
Tracheal air pressure, 97, 352
Tracheal pressure, **106**
Tracts
    Ascending projection, 606–607
    Association, 598
    Descending projection, 602–603
    Vocal, 297–324
Transient noise production, 99
Transverse arytenoid muscle, 80, 81
Transverse plane, 581
Transversus abdominis muscle, 19, 59
Transversus thoracis muscle, 16, 59
Trapezius muscle, 629
Traumatic brain injury (TBI), 597
Trigeminal nerve (*see* Cranial nerves)
Trochlear nerve (*see* Cranial nerves)
Tuning curves (*See* Psychoacoustical tuning curves (PTCs))
Tunnel of Corti, 528–529, 541
Turbulent flow (turbulence), 343
Tympanic membrane (eardrum), 511

U

Ultrasonic imaging, 232
Ultrasonography, 692
Utterance position, 407–408
Uvulus muscle, 148, 160

V

Vagus nerve (*see* Cranial nerves)
Velar, 195
Velopharyngeal-nasal apparatus and speech production
    Running speech activities, 154–156
    Sustained utterances, 152–153
Velum, 144
Ventilation, 60
    Breathing apparatus, 57–58
Ventricles, 650–652
    Cerebral aqueduct, 652
    Fourth ventricle, 652
    Lateral ventricle, 655
    Third ventricle, 651–652
Ventricular folds, 89–90
Vertical phase difference, 102–103
Vestibular system, 522–525
VG (glottal flow function), 291, **292**
VG waveforms, 294–296
Vibration, **101**
Videoendoscopy, 222

Videofluorscopy, 688–689
Videostoboscopy, 222
Vital capacity (VC), 27
Vocal fold abduction, 86–87, **87**
Vocal fold adduction, 87–89
Vocal folds, 72–75, 86
    Effective mass, 95
    Length change, 89, 114–115
    Stiffness, 94
    Vibration, 101–104
Vocal tract, 297–303
    Input signal and, 303–309
    Tube constriction and, 309–324
Voice-onset time (VOT), 353, 356, 360–361, 381n5, 442–445, **568**
Voice range, 107
Voice registers, 108–111
    Loft, 109–111
    Modal, 109
    Pulse, 109
Voicing, 195
von Békésy, Georg, 530, 541
von Helmholtz, Herman, 363–365

VOT (*see* Voice-onset time (VOT))
Vowel durations
    Extrinsic factors affecting, 407–408
    Intrinsic, 406–407
Vowels, 391–398. *see also* Acoustic theory of vowel production
    Coding schemes, 192–194
    null context, 401

W

Wada test, 587
Waveform, 252
Wavelength, 254–255
Weber's law, 557
Wernicke-Geshwind model, 600–601
Wernike's area, 595–596, 601
White matter, 584, 585

X

X-ray imaging, 230–231
X-ray microbeam imaging, 232–234